Oxford Specialty Training:
Training in Paediatrics

The recent upheaval in training and education has left junior doctors with much to contend with, including a new career structure, online curricula, and workplace-based assessments. The need for resources that reflect these changes is great. Other books have become outmoded and although the Internet offers access to boundless medical material, little is tailored to the needs of specialty trainees. Fear not, change is coming; the **Oxford Specialty Training Series** has arrived.

The series encompasses core specialty books as well as basic science and revision texts that directly follow their respective Royal College curriculum. **Training in Paediatrics** exemplifies their compact, but comprehensive style. It has self-contained double-page spreads with a clear layout incorporating high quality illustrations. These features make information easy to access and digest. In addition, the editorial team and contributing authors are drawn from both trainees and senior clinicians to ensure the content is both relevant and of a high standard.

The **Oxford Specialty Training Series** should see you through the first few years of specialty training whether on the ward, in the clinic, or revising for specialty exams. I believe that regardless of your specialty, **Oxford SpecialtyTraining** gives you the best possible chance of success in your chosen career.

Matthew D. Gardiner
Series Editor

Visit our website for details of forthcoming self-assessment titles www.oup.com/uk/medicine/ost/

Oxford Specialty Training: Training in Paediatrics

Edited by
Mark Gardiner
Professor of Paediatrics, University College London

Sarah Eisen
Academic Clinical Fellow, Institute of Child Health, University College London

Catherine Murphy
Paediatric SpR, University College London Hospitals NHS Foundation Trust

Foreword by
Andrew Wilkinson
Professor of Paediatrics, John Radcliffe Hospital, Oxford

Series Editor
Matthew D. Gardiner
Research Fellow in Plastic and Reconstructive Surgery, Kennedy Institute of Rheumatology, Imperial College, London

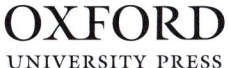

OXFORD
UNIVERSITY PRESS

Great Clarendon Street, Oxford OX2 6DP

Oxford University Press is a department of the University of Oxford.
It furthers the University's objective of excellence in research, scholarship,
and education by publishing worldwide in

Oxford New York

Auckland Cape Town Dar es Salaam Hong Kong Karachi
Kuala Lumpur Madrid Melbourne Mexico City Nairobi
New Delhi Shanghai Taipei Toronto

With offices in

Argentina Austria Brazil Chile Czech Republic France Greece
Guatemala Hungary Italy Japan Poland Portugal Singapore
South Korea Switzerland Thailand Turkey Ukraine Vietnam

Oxford is a registered trade mark of Oxford University Press
in the UK and in certain other countries

Published in the United States
by Oxford University Press Inc., New York

© Oxford University Press 2009

The moral rights of the author have been asserted

Database right Oxford University Press (maker)

Crown copyright material is reproduced under Class Licence
Number C01P0000148 with the permission of OPSI
and the Queen's Printer for Scotland

First published 2009

All rights reserved. No part of this publication may be reproduced,
stored in a retrieval system, or transmitted, in any form or by any means,
without the prior permission in writing of Oxford University Press,
or as expressly permitted by law, or under terms agreed with the appropriate
reprographics rights organization. Enquiries concerning reproduction
outside the scope of the above should be sent to the Rights Department,
Oxford University Press, at the address above

You must not circulate this book in any other binding or cover
and you must impose the same condition on any acquirer

British Library Cataloguing in Publication Data

Data available

Library of Congress Cataloging in Publication Data

Data available

Typeset by Cepha Imaging Private Ltd, Bangalore, India
Printed in Italy
on acid-free paper by
LEGO SpA – Lavis, TN

ISBN 978-0-19-922773-0

1 3 5 7 9 10 8 6 4 2

Foreword

Here is a book specifically written for every trainee in Paediatrics and Child Health.

Paediatrics has always been a great challenge to new graduates because of the diversity of the speciality. Experience as a student may ignite a genuine interest, but the time that most medical schools allocate to paediatrics is too short to give more than a glimpse of this rewarding branch of medicine.

Advances in clinical science as well as social demands give the impression that the range of knowledge needed by a paediatrician is vast. From neonatology to adolescent medicine; from genetics to child protection and all other branches of the discipline, the amount to be understood can be daunting.

Recent developments in the structure of postgraduate training require a change in approach to learning. No longer is the Royal College Membership examination (MRCPCH) dictated by the whims of the examiners. They now know, along with trainees, that there is a well-defined curriculum. Following this requires attention to the details which have been carefully planned.

A wide range of activities is involved in training and assessment. In addition to clinical experience gained at the bedside, there are practical skills and diagnostic procedures to be performed and observed. Resuscitation Council (UK) training courses give experience in team work at critical times. Special tutorials cover child protection issues, communication skills, and research methodology. The objectives are clear. The aim is to make the content and the process transparent and fit for the purpose of identifying competence in trainees.

A great deal must be achieved by self-directed learning, and there is no better way to approach this than to have an up-to-date, comprehensive, and affordable book to read and re-read. *Training in Paediatrics* has been written specifically with your needs in mind. The editors have chosen a style which emphasizes the essentials of every aspect of clinical paediatrics and clearly presents the knowledge in a consistent format. Chapters end with examples of case-based discussions which illustrate and complement those needed to fulfil the work-based assessments during training.

This book should more than satisfy the needs of trainees preparing for the examinations. In addition to covering everything you might expect to find, there are chapters on pharmacology, statistics, and evidence-based medicine, all of which should be essential reading.

I predict that this will soon be regarded as the essential text for paediatric trainees, and no doubt their trainers will also find it invaluable.

Andrew R Wilkinson
Professor of Paediatrics
University of Oxford
John Radcliffe Hospital
Oxford

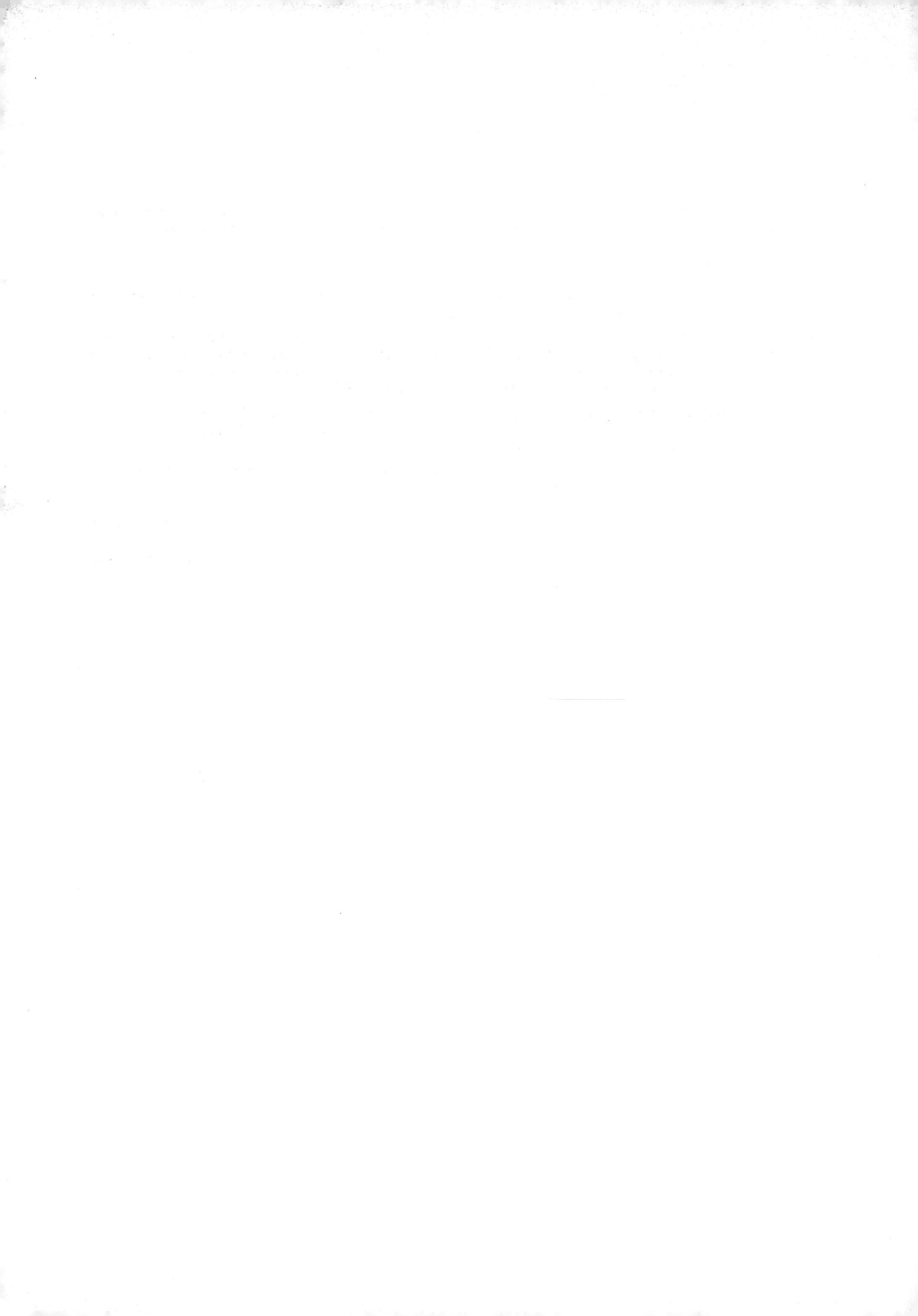

Preface

In current educational jargon reading a book can be described as an 'informal learner directed strategy for delivering the knowledge component of a competency based curriculum.' The great physician and teacher Sir William Osler put it more succinctly:

'He who studies medicine without books sails an uncharted sea, but he who studies medicine without patients does not go to sea at all'

No book can provide the wise head and warm heart that comes only from clinical experience. Yet knowledge is generally preferable to ignorance and, despite all the advances in information technology, is still found most easily between the covers of a book.

This book, written by a group of highly experienced clinicians at the forefront of their specialty will, we believe, provide a useful chart for young paediatricians navigating the sea of paediatrics and child health. Its content has been informed by the paediatric curriculum as defined by the Royal College of Paediatrics and Child Health (RCPCH) with particular emphasis on the requirements of those undergoing Level 1 training leading up to the examination for Membership of the RCPCH.

Each chapter (where appropriate) opens with a brief review of some of the basic science relevant to clinical practice and closes with case-based discussions. Topics are arranged in a uniform format and presented at a level which we hope is neither too brief nor too detailed. Illustrations have been selected to enhance understanding and complement clinical experience.

We hope that you enjoy and benefit from this book and welcome feedback on how it may be improved in the future. Comments or suggestions should be emailed to ost@oup.com.

Mark Gardiner
Sarah Eisen
Catherine Murphy

Acknowledgements

We wish to thank all our contributors for their hard work and patience and for undertaking the significant additional burden of writing in addition to their normal and demanding clinical duties.

We would like to thank the team at Oxford University Press, including in particular Andrew Sandland, Fiona Goodgame, and Marionne Cronin, who have given endless support and have been a pleasure to work with. Many anonymous reviewers have provided valuable feedback and guidance and a number of friends and colleagues have kindly commented on the manuscript, including Janet Rennie, Tim Chambers, Chris Verity, Nick Barnes, John Tripp, and Bob Dinwiddie.

Emma Laxton and Beth Dumonteil did a wonderful job of converting early drafts into perfectly organised word documents and in creating order out of chaos with the image bank. The book would not have been possible without their unfailing hard work and good humour.

Lastly we are grateful to the series editor, Matthew Gardiner, for the original conception and for his helpful advice and support along the way and to our families for their unstinting support.

Mark Gardiner
Sarah Eisen
Catherine Murphy

Contents

Detailed contents *xi*
List of contributors *xv*
Abbreviations and acronyms *xvii*

1 **Neonatology** *1*
Kevin Ives and Topun Austin

2 **Accidents and emergencies** *29*
Julian Sandell

3 **Respiratory medicine** *53*
Eddie Chung

4 **Cardiology** *73*
Nick Archer and Nick Barnes

5 **Gastroenterology and nutrition** *93*
Peter Sullivan

6 **Nephrology and urology** *119*
Stephen Marks and Anja Lehnhardt

7 **Neurology and neurodisability** *143*
Richard Newton and Rob Forsyth

8 **Ophthalmology** *175*
Majeed Jawad

9 **Dermatology** *193*
Edward Seaton

10 **Endocrinology** *209*
Heather Mitchell

11 **Metabolic medicine** *233*
John Walter and Simon Jones

12 **Genetics** *247*
Frances Elmslie, Helen Hanson, and Emma Baple

13 **Haematology** *269*
Owen Smith and Jonathan Bond

14 **Oncology** *291*
Maria Michelagnoli

15 **Infection and immunity** *307*
Nigel Klein, Olaf Neth, and Sarah Eisen

16 **Musculoskeletal disorders** *345*
Clarissa Pilkington, Deborah Eastwood, and Louise Michaelis

17 **Mental health** *369*
Colette Lewin

18 **Community child health** *381*
Deborah Hodes

19 **Adolescent medicine** *407*
Russell Viner

20 **Pharmacology** *425*
Nagi Barakat

21 **Statistics and evidence-based medicine** *449*
Ashley Reece

Index *461*

Detailed contents

List of contributors *xv*
Abbreviations and acronyms *xvii*

1 Neonatology *1*
1.1 Antenatal life *2*
1.2 Birth: adaptation and resuscitation *4*
1.3 Neonatal physiology *6*
1.4 The term newborn infant *8*
1.5 Birth asphyxia and birth injury *10*
1.6 Respiratory disorders in the newborn *12*
1.7 Neurological disorders in the newborn *14*
1.8 Problems in the preterm infant *16*
1.9 Bacterial infection in the newborn *18*
1.10 Viral and congenital infections in the newborn *20*
1.11 Neonatal jaundice *22*
1.12 Metabolic disorders *24*
1.13 Congenital anomalies *26*
1.14 Case-based discussions *28*

2 Accidents and emergencies *29*
2.1 The seriously ill child: physiology *30*
2.2 The seriously ill child: clinical assessment *32*
2.3 Cardiopulmonary arrest *34*
2.4 Accidental injuries: trauma and burns *36*
2.5 Head injury and drowning *38*
2.6 Poisoning *40*
2.7 Respiratory emergencies *42*
2.8 Septicaemia and septic shock *44*
2.9 Anaphylaxis *46*
2.10 Diabetic ketoacidosis *48*
2.11 Convulsions and coma *50*
2.12 Case-based discussions *52*

3 Respiratory medicine *53*
3.1 Respiratory system: anatomy and physiology *54*
3.2 Respiratory system: clinical skills *56*
3.3 Ear, nose, and throat (ENT) *58*
3.4 Upper airways obstruction: stridor *60*
3.5 Pneumonia and pertussis *62*
3.6 Bronchiolitis and pulmonary tuberculosis *64*
3.7 Asthma *66*
3.8 Cystic fibrosis *68*
3.9 Chronic lung disease, bronchiectasis, and sequelae of neurodisability *70*
3.10 Case-based discussions *72*

4 Cardiology *73*
4.1 Basic and clinical cardiology *74*
4.2 Cardiac investigations *76*
4.3 Congenital heart disease *78*
4.4 Acyanotic heart defects: left-to-right shunts *80*
4.5 Acyanotic heart defects: obstructions *82*
4.6 Cyanotic heart defects *84*
4.7 Rheumatic fever and Kawasaki disease *86*
4.8 Infective endocarditis, myocarditis, and pericarditis *88*
4.9 Cardiomyopathy and arrhythmias *90*
4.10 Case-based discussions *92*

5 Gastroenterology and nutrition *93*
5.1 Gastrointestinal system *94*
5.2 Nutrition *96*
5.3 Congenital anomalies and Hirschsprung disease *98*
5.4 Oesophageal and gastric disorders *100*
5.5 Acute gastroenteritis and intussusception *102*
5.6 Coeliac disease and short bowel syndrome *104*
5.7 Inflammatory bowel disease *106*
5.8 Functional gastrointestinal disorders *108*

5.9 Functional abdominal pain and constipation *110*
5.10 Pancreatic and gallbladder disease *112*
5.11 Neonatal liver disease *114*
5.12 Childhood liver disease *116*
5.13 Case-based discussions *118*

6 Nephrology and urology *119*

6.1 The urinary system *120*
6.2 Clinical nephrology *122*
6.3 Urinary tract infection *124*
6.4 Glomerulonephritis *126*
6.5 Nephrotic syndrome *128*
6.6 Renal failure *130*
6.7 Congenital anomalies of the urinary tract *132*
6.8 Renal anomalies and inguinoscrotal disorders *134*
6.9 Cystic disease and tubulopathies *136*
6.10 Genetic syndromes and HUS *138*
6.11 Hypertension, urolithiasis, and nephrocalcinosis *140*
6.12 Case-based discussions *142*

7 Neurology and neurodisability *143*

7.1 The nervous system *144*
7.2 Clinical paediatric neurology *146*
7.3 Neural tube defects and hydrocephalus *148*
7.4 Cortical and cranial vault malformations *150*
7.5 Neurodegenerative disorders *152*
7.6 The cerebral palsies *154*
7.7 Childhood epilepsies: diagnosis and management *156*
7.8 Childhood epilepsies: causes and classification *158*
7.9 Movement disorders *160*
7.10 Headache *162*
7.11 Neuromuscular disorders: overview *164*
7.12 Specific neuromuscular disorders *166*
7.13 Muscular dystrophies *168*
7.14 Infection and injury *170*
7.15 Inflammatory disorders and stroke *172*
7.16 Case-based discussions *174*

8 Ophthalmology *175*

8.1 Eye anatomy and clinical ophthalmology *176*
8.2 Eye symptoms and signs *178*
8.3 Developmental anomalies and visual impairment *180*
8.4 Strabismus and nystagmus *182*
8.5 Eye infections and inflammations *184*
8.6 Childhood cataract and glaucoma *186*
8.7 Retinal and optic nerve disorders *188*
8.8 Genetic eye disease *190*
8.9 Case-based discussions *192*

9 Dermatology *193*

9.1 Skin: anatomy, development, and function *194*
9.2 Clinical dermatology *196*
9.3 Neonatal dermatology *198*
9.4 Eczema *200*
9.5 Skin infections and infestations *202*
9.6 Inflammatory dermatoses *204*
9.7 Hair, nails, mouth, and pigmentation *206*
9.8 Case-based discussions *208*

10 Endocrinology *209*

10.1 Hormones *210*
10.2 Hypothalamus and pituitary gland *212*
10.3 Hypopituitarism, diabetes insipidus, and SIADH *214*
10.4 Growth and its disorders *216*
10.5 Puberty and intersex *218*
10.6 Thyroid disorders *220*
10.7 Adrenal gland *222*
10.8 Adrenal disorders *224*
10.9 Calcium disorders *226*
10.10 Type 1 diabetes mellitus *228*
10.11 Type 2 diabetes mellitus and hypoglycaemia *230*
10.12 Case-based discussions *232*

11 Metabolic medicine *233*

11.1 Metabolic pathways *234*
11.2 Inborn errors of metabolism *236*

- 11.3 Disorders of carbohydrate and fat metabolism *238*
- 11.4 Disorders of amino acid metabolism *240*
- 11.5 Mitochondrial and peroxisomal disorders *242*
- 11.6 Lysosomal storage diseases *244*
- 11.7 Case-based discussions *246*

12 Genetics *247*
- 12.1 Genetics and genomics *248*
- 12.2 Human genetic disease *250*
- 12.3 Paediatric clinical genetics *252*
- 12.4 Trisomies: Down, Edwards, and Patau syndromes *254*
- 12.5 Turner and Klinefelter syndromes *256*
- 12.6 Microdeletion syndromes: DiGeorge, Williams *258*
- 12.7 Marfan, Crouzon, and other syndromes *260*
- 12.8 Neurofibromatosis type 1 and tuberous sclerosis *262*
- 12.9 X-linked disorders: Fragile X and Rett syndrome *264*
- 12.10 mtDNA and imprinted gene disorders *266*
- 12.11 Case-based discussions *268*

13 Haematology *269*
- 13.1 Blood cells: formation and function *270*
- 13.2 Haemostasis *272*
- 13.3 Clinical haematology *274*
- 13.4 Investigations, transfusion, and transplantation *276*
- 13.5 Iron deficiency anaemia and aplastic anaemia *278*
- 13.6 Haemolytic anaemias *280*
- 13.7 Sickle cell disease and thalassaemia *282*
- 13.8 Haemophilia and von Willebrand disease *284*
- 13.9 Coagulation disorders and thrombophilia *286*
- 13.10 Platelet and white cell disorders *288*
- 13.11 Case-based discussions *290*

14 Oncology *291*
- 14.1 Cancer in childhood *292*
- 14.2 Treatment of childhood cancer *294*
- 14.3 Acute leukaemias *296*
- 14.4 Lymphomas *298*
- 14.5 CNS tumours, retinoblastoma, and germ cell tumours *300*
- 14.6 Wilms tumour, neuroblastoma, and STS *302*
- 14.7 Bone tumours and LCH *304*
- 14.8 Case-based discussions *306*

15 Infection and immunity *307*
- 15.1 Immune system *308*
- 15.2 Pathogens: infectious disease *310*
- 15.3 The feverish child: aetiology and assessment *312*
- 15.4 The feverish child: management *314*
- 15.5 Immunodeficiency *316*
- 15.6 Specific primary immunodeficiencies *318*
- 15.7 Measles, mumps, and rubella *320*
- 15.8 Enterovirus and parvovirus infection *322*
- 15.9 Herpesvirus infections: HSV and VZV *324*
- 15.10 Herpesviruses: EBV, CMV, and HHV-6, 7, and 8 *326*
- 15.11 Human immunodeficiency virus: HIV/AIDS *328*
- 15.12 Tuberculosis *330*
- 15.13 Staphylococcal and streptococcal infections *332*
- 15.14 Pneumococcal and meningococcal infections *334*
- 15.15 Zoonoses *336*
- 15.16 Malaria and typhoid *338*
- 15.17 Allergy *340*
- 15.18 Henoch–Schönlein purpura and Kawasaki disease *342*
- 15.19 Case-based discussions *344*

16 Musculoskeletal disorders *345*
- 16.1 Musculoskeletal system *346*
- 16.2 Musculoskeletal system: clinical skills *348*
- 16.3 Orthopaedics: congenital disorders *350*

16.4	Orthopaedics: acquired disorders *352*	19.3	Adolescent health *412*
16.5	Osteogenesis imperfecta and achondroplasia *354*	19.4	Adolescent health promotion *414*
16.6	Osteopetrosis, osteoporosis, and rickets *356*	19.5	Depression, suicide, and self harm *416*
16.7	Juvenile idiopathic arthritis (JIA) *358*	19.6	Somatic symptoms and fatigue *418*
16.8	Reactive arthritis and transient synovitis *360*	19.7	Eating disorders and obesity *420*
16.9	Systemic lupus erythematosus (SLE) *362*	19.8	Sexual health and substance misuse *422*
16.10	Connective tissue disorders *364*	19.9	Case-based discussions *424*

20 Pharmacology *425*

- 20.1 Clinical pharmacology *426*
- 20.2 Paediatric prescribing *428*
- 20.3 Gastrointestinal and musculoskeletal systems *430*
- 20.4 Cardiovascular and respiratory systems *432*
- 20.5 Central nervous system *434*
- 20.6 Antibiotics *436*
- 20.7 Antifungals, antivirals, and antiprotozoals *438*
- 20.8 Endocrine system *440*
- 20.9 Malignancy, immunosuppression, and blood *442*
- 20.10 Nutrition *444*
- 20.11 Fluids and electrolytes *446*
- 20.12 Case-based discussions *448*

16 (continued)

- 16.11 Osteomyelitis and septic arthritis *366*
- 16.12 Case-based discussions *368*

17 Mental health *369*

- 17.1 Paediatric mental health *370*
- 17.2 Common emotional and behavioural problems *372*
- 17.3 Developmental disorders *374*
- 17.4 Attention deficit and conduct disorder *376*
- 17.5 Anxiety, depression, and psychosis *378*
- 17.6 Case-based discussions *380*

18 Community child health *381*

- 18.1 Community child health *382*
- 18.2 Child public health *384*
- 18.3 Child health promotion *386*
- 18.4 Immunisation *388*
- 18.5 Immunisation: the vaccines *390*
- 18.6 Child development *392*
- 18.7 Neurodevelopmental disorders *394*
- 18.8 Hearing loss and communication disorders *396*
- 18.9 Child maltreatment *398*
- 18.10 Child physical abuse *400*
- 18.11 Emotional abuse, sexual abuse, neglect, and FII *402*
- 18.12 Management of suspected child maltreatment *404*
- 18.13 Case-based discussions *406*

19 Adolescent medicine *407*

- 19.1 Adolescence: from child to adult *408*
- 19.2 Clinical skills in adolescent medicine *410*

21 Statistics and evidence-based medicine *449*

- 21.1 Statistics: describing data and testing confidence *450*
- 21.2 Statistics: differences, relationships, risk, and odds *452*
- 21.3 Statistics: clinical test analysis and study design *454*
- 21.4 Evidence-based medicine (EBM) *456*
- 21.5 EBM: critical appraisal and implementation *458*
- 21.6 Critical appraisal exercise *460*

Index *461*

Contributors

Nick Archer
Consultant Paediatric Cardiologist
Department of Paediatrics, John Radcliffe Hospital
Oxford, UK

Topun Austin
Consultant in Neonatology
Cambridge University Hospitals NHS Foundation Trust
Cambridge, UK

Emma Baple
Specialist Registrar in Clinical Genetics
St George's Healthcare NHS Trust
London, UK

Nagi Barakat
Consultant Paediatrician
Hillingdon Hospital NHS Trust
London, UK

Nick Barnes
Consultant Paediatrician
Northampton General Hospital
Northampton, UK

Jonathan Bond
Clinical Research Fellow
MRC Clinical Sciences Centre
Imperial College
London, UK

Eddie Chung
Consultant Paediatrician
University College London Hospitals NHS Foundation Trust,
Senior Lecturer
University College London
London, UK

Deborah Eastwood
Consultant Orthopaedic Surgeon
Great Ormond St Hospital for Children NHS Trust and
Royal National Orthopaedic Hospital,
Hon Senior Lecturer, University College London
London, UK

Sarah Eisen
Academic Clinical Fellow
Institute of Child Health
University College London
London, UK

Frances Elmslie
Consultant Clinical Geneticist
St George's Healthcare NHS Trust
London, UK

Rob Forsyth
Consultant and Senior Lecturer in Paediatric Neurology
Newcastle upon Tyne Hospitals NHS Trust
Newcastle upon Tyne, UK

Helen Hanson
Specialist Registrar Clinical Genetics
St George's Healthcare NHS Trust
London, UK

Deborah Hodes
Consultant Community Paediatrician
Greenland Road Children's Centre
London, UK

Kevin Ives
Consultant Neonatologist and Honorary Senior Lecturer in Paediatrics
John Radcliffe Hospital
Oxford, UK

Majeed Jawad
Consultant Paediatrician
Surrey & Sussex Healthcare NHS Trust
Surrey, UK

Simon Jones
Consultant in Paediatric Inherited Metabolic Disease
Royal Manchester Children's Hospital
Manchester, UK

Nigel Klein
Consultant in Paediatric Infectious Disease
Institute of Child Health and Great Ormond Street Hospital for Children NHS Trust
London, UK

Anja Lehnhardt
Clinical Fellow in Paediatric Nephrology
Great Ormond Street Hospital for Children NHS Trust
London, UK

Colette Lewin
Consultant Child and Adolescent Psychiatrist
Bristol Royal Hospital for Children
Bristol, UK

Stephen Marks
Consultant Paediatric Nephrologist
Great Ormond Street Hospital for Children NHS Trust
London, UK

Maria Michelagnoli
Consultant in Paediatric and Adolescent Oncology
University College London Hospitals NHS Foundation Trust
London, UK

Louise Michaelis
SpR in Immunology
Institute of Child Health and Great Ormond Street Hospital for Children NHS Trust
London, UK

Heather Mitchell
Consultant Paediatrician
Watford General Hospital
Watford, UK

Olaf Neth
SpR in Infectious Disease and Immunology
Institute of Child Health and Great Ormond Street Hospital for Children NHS Trust
London, UK

Richard Newton
Consultant Paediatric Neurologist
Royal Manchester Children's Hospital
Manchester, UK

Clarissa Pilkington
Consultant Paediatric Rheumatologist
Great Ormond Street Hospital for Children NHS Trust
London, UK

Ashley Reece
Consultant Paediatrician
Watford General Hospital
Watford, UK

Julian Sandell
Consultant in Emergency Paediatrics
Poole Hospital NHS Trust
Poole, UK

Edward Seaton
Consultant Dermatologist
Royal Free Hampstead NHS Trust
London, UK

Owen Smith
Professor of Haematology
Trinity College, University of Dublin,
Consultant Paediatric Haematologist
Our Lady's Hospital for Sick Children
Dublin, Ireland

Peter Sullivan
Consultant Paediatric Gastroenterologist
John Radcliffe Hospital
Oxford, UK

Russell Viner
Consultant in Adolescent Medicine
University College London Hospitals NHS Foundation Trust
London, UK

John Walter
Consultant Paediatrician
Willink Biochemical Genetics Unit
Royal Manchester Children's Hospital
Manchester, UK

Abbreviations and acronyms

ABPM	ambulatory blood pressure monitoring		AST	aspartate aminotransferase
ACD	anaemia of chronic disease		AT	antithrombin
ACE	angiotensin converting enzyme		ATD	antithyroid drug
ACF	asymmetric crying facies		AV	atrioventricular
ACS	acute chest syndrome		AVP	arginine vasopressin
ACTH	adrenocorticotropic hormone		AVSD	atrioventricular septal defect
AD	autosomal dominant		AZT	zidovudine
ADD	attention deficit disorder		BAL	bronchoalveolar lavage
ADEM	acute disseminated encephalomyelitis		BBB	blood–brain barrier
ADH	anti-diuretic hormone		BCG	bacille Calmette–Guerin
ADHD	attention-deficit hyperactivity disorder		BFIS	benign familial infantile seizures
ADPKD	autosomal dominant polycystic kidney disease		BFNS	benign familial neonatal seizures
AED	automatic external defibrillator; antiepilepsy drug		BHR	bronchial hyper-reactivity
AEFI	adverse event following immunisation		BJHS	benign joint hypermobility syndrome
AFB	acid-fast bacilli		BLS	basic life support
AFLP	acute fatty liver of pregnancy		BMD	Becker muscular dystrophy
AFP	α-fetoprotein		BMI	body mass index
AgRP	Agouti-gene related peptide		BMT	bone marrow transplantation
AIDS	acquired immunodeficiency syndrome		BMZ	basement membrane zone
AIS	arterial ischaemic stroke		BP	blood pressure
AKI	acute kidney injury		BPD	bronchopulmonary dysplasia
ALCL	anaplastic large-cell lymphoma		BPS	biophysical profile score
ALL	acute lymphoblastic leukaemia		BSA	body surface area
ALT	alanine aminotransferase		BSE	bovine spongiform encephalopathy
ALTE	apparent life threatening event		BWS	Beckwith–Wiedemann syndrome
AMC	arthrogryposis multiplex congenital		CAA	coronary artery aneurysm
AML	acute myeloid leukaemia		CAE	childhood absence epilepsy
AMLS	angiomyolipomas		CAF	Common Assessment Framework
AN	anorexia nervosa		CAFS	conotruncal anomaly face syndrome
ANCA	anti-neutrophil cytoplasmic antibodies		CAH	congenital adrenal hyperplasia
ANOVA	analysis of variance		CAKUT	congenital anomalies of the kidney and urinary tract
AOM	acute otitis media		CAMH	child and adolescent mental health
AP	anteroposterior		CAP	community acquired pneumonia
APTT	activated partial thromboplastin time		CART	cocaine and amphetamine regulated transcript
AR	autosomal recessive		CAT	common arterial trunk
ARC	arcuate nucleus		CBAVD	congenital bilateral absence of the vas deferens
ARI	acute respiratory infection		CBF	cerebral blood flow
ARN	arcuate nucleus		CBT	cognitive behavioural therapy
ARP	Agouti-related peptide		CD	Crohn's disease; conduct disorder
ARPKD	autosomal recessive polycystic kidney disease		CDC	children in difficult circumstances
ARR	absolute risk reduction		CDGP	constitutional delay of growth and puberty
ART	antiretroviral therapy		CdLS	Cornelia de Lange syndrome
AS	aortic stenosis		CDT	Child Development Team
ASD	atrial septal defect; anterior segment dysgenesis; autism spectrum disorders		CF	cystic fibrosis
			CFAP	childhood functional abdominal pain
ASL	airway surface liquid		CFM	cerebral function monitor
ASRT	asthma-related traits			

CFS	chronic fatigue syndrome		DLBL	diffuse large B-cell lymphoma
CGD	chronic granulomatous disease		DM	dermatomyositis
CHD	congenital heart disease		DMARD	disease-modifying antirheumatic drug
CHOP	cyclophosphamide, doxorubicin, vincristine, and prednisolone		DMD	Duchenne muscular dystrophy
CHPP	Child Health Promotion Programme		DPG	diphosphoglycerate
CI	confidence intervals		DSCR	Down syndrome critical region
CK	creatine kinase		DWI	diffusion weighted imaging
CLD	chronic lung disease		EAR	estimated average requirement
CMD	congenital muscular dystrophies		EB	epidermolysis bullosa
CML	chronic myeloid leukaemia		EBM	evidence-based medicine
CMS	congenital myasthenic syndromes		EBV	Epstein–Barr virus
CMT	Charcot–Marie–Tooth		ECG	electrocardiography
CMV	cytomegalovirus		ECMO	extracorporeal membrane oxygenation
CNS	central nervous system; coagulase-negative staphylococci		EDMD	Emery–Dreifuss muscular dystrophy
CNV	copy number variation		EDS	Ehlers–Danlos syndrome
COA	coarctation of aorta		EEG	electroencephalography
COMP	cyclophosphamide, vincristine, methotrexate, and prednisolone		EEV	elastic equilibrium volume
CONS	coagulase-negative staphylococcus		ELBW	Extremely low birthweight
COX	cyclo-oxygenase		EM	erythema multiforme
CP	cerebral palsy		EMA	eosin-5-maleimide; European Medicines Agency
CPAP	continuous positive airways pressure		EMG	exomphalos–macroglossia–gigantism
CPP	cerebral perfusion pressure; central precocious puberty		EMS	external masculinization score
CPR	cardiopulmonary resuscitation		ENS	enteric nervous system
CRH	corticotropin-releasing hormone		ENT	ear, nose and throat
CRMO	chronic recurrent multifocal osteomyelitis		EOG	electro-oculography
CRP	C-reactive protein		EPCR	endothelial protein C receptor
CRT	capillary refill time		EPI	Expanded Programme on Immunisation
CSA	central sleep apnoea		EPO	erythropoietin
CSE	convulsive status epilepticus		ERCP	endoscopic retrograde cholangiopancreatography
CSF	cerebrospinal fluid; colony stimulating factor		ERG	electroretinography
CSOM	chronic suppurative otitis media		ERT	enzyme replacement therapy
CT	calcitonin		ERV	expiratory reserve volume
CTEV	congenital talipes equinovarus		ESFT	Ewing sarcoma family of tumours
CVI	cortical visual impairment		ESR	erythrocyte sedimentation rate
CVID	common variable immunodeficiency		ESRF	end-stage renal failure
CVS	cardiovascular system; chorionic villus sampling		ESWL	extracorporeal shock wave lithotripsy
CXR	chest radiography		EUA	examination under anaesthetic
DALYs	disability adjusted life years		FA	Fanconi anaemia
DAT	direct antibody test		FBAO	foreign body airway obstruction
DBA	Diamond–Blackfan anaemia		FBC	full blood count
DCM	dilated cardiomyopathy		FCMD	Fukuyama-type congenital muscular dystrophy
DDH	developmental dysplasia of the hip		FEF	forced expiratory flow
DEB	dystrophic epidermolysis		FENa	fractional excretion of Na^+
DEXA	bone mineral density scan		FEV1	forced expiratory volume in 1 s
DGCR	DiGeorge critical region		FFA	free fatty acids
DGS	DiGeorge syndrome		FFP	fresh frozen plasma
DHEA-S	dehydroepiandrosterone sulfate		FGF	fibroblast growth factor
DIC	disseminated intravascular coagulation		FGID	functional GI disorder
DIOS	distal intestinal obstruction syndrome		FH	familial hypercholesterolaemia
DKA	diabetic ketoacidosis		FHI	familial hyperinsulinism of infancy
			FII	fabricated or induced illness
			FISH	fluorescence in situ hybridization
			FLAIR	fluid attenuated inversion recovery

fMRI	functional MRI		HIE	hypoxic-ischaemic encephalopathy
FPIE	food protein-induced enterocolitis syndrome		HIGM	hyper-IgM syndrome
FRC	functional residual capacity		HIT/HITTS	heparin-induced thrombocytopenia/ thrombosis syndrome
FSGS	focal segmental glomerulosclerosis		HIV	human immunodeficiency virus
FSH	follicle-stimulating hormone		HKD	hyperkinetic disorder
FSHMD	facioscapulohumeral muscular dystrophy		HL	Hodgkin lymphoma
fT_4	free T4		HLA	human leucocyte antigen
FVC	forced vital capacity		HLHS	hypoplastic left heart syndrome
FXS	fragile X syndrome		HMD	hyaline membrane disease
FXTAS	fragile X-associated tremor/ataxia syndrome		HMSN	hereditary motor and sensory neuropathies
G6PD	glucose-6-phosphate dehydrogenase		HPA	hyperphenylalaninaemia
GABA	gamma-aminobutyric acid		HPI	haemorrhagic parenchymal venous infarction
GABH	group A beta-haemolytic streptococci		HPL	human placental lactogen
GAG	glycosaminoglycan		HPLC	high performance liquid chromatography
GALT	gut-associated lymphoid tissue		HR	heart rate
GAS	group A β-haemolytic streptococi		HRCT	high-resolution computed tomography
GBS	group B β-haemolytic streptococci; Guillain–Barré syndrome		HS	hereditary spherocytosis
GCE	glycine encephalopathy		HSC	haemopoietic stem cells
GCS	Glasgow Coma Scale		HSE	herpes simplex encephalitis
GCSF	granulocyte-colony stimulating factor		HSMNIV	hereditary sensorimotor neuropathy type IV
GCT	germ cell tumour		HSP	heat shock protein; Henoch–Schönlein purpura
GEFS+	generalized epilepsy with febrile seizures+		HSV	herpes simplex virus
GFD	gluten-free diet		HUS	haemolytic uraemic syndrome
GFR	glomerular filtration rate		HVA	homovanillic acid
GH	growth hormone		IBD	inflammatory bowel disease
GHRH	growth hormone releasing hormone		IC	indeterminate colitis; inspiratory capacity
GI	gastrointestinal		ICC	interstitial cells of Cajal
GN	glomerulonephritis		ICP	intracranial pressure
GnRH	gonadotropin-releasing hormone		ICU	intensive care unit
GOR	gastro-oesophageal reflux		IDA	iron deficiency anaemia
GORD	gastro-oesophageal reflux disease		IE	infective endocarditis
GPCR	G-protein coupled receptor		IEF	isoelectric focusing
GSD	glycogen storage disorder		IEM	inborn error of metabolism
GTCS	generalized tonic-clonic seizures		IEP	Individual Education Plan
GU	genitourinary		IFN	interferon
GVH	graft vs host		IGAD	selective IgA deficiency
GVHD	graft vs host disease		IGE	idiopathic generalized epilepsy
HAART	highly active antiretroviral therapy		IGF	insulin-like growth factor
HAE	hereditary angio-oedema		IHPS	infantile hypertrophic pyloric stenosis
HAS	human albumin solutions		ILAR	International League of Associations for Rheumatology
HBC	hepatitis C		IM	intramuscular
HBIG	hepatitis B immunoglobulin		IMR	infant mortality rate
HBV	hepatitis B virus		INR	international normalization rate
hCG	human chorionic gonadotropin		INSS	international neuroblastoma staging system
HCM	hypertrophic cardiomyopathy		IP	incontinentia pigmenti
HDL	high density lipoprotein		IPPV	intermittent positive-pressure ventilation
HDN	haemorrhagic disease of the newborn		IPV	inactivated polio vaccine
HELLP	haemolysis, elevated liver enzymes, low platelets		IRV	inspiratory reserve volume
HFI	hereditary fructose intolerance		ITP	immune thrombocytopaenic purpura
HFOV	high-frequency oscillatory ventilation		IUGR	intrauterine growth retardation
HHF	hyperinsulinaemic hypoglycaemia, familial		IV	ichthyosis vulgaris; intravenous
HHV	human herpesvirus			

IVC	inferior vena cava	MHRA	Medicines and Healthcare Products Regulatory Agency
IVIG	intravenous immunoglobulin		
JAE	juvenile absence epilepsy	MIBG	^{123}I-meta-iodo-benzyl-guanidine
JIA	juvenile idiopathic arthritis	miRNA	micro RNA
JME	juvenile myoclonic epilepsy	MMR	measles, mumps, and rubella
KAFO	knee–ankle–foot orthoses	MMUD	mismatched unrelated donor
KD	Kawasaki disease	MN	medial nucleus
LA	left atrium	MODY	maturity-onset diabetes of the young
LABA	long-acting β-agonists	MPA	main pulmonary artery
LAM	lymphangiomyomatosis	MPGN	membranoproliferative glomerulonephritis
LBP	lipopolysaccharide-binding protein	MPS	mucopolysaccharidoses
LBW	low birthweight	MRCP	magnetic resonance cholangiopancreatography
LCA	Leber congenital amaurosis	MRD	minimal residual disease
LCAD	long-chain acyl CoA dehydrogenase	MRI	magnetic resonance imaging
LCH	Langerhans cell histiocytosis	mRNA	messenger RNA
LCHAD	long-chain hydroxyl-acyl-CoA dehydrogenase deficiency	MRSA	methicillin-resistant *Staph. aureus*
		MSH	melanocytic stimulating hormone
LDH	lactate dehydrogenase	MSUD	maple syrup urine disease
LDL	low density lipoprotein	MTCT	mother to child transmission
LFT	liver function test	mtDNA	mitochondrial DNA
LGMD	limb girdle muscular dystrophy	MUD	matched unrelated donor
LH	luteinizing hormone	MV	mitral valve
LHA	lateral hypothalamic area	NAFLD	non-alcoholic fatty liver disease
LOH	loss of heterozygosity	NAHI	non-accidental head injury
LP	lumbar puncture	NAI	non-accidental injury
LPS	lipopolysaccharide	NBT	nitroblue tetrazolium test
LQTS	long QT syndrome	NCPAP	nasal continuous positive airways pressure
LR	likelihood ratio	NEC	necrotizing enterocolitis
LSD	lysosomal storage disease	NF1	neurofibromatosis type 1
LV	left ventricle	NHL	non-Hodgkin lymphoma
MA	microalbuminuria	NICE	National Institute for Health and Clinical Excellence
MABP	mean arterial blood pressure		
MALT	mucosa-associated lymphoid tissue	NIDDM	non-insulin dependent diabetes mellitus
MBL	mannan-binding lectin	NK cells	natural killer cells
MBTS	modified Blalock–Taussig shunt	NMR	neonatal mortality rate
MCADD	medium chain acyl-CoA dehydrogenase deficiency	NNH	number needed to harm
MCDK	multicystic dysplastic kidneys	NNRTIs	non-nucleoside reverse transcriptase inhibitors
MCH	mean corpuscular haemoglobin	NNT	number needed to treat
MCNS	minimal change nephrotic syndrome	NO	nitric oxide
MCTD	mixed connective tissue disease	NPA	nasopharyngeal aspirate
MCUG	micturating cysto-urethrogram	NPS	nail–patella syndrome
MCV	mean corpuscular volume	NPV	negative predictive value
MD	myotonic dystrophy	NPY	neuropeptide Y
MDGs	Millennium Development Goals	NRTIs	nucleoside reverse transcriptase inhibitors
MDMA	methylenedioxymethamphetamine	NSAIDs	non-steroidal anti-inflammatory drugs
ME	median eminence, myalgic encephalomyelitis	NSE	neuron specific enolase
MEB	muscle–eye–brain disease	NSF	National Service Framework
MELAS	mitochondrial encephalomyopathy, lactic acidosis, stroke-like episodes	NTDs	neural tube defects
		OCN	optic chiasm nucleus
MEN	multiple endocrine neoplasia	OCA	oculocutaneous albinism
MERRF	myoclonic epilepsy with ragged-red fibres	OCD	obsessive-compulsive disorder
MFS	Marfan syndrome; Miller–Fisher syndrome	OFC	occipitofrontal circumference
MG	myasthenia gravis	OI	osteogenesis imperfecta

OME	otitis media with effusion		PTSD	post-traumatic stress disorder
OR	odds ratio		PTV	patient triggered ventilation
ORS	oral rehydration solution		PUD	peptic ulcer disease
OSA	obstructive sleep apnoea		PUJ	pelvi-ureteric junction
PA	postero-anterior		PUO	pyrexia of unknown origin
PAMP	pathogen-associated molecular pattern		PVL	periventricular leukomalacia
PANDAS	paediatric autoimmune neuropsychiatric disorder associated with streptococcal infection		PVN	paraventricular nucleus
			PVR	pulmonary vascular resistance
PBD	peroxisomal biogenesis disorder		PWS	Prader–Willi syndrome
PBSCT	peripheral blood stem cell transplantation		QF-PCR	quantitative fluorescence PCR
PC	protein C		RA	right atrium
PCHR	personal child health record		RAST	radioallergenosorbent test
PCP	*Pneumocystis carinii* pneumonia		RB	retinoblastoma
PCR	polymerase chain reaction		RBBB	right branch bundle block
PCV	pneumococcal conjugate vaccine		RCT	randomized controlled trial
PD	peritoneal dialysis		RDS	respiratory distress syndrome
PDA	patent ductus arteriosus		RES	reticuloendothelial system
PDGF	platelet-derived growth factor		RF	rheumatic fever
PEA	pulseless electrical activity		RMS	rhabdomyosarcoma
PEEP	positive end expiratory pressure		ROP	retinopathy of prematurity
PEFR	peak expiratory flow rate		RP	retinitis pigmentosa
PEM	protein-energy malnutrition		RPA	right pulmonary artery
PET	positron emission tomography		RPD	renal pelvis dilation
PFD	personal flotation device		RPGN	rapidly progressive glomerulonephritis
PFIC	progressive familial intrahepatic cholestasis		RR	relative risk
PFO	patent foramen ovale		rRNA	ribosomal RNA
PHA	pseudohypoaldosteronism		RRR	relative risk reduction
PHN	posterior hypothalamic nucleus		RS	Reed–Sternberg
PHPV	persistent hyperplastic primary vitreous		RSV	respiratory syncytial virus
PI	pancreatic insufficiency		RTA	renal tubular acidosis; road traffic accident
PID	primary immunodeficiency disease		RTK	receptor tyrosine kinase
PIE	pulmonary interstitial emphysema		RV	residual volume; right ventricle
PI	protease inhibitors		RVH	right ventricular hypertrophy
PKD	pyruvate kinase deficiency		RVOTO	right ventricular outflow tract obstruction
PKU	phenylketonuria		SAD	separation anxiety disorder
PLIC	posterior limb of the internal capsule		SADDAN	severe achondroplasia with developmental delay and acanthosis nigricans
PMDI	pressurized metered dose inhaler			
PMN	polymorphonuclear cell		SBS	short bowel syndrome
PMR	perinatal mortality rate		SCA	spinocerebellar ataxias
PN	parenteral nutrition		SCD	sickle-cell disease
PNET	primitive neuroectodermal tumour		SCFE	slipped capital femoral epiphysis
PNH	periventricular nodular heterotopia		SCID	severe combined immunodeficiency
POMC	pro-opiomelanocortin		SD	standard deviation
PP	pancreatic polypeptide		SDS	Shwachman–Diamond Syndrome
PPHN	persistent pulmonary hypertension of the newborn		SEM	standard error of the mean
			SEN	special educational needs
PPI	proton pump inhibitors		SGA	small for gestational age
PPV	pneumococcal polysaccharide vaccine; positive predictive value		SIADH	syndrome of inappropriate ADH secretion
			SIMV	synchronous intermittent mandatory ventilation
PRH	parathyroid hormone		SJS	Stevens–Johnson syndrome
PRL	prolactin		SLE	systemic lupus erythematosus
PS	pulmonary stenosis		SMA	spinal muscular atrophy
PT	prothrombin time		SMEI	severe myoclonic epilepsy of infancy
PTH	parathyroid hormone		SMS	Smith–Magenis syndrome

SNHL	sensorineural hearing loss	TV	tidal volume; tricuspid valve
SON	supraoptic nucleus	U&Es	urea and electrolytes
SP	surfactant protein	UC	ulcerative colitis
SPA	suprapubic aspiration	UCD	urea cycle disorder
SPDA	symptomatic patent ductus arteriosus	UDPGT	uridine diphosphoglucuronosyl transferase
SPECT	single photon emission computed tomography	UNCRC	United Nations Convention on the Rights of the Child
SPT	Skin prick test	UPD	uniparental disomy
SRS	Silver–Russell syndrome	URTI	upper respiratory tract infection
SSNS	steroid-sensitive nephrotic syndrome	USS	ultrasound scan
SSRI	selective serotonin re-uptake inhibitor	UTI	urinary tract infection
SSSS	staphylococcal scalded skin syndrome	VA	ventriculoarterial; visual acuity
STI	sexually transmitted infection	VACTERL	vertebral, anal, cardiac, tracheal, esophageal, renal, limb
STS	soft tissue sarcoma	VAPP	vaccine associated paralytic polio
SUDI	sudden unexpected death in infancy	VATS	video-assisted thoracoscopic surgery
SVAS	supravalvular aortic stenosis	VC	vital capacity
SVC	superior vena cava	VCFS	velocardiofacial syndrome
T1DM	type 1 diabetes mellitus	vCJD	variant Creutzfeld–Jacob disease
T2DM	type 2 diabetes mellitus	VEP	visual evoked potential
TAPVD	total anomalous pulmonary venous drainage	VF	ventricular fibrillation
TAR	thombocytopenia absent radius syndrome	VIP	vasoactive peptide
TB	tuberculosis	VLBW	very low birthweight
TBI	traumatic brain injury	VLCAD	very-long-chain acyl-CoA dehydrogenase deficiency
TBM	tuberculous meningitis	VLDL	very low density lipoprotein
TBSA	total burn surface areas	VMA	vanillylmandelic acid
TCA	tricarboxylic acid	VMN	ventromedial nucleus
TCR	T-cell receptor	VPD	vaccine-preventable death
TF	tissue factor	VSAA	very severe aplastic anaemia
TFPI	tissue factor pathway inhibitor	VSD	ventricular septal defect
TGA	transposition of great arteries	VTE	venous thrombo-embolism
TGF	transforming growth factor	VUJ	vesicoureteric junction
THI	transient hypogammaglobulinaemia of infancy	VUR	vesicoureteric reflux
TI	therapeutic index	vWD	von Willebrand disease
TLC	total lung capacity	vWF	von Willibrand factor
TM	thrombomodulin	VZIG	varicella zoster immune globulin
TOF	tetralogy of Fallot; tracheo-oesophageal fistula	VZV	varicella zoster virus
TPN	total parenteral nutrition	WAGR	Wilms tumour, aniridia, genitourinary abnormalities, retardation
TPO	thrombopoietin	WAS	Wiskott–Aldrich syndrome
TRALI	transfusion-related acute lung injury	WCC	white cell count
TRH	thyrotropin-releasing hormone	WHO	World Health Organization
tRNA	transfer RNA	WMI	white matter injury
TS	transient synovitis	WPW	Wolff–Parkinson–White
TSC	tuberous sclerosis complex	WWS	Walker–Warburg syndrome
TSE	transmissable spongiform encephalopathy	X-ALD	adrenoleucodystrophy
TSH	thyroid-stimulating hormone	XLA	X-linked agammaglobulinaemia
TSLS	toxic-shock-like syndrome	XLD	X-linked dominant
TSS	toxic shock syndrome	XLR	X-linked recessive
TT	thrombin time	ZWS	Zellweger syndrome
TTH	tension-type headache		
TTN	transient tachypnoea of the newborn		
TTP	thrombotic thrombocytopenic purpura		
TTTS	twin–twin transfusion syndrome		

Chapter 1
Neonatology

1.1 Antenatal life 2
1.2 Birth: adaptation and resuscitation 4
1.3 Neonatal physiology 6
1.4 The term newborn infant 8
1.5 Birth asphyxia and birth injury 10
1.6 Respiratory disorders in the newborn 12
1.7 Neurological disorders in the newborn 14
1.8 Problems in the preterm infant 16
1.9 Bacterial infection in the newborn 18
1.10 Viral and congenital infections in the newborn 20
1.11 Neonatal jaundice 22
1.12 Metabolic disorders 24
1.13 Congenital anomalies 26
1.14 Case-based discussions 28

1.1 Antenatal life

Fetal growth and development

Placental function
The placenta develops from the trophoblastic cells of the blastocyst and is of fetal origin, except for the decidua. The placenta has three main functions:

- *Endocrine:* hormones produced include:
  - human chorionic gonadotrophin (HCG): sustains production of progesterone and oestrogen by the corpus luteum prior to implantation. HCG in maternal urine forms the basis of the pregnancy test.
  - progesterone and oestrogen: the latter is dependent on enzymes of the fetal liver and adrenal gland.
  - human placental lactogen (HPL): has several effects including preparation of the breasts for lactation.
- *Exchange:* the placenta provides the fetus with oxygen, water, and nutrients and removes CO_2 and other waste products.
- *Protection:* maternal and fetal blood come into close proximity but do not mix. The trophoblastic cells form a non-antigenic barrier between mother and fetus.

Fetal growth and well-being
A pregnancy may be classified as *'low-risk'* or *'high-risk'* depending on maternal health, results of routine screening, and assessment of fetal health. Fetal health is assessed by monitoring for fetal movements. In a high-risk pregnancy, more detailed assessment includes:

- *Measurement of fetal growth:* serial measurements of abdominal and head circumference and femur length.
- *Amniotic fluid volume measurement:* both oligo- and poly hydramnios are associated with fetal pathology.
- *Fetal umbilical artery Doppler assessment:* abnormality can indicate poor placental function. Absent or reversed end diastolic blood flow velocity is associated with increased perinatal mortality.

If any of these are abnormal, acute assessments include:

- *Biophysical profile score (BPS):* assessment of fetal breathing, cardiotocography: (fetal tachycardia with reduced variability suggests fetal hypoxia), gross body/limb movements, fetal tone, and amniotic fluid volume. In a high-risk pregnancy fetal mortality is low with a normal score.

Intrauterine growth restriction (IUGR)

IUGR is the failure of a fetus to achieve genetic growth potential. Most are *'small for gestational age'* (SGA), i.e. below either the 10th or 3rd weight centile for gestational age. However, a naturally large infant may have IUGR yet *not* be SGA as their weight is above the 10th centile.

Aetiology and pathogenesis
Fetal growth is determined by genetic potential, maternal health, and placental function. IUGR is classified as:

- *Symmetric:* growth failure early and affecting weight, height and head size
- *Asymmetric:* growth failure late with head (brain) growth relatively preserved.

There is overlap, but the causes are different:

Symmetrical IUGR
- *Chromosomal disorders:* trisomy 13, 18, 21; Turner syndrome
- Congenital malformations
- *Intrauterine infection:* CMV, rubella, toxoplasma.

Asymmetrical IUGR
Maternal disease:
- *Undernutrition:* famine, eating disorders
- *Chronic disease:* CVS, diabetes, hypertension
- *Substance misuse:* alcohol, drugs, tobacco
- Low socio-economic status.

Placental insufficiency
- Maternal vascular supply: pre-eclampsia, BP+, diabetes
- *Infarction:* lupus anticoagulant, sickle cell disease
- Multiple gestation.

Asymmetric IUGR is caused by utero-placental insufficiency and fetal hypoxia. Blood supply to vital organs such as brain and heart is preserved but reduced supply to the liver and kidneys causes reduced glycogen stores and oligohydramnios. Progression to fetal acidaemia and death is a risk.

Management
Intensive surveillance of fetal growth is designed to maximize gestation while avoiding fetal compromise. A detailed anomaly scan, karyotyping, and screening for congenital infection is undertaken to identify a cause.

IUGR infants are prone to problems in the neonatal period:
- *Hypothermia:* reduced weight and subcutaneous fat
- *Hypoglycaemia:* reduced glycogen stores
- *Polycythaemia:* chronic hypoxia induces erythropoiesis.

Multiple pregnancies

The rates for spontaneous multiple gestations in the white population are:
- 1 in 89 for twins
- 1 in 8000 for triplets
- 1 in 700 000 for quadruplets.

The number of multiple gestations has increased because of assisted reproduction pregnancies, 20% of which are multiple. 1 in 69 births is now a multiple birth.

Twins
The incidence of twins in the UK is about 15 per 1000 live births. Determining zygosity is important as monozygotic twins have increased morbidity and mortality, particularly in the context of twin–twin transfusion syndrome.

The main pregnancy complications of twins are:
- *Preterm delivery:* 6 times more common in twins.
- *Intrauterine growth restriction:* affects 20% of dichorionic and 40% of monochorionic twins.
- *Congenital abnormalities:* risk 4 times normal in monochorionic twins.
- *Twin–twin transfusion syndrome (TTTS):* the donor develops anaemia, hypovolaemia, oliguria, and oligohydramnios and the recipient experiences the reverse. Preterm labour or intrauterine death may occur.

- *Death of a fetus:* intrauterine death of a monozygotic twin may result in preterm labour with neurological impairment in the survivor.

Prepregnancy care

Pregnancies at increased risk of fetal abnormality can be identified in advance and advice given to optimize chances of a healthy baby. Examples include genetic counselling; management of maternal illness such as diabetes mellitus or epilepsy; avoidance of maternal smoking, alcohol, drug misuse and exposure to toxoplasmosis and listeria; folic acid supplements to reduce risk of neural tube defects.

Prenatal screening and diagnosis

Maternal blood tests
- Blood group and antibodies for rhesus and other antigens
- Hepatitis B and C, rubella, syphilis, HIV
- Serum alphafetoprotein (AFP) for neural tube defects
- 'Triple test' for trisomy 21: AFP, ß-HCG, and estriol.

Utrasound
A dating scan and 18–21 week anomaly scan are recommended. Ultrasound scanning provides information on:
- *Gestational age:* reliable at <20 weeks.
- *Multiple pregnancies:* chorionicity determined.
- *Structural malformations:* 60% of major congenital malformations are identified on the routine anomaly scan.
- *Nuchal translucency:* at 11–14 weeks. Increased in trisomy 21 and other genetic disorders.
- *Fetal growth:* serial measurement of abdominal and head circumference and femur length.
- *Oligohydramnios:* with reduced fetal urine production, placental insufficiency or prolonged rupture of the membranes may result in lung hypoplasia and positional deformities.
- *Polyhydramnios:* associated with fetal bowel obstruction, CNS anomalies, multiple births, and maternal diabetes.
- *Maternal and fetal circulation:* Doppler studies.

Screening tests are non-invasive but only provide an estimate of risk. Diagnostic tests such as chorionic villus sampling (CVS) and amniocentesis provide definitive results but carry a risk of miscarriage.

Maternal disorders

Hypertension
Hypertension in pregnancy is defined as a blood pressure >140/90 mmHg and may be classified as:
- *Essential or secondary:* hypertension before pregnancy
- *Pregnancy-induced hypertension and pre-eclampsia.*
- Complications of pre-eclampsia include eclampsia and HELLP (**H**ypertension, **E**levated **L**iver enzymes, **L**ow **P**latelets) syndrome and are indications for immediate delivery.

Diabetes mellitus type 1 (T1DM)
Maternal T1DM increases fetal morbidity and mortality and causes a specific array of neonatal problems. Good diabetic control from preconception onwards is the aim.

Fetal problems
- *Congenital malformations:* in 6%, cardiac defects, caudal regression syndrome or sacral agenesis.
- Increased risk of miscarriage and intrauterine death
- *Macrosomia:* in 25% due to hyperinsulinaemia
- Polyhydramnios.

Neonatal problems
- *Preterm labour:* occurs in 10%, natural or induced
- *Macrosomia:* predisposes to birth injury
- *Hypoglycaemia:* in first 48 h due to hyperinsulinism
- *Polycythaemia:* plethoric appearance and jaundice
- *Respiratory distress syndrome:* increased risk.

Red blood cell isoimmunisation
Maternal antibodies to red cells antigens including rhesus D, Kell, and ABO group. Anti-D prophylaxis has almost eliminated rhesus haemolytic disease. Severe disease may require intrauterine blood transfusion and delivery preterm.

Neonatal alloimmune thrombocytopaenia
Antibodies against fetal platelets, HPA-1a in 80%, cross the placenta and cause fetal thrombocytopaenia which may be associated with intracranial haemorrhage. Compatible platelet transfusions may be given pre- or postnatally.

Maternal autoimmune diseases
Thyroid disease
- *Maternal hyperthyroidism:* in 10% of mothers with Graves disease antibodies to TSHr cross the placenta and cause fetal hyperthyroidism or transient neonatal hyperthyroidism. Maternal antithyroid drugs can cause neonatal hypothyroidism.
- *Autoimmune thrombocytopaenia:* maternal autoimmune thrombocytopaenia may result in transplacental passage of IgG and fetal thrombocytopaenia.
- *Systemic lupus erythematosus (SLE):* maternal SLE is associated with increased risk of miscarriage and may cause neonatal lupus syndrome with a rash and heart block.
- *Myasthenia gravis:* transplacental passage of anti-AChR antibodies cause transient neonatal myasthenia gravis.

Maternal smoking, alcohol and substance abuse
- *Smoking:* maternal cigarette smoking is associated with an increased risk of IUGR, miscarriage, and stillbirth.
- *Alcohol:* excess alcohol over a period causes fetal alcohol syndrome characterized by: typical facies, micrognathia, symmetric IUGR, cardiac defects and developmental delay.
- *Substance misuse:* cocaine causes placental infarction leading to IUGR, fetal death and placental absorption, or fetal cerebral infarction *in utero*.

Neonatal abstinence syndrome occurs in infants of mothers on opiates or methadone. Signs of opiate withdrawal: high-pitched cry, sneezing, hiccups, vomiting, diarrhoea, seizures, and poor feeding appear in the first few days of life. Methadone withdrawal can be delayed for 2 weeks. Treatment is with oral morphine sulfate in a tapering dose.

1.2 Birth: adaptation and resuscitation

Epidemiology

Definitions

- A *'term'* infant is one that has completed 37–41 weeks of gestation at birth.
- Preterm: <37 completed weeks of gestation.
- Post-term: ≥42 completed weeks of gestation.

Birthweight is classified as:
- Low birthweight   (LBW):   <2500 g
- Very low birthweight   (VLBW):   1500 g
- Extremely low birthweight (ELBW): <1000 g.

Mortality and mortality rates

- *Live birth:* a baby born at any gestation with signs of life including breathing, a heartbeat and voluntary movement.
- *Stillbirth:* a fetus born after 24 weeks of gestation who shows no signs of life. Definitions vary between countries. In the USA, a fetus born with no signs of life after 20–28 weeks gestation or birthweight >350–≥500 g.
- *Maternal mortality:* maternal deaths, during pregnancy or up to 42 days postpartum, per 100 000 live births.
- *Stillbirth rate:* number of fetuses born dead after 24 weeks gestation per 1000 live births and stillbirths.
- *Neonatal mortality rate (NMR):* number of liveborn babies who die within the first 4 weeks or 27 completed days of life per 1000 live births.
- *Perinatal mortality rate (PMR):* stillbirth rate plus early neonatal deaths up to 6 completed days of life per 1000 live and stillbirths.
- *Post-neonatal mortality rate:* deaths from 28 days until 1 year per 1000 live births.
- *Infant mortality rate:* deaths in the first year of life per 1000 live births.

Mortality rates are useful measures which allow comparison between countries and monitoring of changes over time.

Preterm and low birth weight infants

Mortality
Two thirds of all infant deaths occur in the 8% of LBW infants, and half are among the 1.4% born with VLBW.

Table 1.1. Neonatal mortality rates correlate with birthweight. Figures from USA, 2000		
Birthweight (g)	% Births	Neonatal mortality rate (per 1000 live births)
>2500	92.4	0.9
<2500 (LBW)	7.6	48
<1500 (VLBW)	1.4	214

In VLBW infants there is a strong correlation between birthweight and mortality.

Morbidity
The most important sequelae of preterm birth are those affecting the brain and influencing neurodevelopment. Chronic lung disease develops in 37% of VLBW infants and is a major cause of morbidity and mortality in the first years.

Impaired neurodevelopmental outcome includes children who develop cerebral palsy and is associated with a wide spectrum of disability ranging from mild to severe.

Two studies of mortality and disability in infants born alive at 22–26 weeks gestation in the UK in 1995 and 2006 have been carried out: EPICure1 and 2 (Fig 1.1). These show a high rate of morbidity and mortality in infants born at <24 weeks of completed gestation.

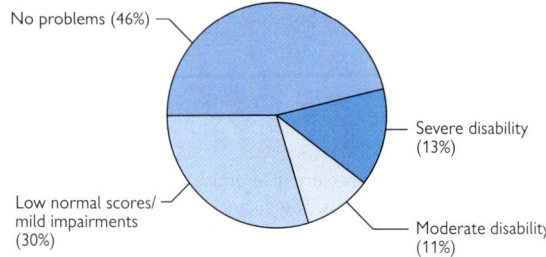

Fig 1.1 Proportion of survivors of infants born alive at 22–25 weeks gestation with disability at age 6 years using standard definitions. EPICure 1 Study.

EPICure 2 showed an increase in overall survival rate for 952 babies born before 26 weeks gestation from 40% in 1995 to 52% in 2006. By gestational age the survival figures were:
- *25 weeks:* increase from 54% to 67%
- *24 weeks:* increase from 35% to 47%
- *<24 weeks:* no statistically significant change.

There was no change in the proportion of 13% with serious brain abnormalities and the proportion of 74% dependent on oxygen on their expected date of delivery.

Birth statistics: a global perspective

There is a striking disparity between the health of mothers and newborn infants in the developing and developed world. Of the 130 million babies born every year there are about 4 million neonatal deaths and 4 million stillbirths.

The most common cause of neonatal mortality globally is infection followed by the complications of prematurity. Half of these infants die after a home birth without any health care. Newborn deaths account for 40% of all deaths among children <5 years.

These infants lack 'essential newborn care': clean delivery practices, temperature maintenance, infection control, exclusive breast-feeding, early detection of problems, and appropriate care seeking.

Adaptation to extrauterine life

Lungs
Before birth the fetal lung is filled with liquid actively secreted by the alveolar epithelium which is important for normal lung growth. During spontaneous labour lung liquid is reabsorbed and squeezing of the chest extrudes some lung liquid from the trachea. Persistence of lung liquid causes transient tachypnoea of the newborn (TTN) which is more common after birth by Caesarean section.

Surfactant is produced by type II alveolar cells from 20 weeks. Surfactant lowers surface tension and allows alveolar expansion.

Circulation
In the fetus the placenta is the main organ of gas exchange so blood bypasses the lungs via the foramen ovale and ductus arteriosus. Pulmonary vascular resistance is high. Oxygenated blood from the placenta passes via umbilical vein, ductus venosus, inferior

vena cava (IVC), and right atrium into the left atrium through the foramen ovale. This oxygenated blood passes to the left ventricle and ascending aorta to supply coronary and carotid arteries. Deoxygenated blood enters the aortic arch through the ductus arteriosus. Both ventricles support the systemic circulation.

Reflex gasping at birth generates a high intrathoracic pressure (>50 cmH$_2$O) which allows air to enter the lungs. Three principle components of the circulatory changes at birth are:
- *Pulmonary vasodilatation:* caused by rise in PaO$_2$, fall in PaCO$_2$, and mechanical stretching
- *Closure of foramen ovale:* increase in blood returning via the pulmonary veins causes a rise in left atrial pressure
- *Closure of ductus arteriosus:* cord clamping removes the low resistance placental circulation and the rise in systemic blood pressure coupled with the fall in pulmonary vascular resistance abolishes the pressure differential and allows bidirectional flow in the ductus. The ductus arteriosus contracts in response to the raised PaO$_2$ of the blood in its lumen.

In addition, the ductus venosus and umbilical arteries constrict.

Metabolism
The fetus is entirely dependent on transplacental nutrient transfer. Blood glucose concentration falls rapidly after birth to a low at 1 h, rising again by 3 h. Insulin levels fall and a surge of glucagon, secondary to a corticosteroid mediated stress response, mobilizes liver glycogen. Ketone body production increases to high levels within 12 h.

Neonatal resuscitation
Assessment of the newborn: the Apgar score
This was devised by Dr Virginia Apgar in 1953. Five clinical features are scored from 0 to 2 at 1 and 5 min after birth.

	Score	0	1	2
A	Appearance	White	Blue extremities	Pink
P	Pulse (bpm)	Absent	<100	>100
G	Grimace	Nil	Some	Cry
A	Activity	Limp	Some flexion	Active
R	Respiration	Absent	Hypoventilation	Good

The Apgar score provides an overall measure of the baby's condition and is assigned irrespective of resuscitation being performed. However, it is of limited prognostic value and a Sarnat score at 48 h is more useful in predicting long term outcome.

Resuscitation
Only 5–10% of all newborns require any resuscitation and <1% require intubation in the delivery room.

Deliveries which should be attended by a paediatrician include: gestation <36 weeks, instrumental or surgical deliveries, malpresentations, multiple pregnancies, fetal distress or meconium staining, antenatal diagnosis of malformation or Rhesus disease.

Factors other than intrapartum asphyxia may delay onset of respiration and may co-exist in a single baby. They include drugs causing CNS depression, prematurity, birth trauma, sepsis, severe anaemia or congenital malformations such as congenital diaphragmatic hernia.

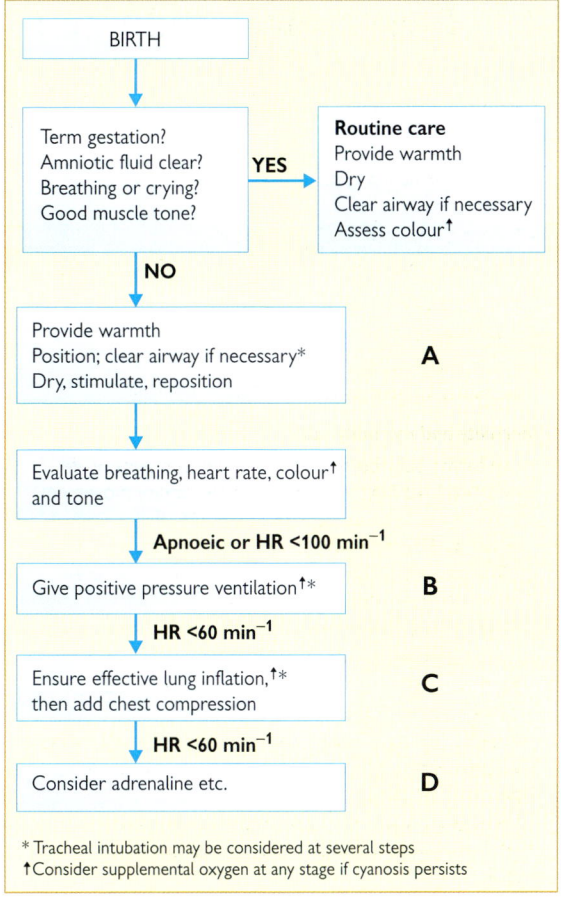

Fig 1.2 Algorithm from Resuscitation Guideline (UK). Courtesy of the Resuscitation Council UK.

Initial assessment and actions
Before delivery introduce yourself to parents, review obstetric records and check all equipment is functional.

At birth, start clock and assess the infant who is likely to fall into one of four main groups:
- Fit, healthy term infant, crying lustily >90%
- Irregular respirations, HR >100 bpm 5%
- Pale, limp, apnoeic, HR <60 bpm 0.5%
- Dead but rescuscitatable <0.1%.

Resuscitation follows the guidelines shown in Fig 1.2.
- *If baby >2 kg with inadequate respiration, HR 80–100 bpm:* administer air by face mask, give peripheral stimulus to breathing.
- *If poor response:* administer mask ventilation attached to a self-inflating bag or a mechanical ventilator via a T-piece using 100% oxygen for term infants or air-oxygen mixture if <32 weeks gestation. Give five breaths at a pressure of 30–40 cmH$_2$O for 2–3 s each to expand the lungs (check chest is moving) and continue at 40–60 breaths/min. Stop when heart rate >100 beats/minute and spontaneous breathing established. Indications for intubation and circulatory support are described in section 1.6.

1.3 Neonatal physiology

The physiological homeostatic challenges faced by newborn infants are all more severe in the preterm infant.

Temperature control

Maintenance of body temperature is a challenge for all newborn babies primarily because their large surface area to body mass causes rapid heat loss. In preterm infants additional factors increase the risk of hypothermia.

Physiology

Heat is lost in four ways:

- *Conduction:* small losses unless baby laid on a cold, uninsulated surface
- *Evaporation:* caused by evaporation of surface water and depends on skin thickness. Trans-epidermal loss is increased in preterm infants by exposure to drying factors such as radiant heaters
- *Convection:* minimal unless infant exposed to cool draft
- *Radiation:* depends on temperature difference between skin and surrounding surfaces such as incubator walls.

Infants are able to conserve and produce heat by:

- *Heat conservation:* a curled-up posture and insulation provided by subcutaneous fat and skin vasoconstriction all reduce heat loss but are less effective in preterms
- *Heat production:* non-shivering thermogenesis by hydrolysis of triglycerides in brown fat is the main mechanism. Shivering occurs at an ambient temperature <15°C in term infants but does not occur in pre-term infants until age 2 weeks.

Management of temperature control

Infants should be nursed in a neutral thermal environment which is the temperature at which heat production and oxygen consumption is minimal and core temperature is close to 37°C.

In order to prevent hypothermia the preterm infant should be:

- Resuscitated under an overhead radiant heater on a pre-warmed resuscitaire in a draught-free area
- Placed in a plastic bag or wrapped in clingfilm to minimize evaporative losses. A hat on the head reduces radiant heat loss
- Transported to the neonatal unit rapidly, avoiding convective heat loss
- Nursed in a double-glazed incubator in a flexed position covered with an insulating fabric under a radiant heat shield with minimal handling
- Ventilated with warm, humidified gases.

Thermal stress

Hypothermia (temperature <35°C) in the newborn infant, increases mortality and morbidity and is associated with:

- Increased oxygen consumption with hypoxia, hypoglycaemia, and metabolic acidosis
- Apnoea
- Failure to gain weight
- Neonatal cold injury or sclerema
- Reduced blood coagulability.

Hypothermia may reflect poor control of the thermal environment or be a sign of serious illness such as sepsis or brain damage.

Overheating by incubator/room temperature too high or over-swaddling may cause fluid loss and hypernatraemia, and apnoea. Pyrexia (temperature >38.0°C) may also be a sign of infection, dehydration, or brain damage to hypothalamic centres.

Respiratory system

Immaturity of the lungs associated with respiratory distress syndrome (RDS) dominates the problems associated with preterm birth.

Lung development

See Chapter 3. The lungs enter the saccular phase at about 24 weeks gestation during which terminal sacs, alveolar ducts and alveoli form. Surfactant production by Type II pneumocytes begins from 23 weeks.

Surfactant is 90% lipids (phosphatidylcholine, phosphatidylglycerol, neutral lipids) and 10% protein (surfactant proteins SP-A, SP-B, SP-C, SP-D). It is a surface tension lowering agent which prevents alveolar collapse and improves lung compliance.

Surfactant deficiency causes RDS in which the opening pressure required to initiate inflation is high and alveoli collapse to zero volume during expiration.

Respiratory support

Strategies include antenatal corticosteroids, surfactant therapy, supplemental oxygen, continuous positive airway pressure (CPAP), positive pressure ventilation, inhaled nitric oxide (NO), and extracorporeal membrane oxygenation (ECMO). See Section 1.6.

Cardiovascular system

The circulatory blood volume of a newborn infant is ~90 mL/kg. Preterm infants, especially with severe RDS, are often hypotensive due to a combination of hypovolaemia and depressed cardiac function.

Continuous blood pressure monitoring can be achieved from an indwelling umbilical or peripheral arterial cannula. Blood pressure varies with gestational age. While a useful rule of thumb is to aim to keep the mean arterial blood pressure (MABP) above a value equal to the baby's gestational age in weeks, blood flow and oxygen delivery to vital organs is more important than the absolute BP value.

Options for treatment of hypotension depend on aetiology and include:

- *Hypovolaemia:* 10–20 mL/kg of saline or blood (if PCV <40%).
- *Inotropic support:* dopamine increases vascular resistance (useful in sepsis). Dobutamine is useful if cardiac contractility needs support.

Rapid fluctuations in MABP should be avoided. Blood sampling should be minimized and recorded so that appropriate replacement transfusions are given.

Fluid and electrolyte balance

The preterm infant in particular has difficulty in regulating fluid and electrolyte balance because of:
- *Immature renal function:* human nephrogenesis is complete by 35 weeks gestation but the newborn GFR is low compared to an adult: preterm 0.5 mL/kg per min, term 1.5 mL/kg per min, adult 2 mL/kg per min.
- *Insensible water loss:* transepidermal water loss is very high in preterm infants but respiratory tract loss may account for up to half of insensible losses. These losses are minimized by high ambient humidity and humidification of respiratory gases.

Part of normal adaptation to extrauterine life is a marked reduction in body water, especially extracellular fluid, which accounts for the early fall in body weight. A diuretic and natriuretic phase occurs after 12–24 h. Sodium is not added to IV fluids until after this has occurred.

Preterm infants may accumulate excess fluid or become dehydrated without careful attention. Weight and serum sodium concentration are the key indicators.

Excess fluid

Caused by fluid overload or fluid retention:
- *Fluid overload:* excess maintenance fluid, when normal diuresis/natriuresis delayed e. g. boluses of dextrose, plasma, blood given and not allowed for.
- *Fluid retention:* renal failure, cardiac failure (e. g. with patent ductus arteriosus, PDA), inappropriate ADH secretion, leaky capillaries.

In the first week excess fluid is indicated by weight loss of <1% per day or weight gain, and after the first week a weight gain of >20 g/kg per 24 h. Oedema may be hidden around the back and flank of a baby nursed supine.

Excess fluids may cause heart failure, pulmonary oedema, an increased incidence of PDA, hyponatraemia and cerebral oedema if there is coexisting encephalopathy.

Treatment depends on aetiology but fluid restriction usually suffices.

Dehydration

Causes include high transepidermal water loss, osmotic diuresis due to hyperglycaemia, gut losses, inadequate intake, over use of diuretics or pyrexia.

In the first week dehydration is indicated by a weight loss ≥3% per day. Signs to recognize are: decreased skin turgor, sunken eyes, depressed fontanelle and reduced urine output.

The effects include hypovolaemia leading if severe to acidosis and uraemia. Jaundice is exacerbated and hypernatraemia common.

Fluid intake according to weight and postnatal age		
Postnatal age (days)	Fluid intake (mL/kg per 24 h)	
	<2.5 kg	>2.5 kg
1	60–100	40–80
2	90–120	60–100
3	120–150	90–120
4	150	120–150
5	150–180	150

Nutrition

Energy and nutrient requirements of the preterm infant are high to maintain the rapid growth which was occurring *in utero*, 15 g/kg per day between 24 and 36 weeks gestation, and to offset the catabolic effects of the stress of preterm birth. Enteral feeding is the best route to deliver nutrition, but total parenteral nutrition (TPN) may be necessary.

Nutrient requirements

An energy intake of 120–140 kcal/kg per day is required to meet energy needs of essential body functions and growth. Fat is the main energy source and should provide 30% of the total caloric intake. A protein intake of 3–4.0 g/kg per day is recommended. Additional sodium, calcium, and phosphorus is required by LBW infants.

Enteral feeding

Preterm infants <34 weeks gestation are unable to coordinate sucking and swallowing and require tube feeding. The tube may be orogastric, which is difficult to fix, or nasogastric, which increases airway resistance. Continuous infusion may be preferable to bolus feeds in VLBW neonates.

Minimal enteral, non-nutritive, feeding may be given initially at 10–20 mL/kg per day. This encourages gut hormone secretion, aids intestinal maturation and gallbladder function, and helps in the earlier achievement of full enteral feeds.

Breast milk is the milk of choice, either mother's own or from a donor. LBW infant formulas have been developed to supply the increased energy, protein, sodium, and phosphate required by LBW infants.

Complications of enteral milk feeding in preterm infants include:
- Pooling in stomach with regurgitation and aspiration
- Compromise of respiratory function by gastric distension and nasogastric tube obstruction with recurrent apnoea
- *Infection:* gastroenteritis or necrotizing enterocolitis
- *Electrolyte imbalance:* hyponatraemia, hypophosphataemia (with breast milk).

Parenteral nutrition

Parenteral nutrition may be total (TPN) or supplementary. It can be life saving but has complications and should be regarded as second best to enteral nutrition. Full TPN provides all the fat, protein, carbohydrate, vitamins, minerals, and calories to support normal growth.

TPN should be considered in VLBW infants after 2–3 days if enteral feeding is not tolerated. It is usually given via a central venous line but can be given via a peripheral vein although thrombosis and extravasation are potential hazards.

Complications of TPN include:
- *Infection:* the major complication, may cause insidious deterioration.
- *Cholestatic jaundice:* 30% of preterm infants receiving TPN for >2 weeks develop conjugated hyperbilirubinaemia which usually resolves with enteral feeding.
- *Hyperglycaemia:* common, sometimes requiring insulin
- *Catheter related:* thrombosis from central lines, tamponade risk if malpositioned in the right atrium, chemical burns from peripheral extravasation.

1.4 The term newborn infant

Examination of the newborn infant

A comprehensive examination, ideally within the first 24 h, and certainly by 72 h, is performed in order to:

- *Detect congenital abnormalities:* present in 1–2% of newborn infants.
- Confirm and consider management of abnormalities detected antenatally.
- *Identify common problems:* such as jaundice, pallor, plethora, cyanosis, respiratory distress.

At the same time, the opportunity is taken to provide care and support for the parents and consider problems related to maternal pregnancy history or familial disorders, answer any questions, provide health promotion information and identify any concerns about the care of the infant after discharge. See http: //nipe.screening.nhs.uk

Examination

Examine in a warm environment, on a firm mattress or in a cot, with both parents present if possible. At some point the infant must be completely undressed, including nappy removal. Examination should be opportunistic but systematic and complete. Inspection is followed by a 'top to tail' progression, finishing with examination of the hips.

General inspection
- *Dysmorphic features:* unusual appearance of face, hands, feet
- *Growth parameters:* evidence of macrosomia or IUGR
- *Colour:* pallor, plethora, jaundice, cyanosis
- *Skin lesions:* Mongolian blue spot, stork marks
- *Tone, posture, and movements*: flexed posture, symmetrical movements.

Head
- *Cranium:* occipitofrontal circumference (OFC), fontanelle, soft tissues
- *Eyes:* check red reflex, iris, sticky eyes, subconjunctival haemorrhage, cataracts
- *Palate:* inspect and palpate to identify cleft

Chest
- *Observe:* for respiratory distress: rate, retractions, grunting, nostril flaring
- *Auscultate heart:* heart rate, murmurs
- *Palpate: apex,* brachial, and femoral pulses.

Abdomen, genitalia, and anus
- Umbilical hernia, liver (normal 1–2 cm), spleen tip, and left kidney may be palpable. Any masses?
- Palpate femoral pulses
- Check testes in scrotum and normal penis in boys, normal anatomy in girls
- *Anus:* check patency.

Spine and hips
- *Spine:* sacral dimples below natal cleft are common and benign. Simple dimples are >2.5 cm from the anus, <5 mm in size midline with no associated vascular or cutaneous stigmata. If proximal, do ultrasound to check for tract and consider MRI. Lesions over spine may indicate spina bifida occulta.

- *Hips:* aim is to identify developmental dysplasia of the hip (DDH). Risk factors include female sex (F: M ratio 9: 1), family history in 20%, breech presentation in 30% and neuromuscular disorders.
  - inspection: asymmetrical skin folds and leg shortening.
  - attempt full abduction of each hip: abduction restricted if hip dislocated.

Barlow manoeuvre: tests for dislocatable hip
The hip is held flexed and adducted. The femoral head is pushed downwards. If dislocatable, the femoral head will be pushed posteriorly out of the acetabulum.

Ortolani manoeuvre: tests for dislocated hip
Abduct hip with upward leverage of femur. A dislocated hip will return with a palpable clunk into the acetabulum.

If examination is questionable hip ultrasound is undertaken at 4–6 weeks of age. Urgent orthopaedic referral is required for a dislocated or dislocatable hip.

Significant congenital anomalies which may be identified on routine examination include trisomy syndromes, cleft lip or palate, congenital heart disease, ambiguous genitalia, hypospadias, undescended testes, umbilical hernia (Fig 1.3), imperforate anus (Fig 1.4), and spina bifida occulta.

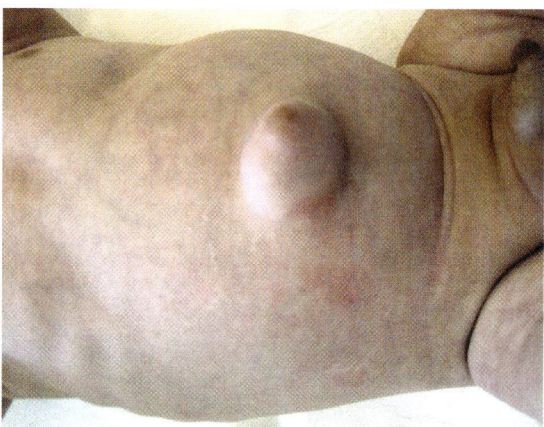

Fig 1.3 Umbilical hernia.

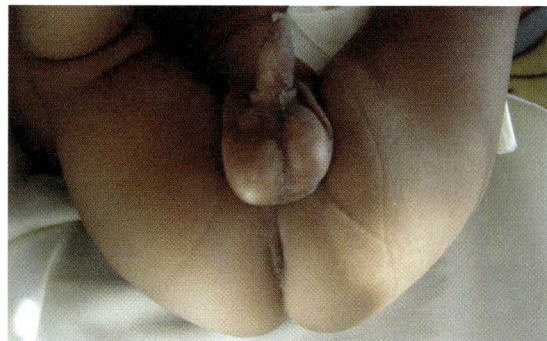

Fig 1.4 Imperforate anus.

Care of the term newborn

Routine aspects of care include:
- Umbilical cord clamped, baby dried and wrapped and handed to mother to allow direct skin-to-skin contact.
- *Vitamin K:* consent given antenatally usually for IM vitamin K as prophylaxis against haemorrhagic disease of the newborn.
- *Vaccinations:* intradermal BCG for infant in high-risk area or ethnic group. Hepatitis B if mother HbsAg positive.
- *Screening:* newborn blood spot screening for phenylketonuria, hypothyroidism, medium chain acyl-CoA dehydrogenase deficiency (MCADD), cystic fibrosis, and haemoglobinopathies: thalassaemia, sickle cell disease.
- *Health promotion:* advice on feeding, immunisation and how to reduce the risk of sudden unexpected death in infancy (SUDI).

Care and support of the parents

The family is always included in the care of the newborn infant but especially so if the infant is very premature, seriously ill, has serious congenital abnormalities, or dies. Promotion of maternal attachment and communication of bad news are important aspects of parental care.

Maternal attachment

Attachment (bonding) between mother, and other family members and the baby is promoted by: prenatal classes and preparation and support during labour, avoiding separation, eye to eye contact after birth (a powerful stimulus), seeing, touching, smelling, and providing care for the baby.

Risk factors for failure of attachment include:
- Family disharmony, unwanted pregnancy, socio-economic disadvantage (single parent, poverty), substance misuse
- Lack of support during labour
- Serious illness in infant, e.g. extreme prematurity, serious congenital malformation
- Separation from infant
- Maternal depression.

Communicating bad news

Parents of an infant with serious malformation or life-threatening illness experience emotional turmoil as they mourn the loss of the expected normal child. Accurate and realistic information must be provided and the parents' anxieties and emotions must be listened to and addressed. It is a role for a senior doctor.

Principles of communication include:
- *The setting:* in private, both parents present, uninterrupted, and unhurried.
- *The start:* establish rapport by using child's name, making eye contact, being open and sympathetic. Establish what the family knows and believes.
- *The information:* establish what has been understood and clarify or repeat important aspects. Mention sources of support such as parent groups. Provide telephone contact and arrange follow up.

Feeding

Breast-feeding is recommended for all term infants for the first 6 months of life: 'breast is best'. All mothers should be encouraged and supported to breast-feed. It takes 24–72 h for breast milk to come in and replace colostrum, a low-volume fluid with high protein content.

Breast-feeding has both advantages and disadvantages for mother and infant.

Composition of breast and formula milk

Compared to formula milk, mature breast milk has a lower concentration of most constituents except carbohydrate.

Human mature breast milk contains:
- 7% carbohydrate, mostly as lactose: formula has 5%
- 1% protein compared to formula 3%
- 4% fat which is similar to the 4% in formula. Fat content in breast milk rises towards the end of the feed. The fat is mainly triglycerides in both milks and provides 50% of the energy intake. Breast milk has five times the content of the essential linoleic acid compared to cow's milk so this is added to formula milk.

The concentration of sodium, potassium, calcium, and phosphate are all lower in breast milk compared to formula.

Advantages of breast-feeding

For the infant
- Ideal nutritional composition, including immune factors
- Reduces risk of gastroenteritis
- May reduce incidence of obesity and asthma
- Promotes mother-infant bonding.

For the mother
- Promotes mother-infant bonding
- Decreased risk of osteoporosis, breast and ovarian cancer
- Increased interval between pregnancies in developing countries.

Disadvantages of breast-feeding

For the infant
- Potentially inadequate milk intake with dehydration and hypernatraemia in first few days.
- Breast milk jaundice
- Vitamin K deficiency bleeding
- *Rickets:* low vitamin D levels if prolonged in at risk infants.
- Iron deficiency if prolonged.

For the mother
- Maternal feelings of inadequacy if unsuccessful
- Breast engorgement, cracked nipples, mastitis.

A small number of contra-indications to breast-feeding exist:
- Maternal HIV (in developed countries) or active TB
- Inborn errors of metabolism, e.g. galactosaemia, PKU
- *Maternal medication with certain drugs:* see BNFC.

1.5 Birth asphyxia and birth injury

Birth asphyxia

Asphyxia is the term used for a state in which respiratory gas exchange is compromised, resulting in hypoxia, hypercarbia, metabolic acidosis, and cardiorespiratory depression. The most important consequence of birth asphyxia is hypoxic-ischaemic injury to the brain resulting in hypoxic-ischaemic encephalopathy (HIE). In developed countries 0.5–1.0/1000 liveborn infants develop HIE.

Aetiology and pathogenesis

Asphyxia may occur before labour (antepartum), during labour (intrapartum) or after delivery (postpartum) or during all of these periods.

Mechanisms may include:
- *Antepartum:*
  - inadequate maternal placental perfusion caused by maternal hypotension or hypertension
  - *compromised fetus:* fetal anaemia, IUGR
- *Intrapartum:*
  - placental failure: prolonged or excessive uterine contractions, placental abruption, ruptured uterus
  - *interruption of umbilical cord blood flow:* cord compression, cord prolapse
- *Postpartum:* failure of cardiorespiratory adaptation at birth, which may itself be a consequence of intrapartum asphyxia or the result of drugs.

Establishing the exact timing and nature of an asphyxial insult can be difficult as the state of the infant during labour can only be assessed indirectly at the time and retrospectively from the condition at birth. This has obvious medico-legal implications and the criteria for establishing that asphyxia has occurred during birth remain controversial.

Neonatal response to asphyxia

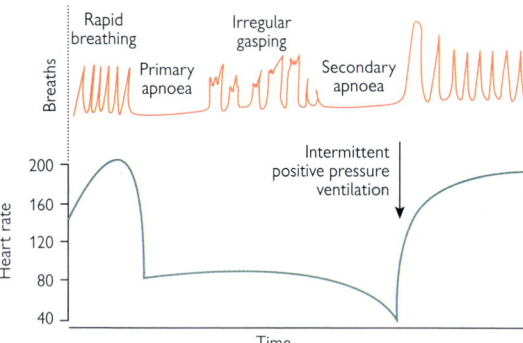

Fig 1.5 Effects of asphyxia.

Sustained severe asphyxia in the newborn leads to:
- Increased respiratory effort.
- Primary apnoea with bradycardia due to vagal stimulation and effect of hypoxia on pacemaker cells but sustained cardiac output and blood pressure due to surge of catecholamines causing peripheral vasoconstriction.
- Irregular gasping followed by terminal apnoea (Fig 1.5).

Worsening acidosis, respiratory and metabolic, is associated with increasing bradycardia (<60/min), hypotension, fall in cardiac output, and hypoxic–ischaemic brain injury.

Severe intrapartum asphyxia may result in the delivery of a baby with severe acidosis (pH<7.0), limp, bradycardic, and in terminal apnoea. Acute severe asphyxia usually causes brain damage within 10–12 min and death after 20–30 min.

The supply of oxygen to the brain is compromised both by failure of gas exchange (hypoxia) and failure of cerebral blood supply (ischaemia) due to circulatory depression. Neuronal death is believed to occur in two phases:

- *Primary neuronal death:* caused by energy depletion with a fall in ATP and phosphocreatine and accumulation of lactic acid with necrosis of neurons
- *Secondary neuronal death:* following re-perfusion of the brain excitatory amino acids are released activating NMDA receptors and causing influx of calcium which triggers neuronal apoptosis.

Neuroprotective measures such as whole body or head hypothermia are designed to prevent secondary neuronal death.

Clinical features

Criteria for identifying an 'asphyxiated' infant include:
- Severe metabolic acidosis: profound acidaemia (pH <7.0) on umbilical cord artery sample
- Apgar score 0–3 for >5 min
- Hypoxic–ischaemic encephalopathy
- Multisystem organ dysfunction.

Management

Involves neonatal resuscitation and leads on to management of HIE (See Section 1.7). Resuscitation of the infant with severe asphyxia may include:

Endotracheal intubation

Laryngoscopy and intubation are indicated if:
- Mask ventilation is ineffective or the infant is still apnoeic or bradycardic at 2 min
- Infant pale, limp, apnoeic. HR <80 bpm, terminal apnoea.

Limit attempts to 20–30 s and mask-ventilate in between. Give IPPV at a rate of 60/min and 30 cmH$_2$O pressure. Oxygen is given as required.

Circulatory support

External cardiac compression is only required if significant bradycardia (<60 bpm) persists despite adequate ventilation. Depress lower third of sternum with both thumbs, grasping the chest with fingers supporting thoracic spine, aiming to reduce AP diameter of chest by one third. Give 60–90 compressions/min, three compressions to one breath.

Drugs

Drugs are only required if there is no response to effective ventilation and cardiac massage.

- *Adrenaline:* IV 10–30 micrograms/kg given IV, preferably via an umbilical venous line
- *Sodium bicarbonate:* 2 mmol/kg IV slowly after prolonged arrest in a baby with severe metabolic acidosis (base deficit >20mmol/L)
- *10% dextrose:* 1 mL/kg IV if there is hypoglycaemia
- *Volume expansion:* 10 mL/kg IV of normal saline or whole blood if there is hypovolaemia from blood loss.

Birth injuries

Severe birth injuries are now uncommon as prolonged labour and difficult instrumental deliveries are avoided by Caesarean section. However, they still do occur after labour involving malpresentations such as breech delivery, shoulder dystocia, instrumental delivery, preterm, or very rapid delivery. They are conveniently classified by location.

Injuries to head
Soft tissue injuries

Scalp swellings and haematomas occur at distinct anatomical levels:
- *Caput succedaneum*: oedema and bruising of presenting part of scalp which crosses suture lines. Resolves within days.
- *Cephalhaematoma* (see Fig 1.6): subperiosteal haemorrhage limited by suture lines associated with prolonged or instrumental labour. May exacerbate jaundice and may calcify. Resolves in days to weeks.

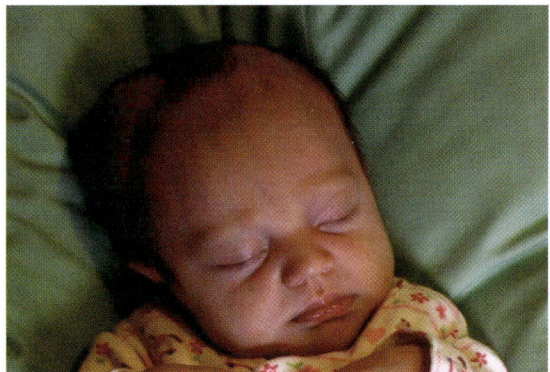

Fig 1.6 Cephalhaematoma.

- *Subaponeurotic (subgaleal) haemorrhage:* a rare bleed beneath the aponeurosis. Risk factors include prematurity, vacuum extraction, and underlying coagulopathy. May progress to hypovolaemic shock.
- *Skull fracture:* uncommon, may involve parietal or occipital bone, good prognosis.

Intracranial haemorrhage
- *Subdural haemorrhage:* asymptomatic subdural haemorrhage is now known to be quite common and resolves on imaging by 3 months. Symptomatic subdural haemorrhage may manifest with hypotonia, seizures, and apnoea, and if large may require surgical intervention.
- *Subarachnoid haemorrhage:* rupture of small blood vessels in the subarachnoid space is not uncommon in traumatic or asphyxial deliveries. Often asymptomatic but may present with seizures. CSF is uniformly blood stained.

If intracranial haemorrhage is suspected, cranial ultrasound is useful initially but definitive diagnosis requires CT or MRI.

Facial palsy

Usually unilateral and caused by forceps delivery or pressure on maternal ischial spine. The eye is involved and remains open. Resolves in 1–2 weeks.

Differential diagnosis includes:
- *Congenital palsy which is bilateral:* Moebius syndrome
- *Asymmetric crying facies (ACF):* usually due to hypoplastic depressor anguli oris muscle, in which the eye can close. May be part of velocardiofacial syndrome.

Injuries to neck and shoulders
Fractured clavicle

May complicate shoulder dystocia or breech delivery. A snap may be heard during delivery. Heals spontaneously.

Brachial plexus injury

Erb's palsy (90%)

Involves C5, C6 ± C7: Incidence 1–2 per 1000 deliveries. There is an association with macrosomia, birthweight >4 kg, and shoulder dystocia. The upper cords of the brachial plexus are contused by excessive traction.

The baby's arm lies limply in the 'waiter's tip' position (Fig 1.7) with absent biceps jerk. The phrenic nerve may be involved with diaphragmatic palsy in 5%. Most resolve spontaneously by 4 months. Physiotherapy ± splints are used to avoid contractures and surgical repair of the plexus using microsurgery is considered if there is no return of biceps function by 6–12 weeks.

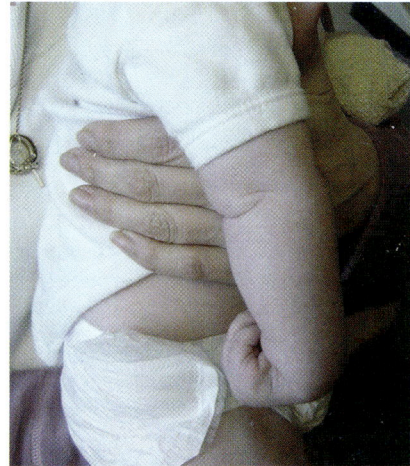

Fig 1.7 Erb's palsy: 'waiter's tip' position.

Klumpke's palsy (<1%)

Involves C8, T1: This rare lesion may complicate breech delivery. A claw hand deformity may be accompanied by Horner syndrome in 30%. Fractures of clavicle, spine, or humerus may accompany brachial plexus injury.

1.6 Respiratory disorders in the newborn

Problems in the term infant

Respiratory distress

Aetiology

The causes of respiratory distress in term newborn infants are usefully classified into common, uncommon and rare:

- *Common:*
  - transient tachypnoea of the newborn (TTN)
- *Uncommon:*
  - pneumonia
  - meconium aspiration
  - pneumothorax
  - cardiac failure
- *Rare:*
  - congenital diaphragmatic hernia,
  - tracheo-oesophageal fistula (TOF)
  - lung malformations, choanal atresia
  - milk aspiration
  - neuromuscular disorders, e. g. myopathy.

Clinical features

Respiratory distress is manifested by tachypnoea, rate >60/min, nasal flaring, grunting, and retractions which may be suprasternal, intercostal, or subcostal. Oxygen saturation is reduced and central cyanosis may be apparent.

Management

A chest radiograph (CXR) is essential to confirm or exclude respiratory disease and diagnose pneumothorax, diaphragmatic hernia, pneumonia or lung malformations. Supplemental oxygen is given to maintain SaO_2 >95%. Treatment depends on cause. Some individual conditions are described in turn:

- *Transient tachypnoea of the newborn (TTN):* caused by delay in absorption of lung liquid, especially after Caesarean section. Usually resolves within 48 h. Oxygen may be required.
- *Pneumonia:* Group B streptococcus most common pathogen. Risk factors include prolonged rupture of membranes, maternal pyrexia, chorioamnionitis. Broad-spectrum antibiotics given after a septic screen.
- *Meconium aspiration:* an asphyxiated infant may gasp and aspirate meconium before delivery, causing a chemical pneumonitis, airway obstruction, and inactivation of surfactant. Assisted ventilation and surfactant therapy is usually required. In severe cases there may be persistent pulmonary hypertension requiring NO or even extracorporeal membrane oxygenation.

Cyanosis/cyanotic spells

Significant causes of central cyanosis include:

- *Cyanotic congenital heart disease:* see Chapter 4
- *Persistent pulmonary hypertension of the newborn:* may be primary or secondary to asphyxia, sepsis, meconium aspiration, or diaphragmatic hernia. Cyanosis occurs due to right to left shunting. Treatment options in addition to oxygen include pulmonary vasodilators (inhaled NO), high-frequency oscillatory ventilation, and extracorporeal membrane oxygenation
- *Respiratory disease:* pneumonia, meconium aspiration, pneumothorax, diaphragmatic hernia, aspiration.

Respiratory distress syndrome (RDS)

Surfactant-deficient RDS, also called hyaline membrane disease (HMD) is a major cause of morbidity and mortality in preterm infants. It affects 50% of infants born <30 weeks and is almost invariable in infants of <27 weeks gestation. It is more common in male infants and in caucasians.

Aetiology and pathogenesis

Important aetiological factors are:

- *Prematurity:* gestational age is a main determinant as surfactant synthesis starts towards the end of the 2nd trimester
- *Perinatal asphyxia:* hypoxia, acidosis, and protein leakage from vessels all inhibit surfactant synthesis
- *Maternal diabetes:* due to delayed surfactant synthesis and elective preterm delivery by Caesarean section
- *Caesarean section:* if carried out pre-labour before 38 weeks gestation there is an increased incidence of RDS and TTN.

Pathogenesis

Interstitial oedema and congestion of alveolar walls leads to necrosis of alveolar epithelial cells. Alveoli become atelectatic but alveolar ducts dilate. Surfactant is inhibited by the leakage of plasma proteins into the alveoli and by an inflammatory response resulting from lung injury.

Pathophysiology

The alveoli collapse and the lungs become stiff and non-compliant, leading to:

- Decreased tidal volume and functional residual capacity
- Increased work of breathing
- Hypoxaemia due to right–left shunts through foramen ovale and ductus arteriosus and intrapulmonary shunts
- Hypoventilation with respiratory acidosis.

The infant attempts to maintain minute volume by increased respiratory rate and to maintain functional residual capacity by contracting the diaphragm against a closed glottis leading to 'grunting' when the air is released.

Hypoxaemia leads to a host of secondary effects including severe metabolic acidosis, hypotension, and impaired perfusion of kidneys, gut and brain.

The natural history of RDS is deterioration over 24–36 h as the infant tires, stabilization, followed by improvement as surfactant reappears at 36–48 h. In VLBW infants surfactant deficiency is compounded by lung immaturity and a complex series of events leads to chronic lung disease.

Clinical features

RDS presents within 4 h of birth with:

- Tachypnoea (>60 breaths/min)
- Sternal retraction, intercostal and subcostal recession
- Expiratory grunting
- Hypoxia and cyanosis (if severe).

Less common causes of respiratory distress in preterm infants include pneumonia, pneumothorax, congenital heart disease, pulmonary hypoplasia, and diaphragmatic hernia.

Management

Prevention

Administration of antenatal corticosteroids reduces the incidence, severity and mortality from RDS. Meta-analysis of RCTs shows a reduction in mortality of 50%. The greatest benefit is when the interval between treatment and delivery is >48 h, but antenatal betamethasone should be considered in all women who threaten to deliver at <34 weeks gestation. Surfactant may be administered prophylactically.

Investigations
Investigations are designed to confirm the diagnosis and to establish baseline values for monitoring progress:
- *CXR*: to confirm RDS and exclude other diagnoses and to define position of ETT and umbilical catheter
- Blood gases
- FBC, U&Es, creatinine, calcium, blood cultures.

Treatment
Supportive treatment depends on severity and includes avoiding hypoxaemia, acidosis, and hypothermia and controlling cardiorespiratory, renal, and electrolyte homeostasis.

Respiratory support is central to management.

Surfactant therapy
Exogenous surfactant therapy has had a major impact on the incidence and severity of RDS, reducing the neonatal mortality by 40%. It is even more effective when combined with antenatal steroids. Natural surfactants are best and prophylaxis is better than rescue treatment.

A prophylactic dose is given down the tracheal tube to infants <30 weeks gestation in the delivery room if intubated for resuscitation or on admission to the intensive care unit. Further doses, up to a maximum of three, may be required if a significant oxygen requirement persists.

Oxygen therapy
Supplemental oxygen may be given via a hood, headbox, or nasal cannulae. In preterm infants the aim is to maintain the PaO_2 in the range 6.00–10.5 kPa (45–80 mmHg) and the oxygen saturation at 88–95%. The maximum FiO_2 should not exceed 95% to avoid oxygen toxicity.

Continuous positive airways pressure (CPAP)
CPAP is designed to prevent alveolar collapse at end expiration using a continuous distending pressure of 4–10 cmH$_2$O. It is usually applied via nasal prongs. Indications include:
- *Moderate RDS:* PaO_2<8 kPa (60 mmHg)
- Recurrent apnoea
- Weaning from mechanical ventilation.

Complications of CPAP include nasal trauma, feeding problems from gaseous distension of stomach, pneumothorax, and failure with need for IPPV (50% of babies <1.5 kg).

Positive pressure ventilation
Babies should be ventilated for the minimum necessary time using the lowest possible mean airway pressure to reduce barotrauma. Options include:
- *Intermittent positive pressure ventilation (IPPV)*: this is given on a background of positive end expiratory pressure (PEEP). Most neonatal ventilators are pressure limited and time-cycled but volume-limited ventilators are used in some units.
- *Patient triggered ventilation (PTV) and synchronous intermittent mandatory ventilation (SIMV)*: these are designed to promote synchrony between the infant's own respiratory efforts and the ventilator. They may decrease the need for sedation.
- *High-frequency oscillatory ventilation (HFOV)*: a continuous pressure is applied and gas exchange occurs via an oscillating pressure waveform applied by an airway vibrator operating at ~10 Hz. HFOV is primarily used as rescue treatment.

Complications of RDS
The main acute complications are air leaks and pulmonary haemorrhage. Longer term sequelae include chronic lung disease and intracranial pathology.

Air leaks
- *Pneumothorax:* occurs in ~10% of infants ventilated for RDS, and is associated with high peak inspiratory pressure, long inspiratory times, and asynchrony. A large tension pneumothorax presents with acute collapse with hypoxaemia and shock. Breath sounds and chest movement are reduced on the affected side. Diagnosis is confirmed by transillumination or CXR (Fig 1.8). Emergency management is by needle aspiration (2nd intercostal space lateral to the mid-clavicular line) followed by chest drain insertion.

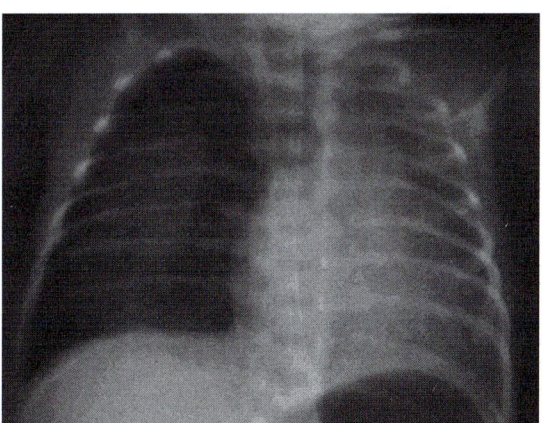

Fig 1.8 Pneumothorax: right side.

- *Pulmonary interstitial emphysema (PIE):* air tracks into the interstitium and perivascular sheaths leading to worsening gas exchange. CXR is diagnostic (Fig 1.9).

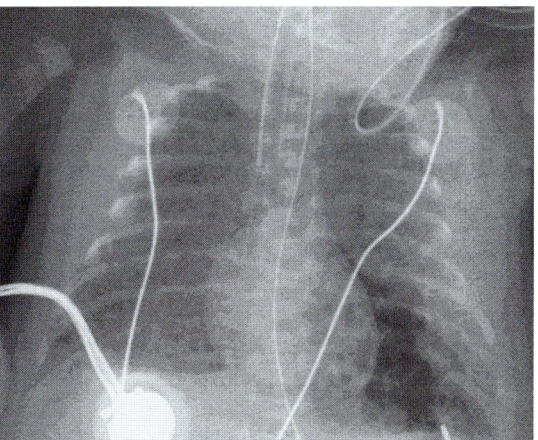

Fig 1.9 Pulmonary interstitial emphysema: left base.

Pulmonary haemorrhage
A haemorrhagic pulmonary oedema may occur with heart failure, e.g. from a large PDA. There is an increased risk (2%) after surfactant therapy. There is blood staining of the tracheal aspirate which may progress to gross haemorrhage and severe disturbance in gas exchange.

1.7 Neurological disorders in the newborn

Hypoxic–ischaemic encephalopathy (HIE)

This is a syndrome of disturbed brain function manifested by altered consciousness, altered tone, and seizures. Other causes of neonatal encephalopathy include metabolic disorders such as bilirubin toxicity or hyperammonaemia, infections, drugs, brain malformations, and stroke.

The neurological manifestations of HIE are classified according to Sarnat staging as:
- *Grade I:* mild
- *Grade II:* moderate
- *Grade III:* severe.

The features in each category are shown in Table 1.2.

Table 1.2. HIE: Sarnat classification			
	Grade I mild	**Grade II moderate**	**Grade III severe**
Alertness	Hyperalert	Lethargy	Coma
Muscle tone	Normal or ↑	Hypotonia	Flaccid
Seizures	None	Frequent	Uncommon
Autonomic function:			
Pupils	Dilated, reactive	Small, reactive	Variable/fixed
Respiration	Regular	Periodic	Apnoeic
Duration	<24 h	2–14 days	Weeks

Multiorgan dysfunction usually accompanies an asphyxial insult severe enough to cause moderate or severe HIE and is manifested by:
- *Myocardial dysfunction:* hypotension, arrhythmias, shock, and metabolic acidosis
- *Renal dysfunction:* tubular or cortical necrosis with oliguria and haematuria
- *Gastrointestinal dysfunction:* bleeding, gut ischaemia, necrotizing enterocolitis, ileus
- *Respiratory failure:* persistent pulmonary hypertension of the newborn (PPHN)
- *Metabolic disorder:* Hypo- or hyperglycaemia, lactic acidosis, hyponatraemia (SIADH)
- *Haematological:* disseminated intravascular coagulation (DIC).

Management
Investigations
- *EEG:* often measured using an amplitude integrated single channel or cerebral function monitor (CFM). This is useful as a measure of severity and indicator of prognosis and demonstrates seizure activity. A persistent low-voltage or burst-suppression pattern is a poor prognostic indicator.

Neuroimaging
- *Cranial ultrasound:* may detect cerebral oedema (loss of sulci, compressed ventricles), hyperechogenic basal ganglia or abnormal cerebral arterial blood flow. It may be useful for prognosis but caution is required in interpretation.
- *MRI:* imaging modality of choice, but may appear normal on day 1–2. Optimal timing is day 7–10. It allows early recognition of basal ganglia, thalamic, internal capsule, white matter, and cortical injury. Myelination of the posterior limb of the internal capsule (PLIC) is a useful guide to prognosis. See Fig 1.10.

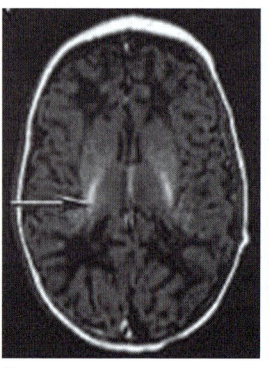 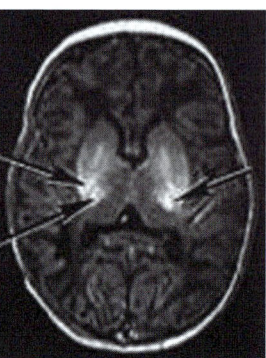

A   B

Fig 1.10 MRI (T1 weighted) in HIE. A. Normal scan with normal signal in posterior limb of internal capsule (PLIC). B. Moderately abnormal scan: loss of signal in PLIC, increased signal in basal ganglia and thalamus. Courtesy of Professor Mary Rutherford, Professor of Perinatal Imaging at Imperial Healthcare.

Blood tests
- FBC and coagulation screen, arterial blood gases
- LFTs, Ca, Mg, U&E, creatinine, lactate, glucose.

Cardiac
- Echocardiography, ECG.

Treatment
Treatment is supportive and focuses on complications arising from multiorgan dysfunction as follows:
- *Circulatory support:* inotropes to maintain blood pressure and renal perfusion
- *Ventilatory support:* maintain normocarbia
- *Fluid balance:* oedema often occurs due to a combination of renal failure, SIADH, heart failure, and leaky capillaries.
- *Seizures:* prompt treatment with phenobarbital, phenytoin, or clonazepam.

Neuroprotective strategies to prevent the secondary neuronal death are under development. Brain cooling or total body cooling both appear promising.

Prognosis in HIE
Mild HIE usually has a normal outcome. Normal neurological examination and establishment of sucking feeds by age 2 weeks often conveys a good prognosis. In infants with grade II or III HIE prognosis is aided by the results of investigations, EEG (at 12–72 h) and MRI. Markers of poor prognosis are:
- *EEG:* background with burst suppression or isoelectric pattern after 12 h of age
- *MRI:* evidence of bilateral basal ganglia involvement and absent signal from myelin in posterior limb of internal capsule.

In addition, persistent seizures or abnormal neurology, delay beyond 2 weeks in feeding orally and poor head growth are all bad signs. In severe HIE the mortality rate is 75% and 80% of survivors have neurological sequelae.

Germinal matrix–intraventricular haemorrhage (GM-IVH)

This type of intracranial haemorrhage occurs in about 20% of VLBW babies (<1500 g).

Aetiology and pathogenesis
- *Vulnerable immature anatomy:* the germinal matrix is a highly vascular layer surrounding the ventricles with little supporting tissue and thin-walled vessels vulnerable to bleeding.
- *Haemodynamic instability:* the cerebral vasculature is vulnerable to fluctuations in arterial blood pressure.

A spectrum of lesions can occur:
- *Isolated germinal matrix haemorrhage:* resolves to form a subependymal pseudocyst.
- *Intraventricular haemorrhage:* without acute ventricular dilatation.
- *Intraventricular haemorrhage: with acute ventricular dilation:* posthaemorrhagic hydrocephalus may ensue due to blockage of CSF flow at level of 3rd ventricle or failure of reabsorption at arachnoid villi. In up to 40% this may persist and require V-P shunt insertion.
- *Haemorrhagic parenchymal venous infarction (HPI):* a large haemorrhage obstructs venous drainage of the deep white matter causing parenchymal venous infarction. The lesion evolves into a porencephalic cyst.

Clinical features
Most bleeds are clinically silent and diagnosed on cranial ultrasound screening. A large haemorrhage may cause apnoea and bradycardia, fits with decerebrate posturing, hypotension, and increased ventilatory requirements.

Management
Investigations
- *Cranial ultrasound:* GMH-IVH is readily diagnosed with cranial ultrasound scanning and all VLBW infants are usually scanned at birth and at 72 h. See Fig 1.11.
- *Laboratory results:* may include a fall in PCV by 5–10%, metabolic acidosis and coagulation abnormalities.

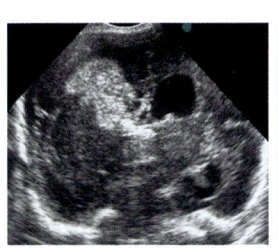

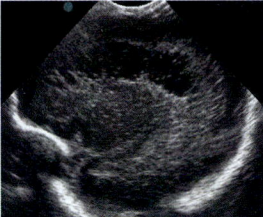

Fig 1.11 A. Coronal USS: large Rt IVH with HPI. B. Parasagittal USS: cystic lesions of PVL.

Treatment
Asymptomatic infants do not need treatment. Those who deteriorate require optimization of ventilation, circulatory support (blood transfusion, inotropes), control of fits with phenobarbital, and correction of coagulation abnormalities.

Prognosis
Infants with uncomplicated GMH-IVH have a good prognosis, with a risk of handicap of about 4%. 50% of babies with posthaemorrhagic hydrocephalus have neurodevelopmental problems, rising to 75% if they require a shunt. A unilateral haemorrhagic parenchymal infarct has a strong association with spastic hemiplegia.

White matter injury (WMI)

The term periventricular leukomalacia (PVL) was applied to focal necrotic lesions identified in the periventricular white matter at autopsy in a high percentage of preterm infants. Cranial ultrasound and MRI are revealing evidence of white matter injury (WMI) during life but the incidence is difficult to quantify.

Aetiology and pathogenesis
The periventricular white matter in the preterm infant is susceptible to a variety of insults resulting in focal necrotic lesions (PVL) or more diffuse injury due to:
- *Hypoxic-ischaemic injury:* WMI has been associated with loss of cerebral autoregulation and hypocarbia (<3 kPa)
- *Inflammation:* there is an association between chorioamnionitis and WMI.

Diffuse WMI associated with loss of oligodendroglia results in loss of white matter volume and mild ventriculomegaly.

Clinical features
Cranial ultrasound screening will detect cystic PVL by age 6 weeks. A persistent 'flare' in the periventricular white matter is found in up to 26% of preterm cohorts and is believed to represent subtle damage which may not lead to cystic change. Bilateral occipital cystic PVL is a reliable predictor of spastic diplegia. Infants with localized cysts or persistent flares without cysts may be normal or develop mild spastic diplegia.

Neonatal seizures

The causes of seizures in the newborn may be:
- *Cerebral:*
  - hypoxic-ischaemic encephalopathy
  - cerebral infarction
  - intracrania haemorrhage
- *Metabolic:*
  - hypoglycaemia, hypocalcaemia,
  - hypo- or hypernatraemia.
  - inborn errors of metabolism
- *Infection:* meningitis or encephalitis
- *Drug withdrawal:* neonatal abstinence syndrome.

Rare causes include brain malformations, pyridoxine deficiency, and benign familial neonatal seizures. 10% are of unknown cause.

Seizures in the newborn may be subtle and manifest as episodes of apnoea and oxygen desaturation, transient eye deviation, altered consciousness, and floppiness as well as generalized or focal clonic or tonic movements.

Investigations to consider include:
- Blood glucose, U&E, calcium, magnesium levels, coagulation screen
- Blood gases, ammonia, lactate, amino acids
- *Septic screen:* FBC, blood cultures, lumbar puncture
- EEG and cerebral function monitoring (CFM)
- *Neuroimaging:* cranial ultrasound, CT or MRI.

Treatment of the underlying cause is combined with control of the fits if they are prolonged or frequent with anticonvulsants: phenobarbital, phenytoin or midazolam. Assisted ventilation may be necessary.

1.8 Problems in the preterm infant

Necrotizing enterocolitis (NEC)

NEC is a serious bowel disorder primarily affecting preterm infants and characterized by inflammation of the bowel which may progress to necrosis and perforation. The incidence is 2–5% in preterm infants <1000 g. It can occur in term infants, usually after asphyxia.

Aetiology and pathogenesis

The aetiology is multifactorial, with several well recognized risk factors:

- *Prematurity:* the main risk factor
- *Enteral feeding:* rapid increase, hypertonic formula, formula rather than breast milk
- *Infection:* infection of ischaemic mucosa by gas-forming or gram-negative organisms. Epidemics of NEC occur.
- *Hypoperfusion and gut ischaemia:* secondary to PDA, cardiac failure, IUGR, or exchange transfusion.

Oedema, haemorrhage, and microvascular sludging in the mucosa causes mucosal ischaemia with probable secondary infection. NEC usually involves the terminal ileum and colon but multiple regions may be involved.

Clinical features

NEC presents classically with abdominal distension, bloody stools, and bilious aspirates. It may however present insidiously with apnoeas or temperature instability or as a rapidly progressive illness with hypotensive shock and DIC. On examination the abdomen may be tender with palpable bowel loops.

Clinical signs of perforation and peritonitis include an abdominal mass, abdominal wall oedema, a tense discoloured abdominal wall and absent bowel sounds.

Bell's staging can be used to guide management: Stage I: suspected, Stage II definite, Stage III advanced.

Management

Investigations

- *Laboratory investigations:* may be consistent with septicaemia, shock, and DIC: raised CRP, hypoxia and acidosis, hyperbilirubinaemia, coagulation abnormalities.
- *Abdominal radiographs:* include lateral horizontal film with infant on left side to detect fluid levels and free intraperitoneal gas. The pathognomonic sign is intramural air (Fig 1.12)

In mild cases the radiographs are normal. Other features include dilated bowel loops, thickened bowel walls, inspissated stool, air in the portal venous system, pneumoperitoneum, and air below the diaphragm or around the falciform ligament.

Treatment

Medical treatment is supportive:

- *'Drip and suck':* nil by mouth, remove all umbilical cannulae, give TPN for 7–10 days
- *IV broad spectrum antibiotics:* ampicillin, gentamicin and metronidazole
- Circulatory and respiratory support as required
- Treat any coagulopathy.

Surgery

Laparotomy is indicated in babies who show no response to conservative management or if there is evidence of perforation or presence of a mass. Peritoneal drainage on the neonatal unit is an initial alternative to laparotomy in very unstable babies.

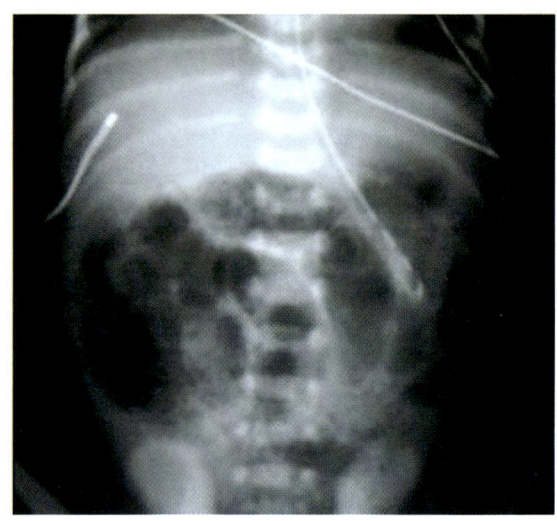

Fig 1.12 NEC: intestinal pneumatosis (intramural air).

At laparotomy non-viable bowel is resected and primary anastamosis or ileostomy/colostomy performed.

NEC is not entirely preventable, but using breast milk, avoiding hyperosmolar feeds, and avoiding rapid increase in feed volume in very immature infants are useful strategies.

Sequelae

Mortality is 20% among infants who perforate. Stricture formation with intestinal obstruction may occur 2–6 weeks after the original illness. Extensive resection can lead to short bowel syndrome causing diarrhoea, failure to thrive, and vitamin B12 deficiency if terminal ileum resected.

Patent ductus arteriosus (PDA)

PDA is a common problem in the preterm infant with symptomatic ducts (SPDA) reported in 50% of infants <800 g.

Aetiology and pathogenesis

In the fetus, ductal patency is maintained by the vasodilatory action of low PaO_2, prostaglandins PGE_2 and PGI_2 and NO. Postnatal ductal constriction is promoted by a rapid increase in PaO_2 which increases production of endothelin-1, a potent vasoconstrictor.

In healthy term and preterm infants functional closure occurs within 72 h of birth and anatomic closure by 2–3 weeks. Risk factors for PDA include:

- Preterm birth
- RDS
- Fluid overload
- Sepsis.

Persistent PDA leads to a left-to-right shunt with increased pulmonary blood flow, pulmonary hypertension and oedema, and biventricular failure.

Clinical features

Duct size and the pressure gradient between systemic and pulmonary circulation determine shunt size and clinical features. The classic signs are:

- Tachycardia with bounding pulses, wide pulse pressure, and an active praecordium.

- *Cardiac murmur:* systolic, loudest at left sternal border. A gallop rhythm and loud P2 may develop. A 'silent' PDA with no murmur is common with a large shunt.
- Hepatomegaly and increased ventilatory requirements.

Management
Investigations
- CXR: cardiomegaly and pulmonary plethora
- *Echocardiography:* this allows direct visualization of patency and size of duct (diameter >1.5 mm), left atrial enlargement (left atrial/aortic root ratio >1.5:1), direction of flow through the duct and aorta.

Treatment
Medical
- Fluid restriction to 100 mL/kg/ per day and diuretics
- *Cyclo-oxygenase (COX) inhibitors:* indomethacin or ibuprofen. Indomethacin in the first 14 days of life closes the duct in up to 70% of symptomatic infants. Side effects include decreased platelet aggregation and gastrointestinal bleeding. Ibuprofen is as efficacious with fewer side effects.

Surgical
If medical treatment fails surgery is the definitive treatment. Video-assisted thoracoscopic surgery is available in some centres. Mortality rate is <1%. Complications include damage to recurrent laryngeal nerve and pneumothorax.

Anaemia

The ill preterm infant may become anaemic because of repeated blood sampling or haemorrhage. Blood transfusion restores and maintains adequate tissue oxygen delivery.

Physiological anaemia of prematurity in VLBW infants occurs with a low of 8 g/dL at 4–8 weeks. It is due to several factors. Erythropoietin (EPO) production switches off after birth and increases slowly thereafter leading to a low red cell mass. Short red cell life span and rapid growth are also factors.

Folic acid deficiency may contribute, but iron deficiency is not a factor in the anaemia of prematurity. Iron deficiency will supervene later if supplements are not given.

Management
A weekly check of Hb and reticulocytes is done in growing preterm babies even if asymptomatic. Indications for blood transfusion remain controversial. Reasonable guidelines for transfusion are:
- *Hb <10 g/dL:* if moderate oxygen requirements
- *Hb <8 g/dL:* if symptomatic with tachycardia, poor weight gain, oxygen requirement
- *Hb <7 g/dL:* if reticulocyte count $<100 \times 10^9$/L, even if asymptomatic.

Osteopaenia of prematurity

This metabolic bone disease occurs at several weeks of age in VLBW survivors of neonatal intensive care. It is primarily caused by phosphate deficiency due to inadequate intake, urinary losses, and increased requirements. It shares radiological and biochemical features with rickets although primary vitamin D deficiency is not the cause.

Clinical manifestations are not usually present although pathological long bone or rib fractures can occur in severe cases. The features are radiological and biochemical.
- *Radiological:* reduced bone mineralization with widening and rachitic cupping of wrists, knees and ribs at age 5–6 weeks
- *Biochemical:* calcium normal or raised, phosphate: low, <1.0 mmol/L, alkaline phospatase raised, >1000 u/L.

It can be prevented by ensuring adequate phosphate intake by using a preterm formula, fortifying expressed breast milk, or by giving oral phosphate 1 mmol/kg per day and vitamin D 400 u/day.

If osteopaenia develops, treatment is with oral phosphate 2 mmol/kg per day and Vitamin D 1000 u/day.

Apnoeas

A clinically significant apnoea is a pause in breathing for more than 20 s, or any apnoea associated with bradycardia or desaturation.

Apnoea is distinguished from periodic breathing, a common occurrence in newborns in which regular breathing is separated by short episodes of apnoea lasting 3–15 s.

Aetiology and pathogenesis

Apnoeic attacks may be symptomatic or due to recurrent apnoea of prematurity. Important causes of symptomatic apnoeic episodes include:
- Infection
- Anaemia
- Cardiac failure
- Metabolic disorders
- Gastro-oesophageal reflux and aspiration.
- Overheating
- Respiratory depression from drugs
- Upper airway obstruction, e.g. from neck flexion.

Recurrent apnoea of prematurity usually develops on day 5 or 6 and resolves by 34–36 weeks gestational age.

Management

Most apnoeic attacks are brief and self-limiting. Any trigger factors causing symptomatic apnoea should be corrected such as anaemia or incubator temperature. Although apnoea may accompany onset of oral feeds, gastro-oesophageal reflux and apnoea are rarely temporally related.

Immediate treatment includes checking the airway and gentle tactile stimulation if breathing has not restarted. Options for recurrent apnoea are:
- *Methylxanthines:* caffeine (orally or IV)
- Low pressure (3–4 cm H_2O) nasal CPAP.

On rare occasions mechanical ventilation may be necessary.

1.9 Bacterial infection in the newborn

Neonatal infection

Infection remains an important cause of morbidity and mortality at all birthweights and gestations but has the highest incidence in VLBW infants.

Pathogens include bacteria, viruses, and fungi. Infection may be acquired transplacentally *in utero*, or by vertical transmission from the birth canal, or acquired at birth.

The term congenital infection is used for infections acquired transplacentally *in utero* from the mother. Maternal infection is usually primary, so there is a lack of maternal immunity, and it is often asymptomatic. Most congenital infections are viral (rubella, CMV, varicella, parvovirus) but non-viral causes include toxoplasmosis and syphilis. Some pathogens such as HSV and HIV can be acquired *in utero* or postnatally.

Neonatal infections are usually hospital-acquired (nosocomial) infections.

Host defences and infection control

Scrupulous attention to hand washing is the most important factor in the prevention of cross-infection. Neonates, especially preterm infants, are deficient in all aspects of immunity: physical, cellular, and humoral.

- *Physical defences:* skin is thin and easily damaged, the umbilical stump becomes necrotic and acts as a locus for infection, insertion of tubes provides a route of entry for pathogens, and there is no protection from resident flora.
- *Cellular immunity:* phagocytic activity of polymorphs from newborn infants is reduced in neonatal serum deficient in immunoglobulins and complement.
- *Humoral immunity:* the normal newborn has virtually no circulating IgA, IgD, IgE, or IgM. IgG is acquired from the mother and in the normal term baby levels are high, falling following delivery with a half-life of 3 weeks to cause transient postnatal hypogammaglobulinaemia which is more severe in preterm infants. Complement levels are low, and even lower in preterm infants.

Bacterial infections

The major bacterial pathogens encountered are:
- Group B β-haemolytic streptococcus (GBS, *Strep. agalactiae*)
- *E. coli*
- *Staphylococcus epidermidis* (coagulase negative staphylococcus, CONS).

Other bacteria which may be responsible for serious infections include gram-negative bacilli (*Pseudomonas aeruginoasa, Klebsiella, Proteus, Enterobacter, Haemophilus*), *Staphylococcus aureus*, Pneumococcus, and *Listeria monocytogenes*.

Bacterial infections may be superficial or systemic causing sepsis. The most important cause of invasive, systemic bacterial infection or sepsis is GBS.

Superficial infections

Umbilicus

Slight redness around the umbilicus is common. Infection with a red flare and local discharge is usually due to staphylococci and *E. coli* and usually responds to topical antibiotics (Fig 1.13).

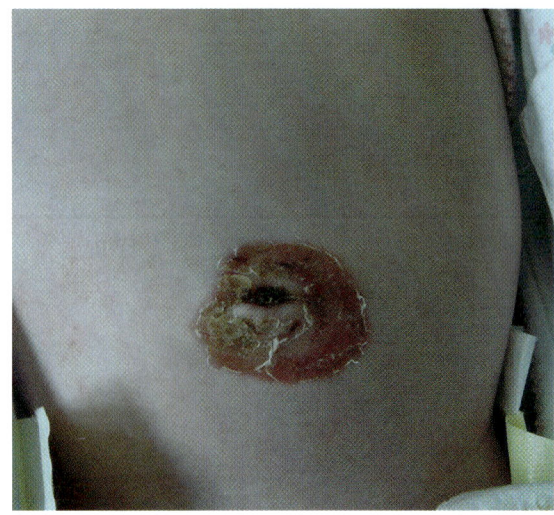

Fig 1.13 Superficial bacterial infection: periumbilical infection.

Skin

Staphylococcal skin infection can cause bullous impetigo or scalded skin syndrome and requires systemic antibiotics: intravenous flucloxacillin.

Conjunctivitis

'Sticky eyes' are common on day 3–5 and usually resolve with sterile water or saline cleaning. If troublesome, topical antibiotic ointment e.g. chloramphenicol is indicated.

Purulent conjunctivitis with eyelid swelling within 48 h of birth is likely to be gonococcal (ophthalmia neonatorum) and requires urgent gram stain and systemic antibiotic treatment with penicillin or cephalosporin.

Chlamydia trachomatis has no distinguishing clinical features and is diagnosed by immunofluorescence testing with monoclonal antibody. Treatment is oral erythromycin for 2 weeks.

Bacterial sepsis

Relative immunodeficiency renders the newborn susceptible not only to invasive bacterial infection but also to rapid dissemination when it does occur. Early diagnosis is essential and initial therapy is started on clinical suspicion rather than laboratory results.

Sepsis is classified as:
- *Early-onset:* within 72 h of birth
- *Late-onset:* after 3–7 days.

The risk factors and aetiology differ for each category.

Early-onset sepsis

This results from vertical infection during birth. Common pathogens include GBS and *E. coli*. Risk factors include:
- Preterm delivery
- Prolonged rupture of membranes
- Maternal pyrexia or infection
- Chorioamnionitis
- Previous infected infant.

Late-onset sepsis

Infections presenting late may be vertically acquired but transmission is more often horizontal by transmission from person to person.

Risk factors include:
- Preterm delivery
- Indwelling catheters (intravascular) or endotracheal tube
- Prolonged antibiotic treatment
- Damage to skin.

CONS is often recovered from the blood stream in infants with indwelling catheters.

Clinical features

The history may reveal risk factors such as maternal pyrexia. A host of symptoms, signs or laboratory findings may be early warnings of sepsis:
- *Temperature change:* temperature <36°C or >37.5°C sustained for >1 h in an appropriate environmental temperature
- *Respiratory:* apnoea or tachypnoea with respiratory distress or increased ventilatory requirements
- *Cardiovascular:* tachycardia, prolonged capillary return (>3 s), pallor, mottled skin
- *Gastrointestinal:* slow feeding, vomiting, abdominal distension, ileus, intestinal obstruction
- *CNS:* lethargy, irritability, hypotonia, seizures
- *Local signs:* pseudoparalysis due to limb pain, tense fontanelle, head retraction.

Diagnosis should be made before late signs emerge such as cyanosis, bilious vomiting, bulging fontanelle, shock, and DIC. Careful clinical examination is mandatory.

Management

Investigations

The standard 'septic screen' includes:
- Full blood count, differential white count
- C-reactive protein (CRP)
- *Microbial samples for culture:* blood, urine, ear and throat swabs, endotracheal tube aspirate (if applicable)
- *Lumbar puncture:* CSF
- *CXR:* unless there is an obvious extrapulmonary focus.

Additional investigations to consider
- Blood gases, U&E, calcium, albumin, coagulation screen
- Maternal vaginal swab culture
- Placental tissue for *Listeria monocytogenes*
- Viral studies.

Interpretation of results

Definitive culture results take too long to obtain to influence the initial decision about whether to treat with antibiotics and the results available within 1–2 h are relied on to influence what is essentially a clinical decision.

Results that mandate early antibiotic treatment include:
- Neutrophilia or neutropaenia
- *Thrombocytopaenia:* platelets <100 × 10^9/L
- Raised CRP (may be normal initially)
- Urine white cells
- *CSF:* >21 × 10^9/L white cells, protein >2 g/L in term infants, glucose <40% blood glucose, organisms seen.

Treatment

In addition to any supportive care, systemic antibiotics are indicated immediately on suspicion of sepsis, after taking cultures.

The initial choice depends on the infant's age and local pathogen incidence and sensitivities. An aminoglycoside such as gentamicin, tobramycin, amikacin, or netilmicin is usually indicated to cover coliforms. A second or third antibiotic is given depending on which organisms are common:
- *GBS:* penicillin G
- *CONS:* flucloxacillin, vancomycin
- *Pseudomonas aeruginosa:* ceftazidime, piperacillin
- *Anaerobes:* metronidazole.

Once culture and sensitivity results are available changes can be made. If blood cultures are negative, CRP remains normal, and signs of sepsis resolve antibiotics are stopped after 48 h. Proven infection is treated for 7–10 days, rising to 14 days in gram-negative infection, 21 days in meningitis, and 3–6 weeks in septic arthritis/osteomyelitis.

Group B streptococcal (GBS) infection

GBS infection is the leading cause of bacterial sepsis in term infants with an incidence of 0.5/1000 live births in the UK. Up to 30% of mothers have rectal or vaginal carriage of GBS, 50% of their offspring will be colonized, and invasive disease occurs in 1–2% of colonized infants.

Prevention

Intrapartum administration of penicillin to mothers at risk reduces neonatal colonization and prevents most cases of GBS sepsis.

Local policies for screening and treatment vary, but intrapartum antibiotics are generally offered to high-risk groups:
- Previous child with GBS disease
- GBS bacteriuria or colonization (but routine culturing of mothers is not recommended)
- Prolonged rupture of membranes >18 h, preterm labour or fever in labour >38°C.

Clinical features

Early-onset sepsis presents with respiratory distress and circulatory collapse with rapid deterioration. 90% present in first 12 h. Late onset sepsis presents with meningitis or focal infection in bones or joints.

Treatment

Infants with early onset GBS sepsis are critically ill and require prompt resuscitation and IV penicillin for at least 14 days.

Mortality is 5% in term infants and 20% in preterm infants. Local practice for investigation, treatment, or observation of infants born to carrier mothers who have received prophylaxis varies, reflecting lack of evidence as to best practice.

Listeria monocytogenes infection

- *Neonatal listeriosis:* now very rare in the UK since advice about avoiding unpasteurized milk, soft cheeses, and undercooked poultry was introduced.
- *Maternal listeriosis:* causes a flu-like illness and can cause fetal infection, preterm labour, with meconium stained liquor, severe early onset sepsis or meningitis. Treatment is with ampicillin and gentamicin.

1.10 Viral and congenital infections in the newborn

Viral infections

Herpes simplex virus (HSV)
Two viruses, HSV1 and HSV2 (HHV1 and HHV2) can infect the newborn with an incidence of 2–5 per 100 000 live births. 85% of infections are with HSV2.

Infection can rarely be transplacental associated with maternal primary infection but is more commonly vertical transmission via the birth canal. The risk of infection is:
- *50% with symptomatic primary maternal infection:* fever, systemic illness, painful genital lesions
- *3% with recurrent infection:* asymptomatic or localized genital lesions.

In 70% of cases maternal infection is undiagnosed.

Clinical features

There are three modes of presentation:
- *Superficial, localized lesions:* vesicles on skin or mouth or keratoconjunctivitis at 10–11 days. Disseminated disease progression is uncommon but many infants go on to have neurodevelopmental delay.
- *Encephalitis:* presents at 7–14 days with lethargy, seizures, and coma.
- *Disseminated disease:* presents in first week with pneumonia, liver failure, disseminated intravascular coagulation. 50% develop encephalitis and 20% have no cutaneous lesions.

Diagnosis

PCR-based DNA analysis of blood, CSF or local lesions. Encephalitis shows characteristic changes on EEG and neuroimaging reflecting the predominant temporal lobe pathology.

Treatment

Intravenous aciclovir for at least 14 days. Recurrence over the first year of life is common and usually responds to further aciclovir. The use of prophylactic, suppressive oral treatment over the first year is unproven.

Delivery by Caesarean section is recommended for mothers with active lesions.

Prognosis

HSV2 infection has the worst prognosis with mortality of 30–60% for disseminated infection, and 10–15% for encephalitis.

Hepatitis
Hepatitis B (HBV) and hepatitis C (HBC) can both be transmitted to the newborn at birth but rarely cause disease until later in life because of the long incubation period.

Hepatitis B, HBV

In the UK, all mothers are screened for hepatitis B surface antigen (HBsAg). The infant is at high risk if the mother is hepatitis B e-antigen positive and e-antibody negative.

All infants at risk are given HBV immunoglobulin as soon as possible after birth, with further doses of vaccine during the first year. This protects 80% of infants. Breast-feeding is not contraindicated.

Of infants who become carriers up to 50% develop chronic HBV liver disease, which progresses to cirrhosis in 10%. There is a long-term risk of hepatocellular carcinoma.

Hepatitis C, HBC

Vertical transmission of HBC is uncommon unless there is co-infection with HIV. Breast-feeding is not contraindicated. Long-term carriage confers risk of liver disease and hepatocellular carcinoma.

Human immunodeficiency virus (HIV) infection
The main route for HIV infection in children is vertical transmission at birth, but transmission also occurs transplacentally and via breast-feeding. The majority of HIV infected infants in the UK are of African origin.

The risk of transmission is highest with:
- Maternal AIDS, high viral load, or low $CD4^+$ count
- Prolonged rupture of membranes (>4 h), preterm delivery
- Vaginal or instrumental delivery.

Interventions have reduced transmission rates from 15–20% to <1%:
- Elective Caesarean section
- Antiretroviral therapy antenatally to mother, postnatally to infant
- Formula feeding instead of breast-feeding.

Clinical features and diagnosis

Symptoms and signs are rare in the newborn and serological diagnosis is complicated by presence of maternal IgG in infant's serum up to age 18 months in absence of infection. Direct assays by HIV culture, PCR detection of proviral DNA and p24 antigen detection are sensitive after ~1 month.

Blood samples are taken on day 1 and repeated at 6 and 12 weeks of age.

Treatment

Infants are started (in the UK) on AZT within 6 h of birth and initial treatment given for 6 weeks. Prophylaxis with co-trimoxazole against *Pneumocystis carinii* pneumonia (PCP) is commenced at 4–6 weeks of age and continued until diagnosis is excluded. An infant <18 months can be considered to be HIV positive if he is seropositive or has had two or more positive direct tests. HIV infection can be excluded if at least two direct tests are negative, with at least one taken after age 4 months.

Unfortunately, millions of infants throughout the world are still acquiring HIV infection. Median survival is 2.5 years.

Congenital infections

Congenital rubella
The incidence in the immunized population of the UK is very low at 2/100 000 live births.

Transmission occurs in 90% of fetuses after maternal viraemia at <16 weeks gestation but both transmission rates and severity fall in the 2nd and 3rd trimester.

Clinical features of congenital rubella syndrome consist of:
- Anaemia, neutropaenia and thrombocytopaenia, hepatosplenomegaly, jaundice
- Deafness
- Microcephaly
- Congenital heart disease
- Osteitis.

Diagnosis is by direct viral culture from urine and detection of IgM in serum. There is no specific treatment. Ophthalmological and audiological assessment should be made. Termination of pregnancy is offered to mothers with positive IgM for rubella.

Congenital cytomegalovirus (CMV) infection

CMV is the most common congenital infection in the UK with an incidence of 3–4/1000 live births, and is more common in developing countries.

Primary infection, shown by seroconversion, occurs in 1–2% of mothers with a transmission rate between 25–40%, higher later in pregnancy. Transmission is much less common after secondary infection (1–2%).

90% of infants are asymptomatic; 5–10% are severely affected. Prognosis is poor if abnormalities are detectable on antenatal ultrasound: microcephaly, periventricular calcification, CNS translucencies, hepatic lesions.

Features at birth include IUGR, hepatosplenomegaly, anaemia, thrombocytopaenia, and chorioretinitis. It is an important cause of sensorineural deafness which is found in 10% of 'asymptomatic' cases. Cerebral calcification (Fig 1.14) confers a high risk of neurodevelopmental delay.

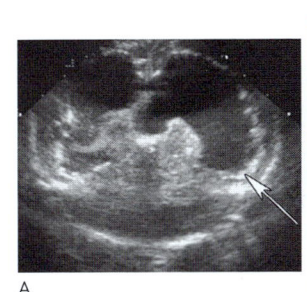

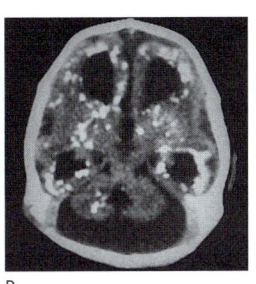

Fig 1.14 Congenital CMV infection: subependymal and basal ganglia intracerebral calcification. A. Coronal cranial US. B. Cranial CT. Reproduced with permission from Ceola AF, Angtuaco TL. Cases of the day: US case of the day. Radio Graphics 1999; 19:1385–1387.

Diagnosis is by virus isolation from urine or saliva, or detection of viral DNA (by PCR) in amniotic fluid, urine or CSF. Protracted postnatal virus shedding can occur.

Severely affected newborns may be treated with ganciclovir which improves acute disease but has an uncertain effect on long-term CNS sequelae.

Varicella zoster virus (VZV) infection

Primary maternal infection in pregnancy is rare (0.7/1000) as most mothers are immune following chickenpox as a child. The effects depend on whether infection occurs early or late in pregnancy:

- *Intrauterine infection:* congenital varicella syndrome. Infection can cause skin scars (in a dermatomal pattern), eye damage (microphthalmia and chorioretinitis), cortical atrophy and calcification, and limb defects.
- *Neonatal chickenpox:* infants born to mothers who develop chickenpox 7 days before or 7 days after delivery are at risk of vertical transmission without the benefit of transfer of any specific maternal antibodies for protection. Varicella zoster immune globulin (VZIG) is given at birth and IV aciclovir started if any sign of infection develops. Disseminated neonatal infection with pneumonitis carries a high mortality.

Parvovirus B19

About 50% of pregnant women are susceptible to infection, the transmission rate is 20–30% and the incidence of infection is 3–7/1000 live births.

The majority of infected babies suffer no ill effects. However, infection in early pregnancy can lead to spontaneous abortion or severe aplastic anaemia, non-immune hydrops (oedema and fetal ascites from heart failure) and fetal loss. Intrauterine transfusion may be required for severe anaemia. In survivors, anaemia may be transient or persist into childhood.

Congenital toxoplasmosis

The incidence of primary maternal infection in pregnancy is 1–2/1000. Infection is from poorly cooked meat, unwashed vegetables, or cat litter. The risk of transmission increases with gestation but the severity of the effects on the fetus diminishes:

- *1st trimester:* transmission rate 15%. In utero death occurs in 35% and the remainder have congenital toxoplasmosis with IUGR, hepatosplenomegaly, jaundice, retinochoroiditis, intracranial calcification (Fig 1.15), epilepsy, and hydrocephalus.
- *2nd trimester:* transmission rate 40%
- *3rd trimester:* transmission rate 60%. 90% are asymptomatic with subclinical disease which may present years later.

Diagnosis is by serology. In a positive mother, treatment with spiramycin, pyrimethamine, and sulphonamides may improve fetal outcome. In infected infants treatment is with spiramycin, sulphadiazine and pyrimethamine for at least a year. Prognosis for mildly affected or asymptomatic infants is good.

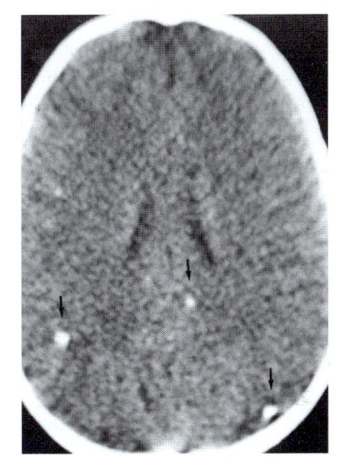

Fig 1.15 Congenital toxoplasmosis: cranial CT. Intracerebral calcification.

Congenital syphilis

In the UK this is rare, although the incidence is increasing. Antenatal screening on maternal blood is done routinely. Transmission rate during primary infection in pregnancy is 100%. Clinical features may not develop for weeks or months and vary in severity from a typical rash on the soles of the feet and organomegaly to systemic illness with bony lesions. Diagnosis is clinical, supported by serology and isolation of spirochaetes from any cutaneous lesions. Negative TPHA (at 6 months) and VDRL (at 1 year) exclude infection. Treatment antenatally or postnatally is with penicillin.

1.11 Neonatal jaundice

Bilirubin metabolism and toxicity

Bilirubin metabolism
Bilirubin is the main breakdown product of haem. Unconjugated bilirubin is lipid soluble, transported in the blood bound to albumin and actively transported into hepatocytes where it is conjugated with glucuronic acid by the enzyme uridine diphosphoglucuronosyl transferase (UDPGT).

The water soluble conjugated bilirubin is excreted as a component of bile. A fraction of this bilirubin is hydrolysed and reabsorbed via the enterohepatic circulation.

Bilirubin toxicity
Unconjugated bilirubin is lipid soluble and able to cross the blood–brain barrier to enter the brain where it exerts a toxic effect in the brain stem, basal ganglia, hippocampus, cerebellum, and acoustic nerve. Bilirubin entry is increased by hypoxia, acidosis, infection, or displacement from albumin.

Bilirubin encephalopathy and kernicterus
Kernicterus describes the yellow staining of basal ganglia seen in infants who have died of acute bilirubin toxicity.

Bilirubin encephalopathy is the clinical state caused by hyperbilirubinaemia and characterized by initial hypotonia and lethargy followed by hypertonicity, opisthotonus, seizures, coma, and death. The sequelae of bilirubin encephalopathy include athetoid cerebral palsy, high-frequency sensorineural hearing loss, paralysis of upward gaze, and learning difficulties.

The relationship between serum bilirubin, bilirubin encephalopathy, and permanent CNS damage is complex, rendering it difficult to establish guidelines for jaundice treatment based on serum bilirubin levels. The risk of toxicity is increased by:
- *Pre-term birth:* short gestation
- Rapidly rising serum bilirubin and prolonged peak
- Hypoalbuminaemia
- Coexisting hypoxia, acidaemia, hypoglycaemia, sepsis.

Physiological jaundice
After birth bilirubin levels rise to a peak between day 3–4, fall quite rapidly for 2–3 days and then decline over 1–2 weeks.

This 'physiological jaundice' is a result of rapid breakdown of haemoglobin and immaturity of liver enzymes.

Physiological jaundice is not clinically apparent in the first 24 h of life and is exacerbated in preterm or breast-fed infants who exhibit a delayed but higher peak in bilirubin levels with a more gradual decline. Physiological jaundice is exacerbated by polycythaemia, bruising, dehydration, and low caloric intake which is more common in breast-fed infants.

Pathological jaundice: early onset

Aetiology
The causes are best classified according to age of onset.

<24 h
Rapidly developing jaundice on the first day is usually caused by haemolysis due to:
- *Isoimmunisation:*
  - *rhesus disease:* now uncommon because of prophylaxis. It is usually identified on antenatal screening tests and if severe can cause anaemia and fetal hydrops.
  - *ABO incompatibility:* now the most common cause of haemolytic jaundice. Although ~20% of pregnancies are 'ABO' incompatible only about 1% result in haemolysis. The most common combination is an ORh+ve mother with an ARh+ve or BRh+ve baby. Maternal IgG anti-haemolysin crosses the placenta and causes haemolysis in the infant. The direct antibody test (DAT, Coombs test) is positive.
- *Red cell defects:*
  - *G6PD deficiency:* X-linked recessive disorder so mostly affects males; severe neonatal jaundice can occur with certain variants
  - *hereditary spherocytosis (HS):* autosomal dominant inheritance with a positive family history in 75%
- *Congenital infection:* an uncommon cause of early onset haemolytic jaundice in the UK.

24 h to 2 weeks
- *Infection:* urinary tract infection
- *Haemolysis:* presenting late, especially G6PD deficiency
- *Extravasated blood:* bruising, cephalhaematoma
- *Polycythaemia:* delayed cord clamping
- *Increased enterohepatic circulation:* bowel obstruction
- *Metabolic disorders:* galactosaemia, tyrosinaemia
- *Hepatic enzyme defects:* Crigler–Najjar, Gilbert syndrome.

Clinical evaluation
Jaundice is detectable clinically when serum bilirubin exceeds 85 micromol/L. Unconjugated hyperbilirubinaemia imparts a light yellow discoloration whereas conjugated hyperbilirubinaemia has a darker, greener hue.

The history should include enquiry about the pregnancy, family history of haemolytic or genetic disease, drug history, associated symptoms, and whether breast or formula fed.

Examination may reveal: pallor due to haemolysis and anaemia, fever or weight loss from infection or dehydration, dysmorphic features, or signs of congenital infection.

Management
Investigations
- *Bilirubin:* measurement of serum bilirubin is indicated if there is jaundice in the first 24 h or significant clinical jaundice.
- Blood group and direct antibody test
- *Full blood count:* reticulocytes, red cell morphology
- *Haemolysis with negative DAT:* tests for HS, G6PD
- *Urine:* microscopy and culture, reducing substances.

Treatment
Treatment options are designed to prevent bilirubin encephalopathy and include phototherapy and exchange transfusion. There is no universal agreement with regard to the precise level of serum bilirubin at which treatment should commence. Tables of guideline thresholds are available which incorporate relevant additional factors including gestational age and weight, postnatal age, well or sick, and bilirubin/albumin ratios.

Phototherapy
Phototherapy is commenced in an infant <24 h with a bilirubin level >100–150 micromol/L and in well term infants with level >300–350 micromol/L at 72 h. Lower thresholds apply to pre-term and sick infants.

Blue light of wavelength 425–475 nm converts unconjugated bilirubin to harmless, water-soluble products. After 4 h, 20% of total bilirubin is in the form of non-toxic isomers.

Intensive phototherapy combines overhead lights with a fibre-optic blanket and can reduce bilirubin levels by 40% or more in 24 h in a non-haemolysing infant.

Disadvantages of phototherapy include parental anxiety and separation, loose stools due to decreased gut transit time, rashes, risk of hypothermia/hyperthermia, and increased fluid loss via skin and gut.

Phototherapy should ideally be continuous. Provided exchange transfusion thresholds are not being approached, infants can 'come out of the lights' for feeds. A rebound is usual after stopping a course of phototherapy and this must be monitored. When phototherapy is used in an infant with an increased conjugated bilirubin component a transient bronze pigmentation of the skin may occur.

Exchange transfusion

This technique not only provides rapid correction of hyperbilirubinaemia but also corrects anaemia and removes haemolytic antibody in haemolytic jaundice due to isoimmunisation. It is now rarely required, but indications include:

- Severe haemolytic disease: bilirubin rising at >10 micromol/L per hour despite phototherapy
- Symptomatic bilirubin encephalopathy.

The infant's blood is removed in aliquots up to a total of twice the blood volume (2 × 80 mL/kg) and replaced with transfused blood. Hazards include thrombosis and embolism, infection, NEC, metabolic abnormalities including hypocalcaemia and hyperkalaemia, and coagulation abnormalities.

Prolonged jaundice

Prolonged jaundice is defined as visibly detectable hyperbilirubinaemia beyond 2 weeks in a term infant and 3 weeks in a pre-term infant. It can be a sign of serious underlying liver disease but the most common cause in term infants is benign, breast-milk related jaundice. See Chapter 5.11 on neonatal liver disease.

Aetiology

The causes of prolonged jaundice are classified according to whether it is unconjugated or conjugated.

Unconjugated hyperbilirubinaemia

Breast milk jaundice is the most common cause. Jaundice persists beyond 14 days in up to 40% of breastfed babies and 9% of breastfed infants are still jaundiced at 28 days of age.

Acute neonatal causes such as haemolysis or low-grade infection may persist beyond 2 weeks.

Less common causes include increased enterohepatic circulation from intestinal obstruction in pyloric stenosis, hepatic enzyme defects, and hypothyroidism or cystic fibrosis which should now be identified on neonatal screening in the UK.

Conjugated hyperbilirubinaemia

- *Obstruction:*
  - *extrahepatic:* biliary atresia, choledocal cyst, inspissated bile/bile plug
  - *intrahepatic:* Alagille syndrome
- Neonatal hepatitis syndrome
- *Metabolic or endocrine:* α1-antitrypsin deficiency, galactosaemia, fructosaemia, tyrosinosis, hypermethioninaemia, glycogen storage diseases, cystic fibrosis, peroxisomal disorders, hypopituitarism, hypoadrenalism
- *Chromosomal disorders:* Turner syndrome, trisomy 13, 18, or 21
- *Infections:* UTI, congenital infections, viral infections.
- *Miscellaneous:* drugs erythromycin, rifampicin, prolonged TPN.

Management

A well breast-fed baby is unlikely to have serious disease but a reliable diagnosis of breast milk jaundice can only be made on exclusion of pathological causes. Jaundice is not an indication for stopping breast-feeding.

Examination to detect anaemia and stool inspection to identify acholic stools is combined with initial screening tests:

- *Total and conjugated bilirubin:* split bilirubin
- Haematocrit/PCV
- Urine dipstick, microscopy, and culture
- G6PD screen in infants of at risk ethnic groups: black, Asian, or Mediterranean.

LFTs are unhelpful as the normal range is wide and borderline or 'raised' values become the focus of unnecessary investigation. Check newborn blood spot results for TFTs.

Conjugated hyperbilirubinaemia >25 micromol/L is always pathological and requires full investigation. One important aim is to distinguish biliary obstruction requiring surgical intervention from intrahepatic causes. The cause may be apparent from history and clinical examination.

Basic initial investigations include:

- Liver function tests: including gamma GT levels
- Coagulation screen, viral serology
- α1-antitrypsin levels, urine for reducing substances
- Plasma and urine organic and amino acids
- Abdominal ultrasound scan.

IM vitamin K should be given prior to transfer for investigation to prevent late-onset haemorrhagic disease.

1.12 Metabolic disorders

Neonatal hypoglycaemia

Neonatal glucose metabolism
In utero, glucose is transferred to the fetus by facilitated diffusion and stored as fat from 28–30 weeks gestation and glycogen in the liver and myocardium from 36 weeks.

Postnatal glucose concentration falls rapidly after birth as it is the main energy source. A rise in glucagon and catecholamine levels stimulates glycogenolysis and gluconeogenesis, producing 4–6 mg/kg per min of glucose. After the first few hours fatty acids become the main energy source and the respiratory quotient falls from 1.0 to 0.7. Insulin levels remain low so there is relative intolerance of intravenous or oral glucose loads.

Aetiology and pathogenesis
A precise definition of hypoglycaemia as a single blood glucose level is impossible as levels as low as 1.5 mmol/L are observed in healthy, asymptomatic infants.

Instead, operational thresholds and therapeutic goals have been proposed as set out below. Glucose levels are lower in whole blood than plasma by 13–18% because of dilution by red cell water.

Aetiology
Transient, early hypoglycaemia occurs either because glycogen stores are depleted or because of hyperinsulinaemia.

Hypoglycaemia due to depleted glycogen stores
- *Small for dates and preterm infants*: low glycogen stores.
- Intrapartum asphyxia and hypoxic-ischaemic encephalopathy
- Hypothermia
- Breast milk insufficiency
- *Serious illness*: sepsis, cardiac disease.

Hypoglycaemia due to hyperinsulinaemia
- *Infants of diabetic mothers*: beta-cell hyperplasia is associated with hyperinsulinism.
- *Rhesus disease*: babies with Rhesus haemolytic disease have islet cell hypertrophy.
- *Maternal glucose infusion*: a large or rapid infusion during labour.

Recurrent or persistent hypoglycaemia may be caused by a number of rare disorders:

Endocrine deficiency
- hypopituitarism, GH deficiency
- congenital adrenal hyperplasia

Syndromes with hyperinsulinism
- Beckwith–Wiedemann syndrome
- Hyperinsulinaemic hypoglycaemia, familial (HHF)

Inborn errors of metabolism
- glycogen storage disease
- galactosaemia
- medium chain acyl-CoA dehydrogenase deficiency.

Pathogenesis: neuroglycopaenia
Brain function is dependent on a continuous supply of glucose from the circulation. Newborn babies can tolerate blood glucose levels of <1.5 mmol/L without any symptoms or sequelae, presumably because alternative fuels such as ketones and lactate are metabolized.

- Neuroglycopaenia leads to a reversible, functional disturbance in brain function manifested as 'symptoms' including:
  - Jitteriness, irritability, high-pitched cry
  - Reduced consciousness, lethargy, hypotonia
  - Apnoea
  - Seizures.

Symptomatic hypoglycaemia implies neuroglycopaenia and if prolonged can lead to brain damage with neurological sequelae including learning difficulties and cerebral palsy. In contrast, asymptomatic hypoglycaemia does not appear to cause brain damage.

Clinical features
Hypoglycaemia may be asymptomatic or associated with symptoms of neuroglycopaenia as described above. Examination may reveal features which provide a clue to aetiology such as IUGR or macrosomia, hepatomegaly, or features of Beckwith–Wiedemann syndrome: large tongue, omphalocele, horizontal earlobe creases.

Management
Blood glucose is monitored in infants known to be at risk of hypoglycaemia, and preventive measures are instituted.

All small for dates, VLBW babies or infants of diabetic mothers should be started on full-strength milk feeds preferably breast milk by 2–4 h of age either orally or via a nasogastric tube. In a well at-risk infant blood glucose should be measured at around 3 h of age, before the second feed.

If enteral feeding is not possible, intravenous 10% dextrose is given starting at 60–70 mL/kg per day, glucose 4–5 mg/kg per min.

Treatment
Recommended operational thresholds for intervention in at risk infants are:
- *<1.0 mmol/L*: in any infant
- *<2.0 mmol/L*: if persistent in asymptomatic infant
- *<3.5 mmol/L*: infants with hyperinsulinism.

A therapeutic goal of blood glucose >2.5 mmol/L is recommended in any systemically unwell infant or infant with abnormal neurological signs.

If asymptomatic hypoglycaemia (i.e. hypoglycaemia without neuroglycopaenia) is detected in an at risk infant not on IV dextrose, the next milk feed due is given immediately (by nasogastric tube) and blood glucose level checked in 1 h. If hypoglycaemia persists, or symptoms develop give a bolus of IV 10% dextrose 2 mL/kg followed by IV 10% dextrose 80–100 mL/kg per day (6–8 mg/kg per min).

Persistent or intractable hypoglycaemia may necessitate further investigations to exclude the causes listed above including endocrine investigations (insulin, pituitary hormone, cortisol levels), metabolic investigations and imaging (cranial MRI, adrenal ultrasound).

Neonatal hyperglycaemia

Iatrogenic hyperglycaemia
LBW infants (<1.5 kg) may have difficulty metabolizing glucose given at rates in excess of 6 mg/kg per min (86 mL/kg per day of 10% dextrose). However, such rates may be necessary to attain adequate fluid volumes or adequate calorie input during TPN.

Hyperglycaemia with osmotic diuresis and dehydration may result. Options then include reducing the concentration of dextrose to 5% or cautiously infusing insulin (0.1 unit/kg per hour).

Neonatal diabetes mellitus
This uncommon condition may represent a delayed maturation of the insulin releasing mechanism of pancreatic β cells. Most cases resolve within a few months.

Inborn errors of metabolism (IEMs)

This group of genetic disorders is considered in detail in Chapter 11. In the UK, newborn blood spot screening includes tests for phenylketonuria (PKU) and medium-chain acyl CoA dehydrogenase (MCAD) deficiency. The introduction of tandem mass spectrometry has greatly extended the range of metabolic disorders for which it is possible to screen and this technique is widely used in the USA.

Incidence
Most of these disorders are inherited in an autosomal recessive manner and have a low incidence. The incidence of autosomal recessive disease is significantly increased in the offspring of consanguineous parents.

Aetiology and pathogenesis
The genes encode enzymes for rate limiting steps in intermediary metabolism. Toxic metabolites are removed in utero by the placenta and many pathways are susceptible to protein loading. Examples of IEMs that may present in the neonatal period include:
- *Amino acid disorders:* urea cycle defects (UCDs)
- *Carbohydrate disorders:* galactosaemia
- *Fatty acid oxidation defects:*
  - long-chain acyl CoA dehydrogenase (LCAD) deficiency
  - medium-chain acyl CoA dehydrogenase (MCAD) deficiency
- Energy metabolism defects.

Clinical features
An IEM should be suspected if a previously well term infant deteriorates acutely at several days of age. Clues in the history include parental consanguinity, a positive family history or a sibling with unexplained illness or neonatal death.

A wide spectrum of presenting clinical features exist which often involve the nervous system:
- *CNS:* neonatal encephalopathy with altered consciousness (lethargy, coma), seizures, hypotonia, poor feeding, vomiting, and apnoea
- *Acid–base disturbance:* metabolic acidosis or less commonly respiratory alkalosis
- *Hypoglycaemia:* severe and persistent
- Acute liver or cardiac disease.

The differential diagnosis includes bacterial sepsis, congenital heart disease, hypoxic–ischaemic or infective encephalopathy, and gastrointestinal obstruction (vomiting).

Management
Immediate management encompasses supportive measures and investigations to establish the diagnosis.

Diagnostic investigations
First line screening tests are done on blood and urine and include:
- *Blood tests:*
  - blood gases, glucose, ammonia
  - lactate, U&E
  - liver function tests
  - FBC and coagulation screen
- *Urine:* reducing substances, ketones.

Second-line investigations may involve more specialized investigations on blood and urine and on CSF, skin fibroblasts, or white cells for enzyme assays and genetic analysis.

If an infant appears moribund or dies, useful samples for further analysis include frozen plasma and urine, blood sample in EDTA for DNA analysis, and biopsies of skin, liver, and muscle.

Treatment
Supportive empirical treatment includes stopping milk feeds to exclude protein and galactose and providing calories with intravenous glucose to avoid a catabolic state.

Hypoglycaemia and metabolic acidosis is corrected and ventilatory or circulatory support given as necessary. Early intervention is important to minimize neurological sequelae. Specific measures may be available for treatment of hyperammonaemia, depending on cause, and dialysis may be life-saving in some conditions

Acid–base imbalance

Metabolic acidosis
Causes depend on whether the anion gap is increased.

Increased anion gap
- *Lactic acidosis:* sepsis, shock, necrotizing enterocolitis
- Inborn error of metabolism
- Renal failure.

Normal anion gap
- *Gastrointestinal HCO_3^- losses:* ileostomy, diarrhoea
- Renal tubular acidosis.

Metabolic alkalosis

Gastric losses
- Vomiting, non-replacement of nasogastric aspirates.

Renal losses
- Thiazide and loop diuretics
- Hypokalaemia.

1.13 Congenital anomalies

Surgical intervention may be required for a range of congenital anomalies which present in the newborn period and range from minor to severe in their effects. Defects affect most systems and are considered in the corresponding chapters.

Prenatal diagnosis is now possible for many of these conditions, allowing parental counselling and advance planning of delivery and management. A selection of the more important are considered here, classified according to the anatomical system involved.

Craniofacial abnormalities

Cleft lip and palate

The incidence is 1/1000 live births. There is familial clustering with polygenic inheritance.

Abnormalities range in severity from bifid uvula or cleft palate or mild unilateral cleft lip to unilateral or bilateral cleft lip and palate. Diagnosis prenatally by ultrasound scanning is increasingly common.

A specialist multidisciplinary team provides care and includes a craniofacial surgeon, orthodontist, specialist nurse, speech and language therapist, and audiologist.

Initial lip repair is carried out a few days after birth or at age up to 3 months and the palate is usually repaired at 6–12 months. A specially moulded palatal prosthesis and special teats allow the infant to feed normally and encourages maxillary growth.

'Before and after' surgery: photographs of previous repairs provide reassurance to parents dismayed by the unsightly deformity. Long-term complications include ear infections, speech delay, and orthodontic problems.

Choanal atresia

A rare anomaly with a bony obstruction occluding the posterior nasal space. Bilateral atresia causes respiratory distress at birth as newborn infants are obligatory nose breathers. An oral airway or endotracheal tube is inserted before surgical correction.

It may occur as part of the CHARGE syndrome: **C**oloboma, **H**eart defects, **A**tresia of choanae, **R**etarded growth, **G**enital hypoplasia (males), **E**ar deformities.

Pierre Robin sequence

The features include micrognathia, posteriorly displaced tongue, and posterior palatal defect. Coexisting anomalies, especially cardiac, are common. Respiratory obstruction may lead to cor pulmonale.

Management strategies include:
- Nurse prone
- Nasal CPAP and nasogastric feeding
- Surgery to posterior palate at 1 year
- ± Tracheostomy if severe.

The problems become less severe with growth of mouth and jaw.

Gastrointestinal obstruction

Aetiology

Mechanical obstruction of the gastrointestinal tract may be caused by:
- Oesophageal atresia
- Duodenal atresia or web
- Malrotation and volvulus
- Meconium ileus
- Hirschsprung disease
- Imperforate anus.

Clinical features

Presentation is within 24–48 h of birth with proximal lesions but may be delayed for several days for distal lesions. Pyloric stenosis does not present at birth as several weeks of enteral feeding are required for hypertrophy of the pyloric smooth muscle to occur.

Clinical features include:
- *Vomiting*: green bile staining if the obstruction is distal to the ampulla of Vater
- Delayed passage of meconium or absent transitional stools
- Abdominal distension with visible loops of bowel or peristalsis.

It is important to distinguish vomiting, the forcible expulsion of gastric contents, from regurgitation or possetting which is the effortless return of small quantities of milk. The differential diagnosis of vomiting due to mechanical obstruction includes:
- *Non-mechanical obstruction*:
  - paralytic ileus due to sepsis, electrolyte disturbance
  - necrotizing enterocolitis
- *Vomiting in systemic illness*:
  - septicaemia, urinary tract infection, meningitis
  - inborn errors of metabolism
  - congenital adrenal hyperplasia
  - drug overdose or withdrawal.

Considering individual conditions:

Duodenal atresia

The incidence is 1/6000 live births. One third of patients have Down syndrome, and other anomalies such as malrotation are common. There may be complete atresia, stenosis due to a duodenal web, or a fibrous cord.

It is often suspected antenatally on account of polyhydramnios and a distended, fluid-filled stomach on ultrasound. Postnatally it usually presents with bilious vomiting in the first 24 h, although stenosis may have a more insidious onset.

The 'double-bubble' appearance on plain abdominal radiograph is diagnostic (Fig 1.16). Surgical repair is carried out after stabilization.

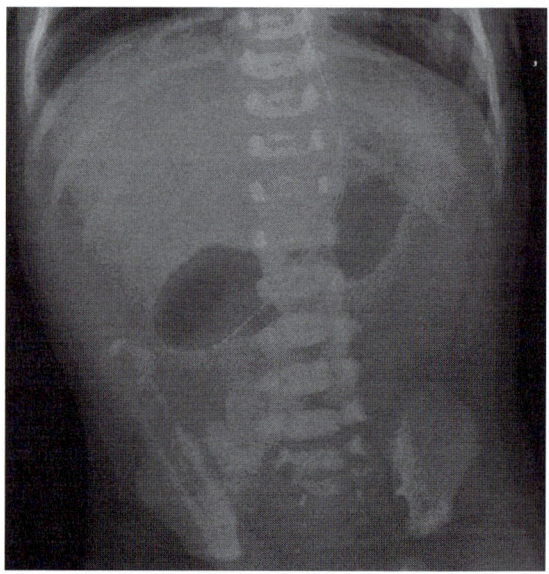

Fig 1.16 Duodenal atresia: 'double bubble'.

Malrotation and volvulus

Malrotation predisposes to midgut volvulus which causes intestinal obstruction and compression of the superior mesenteric artery with small-bowel ischaemia. There is sudden onset of bilious vomiting with abdominal tenderness and shock. Upper gastrointestinal exam (contrast swallow) is diagnostic. Volvulus is a surgical emergency.

Imperforate anus

The incidence is 1/5000. A number of anatomical varieties exist, categorized as 'high' (normal bowel ends above levator ani) or 'low' (bowel terminates just under perineal skin). Fistulas to bladder, rectum, urethra, or vagina are common. Associated anomalies are common, especially in the 'high' variety e. g. present in 80% of infants with VACTERL association.

Management

Diagnostic investigations
- Imaging:
  - plain abdominal radiographs:
  - obstruction: distended loops of bowel with fluid levels
  - perforation: free air under diaphragm, intrahepatic or around falciform ligament.
  - contrast radiographs: to demonstrate malrotation, strictures
- Septic screen
- Biochemistry: urea and electrolytes, LFTs, creatinine, acid-base status

Treatment
- Abdominal decompression: nasogastric tube in situ with frequent aspiration and free drainage
- IV fluids for resuscitation and maintenance
- Preoperative antibiotics
- Evaluate and correct bleeding diathesis.

Respiratory tract

Congenital diaphragmatic hernia

The incidence is 1/4000 births. In 90% of cases there is a left-sided hernia through the foramen of Bochdalek. The remainder are right-sided or through the foramen of Morgagni.

Herniated bowel restricts lung development *in utero* leading to pulmonary hypoplasia and pulmonary arterioles are reduced in number with smooth muscle hypertrophy predisposing to persistent pulmonary hypertension. Associated malformations are found in 30% of liveborn infants including CNS malformations, oesophageal atresia, congenital heart disease and syndromes such as trisomies 13 and 18.

Clinical presentation
- *Prenatal:* the majority are diagnosed on ultrasound screening
- *Failed resuscitation:* deterioration with bag/mask ventilation
- *Respiratory distress:* hours or days after birth if lung well developed.

The classical physical signs are respiratory distress with apex beat displaced to the right, reduced air entry into the left chest and a scaphoid abdomen.

Radiograph of chest and abdomen is diagnostic (Fig 1.17).

Management

The infant should be intubated and a wide-bore nasogastric tube passed to decompress the intrathoracic gut. Operation is deferred usually for 24 h to allow stabilization and maximal reduction in pulmonary vascular resistance.

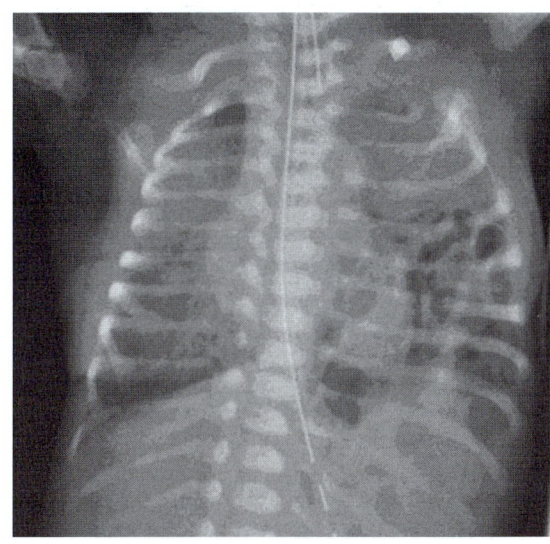

Fig 1.17 Left-sided diaphragmatic hernia: CXR showing abdominal contents in the left hemithorax and right-sided mediastinal displacement.

The main factors influencing outcome are associated congenital anomalies and the degree of pulmonary hypertension. Mortality is high (50%). Long-term sequelae include prolonged oxygen dependency if pulmonary hypoplasia is severe, gastro-oesophageal reflux, and developmental delay.

Inguinoscrotal

Inguinal hernia

Common in preterm infants, especially those with chronic lung disease. More common in males and on the right side (Fig 1.18). It should be repaired before discharge home as there is a high risk of incarceration in the early months of life. An experienced surgeon may be able to reduce an incarcerated hernia by sustained gentle compression with adequate analgesia.

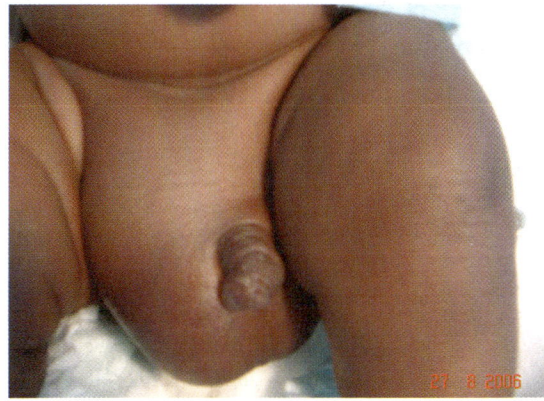

Fig 1.18 Right-sided inguinal hernia in ex-preterm infant.

1.14 Case-based discussions

A term infant with seizures

You are asked to see a term baby age 20 h on the postnatal ward in whom the midwives have observed abnormal movements: clonic movements of his right hand, arm, and face. These initially lasted a few seconds but then became more frequent and prolonged.

His mother went into spontaneous labour at 39 weeks gestation. This is her second pregnancy; the first ended as a miscarriage at 12 weeks. There was no history of prolonged rupture of membranes or maternal pyrexia. He was born by forceps delivery in good condition with Apgars of 9 at 1 min and 10 at 5 min. No active resuscitation was necessary.

On examination the baby appears alert and well perfused and is not tachycardic or tachypnoeic. His fontanelle is soft and he appears to have normal tone and reflexes. You suspect these abnormal movements may be seizures and admit him to the neonatal unit.

What are the causes of neonatal seizures?

The most common cause of neonatal seizures (40%) is hypoxic ischaemic encephalopathy, but there is no history to suggest perinatal asphyxia in this infant. The next most common cause is cerebral arteriovenous infarction (20%) followed by intracranial haemorrhage (12–20%). Birth trauma can result in subarachnoid or subdural haemorrhages.

Hypoglycaemia can cause seizures and a number of inborn errors of metabolism present with seizures, including non-ketotic hyperglycinaemia, maple syrup urine disease, urea cycle defects, and pyridoxine deficiency.

Meningitis must be excluded: the commonest organisms are *group B streptococcus and E. coli*. Herpes simplex encephalitis can also present with fits.

Focal seizures of sudden onset suggest vascular pathology.

Although clinically very well, the baby continues to have focal seizures which become more prolonged. He is started on phenobarbitone IV and a midazolam infusion is commenced after 12 h.

His baseline blood tests are unremarkable: CRP<2 g/dL, glucose 3.4 mmol/L, calcium normal, ammonia 72 micromole/L. He was not acidotic. A lumbar puncture was normal. A cranial ultrasound scan on admission was normal.

72 h after admission his fits had stopped and he was weaned off his anticonvulsants. Neurological examination revealed subtle asymmetry with paucity of spontaneous movement on the right and a palmar grasp that was difficult to elicit. A cranial MRI was consistent with a middle cerebral artery infarction.

What are the causes and prognosis of neonatal stroke?

Before modern neuroimaging it was thought that cerebral infarction was a rare condition. The prevalence is now thought to be around 0.25/1000.

The most common type of neonatal cerebral infarction in the full-term infant is an ischaemic lesion in the territory of the middle cerebral artery, with the left more commonly involved than the right. In the majority of cases no underlying cause is found, although there is an increase in the incidence of heterozygosity for factor V Leiden.

Otherwise healthy babies present with fits, often focal, in the first days of life. There may be some asymmetry on neurological examination, but this is often missed.

Cranial ultrasound examination is often normal although there may be ill defined areas of increased echodensity. MRI is the imaging modality of choice. Diffusion weighted imaging (DWI) shows an increase in signal intensity in the infarcted region.

The prognosis is remarkably good overall with only 1/5 having motor problems in later life, usually a hemiplegia. Involvement of hemisphere, internal capsule, or basal ganglia indicates a poor prognosis.

A term infant with cyanosis

You are called to attend an emergency Caesarean section of a term infant with fetal distress. Following artificial rupture of membranes meconium was noted and the CTG showed prolonged decelerations.

The baby is born floppy and bradycardic and makes no respiratory effort. You suction the oropharynx and under direct vision pass the suction catheter through the larynx. There is some meconium in the oropharynx but none below the vocal cords.

After 5 inflation breaths the heart rate improves but respiratory effort remains poor. At 5 min the baby is intubated. She remains cyanosed despite ventilation in 100% oxygen and is transferred to the neonatal unit.

What is the differential diagnosis?

Both respiratory and cardiac causes must be sought. Although no meconium was seen below the vocal cords one cannot exclude meconium aspiration syndrome as in most cases the baby aspirates *in utero*. Congenital pneumonia, pneumothorax and congenital diaphragmatic hernia must also be considered and it is important to listen for equal air entry.

The baby is put on IPPV with pressures of 20/4 in 100% oxygen. An urgent chest radiograph shows well-inflated clear lung fields with a paucity of vascular markings. An arterial blood gas shows severe hypoxaemia with normocapnia and mild metabolic acidosis. Arterial oxygen saturation in the right hand was 85% and in the left foot was 65%.

What is the further management?

The discrepancies between preductal and postductal arterial oxygen saturations indicate right to left shunting across the ductus arteriosus. The main differential is cyanotic congenital heart disease or persistent pulmonary hypertension of the newborn (PPHN). The history of fetal distress and condition at birth suggests PPHN, but definitive diagnosis must be done on echocardiogram.

An echocardiogram was performed which confirmed a structurally normal heart. There was right to left shunting across the patent ductus arteriosus and foramen ovale. The diagnosis of PPHN was made. The baby was transferred to a specialist centre and put on high-frequency oscillatory ventilation and given inhaled nitric oxide as a selective pulmonary vasodilator.

Chapter 2

Accidents and emergencies

2.1 The seriously ill child: physiology 30
2.2 The seriously ill child: clinical assessment 32
2.3 Cardiopulmonary arrest 34
2.4 Accidental injuries: trauma and burns 36
2.5 Head injury and drowning 38
2.6 Poisoning 40
2.7 Respiratory emergencies 42
2.8 Septicaemia and septic shock 44
2.9 Anaphylaxis 46
2.10 Diabetic ketoacidosis 48
2.11 Convulsions and coma 50
2.12 Case-based discussions 52

2.1 The seriously ill child: physiology

Sudden, unexpected cardiopulmonary arrest is very rare in children. Arrest is nearly always preceded by a period of progressive failure of the respiratory, cardiovascular, or nervous system. Care of the critically ill child therefore requires understanding of how these systems function and how the anatomy and physiology of small infants and children differs from that in adults.

Body size and proportions

Infants and children do not have optimal body proportions overall and the head in particular is disproportionately large. This has several unfortunate consequences:
- *High ratio of body surface area to weight:*
  - rapid heat loss predisposes to hypothermia
  - high fluid turnover increases susceptibility to dehydration.
- *Small body size:*
  - multisystem involvement is more likely in blunt trauma, e.g. a severe pattern of injury in pedestrian road traffic accidents
- *Large head:*
  - tend to fall head first, increasing the likelihood that the head is the point of impact
  - the large head and weak neck of small infants generates large shearing forces if the infant is shaken.

Respiratory system

Airways
- Up to age 6 months infants are obligate nose breathers and do not tolerate nasal obstruction caused by secretions or soft tissue such as adenoids or cannulae.
- The relatively bulky oropharyngeal soft tissues, combined with passive flexion due to larger occiput and shorter neck, renders the oropharyngeal airway easily occluded. The optimal head position is neutral in an infant and 'sniffing' in a child.
- The diameter of the upper airway is the perfect size for complete occlusion by some inhaled objects.
- The internal diameter of all airways are smaller giving rise to a greater rise in airway resistance for any given reduction in diameter by oedema, secretions, or bronchospasm.

Thoracic cage
The ribs and chest wall are elastic and compliant in young infants causing
- Intercostal and subcostal recession
- Pulmonary contusions without rib fracture in chest trauma.

Compliance decreases with skeletal maturation. Recession in an older child indicates a greater degree of respiratory distress. The ribs are positioned more horizontally than in adults and afford less protection to the abdominal contents.

Breathing patterns
The diaphragm is the principle muscle of respiration in infancy. It fatigues easily and air in the stomach, as occurs with bag and mask ventilation, can cause splinting. The sitting position may reduce diaphragmatic work and swallowed air should be decompressed using a nasogastric tube.

Central control of respiration is immature in preterm infants and apnoeic episodes may be spontaneous or provoked by a number of stimuli (see 'Apparent life threatening events', Section 2.7).

Cardiovascular system

Cardiac output and oxygen delivery
The volume of blood expelled from each ventricle during systole is called the 'stroke volume' and depends on:
- *Preload:* the degree of ventricular filling during diastole and contractility of the myocardium.
- *Afterload:* the resistance against which the ventricle pumps.

Cardiac output = heart rate × stroke volume.

The oxygen delivery is the product of cardiac output and arterial oxygen concentration.

Cardiac output is modified by:
- *Intracardiac mechanisms:* stretching of myocardium causes a more forceful contraction (Frank–Starling curve).
- *Extracardiac mechanisms:* sympathetic nervous activity increases cardiac performance by increasing venous return (preload), cardiac contractility and heart rate. It also increases afterload and reduces cardiac output by peripheral vasoconstriction.

Peripheral circulation
Arterial
Whole body oxygen delivery exceeds consumption by a factor of 4, providing a wide safety margin. However, individual organs have different relationships between oxygen delivery and consumption and blood flow to individual organs is influenced by several factors including:
- *Metabolism:* products of local cellular metabolism cause vasodilatation and match oxygen delivery to consumption.
- *Oxygen tension:* reduced oxygen delivery causes relaxation of pre-capillary arterioles with recruitment of capillaries and reduced diffusion distance for oxygen.
- *Autoregulation:* resistance vessels adapt to pressure changes to maintain flow constant.

In addition to local factors, the sympathetic system has a powerful role in acute regulation of the circulation by noradrenaline mediated vasoconstriction of both arterioles and veins.

In the brain and heart local factors can override sympathetically driven vasoconstriction. In contrast, in organs with a blood flow well in excess of their metabolic needs, such as the kidneys or skin, the action of sympathetic vasoconstriction is more pronounced.

Venous
The venous system has a high capacitance and normally contains 75% of the total blood volume. Sympathetic activity tends to reduce venous system compliance and augment venous return. Stretch receptors in the central veins, right atrium, and pulmonary artery mediate enhanced sympathetic activity in response to reduced cardiac filling.

Blood pressure
Blood flow in the circulation is determined by the relationship between pressure gradient and resistance. The blood pressure

changes from aortic root to arterioles and the driving force available to the arterial tree is best expressed as the mean pressure:

Mean pressure = diastolic + 1/3 pulse pressure.

Heart rate
The normal heart rate is higher in small bodies. Increased heart rate increases cardiac output but beyond a certain limit cardiac filling becomes inadequate and cardiac failure ensues.

Following episodes of prolonged and severe hypoxia, a period of bradycardia occurs preceding asystolic cardiac arrest.

Nervous system
Derangements of the nervous system compromise cardiorespiratory function by a variety of distinct mechanisms.

Coma
A child with diminished level of consciousness is vulnerable to respiratory compromise because of inability to protect and maintain the airway and depression of central respiratory drive.

Seizures
A child with convulsive status epilepticus is vulnerable to occlusion of the airway and impaired respiration as a consequence of uncoordinated muscular contractions. In parallel, oxygen consumption of the brain increases. Medications given to control the seizures such as benzodiazepines may cause respiratory depression and apnoea.

Raised intracranial pressure (ICP)
The cranium represents a rigid box with a fixed volume filled by brain, cerebrospinal fluid, and vascular compartments. The normal ICP is <10–15 mmHg. Should the space occupied by brain parenchyma increase, e.g. as a result of oedema or blood from an expanding haematoma, compensatory mechanisms such as decreasing the volume of CSF or venous blood are limited in their effects.

When this capacity to compensate is exceeded, further small increases in volume produce large rapid rises in pressure. A raised ICP affects the cardiovascular system in general and the cerebral circulation in particular:

Cerebral perfusion pressure (CPP) = mean arterial pressure − intracranial pressure (ICP)

Increased ICP reduces CPP and therefore brain blood flow.
- *Cushing's triad:* bradycardia, increased systolic blood pressure, increased pulse pressure. Raised blood pressure and dilatation of cerebral blood vessels causes a further increase in ICP and reduced cerebral perfusion.

Acid–base metabolism

pH
The pH scale was introduced because in the environment [H^+] varies over an enormous scale. In fact, its use is unnecessary in medicine because [H^+] varies over a very small range. pH is the negative logarithm to the base 10 of [H^+] in mol/L. As [H^+] increases, pH reduces and a change in pH of one point corresponds to a 10-fold change in [H^+]. Corresponding values over the physiological range are shown in Table 2.1.

Table 2.1. Values of pH and [H^+] in the physiological range

pH	6.9	7.0	7.1	7.2	7.3	7.4	7.5	7.6	7.7
[H^+] (nmol)	128	100	80	64	50	40	32	25	20

Acids, bases, and buffers
An *acid* is a 'proton donor' and forms hydrogen ions in solution whereas a *base* is a 'proton acceptor' and combines with hydrogen ions in solution. A *buffer* is a compound that limits the change in pH when hydrogen ions are added or removed from a solution.

Production of acid (hydrogen ions)
The processes of metabolism naturally generate hydrogen ions in two principal forms:

CO_2 from oxidative (aerobic) metabolism: respiratory acid
An enormous quantity of CO_2 is produced (15 000 mmol/24 h) which rapidly reacts with water to form carbonic acid which dissociates into hydrogen and bicarbonate (HCO_3^-) ions. This is described by the equation:

$$CO_2 + H_2O = H_2CO_3 = HCO_3^- + H^+$$

Carbonic acid represents an important buffering system in the body.

Metabolic (non-respiratory) acids
Small amounts of metabolic acids (40–80 mmol/24 h) are produced from oxidation of amino acids and anaerobic metabolism of glucose to lactic and pyruvic acid.

Control of hydrogen ion concentrations (pH)
As pH is so critical for many bodily functions it is not surprising that powerful mechanisms exist to maintain pH in the normal range. The main challenge is elimination of acid. Three main mechanisms are:

- *Buffers:* these include bicarbonate, proteins (e.g. albumin) and haemoglobin. Haemoglobin is a powerful buffer which binds both CO_2 and H^+ and has the strongest affinity for these in the deoxygenated state.
- *Respiration:* the respiratory system is the single most important system involved in control of hydrogen ions. The arterial partial pressure of CO_2 ($PaCO_2$) is inversely proportional to alveolar ventilation, so small changes in ventilation have a profound and rapid effect on pH: a rise in $PaCO_2$ of 1.0 k Pa results in a fall in pH from 7.40 to 7.34.
- *Renal handling of bicarbonate and hydrogen ions:* the kidneys secrete hydrogen ions and regenerate bicarbonate ions. Renal handling of electrolytes also influences acid base balance. Bicarbonate ions are freely filtered by the glomerulus and most are reabsorbed in the proximal convoluted tubule. Hydrogen ions are actively secreted in the proximal and distal tubules against a steep concentration gradient and are buffered in the urine by phosphate and ammonia. Channels in the distal tubule controlled by aldosterone exchange sodium for hydrogen or potassium ions. The small capacity of the kidneys for hydrogen ion excretion renders metabolic compensation a slow process.

2.2 The seriously ill child: clinical assessment

Early recognition of respiratory failure, circulatory failure, severe neurological dysfunction or acid–base disturbance allows cardiopulmonary arrest to be anticipated and, if possible, prevented.

Rapid clinical assessment

A structured approach is used:
- Primary assessment
- Resuscitation
- Secondary assessment
- Emergency treatment and stabilization/transfer to ICU.

Primary assessment: ABCDE
- **A**irway: chest movement, breaths, stridor, wheeze, foreign body, airway opening manoeuvre
- **B**reathing:
  - *effort:* rate, accessory muscles
  - *efficacy:* oxygen saturation
  - *effects:* skin colour, conscious level
- **C**irculation: heart rate, pulse volume, blood pressure, capillary refill time (CRT)
- **D**isability: conscious level (AVPU/GCS), posture, pupils: size, symmetry, reaction to light
- **E**xposure: identify rashes

Respiratory rate

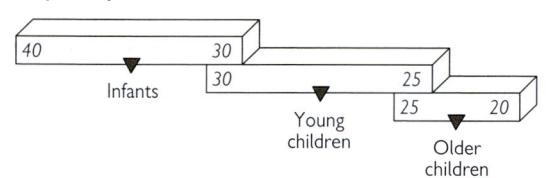

Infants: 40–30
Young children: 30–25
Older children: 25–20

Heart rate

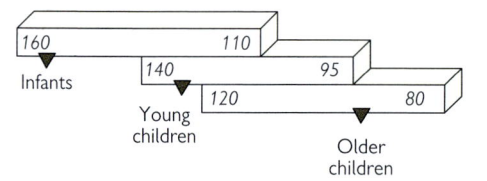

Infants: 160–140
Young children: 140–120 (95)
Older children: 110–80

Systolic blood pressure

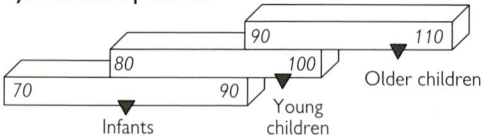

Infants: 70–90
Young children: 80–100
Older children: 90–110

Fig 2.1 Vital signs change with age.

Secondary assessment involves a focused history and full physical examination in order to establish a diagnosis.

Respiratory system

Respiratory failure may be caused by airway obstruction, intrinsic lung disease, or inadequate respiratory effort.

Clinical evaluation should allow recognition of potential respiratory failure. Arterial blood gas analysis is useful to confirm respiratory failure or monitor response to therapy.

Assessment requires evaluation of:

Respiratory rate

The normal rate decreases from 40–60/min in the newborn to 25–35/min in the 1–2 year old and 15–20/min in an adolescent. Abnormalities include tachypnoea, bradypnoea, and apnoea.

- *Tachypnoea:* is usually the first manifestation of respiratory distress in an infant and is accompanied by additional signs of changes in the mechanics of respiration such as recession, grunting. Tachypnoea without these signs ('quiet tachypnoea') suggests metabolic acidosis with respiratory compensation.
- *Bradypnoea:* a slow or irregular respiratory rate in an acutely ill child or infant is more ominous and usually indicates fatigue or CNS depression. A decreasing respiratory rate may indicate deterioration rather than improvement.

Effort of breathing

- Nasal flaring, head bobbing and intercostal, subcostal or suprasternal recession may occur with airway obstruction or alveolar disease and increased work of breathing.
- Stridor is a sign of extrathoracic airway narrowing and may be accompanied by a tracheal tug.
- Wheeze and prolonged expiration is a sign of intrathoracic airway obstruction usually at bronchial or bronchiolar level.
- Grunting is produced by early glottic closure with late expiratory contraction of the diaphragm and maintains functional residual capacity. It occurs in pneumonia or atelectasis.

Efficacy of breathing: air entry and oxygenation

Chest expansion should be bilateral and breath sounds should be equal and easily heard. Hypoxaemia is manifested as central cyanosis. Oxygenation measured by pulse oximetry is a good guide to hypoxaemia.

Effects of respiratory inadequacy

Pallor, mottling, and peripheral cyanosis occur with hypoxaemia, but these signs can also occur if the child is exposed to a cold environment. Hypoxaemia causes tachycardia and delayed peripheral capillary refill initially and if severe leads on to bradycardia and asystole. Cerebral hypoxaemia is associated with agitation or drowsiness.

Cardiovascular system

Shock

Shock is a state in which there is inadequate tissue perfusion; a failure of the circulation to provide adequate oxygen and nutritive substrates to the tissues. It is classified according to the cause and according to the stage reached. It progresses from compensated to decompensated, and then to irreversible shock.

Causes of shock

Shock may be caused by primary cardiac dysfunction or reduced venous return to the heart. Pathological events which cause these circulatory disturbances include:

- *Cardiogenic shock:* pump failure occurs in congenital heart disease, cardiomyopathies, cardiac arrhythmias, myocardial contusion and sepsis.
- *Reduced venous return:* This may be due to:
  - *hypovolaemia:* haemorrhage, burns, dehydration, sepsis.
  - *increased vascular capacitance (distributive):* anaphylaxis, neurogenic shock, sepsis

- *obstruction:* pneumothorax, pulmonary embolism, cardiac tamponade.

Note that 'septic shock' involves several mechanisms: hypovolaemia due to vascular leak, vasodilatation with vasoplegia, and depressed myocardial function.

Stages of shock
Compensated shock
In low-flow states such as hypovolaemic or cardiogenic shock, sympathetic outflow from the medulla causes venoconstriction, arterial vasoconstriction, and tachycardia. Arterial vasoconstriction maintains blood pressure and also diverts blood from non-essential areas such as the skin, kidneys, and splanchnic circulation.

In early septic, or anaphylactic shock, there may be a high flow and high cardiac output state with increased skin blood flow and bounding pulses. However, the cardiac output is unevenly distributed and some tissue beds are inadequately perfused as manifested by oliguria and metabolic acidosis.

Decompensated and irreversible shock
Decompensated shock is heralded by a fall in BP. This may occur if volume loss continues and exceeds 40% of circulating volume or if the circulation cannot meet the demands of the heart itself and myocardial function deteriorates.

Decompensation with hypotension exacerbates tissue hypoperfusion leading to increasing acidosis and inadequate oxygenation of respiratory muscles resulting in respiratory failure. Irreversible alterations occur in the microcirculation and tissues associated with multiple organ failure.

Evaluation of cardiovascular function
Tachycardia is a common response to many types of stress, and hypotension is a late and often sudden sign of cardiovascular decompensation. Skin perfusion varies with environmental temperature. CVS assessment can be difficult and requires evaluation of:

Heart rate
Sinus tachycardia is a common response to anxiety, pain, fever, hypoxia, hypercapnia, hypovolaemia and cardiac impairment. Cardiac output of infants and children is primarily increased by increased heart rate. In neonates, bradycardia may be the initial response to hypoxia, but in older infants and children bradycardia is a late and ominous sign.

Blood pressure
The lower limit or 5th centile of systolic blood pressure in children >1 year is given by the formula:

70 mmHg + (2 × age in years).

Hypotension is a sign of decompensated shock.

Systemic perfusion
This is the best guide to recognition of early, compensated shock and requires assessment of:
- *Pulse volume:* this is related to pulse pressure and is reduced in low cardiac output shock. In early septic shock there may be high output with bounding pulses.
- *Skin perfusion:* decreased skin perfusion may be an early sign of shock and is manifested as pallor, mottling, peripheral cyanosis, and delayed capillary refill time (>2 s). However, skin perfusion may also be reduced by fever or by a cold ambient temperature.
- *Renal perfusion:* urine output of less than 1 mL/kg per hour in a child or 2 mL/kg per hour in an infant indicates poor renal perfusion in the absence of known kidney disease.
- *Brain perfusion:* cortical hypoperfusion may be manifested initially as altered consciousness with confusion, irritability and agitation alternating with lethargy. More profound hypoperfusion produces greater changes, with failure to respond to a pain an ominous sign.

Nervous system
Evaluation of the CNS should include:
- *Conscious level:* the AVPU scale is usually sufficient:
  - **A**lert, response to **V**oice or **P**ain, **U**nresponsive
- *Pupils:* size, symmetry and reaction to light
- *Posture:* hypotonia, opisthotonus, decorticate (flexed arms, extended legs), or decerebrate (extended arms and legs) may be apparent.

Acid–base disorders

Respiratory acid–base disturbances
Primary respiratory acidosis occurs when the $PaCO_2$ is above normal, i.e. >6 kPa, and is due to alveolar hypoventilation. Primary respiratory alkalosis occurs when the $PaCO_2$ is <4.5 kPa and is due to alveolar hyperventilation.

Renal compensation in either state is slow. In persistent respiratory acidosis, the most common scenario, renal conservation of bicarbonate occurs, with base excess positive >+2.2.

Metabolic acid–base disturbances
Metabolic acidosis
This may result from excess acid production or reduced buffering capacity due to a low concentration of bicarbonate. The pH is too acid for the level of $PaCO_2$ observed.

The *anion gap* allows these two mechanisms to be distinguished. The anion gap is calculated as the difference between the sum of major cations and anions:

$$(Na^+ + K^+) - (Cl^- + HCO_3^-) = \text{anion gap in mmol/L}$$
$$140 \quad 5 \quad\quad 100 \quad 20$$

It estimates unmeasured anions in plasma and is normally 10–20 mmol/L. The anion gap is increased when acidosis is caused by production of unmeasured acids e.g. lactate, ketoacids, phosphate and sulphate. It is normal when acidosis is caused by excess bicarbonate losses from the GI tract or kidneys or when renal secretion of H^+ ions fails.

Causes of metabolic acidosis include:
- *Excess H^+ production:* tissue hypoxia causing anaerobic metabolism and lactate/pyruvate production as in shock, inborn errors of metabolism, diabetic ketoacidosis
- *Inadequate renal function:* renal failure, renal tubular acidosis, hypoaldosteronism
- *Excessive bicarbonate loss:* diarrhoea, fistulae, ureteric implantation into colon

Metabolic alkalosis
This may result from excessive loss of H^+, excessive reabsorption of bicarbonate or even ingestion of alkalis. It is uncommon in childhood but may be seen in:
- *Pyloric stenosis:* metabolic alkalosis is caused by vomiting stomach (not duodenal) contents and loss of H^+ ions and Cl^- ions
- *Hypokalaemia:* potassium depletion augments renal excretion of hydrogen ions, and causes shift of hydrogen ions into cells. Metabolic alkalosis in turn exacerbates hypokalaemia as urine alkalinization requires potassium excretion.
- *Diuretics:* thiazide and loop diuretics.

Respiratory compensation may occur with hypoventilation.

2.3 Cardiopulmonary arrest

Cardiopulmonary resuscitation (CPR)
Paediatric cardiopulmonary arrests are uncommon and usually secondary to respiratory compromise and hypoxia, as may occur in severe airways obstruction with inhaled foreign object, epiglottitis, asthma, suffocation, drowning, or major trauma. The precise mechanisms in sudden unexpected death in infancy (SUDI) are unknown.

The hypoxic myocardium becomes increasingly bradycardic before progressing to asystole, the most common rhythm found in out-of-hospital arrests.

Primary cardiac arrest is seen in children with underlying cardiac disease. In this case ventricular fibrillation is the most common arrhythmia and early defibrillation is the main determinant of survival.

Resuscitation Council guidelines are provided for:
- *Paediatric Basic Life Support:* actions of a single rescuer with no equipment.
- *Paediatric Advanced Life Support:* management in a hospital setting.

Paediatric basic life support (BLS)
BLS is outlined in the algorithm in Fig 2.2. Start by checking responsiveness. Do not shake if suspected cervical spine injury.

A. Open airway
Hand on forehead to tilt head gently backwards (neutral position in infant, 'sniffing position' in child) and lift chin with fingertips placed under chin. If this does not open airway, or there is suspected neck injury, perform jaw thrust manoeuvre: lift jaw upwards with two fingers under the angle of the mandible bilaterally.

B. Check breathing
- Look for chest movements
- Listen at nose and mouth for breath sounds
- Feel for air movement on your cheek.

If breathing normally, place in recovery position.

Rescue breaths
If not breathing, or making agonal gasps (infrequent, irregular breaths) give five initial rescue breaths.
- *Rescue breaths for an infant:* ensure a neutral head position, take a breath and cover the mouth and nasal apertures with your mouth, blow steadily over 1–1.5 s.
- *Rescue breaths for a child >1 year:* ensure head tilt and chin lift, pinch the nose closed, place lips around mouth and blow steadily over 1–1.5 s.

The chest should be seen to rise. If it does not, the airway is not clear. Readjust the head tilt/chin lift position. If this fails try jaw thrust, and if this fails check for visible obstruction in the mouth.

C. Check for circulation
Check a central pulse for 10 s:
- *In an infant:* feel for brachial or femoral pulse
- *In a child:* feel for carotid pulse.

Start chest compressions if there are **no** signs of circulation (movement, coughing, normal breathing)
or no pulse
or bradycardia (pulse 60/min with poor perfusion)
or you are not sure (it does no harm).

```
UNRESPONSIVE ?
      ↓
Shout for help
      ↓
Open airway
      ↓
NOT BREATHING NORMALLY ?
      ↓
5 rescue breaths
      ↓
STILL UNRESPONSIVE ?
(no signs of a circulation)
      ↓
15 chest compressions
2 rescue breaths
```
After 1 minute call resuscitation team then continue CPR

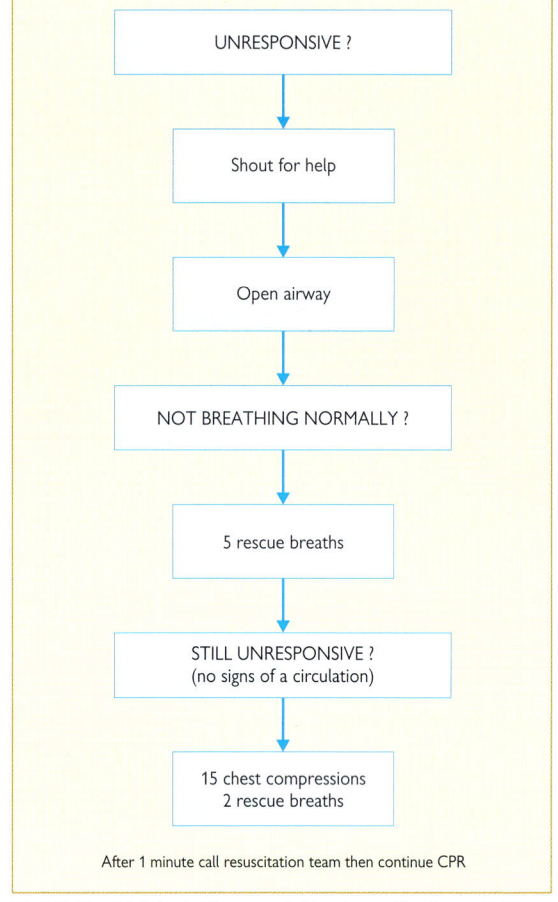

Fig 2.2 Paediatric basic life support. Courtesy of the Resuscitation Council UK.

Chest compression
The child should be flat on their back on a hard surface. Chest compressions should compress the lower third of the sternum, one finger's breadth above the xiphisternum, and should depress the sternum by one third of the depth of the chest.

Compression rate is 100/min and ratio of compressions to breaths is 15:2. Lay rescuers who are assumed to be acting alone are taught a ratio of 30:2.

Technique varies with size and number of rescuers:
- *Infant:* lone rescuer uses two finger tips placed one finger breadth above the xiphisternum. Two or more use hand-encircling approach with both thumbs on lower third of sternum.
- *Child:* place heel of one hand over lower third of sternum, lift fingers, position vertically over chest with arm straight. For larger children (or smaller rescuers) both hands may be used with fingers interlocked.

'Phone first' or 'phone fast'?
- *'Phone fast:'* a lone rescuer should call emergency services after 1 min of CPR.
- *'Phone first':* if there is a sudden, witnessed collapse, rendering ventricular fibrillation a possible cause a lone rescuer should phone first as defibrillation may be necessary.

Paediatric advanced life support

This is the management of cardiopulmonary arrest in a hospital setting (see Fig 2.3 for algorithm) and focuses on the procedures necessary *after* basic life support has been instituted. This may have included intubation and ventilation and gaining intraosseous circulatory access.

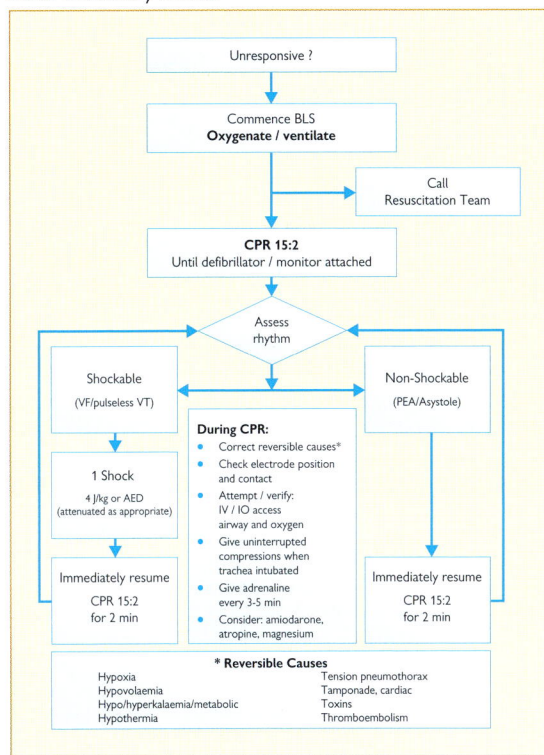

Fig 2.3 Paediatric advanced life support algorithm. Courtesy of the Resuscitation Council UK.

The next step is to assess the rhythm and categorize it as non-shockable or shockable:

- *Non-shockable*:
  - asystole
  - pulseless electrical activity (PEA)
- *Shockable*:
  - ventricular fibrillation
  - pulseless ventricular tachycardia.

Non-shockable rhythms
These predominate and include asystole and PEA. Asystole appears as a 'flatline' on ECG: check the connections and the gain on the ECG monitor. PEA, as the name implies, is the absence of a palpable pulse despite recognizable complexes on ECG. It often precedes asystole and is treated in the same way.

Management of asystole/PEA
Adrenaline 10 micrograms (0.1 mL of 1:10 000 solution) per kg is given intravenously or intraosseously, followed by a normal saline flush 2–5 mL. This stimulates the myocardium and increases aortic diastolic pressure. Continue CPR, pausing every 2 min to assess rhythm and circulation. If no response, repeat adrenaline at 10 micrograms/kg every 4 min. If sinus rhythm and circulation returns, continue post-resuscitation care.

Routine use of sodium bicarbonate is not recommended but should be considered in a patient with prolonged cardiac arrest or cardiac arrest associated with severe metabolic acidosis, hyperkalaemia or tricyclic antidepressant overdose. The dose is 1 mL/kg of 8.4% sodium bicarbonate (1 mmol/kg).

Calcium is only indicated for hypocalcaemia, hyperkalaemia, hypermagnesaemia, or calcium channel blocker overdose.

Shockable rhythms
Ventricular fibrillation and pulseless ventricular tachycardia are uncommon but may occur in cardiac disease, hypothermia or tricyclic antidepressant poisoning. Sudden collapse occurs and rescue depends on defibrillation.

The protocol (see Fig 2.3) is the same for either rhythm:

1 Asynchronous DC shock of 4 J/kg
An automatic external defibrillator (AED) can be used in children over 1 year. Paediatric paddles are required for children <10 kg when using a manual defibrillator. Resume CPR.

2 Second DC shock of 4 J/kg
After 2 min of continued CPR, if monitor still shows VF/VT when compressions paused. Immediately resume CPR for further 2 min. Consider and correct reversible causes (4Hs and 4Ts).

3 Adrenaline 10 micrograms/kg IV or IO
And third DC shock of 4 J/kg
After 2 min of continued CPR if rhythm still VF/VT

4 Amiodarone 5 mg/kg IV
And fourth DC shock of 4 J/kg
After 2 min of continued CPR if rhythm still VF/VT.

Continue giving shocks every 2 min with adrenaline before every other shock. Magnesium is given for hypomagnesaemia or torsades de pointes, seen in long QT syndrome.

Reversible causes
As CPR proceeds, reversible causes should be considered and treated. These are the 4 'H's and 4 'T's (see box)

Reversible causes of cardiopulmonary arrest	
Hypoxia: the usual cause	**T**oxic substances: iatrogenic, accidental, deliberate
Hyper/hypokalaemia: in renal failure, DKA	**T**ension pneumothorax
Hypovolaemia: sepsis, anaphylaxis	**T**amponade
Hypothermia: drowning	**T**hromboembolism: rare

When to stop resuscitation
Successful outcome from resuscitation is not common. Resuscitation attempts may be discontinued if there is no return of spontaneous circulation after 30 min of cumulative life support. Exceptions are recurring or refractory VF/VT, a primary hypothermic insult, or patients with a history of poisoning. The team leader, not the parents (if present) decides when to stop.

Recovery position
The important principles are:
- Place child in lateral position with mouth dependent to allow free drainage of fluid such as saliva or vomitus
- Position should be stable: support back with pillow
- No pressure on chest that impairs breathing
- Airway accessible and easily observed.

2.4 Accidental injuries: trauma and burns

An accident is an 'unforeseen event', but although individually unforeseen, many childhood accidents can be both predicted and prevented. The main varieties of accidental injuries include:
- *Trauma:* falls, transport accidents
- *Burns and scalds:* exposure to smoke, fire, hot liquids
- Drowning, choking, suffocation
- Poisoning.

Inflicted (non-accidental) injury is often an important differential diagnosis and is discussed in Chapter 18.

Childhood accidents
Epidemiology and aetiology
The type and location of childhood accidents relate closely to age and development stage. Babies and toddlers have most accidents at home as this is where they spend their time. Pre-mobile infants may be dropped or fall from elevated surfaces if left unattended. This is a risk from birth as uncoordinated limb movements may be sufficient to cause a fall. Rolling is not a prerequisite. By school age more accidents are occurring on the roads, at play, and at school.

Boys are twice as likely as girls to have accidents. Boys may be more exposed to risks as they may be more active and adventurous and more subject to peer pressure.

Children in lower socio-economic classes are estimated to be up to four times more likely to die in accidents than other children.

Accident statistics
Accidental injury is the leading cause of death in children over the age of one year in the developed world. In the UK in 2005, 251 children aged <5 died as the result of injury or poisoning.

The number of children attending hospital emergency departments after accidental injury is almost 1 million/year. The breakdown by type of accident is:
- *Falls at home:* 390 000
- *Sporting injuries:* 180 000
- *Poisoning:* 52 000
- *Burns and scalds:* 37 000
- *Playground injuries:* 33 000
- *Road and traffic accidents:* 29 000.

Trauma
Most minor trauma care lies outside the direct responsibility of the paediatrician. This section deals with the management of pain and the basic management of major multiple trauma.

Pain
The recognition and assessment of acute pain in infants and children must be adapted to the age and development stage of the child. Infants, including preterm infants, demonstrate measurable behavioural and physiological responses to pain.

Changes in a child's behaviour such as silent withdrawal, fighting behaviour, appearance, activity level, and vital signs (heart rate, respiratory rate) may indicate the presence of pain. Behavioural tools allow pain assessment in young children, including assessment of facial expression, leg posture, activity, and cry. Self-reporting tools in common use include the Wong and Baker 'faces' pain scale used for children >3, and the visual analogue 'pain-ladder' scale for children >7:

0	2	4	6	8	10
No hurt	Hurts little bit	Hurts little more	Hurts even more	Hurts whole lot	Hurts worse

Analgesia should be given orally if possible, given regularly, and titrated to pain severity.
- *Mild:* paracetamol, with or without NSAID
- *Moderate:* add dihydrocodeine
- *Severe:* add opiate or Entonox.

The seriously injured child
A structured approach to clinical evaluation and management is based on primary, secondary and tertiary surveys.

Primary survey
This is directed towards identification of life-threatening injuries and implementation of resuscitation according to the **ABCDE** paradigm (see Section 2.2).

Life-threatening injuries which should be identified and treated in the primary survey include:
- *Respiratory system:* airway obstruction, tension pneumothorax, open pneumothorax, haemothorax, flail chest
- *Cardiovascular system:* cardiac tamponade
- *CNS:* extradural haematoma.

Resuscitation measures include:
- Airway opening manoeuvres and high flow oxygen
- Control of external haemorrhage
- Intravenous access and volume resuscitation
- Nasogastric tube and urinary catheter placement
- Monitoring ECG, blood volume, oxygen saturations
- *Investigations:* baseline bloods and crossmatch specimens. Imaging: chest XR, lateral C-spine, pelvis.

Secondary survey
A detailed physical examination to identify all injuries. 'Log-rolling' manoeuvre required to enable survey of the neck, spine, back, and rectum. Any additional investigations (blood tests, imaging, special investigations) are then requested.

Tertiary survey
All injuries are reviewed and definitive treatment instigated. Investigation results are reviewed and emerging trends identified.

Burns and scalds
About 40 000 children <15 years are injured in burn or scald accidents in the UK each year, the majority (75%) being <5 years. Of these about 1/7 are admitted and 500 have severe burns. 95% of thermal injuries happen at home and half of all severe injuries in the kitchen.

Aetiology
Accidental thermal injuries are most commonly scalds caused by hot drinks, hot tap water, hot oil or fat, and steam or water from kettles. Burns occur after contact with open fires, cookers, irons, fireworks, candles, etc. Young children are vulnerable to sunburn. Most burns are preventable.

Non-accidental burn injuries also occur, although the true incidence is uncertain. Features suggesting a non-accidental injury are discussed in Chapter 18.

Pathogenesis

Most thermal injuries affect the skin and are defined by the total burn surface areas (TBSA) involved, their anatomical location and their thickness. The thickness is a major determinant of healing and is classified into:

Partial thickness

- *Superficial:* affects epidermis only. Erythematous, painful, heals rapidly.
- *Superficial dermal:* affects epidermis and upper dermis. Blistering and intense pain.
- *Deep dermal:* affects epidermis and deep dermis. Mottled, cherry red colour, dry, non-blanching. Painless.

Full thickness

Involves all of epidermis and dermis, and may involve muscle and bone. Pearly white, dry skin with no hair, no sensation and no capillary return. Regenerative elements are destroyed but spontaneous healing can occur in healthy skin at the burn margin with considerable scarring. Excision and grafting is required for all but smallest injuries.

Clinical evaluation

Assess TBSA and depth. For TBSA, remember the 'rule of nines' does not apply to children <14 years because they have a relatively larger head surface area and smaller surface area of the extremities. Lund and Browder charts are used (Fig 2.4).

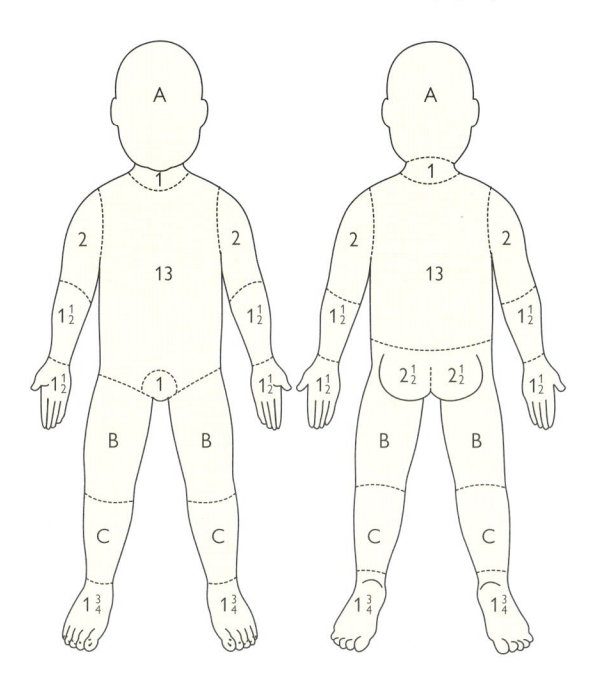

	Surface area at			
Area indicated	1 year	5 years	10 years	15 years
A	8.5	6.5	5.5	4.5
B	3.25	4.0	4.5	4.5
C	2.5	2.75	3.0	3.25

Fig 2.4 Lund and Browder chart. Adapted Land Browder chart reproduced from Illustrated Paediatrics; Lissauer and Clayden, with permission from Elsevier (© 2001).

Attention should also be directed towards:

- *Anatomic location:* involvement of face and upper airway may compromise the upper airway due to laryngeal oedema with stridor, hoarseness and dyspnoea.
- Circumferential full thickness chest or limb burns may impair ventilation and perfusion respectively. Escharotomy (an eschar is a deep, cutaneous slough or scab caused by a thermal burn) should be considered to lessen the pull on surrounding tissues.
- Coexistent smoke or carbon monoxide inhalation
- Life-threatening or spinal injuries
- Occult blood loss causing circulatory compromise.

Management

Initial management of all burns includes:

- Remove heat source and apply active cooling for 20 min
- *Analgesia:* opiates may be necessary
- *Dressing:* clingfilm is sterile and non-adherent
- Elevate limbs to reduce oedema
- Check tetanus status

Major burns require application of the **ABCDE** paradigm with the addition of **F** for fluid.

Fluid resuscitation

IV fluid replacement is required for burns involving TBSA > ≥10%, or 5% in infants <6 months. The Parkland formula is used to calculate the volume of Hartmann's fluid to be given over 24 h:

$$\text{Volume (mL)} = 4 \times \% \text{ TBSA} \times \text{weight (kg)}$$

Give 50% in the first 8 h and 50% in next 16 h from time of injury.

Maintenance fluid is given in addition as 0.45% NaCl/5% dextrose. The rate should be titrated to maintain urine output at 1.0–1.5 mL/kg per hour although some centres accept 0.5 mL/kg per hour if electrolytes are normal.

Assessment of adequacy of fluid resuscitation can be difficult. Poor capillary refill time, a core–peripheral temperature gap, and metabolic acidosis are indicators of circulatory compromise. Excessive fluids may cause pulmonary oedema and hyponatraemia with cerebral oedema and seizures.

Transfer to a specialist burns facility should be considered in children <5 years, full thickness burns >5% or if there are complications such as circumferential burns or inhalation injury.

Complications

Sepsis

The most important cause of morbidity. Diagnosis can be difficult as fever is not a specific predictor of infection in burned children. Although children with sepsis usually have a fever >38 °C, 73% of those without infection also have a fever due to the inflammatory response to the burn. The most useful indicators of sepsis are intolerance of enteral feeding and a rise in CRP.

Toxic shock syndrome (TSS)

This can complicate even small, 'clean' burns. It is caused by toxic shock toxin-1 (TSST-1) from strains of *Staphylococcus*. A sudden deterioration occurs with fever (>39 °C), diarrhoea, vomiting, and rash accompanied by circulatory failure. Treatment includes antibiotics and anti-TSST1 antibodies (human immunoglobulin or fresh frozen plasma). Mortality is up to 50%.

2.5 Head injury and drowning

Head injury

Up to 500 000 children attend emergency departments with head injury each year in the UK. A fatal outcome is fortunately rare, about 1/500, but head injuries account for 40% of injury-related deaths in childhood.

Aetiology and pathogenesis

The causes of head injuries vary markedly with age:

- <2 years: inflicted, non-accidental injury is the most common cause, accounting for up to 25%. In addition, babies may be accidentally dropped or fall from elevated surfaces such as changing tables.
- 1–4 years: falls
- 5–15 years: road traffic accidents. Pedestrians most commonly, followed by cyclists and car passengers
- >15 years: sports injuries, assaults.

There is a peak incidence in summer, in children <10 years, and in late afternoon and early evening.

Dynamics of falls

Factors that determine injury severity include:

- *Distance fallen and impact surface:* most domestic falls are short (<1.5 m), and very rarely cause death or serious injury. However, a fall of 1 m may be sufficient to cause skull fracture and falls >1.5 m can cause serious injury. The impact surface is critical. A soft surface provides slower deceleration and absorbs more kinetic energy, reducing the peak forces acting on the head.
- *Whether the fall was 'broken':* protective reflexes may break the fall, but do not operate in babies or in backwards falls.
- *Impact area: focal or diffuse:* the fall may be on to a point or edge, or more commonly on to a flat, blunt surface.
- *Impact part:* the disproportionate large head size in infants and young children makes them fall 'head first'.

Intracranial pathology

Intracranial pathology or traumatic brain injury (TBI) is classified as primary or secondary and focal or diffuse.

Primary pathology: direct result of trauma

- Focal:
  - cerebral contusions and lacerations which may occur under or opposite (contre-coup) the site of impact.
  - intracranial bleeding which may be extradural (very uncommon), subdural, or intracerebral.
- *Diffuse:* shearing forces cause immediate axonal damage.

Secondary pathology: indirect consequence of primary insult

- *Focal:* ischemia due to intracerebral haematoma
- *Diffuse:* brain ischaemia due to hypoxia or impaired cerebral perfusion due to raised ICP secondary to brain oedema, hypercapnia, and impaired 'autoregulation' or hypotension.

Infection may occur with a compound depressed fracture or basal skull fracture causing meningitis or brain abscess.

Clinical evaluation

History and examination aims to identify the minority of patients at high risk of significant intracranial pathology. Risk features indicating a need for cranial CT include:

History

- Mechanism consistent with severe injury: high-speed RTA as pedestrian, cyclist, or car occupant; fall from >3 m; injury from high-speed projectile or object.
- Witnessed loss of consciousness lasting >5 min
- Amnesia, antegrade or retrograde, lasting >5 min
- Abnormal drowsiness
- Three or more discrete episodes of vomiting
- Post-traumatic seizure but no history of epilepsy
- Clinical suspicion of inflicted, non-accidental injury.

Examination

- Age >1 year: GCS <14 in emergency department
- Age <1 year: GCS < 15 in emergency department or tense fontanelle; bruise, swelling or laceration >5 cm on head
- Suspicion of open or depressed skull injury
- *Signs of basal skull fracture:* these include blood or CSF from ear or nose, bilateral periorbital haematomas (panda eyes), Battle's sign (bruising over mastoid, may take 24 h to develop), haemotympanum
- *Focal neurological deficit:* additional features may include history of drug or alcohol intoxication, history of neurosurgery, presence of a bleeding diathesis such as haemophilia or anticoagulant medication.

Management

A child who has had a minor head injury and has none of the risk factors listed above, is fully conscious and has no adverse medical or social factors, does not require hospital admission. A clear written advice sheet should be provided with criteria for seeking medical advice again.

The child with a severe head injury and GCS ≤8 requires intubation and ventilation with full cervical spine immobilization (cervical spine injury is present in 10% of patients with severe head injury). Cranial CT with scanning of the cervical spine down to C2 should be done within 1 h.

Children with the risk factors listed above should undergo cranial CT combined with a period of observation. Skull radiographs are not generally indicated. Although the presence of a skull fracture increases the likelihood of intracranial pathology fourfold, significant intracranial pathology can exist in the absence of a fracture, especially in injuries inflicted by shaking. If non-accidental injury is diagnosed, early cranial MRI is indicated to assist in clarifying the timing and mechanism of any injury (see Chapter 18).

Consultation with a neurosurgical unit is indicated for:

- Intracranial pathology on cranial CT
- A compound depressed or basal skull fracture
- Coma persisting for >4 h or deteriorating level of consciousness
- Progressive focal neurological signs.

Prevention by individual, local, and national policy is of course most important. Children with significant head injury should be followed up by a specialist multidisciplinary team and both the school medical service and primary health care team should be notified.

Drowning

Drowning describes the process of primary respiratory impairment from immersion in a liquid medium. The final outcome, whether alive or dead, is not part of the definition so the distinction between near-drowning with survival and drowning with a fatal outcome is no longer made.

Accidental drowning is the third most common cause of accidental death in childhood in the UK, after road traffic accidents and burns. In 2005, 26 children <15 years were drowned in the UK.

Epidemiology

Drowning is more common in children aged 4 years or less (60%) and in boys (male:female ratio 4:1). One third of drownings occur in the summer. The location is age dependent:

- *<1 year:* bathtubs and buckets
- *1–4 years:* home settings: garden ponds, pools
- *5–14 years:* open water sites: lakes, rivers and seas.

Many drownings are preventable by active adult supervision, safe water environments such as isolation fencing and use of personal flotation devices (PFDs). There is no conclusive evidence that drowning rates are higher for less experienced swimmers. 80% of childhood drowning accidents occur in unsupervised children.

Pathophysiology

Drowning can happen in as little as 2.5 cm (1 inch) of water and is usually quick and silent. Most children who survive are discovered within 2 min of submersion and most who die are found after 10 min. Submersion of >3 min confers a poor outcome.

The sequence of events following submersion is:

- *Voluntary breath holding and reflex bradycardia:* the diving reflex
- Hypoxia, hypercarbia, and acidosis stimulates compensatory mechanisms with tachycardia and hypertension
- After at most 2–5 min involuntary breathing occurs and inhaled fluid causes laryngeal spasm on touching the glottis which initially protects the lower airway.
- Secondary apnoea gives way to further respiratory efforts with inhalation of water and debris into lower airways.
- Bradycardia, arrhythmia, and cardiac arrest occur.

If this sequence of events can be interrupted and the child survives, additional complications include:

- *Respiratory:* surfactant depletion, pulmonary oedema, pneumonia
- *CVS:* arrhythmias, pulmonary hypertension
- *Metabolic:* hyponatraemia, hypernatraemia
- *Hypothermia:* is common and classified according to deep body temperature (rectal or oesophageal) into mild (>34 °C), moderate (30–34 °C) and severe (<30 °C)
- Spinal injury (diving injury)
- Multiorgan failure from hypoxia/ischaemia.

Management

Primary survey and resuscitation

Airway and breathing

Tracheal intubation and gastric decompression must be performed early to avoid aspiration of stomach contents. The stomach is usually full of water and debris.

In diving accidents, the cervical spine needs to be immobilized until injury is excluded.

Circulation

Cardiac arrest may be due to asystole, PEA, ventricular tachycardia, or ventricular fibrillation (VF). Arrhythmias such as VF are not only more common in hypothermia, but also refractory at temperatures <30 °C.

Exposure: hypothermia

Drowning in icy water can provide some protection against the effects of hypoxia on the heart and brain.

External re-warming is sufficient for temperatures >32 °C, but below this active core re-warming should also be used. Anticipate the need for volume replacement to counter the 'rewarming shock' which occurs to peripheral vasodilatation.

External re-warming

- Remove cold, wet clothing
- Apply warm blankets
- Infrared radiant lamp
- Forced air re-warming blanket, e.g. Bair Hugger.

Core re-warming

- Warm intravenous fluids to 39 °C
- Warm ventilator gases to 42 °C
- Gastric or bladder lavage with 0.9% saline at 42 °C
- Lavage of peritoneum, pleura or pericardium and extracorporeal blood warming are extreme measures.

Resuscitation should be continued until core temperature is ≥32 °C or cannot be raised despite active measures. Careful monitoring of cardiovascular function is vital.

Secondary survey

This should include a careful survey for injuries that may have occurred preceding submersion, especially spinal injuries. Investigations to consider include:

- Blood glucose, gases, electrolytes
- Coagulation screen
- CXR, cervical spine imaging
- Blood and sputum cultures.

Fever >24 h post drowning suggests systemic infection, e.g. with gram-negative organisms such as *Pseudomonas* spp., and broad-spectrum antibiotics should be given.

Prognosis

A poor prognosis is conferred by submersion for more than 3–8 min, no gasp after 40 min of full CPR, rectal temperature >33°C on arrival, persisting coma, acidosis (pH <7.0) or hypoxia (PaO_2 <8.0 kPa).

70% of children survive when early basic life support is provided at the waterside. Of those who survive 25% have mild neurological sequelae and 5% are severely disabled. 75% make a full recovery.

2.6 Poisoning

About 52 000 children attend hospitals with suspected poisoning in the UK each year.

Types of poisoning
Poisoning may be:
- *Accidental:* common in toddlers, mean age 2.5 years
- *Intentional:*
  - deliberate self-harm is most common in adolescents
  - fabricated or induced illness (FII) may involve administration of poisons
  - drug misuse involving alcohol, solvents or opiates occurs in adolescents
- *Iatrogenic:* poisoning usually involves dosage errors rather than wrong drug or route.

The poisonous substances include drugs, household chemicals, alcohol, cosmetics, plants, berries, and mushrooms.

Pathophysiology
Most poisons are ingested and exert their ill effects following enteral absorption, but some caustic agents cause local damage and inhalation of volatile agents can cause direct damage to the respiratory system.

Specific effects reflect the toxic actions of specific poisons and are considered below. However, many poisons act via important final common pathways such as CNS depression and recognizable poison syndromes do exist.

Important systemic effects in poisoning include:
- *Central nervous system (CNS):* a reduced level of consciousness is the most common problem and impairs respiration by causing airway obstruction and central depression of respiratory drive. Convulsions may also occur.
- *Cardiovascular system (CVS):* hypotension is common in poisoning with CNS depressants. Hypertension, usually transient, is less frequent but occurs with sympathomimetic drugs. Cardiac conduction defects and arrhythmias may occur especially in poisoning with tricyclic antidepressants.
- *Body temperature:* hypothermia may develop in prolonged coma, especially after overdose with barbiturates or phenothiazines. Hyperthermia can develop in children taking CNS stimulants or antimuscarinic drugs.

Recognizable poison syndromes include those resulting from altered autonomic nervous system activity (sympathomimetics, parasympathomimetics, anticholinergics), metabolic acidosis, chemical pneumonia, acute cerebellar dysfunction, methaemoglobinaemia, renal failure, and violent emesis.

Clinical evaluation
The constituents of the substance ingested, the timing and the dosage per kg body weight should be identified as accurately as possible. Some idea of the maximum possible amount can be estimated from comparing the number of tablets or volume of liquid remaining with the total described on packaging. Ingestion may have been unobserved and in older children may not be disclosed.

In the UK, the National Poisons Information Service maintains an online database, TOXBASE and telephone advice which is freely available to NHS hospitals (www.toxbase.org)

Examination
Primary assessment should follow the **ABCDE** paradigm (see Section 2.2).

Further examination is directed towards recognition of poisoning syndromes with particular attention to autonomic function including pupillary constriction or dilatation.

Management
Management encompasses primary assessment and resuscitation, initial investigations, measures to prevent absorption or enhance excretion, and specific measures if available.

Resuscitation
Attention to obstructed airway with airway opening measures and insertion of oropharyngeal or nasopharyngeal airway, administer high-flow oxygen and use bag–valve–mask device for assisted ventilation. Intubation and ventilation should be considered if GCS ≤8, airway protection inadequate, or respiration depressed. Treat hypotension by tilting head down and volume replacement with normal saline.

Baseline investigations and monitoring
- *Blood glucose:* hypoglycaemia in alcohol poisoning
- *U&E:* hypokalaemia with β-agonists
- *Hyperkalaemia:* digoxin
- *Blood gases:* metabolic acidosis in carbon monoxide poisoning, salicylates
- *LFTs, coagulation:* hepatotoxicity with paracetamol
- *Drug levels:* paracetamol, salicylates, iron, digoxin
- *Urine:* toxicology screen.

Monitoring in addition to standard nursing observations and neuro observations should include ECG and pulse oximetry.

Preventing absorption
Induction of emesis is not recommended. Gastric lavage is rarely required but may be considered for life-threatening amounts of certain drugs including iron and lithium ingested within the previous hour. It is contraindicated if a corrosive substance or petroleum product has been ingested.

Activated charcoal may be useful in prevention of absorption of poisons toxic in small amounts, e.g. antidepressants. It may be effective up to 1 h after ingestion. Repeated doses may be used as an active elimination technique.

Enhancing excretion: active elimination
This is rarely performed, but may be useful in cases of prolonged, high concentration exposure to dangerous toxins. Methods include:
- Repeated doses of activated charcoal for quinine, theophylline, carbamazepine, phenobarbital
- Whole bowel irrigation for enteric-coated drugs, iron
- Urine alkalinization for salicylates.

Specific poisons

Antidotes are available for certain poisons: see Table 2.2. Management of specific poisons is considered in turn.

Table 2.2. Specific poisons and their antidotes

Toxin	Antidote
Iron	Desferrioxamine
Opiates	Naloxone
Paracetamol	N-acetylcysteine
Digoxin	Digoxin antibodies
Carbon monoxide	Oxygen

Alcohol

Alcohol intoxication occurs in toddlers and adolescents. The main risks are respiratory depression, vomiting with aspiration, and hypoglycaemia. It is potentially fatal.

Paracetamol

Most cases of paracetamol poisoning occur as episodes of self-harm in adolescents. As little as 150 mg/kg of paracetamol taken within a 24 h period may cause severe hepatocellular necrosis. If it is certain that the dose ingested is <150 mg/kg, no further action is required. Children seem less sensitive to the hepatotoxic effects.

Initial symptoms of nausea and vomiting settle within 24 h. Persistence beyond 24 h associated with right subcostal pain and tenderness indicates development of hepatic necrosis which is maximal 3–4 days after ingestion.

Administration of activated charcoal should be considered if a toxic dose has been ingested within the previous hour.

Children at risk and requiring treatment are identified by a single measurement of the plasma paracetamol concentration taken not less than 4 h after ingestion. Patients whose concentration is above the *'normal treatment line'* are treated with acetylcysteine by intravenous infusion (Parvolex), or if acetylcysteine cannot be used, with oral methionine provided it is within 12 h of ingestion.

A lower treatment threshold, 50% of the standard concentration threshold (*'high-risk treatment line'*) is used for high risk groups which include malnourished children and those on enzyme-inducing drugs (e.g. carbamazepine, phenobarbital). Patients who have taken a staggered overdose should be treated regardless of initial paracetamol concentration.

All patients require baseline measurements of electrolytes, creatinine (renal necrosis can occur), liver enzymes, and INR.

Normal results at 48 h exclude hepatic damage. ALT levels >1000 IU/L indicate significant injury and serial measurements of INR provide an important guide to residual liver function.

Opioids and compound analgesics, antimotility drugs

Opioids cause coma, respiratory depression, and pinpoint pupils. The specific antidote naloxone is indicated if there is coma or depressed respiration. Its effects are immediate but short-lived (2 h) and an IV infusion may be optimal. Opioids such as methadone have a very long duration of action. Opioids are also encountered in antimotility drugs: Co-phenotrope (as Lomotil) is the most common and dangerous. The delayed gastric emptying may delay symptoms of severe opioid poisoning for up to 36 h.

Co-proxamol, a combination of dextropropoxyphene and paracetamol, is dangerous as the former has direct cardiotoxic effects and arrhythmias may occur for up to 12 h.

Aspirin

Salicylate poisoning is now uncommon. Symptoms include tinnitus, deafness, dizziness, pyrexia, nausea, vomiting, and metabolic acidosis. Asymptomatic children who have consumed <120 mg/kg of aspirin do not require treatment. Treatment options depending on severity include activated charcoal, urinary alkalinization, and haemodialysis.

NSAIDs

This group includes ibuprofen, mefenamic acid, and diclofenac. Toxicity is generally low. Ibuprofen may cause vomiting, epigastric pain, and tinnitus. Activated charcoal is indicated for ≥ 400 mg/kg taken within the preceding hour.

Antidepressants: tricyclic compounds, monoamine oxidase inhibitors, and selective serotonin re-uptake inhibitors (SSRIs)

Tricyclic compounds cause anticholinergic effects, ataxia, coma and convulsions, hypotension, cardiac conduction defects, and arrhythmias. Activated charcoal should be given and an ECG performed. A prolonged QRS (>0.1 s) is the best indicator of risk for cardiac toxicity. Intravenous infusion of sodium bicarbonate can treat compromising arrhythmias or prevent them in those with a long QRS duration. The use of antiarrhythmic drugs is best avoided.

SSRI poisoning can cause vomiting, agitation, tremor, and rarely convulsions. Severe poisoning results in the 'serotonin syndrome': hyperpyrexia, convulsions, rhabdomyolysis.

Iron

Early features of iron poisoning are gastrointestinal and include nausea, vomiting, abdominal pain, and gastrointestinal haemorrhage. Signs of multiorgan failure, with fulminant hepatic failure, develop 12–48 h after ingestion.

Asymptomatic children with a definite history of consuming <30 mg/kg of elemental iron require no further treatment. If >30 mg/kg may have been ingested an abdominal radiograph is done. If tablets are confined to the stomach repeated gastric lavage or endoscopic removal are options. If large quantities are visible, whole bowel irrigation should be undertaken. Serum iron concentrations are measured 4 h post ingestion (8 h for sustained release preparations). Further treatment depends on levels: if ≥90 micromole/L, intravenous desferrioxamine is given.

Treatment is continued until symptoms have abated and urine discoloration clears. In multiorgan failure higher dose may be required and haemodialysis may be indicated.

Stimulants: ecstasy

Ecstasy (methylenedioxymethamphetamine, MDMA) can cause severe idiosyncratic reactions including coma, convulsions, arrhythmias, hyperthermia, and rhabdomyolysis. Asymptomatic children should receive activated charcoal. Blood levels can confirm exposure.

Bleach

Household solutions are 10% sodium hypochlorite. Ingestion of >100 mL can cause nausea, vomiting, and diarrhoea. Give milk and fluids. Industrial bleaches, 50% sodium hypochlorite, or large volumes can cause oesophageal damage. Endoscopy and gastric aspiration should be considered.

2.7 Respiratory emergencies

Respiratory emergencies include upper airway obstruction and respiratory failure caused by airway obstruction, intrinsic lung disease, or inadequate respiratory effort. So-called 'apparent life threatening events' (ALTEs) are considered here as disturbed respiration appears to be a common final pathway, although there are many causes.

'Apparent life threatening events'

An ALTE is defined as an episode that is frightening to an observer and characterized by some combination of:
- Apnoea, central or occasionally obstructive
- Change in muscle tone, usually limpness.
- Choking or gagging, observed or heard.

Despite the alarming term, few episodes fulfilling this definition actually require cardiopulmonary resuscitation. The incidence is 0.6/1000 live births and ALTEs account for almost 1% of emergency visits for infants. The peak age incidence is between 1 week and 2 months and two thirds are <10 weeks.

Aetiology

This cluster of symptoms and signs has many causes, but no cause is identified in about half of cases. The three most common identified causes are:
- *Gastro-oesophageal reflux disease, GORD*: 30%
- *Seizures from hypoglycaemia, hypocalcaemia*: 11%
- *Lower respiratory tract infection*: 8% (This includes pertussis, bronchiolitis and pneumonia.)

A number of less common causes exist which should be considered especially if ALTEs are recurrent, severe or in an older infant. These include:
- ENT or airway problems
- Urinary tract infection
- Inborn errors of metabolism
- Cardiac arrhythmia
- Breath-holding attacks
- Fabricated or induced illness (FII).

FII should be considered especially in recurrent ALTEs and may be a feature of fabrication, repeated smothering, or deliberate poisoning.

Clinical evaluation

The history should establish the exact description of the episode and its relationship to feeding. Physical examination is often normal but careful examination for respiratory infection is appropriate. SaO_2 should be measured and fundoscopy considered to identify non-accidental head injury.

Management

A single, short, self-correcting episode associated with feeding in a well infant with no abnormal physical findings requires no action other than addressing parental anxiety and arranging follow-up and health visitor input.

A more significant episode or recurrent episodes warrants admission and cardiorespiratory monitoring for 24 h. Investigations are dependent on whether a likely cause is identified clinically but may include:
- Full blood count, C-reactive protein
- *Biochemistry*: urea and electrolytes, calcium, magnesium, glucose, lactate
- *Microbiology*: urine microscopy and culture; per-nasal swab for pertussis
- CXR
- ECG rhythm strip including QTc interval
- EEG, USS brain
- Blood and urine for toxicology and metabolic studies
- Investigation for GORD.

It is important to empathize with the high level of parental anxiety and provide adequate support. Resuscitation training may be considered but home apnoea monitoring is not of proven value. Any association of ALTEs with SUDI is very weak if indeed it exists at all.

Upper airway obstruction

Obstruction to the upper airway is always potentially life threatening. Each year in the UK about 70 children die from suffocation, strangling, or choking (foreign body airway obstruction). A proportion of these episodes are inflicted (non-accidental) and most deaths are out of hospital. See Chapter 3.4 for a discussion of acute stridor.

Aetiology

Important causes of upper airways obstruction (apart from suffocation and strangulation) include:
- *Foreign body airway obstruction (FBAO)*: 'choking'
- *Infections*:
  - croup
  - acute epiglottitis
  - bacterial tracheitis
  - retropharyngeal abscess
  - diphtheria (rare in the UK)
  - peritonsillar abscess (quinsy)
- Angio-oedema
- Smoke inhalation.

In addition, patients with chronic upper airway obstruction may decompensate acutely, particularly with superadded infection. This may occur with subglottic stenosis, vascular rings, tracheomalacia, Pierre–Robin syndrome, and laryngeal webs.

Clinical evaluation

History

The length of history provides a guide to aetiology.

Inhaled foreign bodies cause acute symptoms with choking. Angio-oedema develops over minutes and acute epiglottitis over a few hours.

Croup and retropharyngeal abscess have a prodromal history lasting several days although progression may occur over several hours.

Examination

Specific signs occur in some disorders. A 'barking cough' and hoarse voice reflects the laryngeal inflammation present in croup. Drooling and dysphagia are caused by the painful swelling of epiglottitis or retropharyngeal abscess. Systemic toxicity occurs in bacterial infection: epiglottitis, bacterial tracheitis, retropharyngeal abscess.

Severity of obstruction is evident clinically. Marked stridor, tracheal tug, and prolonged inspiratory phase all indicate severe obstruction. Hypoxia is a late sign.

Management
This depends on cause but is always a matter of urgency. Active treatment is indicated. Investigations are not indicated initially.

Foreign body airway obstruction (FBAO)
Most choking episodes occur in preschool children during play or while eating. If the diagnosis is clear cut the strategy depends on whether an effective cough is present, conscious state, and age of the child (see Fig 2.5).

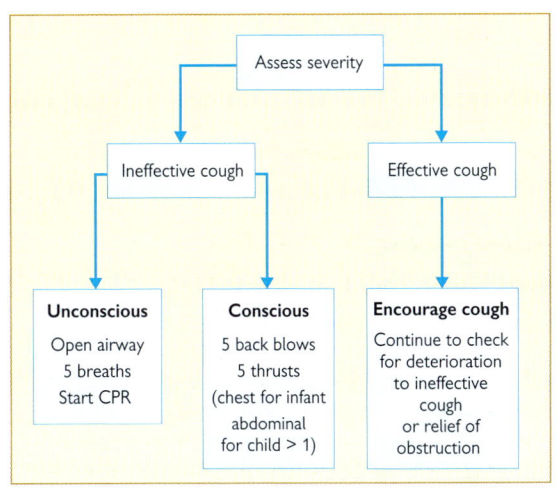

Fig 2.5 Resuscitation Council UK 2005 guideline for relief of foreign body airway obstruction (FBAO). Courtesy of the Resuscitation Council UK.

```
                    Assess severity
                    /            \
            Ineffective cough    Effective cough
            /          \              |
      Unconscious    Conscious    Encourage cough
      Open airway   5 back blows  Continue to check
      5 breaths     5 thrusts     for deterioration
      Start CPR     (chest for    to ineffective
                    infant        cough
                    abdominal     or relief of
                    for child > 1) obstruction
```

If the child is coughing effectively, this should be encouraged: a spontaneous cough is more likely to be effective than any external manoeuvre.

If coughing is ineffective, and the child unable to vocalize, or has a silent cough or cyanosis and the child is conscious five back blows should be given, followed if necessary by five chest thrusts in an infant or abdominal thrusts in a child. In an unconscious child, proceed with basic life support after opening the mouth to look for any obvious removable object.

Croup
See Chapter 3 for details. Principles include:
- Keep child upright and comfortable; minimize upsetting procedures
- Oxygen to keep SaO_2 >93%
- Steroids in all but mildest cases. Options include:
  - oral dexamethasone 0.15 mg/kg to maximum 12 mg
  - oral prednisolone 1 mg/kg
  - nebulized budesonide 2 mg
- Nebulized adrenaline for significant respiratory distress. Use 1 in 1 000 (1 mg/mL) solution in a dose of 400 micrograms/kg (to maximum 5 mg) repeated after 30 min if necessary.

Symptomatic relief may begin within 10 min and lasts up to 1 h. Intubation and ITU admission is required in <2% of hospital admissions.

Epiglottitis
Suspected epiglottitis is an indication for urgent examination under anaesthetic (EUA) with full anaesthetic and ENT senior support.

Respiratory failure
Respiratory *failure* is not the same as respiratory *distress*.
- *Respiratory distress* describes an increase in the work of breathing as manifested by tachypnoea, nasal flaring, recession, use of accessory muscles, grunting, and if airway obstruction is present stridor (upper airway) or wheeze (lower airway). In respiratory compensation for metabolic acidosis there is tachypnoea but no other signs of respiratory distress and this is an important differential.
- *Respiratory failure* describes inadequate oxygenation and or ventilation. Although often accompanied by respiratory distress this may be absent if there is respiratory depression due to coma or exhaustion.

Clinical signs of hypoxia include cyanosis, tachycardia, circulatory failure and ultimately bradycardia followed by asystole. A raised arterial PCO_2 generates no easily detectable clinical signs but lack of adequate chest movements or obvious exhaustion provides a clue to inadequate ventilation. In children, a mixture of hypoxaemia and hypercapnia usually coexists and is confirmed on blood gas analysis.

Aetiology
The most common context in which respiratory failure occurs in infants and children is primary respiratory disease:
- Acute asthma (severe)
- Bronchiolitis
- Pneumonia
- Croup (severe).

Respiratory depression is less common but may be seen e.g. in poisoning by opiates or Guillain–Barré syndrome.

Investigations
A CXR is indicated and a measurement of blood gases: arterial, capillary, or venous.

Management
In addition to specific measures supportive treatment involves:
- *Oxygen:* supplemental oxygen is prescribed to provide a FiO_2 in the range of up to 100%. Oxygen toxicity is not a risk in infants and children. Delivery systems vary with age and include:
  - nasal cannulae
  - face mask
  - head box.
- Continuous positive airways pressure (CPAP)
- Assisted ventilation.

Endotracheal intubation and intermittent positive pressure ventilation should be instituted if progressive respiratory failure is diagnosed.

2.8 Septicaemia and septic shock

Invasive bacteraemia triggers a series of inflammatory and immune mediated metabolic and circulatory changes, the clinical manifestations of which are called sepsis or septicaemia. Septic shock is the end point in which tissue perfusion is compromised.

The incidence has been reduced by the introduction of vaccination against causative pathogens: *Haemophilus influenza* (Hib), *Neisseria meningitidis* (Men C), and *Streptococcus pneumoniae*.

Aetiology and pathogenesis

The main pathogens causing septic shock are:
- *Gram-negative bacteria*: E. coli, Pseudomonas, Meningococcus
- *Gram-positive bacteria*: Pneumococcus, Haemophilus influenzae, Staphylococcus aureus.

Meningococcal septicaemia remains the most common infectious cause of death in childhood in developed countries (see Chapter 15.14).

Pathogenesis

There are several overlapping phases:

Invasion of the blood stream
The mechanisms by which organisms which reside in the nasopharynx in a harmless fashion invade the circulation remain uncertain but are assumed to reflect both factors in the pathogen and host susceptibility.

Septicaemia
Transient bacteraemia which is rapidly cleared is not uncommon in febrile children. Continued replication and septicaemia occurs in a minority and may reflect factors in the host immune response.

Septic shock
Bacterial toxins activate a series of inflammatory cascades, the systemic inflammatory response syndrome. Endotoxin, a cell wall constituent of gram-negative bacteria, causes release of mediators such as tumour necrosis factor alpha and interleukin-1. These responses cause shock by a variety of mechanisms which are initially 'distributive' ('warm' shock) and progress to a combination of hypovolaemic and cardiogenic shock. These include:
- *Vasodilatation*: high cardiac output state
- *Capillary leak*: increased microvascular permeability is associated with massive fluid loss from the circulation and hypovolaemia due to 'redistribution'
- *Tissue hypoxia*: metabolic acidosis due to raised plasma lactate levels
- *Myocardial depression*: a combination of hypoxia, acidosis and other mechanisms depresses myocardial function and impairs cardiac output
- *Cellular metabolism*: progressive deterioration in cellular oxygen consumption heralds multiple organ failure and irreversible shock
- Disseminated intravascular coagulation (DIC).

Clinical assessment

Early recognition of the 'septic' infant or child remains a major challenge especially because of the potentially fulminant course.

A high fever causes tachycardia and peripheral vasoconstriction which is difficult to distinguish from early compensated shock. In meningococcal septicaemia signs of an associated meningitis (if present) may assist diagnosis and a non-blanching petechial or purpuric rash is a well known and subtle early sign. However, in 30% of cases the rash is blanching and maculopapular.

Signs of early 'compensated' shock are listed in the algorithm.

The differential diagnosis in the infant with unequivocal signs of 'shock' includes
- *Cardiac disease*: supraventricular tachycardia, congenital heart disease, cardiomyopathy, myocarditis
- Inborn errors of metabolism
- *Gastrointestinal obstruction*: intussusception, volvulus
- Inflicted injury, non-accidental head injury
- Toxic shock syndrome and HUS.

Management

Investigations: the septic screen
- Full blood count and differential, C-reactive protein
- Urea and electrolytes, glucose, Ca, phosphate, LFTs
- Coagulation screen, blood gases
- Microbiology: blood cultures, urine cultures, etc.
- *Lumbar puncture*: this is unnecessary and even contraindicated in septic shock or if there are signs of raised intracranial pressure.
- CXR.

A CRP of <0.5 mg/dL renders sepsis less likely and either leucopaenia or leucocytosis render invasive bacterial disease more likely.

The management of meningococcal septicaemia is set out in the algorithm in Fig 2.6.

An intravenous broad-spectrum antibiotic, e.g. cefotaxime, is indicated for suspected invasive bacterial disease. A 'wait and see' policy is often inadvisable, but it is reasonable to await investigation results in a well child with concern generated by a localized petechial rash.

Initial management of septicaemic shock includes:
- Oxygen by face mask
- Insertion of two large cannulae (IV or intraosseous)
- *Antibiotics*: IV cefotaxime
- *Fluids*: bolus of colloid (4.5% human serum albumin) at 20 mL/kg. Repeat if necessary.

Further management depends on clinical response as judged by cardiovascular and respiratory parameters and the presence or absence of raised intracranial pressure.

Circulatory support

A total of 60 mL/kg (or more) of colloid should be administered if signs of shock persist. It is increasingly recognized that a massive capillary leak may exist with a corresponding high requirement for fluid volume replacement.

Inotropic support is indicated if poor perfusion persists despite fluid replacement. Dopamine (up to 10 micrograms/kg per minute) is first line. Dobutamine may be added but should not be used alone.

Metabolic derangements

If severe metabolic acidosis (pH <7.15) persists despite adequate fluid replacement, sodium bicarbonate may be necessary.

Hypoglycaemia, hypocalcaemia, hypokalaemia, hypomagnesaemia should be sought and corrected.

Coagulopathy
DIC is treated with fresh frozen plasma (10 mL/kg).

Respiratory support
Elective intubation and ventilation is indicated if shock persists following adequate fluid replacement or requires >60 mL/kg of fluid.

Clinical features of meningitis may or may not coexist with signs of raised intracranial pressure (ICP). This is managed as shown in Fig 2.6).

Early Management of Meningococcal Disease in Children*

6th Edition

RECOGNITION
May present with predominant SEPTICAEMIA (with shock), MENINGITIS (with raised ICP) or both. Purpuric/petechial non-blanching rash. Rash may be atypical or absent in some cases.

- Call consultant in A&E, Paediatrics, Anaesthesia or Intensive Care
- Initial assessment, looking for features of early shock/raised ICP
- DO NOT ATTEMPT LUMBAR PUNCTURE
- IV Cefotaxime (50mg/kg tds) or Ceftriaxone (80mg/kg od) but note MHRA Safety Update - avoid first line use where calcium infusion may be used http://www.nelm.nhs.uk/Record%20Viewing/viewRecord.aspx?id=587080

Published by

Meningitis Research Foundation
Registered Charity No 1091105

SIGNS OF EARLY COMPENSATED SHOCK ?
- Tachycardia
- Cool peripheries/pallor
- Increased capillary refill time (> 4 sec)
- Tachypnoea/pulse oximetry < 95%
- Hypoxia on arterial blood gas
- Base deficit (worse than -5 mmol/l)
- Confusion/drowsiness/decreased conscious level
- Poor urine output (< 1ml/kg/hr)
- Hypotension (late sign)

NO →

RAISED INTRACRANIAL PRESSURE ?
- Decreasing or fluctuating level of consciousness
- Hypertension and relative bradycardia
- Unequal, dilated or poorly reacting pupils
- Focal neurological signs
- Abnormal posturing or Seizures
- Papilloedema (late sign)

YES ↓

- ABC and Oxygen (10 l/min), bedside glucose
- Insert 2 large i.v. cannulae (or intra-osseous)

VOLUME RESUSCITATION
- Boluses of 20ml/kg of colloid (preferably 4.5% albumin) or crystalloid solutions over 5-10 minutes and review
- Repeat fluid bolus if necessary over 5-10 minutes
- Observe closely for response/deterioration
Do not attempt lumbar puncture

YES ↓

- ABC and Oxygen (10 l/min), bedside glucose
- Give Mannitol (0.25 g/kg) bolus over 5 minutes followed by Frusemide (1 mg/kg)
- Steroids (Dexamethasone 0.4 mg/kg bd x 2 days)
- Treat shock if present
Call anaesthetist and contact PICU
- Intubate and ventilate to control PaCO$_2$ (4-4.5 kPa)
- Urinary catheter and monitor output, NG tube
Do not attempt lumbar puncture

NO →

CLINICAL FEATURES OF MENINGITIS ?

YES ↓

After 40 ml/kg to 60 ml/kg fluid resuscitation STILL SIGNS OF SHOCK ?

NO → Repeated Review

YES ↓

WILL REQUIRE ELECTIVE INTUBATION AND VENTILATION
Call anaesthetist and contact PICU
- Continue boluses of 10-20 ml/kg of colloid or crystalloid with review
- Start peripheral inotropes (Dopamine, Dobutamine)
- Nasogastric tube and urinary catheter
- ET tube (cuffed if possible) and CXR
- Anticipate pulmonary oedema (ensure PEEP)
- Central venous access
- Start Adrenaline infusion (central) if continuing need for volume resuscitation and peripheral inotropes

NEUROINTENSIVE CARE
- 30° head elevation, midline position
- Avoid internal jugular lines
- Repeat Mannitol and Frusemide if indicated
- Sedate (muscle relax for transport)
- Cautious fluid resuscitation (but correct coexisting shock)
- Minimal handling, monitor pupillary size and reaction

NO → Dexamethasone (0.4mg/kg bd x 2 days)

Anticipate, monitor and correct:
- Hypoglycaemia
- Acidosis
- Hypokalaemia
- Hypomagnesaemia
- Hypocalcaemia
- Anaemia
- Coagulopathy (fresh frozen plasma 10 ml/kg)
- Raised intracranial pressure

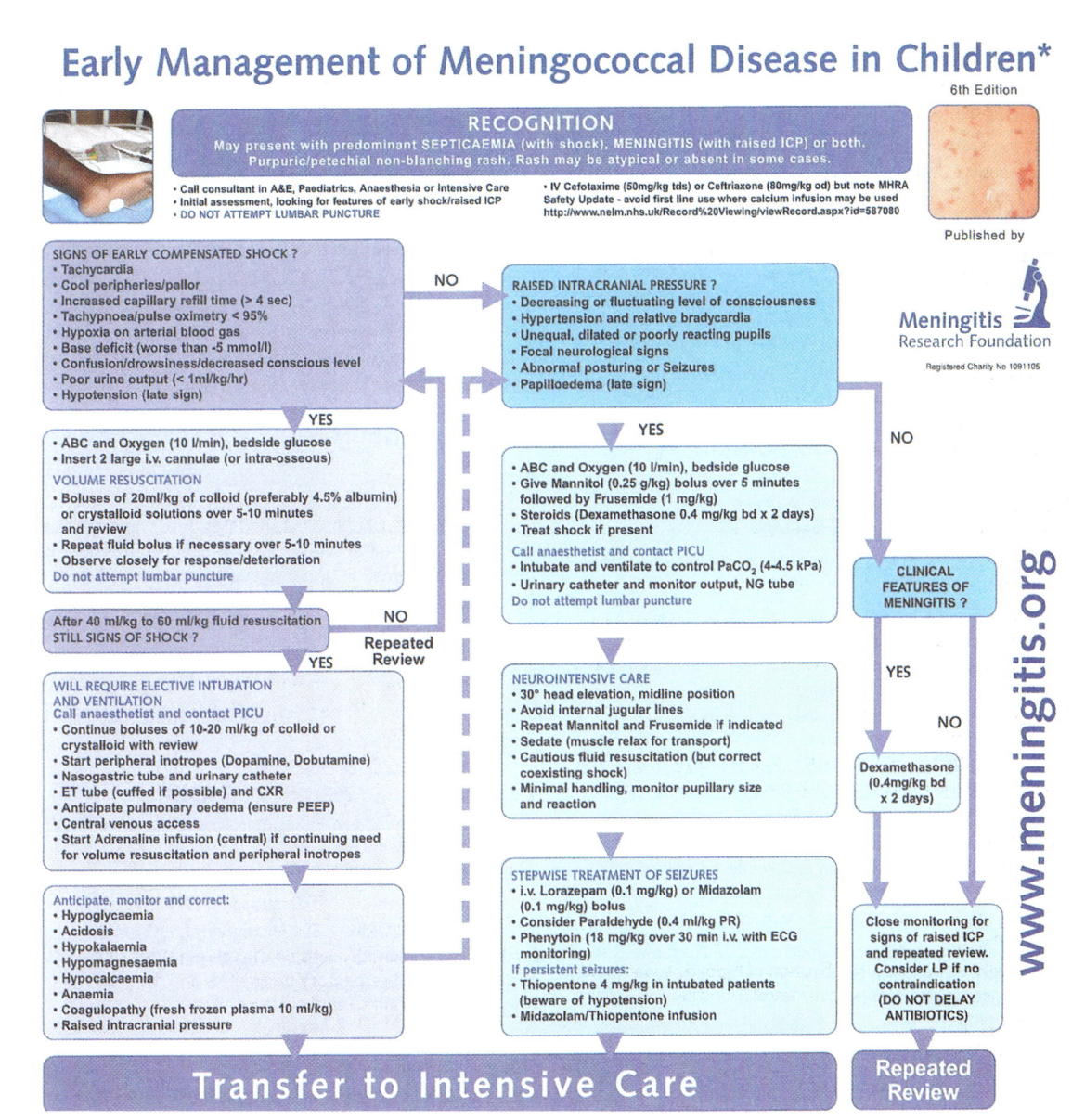

STEPWISE TREATMENT OF SEIZURES
- i.v. Lorazepam (0.1 mg/kg) or Midazolam (0.1 mg/kg) bolus
- Consider Paraldehyde (0.4 ml/kg PR)
- Phenytoin (18 mg/kg over 30 min i.v. with ECG monitoring)
If persistent seizures:
- Thiopentone 4 mg/kg in intubated patients (beware of hypotension)
- Midazolam/Thiopentone infusion

Close monitoring for signs of raised ICP and repeated review. Consider LP if no contraindication (DO NOT DELAY ANTIBIOTICS)

Transfer to Intensive Care

Repeated Review

www.meningitis.org

Fig 2.6 Early management of meningococcal disease in children (6th edition). Courtesy of the Meningtis Research Foundation.

2.9 Anaphylaxis

The terms anaphylaxis or anaphylactic reaction are best reserved for a severe multisystem allergic reaction caused by interaction of a soluble antigen with IgE bound to mast cells and basophils leading to degranulation and release of histamine and other substances, a type I allergic reaction.

Anaphylactoid reactions are clinically indistinguishable from anaphylaxis but are mediated by a drug or substance acting on mast cells *directly* and not via sensitized IgE antibodies.

No reliable epidemiological data on incidence are available because of difficulty in the exact definition of anaphylactic reactions. However, fatal allergic reactions to food account for about 1 death in children <16 years each year in the UK.

Aetiology and pathogenesis

The antigen interacts with specific IgE molecules fixed to mast cells and basophils leading to influx of calcium and degranulation with release of preformed (histamines and tryptase) and newly generated (thromboxane, leukotrienes and platelet activating factor) mediators. These induce reactions in several systems:

- *Respiratory:* bronchospasm, mucosal oedema, upper airway obstruction from oedema of glottis and tongue (angio-edema)
- *Cardiovascular:* vasodilatation and increased capillary permeability
- *Gastrointestinal:* abdominal pain, vomiting
- *Skin:* flushing, erythema, urticaria.

The leading causes of anaphylaxis in childhood differ from those in adults:

- *Foods:* account for >95% of cases and 41% of hospital admissions. Peanuts, tree nuts and seeds, milk, eggs, fish, shellfish, soya, and wheat account for 90% of food-induced cases.
- *Drugs:* B-lactamase antibiotics (e.g. penicillin), vaccines (e.g. MMR)
- *Insect venom:* Hymenoptera (bee and wasp) stings are a rare cause. Children with venom allergy have a high rate of spontaneous improvement.
- *Latex:* a rare cause in childhood and usually in children requiring frequent surgical procedures or indwelling catheters. Cross-reaction to banana, melon, and avocado occurs.

Rare causes of anaphylaxis include exercise (sometimes food dependent) and physical pressure on the skin or cold such as after swimming in cold water.

Anaphylactoid reactions

Activation of mast cells and basophils by IgE-independent mechanisms cause 'anaphylactoid' reactions with an identical clinical picture. Mechanisms include inhibition of prostaglandin synthetase by NSAIDs, complement activation producing C3a and C5a by pooled immunoglobulin in IgA deficient patients, and direct activation by opiates or hyperosmolar compounds such as radiocontrast media and mannitol.

Clinical features

There may be a history of atopy, food allergy, or previous severe reactions. Episodes range from minor to life threatening. Onset may be within seconds of exposure or delayed by 15–30 min or even 1 h. A biphasic response may occur 4–12 h later.

Symptoms and signs usually evolve, affecting the skin, respiratory and cardiovascular system in succession.

- *Skin:* itching with flushing of skin and an urticarial rash (hives)
- *Angio-oedema:* swelling of mouth, lips, face and upper respiratory tract (laryngeal oedema) causing stridor, hoarseness and drooling.
- *Bronchospasm and oedema:* cough, wheeze, dyspnoea and cyanosis
- *Cardiovascular collapse:* faintness and dizziness followed by syncope with pallor, tachycardia and hypotension i.e. shock.

Diagnosis is clinical and is usually not in doubt. It is rare for children to present with syncope, in which case an arrhythmia should be excluded. It may be mistaken for severe acute asthma and panic attacks can cause confusion, especially in victims of previous anaphylaxis.

Management

Prevention

Prevention of further attacks by allergen avoidance is the cornerstone of treatment. Referral should be made to a specialist allergy clinic where the allergen can be identified by skin prick tests, serum testing, or oral challenge if necessary. Advice is given on allergen avoidance and injectable adrenaline (Epipen, Anapen) provided with training.

Treatment of acute severe anaphylaxis

See algorithm in Fig 2.7.

Timely administration of IM adrenaline is life saving but complete management includes:

- Stop administration of causal agent
- Maintain airway and administer 100% oxygen
- Lie flat with leg elevation if hypotensive (unless respiratory distress increased)
- IM adrenaline 1:1000 solution:
    - child <6 years   150 micrograms IM (0.15 mL)
    - child 6–12 years   300 micrograms IM (0.3 mL)
    - >12 years   500 micrograms IM (0.5 mL)
- Repeat in 5 min if no improvement.

Additional measures may include:

- *IV hydrocortisone:* for all severe or recurrent reactions and patients with severe asthma
- *Nebulized salbutamol:* for severe bronchospasm or anaphylaxis in an asthmatic
- *IV or IM antihistamine (chlorpheniramine):* may be helpful and unlikely to be harmful, but IV injection must be slow
- *IV normal saline 20 mL/kg:* rapid infusion if shock does not respond to drug treatment.

```
                    ┌─────────────────────────┐
                    │  Anaphylactic reaction?  │
                    └─────────────────────────┘
                                 ↓
          ┌──────────────────────────────────────────────┐
          │ Airway, Breathing, Circulation, Disability, Exposure │
          └──────────────────────────────────────────────┘
                                 ↓
```

Diagnosis - look for:
- Acute onset of illness
- Life-threatening Airway and/or Breathing and/or Circulation problems[1]
- And usually skin changes

- **Call for help**
- Lie patient flat
- Raise patient's legs

Adrenaline[2]

When skills and equipment available:
- Establish airway
- High flow oxygen
- IV fluid challenge[3]
- Chlorphenamine[4]
- Hydrocortisone[5]

Monitor:
- Pulse oximetry
- ECG
- Blood pressure

[1]**Life-threatening problems:**
Airway: swelling, hoarseness, stridor
Breathing: rapid breathing, wheeze, fatigue, cyanosis, SpO_2 < 92%, confusion
Circulation: pale, clammy, low blood pressure, faintness, drowsy/coma

[2]**Adrenaline** *(give IM unless experienced with IV adrenaline)*
IM doses of 1:1000 adrenaline (repeat after 5 min if no better)
- Adult: 500 micrograms IM (0.5 mL)
- Child more than 12 years: 500 micrograms IM (0.5 mL)
- Child 6-12 years: 300 micrograms IM (0.3 mL)
- Child less than 6 years: 150 micrograms IM (0.15 mL)

Adrenaline IV to be given **only by experienced specialists**
Titrate: Adults 50 micrograms; Children 1 microgram/kg

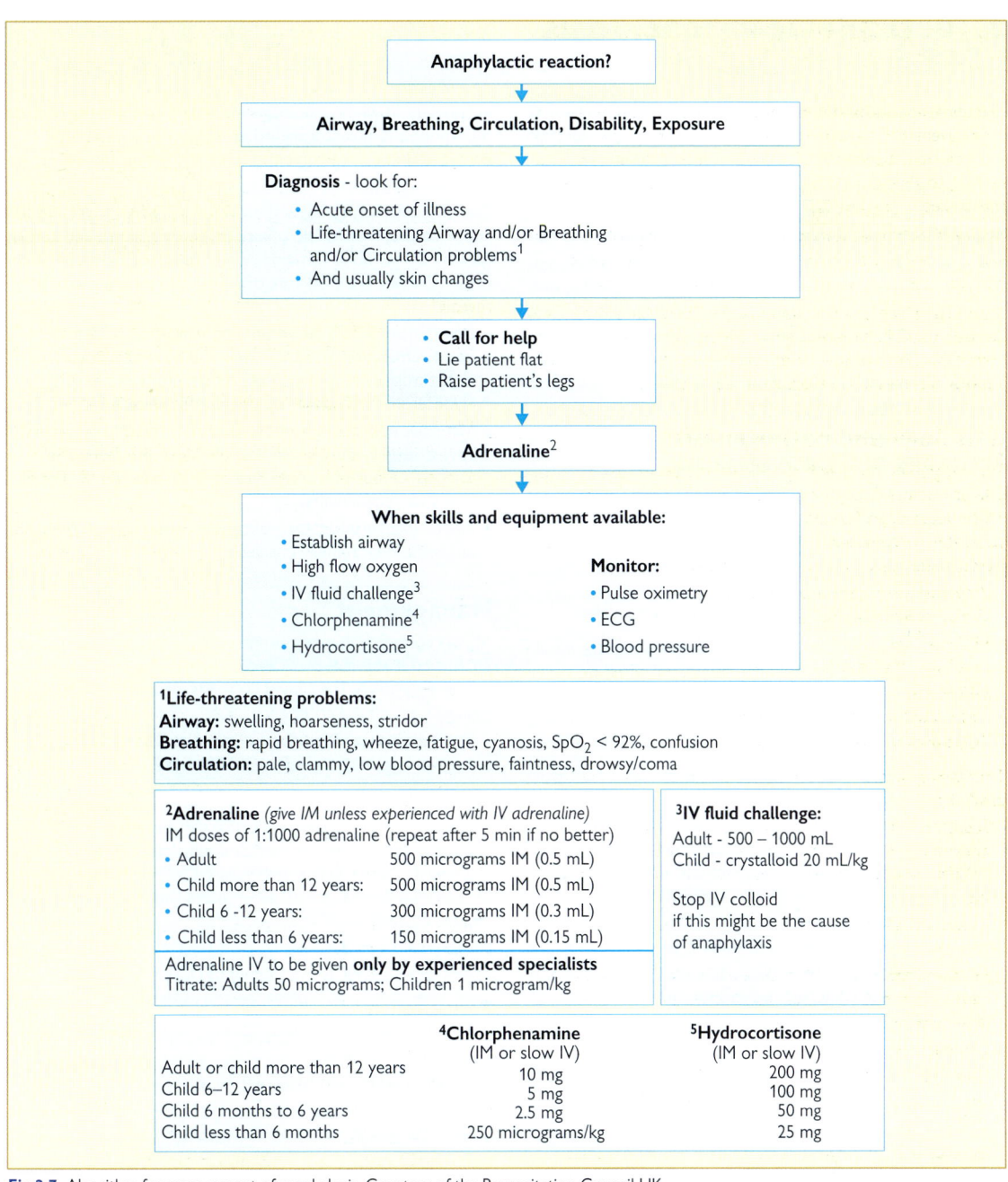

[3]**IV fluid challenge:**
Adult - 500 – 1000 mL
Child - crystalloid 20 mL/kg

Stop IV colloid if this might be the cause of anaphylaxis

	[4]**Chlorphenamine** (IM or slow IV)	[5]**Hydrocortisone** (IM or slow IV)
Adult or child more than 12 years	10 mg	200 mg
Child 6–12 years	5 mg	100 mg
Child 6 months to 6 years	2.5 mg	50 mg
Child less than 6 months	250 micrograms/kg	25 mg

Fig 2.7 Algorithm for management of anaphylaxis. Courtesy of the Resuscitation Council UK.

Important considerations

Adrenaline causes α-receptor effects (vasoconstriction) and β-receptor effects (bronchodilation, enhanced myocardial contraction, suppression of histamine release). It should be given IM to all patients with clinical signs of shock, airway swelling, or breathing difficulty. Intravenous adrenaline is hazardous and used only in profound, life-threatening shock by experienced personnel. Hydrocortisone appears to be of particular importance for asthmatics and must be given if they have been treated previously with corticosteroids.

Recurrence may occur for up to 24 h and observation for this period is indicated in asthmatics, episodes in which continued allergen exposure is possible, or patients with a previous history of biphasic reactions.

A blood sample (clotted) should be taken up to 1 h after onset for mast cells tryptase measurement and serum specific IgE levels to suspected allergens.

2.10 Diabetic ketoacidosis

Diabetic ketoacidosis (DKA) is a clinical state caused by absolute or relative deficiency of insulin and characterized by dehydration and metabolic acidosis.

Biochemical criteria for diagnosis of DKA include hyperglycaemia, blood glucose >11 mmol/L and metabolic acidosis, pH <7.3, HCO_3^- <15 mmol/L with associated glycosuria and ketonuria.

The exact incidence of DKA is uncertain. Hospitalization rates for DKA in established and new cases with type 1 diabetes mellitus (T1DM) are stable at about 10 per 100 000 children. DKA at onset of T1DM is more common in younger children <4 years. The risk of DKA in established T1DM is up to 10% per patient per year. The mortality rate is about 1/300 with cerebral oedema accounting for the majority of deaths.

Aetiology and pathogenesis

DKA is the end stage of a period of absolute or relative insulin deficiency and is more common in T1DM, occurring both at onset and in established T1DM.

DKA at onset is more common in younger children, those without a first degree relative with T1DM and those from families of lower socio-economic status.

DKA in established T1DM is usually due to inadequate insulin therapy during intercurrent illness, treatment error, or insulin omission. Risk is increased in children with poor control or previous episodes of DKA, adolescent girls, children with psychiatric disorders including eating disorders, and those with difficult family circumstances.

Pathophysiology

Insulin deficiency leads to hyperglycaemia which causes an osmotic diuresis with excessive loss of free water and electrolytes. This is compensated by increased oral intake until vomiting occurs, at which point severe dehydration rapidly develops with hypovolaemia and poor tissue perfusion.

Glucagon stimulates lipolysis with formation of keto-acids and poor tissue perfusion leads to lactic acidosis. At presentation a patient with severe DKA has:

- *Dehydration:* 5–10% body weight loss
- Depletion of whole body sodium and potassium.

Measured plasma Na^+ and K^+ concentrations are determined by a variety of factors:

- *Na^+:* hyponatraemia is common because of a dilutional effect as free water shifts extracellularly. In addition hyperlipidaemia, if present, causes an artefactual reduction.
- *K^+:* serum potassium may be high, normal, or low, depending on renal function and the degree of metabolic acidosis. Acidosis and reduced renal function tends to cause hyperkalaemia.
- *Metabolic acidosis:* due to a combination of keto-acid formation from lipolysis and lactic acidosis due to poor tissue perfusion.

Clinical evaluation

In DKA complicating onset of T1DM the classical history is several weeks of polyuria, polydipsia, malaise, and weight loss. Vomiting often heralds the onset of DKA and abdominal pain is a common symptom. Classical symptoms are often absent in toddlers in whom the diagnosis is easy to miss, especially if tachypnoea is misinterpreted as respiratory pathology. In a known diabetic, intercurrent infection or poor adherence are common precipitants.

The physical findings depend on whether DKA is mild, moderate or severe. In mild DKA there is hyperglycaemia and ketosis (pH >7.30) without vomiting or significant dehydration. Most cases, however, are moderate or severe and clinical examination reveals:

- *Dehydration:* 5–10% dehydration is manifested by dry mucous membranes, sunken eyes and signs of hypovolaemia: tachycardia, increased capillary refill time, poor perfusion. Hypotension indicates decompensated shock.
- *Metabolic acidosis:* tachypnoea (Kussmaul breathing) occurs as respiratory compensation develops for the metabolic acidosis. Odour of ketones may be detectable on the breath (like pear-drop sweets).
- *Altered mental status:* level of consciousness may be reduced but coma is extremely unusual.

Management

Always consult with a more senior doctor on call if you suspect DKA even if you feel confident of your management. Children can die from DKA. The clinical diagnosis is confirmed by demonstrating biochemical criteria for DKA:

- *Hyperglycaemia:* blood glucose >11 mmol/L
- *Acidaemia:* pH <7.3, bicarbonate <15 mmol/L
- *Ketonuria.*

Children who are clinically well, <5% dehydrated, and tolerating oral fluids can be managed with oral rehydration and subcutaneous soluble insulin. Those with severe DKA or at increased risk of cerebral oedema should be considered immediately for treatment in a paediatric ICU.

Management of moderate (pH <7.2, HCO_3^- <10 mmol/L) to severe (pH <7.1, HCO_3^- <5 mmol/L) DKA is as follows.

Resuscitation

- If decreased conscious state, or recurrent vomiting an oral airway and nasogastric tube should be inserted. Aspirate nasogastric tube and leave on free drainage.
- Give 100% O_2 by face mask
- Insert IV cannula.

Take blood samples for glucose, U&E, PCV, FBC, and arterial, capillary, or venous sample for blood gases. If shocked with poor capillary return and tachycardia and/or hypotension give 10 mL/kg 0.9% normal saline as a bolus and repeat as necessary to a maximum of 30 mL/kg.

Fluids

Volumes

Once circulating blood volume has been restored using up to 30 mL/kg of 0.9% saline calculate fluid requirement as deficit plus maintenance and give the total volume evenly over 48 h.

Deficit (litres) = % dehydration × body weight (kg)

Maximum estimate of deficit is 10%. Allow for initial resuscitation volume.

> **Worked example**
>
> 20 kg 6 year old 10% dehydrated given 20 mL/kg 0.9% saline
>
> Deficit = 10% × 20 kg = 2000 mL (2 L)
>
> Minus resus fluid = 20 mL × 20 kg = 400 mL
>
> Deficit = 1600 mL
>
> 20 kg boy aged 6 years
>
> Maintenance = 60 mL × 20 kg/24 h = 2400 mL over 48 h
>
> This boy requires a total of 4000 mL over 48 h (see Table 2.3). Excessive urinary losses are not included in calculations.

Table 2.3 Fluid maintenance requirements

Age (years)	mL/kg per 24 h
0–2	80
3–5	70
6–9	60
10–14	50
>14	30

Type of fluid
Initially use 0.9% saline. Add KCl at 40 mmol/L to rehydration fluid after initial volume repletion unless anuria is suspected (failure to micturate is not the same as anuria). Plasma levels of K^+ will fall once insulin therapy is commenced. Add dextrose to fluid when blood glucose has fallen to 14–17 mmol/L. In first 6 h this may be 0.9% saline/5% dextrose. After first 6 h, if plasma sodium stable, use 0.45% saline/5% dextrose. Administration of bicarbonate or phosphate is rarely indicated.

Insulin

Soluble insulin is given at a rate of 0.1 u/kg per hour.

Make up a solution of 1 u/mL by adding 50 u insulin to 50 mL 0.9% saline in a syringe pump.

Try to maintain insulin at this rate and keep glucose levels in range of 4–12 mmol/L by increasing the dextrose concentration in fluids up to 10%, until the pH is >7.3.

Once pH is >7.3 and dextrose-containing fluid has been started, consider reducing insulin infusion rate to 0.05–0.1 u/kg per hour.

Monitoring and investigations

This should include
- Hourly BP, HR, and respiratory rate
- Neuro observations
- *ECG:* monitor T waves for hyper- or hypokalaemia
- Initial weight and twice daily thereafter
- *Fluid balance:* hourly input/output
- Hourly blood glucose (capillary) measurement
- *Electrolytes and blood gases:* 2 h after onset of IV therapy then 4 hourly, or more frequent if unstable.

Principles of DKA management

Understanding the basic pathophysiology allows rational management of this challenging condition.

Fluid and electrolytes
All patients with moderate to severe DKA have a significant whole-body deficit of Na^+ and K^+ and dehydration with some hypovolaemia. Rapid volume expansion to restore circulation is the most important initial step, usually requiring 10–20 mL/kg of 0.9% saline. Subsequent fluid management aims to restore the deficit slowly over 48 h.

Acidosis
Even severe acidosis will respond to insulin and fluid replacement, as keto-acids are metabolized and tissue perfusion is improved.

Insulin and dextrose
An infusion rate of 0.1 u/kg per hour equates to 2.4 u/kg per day, which is about twice the usual requirement in established T1DM (1.0 u/kg per day). It is essential to include dextrose in the IV fluids when blood glucose is in the range 14–17 mmol/L or if blood glucose levels fall faster than 5 mmol/L per hour. While acidosis persists it is better to increase dextrose administration than reduce insulin infusion rates.

It is vital to carefully monitor all therapy. Do not write fluid and insulin prescriptions and walk away, as delays or mistakes in administration can occur and be life threatening.

Complications of DKA

The most important is cerebral oedema, but hypokalaemia, aspiration pneumonia, and hypoglycaemia may also occur.

Cerebral oedema in DKA

Cerebral oedema is rare, occurring in <1% of cases of DKA, but the mortality rate is ~25% and it accounts for ~75% of all deaths. Risk factors include young age, newly diagnosed T1DM, and longer duration of symptoms, all of which correlate with greater likelihood of severe DKA.

The causes are complex and multifactorial but probably relate to osmotic disequilibrium between plasma and brain extracellular fluid. The brain has equilibrated with hyperosmolar plasma and as plasma osmolarity falls water shifts into the brain. Epidemiological associations exist with severity of acidosis, greater hypocapnia, and high urea levels but not with the degree of hyperglycaemia.

Clinical features
Onset is typically 4–12 h after initiation of treatment but cerebral oedema may occur at any time. Symptoms and signs variable but may include:
- Headache, restlessness, irritability, reduced level of consciousness
- Bradycardia and rising BP
- Focal neurological signs: altered pupillary responses, cranial palsies
- Abnormal posturing.

Management
If cerebral oedema is suspected inform senior staff and arrange intensive care transfer. Immediate measures while awaiting transfer:
- Exclude hypoglycaemia as cause of CNS signs
- Reduce IV fluids to two-thirds maintenance and replace deficit over 72 h rather than 48 h
- Give IV 2.5–5 mL/kg of mannitol 20% over 15 min. Repeat after 2 h if no response
- Nurse in head-up position
- When stable arrange cranial CT to exclude other causes of raised ICP (thrombosis, haemorrhage)
- Neurointensive care may be necessary including intubation and ventilation to control arterial PCO_2.

2.11 Convulsions and coma

Convulsive status epilepticus (CSE)

Generalized convulsive (tonic-clonic) status epilepticus (CSE) is defined as a generalized convulsion lasting 30 min or more, or repeated convulsions occurring over a 30 min period without recovery of consciousness. However, the management approach is the same for any child with a tonic-clonic seizure lasting >5 min.

The outcome is mainly determined by the cause. Neurological sequelae are age dependent: 29% in those under a year but only 6% in those >3 years. Overall mortality is 4%.

Aetiology and pathogenesis

The most common cause of a generalized tonic-clonic seizure lasting >5 min is a febrile seizure. Other less common causes include:
- Epilepsy
- *Intracranial infection:* encephalitis or meningitis
- *Metabolic disorders:* e.g. hypoglycaemia
- Poisoning
- *Traumatic brain injury:* accidental or non-accidental.

A generalized seizure causes an increase in brain metabolic rate and oxygen and glucose requirement which is met by compensatory mechanisms which are effective for at least 30 min unless there is hypoglycaemia or the seizure compromises ventilation. Beyond 30 min decompensation occurs and additional complications may arise such as hypoxia and aspiration, cardiac arrhythmias, hypotension, and reduced cardiac output.

Clinical evaluation

Primary assessment and resuscitation (see below) obviously precedes history taking and examination which are an important component of the secondary assessment.
Important points in history are:
- Duration and nature of any current seizure activity
- Treatment given pre-hospital
- Prior history of seizures including medication
- Recent intercurrent illness
- Recent head injury or toxic exposure
- *Conditions associated with hypoglycaemia:* T1DM, congenital adrenal hyperplasia, ethanol ingestion.

Physical examination should be directed towards identifying:
- *Fever:* fever suggests a febrile seizure, intercurrent illness, or intracranial infection
- *Intracranial infection:* signs of meningitis or encephalitis
- *Intracranial pressure:* bulging fontanelle in an infant, bradycardia and hypertension.
- *Traumatic brain injury:* soft tissue swelling of scalp, retinal haemorrhages
- *Neurocutaneous syndromes:* depigmented macules of tuberous sclerosis complex (TSC)
- Focal or asymmetrical neurological signs.

Management

Protocols for management of CSE differ only in detail. Primary assessment and resuscitation follows the standard **ABC** routine:
- **A***irway:* ensure airway is patent. Put child in recovery position.
- **B***reathing:*
  - assess respiratory rate, O_2 saturation
  - give high flow oxygen via a non-rebreathe face mask; support hypoventilation with oxygen via a bag–valve–mask device and consider intubation.
- **C***irculation:*
  - assess heart rate, blood pressure, capillary refill time
  - establish intravenous or intraosseous access
  - blood tests: capillary glucose testing, FBC, urea and electrolytes, calcium, magnesium, blood gases, blood cultures.
  - Treat hypoglycaemia with 5 mL/kg of 10% dextrose IV.

Seizures are treated in a series of steps as shown in Fig 2.8.

Step 1: benzodiazepines: lorazepam 0.1 mg/kg IV or IO or, if no vascular access, diazepam 0.5 mg/kg PR or, midazolam by buccal or intranasal route.

Step 2: if the convulsion has not stopped after 10 min a second dose of lorazepam 0.1 mg/kg IV/IO is given or, if there is still no vascular access, paraldehyde 0.4 mL/kg PR

Step 3: if convulsions still persist after a further 10 min a longer acting antiepilepsy drug is indicated. Phenytoin 18mg/kg IV or IO is given over 20 min. If child already on phenytoin, use phenobarbital 20 mg/kg IV or IO over 10 min.

Step 4: if 20 min after step 3 has commenced the child remains in CSE, then rapid sequence of anaesthesia is performed with thiopentone 4 mg/kg IV or IO.

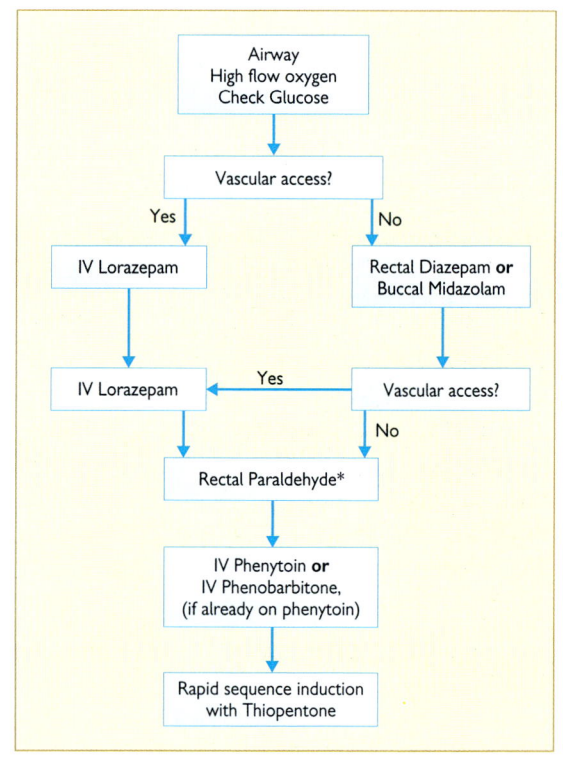

Fig 2.8 Algorithm for convulsive status. Courtesy of the APLS Working Group.* Paraldehyde is no longer used in most centres.

Decreased conscious level: coma

Decreased conscious level is defined as a modified Glasgow Coma Score (GCS) <15, or being responsive only to voice or pain or being unresponsive on the AVPU scale. Coma is a state of profoundly reduced conscious level.

Aetiology
Specific causes other than sepsis or shock include:
- *Traumatic brain injury:* accidental and non-accidental
- *Intracranial infection:* meningitis, tuberculous meningitis, brain abscess, herpes simplex encephalitis
- *Seizures:* ictal or post-ictal states
- *Metabolic disorders:* hypoglycaemia, hyperammonaemia
- *Poisoning:* opiates, barbiturates, tricyclic antidepressants
- *Raised intracranial pressure:* hypertension.

Clinical assessment
Important points in history include:
- *Prodromal illness:* headache, vomiting, fever, or seizures
- *Speed of onset, head trauma:* remember that inflicted trauma such as shaking will not usually be disclosed.
- *Ingestion of medications:* accidental or deliberate,
- Family history of metabolic disorders, previous history of epilepsy, diabetes mellitus.

Primary assessment is focused on **A**irway, **B**reathing, and **C**irculation but secondary assessment should focus on clues to aetiology.
- *General examination:* fever (absence makes intracranial infection unlikely), trauma: bruising or scalp swellings
- *Neurological examination:* level of consciousness: GCS or AVPU score', signs of meningism or raised intracranial pressure, fundi (papilloedema or retinal haemorrhages), focal neurological signs, or abnormal posturing.

Glasgow Coma Scale

Best Eye Response (4)
1. No eye opening
2. Eye opening to pain
3. Eye opening to verbal command
4. Eyes open spontaneously

Best Verbal Response (5)
1. No vocal response or grimace response to pain
2. Occasional whimpers (mild grimace) to pain
3. Cries (vigorous grimace) to pain only
4. Spontaneous irritable cry
5. Alert, babbles, coos, words or sentences

Best Motor Response (6)
1. No motor response to pain
2. Abnormal extension to pain (decerebrate)
3. Abnormal flexion to pain (decorticate)
4. Withdrawal to painful stimuli
5. Localizes to painful stimuli or withdraws to touch
6. Obeys commands / normal spontaneous movements

Management
Initial management follows the **ABC** paradigm for the sick child. A capillary blood glucose should be checked immediately as hypoglycaemia is an important remedial cause of altered consciousness.

Investigations
- Blood:
  - glucose, gases, urea and electrolytes
  - LFTs, plasma ammonia, plasma lactate
  - full blood count, coagulation screen
  - blood culture
- *Plasma/serum/urine:* save for later analysis
- Plasma/urine for toxicology, organic, and amino acids.

Consideration is given to:

Cranial imaging
A cranial CT should be considered when the patient is stable if the working diagnosis is raised intracranial pressure, intracranial abscess, traumatic brain injury, or the cause of altered consciousness remains uncertain.

Lumbar puncture (LP)
An LP should be performed, if no contraindications exist, if the working diagnosis is intracranial infection (meningitis, encephalitis) or the cause remains uncertain. CSF should be analysed by gram staining and microscopy, culture, protein, glucose, PCR for HHV1 and other viruses.

Contraindications to performing an LP include:
- Clinical evidence of systemic meningococcal disease, e.g. shock
- GCS ≤8 or deteriorating
- Pupillary abnormalities
- Focal neurological signs, abnormal posturing
- Signs of raised intracranial pressure
- Bleeding diathesis.

A normal cranial CT does not exclude acute raised intracranial pressure. The decision to perform an LP in a child with reduced conscious level should be made by an experienced paediatrician who has examined the child.

If the cause remains obscure, after reviewing initial core investigations, further helpful investigations might include:
- EEG: detects non-convulsive status epilepticus
- Acyl-carnitine profile (on Guthrie card)
- ESR and autoimmune screen (cerebral vasculitis).

Further management depends of course on whether a cause for which specific treatment exists has been identified. If no obvious cause can be identified, consideration is given to starting antibiotics and intravenous aciclovir.

Intubation
Indications for intubation include:
- GCS <8 or deteriorating
- *Airway compromise or inadequate respirations:* O_2 sat <92% despite high flow O_2 therapy and airway opening manoeuvres
- *Shock:* persisting despite volume replacement >40 mL/kg
- Signs of raised intracranial pressure.

2.12 Case-based discussions

A child in convulsive status
A 3 year old child is brought into the hospital emergency department by ambulance. The child has been convulsing for almost 15 min.

What is your initial management?
Management should follow the **A**irway, **B**reathing, **C**irculation sequence. The child is placed in the recovery position and oxygen should be given by face mask. Blood glucose should be checked as hypoglycaemia is an easily treatable cause of seizures and will cause brain damage if unrecognized and untreated.

Diazepam may be given rectally 0.5 mg/kg, or buccal midazolam at the same dose if vascular access is not obtained. If vascular access is obtained, lorazepam should be given intravenously at 0.1 mg/kg.

The blood glucose was normal. A dose of lorazepam was given, but the seizures continued. After 10 min, a further dose was given, to no avail.

What is your subsequent management?
The child should be loaded with phenytoin, followed by a phenytoin infusion, with blood pressure and ECG monitoring. If seizures are not controlled, the next step is rapid sequence induction with thiopentone, followed by mechanical ventilation.

What secondary assessment and investigations might be appropriate?
Secondary assessment is focused on identifying a cause. Enquiry should be made about any history of previous seizures, recent intercurrent illness, or head trauma.

General examination should assess whether the child is febrile or has any evidence of head trauma. The child should be inspected for features suggesting known epilepsy (Medicalert bracelet, helmet). Features of a neurocutaneous syndrome should also be sought.

Neurological examination for evidence of meningism, raised intracranial pressure, focal neurological signs. Blood tests should be sent to investigate for sepsis, electrolyte abnormalities and toxicology.

The child was apyrexial with no circulatory or respiratory compromise. There were no signs of meningism or focal neurological signs. Several small hypopigmented lesions were seen on his limbs (Fig 2.9).

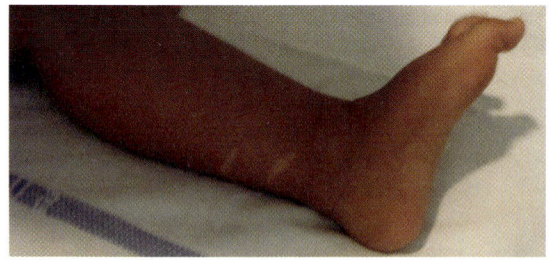

Fig 2.9 Hypopigmented macules on limb

What diagnosis is suggested by these features?
A diagnosis of tuberous sclerosis complex is likely. Seizures may occur due to the presence of tubers in the brain, and are often difficult to control. The skin should be carefully inspected in any child with seizures.

Sudden unexpected death in an infant
A 3 month old baby boy is brought by ambulance to the hospital emergency department having been found in his cot blue and not breathing. Parents tried mouth-to-mouth resuscitation when they found him, while waiting for the ambulance to arrive. After 30 min there has been no response and resuscitation is discontinued.

When and what samples do you collect?
This is a sudden unexplained death in infancy (SUDI) and the Department of Health guidelines in *Working Together 2006* need to be followed:

- A full physical examination must be carried out, with documentation of all lesions and abnormalities, including any iatrogenic lines and tubes.
- If possible take specimens before child declared dead; if not, obtain the permission of the coroner.
- Blood samples can be taken from a venous or arterial site. A larger gauge needle may be necessary. The femoral vein can be used for sampling blood. Cardiac puncture should be avoided if possible as this may damage intrathoracic structures.
- Record the site from which all samples were taken and document all samples.
- Retain infant's clothes and nappy in labelled bags.

Sample	Test
Blood	Toxicology, culture, chromosomes, metabolic screen
Cerebrospinal fluid	MC&S
Nasopharyngeal aspirate	Viral/bacterial cultures, immunofluorescence
Swab lesions; throat swab	Culture and sensitivity
Urine (if available from SPA)	Toxicology, organic/amino acids

Whom do you inform?
Coroner (post-mortem), police child abuse investigation team, social work team, GP, health visitor, designated doctor for SUDI, and consultant in charge must all be informed.

What happens to the parents?
Good practice is that within 24 h, they will have a joint police/paediatric home visit, preferably and if possible with the consultant paediatrician. Support, advice and information for parents may include details of the Foundation for the Study of Infant Deaths (FSID, www.sids.org.uk/fsid), Child Death Helpline and Cruse: Bereavement Support and Advice.

The consultant should arrange to meet with the parents a few days after the post-mortem has been performed to provide preliminary results and meet the parents again 2 months later to provide his/her views on the cause of death.

Subsequent infants of these parents may be placed on the Care of the Next Infant Scheme (CONI) for parental support (see also Chapter 18.13).

Chapter 3
Respiratory medicine

3.1 Respiratory system: anatomy and physiology *54*
3.2 Respiratory system: clinical skills *56*
3.3 Ear, nose, and throat (ENT) *58*
3.4 Upper airways obstruction: stridor *60*
3.5 Pneumonia and pertussis *62*
3.6 Bronchiolitis and pulmonary tuberculosis *64*
3.7 Asthma *66*
3.8 Cystic fibrosis *68*
3.9 Chronic lung disease, bronchiectasis, and sequelae of neurodisability *70*
3.10 Case-based discussions *72*

3.1 Respiratory system: anatomy and physiology

Lung development
The respiratory tract develops from endoderm which undergoes extensive branching morphogenesis and alveolization together with angiogenesis and vascularization from about 28 days of gestation. Lung maturity is of course a critical limiting factor in determining postnatal viability in infants born preterm (see Chapter 1).

The five main periods are shown in Fig 3.1:
- *Embryonic, up to week 7:* the primitive trachea separates dorsoventrally from the primitive oesophagus. The primary bronchial branches arise and the lobar airways lined with endoderm are established.
- *Pseudoglandular, weeks 7–17:* airway formation, including all pre-acinar airways, is completed during this period.
- *Canalicular, weeks 17–27:* the branching of peripheral airways is completed by about 24 weeks and the peripheral airways enlarge and are lined by thinned epithelium which eventually forms type I and II pneumocytes.
- *Saccular, weeks 28–36:* the sac-shaped distal airways extend to form cup-shaped alveoli.
- *Alveola, weeks 36 onwards:* alveoli multiply. At birth, 30–50% of the adult number are present.

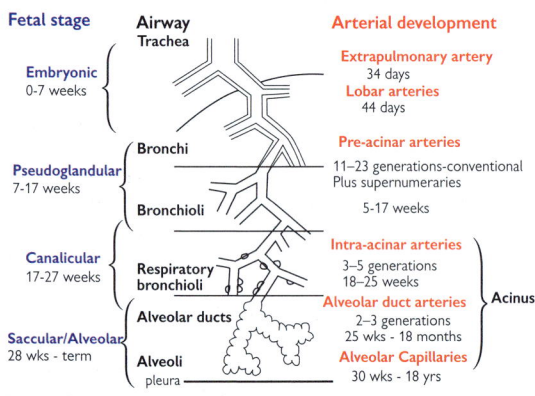

Fig 3.1 Lung development *in utero*. Reproduce with permission from Paediatric Respiratory Reviews (2005) 6, 35–43.

Postnatal lung growth
A 10-fold increase in alveolar numbers occurs from birth to age 3 years. Subsequent lung growth occurs by alveolar enlargement. Until puberty, girls have larger airways than boys; after puberty this is reversed. In boys, lung growth continues for 2–3 years after skeletal maturity.

Respiratory physiology
Mechanics of breathing
Newborn infants have an abdominal breathing pattern. Descent of the diaphragm during inspiration is accompanied by outward displacement of the abdominal wall. As the chest wall becomes less compliant with age it becomes the primary mechanism of increasing intrathoracic volume during inspiration.

Lung volumes and capacities
Volumes
- *Tidal volume (TV):* volume of air inspired and expired during quiet normal breathing
- *Inspiratory reserve volume (IRV):* maximum volume that can be inhaled after a normal tidal volume inspiration
- *Expiratory reserve volume (ERV):* maximum volume that can be exhaled after a normal tidal volume expiration
- *Residual volume (RV):* volume of air remaining in lungs after a maximum expiration.

Capacities (sum of more than one volume)
- *Total lung capacity (TLC):* volume in lungs after maximal inspiration:

  TLC = IRV + TV + ERV + RV.
- *Functional residual capacity (FRC):* volume in lungs at end of a TV expiration:

  FRC = ERV + RV.
- *Inspiratory capacity (IC):* maximum volume that can be inhaled from end of a TV expiration:

  IC = IRV + TV.
- *Vital capacity (FC):* volume of air that can be exhaled after a maximum inspiration:

  VC = IRV + TV + ERV.

In children with healthy lungs, the elastic force of the chest wall is balanced by the elastic recoil of the lungs at the end of a TV expiration. This is called the elastic equilibrium volume (EEV) and FRC coincides with EEV. The closing volume is the lung volume at which airways begin to close spontaneously during expiration. In newborn infants the EEV may be below the closing volume.

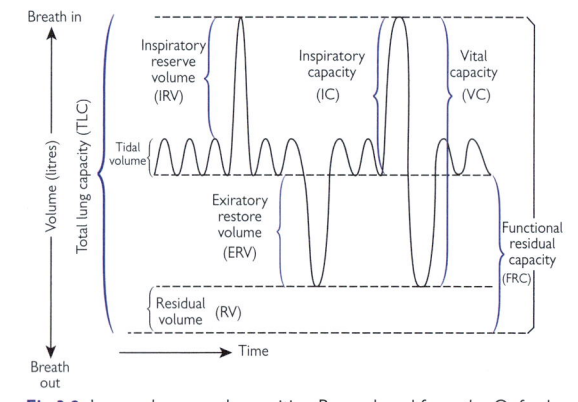

Fig 3.2 Lung volumes and capacities. Reproduced from the Oxford Handbook of Respiratory Nursing (Robinson and Scullion), with permission from OUP.

Lung function tests
Lung function tests measure several aspects of pulmonary function, including:
- Airway function
- Lung volumes
- Gas exchange.

They are rarely used for diagnosis, but are useful for:
- Detection and measurement of severity of lung dysfunction
- Evaluating response to treatment
- Monitoring progression and predicting prognosis (e.g. in cystic fibrosis and myopathies)
- Measuring effects of exposure to allergens
- Assessing risks for surgery
- Distinguishing between obstructive and restrictive disorders.

Spirometry, the measurement of the pattern of air movement into and out of the lungs during controlled ventilatory manoeuvres is the most common test used. It can be performed in most children aged >5 years.

Spirometry
The child is asked to take a maximal breath in (i.e. inspire to TLC) and then to breathe out into a mouthpiece as hard, as fast, and as long as they can (i.e. maximal forced expiration to RV). Three attempts are made, the best of which is recorded.

The volume of air shifted by this manoeuvre is the FVC. The volume of gas expired (as %FVC) and the flow rate (L/s) is measured using a spirometer.

Data is presented as a flow–volume curve which has a characteristic and sometimes diagnostic shape. The first third of expiration (including PEF and F75) is effort dependent, but the remaining two thirds is effort independent and related to airway resistance, declining linearly with lung volume.

In healthy children there is a rapid rise to the highest flow (peak expiratory flow rate, PEFR) immediately after the start of expiration, followed by a linear decline in flow rate as the lung empties. The measurements usually made are:
- *FVC*: forced vital capacity
- *FEV1*: forced expiratory volume in 1 s
- *FEF1/FVC*: normal ratio 75–80%
- *FEF$_{25-75}$*: forced expiratory flow over the middle 50% of vital capacity (an index of small airway function)
- *PEFR*: peak expiratory flow rate (quite effort dependent, can underestimate small airway obstruction).

Flow–volume curves during inspiration and expiration are combined to form a flow–volume loop (Fig 3.3). All results are compared with normal values for children of similar age, height, ethnicity, and sex. Abnormalities found in obstructive, restrictive or mixed lung disease are as follows.

Obstructive lung disease (airflow limitation)
The flow curve during expiration has a lower peak and a scalloped appearance as small airway obstruction becomes more severe. There is a decreased FEV1, FEF$_{25-75}$, and FEV1/FVC ratio (<80%). TLC is normal or increased.
Examples: asthma, cystic fibrosis, bronchiectasis.

If obstruction is shown it is useful to determine its reversibility with bronchodilators by repeating spirometry 15–20 min after a bronchodilator (e.g. salbutamol). An increase of FEV1 of 15% indicates reversibility.

Restrictive lung disease (diminished lung volumes)
The FVC and expiratory flows are proportionately reduced generating a flow-volume loop of normal shape but proportionately small. The FEV1/FVC ratio is normal or increased (due to increased elastic recoil). TLC and FVC are decreased.

Examples: interstitial lung disease (pneumonitis, fibrosing alveolitis), chest wall deformity (scoliosis), neuromuscular disease (muscular dystrophy).

A mixed obstructive and restrictive pattern of lung disease may exist. For example, in severe cystic fibrosis, bronchiectasis causing airway obstruction may coexist with fibrosis and collapse causing a restrictive element.

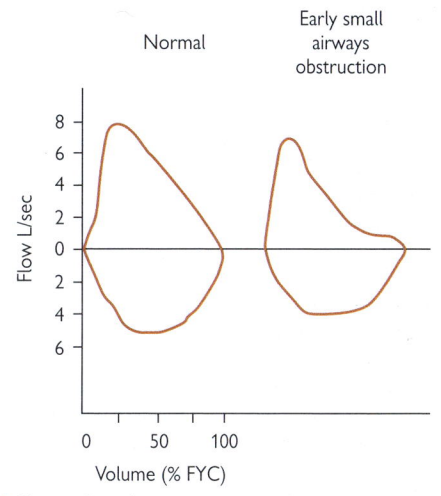

Fig 3.3 Flow–volume loops: expiration and inspiration.

Defence mechanisms and immunity

The frequency of respiratory tract infection in childhood is a reflection of the intrinsic vulnerability caused by continual exposure of a large, moist, warm, permeable surface area to a host of microbes, combined with an immature and relatively unexposed immune system. The main defences comprise the physical barriers of mucus secretion and ciliary action together with innate and acquired immune mechanisms.

Mucus acts as a physical barrier to which particles and organisms adhere. Motile cilia line the respiratory tract and propel the overlying mucus to the oropharynx where it is either expectorated or swallowed. Disruption of these defences occurs in cystic fibrosis and primary ciliary dyskinesia (Kartagener syndrome).

Innate immunity is mediated by cells and proteins which recognize invading pathogens in a non-specific manner. Components include complement, lysozyme, collectins, and B-defensins. Acquired immunity is mediated by T-helper (CD4$^+$) and T-cytotoxic (CD8$^+$) lymphocytes together with B lymphocytes which secrete immunoglobulins.

Excessive inappropriate inflammatory responses may themselves be harmful, e.g. in chronic asthma.

3.2 Respiratory system: clinical skills

History
In most cases the history equates to observations by the parents of cough, noisy breathing, or altered breathing patterns. Features to establish for each symptom include:

- *Cough:* Dry or productive? Paroxysmal? Relationship to feeding or vomiting in infants?
- *Noisy breathing:* parents may be able to hear a variety of noises associated with breathing including snoring, nasal airway noise, stridor, wheeze, and grunting (see Table 3.2) but usually refer to them all as 'wheeze'.
- *Altered breathing:* parents may note rapid breathing, intercostal or subcostal recession, use of accessory muscles.

The differential diagnosis of a recurrent or persistent cough is shown in Table 3.1.

Table 3.1. Causes of a chronic cough
Infection: TB, pertussis, *Mycoplasma pneumoniae*
Asthma
Gastro-oesophageal reflux/aspiration
Cystic fibrosis
Inhaled foreign body
Postnasal drip
Rarities: primary ciliary dyskinesia, immunodeficiency, habit

Examination
The respiratory system is unusual in generating acoustic as well as visual signs of disease. The definition and nature of the common respiratory noises is shown in Table 3.2.

Table 3.2. Common respiratory noises	
Wheeze	A high pitched noise caused by narrowing of the intrathoracic airways. Louder on expiration (when intrathoracic airways tend to collapse)
Stridor	A noise caused by narrowing of the extra-thoracic airways (larynx, upper trachea). Louder on inspiration (when extrathoracic airways tend to collapse)
Cough	Sudden expulsion of air from the lungs due to spasmodic contraction of the thoracic cavity. Bronchiolitis, pertussis and croup all generate distinct and characteristic coughs
Grunting	An end-expiratory noise caused by breathing out against a partially closed glottis
Snoring	The noise produced by vibration of the soft palate and uvula which occurs when there is any blockage to the flow of air in the back of the mouth or nose
Snuffles	The noise produced by breathing through narrowed nasal passages (e.g. a blocked nose)
Rattle	The noise produced by breathing through secretions in the hypopharynx, trachea, or large bronchi

The emphasis in examination is very age dependent. Inspection provides 90% of useful information in infants; palpation and percussion are of more value in the older child.

Inspection
- Cyanosis and oxygen saturation
- *Increased work of breathing:*
  - respiratory rate, nasal flaring
  - recession: intercostal, subcostal, tracheal tug
- *Thoracic cage* (see Fig 3.4):
  - asymmetry, scoliosis or kyphosis
  - hyperinflation: increased AP diameter (barrel chest)
  - Harrison sulcus
  - pectus excavatum or carinatum
- Scars and clubbing

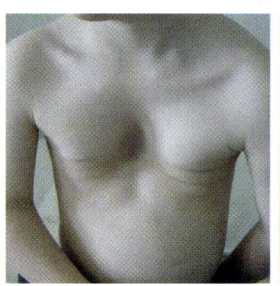

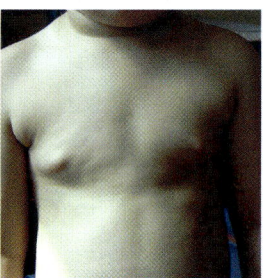

Fig 3.4 Thoracic cage signs: A. Pectus excavatum. B. Harrison sulci.

Palpation
In the older child, feel the trachea, palpate cervical nodes, localize the apex beat, and observe chest expansion.

Percussion
Warn the child, e.g. 'I'm going to make you sound like a drum'. Compare right with left. Percuss the upper border of the liver (6th intercostal space anteriorly).

Auscultation
Listen and note the breath sounds and any added sounds. Normal breath sounds are 'vesicular' and fade quickly in the first third of expiration. Breath sounds may be diminished or absent, the expiratory phase may be prolonged, or the sounds may be 'bronchial' rather than 'vesicular'. If bronchial breathing is noted (a sign of consolidation) check for vocal resonance. Ask the child to say '99' while auscultating. The sound is louder over an area of consolidation.

Added sounds include: wheezes (narrowing of intrathoracic airways, usually louder on expiration), crackles (fluid in small airways or alveoli), pleural rub.

Investigations
Imaging, pulse oximetry and blood gas analysis, lung function tests, and bronchoscopy are all important investigations. Imaging modalities include radiography (CXR, CT scan), ultrasound scanning, ventilation–perfusion scan and MRI. However, the CXR is the most common and important investigation.

Paediatric chest radiograph (CXR)

Systematic approach

1 Check patient name, date of birth
Date of radiograph, side marker (left or right).

2 Review
Projection, lung volumes (inspiratory/expiratory), positioning.
- *Projections used:*
  - supine, antero-posterior (AP) for most babies (this projection makes the heart shadow and mediastinum appear larger and makes air or fluid in the pleural space more difficult to detect)
  - erect, antero-posterior (AP) for toddlers
  - erect, postero-anterior (PA) for the older child
- *Lung volumes:* the ideal radiograph is taken at end inspiration, but this is difficult in an uncooperative or tachypnoeic infant. A good inspiratory film should have the anterior 6th rib meeting the mid-diaphragm (Fig 3.5).
- *Positioning:* check for rotation by seeing if the anterior ends of the ribs are equidistant from the spine and clavicles are symmetrical.

3 Systematic review of:
- Lung fields and pleural space
- Trachea, bronchi, and hilar regions
- Superior mediastinum
- Heart and pulmonary vasculature
- Bones (ribs, scapulae, clavicles)
- Tubes, lines, soft tissue shadows.

Lung fields and pleural space
Divide the lung fields into upper, middle, and lower zones and compare the two sides looking for increased translucency (dark) or increased opacification (white).
- *Increased translucency:* symmetrical increased translucency with low flattened diaphragms and narrow cardiothymic shadow indicates hyperinflation or air-trapping. Asymmetrical translucency occurs in localized hyperinflation (e.g. inhaled foreign body) and pneumothorax.
- *Increased opacification:* usually in the lung (consolidation, collapse, oedema) or pleural space (pleural effusion)
  - *consolidation:* inflammatory exudate (or blood) in the alveolar spaces is associated with preservation of lung volume and air bronchograms. It may be lobar or patchy
  - *collapse:* may occur with airway obstruction or extrinsic compression. there is loss of lung volume which may be associated with displacement of horizontal fissure, diaphragm elevation, mediastinal shift, tracheal deviation, or compensatory hyperinflation
  - *oedema:* a 'bats wing' distribution extending from hilar regions with fluid in fissures and interlobular septa
  - *pleural fluid:* pleural fluid produces a generalized hazy opacification in the supine position with lung markings visible through the fluid. An ultrasound examination will confirm and determine the nature of the fluid (effusion, loculated).

Trachea, bronchi, and hilar regions
- A lateral view may reveal subglottic narrowing of the trachea, which may occur in croup or extrinsic compression (e.g. vascular ring).
- Bronchial wall thickening is shown by 'tram track' parallel lines at the hila and is found in asthma and cystic fibrosis.
- Hilar lymphadenopathy is seen in viral pneumonia, cystic fibrosis and if very prominent raises the possibility of TB or malignancy.

Superior mediastinum
The thymus gives rise to an anterior mediastinal shadow in infancy which varies in size and is recognized by the 'sail' shape (right lobe resting on horizontal fissure) and wavy margins. It becomes less evident between 2 and 8 years. Other mediastinal masses are rare: lymphoma, bronchogenic cyst, and neurogenic tumour.

Heart and pulmonary vasculature
The cardiothoracic ratio may approach 60% in the first year and is normally 50% thereafter. Atrial and visceral situs is established by observing cardiac apex, aortic arch and gastric air bubble, all normally on left.

The pulmonary vasculature should be assessed:
- Increased pulmonary blood flow (pulmonary plethora) is characterized by pulmonary artery branches in the peripheral third of the lung.
- Decreased blood flow (pulmonary oligaemia) is characterized by non-visualization of pulmonary vessels centrally.
- Dilated proximal pulmonary arteries with peripheral 'pruning' indicates pulmonary hypertension.

Bones
Check for rib fractures (possible non-accidental injury), the expanded anterior rib ends of a rickety rosary, and the short or broad ribs of skeletal dysplasia.

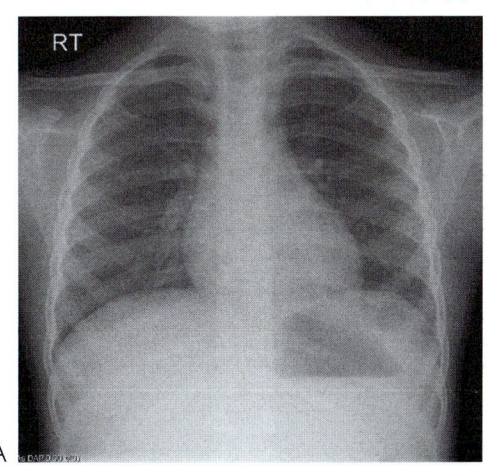

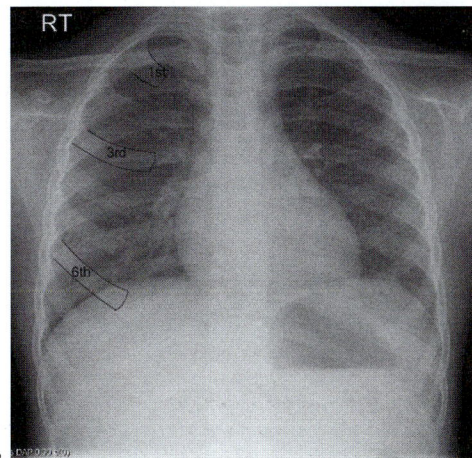

Fig 3.5 A. Normal CXR: good inspiratory film. B. 1st, 3rd, and 6th ribs outlined.

3.3 Ear, nose, and throat (ENT)

ENT disorders encompass several common infections of the upper respiratory tract (acute otitis media, coryza, tonsillitis), conditions affecting respiration during sleep (obstructive sleep apnoea), and a number of rare congenital defects.

Otitis media

Acute otitis media (AOM)
AOM affects an estimated 70% of children by the age of 2 years with a peak incidence between 6 and 24 months.

Aetiology
Risk factors include structural abnormalities of the upper airway that affect drainage of the middle ear via the eustachian tube, e.g. Down syndrome, cleft lip and palate.

Common pathogens include respiratory viruses and bacteria: *Pneumococcus, Haemophilus influenza,* β-haemolytic streptococci, and *Moraxella catarrhalis*.

Clinical features
Young children with AOM often present with non-specific features of fever, irritability, and vomiting. An older child may complain of earache and a younger child may pull at the affected ear or bang their head on the cot.

The tympanic membranes must be examined in every febrile child. In AOM the eardrum may appear injected or bulging with loss of the normal light reflex. A purulent discharge may be present if perforation of the eardrum has occurred.

Complications (mastoiditis, meningitis) are now rare.

Management
Clinical distinction between viral and bacterial AOM is not usually possible although unilateral disease is more likely to be bacterial than is bilateral. Antipyretics and analgesics are recommended in all cases, but decongestants and antihistamines are not indicated.

The use of antibiotics remains a matter for debate, the evidence base being stronger in children >2 years of age. A reasonable approach is to prescribe an oral antibiotic such as amoxicillin for all cases of definite AOM aged <2 years and for children >2 years with severe AOM. Most children >2 years will improve spontaneously and if not severe a policy of delayed antibiotic usage may be adopted, i.e. antibiotics to be collected at parents' discretion if no improvement at 72 h.

Otitis media with effusion (OME)
Recurrent AOM may lead to otitis media with effusion (OME): middle ear effusion without signs of active infection. This was previously called 'glue ear' or chronic secretory otitis media.

OME has a cumulative incidence of 80% by the age of 4 years and like AOM is more common in children with structural ENT abnormalities. It is the most common cause of conductive hearing loss in children. Inspection of the tympanic membrane shows retracted drum and loss of light reflection and hearing assessment a conductive loss of 25–30 dB.

Management
Spontaneous resolution within 3 months occurs in the majority of children but some go on to develop language delay and behavioural problems. Watchful waiting for 3 months is appropriate for children <3 years of age, hearing loss of ≤25 dB and no speech and language or behavioural problems.

Medical therapy including decongestants, mucolytics, antihistamines, antibiotics, and steroids are not of proven benefit.

Children with persistent bilateral OME who are aged >3 years or have speech and language or behavioural problems warrant ENT referral for consideration of surgical options. These include insertion of aeration tubes (grommets), adenoidectomy, or both. The benefits of grommets are not well established, especially after the first year.

Chronic suppurative otitis media (CSOM)
In CSOM there is a chronic middle ear infection with intermittent or persistent ear discharge from a perforated eardrum. ENT assessment is indicated. Two categories are recognized:
- 'Safe' CSOM: central perforation
- 'Unsafe' CSOM: marginal perforation with risk of cranial nerve palsy or intracranial complications.

Coryza, allergic rhinitis, epistaxis

Coryza (common cold)
Corzya is the most common childhood infection and is caused by a variety of viruses: rhinoviruses, coronaviruses, influenza viruses, and respiratory syncytial virus (RSV).

Nasal discharge is accompanied by fever, lethargy, headache, and poor feeding (in infants). Most are self-limiting within 2–3 days. Complications include nasal obstruction which causes breathing and feeding difficulties, especially in young infants who are obligate nose breathers. Infection may spread to the middle ear.

Management is symptomatic, with antipyretics and topical nasal saline drops or decongestant before feeds in young infants.

Allergic rhinitis
Allergic rhinitis is a common feature of atopy. Inflammation of the nasal mucosa is mediated through an IgE-mediated response to allergens and may be seasonal (pollens) or perennial (house dust mite, animal danders).

Clinical features include nasal discharge, itching, excessive sneezing, postnasal drip with cough, nosebleeds, and otitis media with effusions (glue ear). Mouth breathing and snoring with sleep disturbance are common. Nasal polyps are uncommon and their presence should prompt suspicion of cystic fibrosis or primary ciliary dyskinesia.

Management options include avoidance of trigger factors, non-sedating antihistamines, and inhaled nasal steroids.

Epistaxis
Nosebleeds are extremely common and arise in 90% of cases from Little's area where the venous plexus forms on the anterior septum. Acute bleeds result from trauma (e.g. nose picking) but recurrent bleeding should prompt consideration of a bleeding diathesis, especially if there is abnormal bruising or bleeding or a relevant family history.

Bleeding with an offensive discharge may be caused by a retained foreign body. Treatment options for an acute bleed include local pressure or insertion of a nasal pack. Cauterization of a bleeding point may be performed for recurrent bleeding.

Tonsillitis

Inflammation of the mucous membranes and underlying structures of the pharynx and tonsils, usually secondary to viral or bacterial infection, is termed tonsillitis or pharyngitis. Acute tonsillitis is common in children aged >2 years.

Aetiology and pathogenesis

Viral aetiology is more common in younger children. Adenoviruses, influenza A and B, and parainfluenza viruses are common pathogens and Epstein–Barr virus (EBV) is important in older children.

Bacterial pathogens include group A β-haemolytic streptococci (GABH, *Streptococcus pyogenes*). *Corynebacterium diphtheriae* infection is rare in developed countries.

Prognosis is excellent. Post-streptococcal acute rheumatic fever and acute glomerulonephritis are now rare. Recurrent tonsillitis associated with tonsillar enlargement may be associated with obstructive sleep apnoea.

Clinical features

A history of fever and sore throat are the usual presenting features. There may be pain and difficulty in swallowing.

On examination, typical findings include fever and tender cervical lymphadenopathy with moderate to severe pharyngeal erythema and tonsillar enlargement. Erythema may be associated with petechiae, exudates or ulceration. Resistance to neck movement may mimic meningism.

A scarlatiniform rash suggests streptococcal infection and splenomegaly, generalized lymphadenopathy and palatal petechiae suggests EBV infection.

Examination can not be relied on to allow a clear distinction between viral or bacterial aetiology.

Investigations

- *Throat swab:* culture for GABH
- Monospot, EBV IgM
- Antistreptolysin-O antibody titres.

Management

Treatment is supportive for most patients with analgesia and antipyretics (paracetamol) and adequate hydration.

Antibiotic treatment is reasonable in children with marked constitutional disturbance or pus on the tonsils but is not indicated for symptomatic relief only or to prevent sequelae or complications.

Oral penicillin V (or a macrolide if penicillin allergic) is the antibiotic of choice (amoxicillin can precipitate a rash in those with EBV infection).

Recurrent tonsillitis is common and may prompt consideration of adenotonsillectomy. Recurrent URTIs and tonsilllar hypertrophy in themselves are not indications for tonsillectomy as many large normal tonsils will regress spontaneously. However, disabling episodes of sore throat due to tonsillitis occurring 5 or more times over at least a year merit consideration for this operation which has appreciable perioperative morbidity.

Snoring and sleep apnoea

A number of conditions predispose both to snoring and to the obstructive variety of sleep apnoea.

Snoring

Snoring is a sound made during breathing while asleep and is generated by vibration of the soft palate and uvula. It is common: 20% of normal children snore occasionally and up to 10% do so every night. Predisposing factors include:

- *Airway obstruction:* obstruction of nasal passages (by coryza, allergic rhinitis, or anatomical deformity) creates a vacuum in the pharynx during inhalation tending to pull the floppy tissues together
  - adenotonsillar hypertrophy, a large uvula or large tongue obstructs the pharyngeal airway
  - a small jaw, e.g. Pierre Robin sequence or the relatively large tongue in Down syndrome obstructs the airway
- *Muscular hypotonia:* poor muscle tone allows the tongue to fall back. This may occur during deep sleep and is a factor in Down syndrome and Prader–Willi syndrome
- *Obesity:* easily overlooked.

Sleep apnoea

There are three types of sleep apnoea: obstructive, central, and mixed.

Obstructive sleep apnoea (OSA)

This occurs when a snoring child experiences episodes of complete airway obstruction. Increased respiratory efforts (loud snoring) are followed by episodes of apnoea lasting up to 5–10 s and associated with significant hypoxia and hypercapnoea. This is followed by snorting, gasping for air or waking up before normal breathing resumes.

The sequelae of significant OSA include poor-quality sleep and excessive sweating during sleep. Sleep deprivation can lead to daytime somnolence, morning headaches, reduced school performance, and behavioural problems.

Predisposing factors include those listed under snoring. If OSA is suspected a full ENT examination should be combined with sleep studies with monitoring of oxygen saturation, and respiratory movements and heart rate or full polysomnography (EEG, end-tidal CO_2, electro-oculograms, and recording of breathing movements).

Management

This depends on the cause, but options include:

- *Medical:* weight loss, nasal corticosteroids, nasal continuous positive airways pressure (NCPAP)
- *Surgical:* adenotonsillectomy, uvulopalatopharyngoplasty, tracheotomy.

Central sleep apnoea (CSA)

This is uncommon. Congenital central hypoventilation syndrome (Ondine's curse) is caused by mutations in *PHOX2B* or any of five other genes. Secondary central hypoventilation is associated with raised intracranial pressure and hypothalamic disorders.

Mixed sleep apnoea

Children with Prader–Willi syndrome may have obstructive sleep apnoea due to obesity and central hypoventilation.

3.4 Upper airways obstruction: stridor

The narrow lumen of the upper airway in children is vulnerable to obstruction. Small reductions in diameter cause a large increase in airway resistance. Upper airways obstruction may be acute and life threatening. The clinical hallmark is stridor which is usefully classified as acute or chronic.

Acute stridor

Aetiology
The causes include:
- *Infection:*
    acute laryngotracheobronchitis (croup)
    bacterial tracheitis
    epiglottitis, retropharyngeal abscess
- Angio-oedema
- Inhaled foreign body.

Clinical evaluation
History and examination usually allows a clinical diagnosis. The speed of onset is helpful. Croup has a prodrome of several days whereas epiglottitis develops over hours and inhalation of a foreign body presents with sudden choking.

On examination a 'barking' cough suggests laryngeal involvement (croup) whereas drooling and systemic toxicity suggests epiglottitis or bacterial tracheitis.

Severe obstruction is indicated by:
- Stridor at rest: inspiratory and expiratory
- Tachypnoea
- Tracheal tug and subcostal recession
- Tachycardia, pallor, and hypoxaemia.

Investigations such as lateral cervical radiographs are not generally useful and may be dangerous in epiglottitis.

Acute laryngotracheobronchitis (croup)
Croup is a common viral respiratory tract infection and the most common cause of acute upper airways obstruction in children. It affects the age range 6 months to 6 years with a peak incidence in the second year of life.

Aetiology and pathogenesis
Common pathogens include parainfluenza virus, influenzae and adenovirus, and RSV. Recurrent episodes occurring typically at night in atopic children are sometimes designated 'spasmodic' croup. Inflammation affects the larynx, trachea, and bronchi.

Clinical features
Typical viral croup is preceded by 12–72 h of coryza, fever, and cough. The characteristic signs of 'barking' cough and hoarseness (indicating laryngeal involvement) and harsh inspiratory stridor often develop quite suddenly, along with a variable degree of respiratory distress.

High fever or systemic toxicity suggests bacterial tracheitis or epiglottitis and 'croup' under the age of 4 months should raise suspicion of a congenital airway abnormality.

Categorization into mild, moderate, or severe provides a useful guide to management:
- *Mild*: active child, stridor with agitation, minimal increased breathing effort
- *Moderate:* stridor, retractions and decreased air entry
- *Severe:* stridor at rest with expiratory component, marked increased breathing effort: tachypnoea, retractions, agitation, pallor, tachycardia.

Deterioration with severe airways obstruction is accompanied by quieter stridor, hypoxia, and exhaustion

Management
In most children croup is mild and runs a 3 day course, worsening at night and settling during the day. Such cases can be observed at home, the only active management being domestic use of the 'steamy bathroom'.

Treatment for moderate or severe croup includes:
- *Steroids:* oral dexamethasone (0.15 mg/kg) or nebulized budesonide (2 mg) have been shown to be equally effective in treating children with mild, moderate, or severe croup. Steroid use improves clinical parameters, decreases duration of hospital stay and reduces need for nebulized adrenaline. Most children improve within 2 h and relapse is uncommon.
- *Nebulized adrenaline:* use 1 in 1000 (1 mg/mL) adrenaline in a dose of 400 microgram/kg (max 5 mg) in severe croup. Circumoral pallor and tachycardia occur but no serious side effects have been documented. Alpha-receptor mediated vasoconstriction causes decreased mucosal oedema with a duration of action of 20 min to 3 h. Adrenaline buys time for steroids to act or intubation to be organized. A rebound effect can occur and close monitoring is required despite apparent improvement.
- *Humidified oxygen:* guided by saturations.
- *Intubation:* the intubation rate for hospitalized children is 1–2%. The indication is worsening obstruction or impending exhaustion.

Epiglottitis
Epiglottitis in children is usually caused by invasive *Haemophilus influenzae B* (Hib) infection and has become rare in the UK since the introduction of the Hib vaccine in 1992.

Severe oedema of the loose mucosa on the lingual surface of the child's epiglottis causes supraglottic obstruction. Clinical presentation is summarized by the four **D**s:
- **D**ysphagia
- **D**rooling: caused by the painful epiglottis
- **D**ysphonia: soft, muffled voice, soft inspiratory stridor
- **D**yspnoea: supraglottic obstruction.

High fever and systemic toxicity, the older age (1–7 years), short history and absence of a 'barking' cough (no laryngeal inflammation) allows distinction from croup.

This is an emergency as sudden complete airway obstruction may supervene, especially if invasive manoeuvres such as IV access are attempted. Examination under anaesthesia for diagnosis and elective intubation is arranged urgently. Blood cultures are then taken and IV ceftriaxone administered.

Bacterial tracheitis
Bacterial tracheitis is now more common than epiglottitis, except in unvaccinated children. The most common pathogen is *Staphylococcus aureus*. It should be considered in the sick, toxic older child with high fever and stridor. Management includes intubation and systemic IV antibiotics.

Chronic stridor

Persistent stridor is most common in young infants.

Aetiology
Laryngomalacia is the most common cause, but a variety of rare anomalies must also be considered (see Box)
The main clinical entities are considered in turn.

Causes of persistent stridor
Laryngomalacia
External compression: vascular ring
Vocal cord paralysis: unilateral or bilateral
Subglottic stenosis: congenital or acquired
Laryngeal web, haemangiomata, papillomatosis
Hypocalcaemia

Laryngomalacia
Laryngomalacia (literally 'soft larynx') is a congenital disorder in which the supraglottic larynx (the part above the vocal cords) is tightly curled with shortened aryepiglottic folds (bands holding the anterior epiglottis to the posterior arytenoids) creating an 'omega' shape in cross-section.

The upper larynx collapses inwards during inspiration causing partial airway obstruction. It is more common in Down syndrome.

Infants with laryngomalacia have a higher incidence of gastro-esophageal reflux, presumably as a result of more negative intrathoracic pressures.

Conversely, children with gastro-esophegeal reflux may have pathologic changes in the larynx similar to laryngomalacia.

Clinical features
Although the condition is congenital, stridor may not become apparent until 4–6 weeks of age when inspiratory flow rates become high enough to generate airway sounds.

Stridor tends to be worse when the baby is on his or her back, during viral URTIs, and during crying and agitation. It may get louder over the first year as air is moved more vigorously.

The noise is purely inspiratory and the cry is normal unless reflux laryngitis is present An abnormal cry suggests pathology at the vocal cords. Occasional coughing and choking with feeding may be noted if reflux coexists.

Management
This is a benign condition in most (99%) cases with spontaneous resolution by the second year of life as the cartilage hardens. In severe cases, or if the diagnosis is in doubt, further investigations may include:
- *CXR:* right-sided aortic arch in vascular rings
- *Laryngoscopy:* direct visualization of the airway reveals an omega shaped epiglottis that prolapses over the larynx during inspiration.

Treatment
- Anti-reflux treatment is indicated if there is evidence of significant gastro-oesophageal reflux.
- Supplemental oxygen is given for significant hypoxaemia (resting O_2 saturation <90%) as there is a small risk of pulmonary hypertension.
- Surgery (aryepiglottoplasty) is only indicated for severe cases with failure to thrive and/or severe apnoeas.

External compression: vascular ring
Vascular rings are congenital anomalies of the aortic arch and great vessels. Double aortic arch and right aortic arch with left ligamentum arteriosum account for 90% of cases.

Clinical features arise from compression of the airways and oesophagus. Persistent biphasic stridor is associated with feeding difficulties.

A right aortic arch on CXR should raise suspicion of a vascular ring in a symptomatic infant. A barium oesophagram is diagnostic in most cases. Treatment is surgical.

Subglottic stenosis
The subglottic region extends from below the true cords to the lower cricoid cartilage and is the narrowest part of the child's upper airway. Stenosis may be congenital or acquired:
- *Congenital* subglottic stenosis is classified as membranous (submucosal hypertrophy) or cartilaginous (abnormal cricoid cartilage).
- *Acquired* subglottic stenosis is a complication of tracheal intubation and is less common since changes in neonatal ventilation techniques.

Mild to moderate subglottic stenosis may only be manifest when a viral upper respiratory tract infection causes further narrowing. Severe stenosis causes biphasic stridor and dyspnoea.

Plain radiographs, lateral or anteroposterior, demonstrate the narrowing and bronchoscopy confirms the diagnosis. Most cases improve as the child grows. Severe cases may require intubation, tracheostomy and laryngotracheoplasty.

3.5 Pneumonia and pertussis

The overall incidence of lower respiratory tract infection is 30–40 cases per 1000 children per year in the UK. Distinct clinical entities include pneumonia, pulmonary TB, and bronchiolitis. The term 'chest infection' is sometimes used as a synonym but clinical evaluation should allow a more precise diagnosis.

Pneumonia

Pneumonia is an infection of the lower respiratory tract associated with inflammation involving the alveoli. Childhood pneumonia is very common and accounts for up to 3 million deaths annually in developing countries. A community acquired pneumonia (CAP) is a pneumonia in a previously well child due to an infection acquired outside hospital.

Aetiology and pathogenesis

CAP can be caused by a wide variety of pathogens including viruses and bacteria. A microbiological diagnosis is often difficult to establish in clinical practice. The causative organisms are to some extent age-related, with viruses more common in children <5 years and bacteria in children >5 years of age.

In infants and toddlers, viruses account for 90% of lower respiratory tract infections. RSV is most common, but others include adenovirus, influenza, parainfluenza, and metapneumovirus.

The most common bacterial pathogens are *Strep pneumoniae* and *H. influenzae type B* (in unimmunized children). Higher rates of infection with *Mycoplasma pneumoniae* in children >5 years of age have been reported. *Bordetella pertussis*, *Chlamydia trachomatis*, *Staph. aureus*, and *Mycobacterium tuberculosis* can also cause pneumonia.

The distribution of pathological changes varies with pathogen but an alveolar inflammatory exudate with air loss and consolidation is the hallmark. Pneumonia may be lobar or diffuse and patchy with airway involvement (bronchopneumonia). Tidal volume is reduced and ventilation-perfusion mismatch causes hypoxaemia.

Clinical features

Presenting features vary with age, infectious agent, and severity or stage of the illness. Fever, cough, and difficulty breathing are common presenting symptoms, often preceded by signs of a minor upper respiratory tract infection.

Examination
This includes assessment for:
- *Fever:* > 38.5 °C is a feature of bacterial pneumonia
- *Oxygenation:* cyanosis indicates severe illness. Pulse oximetry identifies significant hypoxaemia (SaO_2 <92% in air)
- *Respiratory rate:* tachypnoea is a useful indicator of pneumonia. Rates defined by the WHO provide a 74% sensitivity for radiologically defined pneumonia:

Age	
<2 months	>60 breaths/min
2–12 months	>50 breaths/min
>12 months	>40 breaths/min

- *Work of breathing:* chest recession, nasal flaring and grunting are most sensitive in children aged <3 years.
- *Percussion and auscultation*

Dullness to percussion indicates either consolidation if there is bronchial breathing or a pleural effusion if breath sounds are diminished. Crackles on inspiration are a sign of pneumonia. Wheeze may be heard if there is bronchial inflammation and narrowing.

It may be difficult to distinguish viral from bacterial pneumonia but certain clinical features provide an indication of causal organism:
- Fever >38.5 °C, recession and tachypnoea >50 breaths/min in a child <3 years suggests a bacterial pneumonia.
- Conjunctivitis (or history of sticky eyes) in infants <3 months with prominent cough suggests *Chlamydia trachomatis*.
- Wheeze and hyperinflation from airway inflammation is more commonly seen in viral or mycoplasma infection.

Staphylococcal pneumonia is uncommon in developed countries but more likely in an infant, post-measles or varicella, in cystic fibrosis and if abscesses or pneumatocele are present. Pneumonia can be overlooked in certain circumstances:
- Infant with features of generalized sepsis but no respiratory signs
- Absence of tachypnoea early in illness (first 3 days)
- Children with co-morbid conditions e.g. asthma
- Abdominal pain caused by diaphragmatic irritation, especially in right lower lobe pneumonia.

Initial management

Many infants and children with a diagnosis of lower respiratory tract infection including CAP are managed at home with fluids, antipyretics and oral antibiotics if a bacterial cause is suspected. Indications for hospital admission are:
- Oxygen saturation < 92% in air
- *Respiratory rate:*
  - > 70 breaths/min in infants
  - > 50 breaths/min in older children
- *Signs of breathing difficulty:* recession, nasal flaring, grunting, apnoea
- Not tolerating oral feeds and signs of dehydration
- *Social concerns:* family unable to provide support.

Investigations

Most clinicians undertake investigations to confirm the diagnosis and clarify aetiology, although the published evidence base for their usefulness is surprisingly weak. Investigations to consider include:

Full blood count and acute phase reactants
Total leukocyte and neutrophil count, C-reactive protein, and ESR have poor sensitivity and specificity for distinguishing between viral and bacterial pneumonia.

Microbiological investigations
- *Blood cultures:* the yield is low and a positive result takes 48–72 h. Positive in 10–15% of patients with pneumococcal pneumonia.
- *Respiratory tract samples:* sputum for culture is rarely available and samples are frequently contaminated. Nasopharyngeal aspirate (NPA) for viral immunofluorescence assay or PCR is useful in infants. Bronchoscopy or pleural fluid aspiration may provide samples.

- *Serology:* paired serology 14 days apart is available for diagnosis of mycoplasma but treatment is usually given on empirical grounds.

Imaging

- *CXR:* the appearance of consolidation on CXR is reliable for the diagnosis of pneumonia (Fig 3.6) but CXR appearances are not reliable for distinguishing between viral and bacterial infection as there is considerable overlap. The CXR may appear normal early in the disease. However, as an approximate guide:
  - *viral pneumonia:* patchy perihilar infiltration, hyperinflation, atelectasis
  - *bacterial pneumonia:* lobar consolidation (air bronchogram) occasionally with parapneumonic effusion. pneumatocoele and abscesses suggest staphylococcal pneumonia
  - *mycoplasma pneumonia:* patchy, segmental consolidation with hilar lymphadenopathy.

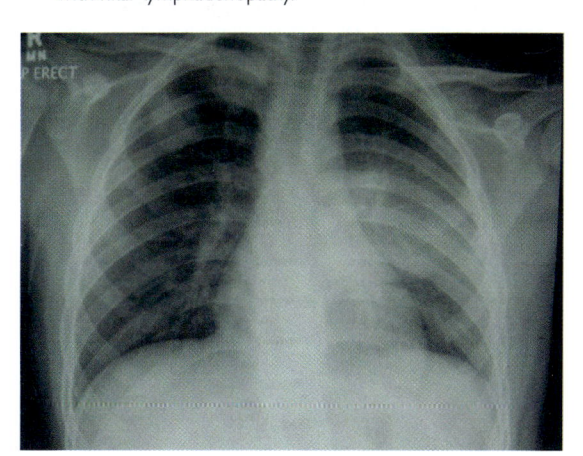

Fig 3.6 Lobar pneumonia: CXR left lower lobe.

- *Ultrasound:* this is most useful if a pleural effusion is suspected on CXR. It can differentiate between clear fluid and fibrino-purulent effusions
- *CT scan:* provides more detailed imaging of suspected abscess or empyema.

Treatment

As viral and bacterial pneumonia are often difficult to distinguish treatment including use of antibiotics is based on age and severity.

Treatment may include:
- *Oxygen:* to maintain SaO_2 >92%
- *Fluids:* restrict to 80% maintenance as hyponatraemia secondary to inappropriate ADH secretion is common.
- Antipyretics
- Antibiotics:
  - <5 years: amoxicillin is first choice oral antibiotic, alternatives include co-amoxiclav and macrolides
  - >5 years: a macrolide (erythromycin, clarithromycin or azithromycin) is the first choice oral antibiotic as mycoplasma infection is more likely.

Oral antibiotics are safe and effective for many children with CAP, but in severe cases with sepsis, consolidation with effusion, failed response or intolerance to oral antibiotics IV treatment is indicated with a third-generation cephalosporin (e.g. cefuroxime) or ampicillin. A change to oral antibiotics can then be made if there is clear improvement. Treatment duration is between 5 and 10 days depending on severity.

- *Physiotherapy:* not indicated in the normal child.

Complications

Most children with CAP improve without complications, but an unexplained trend of increased complications of bacterial pneumonia has been seen worldwide. Treatment failure (antibiotic resistance), lung abscess, metastatic infection, and pleural infection (effusion or empyema) are all recognized complications.

Pleural effusion or empyema

Persistent or recurrent fever after 48 h treatment for pneumonia should raise suspicion of a parapneumonic effusion or empyema (Fig 3.7). An AP or PA CXR and ultrasound should allow diagnosis and evaluation of the nature of pleural fluid.

A small unloculated effusion may resolve with IV antibiotics alone. A diagnostic pleural tap is usually unnecessary. A large loculated empyema with obvious pus and thickened pleura will require drainage.

Options include a pigtail chest drain with intrapleural fibrinolytics, video-assisted thoracoscopic surgery (VATs) or early mini-thoracotomy following chest CT scan.

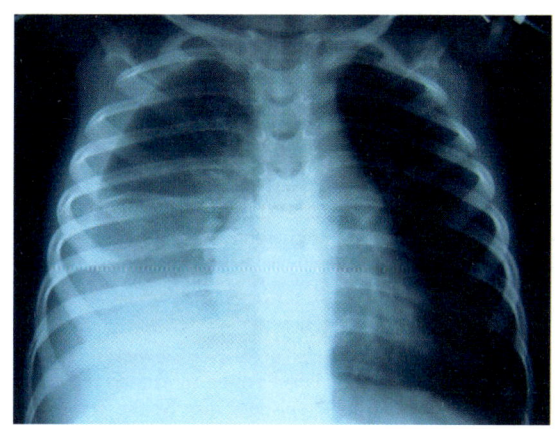

Fig 3.7 Empyema: CXR right hemi-thorax.

Prevention

The new pneumococcal conjugate vaccine will reduce the rate of pneumonia and offers protection against most drug resistant strains.

Pertussis (whooping cough)

Pertussis is a respiratory tract infection characterized by paroxysmal cough associated with inspiratory whoop. It is caused by infection with *Bordetella pertussis*. In the UK vaccination programmes provide up to 90% protection.

- An early catarrhal stage is followed by the paroxysmal cough which can persist for up to 12 weeks (the 'hundred day cough').
- The incidence is highest <5 years of age and infants <12 months are more severely affected. Apnoeas and cyanotic episodes are more frequent and complications can include pneumonia, encephalopathy and bronchiectasis.
- Diagnosis is confirmed by culture *of B. pertussis* on a per-nasal swab. A lymphocytosis may be associated.
- Oral erythromycin eradicates carriage and reduces spread but does not alter the course of the illness.

3.6 Bronchiolitis and pulmonary tuberculosis

Bronchiolitis

Bronchiolitis is an acute viral lower respiratory tract infection associated with inflammation of the small airways (bronchioles). It occurs primarily in babies aged 2–12 months.

Bronchiolitis is common with an annual incidence of 11% <1 year and 6% in those aged 1–2 years. Incidence peaks at age 2–8 months. 75% of cases occur in infants <1 year and 95% in children <2 years. Bronchiolitis is slightly more common in boys. Peak incidence occurs during the winter months in temperate climates and the rainy season in tropical climates.

Aetiology and pathophysiology
RSV is the most common pathogen (75%) but other viruses which cause a similar clinical picture include adenoviruses, influenza and parainfluenza viruses, and human metapneumovirus which tends to affect older infants. RSV is highly infectious and spreads by contagion as well as droplets.

Initial infection is confined to the upper respiratory tract but spreads to the lower respiratory tract occurs in 40% where infection of bronchiolar respiratory and ciliated epithelial cells causes increased mucus secretion, cell death, and sloughing followed by lymphocytic infiltration around the bronchioles and submucosal oedema.

Mucus secretion, debris, and oedema cause narrowing of the small airways with ventilation/perfusion mismatching and hypoxia. Dynamic narrowing of airways during expiration causes air trapping and increased end-expiratory lung volume with decreased lung compliance causes increased work of breathing. Recovery of pulmonary epithelial cells begins to occur after 3–4 days.

Clinical features
Coryza and low-grade fever progress over a few days to cough and difficulty breathing as inflammation spreads to the lower respiratory tract. Apnoeic episodes may be the presenting feature in infants <6 weeks of age.

Examination
Findings vary with stage and severity but typically include:
- Low grade fever 38.5–39 °C
- Hypoxaemia
- Tachypnoea >50–60 breaths/min
- Nasal flaring, intercostal recession, cough
- Diffuse bilateral inspiratory crackles and expiratory wheeze
- Palpable liver (hyperinflation depresses the diaphragm).

Management
Diagnosis is often straightforward especially during epidemics. Useful investigations include:
- *CXR*: findings are non-specific and include hyperinflation, patchy infiltration, focal atelectasis. It is not routinely indicated but useful in severe cases or if diagnosis uncertain.
- *Nasopharyngeal aspirate* for direct fluorescent antibody test for RSV. Sensitivity 87–91% and specificity >96% for RSV and other common respiratory viruses. PCR.
- Pulse oximetry.

Treatment is supportive and depends on severity. In many infants this is a mild, self limiting illness and can be managed at home.

Risk factors for more severe disease include:
- Infants <8 weeks
- Infants born at <35 weeks gestation
- Chronic lung disease of prematurity
- Congenital heart disease.

Hospital admission is advisable if risk factors are present or there is clinical evidence of moderate or severe disease such as SaO_2 <94% in air, respiratory rate > 60 breaths/min with recession, and poor feeding.

Management may then include:
- *Oxygen*: administered via nasal cannulae, face mask, or head box
- *Fluids*: oral feeds, nasogastric tube or IV fluids depending on severity. Fluid restriction to avoid hyponatraemia is advisable in severely affected infants.
- Apnoea monitoring
- *Nasal continuous positive airways pressure (NCPAP)*: this reduces work of breathing and aids oxygenation in severely affected infants or those at risk
- *Intubation and assisted ventilation*: severely ill infants (1% of hospital admissions) may require assisted ventilation in an ICU.

A respiratory rate >60 breaths/min and FiO_2 requirement >60% are indicators of an infant at risk of respiratory failure. Capillary blood gas estimation for $PaCO_2$ may guide PICU referral.

Infants should be isolated or cohorted. There is no evidence to support the use of physiotherapy, steroids, nebulized bronchodilators (β_2 agonists, ipratropium), nebulized adrenaline, or ribavirin.

Complications
Otitis media is common. Secondary bacterial infection can occur and antibiotics should be considered if an infant deteriorates with high fever, toxic appearance and focal lobar infiltrates on CXR.

Prognosis
Most children, regardless of severity, recover within 7–10 days. There is an association between RSV bronchiolitis and subsequent wheezing illness in childhood. It remains unclear whether this is causal (by selective promotion of helper T cell subsets) or whether children genetically predisposed to wheezing are more likely to develop bronchiolitis. Reinfection can occur despite the presence of serum antibodies.

Prevention
Palivizumab, a monoclonal antibody against RSV, is effective as prophylaxis against RSV bronchiolitis.

A course of IM injections at intervals of several weeks is given and is currently recommended in at-risk groups such as infants with chronic lung disease of prematurity on home oxygen.

Pulmonary tuberculosis (TB)

TB remains one of the major diseases afflicting children with an estimated 1 million new cases annually About 60% of cases are in infants and children <5 years and rates increase again in late childhood and adolescence. TB is also discussed in Chapter 15.12.

Aetiology and pathogenesis

Infection is acquired by inhalation of *Mycobacterium tuberculosis* in airborne mucous droplets from an adult with pulmonary TB. The tubercle bacilli multiply within the alveoli and alveolar ducts and depending on the subsequent course of events this leads either to tuberculous infection or tuberculous disease. Confusingly, the term 'tuberculosis' is often used for both these states.

Tuberculous infection

The primary complex consists of local reaction in the lung parenchyma and inflammatory reaction in the hilar lymph nodes. The child is often asymptomatic. Tuberculin sensitivity develops over 3–12 weeks. Most have a normal CXR.

Tuberculous disease

Early haematogenous dissemination leading to miliary TB or TB meningitis occurs in only 0.5–2% of infected children. Pulmonary tuberculous disease may develop. Enlarging nodes cause partial bronchial obstruction or erode through the bronchus transmitting infection to the lung parenchyma. A combination of collapse and consolidation generates segmental lesions. Extrapulmonary disease develops in about 30% of cases (e.g. cervical lymphadenopathy).

Clinical features

Tuberculous infection

Most children develop no signs or symptoms following infection although transitory fever, cough, malaise may occur.

Tuberculous disease: pulmonary

The clinical manifestations of intrathoracic pulmonary TB disease are often subtle and tend to vary with age of onset. Infants and adolescents are likely to have significant symptoms and signs whereas school-age children are often clinically silent.

Infants may have cough, tachypnoea, and failure to thrive. Older children and adolescents are more likely to develop adult-type classical features of fever, malaise, weight loss, night sweats, and productive cough.

Management

Diagnostic investigations

- *Diagnosis of TB infection* hinges on the demonstration of a positive tuberculin skin test. Diagnosis of *TB disease* is based on CXR changes and the tuberculin skin test. Definitive diagnosis by histology or culture of *M. tuberculosis* is often difficult in children and is not a prerequisite for the initiation of treatment (see below).
- *Tuberculin sensitivity (Mantoux test):* Purified protein derivative is inoculated intradermally and read 48–72 h later. The area of induration (not erythema) is measured. The threshold size for positivity is:
  - *15 mm:* child >4 years with no risk factors
  - *10 mm:* child <4 years with risk factor
  - *5 mm:* immunosuppressed or history of TB contact
  Sensitivity is reduced in young or malnourished children or HIV co-infection. It takes up to 12 weeks to develop.
- *CXR:* radiographic hallmarks include hilar lymphadenopathy and segmental lesions of collapse and consolidation.
- *Microbiology:* acid-fast stain and culture of sputum is optimal, but sputum is rarely available from young children. Early morning gastric aspirates x 3 (to capture sputum swallowed overnight) should be sent for AFB stain and culture, and PCR if available. Culture positivity may take 6 weeks.
- *Biopsy:* biopsy of a lymph node or pleura may provide typical histology of granuloma and material for culture.

Treatment

Treatment with anti-TB drugs is given for children with evidence of TB disease. The standard regimen is an initial phase of 2 month treatment with isoniazid, rifampicin, and pyrazinamide followed by a continuation phase of 4 months isoniazid and rifampicin. Ethambutol is included only if the risk of isoniazid resistance is high. Longer treatment may be necessary for resistant organisms.

Chemoprophylaxis is given for infants or children exposed to a risk of infection or who have evidence of latent infection. Isoniazid and rifampicin are given for 3 months.

Diagnosis of a case of childhood tuberculous disease should precipitate contact tracing and screening.

Respiratory infection in the immunocompromised host

Pulmonary infection is a common presenting feature of immunodeficiency.

Aetiology and pathogenesis

Immunodeficiency is considered in detail in Chapter 15.5. Acquired causes are most common and include treatment with myelosuppressive or immunosuppressive drugs. Primary immune deficiencies are genetic and may predominantly affect humoral or cellular immunity or both. Primary ciliary dyskinesia interferes with the ciliary defence mechanisms of the respiratory epithelium.

Clinical features

Immunocompromise should be considered if any of the following features are present. Several occur in cystic fibrosis, a diagnosis which should be considered first.

- Chronic cough *without wheeze*
- Pulmonary suppuration/recurrent pneumonia
- Bronchiectasis
- Recurrent sino-pulmonary infection
- Respiratory infection with unusual pathogens.

Additional features may be present: a family history of immunodeficiency, consanguinity, failure to thrive, invasive infections in more than one system, hepatosplenomegaly.

Management

Initial screening investigations should include:

- Full blood count and WCC differential
- Lymphocyte subsets
- Immunoglobulin levels, IgG subclasses
- Tetanus, HiB and pneumococcal antibodies (>2 y)
- CXR.

Treatment depends on cause.

3.7 Asthma

Asthma is a chronic inflammatory disorder of the small airways characterized by recurrent episodes of cough and wheeze. The incidence has increased in recent years and asthma now affects 10–15% of school-age children in the UK.

Aetiology and pathogenesis

Asthma is caused by an interaction between genetic and environmental factors. Family and twin studies demonstrate that asthma is inherited as a multifactorial trait.

Asthma genes

Multiple genes have been implicated in the causation of asthma and asthma-related traits (ASRT). ASRT include atopy, atopic dermatitis (eczema), and endophenotypes such as bronchial hyper-responsiveness and serum IgE levels.

Environmental triggers

Episodes of acute asthma, as well as chronic inflammation, are provoked by a number of factors including: respiratory infections (viral infections including rhinoviruses, bacterial infections e.g. *Mycoplasma pneumonia*, and aspergillosis), allergens (household inhalants, animal dander, house dust mites, seasonal outdoor allergens: pollens, grass); irritants: (tobacco smoke, cold air), weather changes (in atmospheric temperature, pressure and humidity), exercise, and emotional factors.

In addition, gastro-esophageal reflux can increase airway reactivity, mediated via vagal or other reflexes. Allergic rhinitis or sinusitis may aggravate asthma. Variation in allergen exposure, posture-related irritation, respiratory drive, and circadian variation in lung function and inflammatory mediator release may all contribute to nocturnal asthma.

Airway inflammation

Imbalance between populations of Th1 and Th2 lymphocytes is proposed to have a central role. Th1 cells are critical in responses to infection whereas Th2 cells generate a family of cytokines (IL-4, IL-5, IL-13) that mediate allergic inflammation. The 'hygiene hypothesis' suggests that asthma arises when reduced environmental exposure to infection fails to activate Th1 responses with persistence of the newborn skew towards Th2 cytokine generation.

Inflammation leads to airway narrowing on account of mucus secretion, mucosal oedema and bronchial hyper-reactivity with bronchospasm.

Clinical features

The diagnosis of asthma is clinical. It is usually straightforward but can be difficult in younger children (<2 years).

History

The history is of recurrent episodes of cough, difficulty in breathing and wheeze. Note that parents may use the term 'wheeze' for any noise associated with breathing and this is a potential source of confusion. Cough may be the only symptom, especially in exercise-induced or nocturnal asthma. The presence of other features of atopy or a family history of atopy or asthma is supportive evidence. Enquiry should be made about seasonal or circadian variation in symptoms, pets, and parental smoking habits.

Examination

Physical findings in between acute exacerbations varies with severity. In mild asthma examination is normal. In moderate or severe asthma there may be signs of hyperinflation (increased antero-posterior chest diameter) and chronic obstruction with recession (Harrison sulci). Features of atopy (allergic rhinitis, eczema) may be present.

Auscultation may reveal prolongation of the expiratory phase, expiratory wheezing or unequal breath sounds. Finger clubbing is not a feature of chronic asthma.

Examination during an acute phase reveals findings which vary depending on whether the episode is mild, moderate or severe:
- *Mild*: tachypnoea, end expiratory wheeze, SaO_2 >95% in air
- *Moderate*: tachypnoea, use of accessory muscles, suprasternal retraction, wheeze expiratory and inspiratory, SaO_2 reduced to 92–95% in air, tachycardia, ± pulsus paradoxus
- *Severe*: as above; pulsus paradoxus often present, SaO_2 <92% in air.

As respiratory muscle fatigue supervenes wheezing may diminish as airflow lessens (the 'silent chest'), pulsus paradoxus disappears, and hypoxaemia may cause bradycardia.

Differential diagnosis

'All that wheezes is not asthma'. A number of conditions cause chronic respiratory symptoms similar to those of asthma and alternative diagnoses to consider include:
- *Upper airway disease*: rhinitis, sinusitis, adenotonsillar hypertrophy, postnasal drip
- *Viral bronchitis*: recurrent episodes of viral associated wheezing are common in infants <2 years
- *Gastro-esophageal reflux* with recurrent aspiration
- *Congenital anomalies*: structural disease of bronchi (cysts, webs) vascular rings, H-type fistula, bronchomalacia
- *Chronic bronchial sepsis*: cystic fibrosis, primary ciliary dyskinesia, immunodeficiency
- *Pulmonary TB*: bronchial compression by lymph nodes.

Signs raising suspicion of an alternative diagnosis include clubbing, weight loss, productive cough, upper airway disease (adenotonsillar hypertrophy, nasal polyps), severe chest deformity, asymmetric wheeze, stridor. Foreign body inhalation and cardiac failure can mimic acute asthma.

Investigations

The only investigations required in the initial work-up are CXR and measurement of peak expiratory flow rate (PEFR). The typical CXR findings include hyperinflation and increased bronchial markings. A CXR is also helpful in excluding alternative diagnoses such as congenital anomalies, pulmonary TB and inhaled foreign body.

The PEFR in L/min can be measured with a handheld device (in children >5 years) and gives an indication of large airway obstruction.

Average PEFR (l/min) = $(5 \times \text{height in cm}) - 400$

Additional investigations at specialist centres may be helpful if there is diagnostic uncertainty or failure to respond to therapy:
- *Spirometry*: is possible in children aged >5 years and should show an obstructive defect in asthma: decreased FEV_1, FEF_{25-75} and FEV_1/FVC ratio (<80%) and a concave flow-volume loop.

- *Allergy testing:* eosinophil counts and IgE levels may help if allergic factors are prominent. Skin prick testing can be undertaken for suspected allergens.

Medical care

Non-pharmacological measures

Primary prophylaxis

Breast-feeding should be encouraged as it confers a protective effect in relation to wheezing in infancy. Parents who smoke should be offered support to stop.

Secondary prophylaxis
- *Allergen avoidance:* house dust mite control measures are recommended in families with evidence of mite allergy, including complete barrier bed-covering systems and regular washing of bedlinen. Avoidance of exposure to animal allergens, particularly cats and dogs, in those with evidence of allergy.
- *Environmental factors:* exposure to tobacco smoke contributes to the severity. Parents who smoke should be advised of the dangers and offered support to stop.
- *Dietary manipulation:* weight reduction if obese.

Pharmacological management

This includes control of chronic symptoms and treatment of acute asthmatic episodes. These are considered in turn:

Chronic asthma

A stepwise approach is adopted according to British Thoracic Society guidelines. High level therapy may be initiated to establish prompt control followed by a 'step-down' to the minimum therapy necessary for adequate control. Short-acting B2 agonist bronchodilators are used for quick relief.

Step 1: *mild intermittent asthma*
Inhaled short-acting β_2 agonist as required.

Step 2: *mild persistent asthma*
Add regular preventer therapy: low dose inhaled steroid 200–400 micrograms/day. initiated if inhaled b2 agonists are being used more than a few times per week (consider montelukast in <2 years age group).

Step 3: *moderate persistent asthma*
Increase to medium dose regular inhaled steroids of 400 micrograms/day or add on regular LABA in combination with inhaled steroid and/or leukotriene receptor antagonists.

Step 4: *severe persistent asthma*
Increase inhaled steroid to high dose up to 800 micrograms/day. Consider alternate day prednisolone.

Step-down treatment when good control achieved.

Inhaler devices
- *Nebulizers:* can be used at any age and have the advantage that oxygen can be delivered simultaneously if used as the driving gas.
- *Pressurized metered dose inhalers (PMDIs):* are used with a spacer device in children under about 9 years of age and with a spacer and a mask <4 years. Dry powder inhalers can be used from age 5–6 years.

Acute asthma

The mainstays of treatment are oxygen, bronchodilators and steroids. The strategy is determined by the severity of the asthma and the response to initial measures. Episodes are categorized into mild, moderate, severe and life threatening. A number of general principles apply:
- *Bronchodilator delivery by inhalation:* PMDIs in combination with large volume spacers are as effective as nebulizers in most children. However, < 2 years a nebulizer may be preferred and in moderate to severe asthma there may be insufficient inspiratory flow to move the spacer valve.
- *Steroids:* if indicated, steroids should be given as early as possible. Intravenous and oral steroids are equally effective and begin to work within 3–4 h.
- *Oxygen:* oxygen should be given to maintain measured SaO_2 > 95%. Significant hypoxia may preclude the use of spacers initially.

Treatment according to severity is as follows:
- **Mild:** inhaled salbutamol up to 10 puffs (100 micrograms/puff) via a spacer or 2.5–5.0 mg in 5 mL via a nebulizer. Reassess after 20 min and repeat if needed.
- **Moderate:** inhaled salbutamol: up to 10 puffs (100 micrograms/puff) via a spacer or 2.5–5.0 mg in 5 mL via a nebulizer. Reassess and repeat inhaled salbutamol as required.
  - Oxygen to keep SaO_2 >95%.
  - Oral prednisolone 1–2 mg/kg
- **Severe:** inhaled salbutamol 0.15 mg/kg in 5 mL via a nebulizer given continuously (i.e. ~6 nebulizations/h). Add ipratroprium bromide to third and sixth nebulizer and every 4 h thereafter.
  - Oxygen to keep SaO_2 > 95%
  - IV Hydrocortisone 4 mg/kg 6 hourly
  - IV 0.45% saline, 5% dextrose at 2/3 maintenance

If response to inhaled bronchodilators is poor, IV bronchodilators are the next step. The rationale is that severe bronchoconstriction is preventing inhaled medication reaching its site of action. Options include salbutamol, aminophylline, and magnesium sulfate.

- *Salbutamol:* a bolus of 15 micrograms/kg (>2 years, maximum 250 micrograms) is given over 10 min and is probably best followed with an infusion (1–5 micrograms/kg per minute). Monitor for hypokalaemia.
- *Aminophylline:* a loading dose (if no theophylline given in preceding 24 h) of 5 mg/kg (max 500 mg) over 30 min followed by an infusion (1 mg/kg per hour). Side effects: arrhythmias, convulsions, vomiting, and hypotension.
- *Magnesium sulfate:* a dose of 50 mg/kg (max 2 g) is given over 30 min with blood pressure and ECG monitoring and can be repeated after 12 h. Hypotension is a potential side effect.

If fatigue and exhaustion supervene with inadequate oxygenation and a silent chest, adequate control may be re-established with mechanical ventilation.

3.8 Cystic fibrosis

Cystic fibrosis (CF) is the most common severe autosomal recessive genetic disorder in white people. It is a multisystem disorder characterized by chronic respiratory tract infections and pancreatic enzyme insufficiency.

The carrier rate in whites is 1 in 25 giving an incidence of 1/2500 live births. There are approximately 7000 patients with CF in the UK, about half of whom are adults. Life expectancy is 30–40 years with up to 80% of children now surviving into adulthood. Females are generally more severely affected than males.

Aetiology and pathogenesis

Genetics
CF is caused by mutations in the *CFTR* (cystic fibrosis transmembrane conductance regulator) gene. Over 1000 different mutations have been identified, the most common of which is ΔF508, accounting for 76% of affected chromosomes in the UK. Five classes of mutation are recognized on the basis of their effect on CFTR protein function.

CFTR structure and function
CFTR is a glycoprotein with 1480 amino acids. The protein is found in epithelial cells of the airways, ducts of the pancreas, sweat glands and biliary system, and the vas deferens.

The protein has five domains: two membrane-spanning domains (MSD1 and MSD2) each connecting to a nucleotide binding fold (NBD1 and NBD2) in the cytoplasm, and a single regulatory R domain (Fig 3.8).

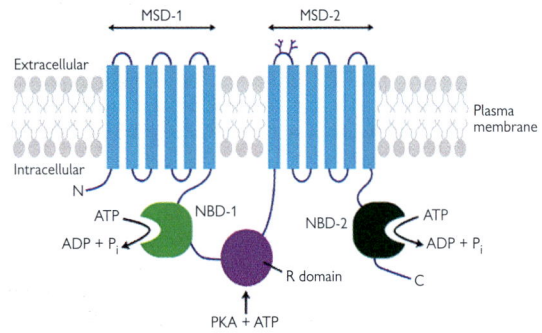

Fig 3.8 Structure of CFTR protein. After Expert Reviews in Molecular Medicine, courtesy of Cambridge University Press.

CFTR functions as a chloride channel which is activated by phosphorylation of the R domain and binding of ATP to the two NBFs. Activation also results in opening of adjacent outwardly rectifying chloride channels (ORCC) and closure of epithelial sodium channels.

Pathogenesis of cystic fibrosis
Loss of function of CFTR leads to decreased secretion of chloride and increased reabsorption of sodium and water across epithelial cells. This results in viscid secretions in the respiratory tract, pancreas, gastrointestinal tract, sweat glands, and other exocrine tissues.

Respiratory tract
There is defective chloride secretion and excess reabsorption of sodium and water. The airway surface liquid (ASL) is reduced in thickness allowing viscid mucus to contract and inhibit ciliary function. This leads to a cycle of chronic infection and inflammation with lung damage.

Gastrointestinal tract, pancreas, and liver
- *Pancreas:* 85% of patients with CF have pancreatic insufficiency (PI) which arises from reduced bicarbonate secretion (disturbing optimal pH for pancreatic enzymes), reduction of water content of secretions, and plugging of ductules and pancreatic acini. Pancreatitis may occur.
- *Gastrointestinal tract:* defective CFTR function leads to reduced chloride and water secretion into the gut. This causes meconium ileus at birth and distal intestinal obstruction syndrome in later life.
- *Liver:* reduced CFTR function in epithelial cells lining the biliary ductules leads to increased bile viscosity and plugging of biliary ductules. This may cause obstructive cirrhosis, portal hypertension, and hypersplenism. Gallstones and cholecystitis are more common in CF.

Sweat ducts
CFTR dysfunction leads to failure of chloride and sodium reabsorption from the sweat ducts. The resulting high sweat salt content forms the basis of the diagnostic sweat test.

Vas deferens
Most males are azoospermic because of agenesis of the vas deferens. Mild mutations in CFTR can cause isolated congenital bilateral absence of the vas deferens (CBAVD).

Clinical features
CF may be diagnosed prenatally or by newborn screening (see below). The classical presentation is with recurrent chest infections, failure to thrive, and steatorrhea but the spectrum of disease is wide. A minority (10%) present in the newborn period with meconium ileus. The presenting features according to system are:

- *Respiratory tract:* chronic or recurrent cough; recurrent lower respiratory tract infections, atypical asthma, recurrent wheezing, recurrent sinusitis, nasal polyps
- *Gastrointestinal, pancreatic, and hepatobiliary tracts:*
  - neonatal: CF may present with intestinal obstruction at birth due to meconium ileus (7–10% of patients with CF), volvulus or intestinal atresia. Passage of meconium may be delayed and there may be prolonged cholestatic jaundice.
  - Infants and children: failure to thrive, flatulence, recurrent abdominal pain and abdominal distension. Malabsorption of fats is accompanied by steatorrhea (frequent, foul smelling, bulky stools). Intussusception and rectal prolapse may occur.

On examination
Physical signs depend on systems involved and progression of the disease and may include:

- *Respiratory system:* rhinitis, sinusitis and nasal polyps, clubbing, cyanosis, increased AP diameter of chest, cough, tachypnoea and recession, wheezes or crackles on auscultation.
- *Gastrointestinal tract:* signs of malnutrition: low weight, anaemia, dry skin (vitamin A deficiency) skin rash (zinc deficiency), abdominal distension, hepatosplenomegaly, rectal prolapse.

Management

Diagnostic investigations

Sweat test

The sweat test remains the first-line diagnostic test in suspected CF. The quantitative pilocarpine iontophoresis test is preferred. A minimum of 100 mg of sweat should be collected on to filter paper for estimation of sweat chloride and sodium. Sodium should not be interpreted without a chloride result. The following definitions are used for interpretation:

- Negative (normal) test: Cl^- <40 mmol/L
- Borderline (suggestive) test: Cl^- 40–60 mmol/L
- Positive (supportive) test: Cl^- >60 mmol/L.

Sweat tests can be performed after 2 weeks of age in infants weighing >3 kg who are normally hydrated. A sweat test should be repeated to confirm positive results and if negative in the presence of strongly suggestive clinical features.

There are several rare conditions which give a false positive sweat test including adrenal insufficiency, ectodermal dysplasia, glycogen storage disease, and familial hypoparathyroidism.

Genotyping: DNA analysis

CFTR analysis for ΔF508 and up to 30 other mutations is widely available, accounting for up to 90% of all CF mutations in a particular population. Detection rate is lower in non-white populations and children with atypical disease or borderline sweat chloride levels. A negative result reduces the likelihood of CF but does not exclude it.

Baseline investigations

- *Imaging:* CXR shows hyperinflation and peribronchial thickening initially. These progress to patchy infiltration and atelectasis, bronchiectasis and marked hyperinflation.
- *Microbiology:* sputum culture/cough swab. The most common bacterial pathogens are Staphylococcus aureus, Pseudomonas aeruginosa, Klebsiella pneumonia, Burkholderia cepacia, and Haemophilus influenzae.
- *Blood tests:*
  - full blood count, coagulation screen, immunoglobulins
  - urea and electrolytes, liver function tests
  - vitamin A, D, and E levels.

Treatment

The main aims are to prevent progression of lung disease, maintain adequate nutrition, monitor for and treat complications, and provide psychological support.

Respiratory

- *Physiotherapy:* twice daily physiotherapy comprising postural drainage and percussion in infants and children and independent airway clearance devices with deep breathing exercises in older children. Regular physical exercise should be encouraged.
- *Antibiotics:* most UK centres start prophylactic oral flucloxacillin at diagnosis. Acute infections are treated with antibiotics to which the organisms are sensitive and may require one or more antibiotics given PO, IV, or by inhalation. Ciprofloxacin given orally is effective against most organisms encountered. In patients colonized with P aeruginosa oral azithromycin three times per week or aerosolized antibiotics (gentamicin, colomycin, tobramycin) given long term may reduce infective exacerbations.
- *Mucolytics:* neutrophil-derived DNA increases sputum viscosity. DNAase increases mucociliary clearance and improves lung function.
- *Inhaled bronchodilators and steroids:* bronchial hyperactivity with reversible airway obstruction is present in 30% of CF patients and may benefit from treatment with bronchodilators and steroids.

Nutrition

- *Pancreatic enzymes:* pancreatic insufficiency is present or develops in 90% of patients and is treated with oral pancreatic enzyme supplements e.g. Creon, containing lipase, amylase, and protease in enteric-coated microspheres within a gelatin capsule. The current recommended dose is 10 000 units lipase/kg daily. Excessive dosage may be associated with fibrosing colonopathy.
- *Proton pump inhibitors:* may compensate for defective pancreatic bicarbonate secretion and increase efficacy of pancreatic enzyme supplements.
- *Vitamin supplements:* regular supplements of fat soluble vitamin (A, D, E, K) are required.
- *Diet:* a high-fat, high-calorie diet is recommended to meet the above average energy requirements and compensate for malabsorption. Continuous overnight enteral feeding via a nasogastric tube or gastrostomy may be necessary.

Management of complications

Increased long-term survival is accompanied by an increased rate of complications including:

- *Gastrointestinal:* distal intestinal obstruction syndrome (DIOS), hepatic cirrhosis, cholecystitis, gallstones
- *Respiratory:* haemoptysis, cor pulmonale
- *Metabolic:* glucose intolerance and insulin-dependent diabetes mellitus, bone disease. Heat stroke.
- *Reproductive:* delayed puberty and reduced fertility are common. Most males are azoospermic but female fertility is only mildly impaired.
- *Psychological:* psychological and emotional support is essential for children and parents.

New management strategies

Lung transplantation can enhance quality of life and prolong survival. Decisions about the need for transplantation should be addressed well in advance: CF patients have reasonable post-transplant survival rates (50% at 5 years). An FEV1 of <30% predicted is associated with a 50% 2 year mortality and is used as one benchmark for referral. Gene therapy trials are still under way.

Prenatal diagnosis and screening

Prenatal diagnosis can be offered to mothers with a family history. Carrier screening is offered in families of an affected child and is offered in some centres to mothers booking in early pregnancy.

Newborn screening: all newborn infants in the UK are now offered screening for CF by measurement of immunoreactive trypsinogen (IRT) as part of the existing blood spot screening programme. Mutation analysis is carried out in infants with IRT > 99.5th centile. Evidence of benefit is strongest for nutritional and cognitive effects.

3.9 Chronic lung disease, bronchiectasis, and sequelae of neurodisability

Significant structural damage to the lungs may be a sequela of preterm birth, chronic lung disease of prematurity, or suppurative lung infection, bronchiectasis. The respiratory consequences of neuromuscular disorders such as muscular dystrophy are often a primary determinant of mortality.

Chronic lung disease of prematurity

Chronic lung disease (CLD) is a general term for long-term respiratory problems in infants born preterm. It was previously known as bronchopulmonary dysplasia (BPD). It affects up to 50% of VLB (<1500 g) babies.

Aetiology and pathogenesis

The exact aetiology is uncertain but a combination of the following factors acting on the immature lung have a role:
- *Mechanical ventilation:* alveolar barotrauma and volutrauma causing deranged alveologenesis
- *Oxygen use:* high concentrations of oxygen can cause damage by oxygen free-radicals
- Surfactant deficiency.

Normal lung development is disturbed and activation of inflammatory cascades cause inflammation and scarring. Secondary pulmonary vascular dysfunction may lead to pulmonary hypertension.

Risk factors for CLD include:
- *Preterm birth:* <34 weeks gestation, birthweight <2000 g
- Respiratory distress syndrome (surfactant deficiency)
- Mechanical ventilation and supplemental oxygen
- Pulmonary interstitial emphysema
- Persistent patent ductus arteriosus
- White, male infants.

Clinical features

Diagnostic criteria vary, but most definitions include:
- Use of positive pressure ventilation in first 2 weeks of life for at least 3 days
- Requirement for supplemental oxygen after 28th day of life or 36 weeks post conceptual age
- *Clinical signs of abnormal respiratory function:* tachypnoea, recession, inspiratory crackles, and expiratory wheeze
- *CXR:* characteristic bilateral, diffuse changes, with hyperexpansion, atelectasis and pulmonary interstitial emphysema

Management

Preventive measures include administration of prophylactic steroids to mothers at risk to reduce risk of neonatal RDS, early surfactant administration, management of ventilation to avoid barotrauma and hyperoxia.

Treatment varies according to the stage of the disease. In an infant with persistent hypoxia and difficulty weaning from ventilation, diuretics (furosemide) may provide short-term improvements in lung function.

Long-term treatment includes:
- Supplemental oxygen
- Bronchodilators and inhaled steroids
- Prophylaxis of RSV infection with palivizumab
- Optimization of nutrition
- Emotional support for parents.

Most infants can be weaned from oxygen by the end of their first year. Lung function tends to improve slowly throughout childhood.

Bronchiectasis

Bronchiectasis was originally used as a morphological term to describe dilatation of bronchi with destruction of elastic and muscular components of their walls. It is now used to describe both clinical and radiological disease entities. The advent of high-resolution CT scanning (HRCT) has improved diagnosis.

Aetiology and pathogenesis

Cystic fibrosis is the most common cause. Other causes of non-CF bronchiectasis include:
- Idiopathic
- *Post pneumonia:* accounts for 30%, especially pertussis, measles
- Immunodeficiency with recurrent infection
- Recurrent aspiration
- *Airway obstruction:* intraluminal (foreign body) or extrinsic compression
- Primary ciliary dyskinesia.

The exact pathogenesis remains uncertain. The initial trigger is often infective, setting up a vicious cycle of impaired mucociliary clearance and recurrent infection. Persistent endobronchial infection causes bronchial wall thickening that progresses to bronchial dilatation which may regress or persist and become irreversible. This may be exacerbated by immunodeficiency or anatomical lung abnormalities. Pneumonia in the first year appears more likely to have bronchiectasis as a sequela.

Clinical features

The diagnosis should be considered in a child with a daily productive cough for >6 weeks. In infants and toddlers the cough is 'loose' and followed by swallowing. Haemoptysis is the second most common symptom. The most common misdiagnosis is *'difficult to control asthma'*.

Examination may be normal. Crackles and wheeze on auscultation are the most common physical signs. Digital clubbing is a feature of bronchiectasis with pulmonary suppuration.

Diagnosis

A normal CXR does not exclude bronchiectasis. Diagnosis is established using HRCT, which has a sensitivity and specificity of 90%. Diagnostic HRCT features include bronchi with internal diameter larger than the accompanying artery (signet sign), non-tapering bronchi, and airways visible in the extreme lung periphery.

Investigations to establish the cause include:
- Sweat test for CF
- Full blood count
- Ig levels, IgG subclasses
- Specific antibodies to tetanus toxoid, HiB, pneumococcus
- Nasal brushings for ciliary beat frequency and electron microscopy
- Bacterial culture of sputum or bronchoalveolar lavage (BAL) fluid
- Assessment for aspiration.

Treatment
In addition to treatment of any underlying disorder, medical measures include chest physiotherapy and long term antibiotics on a rotating basis. Surgical resection may be beneficial for severe, well localized disease.

Neurodisability
Children with severe neurological impairment and complex disability have a high incidence of respiratory problems. Pneumonia is a common cause of death.

Aetiology and pathogenesis
The causes of respiratory difficulties in children with cerebral palsy (CP) and neuromuscular disease are multifactorial and include:
- Recurrent aspiration: associated with oesopharyngeal motor problems and gastro-oesophageal reflux.
- Poor cough and airway clearance
- Weakness of respiratory muscles
- Thoracic cage deformity: kyphoscoliosis
- Sleep apnoea
- Bronchial hyper-reactivity (BHR)

These are considered in turn:

Recurrent aspiration
Aspiration may be 'from above' caused by disturbance of the complex choreography involved in swallowing, or 'from below' caused by gastro-oesophageal reflux (GOR). Failure of proper bolus formation, glottic closure, and coordination of swallowing and breathing leads to aspiration especially of thin liquids. GOR is caused by spasticity of abdominal muscles (increasing abdominal pressure) and incoordination of oesophageal and sphincter muscle activity. Recurrent aspiration leads to recurrent infection and chronic inflammation of lower airways and may also provoke apnoea and laryngeal spasm in infants.

Poor cough and airway clearance
The cough mechanism is often unsatisfactory and the cough reflex may be insensitive. This leads to poor protection of and inadequate clearance of lower airway secretions.

Weakness of respiratory muscles
This is a problem in spinal cord lesions and neuromuscular disorders (SMA, Duchenne). Intercostal muscles are affected first, followed by diaphragmatic weakness. Hypoventilation occurs first during sleep. In spinal lesions problems depend on the level and completeness of the lesion.

Thoracic cage deformity: kyphoscoliosis
Kyphoscoliosis is common because of the effects of gravity and asymmetrical muscle tone. Lung function is compromised and unequal lung expansion can cause ventilation/perfusion mismatch.

Sleep apnoea
Obstructive sleep apnoea (OSA) is common in children with CP and pseudobulbar palsy. The pharynx fails to stiffen just before diaphragmatic contraction, causing collapse during inspiration. Failure to thrive and pulmonary hypertension may result. Central sleep apnoea may be a feature of myotonic dystrophy, and in the Chiari malformation central and obstructive apnoea may occur.

Bronchial hyper-reactivity (BHR)
Asthma is common and may coexist with cerebral palsy. In addition, recurrent aspiration and bronchiectasis are associated with bronchial hyper-reactivity.

Clinical features
Significant respiratory problems may be silent or go unnoticed because of difficulties in communication with a disabled child and the limited repertoire of responses. An experienced parent or carer may be acutely sensitive to problems in their child. The common presentations are:
- *Recurrent lower respiratory tract infections*: a feature of recurrent aspiration and bronchiectasis
- *Noisy breathing*: bronchial hyperactivity, obstructive sleep apnoea
- *Chronic cough*: recurrent asthma, bronchial hyper-reactivity, bronchiectasis
- *Apparent life threatening episodes (ALTEs)*: aspiration, GOR, obstructive sleep apnoea
- *Respiratory failure during respiratory infections*: reduced reserve with respiratory muscle weakness, scoliosis

Management
Investigations obviously depend on the precise diagnosis but may include:
- *Imaging*: CXR, CT scan, videofluoroscopy
- *Lung function tests*: these maybe difficult in a disabled child
- *Overnight oximetry* is a useful screening tool for OSA.

Treatment options may include:
- Trial of anti-reflux therapy, speech therapy input, nasogastric or gastrostomy feeding. Surgical fundoplication
- Trial of bronchodilators and/or inhaled steroids
- Trial of prophylactic antibiotics during winter
- Respiratory support: trial of nasal mask CPAP in children with Down syndrome or cerebral palsy and OSA (not improved by adenotonsillectomy). Early institution of nasal mask bi-level positive pressure support is advisable in type II spinal muscular atrophy and in patients with Duchenne muscular dystrophy. The extent of treatment in the event of deterioration is best discussed in advance in children with progressive disease. Consent to intervention is obviously problematic in children with communication difficulties.

3.10 Case-based discussions

A child with acute stridor

An 11 month old infant presents to the emergency department with noisy breathing and a harsh 'barking' cough in the early hours of the morning. Over the past 3 days he has had rhinorrhea, low grade fever, and a mild cough. Past medical history is unremarkable. He is fully immunized.

On examination:
- Alert but tired. Temperature 38.0 °C, HR 130/min
- He has a sealion-like barking cough and episodic stridor on inspiration. There is a marked tracheal tug and chest wall recession. He is not toxic and there is no drooling.
- RR 45/min, oxygen saturation 92% in room air.
- Breath sounds are generally reduced on auscultation.

What is the likely diagnosis?
Acute viral laryngotracheobronchitis (croup) is the most probable diagnosis. The characteristic barking cough, stridor, and respiratory distress are often preceded by cough and coryzal symptoms. Deterioration during the night is typical, perhaps because mouth breathing during sleep dries out secretions. The barking cough is a key indicator of laryngeal inflammation, which does **not** occur in epiglottitis.

What is your immediate management?
The diagnosis is made clinically and no investigations are required. Radiographs of the chest or neck are not indicated. The degree of upper airway obstruction is moderate to severe and there is an oxygen requirement. Hospital admission is indicated.

Humidified oxygen should be given by face mask to maintain oxygen saturations >95%.

In the hospital setting, treatment with steroids should be considered. Steroids have been shown to reduce the rate and duration of hospitalization and intubation, the rate of return to medical care and the duration of symptoms in children with mild, moderate, and severe symptoms. Oral dexamethasone or nebulized budesonide are both effective and he is given a single dose of oral dexamethasone.

Two hours after admission his condition deteriorates with an increased oxygen requirement, continuous stridor, and signs of exhaustion.

What is your continuing management?
A minority of children with croup develop severe airways obstruction requiring intubation. The anaesthetic and ENT teams on call should be alerted to his condition and nursing should be in a high dependency unit.

Nebulized adrenaline can give a temporary improvement in airway obstruction by shrinking oedematous inflamed airway membranes. Onset of action is rapid but the effect may be transitory.

Nebulized adrenaline is given and his condition improves.

He continues to improve and by breakfast time is in air with minimal stridor and normal vital signs.

A girl with persistent cough

A girl aged 17 months presented with a 1 month history of worsening cough accompanied by wheezing. Two courses of antibiotics from the GP had been given with no effect. Her appetite had diminished and her mother had noted undigested food in the stools. Further questioning revealed a persistent cough since birth. Her mother smoked 20 cigarettes a day and there was a strong family history of asthma. She was the first child of unrelated white parents.

Her birth weight was 2300 g at 39/40 gestation and there were no perinatal problems.

On examination:
- Weight 7.2 kg, << 0.4th centile
- Apyrexial. RR 40/min. No recession. Bilateral scattered wheeze.

What is the most likely diagnosis?
The combination of persistent cough and failure to thrive makes cystic fibrosis an important diagnosis to exclude. Asthma and the effects of passive smoking are possible explanations of persistent cough, but failure to thrive and stool abnormalities would not be expected.

What investigations are indicated?
A full screen for failure to thrive including immunoglobulin levels and CXR. A sweat test is required to exclude cystic fibrosis.

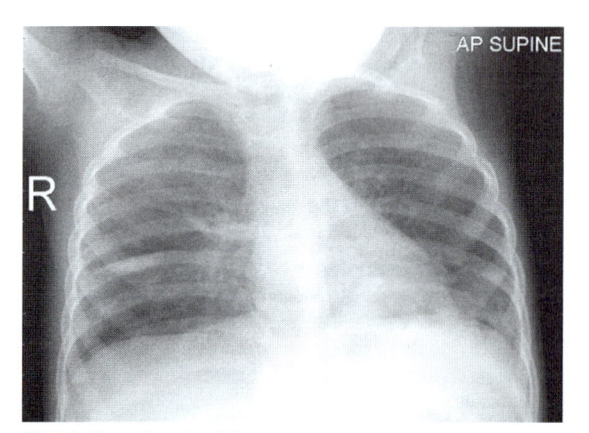

Fig 3.9 Cystic fibrosis: CXR.

All investigations were normal except for:
- *CXR: bilateral patchy linear shadowing (Fig 3.9)*
- *Sweat test: sodium 97 mmol/L, chloride 118 mmol/L*
- *Repeat test: sodium 102 mmol/L, chloride 117 mmol/L*

What is the management?
The diagnosis of CF was later confirmed by DNA analysis which revealed that she was homozygous ΔF508. She was started on Creon, vitamin supplements (Dalivit, vitamin E), prophylactic oral flucloxacillin, and twice daily physiotherapy. Her parents were offered genetic counselling.

Chapter 4
Cardiology

- 4.1 Basic and clinical cardiology 74
- 4.2 Cardiac investigations 76
- 4.3 Congenital heart disease 78
- 4.4 Acyanotic heart defects: left-to-right shunts 80
- 4.5 Acyanotic heart defects: obstructions 82
- 4.6 Cyanotic heart defects 84
- 4.7 Rheumatic fever and Kawasaki disease 86
- 4.8 Infective endocarditis, myocarditis, and pericarditis 88
- 4.9 Cardiomyopathy and arrhythmias 90
- 4.10 Case-based discussions 92

4.1 Basic and clinical cardiology

Embryology and anatomy

Cardiac development
The cardiovascular system (CVS) develops from the mesodermal germ layer and is the first major system to function in the embryo. The primordial heart and vascular system appear in the 3rd week of gestation and the heart functions from the beginning of the 4th week.

The critical period of heart development is from the 4th to 7th weeks of gestation, during which time the heart becomes partitioned into four chambers. As the pharyngeal arches form during the 4th and 5th weeks they are penetrated by the aortic arches arising from the aortic sac.

Anatomy: nomenclature
The complex developmental abnormalities of cardiac anatomy can be described in a number of ways. In Europe an approach designated 'segmental and sequential' has been adopted, based on morphological description of heart chambers rather than their embryology or anatomical position.

Any cardiac anomaly can then be described by characterizing the following features:

Visceroatrial situs

The term 'situs' means position or site and the normal arrangement is called 'situs solitus'. This encompasses normal arrangement of the left and right atria and normal asymmetry of the abdominal viscera and a trilobed right and bilobed left lung.

Abnormalities include:
- *Situs inversus*: mirror image arrangement of atria, bronchi, and abdominal viscera
- *Situs ambiguus*: liver in midline with either *right* isomerism (with asplenia) or *left* isomerism (with polysplenia). Various cardiac defects, bowel malrotation and biliary atresia may be associated.

Atrioventricular (AV) connections
- *Concordant*: left atrium to left ventricle, right atrium to right ventricle (the normal arrangement)
- *Discordant*: left atrium to right ventricle, right atrium to left ventricle
- *Univentricular*: one ventricle functionally, with many different subtypes. The practical implication of this is that repair to form a biventricular circulation is often not possible.

Ventriculoarterial (VA) connections
- *Concordant*: the normal arrangement
- *Discordant*: transposition of the great arteries
- *Double outlet*: both great vessels arise from the same ventricle
- *Single outlet*: a common trunk (truncus arteriosus)
- *Atresia*: either the aortic or pulmonary valve is not patent.

Circulatory physiology

Circulatory changes at birth
This is considered in detail in Chapter 1.1. In the fetus the placenta is the organ of gas exchange and most blood bypasses the lungs by shunting 'right to left' through the foramen ovale and ductus arteriosus. At birth the lungs become the organ of gas exchange and the following circulatory changes occur:

- *Pulmonary vasodilatation*: this causes a fall in pulmonary vascular resistance which occurs rapidly in the first few breaths and continues until 3 months of age
- Closure of the foramen ovale as a result of increased pulmonary venous return and left atrial pressure
- Closure of the ductus arteriosus, ductus venosus and umbilical arteries.

Cardiac output
Cardiac output is determined by stroke volume and heart rate. Factors influencing stroke volume are:
- *Preload*: the degree to which the ventricle is stretched before contraction. This depends on venous pressure, length of diastole, and the force of atrial contraction.
- *Myocardial contractility*: this is enhanced by sympathetic or inotropic drive and may be reduced by metabolic or electrolyte imbalance and intrinsic myocardial dysfunction.
- *Afterload*: this is determined by systemic resistance and reflects aortic and peripheral vascular resistance.

Cardiac failure
This occurs when the cardiac output no longer meets the metabolic demand of the body. The aetiology in infants and children includes pressure overload, volume overload, myocardial dysfunction and rhythm abnormalities (see Table 4.1).

Table 4.1. Aetiology of cardiac failure	
Pressure overload	Obstructive lesions: left sided, e.g. coarctation of aorta, hypertension (Critical left heart obstruction with circulatory collapse is most important cause in the newborn)
Volume overload	Left-to-right shunts, e.g. VSD, PDA (Failure occurs after the neonatal period as the fall in pulmonary vascular resistance leads to increase in shunt volume) Valvular regurgitation A-V malformation, e.g. giant haemangioma
Myocardial dysfunction	Myocarditis Cardiomyopathy Sepsis, ischaemia, acidosis Pericardial effusion/cardiac tamponade
Cardiac arrhythmias	Tachycardia: of supraventricular, junctional, or ventricular origin Bradycardia, e.g. complete (3rd degree) heart block

Clinical cardiology

Paediatric heart disease presents in diverse ways, from the severely ill newborn requiring intensive care to the asymptomatic child with a murmur heard on routine examination.

Natural changes in cardiovascular physiology often determine the timing of presentation of structural heart disease, e.g. ductal closure in critical left-sided obstructive lesions; the fall in pulmonary vascular resistance in left-to-right shunts.

History

Key features include details of pregnancy and birth, a family history of congenital heart disease, and cardiac symptoms which vary with age (Table 4.2):

- *Infants:* central cyanosis, symptoms of cardiac failure: breathlessness, sweating, or fatigue on feeding and poor weight gain; circulatory collapse with hypotension and acidosis
- *Children:* palpitations, dizziness/syncope on exertion, exercise limitation, and (very rarely) chest pain.

Table 4.2. Common cardiac symptoms: differential diagnosis

Chest pain	Musculoskeletal: 'stitch', costochondritis (*very common*)
	Psychogenic: anxiety, panic attacks (*very common*)
	Gastrointestinal: oesophagitis, retrosternal or epigastric pain (*common*)
	Respiratory: pleuritic pain, tightness in asthma, sickle crisis
	Nervous system: shingles (*rare*)
	Cardiac:
	    pericardial (central, sharp, worse when supine)
	    ischaemic (crushing, radiation to neck, jaw, arms)
	    induced by exercise (*very rare*)

Palpitations	Awareness of benign ectopic beats Sinus tachycardia: anxiety, anaemia, hyperthyroidism Cardiac arrhythmia: sudden stop and start and associated with pallor, chest pain, dyspnoea or syncope. May be of supraventricular, junctional, or ventricular origin.
Syncope	Vasovagal syncope (faint): *very common* Cardiac arrhythmia: most commonly associated with exercise, occurs without warning (*very rare*)

Examination

Inspection
Growth/stature, central cyanosis, dysmorphology, clubbing (after infancy), breathlessness, scars. Pulse oximetry is part of examination as mild desaturation is difficult to detect clinically, especially in Asian or Afro-Caribbean children.

Palpation
Check four limb pulses are equal, assess volume, character, rate, regularity; blood pressure; precordial palpation: locate apex beat, note presence of heaves and thrills.

Auscultation
- *Heart sounds*: First heart sound caused by closure of mitral and tricuspid valves. Second sound (S2) generated by closure of aortic (A2) and then pulmonary (P2) valves. A2–P2 interval widens during inspiration. P2 is loud in pulmonary hypertension. S2 is widely split and fixed with an atrial septal defect and right bundle branch block. S2 is single in aortic or pulmonary atresia, transposition of great arteries, truncus arteriosus and severe pulmonary stenosis.
- *Ejection click* with aortic or pulmonary stenosis, bicuspid aortic valve, truncus arteriosus
- *Third or fourth heart sound* (gallop rhythm) in cardiac failure.

Murmurs
A murmur should be assessed for:
- *Intensity:* (grades 1–6); >3/6 have a palpable thrill
- *Timing:* systolic (early, mid, late or pan systolic), diastolic (early, middle, late) or continuous (begins in systole, carries on through S2 into diastole)
- *Character:* harsh, vibratory, blowing or scratchy
- *Location:* where it is heard loudest
- *Radiation:* to the back, axillae, neck, sides of chest.

Causes of specific murmur types include:
- *Early to mid-systolic:* innocent (Still's type) murmur (vibratory or musical quality)
- *Mid-systolic (crescendo-decrescendo, ejection):* generated by turbulent flow in ventricular outflow tracts e.g. aortic or pulmonary stenosis, ASD, tetralogy of Fallot
- *Pansystolic:* (lower left sternal edge); VSD, tricuspid regurgitation (rarer); apex, mitral regurgitation
- *Early diastolic:* aortic or pulmonary regurgitation
- *Mid-diastolic:* anatomic or relative stenosis of mitral or tricuspid valve; low-frequency murmurs
- *Continuous:* patent ductus arteriosus, Blalock–Taussig shunt, venous hum, coarctation of the aorta.

Innocent murmurs
Audible in the absence of an anatomical abnormality, occur in ≥80% of normal children at some point in childhood, and are brought out or accentuated by febrile illness. Usually systolic and quiet with no associated symptoms and an otherwise normal cardiovascular examination. They include:

- *Still's murmur:* usually preschool child, mid-systolic, vibratory, loudest between lower left sternal edge and apex, better heard supine and with the bell
- *Venous hum:* continuous, best heard at the upper sternal edge sat upright, inaudible supine and with unilateral pressure on the neck
- *Pulmonary flow murmur:* in neonates, physiological flow across a branch pulmonary artery accounts for a significant proportion of systolic murmurs; in adolescents, may be a mid-systolic murmur at the upper left sternal edge
- *Carotid bruit:* heard over neck/supraclavicular fossa.

Echocardiography is mandatory if clinical uncertainty exists (particularly in infants and teenagers).

Signs of cardiac failure
Signs of cardiac failure are a result of:
- *Increased sympathetic drive:* tachycardia, pallor, sweating
- *Myocardial failure:* gallop rhythm, ventricular heave, poor peripheral perfusion, hepatomegaly, pulmonary congestion with tachypnoea and crepitations.

Signs of the underlying aetiology may also be apparent.

4.2 Cardiac investigations

Chest radiography (CXR)
The appearance of the cardiac silhouette and lung fields can be a useful guide diagnostically. However, a normal CXR does not exclude major congenital heart disease. The most common use now is to assess heart size and pulmonary vascularity.

Cardiac silhouette
The radiographic position of normal right and left heart structures are shown in Figs 4.1–4.2 and characteristic CXR findings in congenital heart disease are considered with each lesion.
A globular heart may indicate a pericardial effusion. The position of abdominal viscera, heart, cardiac apex, aortic arch, and bronchial/lung morphology should also be defined.

Lung fields
- *Pulmonary plethora:* left-to-right shunts, transposition of great arteries, pulmonary venous engorgement of any cause. (See Fig 4.3.)
- *Oligaemia:* reduced pulmonary blood flow is seen in tetralogy of Fallot, Ebstein's anomaly, pulmonary hypertension. (See Fig 4.4.)

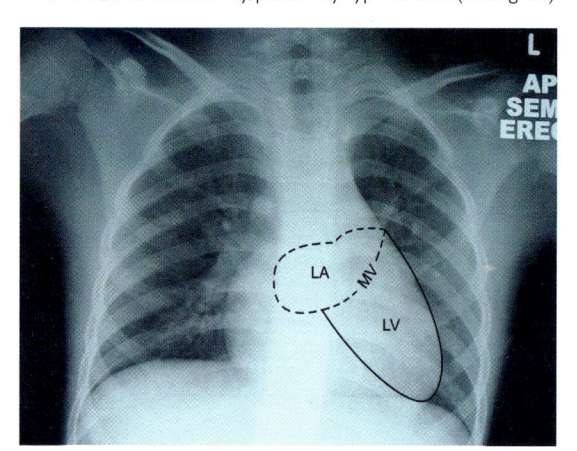

Fig 4.1 Position of left heart structures: normal CXR. LA, left atrium; MV, mitral valve; LV, left ventricle.

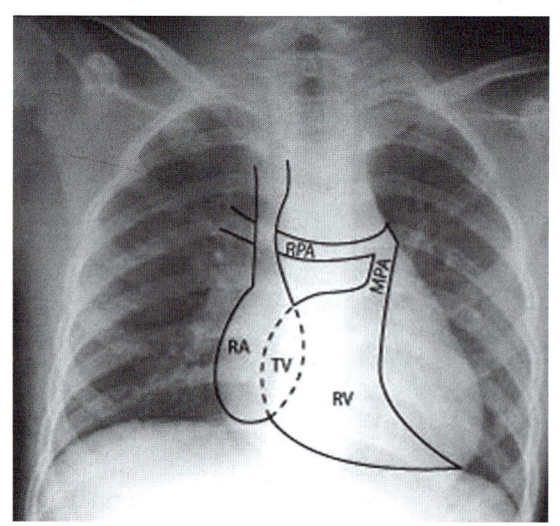

Fig 4.2 Position of right heart structures: normal CXR. RA, right atrium; TV, tricuspid valve; RV, right ventricle; MPA, main pulmonary artery; RPA: right pulmonary artery.

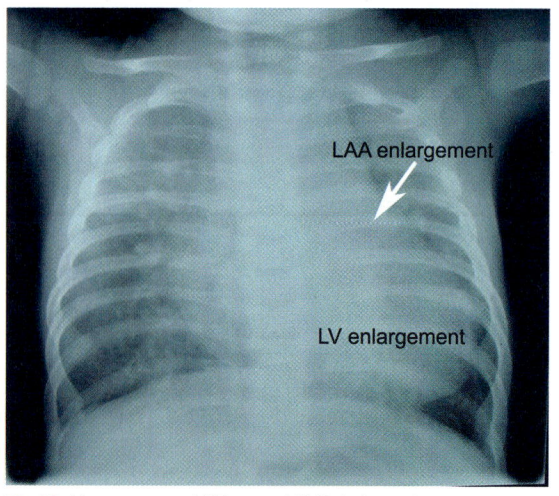

Fig 4.3 Non-restrictive VSD: typical CXR. Left atrial appendage and LV enlargement with increased pulmonary vascular markings.

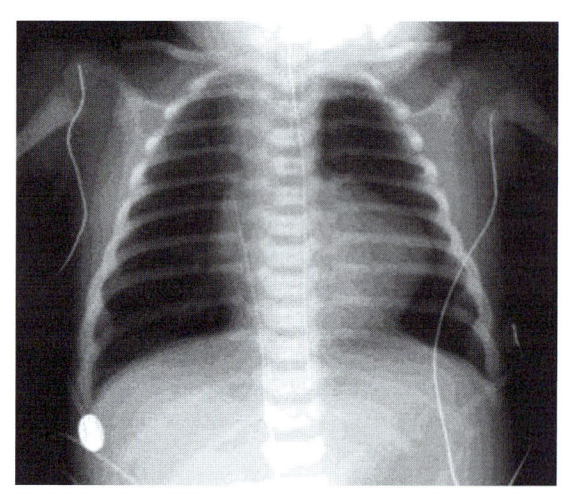

Fig 4.4 Tetralogy of Fallot: typical CXR appearances. Decreased pulmonary vascular markings, boot-shaped heart and a concave main pulmonary artery segment.

Echocardiography
Ultrasound of the heart in a child or fetus outlines cardiac anatomy and function and can include Doppler estimation of intracavitary pressure and transvalvar pressure gradients. Types include transthoracic, transoesophageal, intra-cardiac and fetal (maternal transabdominal). Transoesophageal echo is particularly useful in providing a clearer view of posterior heart structures in larger adolescents, e.g. atrial septum.

Cardiac catheterization
Increasingly sophisticated echocardiography is diminishing the need for 'diagnostic' catheterization. Up to 80% of catheterization procedures are now 'interventional', a development that has revolutionized the treatment of congenital heart disease (CHD). See Section 4.3.

Catheterization facilitates the measurement of local O_2 saturation and pressure and the calculation of pulmonary and systemic vascular resistance. Normal right-sided O_2 saturations are 60–70%, left-sided are typically 95–100%. A change in saturations between atrium and ventricle on either side may indicate a shunt.

LV systolic pressure should be same as measured arterial BP, and RV pressure approximately 25% of LV pressure.

Electrocardiography (ECG)

Normal changes in cardiac physiology between fetal life and childhood are reflected in the ECG, particularly the switch from right ventricular to left ventricular dominance over the first 12–18 months of life. In addition, the chest wall becomes thicker and the normal heart rate slows.

Age-related changes include:

- QRS axis: changes from a range of +60° to +190° at birth to +10° to +100° at 1 year
- T wave: upright in VI at birth but inverts by 48 h and remains inverted to age 7–10 years
- PR interval: increases with age
- QT interval: longest in infancy, decreases from 6 months, shortens with tachycardia.

A standard ECG is recorded at 25 mm/s (5 large squares/s) and a voltage of 10 mm/mV. 300 large squares is 1 min and rate is calculated by 300/R–R interval in large squares. Each small square is 0.04 s or 40 ms.

Interpretation should follow a systematic approach:
1 Rate
2 Rhythm
3 P wave morphology and axis
4 Mean QRS axis
5 QRS complexes
6 T waves and ST segments
7 Intervals PR and QT

- *Rate:* typically 140/minute at birth, 120/m at 1 year and 100/m at 5 years. Sinus tachycardia rarely exceeds 180–200/m except in severely ill young infants.
- *Rhythm:* in sinus rhythm a P wave precedes each QRS complex and the P wave is upright in leads I and aVF.
- *P wave:* wide biphasic P waves > 120 ms indicate left atrial enlargement and peaked P waves ≥3 mm in any lead indicate right atrial enlargement.
- *Mean QRS axis:* the mean frontal QRS axis is determined graphically (Fig 4.5) by plotting net RS deflection for lead I and aVF. A dominant S wave in aVF (a 'superior' axis) strongly suggests structural cardiac disease.

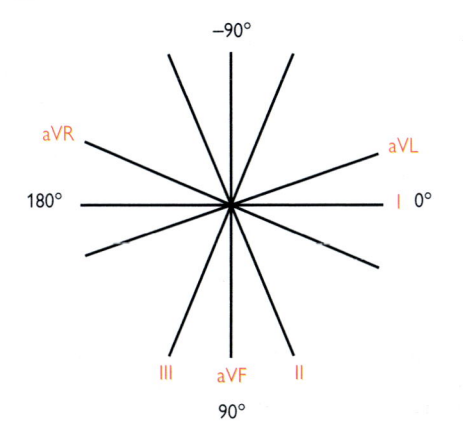

Fig 4.5 Hexaxial reference system for mean QRS axis. (See 'How to read paedietric ECGs', Park M, for complete account).

- QRS complexes: normal duration increases with age. Increased R and S wave amplitudes indicate right or left ventricular hypertrophy, with tall R waves in leads 'viewing' the hypertrophied ventricle and deep S waves in the inverse leads. A slurred R wave upstroke (delta wave) suggests an accessory pathway and PR interval is usually shortened. QRS duration >80–120 ms can be either right or (more rarely) left bundle branch block and indicates structural (usually postoperative) heart disease or heart muscle disease.
- *T waves and ST segments:* persistence of an upright T wave in VI beyond 48 h of age up to 7 years indicates right ventricular hypertrophy. Hyperkalaemia causes high-voltage, tent-shaped T waves; simple inversion occurs in leads V4–V6 in myocarditis. ST segment elevation may occur in pericarditis and depression in myocardial damage.
- *PR interval* (start of P wave to start of QRS complex): normal range in children is 0.08–0.19 s (2–4 small squares).
  - short PR interval: pre-excitation termed Wolff–Parkinson–White syndrome if accompanying arrhythmia (may be isolated or accompanying Ebstein's malformation, Pompe disease)
  - long PR interval (1st degree heart block): myocarditis, ASD, AVSD, Ebstein's malformation, rheumatic fever, hyperkalaemia, digoxin toxicity
- *QT interval* (onset of QRS complex to end of T wave): reflects ventricular depolarization and repolarization time and is rate variable.
  - Corrected QT (QTc) = $QT/\sqrt{(R\text{-}R\ interval)}$. A QTc up to 0.45 may be normal in the first 6 months of life; after this it should not exceed 0.40 s.
  - long QT interval: long QT syndrome (LQTS), a genetic disorder caused by mutations in several different ion channel genes, hypokalaemia, drugs (erythromycin, flecainide).

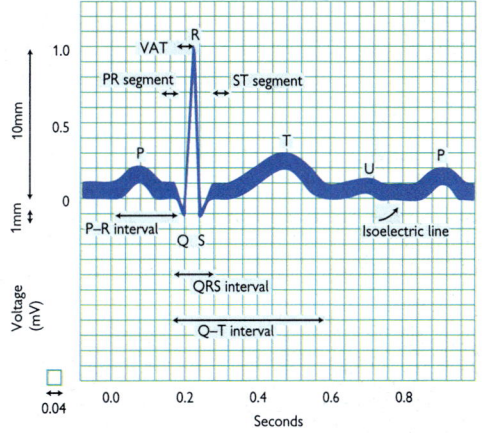

Fig 4.6 ECG: intervals and segments.

Common ECG abnormalities

- *Superior QRS axis:* atrioventricular septal defect, ostium primum ASD, tricuspid atresia.
- *Right ventricular hypertrophy (RVH):* upright T waves in VI (from aged 2 days to 7 years), marked right axis deviation, Q wave in VI, R waves >20 mm in VI
- *Left ventricular hypertrophy (LVH):* Left axis deviation, R in I, II, III, aVL, aVF, V5 or V6 >normal, S in V1 or V2 >normal, Q in V5 and V6 ≥5 mm.

4.3 Congenital heart disease

Congenital heart disease (CHD) is the most common congenital abnormality, with an approximate incidence of 1% of live births.

Aetiology

Identified causes include genetic defects and maternal illnesses or medications but in most cases no aetiology is apparent. Maternal factors include:

- *Infections:* e.g. rubella
- *Disease:* e.g. type 1 diabetes mellitus, phenylketonuria, systemic lupus erythematosus
- *Medication:* anti-epilepsy drugs, lithium (Ebstein's anomaly).

Genetics of congenital heart disease (CHD)

The majority of cases are multifactorial: multiple genes interact with environmental factors. In a minority of cases a clear genetic cause is identified. The genetic mechanism may be a chromosomal deletion or mutation in a known single gene and the heart defect may occur in the context of a recognizable syndrome or in isolation. Recognition is helpful in directing genetic counselling and in predicting co-morbidity and prognosis.

In the absence of a specific syndrome or pattern, empiric data shows there is a small increased risk to siblings of an affected child (1.5–4%), and to offspring of an affected parent (1.5–7%). This risk varies with defect (higher for left-sided obstructive defects, e.g. aortic stenosis) and is higher if the mother is the affected parent.

Fetal echocardiography can be performed at 18–20 weeks gestation to detect major heart defects; overall sensitivity for all CHD is approximately 70% with targeted scanning by experienced personnel.

Syndromic CHD

Table 4.4 outlines some examples of syndromes with cardiac defects. Most are caused by chromosomal abnormalities but some are single-gene disorders. In chromosomal microdeletions the gene responsible for the cardiac defect is known in some cases.

Cardiac defects are also present in numerous other syndromes which are uncommon and may have a short life expectancy: Edward's (trisomy 18), Patau's (trisomy 13), cri-du-chat, Wolf–Hirschorn, Pierre Robin, Cornelia de Lange; and in two associations: VACTERL and CHARGE.

More recently, several genes have been identified which cause non-syndromic cardiac defects and segregate in autosomal dominant fashion: *GATA4* (septal defects), *NKX2.5* (atrial septal defects), *TBX20* (septal and valve defects).

Classification

Over 100 anatomically distinct congenital heart defects exist. A handful account for the majority of cases (see Tables 4.3 and 4.4).

Table 4.3. Congenital heart defects: classification and frequency		
Acyanotic left-to-right shunts	Ventricular septal defect (VSD)	20%
	Persistent ductus arteriosus (PDA)	12%
	Isolated atrial septal defect (ASD)	7%
Obstructions	Pulmonary stenosis (PS)	10%
	Aortic stenosis (AS)	5%
	Coarctation of aorta (COA)	8%
Cyanotic	Tetralogy of Fallot (TOF)	10%
	Transposition of great arteries (TGA)	5%
	Total anomalous pulmonary venous connection (TAPVC)	1%

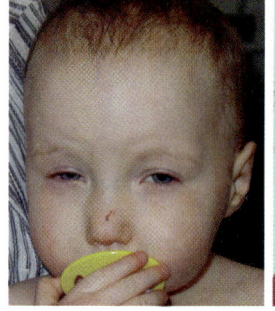

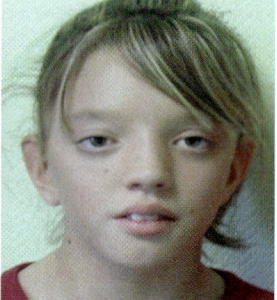

Fig 4.7 A. Di George syndrome: telecanthus, bulbous nose. B. Noonan syndrome : ptosis, webbed neck, hypertelorism.

Table 4.4. Syndromic congenital heart disease				
Syndrome	Genetic defect		% CHD	Cardiac defects
	Chromosome	Gene		
Down	Trisomy 21		40	AVSD, VSD, tetralogy of Fallot (TOF), ASD,
Turner	45, X		35	COA, Aortic stenosis (AS), ASD
Noonan	12q	PTPNII	100	Pulmonary stenosis (PS,) VSD, septal hypertrophy (Fig 4.7)
Williams	del7q11.23	ELN	>80	Supravalvar AS, COA, peripheral PS
Holt–Oram	12q	TBX5	95	ASD, VSD
Marfan	15q	FBN1	30	Aortic root dilation/dissection, mitral valve prolapse
Di George	del22q11.2	TBX1	85	Interrupted aortic arch, truncus arteriosus, TOF, pulmonary atresia (Fig 4.7)
Alagille	del20p12	JAG1	90	Peripheral PS, TOF, COA

Haemodynamics

Left-to-right shunts
Shunt magnitude is determined by the level and size of the defect connecting the systemic circulation to the pulmonary circulation and the relative resistances of the systemic and pulmonary vasculature. The natural fall in pulmonary vascular resistance after birth is an important influence on the development of symptoms associated with larger defects. Large shunts result in pulmonary hypertension.
- *ASD:* low right ventricular pressure favours volume-loading of the right heart. ASDs are virtually never symptomatic in infancy and only rarely cause symptoms in early childhood.
- *VSD:* in small defects shunt is limited by defect size, in large defects by pulmonary vascular resistance (PVR). Large defects present at 4–6 weeks of age when PVR falls and allows a significant shunt.
- *PDA:* similar to VSD. High PVR limits significant shunting in the first week of life in newborn infants.

Obstructive lesions
The haemodynamics fall into two categories:
- *Minor:* e.g. aortic or pulmonary stenosis which are usually an incidental finding in a well child.
- *Major (duct dependent):* these present acutely in the newborn when the ductus arteriosus closes at ~2 days of age. They include coarctation of aorta, interrupted aortic arch, hypoplastic left heart syndrome, critical aortic or pulmonary stenosis.

Cyanotic lesions
Central cyanosis related to CHD occurs in two main haemodynamic situations:
- Obstruction to pulmonary blood flow accompanied by a right-to-left shunt which permits desaturated systemic venous blood to bypass the lungs and enter the systemic circulation directly, e.g. tetralogy of Fallot, pulmonary or tricuspid atresia, Ebstein's anomaly. There is pulmonary oligaemia.
- Admixture lesions in which there is common mixing of desaturated and oxygenated blood, e.g. truncus arteriosus, total anomalous pulmonary venous drainage, transposition of the great arteries. Pulmonary blood flow may be low, normal, or high depending on any obstruction and pulmonary vascular resistance.

Therapeutic interventions

Medical treatment
Ductus arteriosus
In some conditions the systemic or pulmonary circulation may be 'duct dependent' and IV prostaglandin E1 (alprostadil) or prostaglandin E2 (dinoprostone) may be given to maintain ductal patency in these situations:
- *Duct-dependent systemic circulation:* obstructed left heart, e.g. preductal coarctation of aorta, interrupted arch, critical AS, hypoplastic left heart
- *Duct-dependent pulmonary circulation:* obstructed 'right' heart, e.g. pulmonary atresia with intact ventricular septum, critical pulmonary stenosis
- To promote mixing between parallel circulations, e.g. in transposition of the great arteries.

Conversely, patency of the duct may cause a significant adverse left-to-right shunt, particularly in preterm neonates, and ductal closure may be induced by administering prostaglandin inhibitors, e.g. indometacin, ibuprofen.

Cardiac failure
Medical management of cardiac failure may include:
- *Oxygen:* caution is necessary for duct-dependent lesions as O_2 may trigger ductal closure, and for lesions such as hypoplastic left heart in which an O_2-induced fall in pulmonary vascular resistance may divert blood from the systemic circulation. Air may be used to resuscitate these infants.
- *Diuretics:* reduce preload; usually use a combination of a loop diuretic (furosemide) with a potassium-sparing (aldosterone antagonist) diuretic (e.g.spironolactone).
- *Inotropes* dopamine, dobutamine, adrenaline, milrinone.
- *Angiotensin converting enzyme (ACE) inhibitors:* e.g. oral captopril to reduce afterload. Commence at low dose and monitor for hypotension and renal impairment.

Interventional cardiology
Occlusions
Transcatheter occlusion of intracardiac (secundum ASD, some VSDs) and extracardiac (e.g. PDA) communications has been revolutionized by the development of devices made from Nitinol wire mesh. Complications include device migration (2%) and transient arrhythmias (1–2%).

Dilatations
Balloon devices are used for atrial septostomy, valvuloplasty, and angioplasty. Atrial septostomy improves mixing in patients with transposition of the great arteries (TGA). Valvuloplasty is the initial treatment of choice for pulmonary valve stenosis in all age groups and in non-calcific aortic stenosis. Angioplasty (±stent insertion) is used in both native and postsurgical coarctation of aorta.

Electrophysiology
Transvenous/epicardial pacemaker implantation, radiofrequency ablation and implantable cardioverter defibrillators are all available for children.

Cardiac surgery
Non-bypass surgery
Procedures include pulmonary artery banding, arterial duct ligation, coarctation of the aorta repair, modified Blalock–Taussig (BT) shunt insertion (a subclavian artery–branch pulmonary artery conduit that increases lung blood flow).

Bypass surgery (open-heart surgery)
- *Arterial switch:* for isolated TGA. 1 year survival 97%.
- *Norwood procedure:* used to initially palliate hypoplastic left heart syndrome (HLHS).
- *Fontan procedure:* diverts systemic venous return directly to the pulmonary circulation, with or without placing a connection to the right atrium. Used in children with only a single effective ventricle, e.g. tricuspid or pulmonary atresia.
- *Rastelli procedure:* (indication TGA/VSD/PS). An RV-pulmonary artery conduit is placed and an intracardiac tunnel connects LV to aorta. VSD is patched.

4.4 Acyanotic heart defects: left-to-right shunts

Atrial septal defect (ASD)
ASDs comprise 10% of all CHD. Up to 50% of cases of CHD include an ASD as a component.

Anatomy and pathophysiology
There are three types:
- *Ostium secundum ASD (60%)*: failure of development of the septum secundum or excessive resorption of the septum primum leaves a hole in the mid-portion of the atrial septum. Female to male ratio 2:1.
- *Ostium primum ASD (30%)*: incomplete fusion of the endocardial cushions results in a partial atrioventricular septal defect manifest as a gap in the inferior part of the atrial septum and a cleft mitral valve. Common in children with trisomy 21.
- *Sinus venosus ASD (10%)*: a defect located where either the SVC or IVC joins the right atrium. Partial anomalous pulmonary venous drainage is a common association.

Shunt magnitude is determined by defect size and relative compliance of the two ventricles. Left-to-right shunting is favoured by the low pressure and high compliance of the RV leading to volume-loading of the right heart.

Clinical features
Usually asymptomatic in childhood. Primum defects with a significant shunt or mitral regurgitation may develop heart failure in infancy. Large secundum defects may cause exercise intolerance or palpitations in older children or adults.

Examination
Signs of increased flow through the right heart:
- RV heave at the left sternal edge
- S2 widely split and fixed (i.e. no respiratory variation)
- Diastolic flow murmur across tricuspid valve
- Systolic ejection murmur across pulmonary valve (second left intercostal space).

Investigations
- ECG:
  - first degree heart block (PR interval >0.19 s)
  - RV volume overload: rSR in VI, QRS axis deviated to right
  - RA enlargement: tall peaked P waves
- CXR: RA and RV enlargement with prominent pulmonary trunk and increased pulmonary vascular markings (Fig 4.8).
- Echocardiography: 2D imaging confirms diagnosis and Doppler assessment determines the shunt magnitude and presence of AV valve regurgitation.

Management
80% of small secundum defects (3–8 mm) diagnosed in infancy close spontaneously by 18 months. Right heart volume-loading necessitates closure and a majority (60%) can be occluded with a transcatheter device. Patients with isolated ostium primum ASD require elective surgical repair between age 2 and 5 years.

Ventricular septal defect
The most common congenital heart defect, accounting for 20% of all defects; 30% of all cases of CHD include a VSD.

Anatomy and pathophysiology
Defects may occur anywhere in the septum, may vary in size, and may be single or multiple. They may occur in isolation or in association with more complex anomalies. The magnitude of the associated left-to-right shunt determines symptomatology. In small defects shunting is limited by defect size and is independent of PVR. Such defects are termed 'restrictive'. Larger defects offer little local resistance and the degree of shunting is determined by PVR, a lower PVR facilitating a greater shunt. Shunt magnitude (and symptoms) tend to increase over the early weeks of a life as the natural postnatal fall in PVR progresses. Large shunts result in LA and LV volume overload.

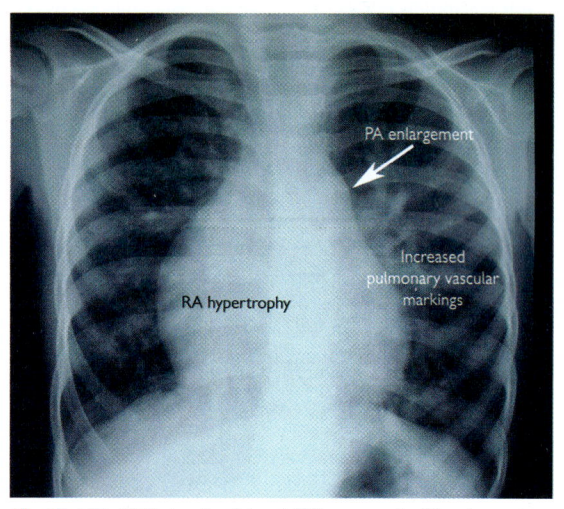

Fig 4.8 ASD: CXR showing RA and RV hypertrophy, PA enlargement, increased pulmonary vascular markings.

Clinical features
Small VSD

These are asymptomatic and are typically found during routine physical examination.

Examination
- Normal growth.
- *Murmur*: grade 1–4/6 pansystolic murmur at lower left sternal edge. A palpable thrill may be present. Not usually audible in first few days of life when PVR is high. The murmur intensity is often louder with the smaller defects as their restrictive nature generates high velocity shunting.
- ECG and CXR are normal.

Moderate to large VSD

As PVR falls and left-to-right shunting increases congestive cardiac failure develops with dyspnoea, feeding difficulties and recurrent pulmonary infections. Poor feeding and the increased energy expenditure associated with tachypnoea result in failure to thrive (inadequate weight gain).

Examination
- Hyperdynamic precordium: forceful LV impulse.
- Increased P2 (if pulmonary hypertension present)
- *Murmurs*: across defect a blowing, pansystolic murmur at lower left sternal edge, less harsh than in a small defect.
- Apical mid-diastolic low-pitched rumble caused by increased flow across mitral valve. Perimembranous and subaortic defects may result in aortic valve cusp prolapse with aortic regurgitation and a diastolic murmur. Signs of congestive cardiac failure may be present.

Investigations
- *ECG:* this mirrors size of shunt and degree of pulmonary hypertension. In large defects there is biventricular hypertrophy and notched or peaked P waves.
- *CXR:* cardiomegaly and pulmonary plethora is directly proportional to magnitude of left-to-right shunt (see Fig 4.3).
- *Echocardiography:* two-dimensional and Doppler colour flow mapping identifies the defect position and size, the degree of left ventricular overload, and whether or not the defect is restrictive.

Management

A significant percentage of small defects (muscular 80%, membranous 35%) close spontaneously in the first 2 years. Parents should be reassured of their benign nature.

In symptomatic patients with significant left-to-right shunts medical management is directed towards the control of heart failure, prevention of pulmonary vascular disease and maintenance of normal growth.

Diuretic therapy combines a loop diuretic, e.g. furosemide (reduces circulating volume, reducing preload) with an aldosterone antagonist, e.g. spironolactone. The latter negates the effect of hyperaldosteronism (fluid and salt retention) that usually accompanies congestive cardiac failure. Afterload reduction with the addition of an ACE inhibitor, e.g. captopril, reduces shunt magnitude and augments stroke volume without increasing myocardial O_2 consumption.

Surgical closure
- *Indications:*
  - any large defect with failure of medical treatment
  - large defect in infant aged 6–12 months with reversible pulmonary hypertension even if symptoms are mild
  - aortic regurgitation, progressive subvalvar LV or RV outflow obstruction
- *Complications (1–2%):* heart block, stroke, infection. Endocarditis precautions are still required after closure. Mortality rates are very low (1%).

Palliative pulmonary artery banding with repair in later childhood is reserved for complex cases or multiple defects. Severe secondary pulmonary vascular disease (Eisenmenger syndrome, shunt becomes right-to-left) is very rare, is a contraindication to closure, and necessitates consideration of heart–lung transplant.

Atrioventricular septal defect

30% of affected children have Down syndrome.

There is a common atrioventricular valve with five leaflets. Haemodynamic consequences parallel those of a large VSD, with congestive cardiac failure evident by 1–2 months of age. A murmur is not usually audible at birth.
- *ECG:* superior QRS axis. RVH/RBBB, LVH in many, 1st degree heart block in most
- *CXR:* cardiomegaly and pulmonary plethora once symptomatic.

Management

Initial medical treatment as for large VSD. Corrective surgery at around 4 months of age. Mitral regurgitation is a common postoperative sequel (10%) and complete heart block affects 5%.

Patent ductus arteriosus (PDA)

PDA is most commonly seen in the smallest preterm neonates (see Chapter 1). 5% of CHD cases include a PDA and in some cases either the systemic or pulmonary circulation is actually dependent on a patent ductus.

Anatomy and pathophysiology

The ductus arteriosus normally closes within the first 72 h after birth, partly in response to increased oxygenation. This physiological adaptation may fail in preterm infants: a symptomatic PDA (sPDA) affects 50% of newborns with a birth weight <1500 g.

The haemodynamic consequences are similar to those in VSD. A small PDA restricts left-to-right shunting, but with larger ducts the pulmonary vascular resistance is the main determinant of shunt magnitude. As PVR falls, the shunt increases and volume loading of the left heart develops and lung compliance decreases, increasing the work of breathing and often necessitating respiratory support in preterm infants. In term infants, significant shunting is unusual in the first 4 weeks.

Clinical features

Small PDAs (≤1 mm diameter) are asymptomatic. A large PDA causes recurrent lower respiratory tract infections, failure to thrive, and eventual cardiac failure. Exertional dyspnoea may occur in older children.

Examination
- Bounding peripheral pulses, hyperdynamic precordium and a thrill beneath the left clavicle
- Continuous 'machinery murmur' below left clavicle (which may be limited to only systole in preterm infants)

Investigations
- *ECG:* left ventricular hypertrophy
- *CXR:* cardiomegaly and pulmonary plethora
- *Echocardiography:* identifies ductal size, degree of shunt and left-heart volume loading.

Management

A very small PDA may close spontaneously and requires no treatment or follow up. A large duct is an endarteritis risk while patent and a significant shunt may eventually cause pulmonary hypertension.

For preterm infants with significant left heart volume load, fluid restriction and diuretics provide short-term benefit. Prostaglandin synthetase inhibitors (indomethacin, ibuprofen) achieve closure in 60%. Surgical ligation is reserved for those who fail to respond to medical treatment and have persisting respiratory failure. In infants (as small as 1500 g) and older children most ducts can now be closed by transcatheter occlusion with a success rate close to 100%.

4.5 Acyanotic heart defects: obstructions

Obstructive defects fall broadly into two clinical categories:
- *Obstruction in the sick newborn:* coarctation of aorta (duct-dependent), interruption of aortic arch, critical aortic stenosis, hypoplastic left heart syndrome
- *Obstruction in the well child:* aortic stenosis, pulmonary stenosis, coarctation of aorta (not duct-dependent).

Obstruction in the sick newborn

Coarctation of the aorta (COA)
COA accounts for 5–8% of all CHD. It may occur as an isolated defect or in association with other lesions, most commonly bicuspid aortic valve (30–50%) and VSD. The male: female ratio is 2: 1. 20% of Turner syndrome patients have COA.

Anatomy and pathophysiology
COA is a constricted aortic segment with local medial thickening forming either a shelf-like or curtain-like structure that may be discrete or involve a longer segment. Hypoplasia of the isthmus and aortic arch is typical.

The haemodynamic consequences depend on location and associated defects, but in all cases significant afterload is imposed on the LV. In a minority, the RV supplies the descending aorta through a PDA and postnatal ductal closure precipitates circulatory collapse. Ductal closure increases LV afterload and may be poorly tolerated, with circulatory collapse. Most non-duct-dependent cases are asymptomatic until later life.

Clinical features
Early presentation may be abrupt and acute with ductal closure precipitating circulatory collapse, or less acute with the development of congestive cardiac failure during the first few weeks of life. Presentation can also be at any time through childhood and even occasionally in adult life with hypertension, stroke, a murmur, or abnormal leg pulses.

Examination
Infants may be moribund with signs of congestive cardiac failure. A key feature is reduced or absent lower extremity pulses and BP discrepancy between upper and lower limbs. In severe heart failure all pulses are diminished. Gallop rhythm and a systolic murmur between the shoulder blades and/or over the left infraclavicular area may be heard.

Investigations
- *ECG:* in the neonate or infant—right ventricular dominance (right axis deviation, RVH, RBBB)
- *CXR:* cardiomegaly, pulmonary oedema/congestion
- *Echocardiography:* outlines diagnosis, LV function and any associated intracardiac anomalies.

Management
Medical care includes infusion of prostaglandin E2 (if there is duct dependence) and treatment of cardiac failure with O_2, inotropes, diuretics, and ventilation. Once stabilized, urgent intervention is undertaken, either surgically with a subclavian flap repair or resection and an end-to-end anastomosis, or with the placement of a stent. Lifelong follow-up is mandatory to detect re-coarctation or residual stenosis (20%), usually treatable with balloon angioplasty.

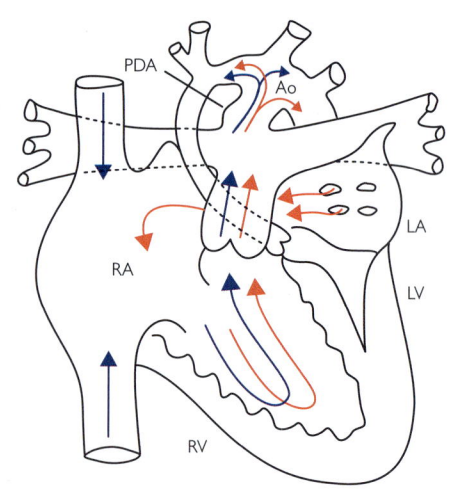

Fig 4.9 Hypoplastic left heart syndrome: anatomy. Adapted courtesy of Eliot May.

Hypoplastic left heart syndrome (HLHS)
This uncommon syndrome accounts for 1% of all CHD (Fig 4.9).

Anatomy and pathophysiology
There is hypoplasia of the left side of the heart with a diminutive left ventricle and ascending aorta and severe stenosis or atresia of the mitral and aortic valves. The systemic circulation is duct dependent and maintained by the right ventricle.

Clinical features
The diagnosis is usually made antenatally. Alternatively, ductal closure in early life precipitates circulatory failure, absent femoral and brachial pulses, signs of heart failure with hepatomegaly but usually no murmur. Severe acidosis is typical. Desaturation is common but often overlooked.

Investigations
- *ECG:* RVH, absent left ventricular forces
- *CXR:* cardiomegaly with pulmonary oedema
- *Echocardiography:* diagnostic.

Management
Antenatal diagnosis creates a choice between termination or continuing to term and undergoing complex palliative surgery. Termination rates show considerable geographic and cultural variation.

Antenatal diagnosis facilitates the prevention of circulatory collapse, with a prostaglandin infusion commenced at birth to maintain ductal patency. Resuscitation and stabilization is required prior to surgical intervention (*Norwood* procedure) at around 3–5 days of age. The three-stage Norwood procedure creates unobstructed RV–aorta flow, with the lungs supplied initially by an aorta–pulmonary artery shunt. At ~6 months of age the superior venocaval return is attached directly to the pulmonary circulation (cavopulmonary *Glenn* shunt, mortality <5%). A *Fontan* circulation is then formed at ~18 months of age, the inferior vena cava being attached to the pulmonary circulation.

Five year actuarial survival is around 60%. The long-term outlook is uncertain; some may require transplantation.

Critical aortic stenosis and interrupted aortic arch

Critical aortic stenosis is often diagnosed antenatally. The systemic circulation is duct-dependent. Clinical presentation and initial non-surgical management is as for HLHS and is followed by early emergency balloon valvuloplasty.

An interruption in the aortic arch may occur at any site from the origin of the innominate artery to left subclavian artery and is more common in the presence of a 22q11 deletion. The systemic circulation is duct-dependent; presentation and initial management is similar to HLHS.

Obstruction in the well child

Aortic stenosis (AS)

AS accounts for 5% of all CHD and is more common in males (male:female ratio 4:1). Supravalvular stenosis is common in Williams syndrome.

Anatomy and pathophysiology

Obstruction may be valvular (70%), subvalvular (25%), or supravalvular. In valvular stenosis there may be one, two (bicuspid), or three aortic valve leaflets which are fused together. Subvalvular stenosis caused by a discrete fibromuscular ring is often associated with other defects, e.g. VSD, PDA, and coarctation. Critical AS causes congestive cardiac failure in the newborn period. Increase in cardiac output throughout childhood may worsen obstruction, as may valve calcification in later life.

Clinical features

Mild to moderate, and some severe cases are asymptomatic but a minority report exercise intolerance. Severe stenosis can cause exertional angina, syncope, and easy fatiguability but symptoms are a poor guide to severity overall.

Examination

- Williams syndrome has a typical facies. Pulse pressure is narrow. There is a systolic thrill at the upper right sternal border, the suprasternal notch, and over the carotids.
- Ejection click (after first heat sound) in valvular stenosis.
- Ejection systolic murmur best heard in 2nd right or left intercostal space, radiating to neck and apex.

Investigations

- ECG: normal (mild stenosis), LVH with strain in severe stenosis.
- CXR: normal or visible post-stenotic dilation (ascending aorta, prominent aortic knuckle), cardiomegaly in severe cases
- Echocardiography: diagnostic, defining valve morphology, severity, left ventricle dimensions, presence of any aortic regurgitation.

Management

Strenuous activity should be avoided in moderate to severe stenosis. Asymptomatic children require long-term serial echocardiography to monitor for progression and need for intervention. A transvalvular Doppler gradient >70 mmHg or a mean gradient of 35 mmHg is a commonly used threshold for intervention. Options include balloon dilatation, valvotomy, Ross procedure (pulmonary root autograft), and valve replacement.

Pulmonary stenosis

More commonly valvular but may be supra- or subvalvular. If valvular, the pulmonary valve leaflets are fused together. Most patients are asymptomatic. Examination may reveal a thrill and an ejection systolic murmur at upper left sternal edge, a quiet P2, and a widely split S2, and in valvular PS an ejection click. ECG indicates right ventricular hypertrophy, as does CXR in moderate-severe cases. Echocardiography is diagnostic.

Balloon dilatation (valvuloplasty) is the treatment of choice in all age groups when the gradient across the valve reaches 60 mmHg.

Coarctation of aorta (COA)

Coarctation is more commonly not duct-dependent. Arterial collateral vessels develop to partially bypass the obstruction. Mechanical obstruction and activation of the renin-angiotensin system results in hypertension.

Clinical features

Patients are usually asymptomatic and present with incidental detection of hypertension or a murmur. Symptoms may include headaches, chest pain, fatigue, or even intracranial haemorrhage. Infective endocarditis may occur.

Examination

- Radiofemoral delay on simultaneous palpation of upper and lower extremity pulses
- Blood pressure: always hypertension in right arm and a pressure difference of >20 mmHg between arms and legs
- Ejection systolic murmur at upper left infraclavicular area and between scapulae/under left scapula. The murmur of collaterals may be continuous.

Investigations

- ECG: normal/left ventricular hypertrophy
- CXR: cardiomegaly. Notching of ribs 4–8 (children >5 years). '3' sign: visible notch in descending aorta at site of constriction
- Echocardiography: is diagnostic and MRI is useful for detailed anatomical delineation prior to intervention.

Management

Hypertension is treated with β-blockers. Options include definitive surgical repair, balloon angioplasty, or an endovascular stent. Mortality or significant morbidity is <1%. Lifelong endocarditis prophylaxis is necessary, as is follow-up for recoarctation (3%).

Vascular rings and slings

These are uncommon anomalies accounting for <1% of CHD. Abnormal or incomplete regression of one of the six embryonic branchial arches creates an anomalous configuration of the arch and associated vessels forming a complete or incomplete ring around the trachea and oesophagus. There is an association with the 22q11 deletion.

The two most common types (85–95% of cases) are:
- Double aortic arch
- Right aortic arch with left ligamentum arteriosum.

Clinical features reflect airway or oesophageal compression and presentation is usual in infancy or early childhood with persistent stridor and feeding difficulties.

CXR may reveal a right-sided aortic arch or lobar emphysema from bronchial compression. Microlaryngobronchoscopy and echocardiography are done to visualize the airways and check for vascular compression. Additional imaging may include CT, MRI, and digital subtraction angiography. A barium or gastrografin swallow can also help make the diagnosis but is not usually definitive.

Treatment is surgical, though tracheomalacia may persist even after successful surgical repair.

4.6 Cyanotic heart defects

Central cyanosis is apparent when there is ≥2.5 g/dL of reduced haemoglobin, corresponding to O_2 saturation <85% in a child with normal Hb levels.

Cyanotic lesions can be categorized broadly into those with obstruction to pulmonary blood flow (reduced pulmonary vascularity) and those that permit admixture of systemic and pulmonary venous return (increased pulmonary vascularity). This classification is not absolute as the presence of additional abnormalities may increase pulmonary blood flow.

- *Cyanosis and pulmonary oligaemia:* tetralogy of Fallot (TOF); pulmonary atresia; Ebstein's anomaly; tricuspid atresia
- *Cyanosis and pulmonary plethora:* transposition of great arteries (TGA); common arterial trunk (truncus arteriosus); total anomalous pulmonary venous connection.

Cyanotic heart disease may manifest at birth or soon after (e.g. TGA) or later in infancy (e.g. TOF).

Tetralogy of Fallot (TOF)

TOF accounts for 5–7% of all CHD and is the most common cyanotic heart defect presenting beyond infancy. Syndromic associations include the 22q11 deletion, VACTERL, and valproate embryopathy. There is a slight male preponderance.

Anatomy and pathophysiology

The 4 primary components of the tetralogy are (Fig 4.10):
1. *VSD:* usually single, large and subaortic
2. *Overriding aorta:* the aortic root is of biventricular origin just above the VSD
3. *Right ventricular outflow tract obstruction (RVOTO):* predominantly infundibular (subvalvar) but may be valvular or supravalvar or occur at multiple sites
4. *RV hypertrophy:* this is secondary to the RV outflow tract obstruction and typically increases with age.

Additional anatomic variations include: right aortic arch (25%), coronary artery abnormalities (5%), atretic pulmonary valve (15%), and atrial septal or atrioventricular defects.

RVOTO tends to increase through infancy, increasing the magnitude of the right-to-left shunt through the VSD. Mild RVOTO allows a small left-to-right shunt with acyanosis ('pink' Fallot) and haemodynamics comparable to a small VSD. By later infancy, moderate RVOTO has usually developed and results in cyanosis and the risk of cyanotic 'spells'.

Clinical features

Presentation is usually with an incidental murmur or cyanosis developing in the first year of life. Neonatal cyanosis is uncommon. Failure to thrive is not uncommon.

Examination

- Cyanosis and clubbing (in untreated older children)
- *Heart sounds:* P2 is soft
- An ejection systolic murmur (±thrill) is heard at the left sternal border: upper (valvular stenosis), mid (infundibular stenosis). Length and intensity is inversely related to degree of stenosis: mild obstruction generates a loud, long murmur; severe obstruction a short quiet murmur. A murmur may be audible at birth.

Investigations

- *ECG:* normal at birth. RVH develops in infancy
- *CXR:* classical 'boot-shaped' heart with concave pulmonary artery and pulmonary oligaemia (Fig 4.4)
- *Echocardiography:* diagnostic and can quantify RVOTO.
- *FBC:* quantiifies degree of polycythemia and iron status.

Management

- *Surgical treatment:* Varies with anatomy and institution. Some require an initial palliative procedure, e.g. modified Blalock–Taussig shunt (MBTS), to increase pulmonary blood flow. Definitive repair is often undertaken in the first year of life. One year survival is 98%. Lifelong endocarditis prophylaxis is imperative.
- *Medical management* is required for hypoxic spells, which tend to become more frequent and severe with age and are less of a problem since earlier surgical repair has become feasible. Immediate expert cardiological advice should be sought in managing acute spells. Propranolol may ameliorate further paroxysms.

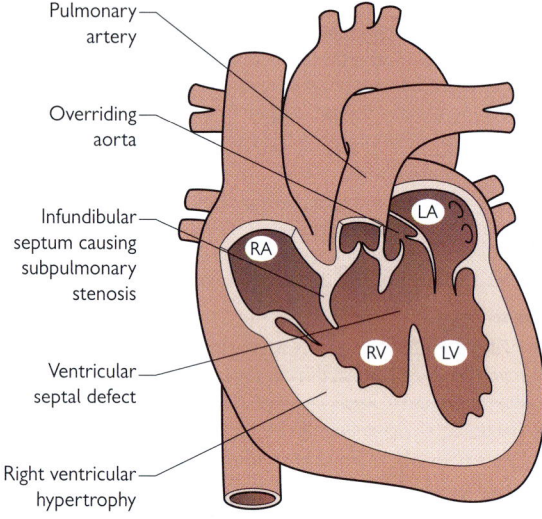

Fig 4.10 Tetralogy of Fallot.

Pulmonary or tricuspid atresia

Severe abnormalities of the tricuspid or pulmonary valves (including atresia) usually present as cyanosis with decreased pulmonary blood flow in the newborn.

Pulmonary atresia

In pulmonary atresia with intact ventricular septum the pulmonary circulation is duct-dependent and cyanosis occurs when the duct closes. There is usually no murmur. Pulmonary atresia with VSD and collaterals (from aorta to lungs) is not duct-dependent and may present with cyanosis or cardiac failure. Management is complex, highly patient-specific, and often involves several surgical and catheter procedures.

Tricuspid valve abnormalities

The tricuspid valve may be hypoplastic, dysplastic, atretic or displaced inferiorly (Ebstein's anomaly). In the latter, severity is related to the degree of displacement of the tricuspid valve. Severe cases present with cyanosis in the 1st week of life. CXR typically shows massive cardiomegaly and pulmonary oligaemia The ECG may have a superior QRS axis.

Transposition of great arteries (TGA)

Complete TGA accounts for 5% of all CHD and has a male: female ratio of 3:1.

Anatomy and pathophysiology

The aorta arises from the RV and the pulmonary artery (PA) from the LV (Fig 4.11). Two parallel circulations exist, an arrangement that is incompatible with life postnatally without a communication at atrial, ventricular, or ductal level.

At birth a patent foramen ovale (PFO) and the ductus provide a communication between the two circuits, but profound cyanosis with an arterial O_2 saturation of 30–50% is typical. An accompanying VSD may facilitate O_2 saturations of 90%.

Clinical features

Cyanosis of variable severity usually appears in the 1st week of life and worsens with ductal closure.

Examination

Cyanosis. S2 single and loud. No murmur (unless VSD or PS present).

Investigations

- *ECG:* normal or right ventricular hypertrophy with right axis deviation
- *CXR:* cardiomegaly with narrow mediastinum ('egg on side') and pulmonary plethora.
- *Echocardiography:* is diagnostic
- Hypoglycaemia and metabolic acidosis are common.

Management

In severe hypoxia, resuscitate with O_2 and correct metabolic acidosis. A prostaglandin E2 infusion to maintain ductal patency will facilitate left-to-right shunting at atrial level by increasing pulmonary venous return and left atrial pressure. This facilitates some mixing of oxygenated blood with the systemic circulation.

Balloon atrial septostomy is done in selected cases and increases interatrial shunting. As pulmonary vascular resistance falls, increased pulmonary blood flow leads to LV overload and cardiac failure, especially in cases with a VSD. Diuretics are therapeutic.

Surgical repair (arterial switch) is usually undertaken in the 1st 2 weeks in infants presenting in the neonatal period without other anomalies. One year survival is 98% and 5 year survival >90%.

Common arterial trunk (CAT)

In CAT, or truncus arteriosus, a single great artery arises from the heart with a single truncal valve which may be stenotic or regurgitant. A large subaortic VSD is always present.

Clinical features include mild cyanosis and heart failure as PVR falls. There is a prominent RV impulse, a single S2, and an ejection systolic murmur, with cardiomegaly and pulmonary plethora on CXR. Management is surgical, with a mortality rate now <10% in many centres.

Total anomalous pulmonary venous drainage (TAPVD)

This uncommon lesion accounts for 1% of all CHD.

Anatomy and pathophysiology

In TAPVD the pulmonary veins drain to a site other than the LA. Three main subtypes exist:

- *Supracardiac:* a common vein drains to the SVC via an ascending vein and the left innominate vein

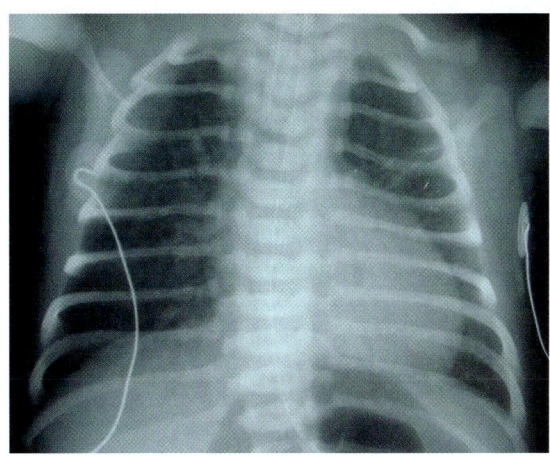

Fig 4.11 TGA in neonate: CXR showing cardiomegaly, pulmonary plethora, narrow mediastinum (aorta anterior to PA).

- *Cardiac:* the pulmonary veins drain into coronary sinus or directly into right atrium
- *Infracardiac (sub-diaphragmatic):* drainage is into the portal vein, hepatic vein, or IVC below the diaphragm.

An ASD or PFO is always present, permitting some of the pulmonary venous return to enter the systemic circulation.

Clinical features

The presence of obstruction to the pulmonary venous return determines the severity and timing of presentation. Most supracardiac and cardiac types are unobstructed, whereas obstruction is common with the infracardiac type.

Without obstruction

Presentation is with cyanosis and cardiac failure or with failure to thrive and recurrent chest infections.

Examination

Mild cyanosis and tachypnoea. RV heave. S2 widely split with loud P2. Ejection systolic murmur and tricuspid diastolic rumble.

- *ECG:* right ventricular hypertrophy
- *CXR:* dilated superior mediastinum (supracardiac), enlarged right heart, pulmonary venous congestion ('snowman in a snowstorm' or 'cottage loaf')

With obstruction

Presentation is usually on day 1 of life with severe cyanosis, respiratory distress, crepitations, and hepatomegaly.

A gallop rhythm is audible but usually no murmur.

- *ECG:* Right ventricular hypertrophy
- *CXR:* Normal cardiac size with marked pulmonary oedema.
- *Echocardiography:* is diagnostic.

Management

Semi-elective surgical correction is possible for non-obstructed cases. With obstruction, resuscitation is with O_2, positive pressure ventilation, diuretics, and correction of acidosis followed by urgent surgery to redirect pulmonary venous return to the LA.

4.7 Rheumatic fever and Kawasaki disease

Inflammaton of the heart may involve all tissue layers as a pancarditis, or variable combinations of endocardium, myocardium, pericardium, and blood vessels. It may be triggered by a response to remote infection (rheumatic fever) or an as yet unidentified pathogen (Kawasaki disease). Direct infection of cardiac tissue by pathogenic microbes may cause endocarditis (infective endocarditis), myocarditis (usually viral), or pericarditis.

Rheumatic fever (RF)

RF is a systemic autoimmune disease that may occur following group A β-haemolytic streptococcal (GAS) infection of the pharynx. Occurring in clusters, the incidence rate after GAS infection is currently around 0.5–3%. Two million children in the world are affected by rheumatic heart disease but it remains a neglected disease of the poor.

Aetiology and pathogenesis
The presence of antibodies to the streptolysin O toxin is a marker of group A beta haemolytic infection. Inflammatory lesions develop in the joints, skin, brain, and heart 2–3 weeks after infection. A pancarditis is typical with pericarditis, myocarditis, and endocarditis affecting particularly the mitral and aortic valves which may become deformed.

Clinical features
The median age for acute RF is 8 years. Sex incidence is equal. A history of an antecedent sore throat is present in 70% of older and 20% younger children. Other symptoms at presentation may include fever, rash, malaise, joint pain, chorea, or neuropsychiatric disturbance.

Examination
The diagnosis is made by use of the Jones criteria and requires evidence of antecedent group A streptococcal infection (throat swab culture, elevated or rising streptococcal antibody titre) together with either 2 major or 1 major and 2 minor manifestations (see Table 4.5).

Table 4.5. Major and minor criteria for acute RF

	Major	Minor
Joints	Polyarthritis	Arthralgia
Cardiac	Carditis	Prolonged PR
CNS	Chorea	
Skin	Erythema marginatum Subcutaneous nodules	
General		Fever ↑Acute phase reactants (ESR, CRP), Previous RF

Major manifestations
- *Arthritis:* painful, migratory large-joint polyarthritis is the most common (70%) and earliest manifestation.
- *Carditis:* pancarditis is the most serious complication and the next most common (50%). Manifestations include tachycardia, cardiomegaly, pericardial rub, gallop rhythm, and murmurs (valve regurgitation). Pericardial effusion with tamponade, cardiac failure, and heart block may occur.
- *CNS:* manifesting initially with emotional lability and personality change, chorea affects 15%, may last up to 18 months, can occur in isolation, and is more common in young girls.
- *Skin:* erythema marginatum occurs in 5–10% patients, is non-pruritic and commonest on the trunk and proximal limbs. Subcutaneous firm, non-tender nodules 1–2 cm in diameter affect 5–10%. They last for weeks and commonly accompany carditis.

Investigations
Evidence of Group A BHS infection
Throat swab culture is usually negative at time of RF. Group streptococcal antigen detection sensitivity is 60–90%. Positive anti-streptococcal antibodies: ASO titre, anti-DNAseB.

Cardiological
- *ECG:* prolonged PR interval or higher AV block, ST elevation in pericarditis.
- *CXR:* cardiomegaly may signify congestive cardiac failure, pericarditis or pancarditis
- *Echocardiography:* useful in identifying valvular regurgitation, ventricular dysfunction and pericardial effusion.

Management
- *Antibiotics:* to eradicate GAS pharyngitis. Options include penicillin (oral or IM), cefuroxime, or a macrolide if penicillin allergic
- *Anti-inflammatory medication:* anti-inflammatory doses of aspirin plus oral prednisolone for significant carditis
- *Cardiac failure:* supplemental O_2, diuretics and ACE inhibitors (e.g. captopril)
- *CNS:* haloperidol for severe chorea.

Secondary prophylaxis with antistreptococcal antibiotics (penicillin V) is indicated but the optimal duration is uncertain.

Kawasaki disease (KD)

KD is a systemic vasculitis with a predilection for cardiac involvement which may be fatal, particularly in unrecognized cases. It is the most common cause of acquired heart disease in children in the developed world. Worldwide the annual incidence varies from 3/100 000 in the UK to 100/100 000 in Japan. It affects predominantly children <5 years with a peak at 18 months. KD and the differential diagnosis is discussed in Chapter 15.18. This section focuses predominantly on the cardiac complications.

Aetiology and pathogenesis
The cause remains uncertain but current evidence favours a bacterial superantigen toxin (as yet unidentified) affecting a genetically predisposed host.

Clinical features
Diagnosis remains clinical. This disease evolves through 3 phases: acute (day 1–10), subacute (day 11–25) and convalescent.

Acute phase
Diagnostic criteria include a fever for at least 5 days together with at least 4 of the following:
1. *Rash:* diffuse, polymorphic, not vesicular, lasts 7 days
2. *Conjunctivitis:* bilateral, without corneal ulceration (anterior uveitis may be present)
3. *Oral mucositis:* strawberry tongue, erythema/cracking of lips and tongue
4. *Cervical lymphadenopathy:* may be a solitary, painful gland
5. *Peripheral extremities:* erythema and oedema (in 1st week).

In 'incomplete' KD (more common in infants) coronary artery vasculitis may be present on echocardiography in the presence of fewer than four of the criteria usually required to make the diagnosis.

Cardiac findings may emerge in the 2nd week manifesting as:
- *Pericarditis:* chest pain, pericardial rub, ST elevation on ECG
- *Myocarditis:* tachycardia, gallop rhythm, tachypnoea, low voltage/ST changes on ECG.
- *Coronary arteritis:* myocardial infarction, arrhythmias, sudden death (<1% risk, peak time weeks 3–6).

Subacute phase
Fever, rash, and lymphadenopathy subside. Thrombocytosis develops. The tips of fingers and toes desquamate. Coronary artery aneurysm (CAA) may cause myocardial ischaemia/infarction and arrhythmias. Aneurysmal change in peripheral arteries (very rare) may cause gangrene and cerebral infarction.

Convalescent phase
Starts once clinical signs disappear, lasts until inflammatory markers normalize.

Investigations
- *FBC:* Leucocytosis with neutrophilia in week 1, later changing to a lymphocytosis. By day 14 there may be a hypochromic anaemia and thrombocytosis (>1000 × 10^9/L).
- ESR, CRP↑
- Exclude differential diagnoses (see Chapter 15.18)
- ECG (to detect ischaemia), CXR and echo.

Echocardiography is most useful in week 1 if there is clinical suspicion of carditis. It may be a useful adjunct to diagnosis in incomplete cases in week 2 and may outline coronary artery dilatation (ectasia) or CAA for the first time at this stage (Fig 4.12). Coronary artery calibre should be recorded with reference to standardized age-defined normal limits, which naturally increase with age. CAA (present in 20% of untreated patients, <1% of treated patients) regress within 12 months in approximately 50–65%. Onset is unusual after 6 weeks from the onset of the disease.

Management
Once the diagnosis has been confirmed clinically the aim of treatment is to suppress the inflammatory process and reduce the likelihood of developing carditis and CAA. Intravenous immunoglobulin (IVIG) therapy is of proven benefit in reducing the incidence of CAA if given within 7–10 days of the onset of symptoms.

Acute phase
- IV immunoglobulin 2 g/kg as single dose over 12 h.
- Aspirin 30 mg/kg per day in 4 divided doses until apyrexial for 72 h and (in some institutions) day 14 of illness.
- Exercise restriction
- If no disease defervescence within 48 h, or disease recrudescence within 2 weeks, repeat IVIG; if persists, consider steroid, e.g. pulsed methylprednisolone.

Subacute phase and convalescence
- Aspirin 2–5 mg/kg per day
- Echocardiography in week 3 and at 6–8 weeks; exercise restriction until evidence of no CAA at 6–8 weeks.

At 6–8 weeks, management depends on coronary artery status:
- *Normal coronary arteries:* stop aspirin, repeat echo at 1 year, discharge if normal.
- *CAA <8 mm, no stenosis:* repeat echo/ECG 6 monthly and discontinue aspirin if dilation regresses and resolves. Lifelong follow-up. Consider exercise test if multiple aneurysms.
- *CAA >8 mm and/or stenosis:* lifelong aspirin 5 mg/kg per day, consider warfarin. Repeat echo/ECG 6 monthly and consider coronary angiography and exercise stress testing. Minimizing atheroma risk factors may reduce the risk of myocardial infarction.

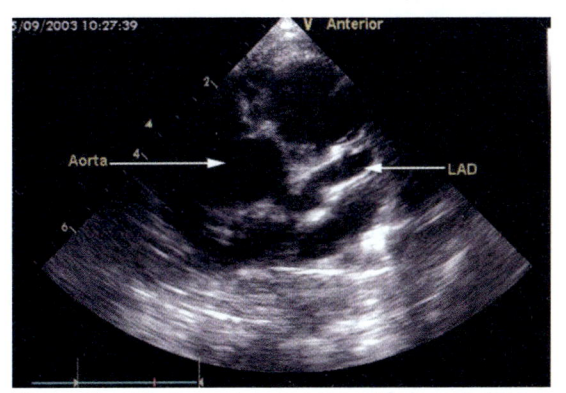

Fig 4.12 Kawasaki disease: short axis echocardiogram at the level of the aortic root illustrating an aneurysm of the left anterior descending coronary artery.

4.8 Infective endocarditis, myocarditis, and pericarditis

Infective endocarditis (IE)
Infection of the endocardial surface of the heart is a rare but serious illness in childhood with an annual incidence of 3–4/1 000 000.

Aetiology and pathogenesis
Most affected children have structural heart disease, although in neonates with central venous lines the condition may occur on normal heart valves. A pressure gradient or turbulent flow causes local endothelial damage and formation of a sterile platelet-fibrin thrombus. This may occur with all congenital heart lesions, except secundum ASD, and with implanted devices such as prosthetic valves. Localized infection may cause bacteraemia and bacterial invasion of the sterile thrombus, followed by accelerated platelet aggregation and fibrin deposition and the formation of a vegetation.

Common pathogens include:
- *Bacteria:*
  - *Streptococcus viridans* (20–50%)
  - *Staphylococcus aureus* (50–60%)
  - Enterococci (after GI procedures)
  - Coagulase negative staphylococci (CONS)
- *Fungi: Candida albicans* (in sick neonates).

The clinical course and complications result from embolization, progressive valvular destruction and distant immune complex deposition.

Clinical features
Onset may be fulminant with features of septicaemia, multiorgan involvement and valvar regurgitation (particularly with *S. aureus*), or more insidious over weeks with fever and non-specific symptoms (*Strep. viridans*, CONS, *Candida*). Predisposing infection such as skin abscess is sometimes identified.

Examination
- A murmur, which may be new or changing, is universal
- Fever (90%)
- Splenomegaly (70%)
- *Peripheral microembolic skin lesions (50%):* these include petechiae of skin or conjunctiva (Fig 4.13), and more rarely nail splinter haemorrhages, Osler nodes (tender, red nodes on tips of fingers and toes; see Fig 4.14) and Janeway lesions (painless erythematous lesions on palms and soles).
- *Distant-organ embolic phenomena (50%):* include hemiparesis/seizures, optic fundus haemorrhage (Roth's spots), lung infarction and haematuria/renal failure
- Signs of heart failure.

Investigations
- *Blood cultures:* 3–5 samples should be drawn over 24 h (ideally before antibiotic therapy), and are positive in 90% if pre-antibiotic therapy and in 50% if child is already on antimicrobials or infected with a fungal organism.
- FBC (anaemia, leucocytosis), elevated ESR
- Urine microscopy/urinalysis (haematuria)
- *Echocardiography:* demonstrates vegetations (but sensitivity is <100%) and valve/myocardial function. Vegetations may be absent early on in fulminant cases. Transoesophageal echocardiography may be required when clinical suspicion is high and transthoracic echocardiography is non-yieldworthy.

Management
Children at risk of IE include those with acquired valvular heart disease, valve replacement, structural congenital heart disease (before and after surgery) except isolated ASD, hypertrophic cardiomyopathy and previous IE.

At-risk patients should be offered information about prevention including the importance of good oral health, symptoms of IE, and the risks of invasive procedures (e.g. body piercing or tattooing). In the UK, NICE guidelines (2008) recommend that antibiotic prophylaxis is **not** offered to people undergoing dental procedures or non-dental procedures in the GI, respiratory, or GU tracts. This is a change to previously established procedure.

The cornerstone of medical therapy is a prolonged course of intravenous bactericidal antibiotics. Initial empirical antibiotic therapy, e.g. benzylpenicillin plus aminoglycoside, can usually be tailored according to the organism isolated. Typical protocols are:
- *Streptococcal endocarditis:* benzylpenicillin + aminoglycoside for 4 weeks.
- *Enterococcal endocarditis:* ampicillin + gentamicin for 6 weeks.
- *Staphylococcal endocarditis:* flucloxacillin + gentamicin for 4 – 6 weeks (the gentamicin course may be truncated).

Mortality is around 10–20% and is higher with *Staph. aureus* or fungal infection. Surgical intervention may be required for valve dysfunction with cardiac failure, the removal of large vegetations, or significant (CNS) embolic episodes.

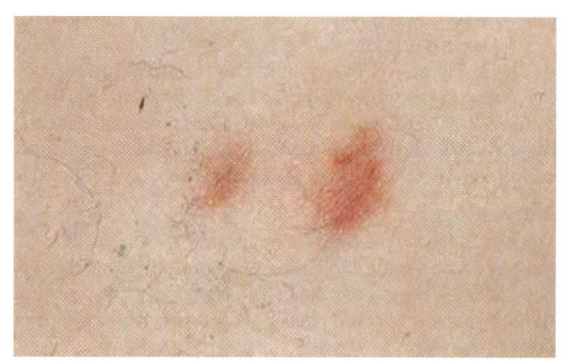

Fig 4.13 Embolic/vasculitic skin lesion in acute endocarditis of aortic valve caused by *Staph. aureus*.

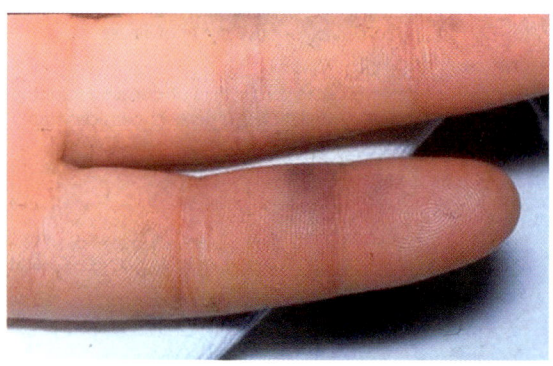

Fig 4.14 Osler node in a child with infective endocarditis caused by *Strep. viridans*.

Myocarditis

Many mild cases probably go unrecognized. Clinically detectable cases are rare and slightly commoner in males. There is clinical overlap with dilated cardiomyopathy and definitive diagnosis may be impossible without biopsy.

Aetiology and pathogenesis
- *Infectious*: (commonest): usually viral (e.g. adenovirus, coxsackie B, EBV, VZV, HIV) though bacterial, protozoan, and other infectious agents may be responsible, e.g. *Trypanosoma cruzi* (Chagas disease), *Borrelia burgdorferi* (Lyme disease)
- *Toxins*: anthracyclines, radiation, diphtheria exotoxin
- *Immune-mediated*: Kawasaki disease, rheumatic fever
- *Connective tissue disorders*: SLE, dermatomyositis.

Myocyte necrosis is followed by a cell-mediated inflammatory infiltration.

Clinical features
Children may complain of non-specific malaise and chest discomfort, palpitations and exertional dyspnoea. Infants may have a more precipitous presentation with vomiting and circulatory collapse which may occur 2 weeks after an antecedent viral illness.

Examination
- Fever (20%)
- Cardiac failure: sweating, respiratory distress, tachycardia, gallop rhythm, murmur (atrioventricular valve regurgitation)
- Severe cases: shock/collapse (secondary to severe muscle dysfunction and/or arrhythmia)
- Hepatomegaly: secondary to hepatitis or cardiac failure.

Investigations
- Elevated creatine kinase (CK), CK-MB, and troponins I and T
- *ECG*: arrhythmias, conduction disturbances, low QRS voltages, ST-T changes
- *CXR*: cardiomegaly with pulmonary venous congestion
- *Echocardiography*: reduced ventricular function, valvular regurgitation, chamber enlargement, ventricular thrombus
- *Endomyocardial biopsy*: in selected cases.

Management
Mild cases recover with supportive care. Cardiac failure may require O_2, diuretics, anti-arrhythmics, inotropes, and even ventilation or extracorporeal membrane oxygenation (ECMO).

The role for IVIG or specific antiviral agents is undetermined, although steroids are of proven benefit in rheumatic carditis. The mortality rate is as high as 75% in symptomatic neonates, and the condition at any age may be a precursor of dilated cardiomyopathy.

Pericarditis

An uncommon condition in childhood, inflammation of the pericardium may be an acute or chronic process and may precipitate the accumulation of a pericardial effusion.

Aetiology and pathogenesis
- *Infection*: may be viral (coxsackie/enteroviruses), bacterial (*Staph. aureus*, *Strep. pneumoniae*), or tuberculous
- *Immune mediated*: cardiac surgery, (post-pericardotomy syndrome), rheumatic fever, collagen vascular disease
- Malignancy
- Uraemia, drugs (e.g. isoniazid).

The degree of associated myocarditis and the speed of fluid accumulation are key determinants of clinical severity. A rapidly developing effusion or an effusion accompanied by myocarditis may cause cardiac tamponade.

Clinical features
There may be a history of antecedent viral infection, heart surgery or a precipitating chronic illness such as renal failure. Chest pain radiating to the back and relieved by sitting forward is the classic symptom.

Examination
- Fever
- Pericardial friction rub, muffled heart sounds
- *Cardiac tamponade*: pulsus paradoxus with hypotension, poor peripheral perfusion, and respiratory distress.

Investigations
- *ECG*: low QRS voltages (effusion), ST segment elevation followed by T wave inversion after 2 weeks (signifying myocarditis). See Fig 4.15.

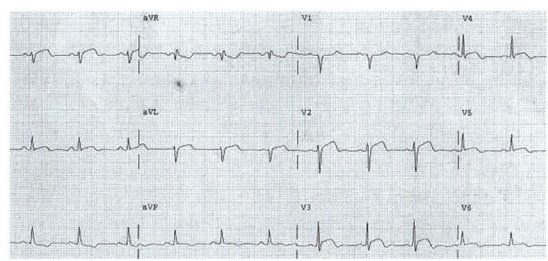

Fig 4.15 Pericarditis: ECG. ST elevation I, II, aVL, V2–V6.

- *CXR*: cardiomegaly, increased vascular markings (if tamponade), pleural effusion may coexist
- *Echocardiography*: quantifies ventricular function and identifies pericardial/pleural effusions, tamponade, and valvar regurgitation.

Management
Identify and treat the underlying cause. Purulent pericarditis requires surgical drainage and IV antibiotics. Urgent pericardiocentesis is required for tamponade of any cause. Non-infective causes may respond to NSAIDS or steroids.

4.9 Cardiomyopathy and arrhythmias

Cardiomyopathies
The cardiomyopathies are a heterogeneous and uncommon group of diseases with a wide variety of causes.

Classification
There are three main types with differing pathophysiology:
- Dilated
- Hypertrophic
- Restrictive.

Dilated cardiomyopathy (DCM)
The most common form.

Aetiology
- *Idiopathic:* (≥60% cases)
- *Familial (genetic):* at least 16 genes have been identified and several other loci mapped (*CMD1A-V*). Inheritance is usually autosomal dominant, but X-linked, recessive and mitochondrial forms exist
- *Extrinsic:* infections (viral, protozoal), storage disorders, nutritional deficiency, mitochondrial diseases, anthracycline therapy, muscular dystrophy, thyroid disease, hypocalcaemia, hypophosphataemia.

Clinical features
There is poor systolic contraction with chamber dilatation and a risk of arrhythmias and intracardiac thrombus. Symptoms and signs of congestive cardiac failure develop, including a gallop rhythm and the murmurs of mitral and tricuspid regurgitation.

Investigations
- *ECG:* sinus tachycardia, LVH, ST-T changes, atrial hypertrophy
- *CXR:* cardiomegaly, pulmonary congestion
- *Echocardiography:* diagnostic; quantifies function and excludes intracardiac thrombus.

Management
Medical therapy includes ACE inhibition (captopril), β-blockade (carvedilol) and interventions such as implantable defibrillators and LV assist devices. End-stage DCM requires cardiac transplantation. Spontaneous recovery can occur (presumed myocarditis). One year survival is 80%.

Hypertrophic cardiomyopathy (HCM)
A heterogeneous disease, HCM is familial in 50% of cases. Cardiac hypertrophy and dysfunction can also occur in association with Noonan syndrome, metabolic syndromes, valve stenosis and hypertension.

Familial hypertrophic cardiomyopathy (HCM)
This disorder has a prevalence of 0.2% and is a leading cause of sudden death in otherwise healthy active young people.

Aetiology and pathogenesis
Mutations in 14 different genes are known to cause autosomal dominant HCM. The genes encode cytoskeletal and sarcomeric proteins such as troponin T, α-tropomyosin, and titin. Left, right, biventricular, or septal hypertrophy may develop and the latter may cause left ventricle outflow obstruction. The LV is 'stiff' with impaired filling and increased pulmonary venous pressure.

Clinical features
Presentation is commonly at age 10–25 years. Symptoms include dyspnoea, exercise limitation, palpitations, chest pain, and syncope. Acute syncope occurs in 15–25% of adults and may cause sudden death. Examination may reveal signs of LV hypertrophy and mitral regurgitation.

Investigations
- *ECG:* abnormal in 90%. LVH, deep Q waves (septal hypertrophy), ST-T changes
- *CXR:* LVH with 'globular'-shaped heart
- *Echocardiography:* ventricular hypertrophy, especially septal, abnormal myocardial reflectivity, mitral regurgitation, left ventricular outflow obstruction, diastolic dysfunction.

Management
Differentiation between physiological hypertrophy secondary to athletic participation and familial HCM may be difficult. Avoidance of strenuous exercise is recommended if the diagnosis is certain. β-Blockers may help outflow obstruction, as may disopyramide (or surgery).

Sudden death (probably secondary to ventricular dysrhythmia) occurs in 6–8% of children referred to tertiary centres. Risk factors include a family history of sudden death, syncope, and exercise-induced hypotension and may be an indication for implanting a cardioverter-defibrillator.

Restrictive cardiomyopathy
This accounts for 5% of cases. It may be idiopathic or complicate storage diseases such as the mucopolysaccharidoses. Stiff ventricular walls elevate diastolic filling pressure with secondary atrial dilatation. Progressive cardiac failure occurs. Diuretics, calcium antagonists, anticoagulation, and anti-arrhythmics or pacing are the mainstays of treatment.

Cardiac arrhythmias
Variations of sinus rhythm include:
- *Sinus tachycardia:* this rarely exceeds 200 beats/min
- *Sinus arrhythmia:* phasic variation in rate with the respiratory cycle with an increase on inspiration
- *Sinus bradycardia:* causes include hypoxia, raised ICP, hypothermia, hypoxia, hypokalaemia, β-blockade and anorexia.

ECG criteria for sinus rhythm are: P wave always followed by a QRS complex, QRS complex always preceded by P wave, and P wave axis 0–90° (upright P waves in I and aVF).

Aetiology
Most children with an arrhythmia do not have a congenital structural heart defect. Causes include: an accessory AV pathway, hyper- and hypokalaemia, hypocalcaemia, drug toxicity, myocarditis, cardiomyopathy, structural heart defects, post surgery, cardiac rhabdomyosarcoma, long QT (LQT) syndrome.

Classification
Arrhythmias can be classified by HR: slow or fast
- *Bradyarrhythmias:* atrioventricular (AV) block, sinus node dysfunction
- *Tachyarrhythmias:* SVT, ventricular tachycardia.

Clinical features
Infants with supraventricular tachycardia may present with congestive cardiac failure or circulatory collapse. Older children may complain of palpitations and chest pain. Syncope *on exertion* at any age has an attendant mortality and should prompt immediate investigation to exclude a precipitating ventricular dysrhythmia.

Investigations and management
A standard 12-lead ECG may be normal if the arrhythmia is episodic, though may indicate pre-excitation with a short PR interval and slurred R wave upstroke ('delta wave'), or a prolonged

QTc interval. Ambulatory ECG, exercise stress testing, and tilt testing may be useful diagnostic adjuncts.

Acute medical interventions are dysrhythmia-specific and may include vagal manoeuvres, anti-arrhythmic drugs, and cardioversion. Prophylactic anti-arrhythmics, radiofrequency ablation, and implantation of a pacemaker or defibrillator each have a role in selected cases.

Specific cardiac arrythmias

Atrioventricular (AV) block

- *1st degree block:* PR interval prolonged (Fig 4.16). May be a harmless variant or associated with structural heart disease or acute inflammatory processes (e.g. Lyme disease, rheumatic fever)

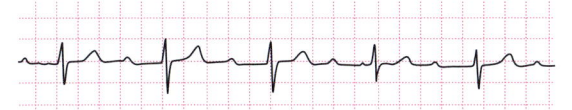

Fig 4.16 1st degree AV block.

- *2nd degree block:*
  - *Mobitz Type I:* increasing PR interval followed by absent QRS complex. Common and usually asymptomatic.
  - *Mobitz Type II:* constant PR interval with random dropping of QRS complexes (Fig 4.17). May be poorly tolerated and requires a search for a precipitant. Causes include: muscular dystrophies, maternal SLE, post cardiac surgery, digoxin toxicity

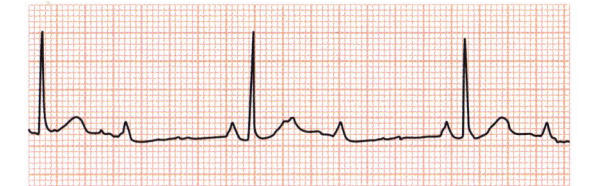

Fig 4.17 Mobitz Type II AV block with 2:1 conduction.

- *3rd degree block:* complete heart block in which atrial and ventricular activity are completely independent.

Supraventricular tachycardia

Accounts for 95% of tachyarrhythmias in children. Most are AV re-entry tachycardias with an accessory pathway from atria to ventricles. If this allows antegrade conduction the ECG shows pre-excitation (Fig 4.18B), and the condition is termed Wolff–Parkinson–White (WPW) syndrome. The rhythm is narrow complex with retrograde P waves.

In teenagers and young adults, SVT is usually due to AV nodal re-entry tachycardia. A narrow complex tachycardia occurs with P waves buried in the QRS complex (Fig 4.18A).

Clinical features
Age dependent:
- *Fetus:* fetal tachycardia, hydrops fetalis
- *Infant:* signs of heart failure or circulatory failure
- *Preschool child:* abdominal pain, palpitations, unexplained episodic pallor and sweating
- *Older child:* palpitations, chest pain.

Investigations
ECG: narrow complex tachycardia; pre-excitation on resting strip (if accessory bundle present).

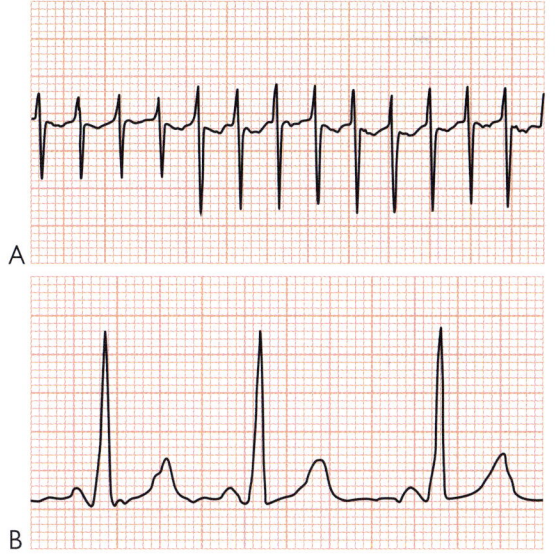

Fig 4.18 SVT: A. Narrow QRS complex tachycardia. B. Pre-excitation of WPW syndrome.

Management
The aim of acute management is to terminate the arrhythmia by slowing conduction through the node by:
- *Vagal stimulation:* in infants, application of a towel soaked in ice-cold water to the 'snout' region of the face. In children, Valsalva manoeuvre or carotid sinus massage
- *IV adenosine:* given as a rapid bolus (short half-life)
- *DC cardioversion:* 1–2 J/kg, used when there is acute circulatory compromise or persisting SVT despite drug treatment.

An ECG strip recorded during intervention may provide useful diagnostic information about the mechanism.

In infants with SVT, 80% are symptom free by 1 year with regression of the accessory pathway. Parents can be taught to auscultate to detect SVT recurrence before cardiac failure develops over hours/days. In older children drugs may be used to reduce recurrence, e.g. β-blockers, flecainide. Radiofrequency ablation is available for older children with recurrent paroxysms.

Long QT syndrome (LQTS)

Mutations in 10 different ion channel genes (including *SCN5A, KCNQ1, CACNA1C*) cause this AD genetic disease.

An abnormally long delay occurs between ventricular depolarization and repolarization and may precipitate syncope or sudden death from ventricular dysrhythmias. Triggers may include exercise, sleep and fever. Romano–Ward and Brugada syndromes are eponymous forms.

ECG diagnosis can be difficult (Fig 4.19). Once confirmed, β-blockade and implantable cardioverter-defibrillators (ICD) are the mainstays of treatment.

Prolongation of the QT interval may also occur as a result of drugs or electrolyte disturbance (hypokalaemia, hypocalcaemia).

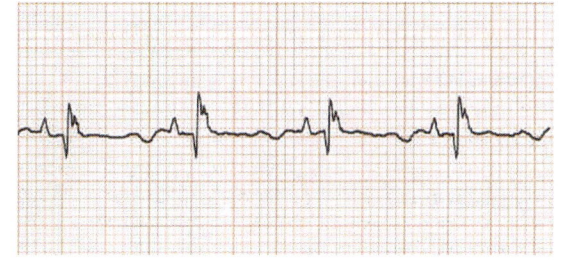

Fig 4.19 LQTS: ECG.

4.10 Case-based discussions

An infant with tachycardia

A 1 month old male infant is brought to the hospital emergency department by his parents with a 36 hour history of poor feeding and increasing lethargy. He was born at term and has been previously well.

On examination he is pale but apyrexial. The heart rate is 250/min. Peripheral pulses are palpable and low volume and the CRT is >4 s.

BP 75/40 mmHg. Cardiac auscultation is normal.

The respiratory rate is 50/min with flaring and mild recession but no grunting. Liver is palpable at 3 cm.

There is no clinical cyanosis and O_2 saturation provides poor pick-up.

What is your initial working diagnosis and management?

The differential includes causes of circulatory failure such as infection and hypovolaemia, but tachycardia and hepatomegaly suggest a primary cardiac cause.

The heart rate strongly suggests supraventricular tachycardia as sinus tachycardia rarely exceeds 200/min even in young infants.

Infants in the first few weeks of life account for about a third of children presenting with SVT. They tolerate arrhythmias less well than older children, as they have less reserve to maintain their cardiac output in the presence of an inefficiently rapid heart rate.

This is most rapidly confirmed by attaching ECG leads. SVT is usually narrow complex, although aberrant conduction pathways may cause a wide complex rhythm.

Initial management is to terminate the arrhythmia. Vagal manoeuvres are appropriate in the first instance. In an infant, an ice pack should be applied to the face for 30 s or facial immersion in ice-cold water for not more than 10s can be attempted. An older child can be asked to hold their nose and breathe out, or to breathe through a narrow straw (to achieve the Valsalva effect). Carotid sinus massage (on one side only!) may also be useful.

When an ice pack is applied to the baby's face, his heart rate remains at 280/min.

How should he be managed now?

Oxygen should be given by mask. IV access should be obtained, and adenosine given (starting dose 150 micrograms/kg) followed by a rapid flush. Adenosine works by blocking atrioventricular nodal conduction and interrupting a re-entry circuit.

It is important to continue ECG monitoring throughout administration, and also to record a rhythm strip, as response to adenosine may be of diagnostic significance: even brief termination of the arrhythmia by adenosine suggests the involvement of the atrioventricular node in a supraventricular re-entrant pathway. Current recommendations for dosage vary, but increasing doses of up to 350 micrograms/kg can be tried in resistant cases.

If pharmacological cardioversion with adenosine is unsuccessful, synchronized DC cardioversion may be required.

What subsequent management is appropriate?

The baby should be admitted and continuous cardiac monitoring performed as the arrhythmia may recur. Blood tests should be taken to exclude electrolyte abnormalities and sepsis as provoking factors. Cardiac failure may require short-term diuretics.

A formal ECG must be performed and an echocardiogram arranged to rule out structural abnormalities. The infant should be referred to a cardiologist who may rarely perform further electrophysiological studies. The commonest cause of SVT in an infant is a re-entry tachycardia with an accessory pathway.

Prophylaxis for some months with flecainide or β-blockade may be given, followed by an attempt at withdrawal which is successful in ~70% of cases. Resistant cases require longer prophylaxis and consideration of electrophysiological studies.

An infant with heart failure

A 10 week old female infant presents with a 4 week history of progressive breathlessness, poor feeding, and failure to thrive.

On examination she is pink. Pulses are all low volume and there is a palpable cardiac impulse. On auscultation, P2 is loud and there is a 2–3/6 harsh pan-systolic murmur maximal at the lower left sternal edge and a 1/6 low-pitched mid-diastolic murmur at the apex. There is tachypnoea (50/min), indrawing but no grunting or flaring The liver is 3 cm palpable, spleen not palpable.

What is your approach to diagnosis?

This presentation with gradual onset and abnormal cardiac signs is much more suggestive of cardiac disease and cardiac failure than respiratory illness.

History and signs suggest a large left-to-right shunt with increased pulmonary blood flow and a high pressure in the pulmonary artery (loud P2). VSD is the most likely diagnosis. PDA (though murmur usually continuous) and AVSD (often associated with Down syndrome) could produce a similar picture. Absence of cyanosis makes a more complex lesion unlikely.

CXR (cardiomegaly and pulmonary plethora) and ECG will give diagnostic clues, e.g. a superior QRS axis is suggestive of AVSD. Echocardiography is mandatory to confirm the precise anatomical diagnosis.

Echocardiography confirms a large isolated VSD.

What is the initial management?

Diuretics will produce short-term clinical improvement. Addition of afterload reduction (ACE inhibitor) and surgical planning for repair of a structural lesion follow echocardiography. Optimizing nutrition is very important.

Surgery is required for large symptomatic lesions. The exact timing varies between institutions.

Chapter 5

Gastroenterology and nutrition

5.1 Gastrointestinal system *94*
5.2 Nutrition *96*
5.3 Congenital anomalies and Hirschsprung disease *98*
5.4 Oesophageal and gastric disorders *100*
5.5 Acute gastroenteritis and intussusception *102*
5.6 Coeliac disease and short bowel syndrome *104*
5.7 Inflammatory bowel disease *106*
5.8 Functional gastrointestinal disorders *108*
5.9 Functional abdominal pain and constipation *110*
5.10 Pancreatic and gallbladder disease *112*
5.11 Neonatal liver disease *114*
5.12 Childhood liver disease *116*
5.13 Case-based discussions *118*

5.1 Gastrointestinal system

The gastrointestinal (GI) tract is the organ system in multicellular animals responsible for ingestion, digestion, and absorption of foodstuffs and elimination of remaining waste.

In addition it has endocrine and immune functions and via the gut–brain axis interacts to regulate food intake and fluid and electrolyte balance.

Embryology and anatomy
Embryology
The primordial gut forms during the 4th week by incorporation of the dorsal part of the yolk sac into the embryo. It is divided into foregut, midgut, and hindgut supplied by coeliac, superior, and inferior mesenteric arteries.

As it elongates, the midgut herniates into the umbilical cord as a U-shaped loop (week 6) and rotates 90° counterclockwise. During week 10 the intestines return to the abdomen, rotating a further 180° in the process.

The hindgut gives rise to the distal transverse colon, descending and sigmoid colon, rectum, and superior part of the anal canal.

Anatomy
At birth the basic anatomy of the human gut is fully developed, although the relative length of each segment is much shorter than that in the adult.

The gut is a tube with four concentric layers: mucosa, submucosa, muscularis externa, and serosa. The mucosa is further divided into epithelium, lamina propria, and muscularis mucosae.

In the small intestine, the surface area is increased by a factor of 300 by valvulae conniventes, villi, and microvilli. Villous cells are responsible for digestive and absorptive functions and crypt cells are predominantly secretory.

Enteric nervous system (ENS)
The ENS is an interdependent part of the autonomic nervous system, containing ~100 million neurons. It is sometimes accorded the status of a 'second brain', being derived from the same neural crest as the CNS. It comprises two major plexuses embedded in the wall:
- *Myenteric plexus (of Auerbach)* located between the longitudinal and circular muscle layers in the bowel wall, primarily controls motility
- *Submucosal plexus (of Meissner)* between the circular muscle and submucosa, regulates blood flow and epithelial cell function.

The ENS controls peristalsis and enzyme secretion. A variety of fibres link the ENS to the rest of the nervous system: vagal connections provide a massive sensory link and sympathetic C fibres transmit visceral pain. ENS ganglia utilize up to 30 different neurotransmitters.

Functional GI disorders
Dysfunction in the gut–brain axis underlies many of the 'functional' disorders of the GI tract. See Section 5.8.

Gut-associated lymphoid tissue (GALT)
The GALT (see Fig 5.1) is one component of the mucosa-associated lymphoid tissue (MALT), a diffuse system of lymphoid tissue found at various sites.

Specialized M cells in Peyer's patches sample, process, and present antigens to subepithelial lymphoid cells. The GALT must respond effectively to microbial pathogens yet tolerate dietary antigens and commensal microbes. Inflammation and allergy emerge when this homeostasis fails.

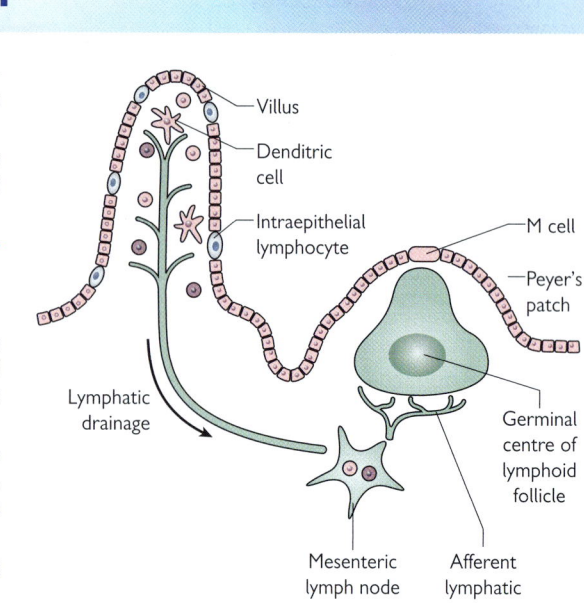

Fig 5.1 Gut associated lymphoid tissue (GALT).

Physiology
Gut motility
Each section has a unique pattern of motility reflecting its particular function. Specialized sphincters regulate the passage of ingested material from one section to another.

Gut motility depends on:
- Intrinsic myogenic activity
- Interstitial cells of Cajal (ICCs)
- Autonomic and enteric nervous systems
- GI hormones.

The ENS generates and propagates coordinated motor events such as peristalsis and controls sphincters. A very wide range of neurotransmitters function in the gut:
- *Inhibitory (relaxation) transmitters:* vasoactive peptide (VIP) and nitric oxide (NO)
- *Excitatory transmitters:* methylcholine and serotonin.

Standing contractions mix food. Peristaltic movements propel food in an anterograde or a retrograde (vomiting, regurgitation) direction. Phasic contractions of sphincters regulate compartmentalization and bursts of contraction progress slowly down the intestine during fasting and particularly at night. Distension of the rectum leads to relaxation of the internal anal sphincter mediated via the myenteric plexus.

Gut motility disorders
Gut motility disorders are common and may present as vomiting, abdominal pain, recurrent obstruction, constipation or diarrhoea. They include gastro-oesophageal reflux, pyloric stenosis, and Hirschsprung disease.

Digestion and absorption
Digestion is the preparation of food for absorption and uptake of the resulting small molecules through the epithelium into the bloodstream. The small intestine is primarily responsible for absorption of water and electrolytes, carbohydrates, proteins, lipids, and fat-soluble vitamins.

- *Water:* is passively absorbed and linked to electrolyte and solute absorption. Sodium is taken up via the NaCl coupled transporter and the Na–glucose co-transporter, SGLT1.
- *Carbohydrate:* digestion has a luminal (via pancreatic α-amylases) and mucosal (brush border membrane hydrolases and saccharidases) phase. Monosaccharides are then absorbed via facilitative transporters.
- *Protein:* digestion starts in the stomach, creating polypeptides which enter the duodenum where pancreatic proteases (trypsin, chymotrypsin, elastase, carbopeptidase) convert them to oligopeptides and free amino acids. These are taken up via Na^+-dependent transporters and a hydrogen–peptide co-transporter.
- *Dietary fat:* 95% long-chain triglycerides, is emulsified in the duodenum and digested by pancreatic lipase and co-lipase in the neutral pH of the duodenum to form monoglycerides and fatty acids. These interact with bile salts to form mixed micelles. After take up and processing in the enterocyte they are incorporated into secretory vesicles and released into the extracellular space from where chylomicrons move to the lymph lacteals and into the lymphatic system which delivers them to the systemic circulation.

Liver function

Table 5.1 summarizes the main functions of the liver.

Table 5.1.	Liver functions
Synthesis	Plasma proteins including albumin, globulins and clotting factors Lipoproteins
Storage	Glycogen, fats, cholesterol Trace metals: iron, copper Vitamins: A, D, K, B12
Excretion	Detoxification and excretion of amino acids, bilirubin, hormones, and exogenous substances: drugs, alcohol
Metabolism	Carbohydrates: glycogenesis, glycolysis, glycogenolysis, and gluconeogenesis Fats: synthesis of lipoproteins, cholesterol phospholipids, metabolism of lipids for lipogenesis or lipolysis Proteins: amino acid deamination and transamination, ammonia metabolism via urea cycle
Bile	Bile contains bile salts, critical for fat digestion, cholesterol, phospholipids, electrolytes and waste products including bile pigments (bilirubin), hormones, drugs
Immunity	Filters and removes bacteria Phagocytes produce acute-phase proteins

Bilirubin metabolism

Bilirubin is the breakdown product of the haem moiety present in haemoglobin and other haemoproteins. Unconjugated bilirubin is lipid soluble because of internal hydrogen bonding and circulates in plasma tightly bound to albumin.

Free unconjugated bilirubin is toxic to neuronal cells. It is conjugated to glucuronides by microsomal glucoronyl transferase (gene UGT1A1) in hepatocytes and then actively transported into the bile canaliculi. Conjugated bilirubin is water-soluble.

Hepatic enzyme activity is low at birth but rapidly matures. Delayed development is an important cause of neonatal unconjugated hyperbilirubinaemia. The small amount of unconjugated bilirubin that appears in bile is partially re-absorbed. Intestinal bacteria degrade bilirubin into urobilinogen which is absorbed and undergoes enterohepatic recirculation.

Appetite control

Major recent advances have been made in understanding the neuroendocrine control of food intake. Circulating peptide hormones affect the neuronal circuitry that regulates how hungry you feel by acting in an orexigenic (appetite stimulating) or anorexigenic (appetite inhibiting) fashion.

Central control (Fig 5.2)

- Neurons in the arcuate nucleus (ARC) project to the paraventricular nucleus (PVN). Neuropeptide Y (NPY) and Agouti-related peptide (AgRP) neurons stimulate appetite via Y1 and Y5 hypothalamic receptors.
- αMSH and CART neurons inhibit appetite via MC3 and MC4 receptors.
- POMC is a precursor of αMSH. AgRP acts as an antagonist at MC3/MC4 receptors.

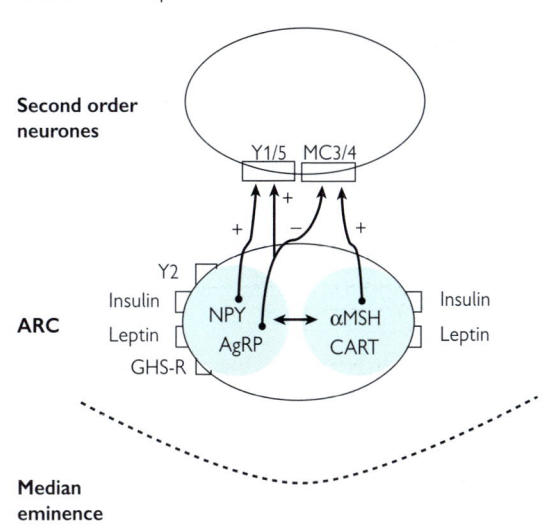

Fig 5.2 Central appetite control. Journal of Endocrinology (2005) 184, 291–318. © Society for Endocrinology. Reproduced by permission.

Peripheral control

Eating releases a number of 'satiety gut hormones' including peptide YY (PYY3–36) and pancreatic polypeptide (PP). These inhibit appetite and inhibit release of the 'hunger hormone' ghrelin, a peptide hormone released from endocrine cells of the stomach (Fig 10.7). In addition, adipocytes release an array of adipocytokines including leptin, adiponectin, and visfatin. Leptin inhibits appetite, but acts only as a reassurance factor. Obese people have high levels.

5.2 Nutrition

Infant feeding
The UK Department of Health recommends:
- Breast milk as the best form of nutrition for infants
- Exclusive breastfeeding for the first 6 months (26 weeks) of an infant's life
- Age 6 months for the introduction of solid foods
- Breast-feeding and/or breast-milk substitutes should continue beyond the first 6 months, along with appropriate solid foods.

The health benefits of breast-feeding have long been recognized (see Box), and can be promoted by various strategies.

Benefits of breastfeeding
Breastfed babies are less likely to develop: • Enteric, respiratory, and urinary tract infections (UTIs)   • Obesity in later childhood   • Atopic disease   • Juvenile-onset IDDM.   Breastfeeding mothers have: • Reduced risk of premenopausal breast cancer   • Increased likelihood of returning to prepregnancy weight.

Introducing solids early (4–6 months) before sufficient development of neuromuscular coordination and of the gut and kidneys can increase the risk of infections and allergies.

Weaning foods and drinks
Salt should not be added, and nut butters should be avoided in infants with a family history of atopy. Breast milk or infant formula should remain the milk drink until the age of 12 months at which time cow's milk can be introduced.

Vitamin supplementation
Breast-fed infants or infants receiving <500 mL of infant formula per day require a vitamin D supplement.

Infants should regain their birthweight by age 2 weeks and thereafter gain about 15–30 g/day. Weight at birth reflects maternal influences in addition to genetic potential, so 'catch up' and 'catch down' is commonly seen in the 1st 2 months.

Normal nutritional requirements
The high surface to volume ratio of infants and children increases their energy needs expressed per kg body weight (Table 5.2). From 1–5 years, take a base of 1000 kcal and add 100 kcal for each year.

Table 5.2. Estimated average requirement (EAR)		
Age (years)	kcal/day	
1–5	1100–1500	
6–8	1400–1600	
9–13	1600–2000 (girls)	1800–2200 (boys)
14–18	2000 (girls)	2200–2400 (boys)

Healthy eating
A mixture of foods, all providing different nutrients, makes up a balanced diet. Food can be categorized into five groups each of which contribute to a balanced diet (Table 5.3). Five portions of fruit and vegetables a day is recommended.

Table 5.3. Food groups	
Food group	Main nutrients
Bread, cereals, and potato	Carbohydrates, fibre, B vitamins, iron, and calcium
Fruit and vegetables	Vitamins, minerals, fibre, potassium
Milk and dairy products	Calcium, protein, riboflavin, vitamins A and D
Meat, fish, eggs, nuts, pulses	Protein, B vitamins, iron, zinc, magnesium
Fat-rich and sugar-rich foods	Fatty acids, vitamins

Certain points are especially relevant for preschool, school age, and teenage children:

Preschool
- *1–2 years*: a higher-fat, lower-fibre diet is appropriate. Full-fat milk products are advised.
- *2–5 years*: a gradual change to a lower-fat, higher-fibre diet. Semi-skimmed milk can be introduced after the age of 2 years. Children <5 years should not be given skimmed milk. Common problems include constipation (increase fibre and water intake) and toddler diarrhoea (restrict sweetened drinks, avoid high fibre intake).

School-age children
It is important that healthy eating habits are established. A recent survey showed excess average intake of saturated fatty acids and excess salt and sugar intakes. Regulations exist on national minimum nutritional standards for schools which opt to provide lunches.

Teenagers
The demand for energy and most nutrients is relatively high. Iron requirements increase especially in girls after menstruation begins. 9% of girls have mild anaemia and an intake of iron below the lower reference nutrient intake Girls on vegetarian or slimming diets are at risk. The rapid increase in bone mass generates a higher calcium requirement. Average daily salt intakes tend to be too high. Inactive teenagers may become overweight or obese.

Salt
Food is often misleadingly labelled with the weight of *sodium*. This must be multiplied by 2.5 to give the weight of *salt* (sodium chloride). See Table 5.4.

Table 5.4. Daily recommended maximum intake of salt		
Age (years)	Salt (g)	Sodium (g)
0–1	<1	<0.4
1–3	2	0.8
4–6	3	1.2
7–10	5	2.0
>11	6	2.5

Malnutrition

Malnutrition remains a major global health problem. Obesity, an excess accumulation of adipose tissue, is a form of malnutrition. The causes of malnutrition are listed in Table 5.5.

Table 5.5. Causes of malnutrition	
Inadequate intake	Starvation: inadequate food supply Anorexia, dietary problems Feeding difficulties: cerebral palsy, cleft palate Eating disorder, diencephalic syndrome Chronic illness
Malabsorption	Pancreatic insufficiency: cystic fibrosis Small intestinal disease: coeliac disease, Cow's milk protein intolerance, Disaccharidase deficiency
Excessive losses	Persistent vomiting Protein losing enteropathy Chronic diarrhoea Chronic illness
Excessive requirements	Thyrotoxicosis, malignancy Cystic fibrosis, congenital heart disease, TB, HIV

Malnutrition is often classified according to whether there is a deficiency of macronutrients, so-called protein-energy malnutrition (PEM), or a deficiency in specific micronutrients, or a combination of both. PEM is further classified into:

- *Kwashiorkor:* malnutrition with oedema and anorexia. Body weight is 60–80% of expected. Often occurs after weaning at 18–24 months. There is muscle wasting but preservation of some subcutaneous fat.
- *Marasmus:* an adaptive response with emaciation and growth failure but preserved appetite. Oedema is not present. Body weight is <60% of expected. In developing countries it is often associated with failure of lactation due to maternal malnutrition. Children are withdrawn and apathetic.

Nutritional assessment

The dietary intake is reviewed and any feeding difficulties or chronic diseases documented.

Clinical examination focuses on pattern of weight gain, current weight, and body mass index (BMI). PEM may be associated with behavioural changes such as apathy, irritability, and decreased social responsiveness. Examination reveals decreased subcutaneous fat, thin sparse hair, angular stomatitis, or cheilosis. Hepatomegaly due to fatty infiltration may be present.

More detailed assessment involves anthropometry. Body fat is assessed by skinfold thickness, an estimate of subcutaneous fat, and the waist-to-hip circumference ratio.

Laboratory evaluation

Tests which measure nutritional status, as opposed to seeking an aetiology for malnutrition include:

- *FBC with red cell indices and film:* identifies anaemias due to iron, folate, B12 deficiency
- *Serum albumin.*

Consequences of malnutrition

Malnutrition affects nearly every organ system, impairing physical growth, cognitive function, and immune responses. Globally it is the most important risk factor for illness and death contributing to >50% of deaths in children worldwide.

Features of specific micronutrient deficiencies include:
- *Vitamin A:* night blindness, xerophthalmia, follicular hyperplasia, and impaired resistance to infection. Vitamin A deficiency increases morbidity and mortality of severe measles
- *Vitamin D:* rickets is discussed in Chapter 16.6
- *Vitamin E:* deficiency is rare and causes ataxia, peripheral neuropathy, and retinitis pigmentosa
- *Vitamin K:* deficiency in the newborn causes haemorrhagic disease and is prevented by vitamin K at birth
- *Iron:* deficiency causes anaemia and may contribute to cognitive impairment
- *Zinc:* deficiency occurs secondary to poor absorption; features include anaemia, hyperpigmentation, immune deficiency, and diarrhoea
- *Iodine:* maternal iodine deficiency is less common since the introduction of iodized salt; it was the most common preventable cause of mental retardation
- *Folate:* deficiency causes megaloblastic anaemia, poor weight gain, and chronic diarrhoea; causes include coeliac disease, drugs, and increased requirements.

Management: nutrition support

A multidisciplinary approach is required. The formula for calculating adequate caloric intake is:

$$\text{kcal/kg} = \text{recommended daily allowance} \times (\text{ideal weight/actual weight})$$

Enteral feeding via the oral route is preferred if possible. If oral feeding is not possible, enteral access at the level of the stomach or jejunum is allowed by tubes inserted via the nose (nasogastric, nasojejunal) or via a gastrostomy (percutaneous endoscopic gastrostomy, PEG tube, button gastrostomy). Indications for gastrostomy tube feeding include:

- Oral feeding difficulties
- Cerebral palsy, bulbar palsy, in conjunction with fundoplication if there is gastro-oesophageal reflux (GOR)
- *Nutritional support in chronic disease:* cystic fibrosis, bronchopulmonary dysplasia, Crohn's disease (see Table 5.6). Parenteral nutrition via a central line is now even possible at home and may be total or combined with enteral feeds.

Table 5.6. Examples of diseases in which parenteral feeding may be necessary	
Congenital abnormalities	Tracheo-oesophageal fistula, Pierre Robin syndrome, cleft palate
Anorexia nervosa	
Severe burns, sepsis, or trauma	
Neuromuscular disorders	Cerebral palsy, muscular dystrophy, myasthenia gravis
Gastrointestinal disorders	Short bowel syndrome, inflammatory bowel disease, chronic liver disease
Malignant disease	
Palliative care, post chemotherapy or radiotherapy	

5.3 Congenital anomalies and Hirschsprung disease

Congenital anomalies

Common developmental abnormalities of the GI tract are listed in Table 5.7. Many are now diagnosed prenatally by ultrasound.

Table 5.7. Congenital anomalies of the GI tract	
Oesophageal atresia and tracheoesophageal fistula (TOF)	
Duodenal atresia/stenosis	
Intestinal malrotation	Volvulus
Meckel diverticulum	
Abdominal wall defects	Gastroschisis
	Omphalocele (exomphalos)
Anal atresia/stenosis	

Oesophageal atresia

The incidence is 1/3500 live births. Associated anomalies are common and may include the VACTERL sequence: **V**ertebral, **A**nal, **C**ardiac, **T**racheal, **E**sophageal, **R**enal, **L**imb.

The most common anomaly is blind-ending upper oesophageal pouch with a gap between it and the distal oesophagus which connects to distal trachea as a tracheo-oesophageal fistula (TOF) but there are several types (Fig 5.3).

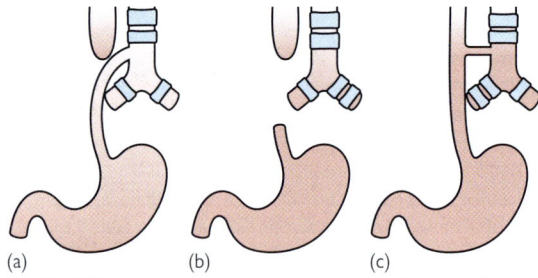

Fig 5.3 Different types of oesophageal atresia: A. Blind oesophagus with TOF between distal oesophagus and trachea (86%). B. Oesophageal atresia without fistula (8%). C. H-type fistula without atresia (4%).

Prenatal presentation is with polyhydramnios and postnatally there is frothing of oral secretions with choking and cyanosis if a feed is given. Diagnosis is made by inability to pass a wide bore orogastric tube, confirmed on radiography.
Management is surgical.

Atresia/stenosis

The duodenum is the most frequent (33% of cases) site of atresia (lack of lumen) or stenosis (narrowing). Down syndrome coexists in up to 30% of affected infants. Duodenal atresia classically presents with bilious vomiting and a 'double-bubble' on plain abdominal radiograph.

Malrotation

This refers to failure of the usual complete 270° rotation as the gut returns to the abdominal cavity (Fig 5.4). It covers a spectrum of abnormalities:
- *Non-rotation*: the duodeno-jejunal loop lies to the right of the spine and the caecum and colon on the left. It rarely causes obstruction and may be associated with diaphragmatic hernia or abdominal wall defects.
- *Malrotation*: obstruction of the duodenum may occur because of Ladd's bands or volvulus rotation of the unfixed midgut loop on its narrow base with ensuing intestinal ischaemia.

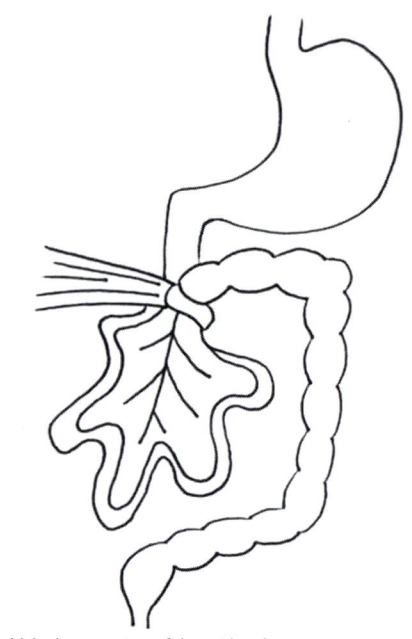

Fig 5.4 Volvulus: rotation of the midgut loop.

Abdominal wall defects
Gastroschisis

Viscera herniate through a small defect in the anterior abdominal wall, usually to the right of the umbilicus. There is no covering membrane (Fig 5.5). It is usually an isolated lesion, but intestinal atresia and significant intestinal malfunction is common. It is increasing in frequency especially among young mothers and lower birthweight babies. Prenatal diagnosis can be made as early as 12 weeks gestation.

Management is surgical. The infant's lower body is placed in a sterile plastic bag and a large-bore nasogastric tube passed to limit passage of air into the bowel.

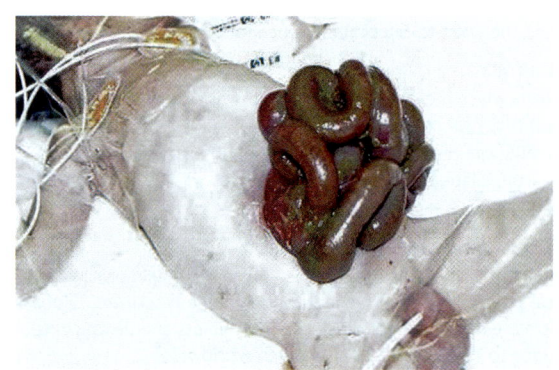

Fig 5.5 Gastroschisis.

Omphalocele

The incidence is 1/5000 fetuses. There is a defect of the umbilicus with herniation of abdominal contents (Fig 5.6). Herniated organs are covered by a sac.

Associated malformations are common, as are syndromes such as Beckwith–Wiedemann and trisomies 13 or 18.

Management

Prenatal diagnosis allows optimal care. Immediate postnatal management includes nasogastric and endotracheal intubation. Prognosis has improved markedly.

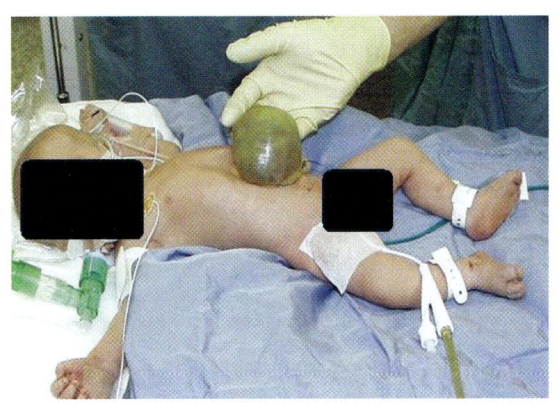

Fig 5.6 Omphalocele.

Hirschsprung disease

Hirschsprung disease (HSCR) or aganglionic megacolon is characterized by an absence of ganglion cells for a variable length of the distal colon resulting in functional colonic obstruction. The incidence is 1/5000 live births and the male to female ratio is 4:1. It can be further classified into:
- *Type 1 (80%):* short-segment disease in which aganglionosis affects only rectum and/or sigmoid
- *Type 2:* long-segment disease in which aganglionosis affects a variable segment of the colon.

Extreme varieties occur including 'ultrashort segment' disease and total intestinal aganglionosis. HSCR may be non-syndromic or occur in association with a number of syndromes (see below).

Aetiology and pathogenesis

HSCR is a genetic trait caused by mutations in up to 10 different genes acting alone or in combination:
- *RET:* the most important gene is *RET* on chromosome 10q encoding the receptor tyrosine kinase. Loss-of-function mutations in *RET* are found in up to 25% of children, especially in familial, long-segment disease.
- *EDNRB* and *ET3:* mutations in the endothelin B receptor gene, *EDNRB*, account for 5% of HSCR cases, and mutations in its ligand endothelin 3, *ET3*, account for 1%.

Hirschsprung disease is also found in a number of syndromes, for some of which the mutated gene is known. These include Down syndrome (HSCR affects 1% of DS children) and rarities such as congenital central hypoventilation, Mowat syndrome, and Shah–Waardenburg syndrome.

Pathogenesis

Enteric ganglion cells are derived from the neural crest. During normal embryonic development neuroblasts appear in the small intestine by the 7th week of gestation and migrate along the colon by the 12th week of gestation.

In HSCR both the myenteric (Auerbach) and submucosal (Meissner) plexuses are absent for a variable distance. Loss of the intrinsic enteric inhibiting nerves leads to an imbalance of control of smooth muscle contractility with excess excitatory input, increased tone, and functional obstruction.

Clinical features

The majority of infants (90%) present in the first week of life with distal bowel obstruction. The classical features include:
- *Delayed passage of meconium:* Hirschsprung disease should be considered in any newborn who fails to pass meconium within 24–48 h
- Positive family history (10%)
- Poor feeding followed by bilious vomiting.

Examination reveals abdominal distension, and withdrawal of the finger after rectal examination may result in explosive passage of gas and faeces.

Hirschsprung-associated enterocolitis, related to stasis and bacterial overgrowth, presents with watery grey stools and may occur in 5–15% of infants. This serious condition may progress to colonic perforation and life-threatening sepsis.

Hirschsprung disease rarely accounts for intractable constipation with onset later in life. However, it may present in later childhood with severe chronic constipation, abdominal distension, and failure to thrive. A careful history usually reveals problems with constipation from early infancy.

It is noteworthy that children with HSCR rarely develop soiling, in contrast to those with intractable functional constipation.

Investigations

Rectal biopsy

Full-thickness rectal biopsy remains the definitive diagnostic test: for infants <6 months a suction biopsy can be done, but >6 months an open rectal biopsy is preferred.

The pathognomonic finding is absence of ganglion cells in the myenteric and submucosal plexuses of the bowel wall. Acetylcholinesterase staining reveals hypertrophied nerve trunks throughout the lamina propria and muscularis propria.

Imaging

A plain abdominal radiograph may show dilated colon. Barium enema has limited usefulness but may be used in the diagnostic work-up of an infant with a meconium obstruction. The classical finding is a narrow distal colon with proximal dilation.

Ano-rectal manometry is used in some specialist constipation clinics.

Treatment

The treatment is surgical. The aim is to remove the aganglionic segment and anastomose healthy innervated bowel close (within ~2 cm) to the dentate line.

A primary pull-through procedure is commonly undertaken, unless there are contra-indications such as enterocolitis, perforation, or massive bowel dilatation. The alternative is a two-stage procedure with a diverting colostomy formed until the child weighs <10 kg. The most commonly performed procedures are the Swenson, Duhamel, and Soave procedures. Recent refinements include laparoscopic approaches and trans-anal pull-through operations.

Prognosis

Most children acquire faecal continence, but significant soiling or persistent obstruction may occur. Children with Down syndrome have lower rates of continence and placement of a permanent colostomy may be necessary.

5.4 Oesophageal and gastric disorders

Gastro-oesophageal reflux and disease

Gastro-oesophageal reflux (GOR)
GOR is the non-forceful reflux of gastric contents into the oesophagus.

Infant regurgitation or 'possetting'
This is one manifestation of GOR (milk being regurgitated from the mouth rather than just refluxed into the oesophagus) and is common and normal in infancy. At least one episode of regurgitation per day, usually after feeding, occurs in 50% of infants aged 0–3 months.

It is due to functional immaturity of the lower oesophageal sphincter and resolves spontaneously by 12–18 months of age as the sphincter matures and the infant adopts a more upright posture and a more solid diet. This benign form of GOR requires no treatment.

Regurgitation must be distinguished from vomiting which involves forceful contraction of diaphragm and abdominal muscles and from gastro-oesophageal reflux disease (GORD: see below).

GOR often presents with a history of regurgitation of feeds, and is often inferred from signs such as squirming which are taken to reflect discomfort related to feeds.

Management
Explanation and reassurance is sufficient for healthy infants with simple GOR and regurgitation: it is a benign condition which will resolve spontaneously. If regurgitation is frequent and troublesome, additional simple measures include:
- *Positioning:* elevate head of cot, left lateral position after feeds
- Frequent, small-volume feeds
- Feed thickeners (Carobel).

Consider a trial of formula free from cow's milk protein if there is uncertainty about diagnosis: GOR or CMPI.

Gastro-oesophageal reflux disease (GORD)
GORD is present when reflux is severe enough to cause complications. These may include:
- *Failure to thrive:* inadequate weight gain
- *Oesophagitis:* manifested by pain and irritability related to feeds and in severe form haematemesis, anaemia or stricture formation. Young children with severe reflux oesophagitis may show a behavioural pattern of back arching and facial grimacing (Sandifer syndrome)
- *Aspiration:* manifested by acute episodes of apnoea or 'acute life-threatening events' (ALTE) or chronic episodes of cough, wheeze, or pneumonia.

Aetiology and pathogenesis
GORD is often a secondary phenomenon and there are a number of important risk factors:
- Prematurity
- *Neurodevelopmental disorders:* cerebral palsy
- Chronic lung disease: cystic fibrosis
- *Post surgical repair:* of oesophageal atresia, congenital diaphragmatic hernia
- Hiatus hernia.

Clinical features
GORD presents with symptoms and signs related to the complications listed above: overt regurgitation (milk coming out of the mouth) may not necessarily be present.

The differential diagnosis includes:
- Causes of true vomiting such as GI tract obstruction (pyloric stenosis)
- Urinary tract infection
- Gastroenteritis
- Metabolic disorders.

In most infants a careful history and examination are sufficient but investigations may be indicated if the diagnosis is unclear or symptoms are severe.

The initial stages of pyloric stenosis may be mistaken for GOR if a careful history is not taken and examination is inadequate.

Investigations
- *Upper GI tract contrast radiography:* is an insensitive test for GOR, but useful to exclude anatomical abnormalities such as malrotation or duodenal web in an infant or hiatus hernia and oesophageal stricture in the older child.
- *Oesophageal 24 h pH study:* the pH of the distal oesophagus is recorded using an intraluminal antimony electrode, episodes of acid reflux corresponding to drops in pH <4.0. It is useful for demonstrating occult reflux, determining a temporal association between symptoms and acid reflux and assessing adequacy of therapy. Studies using intraluminal electrical impedance which detects fluid bolus movements, and therefore detects both acid and non-acid reflux, suggest that most reflux occurs post-prandially with pH >4.0. pH studies may therefore underestimate reflux.
- *Endoscopy:* can assess the presence and severity of oesophagitis.

Management
In addition to the simple measures described above, medical measures include:
- *Sodium alginate preparations (e.g. Gaviscon):* these form a 'raft' that floats on gastric contents and neutralizes acids. Studies show a marginal effect on average height of reflux.
- *Prokinetic agents:* evidence for the efficacy of motility stimulants such as domperidone is unconvincing.
- *Acid blocking agents:* H2-receptor antagonists (H2RAs) such as cimetidine or ranitidine relieve symptoms of oesophagitis and promote healing. Proton pump inhibitors (PPIs) such as omeprazole are used for moderate oesophagitis not responding to a H2RA.
- *Surgery:* anti-reflux surgery (Nissen fundoplication) is considered for selected patients when optimal medical therapy fails. There is a high failure rate and significant risk of morbidity.

Pyloric stenosis

Infantile hypertrophic pyloric stenosis (IHPS) is the most common cause of intestinal obstruction in infancy. The incidence in the UK is 1/1000 live births. Male:female ratio 4:1.

Aetiology and pathogenesis
IHPS is a multifactorial familial disorder. Inheritance is polygenic. Stenosis is not present at birth. Gradual hypertrophy of the muscular wall following initiation of enteral feeding causes obstruction of the pyloric lumen.

Clinical features
History

Infants typically present with vomiting at 2–6 weeks of age. Vomiting is non-bilious and becomes forceful ('projectile') with time. The infant remains hungry and constipation is common. Late presentation occurs up to 12 weeks.

Examination

There may be signs of dehydration, weight loss, and failure to thrive. Jaundice is present in 3%.

Abdominal examination may reveal visible peristalsis and a palpable pyloric 'mass'. This is best performed during a 'test feed'.

Management: investigations
Blood tests

Urea and electrolytes, blood gases

The classical electrolyte and acid–base disturbance of IHPS is a hypochloraemic, hypokalaemic metabolic alkalosis due to vomiting of acidic gastric contents.

IHPS is the only common cause of metabolic alkalosis in infants. The serum HCO_3^- values are usually >25–30 mEq/L.

Imaging

Abdominal ultrasonography is the imaging modality of choice. Diagnostic criteria are:
- Muscle wall thickness >4 mm
- Pyloric canal length >16 mm.

Management: treatment
Initial treatment is rehydration and correction of the electrolyte and acid-base imbalance. IV normal saline with added potassium (20–40 mmol/L) is usually appropriate.

Definitive surgical treatment by Ramstedt pyloromyotomy is then performed by an open or laparoscopic approach. The hypertrophic muscle is split longitudinally. Postoperative complications may include wound infection or dehiscence, but overall the prognosis is excellent.

Peptic ulcer disease

Peptic ulcer disease (PUD) is uncommon in children and is more often duodenal than gastric. PUD is classified into primary, commonly associated with *Helicobacter pylori* infection, and secondary to systemic illness or ulcerogenic drugs.

Primary peptic ulcer disease
Most cases occur after infancy and early childhood. The worldwide annual incidence of primary duodenal ulcers is estimated to be 5/100 000 children, the prevalence increasing during adolescence.

Aetiology: Helicobacter pylori

The majority of primary duodenal ulcers are associated with *H. pylori* (Hp) infection of the gastric antral mucosa. *H. pylori* is almost always acquired in childhood and leads to lifelong infection. The majority of patients with *H. pylori* infection have asymptomatic gastritis, but up to 15% develop PUD and 1% develop gastric adenocarcinoma in later life.

Clinical features

The most common symptom of primary duodenal ulcer disease is chronic and recurrent epigastric pain, frequently associated with vomiting and nocturnal awakening.

Management

Investigations

Upper GI endoscopy is the investigation of choice for suspected peptic ulcer disease. *H. pylori* infection is diagnosed by culture of gastric biopsies and urease testing Non-invasive testing using the ^{13}C-urea breath test for *H. pylori* infection has no role in the initial investigation of possible PUD in children but can be useful in monitoring treatment. Serological tests are unreliable in children <12 years.

Treatment

Medication to reduce acid production (omeprazole, ranitidine, cimetidine) combined with agents that improve mucosal defence (sucralfate) are used initially.

Eradication therapy is recommended for those with PUD and active *H. pylori* infection. Acid suppression is combined with two antibiotics (amoxicillin plus clarithromycin or metronidazole depending on sensitivity) for 2 weeks and acid suppression continued for a further 2 weeks.

Secondary peptic ulcer disease
Aetiology

- *Stress*: acute gastritis with erosions occurs in the severe stress of acute illness such as burns or multiple trauma
- *Drugs and toxins*: corticosteroids and non-steroidal anti-inflammatory drugs (NSAIDs)
- *Crohn disease*: this may present with inflammation of the proximal GI tract such as focal gastritis
- *Zollinger–Ellison syndrome*: a gastrinoma in the pancreas.

Clinical features and management

Prophylaxis with gastric acid-suppressing drugs is indicated in individuals at risk. Secondary ulcers often present acutely with massive haemorrhage or intestinal perforation. Endoscopy is indicated if the diagnosis is in doubt or therapeutic endoscopy or surgical intervention is being considered. Acute bleeding may require transfusion and intervention such as endoscopic diathermy. Adequate doses of omeprazole (IV) should be given.

5.5 Acute gastroenteritis and intussusception

Acute gastroenteritis
Acute diarrhoea, with or without vomiting, due to an infection of the GI tract, is very common. In the UK it accounts for 20% of GP consultations and 16% of emergency department presentations each year in children <5 years. Globally it causes 1 million child deaths each year.

Aetiology
In the UK, viruses account for 80%. Rotavirus is most common (see Box), but other viruses include adenoviruses, astroviruses, and norovirus.

Bacteria account for 10–20% of cases (*Campylobacter* spp., *Salmonella* spp., *Shigella* spp., *E. coli*) and protozoa such as *Giardia lamblia* and *Cryptosporidium* the remainder.

> **Rotavirus**
> - Family Reoviridae
> - RNA virus
> - Classified according to (VP6) epitopes into groups A–E
>
> Group A rotavirus is endemic worldwide and is responsible for 20% of cases of gastroenteritis.

Clinical features
There is acute onset (<7 days) of watery, frequent stools with or without vomiting, abdominal pain and fever.

The differential diagnosis includes:
- *Other GI tract pathology:* intussusception, appendicitis, pyloric stenosis
- *Other infections:* UTI, pneumonia, meningitis, haemolytic uraemic syndrome.

The main danger of this usually self-limiting condition is the risk of dehydration and assessment of the degree is central to clinical examination (see Table 5.8). Hypernatraemic dehydration may cause a 'doughy' feel to the skin.

The WHO now categorizes dehydration according to body weight loss into none (<3%), some (3–8%) and severe (>8%). The corresponding clinical signs are shown in Table 5.8.

Table 5.8. Assessment of dehydration

No dehydration: <3% body weight loss	
	Alert and responsive, moist mucous membranes
	Normal skin turgor
Some dehydration: 3–8% body weight loss	
	Irritable, restless
	Dry mucous membranes, sunken eyes
	Reduced skin turgor: skinfold return prolonged >1 s
Severe dehydration: >8% body weight loss	
	Lethargy, reduced conscious level
	Very dry mucous membranes, sunken eyes
	Skinfold return prolonged >2 s
	Signs of hypovolaemic shock: tachycardia, capillary refill >2 s, acidotic rapid breathing, oliguria or anuria

Management: investigations
Stool microscopy and culture and plasma urea and electrolytes are indicated. The latter is particularly important in order to identify hyper-or hyponatraemia.

Management: treatment
Rehydration
Administration of hypo-osmolar oral rehydration solution (ORS) is the mainstay of therapy for most children. This simple mixture of sugar, salts, and water was one of the most important medical advances of the 20th century and has saved many lives. It exploits the coupled sodium–glucose co-transporter at the intestinal brush border (Fig 5.7).

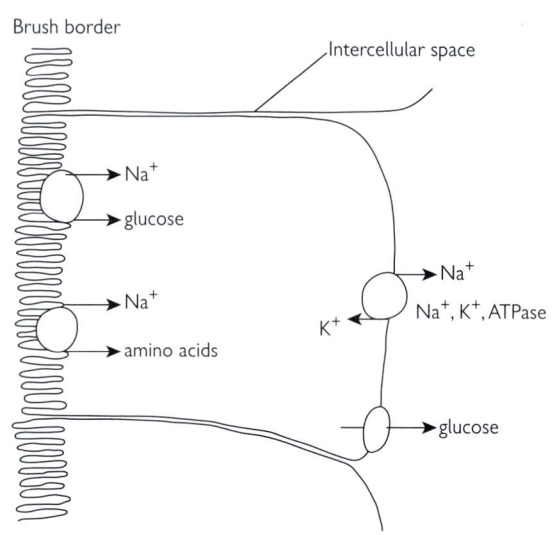

Fig 5.7 Brush border sodium–glucose co-transporter.

The optimal composition of ORS varies. The original WHO-ORS had a high sodium content (90 mmol/L) but European children with diarrhoea have lower stool losses of sodium. In Europe a lower-osmolality solution is optimal, and ORS contains 60 mmol/L sodium, >25 mmol/L chloride, 20 mmol/L potassium, and 74–100 mmol/L glucose.

Oral rehydration clearly depends on a cooperative child who is not vomiting. The enteral route can be accessed via a nasogastric tube if adequate oral amounts are not achieved. The oral route is preferred for moderate hypernatraemic dehydration, plasma Na^+ 150–170 mmol/L, with the deficit replaced slowly over 48 h. This is less likely than IV rehydration to cause an unduly rapid fall in plasma Na^+ concentration leading to brain oedema and seizures.

Those with severe rehydration require restoration of the circulating blood volume by an immediate IV bolus of 20 mL/kg of normal (0.9%) saline which may be repeated after 30 min if necessary. Further provision of deficit, maintenance, and ongoing losses is continued IV, usually with 0.45% saline with 20 mmol/L potassium and 2.5% dextrose.

Feeding
Children with mild to moderate dehydration should have rapid reintroduction of a normal diet after a few hours of oral rehydration. Breastfeeding should continue throughout. Lactose-free formulae are rarely required but can be used if diarrhoea worsens on reintroduction of milk, the stool is acid and contains >0.5% reducing substances.

Drug therapy
Antidiarrhoeal agents are contraindicated and may cause serious side effects. There is no role for antibiotics except in dysentery due to *Shigella*, invasive *Salmonella typhi*, or children who are

immunocompromised. There is some evidence that the addition of probiotics such as *Lactobacillus* GG to ORS is beneficial in acute diarrhoea caused by rotavirus infection.

Giardiasis

Giardiasis caused by *Giardia lamblia* infection is one of the most common causes of waterborne disease.

Clinical features

The illness usually occurs within 5–10 days of infection but it can be up to 25 days before the symptoms appear.

Abdominal cramping, bloating, and flatulence occur in 75% of symptomatic patients. Diarrhoea and malabsorption may lead to weight loss and dehydration. About 15% of cases of giardiasis are asymptomatic, with cyst passage only.

Management

Stool microscopy may aid in diagnosis but the cysts or trophozoites may be missed unless the technique is applied thoroughly. Small-bowel biopsy is definitive.

Treatment is with oral metronidazole 15 mg/kg for 3 days or tinidazole for those >3 years of age.

Intussusception

Intussusception is the telescoping or prolapse of one segment of bowel into the adjacent, distal bowel. It is an uncommon but potentially fatal condition and the most common cause of intestinal obstruction in infants and children aged 3 months–6 years.

The incidence is 1–4/1000 live births with a peak at 6–9 months and a male preponderance overall of 3:1.

Aetiology and pathogenesis

Most cases are 'idiopathic', the lead point being lymphoid tissues from Peyer's patches in the terminal ileum. This explains the relationship to preceding respiratory or GI tract infection and the increased incidence after administration of early versions of rotavirus vaccine.

In older children a mechanical lead point (e.g. Meckel diverticulum, polyp, lymphoma) is more likely and it may complicate Henoch–Schönlein purpura and cystic fibrosis.

Intussusception occurs most commonly at the terminal ileum (ileo-colic). The mesentery of the intussusceptum is compressed leading to obstruction and progressive venous engorgement and ischaemia with bleeding and outpouring of mucus ('redcurrant jelly' stool).

Clinical features

The classical clinical triad of abdominal pain, redcurrant jelly stool, and an abdominal mass is present in less than a third of cases.

Typically there is sudden onset of intermittent bouts of severe abdominal pain occurring every 10–20 min and manifested by inconsolable crying and drawing up of the legs. Abdominal pain usually precedes the vomiting. Stools are initially loose and watery, but within 12–24 h blood or mucus (redcurrant jelly stools) are passed.

On examination

Initially the patient appears well, in between the episodes of pain. As the condition progresses lethargy and irritability followed by signs of shock may supervene.

The abdomen is soft initially and a sausage-shaped mass (the intussusceptum) may be palpable in the right upper quadrant if the intussusception is ileo-caecal.

Management

Investigations

Imaging

A plain abdominal radiograph may be done initially to identify gross pathology such as obstruction or perforation but abnormalities are seen in only about 50% of cases of intussusception (Fig 5.8A).

Abdominal ultrasound is a rapid and non-invasive technique which enables accurate diagnosis with high specificity and sensitivity of >98% (Fig 5.8B).

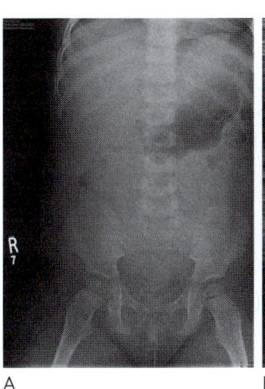

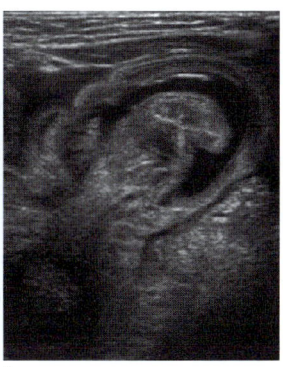

Fig 5.8 Intussusception: A. Plain abdominal radiograph. Paucity of gas in right lower quadrant. Outline of intussusceptus just visible. B. Ultrasound scan. Longitudinal view: 'sandwich' sign of multiple layers of hypoechoic bowel wall and hyperechoic mesentery within the lumen of the distended bowel. An axial view would show the 'doughnut' sign: hypoechoic dark ring of oedematous bowel wall and hyperechoic white centre of intussusceptum.

Treatment

Surgical consultation should be initiated as soon as the diagnosis is suspected.

In a well patient with a short history, pneumatic or hydrostatic reduction under fluoroscopic control should be attempted and is successful in 50–95% of cases. Perforation is the most common complication (1%).

If diagnosis is late and complications have supervened (bowel ischaemia, intestinal haemorrhage or perforation, shock, and sepsis) standard resuscitation measures should be followed by laparotomy for open reduction of the intussusception and resection of any gangrenous bowel.

Prognosis is excellent with early diagnosis, but overall mortality remains 1–2%. Recurrence is more common in older children in whom an anatomical lead point is more likely, and after hydrostatic reduction (5–10%).

5.6 Coeliac disease and short bowel syndrome

Coeliac disease

Coeliac disease is an immune-mediated enteropathy caused by ingestion of gluten-containing cereals such as wheat, rye, and barley in genetically predisposed individuals. The estimated UK prevalence is up to 1/100 (female:male ratio 2:1) if diagnosis is based on serological tests.

Aetiology and pathogenesis
It is a multifactorial genetic trait in which environmental factors include the dietary antigen gluten.

Genetics
The prevalence of coeliac disease in 1st-degree relatives is 10% and the concordance rate is 80–100% in monozygotic and 20% in dizygotic twins. It has the strongest HLA association of any complex disease: 95% of patients are positive for DQ2 and the remainder have DQ8. Non-HLA susceptibility genes have yet to be identified.

Gluten as an antigen
The enteropathy is triggered by dietary exposure to protein present in the white flour component of wheat grains, especially gliadins (wheat), secalins (rye), and hordeins (barley). Oats, derived from a different group within the cereal family, appear to be safe, but commercial preparations may be contaminated with other cereals.

These gluten peptides, which are prolamins, are deamidated by tissue transglutaminase (tTG) and presented by DQ2 and DQ8 molecules on antigen-presenting cells (APCs) to $CD4^+$ cells in the lamina propria.

The exact role if any of antibodies to tissue transglutaminase (tTG) in the pathogenesis is unclear, but it is known to be the autoantigen for anti-endomysial antibody (AEA).

The enteropathy
The disease affects mainly the mucosa of the proximal small intestine, decreasing distally. There is a spectrum of appearances between normal and flat (total villous atrophy). Marsh classified the abnormal mucosal appearances:
- *Stage 0:* pre-infiltrative: normal appearance but positive anti-gliadin antibodies
- *Stage I:* infiltrative: lymphocytic enteritis. Normal mucosal architecture but increase in intraepithelial lymphocytes (IEL)
- *Stage II:* increased IEL, increased crypt depth, no villous atrophy
- *Stage III:* villous atrophy, characteristic but not diagnostic
  - A: partial
  - B: subtotal
  - C: total
- *Stage IV:* hypoplastic, total villous atrophy; an end-stage lesion.

Associated disorders
There are a number of conditions associated with coeliac disease, several of which involve immune dysfunction: type 1 diabetes mellitus, selective IgA deficiency, autoimmune thyroiditis, dermatitis herpetiformis, IgA nephropathy, Sjögren's syndrome, and rheumatoid arthritis. It is also more common in Down, Turner, and Williams syndromes.

Clinical features
Classic coeliac disease presenting with a malabsorption syndrome after weaning and the introduction of cereals is less common now, perhaps due to later weaning.

The diagnosis is now usually made in children with subtle or no GI symptoms. The present situation has been referred to as the 'coeliac iceberg' (Fig 5.9) with a visible tip of manifest symptomatic cases representing only 10% of the total, and the submerged majority represented by:
- *Silent coeliac disease:* asymptomatic, detected on serological screening and mucosal changes which normalize on a gluten free diet.
- *Latent coeliac disease:* patients in whom mucosal changes have not developed despite positive coeliac serology.

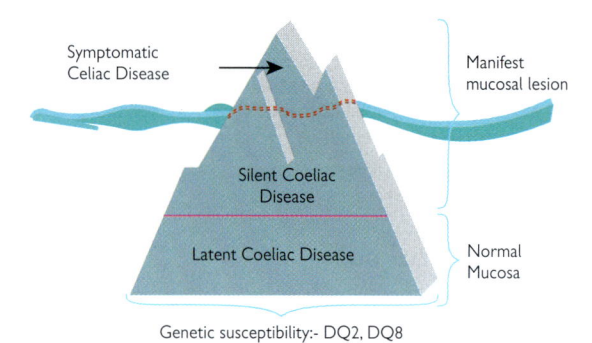

Fig 5.9 The coeliac iceberg. Source: US FDA.

The manifestations can usefully be divided into GI and non-GI:
- *Gastrointestinal:* the 'classic' form presents at age 6–24 months with anorexia, chronic diarrhoea, vomiting with failure to thrive. The stools are pale, offensive, and porridge like. Examination reveals irritability and lethargy, buttock and muscle wasting, hypotonia, and abdominal distension with anaemia and nutritional deficiencies such as rickets if diagnosis is delayed. Presentation at a later age may be with milder GI symptoms such as intermittent diarrhoea and recurrent abdominal pain.
- *Non-GI:* presenting signs in older children may include short stature, delayed puberty, unexplained anaemia or iron deficiency anaemia unresponsive to treatment, recurrent aphthous stomatitis, or dental enamel defects. It is now accepted that dermatitis herpetiformis is a skin manifestation of CD.

Management
Diagnostic and initial investigations
Identification of nutritional deficiencies
- *FBC:* Hb and film
- Albumin, iron, folate, B12 levels.

Serological tests
IgA endomysial antibody (EMA) and tissue transglutaminase antibody (tTGA). Total serum IgA must be measured simultaneously as the tests are IgA dependent and unreliable in the presence of selective IgA deficiency (present in 2%).

Biopsy
The gold standard for definitive diagnosis remains the characteristic mucosal changes seen on endoscopic small-bowel biopsy. Multiple biopsies from the second part of the duodenum or beyond are recommended as histologic changes may be patchy. Gluten intake must be adequate at the time of biopsy.

The diagnostic criteria in a child >2 years are:
- Characteristic histology on biopsy (Marsh stage ≥II) and positive serology: EMA or tTGA.
- Clinical and serological response to gluten-free diet (GFD).

In children <2 years a gluten challenge and re-biopsy after a period on a GFD should be considered as the differential diagnosis in young children with partial villous atrophy is wide and includes cow's milk sensitive enteropathy, post-enteritis enteropathy, and immunodeficiency enteropathy.

Management
A strict GFD for life is the current treatment. This diet excludes wheat, rye, and barley. Pure oats are not toxic in most patients with CD, but commercial oats may be contaminated with gluten-containing grains and it is prudent to exclude oats from the diet.

Children compliant with their GFD show resolution of symptoms, improved growth and normalization of nutritional deficiencies. A long-term GFD protects against morbidity and mortality from osteopaenia and non-Hodgkin's lymphoma of the small intestine.

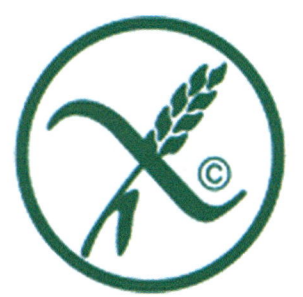

Fig 5.10 Crossed grain symbol: a registered trademark indicating gluten-free products and services (Coeliac UK).

Follow-up is essential to review dietary compliance and monitor growth. tTG levels can be monitored if there is concern about dietary compliance. First-degree relatives should be screened, and patients encouraged to join the charity Coeliac UK(see Fig 5.10).

In the future it may be possible to modify the immune response to gluten or produce genetically modified non-disease-activating cereals.

Short bowel syndrome (SBS)
Loss of >75% of the small bowel is associated with intestinal failure, a requirement for parenteral nutrition support, and decreased overall survival. Loss of >50% is unlikely to lead to major nutritional sequelae.

Aetiology and pathogenesis
Aetiology
The most common cause of SBS is massive surgical resection on account of necrotizing enterocolitis (NEC), intestinal atresias, volvulus, or gastroschisis.

Pathogenesis
Ileal resection severely decreases absorption of water and electrolytes. Loss of the terminal ileum causes malabsorption of bile salts and vitamin B12. Continued loss of bile salts following resection of the terminal ileum leads to fat malabsorption, steatorrhoea, and loss of fat-soluble vitamins.

If the ileocaecal valve can be preserved, intestinal transit is slowed, allowing more time for absorption. If the ileocaecal valve is lost, transit time is faster, and loss of fluid and nutrients is greater.

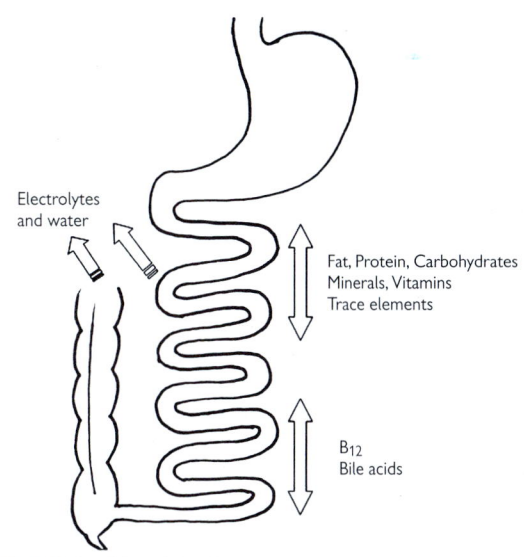

Fig 5.11 Small-bowel function.

Furthermore, colonic bacteria can colonize the small bowel, worsening diarrhoea and nutrient loss.

Increased oxalate absorption may lead to urinary stones and low bile levels are associated with gallstones.

Clinical features
Loss of significant lengths of ileum almost invariably results in diarrhoea, abdominal bloating, weight loss from malabsorption, and fatigue.

Treatment
Good clinical outcome can eventually be achieved with as little as 15 cm of jejunum and ileum with the presence of an ileocaecal valve or 40 cm without the valve.

Parenteral nutrition (PN) is the mainstay of treatment, with continuous attempts to introduce enteral nutrition. Prolonged use of PN is associated with liver abnormalities, including elevated liver enzymes, jaundice, or rarely, progression to liver scarring and liver failure. The majority of children with blood abnormalities and/or jaundice have improvement of their liver function if PN can be safely discontinued and enteral nutrition advanced. These children need the support of a dedicated multidisciplinary nutritional team.

Results of small intestinal transplantation are improving with increasing clinical experience. However, overall survival is poor and this remains a last resort. The overall mortality of infants with SBS who are dependent on PN for >90 days after surgery is ~30%.

5.7 Inflammatory bowel disease

Inflammatory bowel disease (IBD) encompasses two major forms of chronic intestinal inflammation: Crohn's disease (CD) and ulcerative colitis (UC). In about 15% of children with IBD colitis a clear distinction between CD and UC is not possible and these children are designated 'indeterminate colitis' (IC).

The incidence of IBD (especially CD) in children has increased over the last two decades and is currently about 5/100 000 children <16. This means 700 new cases per year in the UK (60% CD, 30% UC, 10% IC).

The median age at diagnosis of IBD is 12 years, but 5% of all cases are diagnosed in children <5 years. It is important to consider IBD, especially UC, in younger children.

Aetiology and pathogenesis
IBD is a multifactorial genetic disorder in which there is a breakdown of immune tolerance to the gut microflora in genetically susceptible individuals. There have been significant recent advances in understanding the molecular genetic basis of IBD, especially of CD.

Genetics
- Family clustering, twin studies, and ethnic variability provide conclusive evidence that IBD is a multifactorial genetic trait. Concordance rates in MZ and DZ twin pairs are 36% (MZ) and 4% (DZ) for CD and 16% (MZ) and 4% (DZ) for UC, indicating a greater genetic contribution in CD.
- Up to 32% of patients with IBD have an affected relative, with siblings at greater risk.
- Eight loci for IBD (*IBD1–IBD8*) have been mapped and at the *IBD1* locus on chromosome 16 sequence variants in the *CARD15* (caspase activating recruitment domain) gene have been associated with susceptibility to CD.
- The *CARD15* gene is expressed in intestinal epithelial cells and monocytes and encodes a protein with a key role in the innate immune response to bacterial antigens.

Pathology
- *Ulcerative colitis*: this is limited to the rectum and colon, although a 'backwash' ileitis can be found in severe pancolitis. The lesions are homogenous with an intense neutrophil infiltrate limited to the mucosa, goblet cell depletion, crypt distortion and crypt abscesses. Childhood onset UC is more likely to be extensive with 60–80% of children having a pancolitis.
- *Crohn disease*: in contrast, CD affects the whole thickness of the bowel wall and can occur anywhere from mouth to anus. In two-thirds there is involvement of terminal ileum, right colon, and transverse colon. The inflammation is focal and patchy. The diagnostic feature is non-caseating granulomas and fissuring ulceration.

Clinical features
Although there is considerable overlap in clinical features, CD and UC presenting features are distinctive. A positive family history of IBD is the most common risk factor. A significant delay of several months between onset of symptoms and diagnosis is unfortunately common.

Crohn disease
The initial symptoms may be subtle and variable. Only 25% have the classical combination of abdominal pain, diarrhoea, and weight loss. Systemic symptoms such as anorexia, lethargy, and pyrexia are present in a minority. Anal pain on defecation should be asked about specifically.

Linear growth failure and pubertal delay are common in CD at presentation. Anal inspection is crucial as abnormalities in the perineum are present in 50% of children with CD including skin tags, fissures, fistulae, and abscesses (Fig 5.12).

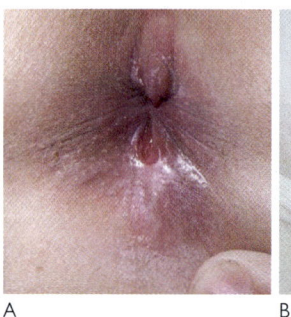

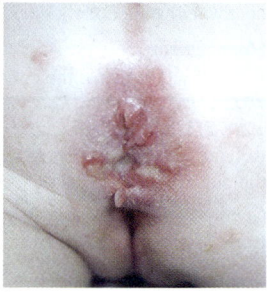

Fig 5.12 Crohn disease: A. Anal fissure; B. Anal skin tags.

Extraintestinal manifestations are more common in CD than in UC (Table 5.9).

Table 5.9. Extraintestinal manifestations of CD	
Dermatological	Erythema nodosum (common) (Fig 5.13) Pyoderma gangrenosum (rare)
Ophthalmological	Conjunctival ulceration Uveitis Episcleritis
Skeletal	Arthritis Arthralgia Ankylosing spondylitis
Hepatic	Hepatitis Primary sclerosing cholangitis

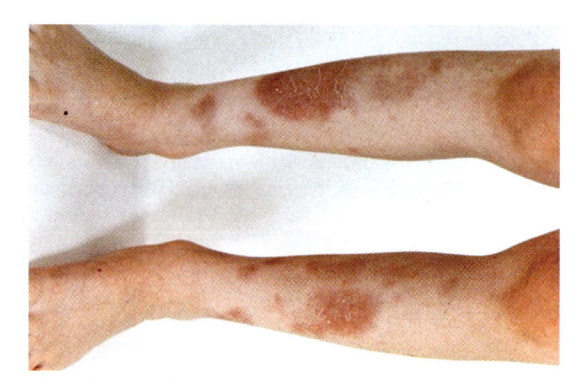

Fig 5.13 CD: erythema nodosum.

Ulcerative colitis
Bloody, mucousy diarrhoea is the hallmark of UC. Initially it may be intermittent and in isolated proctitis (<5%) episodic blood on formed stools may mimic a polyp. The pain of colitis tends to be pre-defecation, cramp-like, suprapubic pain relieved by defecation. Tenesmus is common: straining with passage of blood or bloody mucous.

See Table 5.10 for causes of lower GI tract bleeding.

Toxic megacolon, a medical emergency, should be suspected in the presence of >12 bloody stools in 24 h, abdominal distension and tenderness, tachycardia, and fever.

Systemic symptoms such as growth faltering, pubertal delay, and extraintestinal manifestations are less common in UC.

Diagnosis and investigations

Investigations depend on whether clinical suspicion is low or high:

Low clinical suspicion
- FBC for anaemia and thrombocythaemia
- ESR and CRP
- Albumin, iron/ferritin, Ca, Mg, Zn, folate, vitamin B12.

High clinical suspicion
- *Exclude infective cause:* stools for microscopy, culture and sensitivity, *Clostridium difficile* toxin ova, cysts and parasites
- *If infection excluded and symptoms persist:*
  - *Endoscopy:* tissue diagnosis by endoscopic biopsy is essential. All children should undergo endoscopic examination of the upper and lower GI tract with serial mucosal biopsies.
  - *Imaging:* barium meal and follow-through examination should be undertaken to complete examination of the entire GI tract. In the future greater use will be made of gadolinium-enhanced MRI and video-capsule endoscopy.

If IBD is confirmed, liver function tests, anthropometry, and bone densitometry are done.

Management

The goals of treatment are to induce remission of the active disease and prevent relapse, and to restore nutritional status and promote normal growth and development. An individual treatment plan will consist of one, or a combination of, nutritional therapy, drug therapy and surgery, and psychological support.

Nutritional therapy

Exclusive enteral nutrition for 6 weeks is the first line therapy used by most European centres for induction of remission in CD. There are two types:
- *Elemental:* efficacious but unpalatable; usually administered by nasogastric tube
- *Polymeric:* contains whole proteins and better tolerated orally.

The remission rate is 86% and adverse systemic side effects are less than those for steroids but the duration of remission is shorter. Nutritional deficiencies due to inadequate intake or increased losses are common and must be corrected and dietary supplementation (calories, multivitamins, minerals) is usually required. Exclusion diets do not provide long-term benefits unless the item excluded clearly causes symptoms.

Pharmacological treatment
- *Corticosteroids:* systemic steroids (oral prednisolone) are the mainstay of inducing remission in moderate–severe UC, and are effective in CD. Steroid resistance or dependence may be encountered, and side effects in children who are already growth delayed with poor mineralization are a problem. Budesonide is moderately effective and has fewer side effects.
- *5-Aminosalicylates:* sulphasalazine and mesalazine are effective as monotherapy for inducing remission in mild–moderate UC and prolong remission chronically in UC.
- *Azathioprine:* (or 6-mercaptopurine, its metabolite) is the most frequently prescribed immunomodulator used in both CD and UC and may allow steroid sparing. Bone marrow suppression with leucopaenia occurs and monitoring neutrophil count is mandatory. Pancreatitis may be a side effect.
- More potent immunosuppression with methotrexate or ciclosporin is needed in a few cases. Infliximab, a chimeric monoclonal antibody to TNF-α, is increasingly being used in refractory CD and is efficacious. Non-chimeric biologic agents like adalimulab are used in those with hypersensitivity reactions to infliximab.
- *Antibiotics:* metronidazole and ciprofloxacin are used especially for perianal disease.

Surgery

This may still be necessary in up to 70% of children with CD. Indications for surgery in CD include refractory disease, stricture resection or stricturoplasty, and complications such as intestinal perforation, haemorrhage, obstruction, or abscess.

Proctocolectomy with ileostomy or an ileo-anal pouch anastamosis is curative in UC. The usual indication is steroid dependence despite the use of immunomodulatory drugs.

Psychological considerations

The child or adolescent with IBD carries a heavy burden: decreased physical functioning, frequent relapses, unpleasant symptoms, demanding treatment regimes, and altered physical appearance. Psychological problems such as depression, denial, and non-adherence are common and quality of life is impaired.

Children with IBD and their families need multidisciplinary help including counselling in order to cope. Effective transition to adult care services should be organized.

Table 5.10. Causes of lower GI tract bleeding

Bleeding	Anatomical source	Diagnoses			
		<1 month	1 m–2 years	2–10 years	10–16 years
Bright red on stool	Anus, rectum	Anal fissure	Anal fissure	Anal fissure	Polyp
		Vit K deficiency	Lymphonodular hyperplasia	Polyp	Anal fissure
		Lymphonodular hyperplasia			Haemorrhoids
Bloody diarrhoea	Colon	Vit K deficiency	Food allergy	Infection	Infection
		NEC	Infection	IBD	IBD
		Hirschsprung	Hirschsprung		
		Enterocolitis	Enterocolitis		
Melaena	Small bowel/proximal colon	Duplication cyst	Meckel diverticulum	Meckel diverticulum	Angiodysplasia
		Volvulus	Duplication cyst	Angiodysplasia	
			Volvulus		

5.8 Functional gastrointestinal disorders

Childhood functional GI disorders (FGIDs) encompass variable combinations of chronic or recurrent symptoms which are often age-dependent.

Aetiology and pathogenesis

Although not explained by organic disease of an anatomical, infectious, inflammatory, or neoplastic nature, it is increasingly clear that their aetiology reflects a complex interaction between susceptibility to gut dysfunction and psychosocial factors (Fig 5.14).

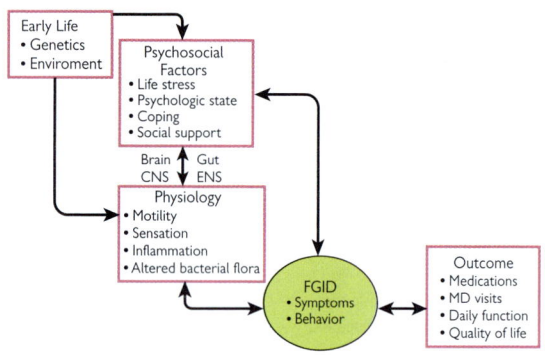

Fig 5.14 FGIDs: conceptual model. Reproduced from Gastroenterology 130 (5): Drossman; The Functional Gasterointestinal Disorders and the Rome III Process, with permission from Elsevier, © 2006.

Functional symptoms may be part of normal development, such as infant regurgitation, or arise from maladaptive behavioural responses to internal or external stimuli as in functional faecal retention from painful defecation or coercive toilet training.

The role of postinfectious inflammatory states and neuroimmune interactions altering visceral sensation and gut motility in cyclical vomiting, recurrent abdominal pain, chronic diarrhoea, and constipation is increasingly recognized.

Clinical classification

Clinical expression of FGIDs depends on the child's autonomic, affective, and intellectual development. Infants and preschool children cannot accurately report symptoms such as nausea and pain.

Disability from a functional symptom is highly dependent on whether adaptive or maladaptive responses occur in the individual and their family. Symptoms may be amplified and a vicious cycle of symptom anxiety and health-care seeking may be set in motion if concerns are dismissed or unnecessary diagnostic studies performed.

The Rome criteria

The Rome criteria are a consensus statement to guide diagnosis of FGIDs which are now in their third iteration (Rome III). A selection of diagnostic categories according to Rome III is set out in Table 5.11. Although grouped into those affecting neonates/toddlers or children/adolescents, several span the age groups including in particular cyclical vomiting and functional constipation. The most important conditions are considered in turn below.

Table 5.11. Rome III FGIDs

Functional disorders: neonates and toddlers
Infant regurgitation
Cyclic vomiting syndrome
Infantile colic
Functional diarrhoea
Infant dyschezia
Functional constipation
Functional disorders: children and adolescents
Vomiting and aerophagia
Adolescent rumination syndrome
Cyclic vomiting syndrome
Aerophagia
Abdominal pain-related
Functional dyspepsia
Irritable bowel syndrome
Abdominal migraine
Childhood functional abdominal pain
CFAP syndrome
Constipation and incontinence
Functional constipation
Non-retentive faecal incontinence

Infantile colic

This is defined as excessive crying in an otherwise healthy baby during the first few months of life.

The 'rule of 3' is useful for diagnosis: crying for at least 3 h per day on at least 3 days per week for at least 3 weeks. Depending on definition it affects 5–25% of infants. Inconsolable crying usually occurs late afternoon/early evening beginning in the first few weeks of life and abating spontaneously by around 3 months of age.

The cause of colic is unknown, although it is generally ascribed to pain arising from the GI tract. GOR is an important differential.

The only proven treatment is time: the behaviour rarely persists beyond 4–6 months of age. Myriad strategies have been proposed, of which available evidence offers tentative support for three:

- A trial of hypoallergenic (protein hydrolysate) formula for bottle-fed infants
- A low-allergen material diet (excluding dairy, wheat, eggs, tree nuts, fish) for breast-fed infants
- Reduced stimulation of the infant.

No good evidence supports drug therapy. Dicyclomine, an antispasmodic, shows an effect but infrequent adverse effects such as apnoea have reduced its use.

The enormous stress colic places on parents and other family members should not be underestimated.

Functional diarrhoea

This is also called 'toddler diarrhoea' and has an onset in infancy or preschool years. Stools often contain mucus and/or visible undigested food. Enquiry should be made about recent enteric infection, laxative or antibiotic use, and diet (excessive consumption of fruit juice, carbohydrates).

Diagnostic criteria:

- Painless passage of three or more large, unformed stools per day during waking hours
- Symptom duration >4 weeks
- Onset age 6–36 months
- No failure to thrive if calorie intake adequate.

Spontaneous recovery occurs and parental reassurance is all that is necessary. Restrictive diets should be avoided, but a daily diet and defecation diary may document a relation to specific foods.

Infant dyschezia

The diagnostic criteria are episodes of at least 10 min of straining and crying before successful passage of soft stools in an infant of <6 months with no other health problems. The infant may turn red or purple. It is assumed to reflect a failure to coordinate increasing abdominal pressure with relaxation of the pelvic floor.

Examination should exclude anorectal abnormalities and parents are mostly happy to accept the explanation that the infant will learn to coordinate bearing down with pelvic floor relaxation.

Adolescent rumination syndrome

This is most common in female adolescents and appears to serve the purpose of self-stimulation in intellectually handicapped children. Psychological disturbances (anxiety, depression, OCD) are present in up to one third of affected children.

Diagnostic criteria

- Repeated painless regurgitation and re-chewing or expulsion of food that begins soon after a meal, does not occur in sleep, and does not respond to standard treatment for GOR
- No retching or evidence of organic disease.

Management strategies include behavioural therapy, tricyclic antidepressants, and postpyloric feeding (if weight loss is significant).

Irritable bowel syndrome (IBS)

Diagnostic criteria

Abdominal discomfort (an uncomfortable sensation not described as pain) or pain associated with two or more of the following at least 25% of the time:

- Improved with defecation
- Onset associated with change in stool frequency (increase or decrease)
- Onset associated with change in stool appearance (hard or loose)
- No evidence of an organic disease.

Criteria fulfilled at least once per week for at least 2 months. Visceral hypersensitivity has been documented in children with IBS, and may be related to infection, inflammation, or allergy compounded by ineffective coping mechanisms.

Management

Triggering events and psychosocial factors should be explored. A confident diagnosis and reassurance combined with advice on coping strategies may be therapeutic. Peppermint oil may provide benefit in some children.

Cyclic vomiting syndrome

Frequency of episodes averages 12 per year, and 80% of patients identify circumstances or events that trigger attacks.

Diagnostic criteria:

- Two or more episodes of intense nausea and unremitting vomiting or retching lasting hours to days
- Return to usual state of health in between for weeks or months.

Episodes tend to start in night or morning and end as rapidly as they begin. A family history of IBS or migraine is common. Accompanying features during an attack may include abdominal pain, headache, fever, tachycardia, salivation, loose stools, skin blotching, hypertension, and leucocytosis. The differential diagnostic list of organic causes of episodic vomiting is long: see Table 5.12.

Table 5.12. Causes of episodic vomiting	
Brainstem glioma	
Obstructive uropathy	
Endocrine/metabolic	Familial dysautonomia Urea cycle disorders Organic acidaemias
Gastrointestinal pathology	Recurrent pancreatitis Intermittent small bowel obstruction Peptic ulcer disease Chronic intestinal pseudo-obstruction
Fabricated or induced illness (FII)	

Management

Management may involve prophylaxis, blockade of the prodrome, and treatment of an established episode:

- *Prophylaxis:* avoid trigger factors and consider treatment with promethazine or pizotifen
- *Blockade of prodrome* (if prodrome recognizable): consider sublingual prochlorperazine and 5HT3 blockade using ondansetron orally or IV
- *Established emetic episode:* hypertension and inappropriate ADH secretion is common. Give IV fluids at 60% maintenance (4% dextrose, 0.45% saline). Continue antiemesis with ondansetron, induce sedation with IV lorazepam (>12 years) or IM chlorpromazine (<12 years) and control BP with labetolol.

5.9 Functional abdominal pain and constipation

Abdominal pain related FGIDs

This includes a cluster of disorders: functional dyspepsia, abdominal migraine, and childhood functional abdominal pain.

In this cluster of FGIDs it is important to ensure that certain 'alarm' features which may indicate organic disease (see Box) are absent:

Alarm features suggesting organic disease

Symptoms
- Persistent right upper or lower quadrant pain
- Pain causing nocturnal waking
- Dysphagia or persistent vomiting
- Nocturnal diarrhoea
- GI tract blood loss
- Family history of IBD, coeliac disease, peptic ulcer

Signs
- Unexplained fever
- Involuntary weight loss or deceleration of linear growth, delayed puberty
- Arthritis
- Perianal disease

Presence of alarm features should prompt further diagnostic testing. Diagnostic criteria all include no evidence of organic disease, i.e. inflammatory, anatomic, metabolic, or neoplastic process. Organic disease accounts for 10% of recurrent abdominal pain (see Box).

Organic causes of recurrent abdominal pain

Gastrointestinal
- Inflammatory bowel disease
- Peptic ulcer disease
- Meckel's diverticulum
- Pancreatitis
- Gallstones or hepatitis

Genitourinary
- Urinary tract infection
- Renal calculi
- Hydronephrosis

Gynaecological
- Dysmenorrhoea
- Ovarian cysts
- Pelvic inflammatory disease

Others
- Lead poisoning
- Sickle cell disease

Functional dyspepsia

Diagnostic criteria
- Persistent or recurrent pain or discomfort centred in the upper abdomen (above the umbilicus)
- Not relieved by defecation or associated with change in stool form or frequency (i.e. not IBS).

Criteria should be fulfilled once per week for at least 2 months and there must be no evidence of organic disease. Upper GI endoscopy is not necessary to make this diagnosis, but is indicated to exclude or confirm *H. pylori* associated disease if there is dysphagia or failure of acid-reducing medications. Disordered gastric motility has been documented.

Management
Therapeutic options, unsupported by evidence, include H2 blockers or PPIs for pain and prokinetics such as domperidone for discomfort.

Abdominal migraine

This is more common in girls than boys (3:2) with an age of onset 7–12 years. It may share pathological mechanisms with cyclical vomiting syndrome and migraine headache.

Diagnostic criteria
- Paroxysmal episodes of intense, acute periumbilical pain lasting >1 h
- Well for weeks or months in between
- Pain interferes with normal activities
- Pain associated with 2 or more of:
  - anorexia, nausea, vomiting
  - headache, photophobia, pallor
- No evidence of organic disease.

Criteria should be fulfilled two or more times in preceding 12 months.

Management
Management includes avoidance of any identified trigger factors such as foods, fasting, or sleep disturbance and consideration of prophylaxis with pizotifen or propranolol for frequent episodes.

Childhood functional abdominal pain (CFAP) and CFAP syndrome

Diagnostic criteria
- Episodic or continuous abdominal pain
- Insufficient criteria for other FGIDs
- No evidence of organic disease (see Alarm features)
- Criteria fulfilled at least once per week for at least 2 months.

A subgroup of children have some loss of daily functioning and additional somatic symptoms (headache, limb pains, difficulty sleeping) and are designated CFAP **syndrome**.

Anxiety, depression, and somatization may coexist in the children and their parents.

Management
In the absence of alarm features it may still be reasonable to undertake limited investigations such as FBC, CRP, ESR, LFTs, urinalysis, and culture.

Management is challenging, especially in those with CFAP(S). It is important to explore the contribution of psychosocial factors. The child and parents should be given reassurance that although the symptoms are real they are not dangerous, and explanation given of interactions between brain and gut. Psychological counselling and behavioural therapy may help if child and family are willing to participate. Success has been achieved with tricyclic antidepressants.

Functional constipation

This encompasses all children in whom constipation does not have an organic aetiology. 40% of children with functional constipation develop symptoms during the 1st year of life, and incidence peaks at 2–4 years with an excess of boys.

Aetiology and pathogenesis
The exact aetiology of functional or 'simple' constipation remains uncertain.

Onset often occurs during one of three periods:
- Infants with hard stools when changed to formula milk or weaned
- Toddlers acquiring toilet skills with painful defecation
- At start of school

Faeces accumulate and stretch the rectum leading to a vicious circle in which the desire to defecate is reduced and passage of infrequent large stools is painful. 'Overflow incontinence' causes soiling.

A variety of maladaptive responses may exacerbate the situation.

Diagnostic criteria
Must include two or more of the following:
- Bowels open twice or less per week
- At least one episode of faecal incontinence per week (after acquisition of toileting skills)
- History of retentive posturing or excessive volitional stool retention
- History of painful or hard bowel movements
- Presence of a large faecal mass in the rectum
- History of large-diameter stools that may obstruct the toilet.

Criteria should be fulfilled at least once per week for at least 1 month (<4 years) or 2 months (>4 years).

This is a clinical diagnosis.

Clinical evaluation
History
History should elicit:
- Time to passage of meconium after birth
- Age of onset of constipation, trigger factors
- Stool characteristics: use Bristol Stool Form Scale (Fig 5.15)
- Associated symptoms such as pain, blood, faecal incontinence, and coexistence of urinary problems.

Examination
Abdominal examination usually reveals a faecal mass. The perineal and perianal region should be examined for fissures and signs of spinal dysraphism or sacral agenesis. Digital rectal examination should be performed at least once but if the prospect elicits a very negative response this can be delayed to facilitate the therapeutic alliance between child and clinician.

A plain abdominal radiograph is useful in determining the presence of a faecal mass in a child who is obese or refuses rectal examination.

Management
Parental education
- Use diagrams (and radiographs) to explain how faeces have accumulated and stretched the rectum leading to a vicious cycle in which the desire to defecate is reduced and passage of infrequent large stools is painful. Explain how overflow incontinence causes soiling, if present.
- Allay myths and fears: explain that there is no blockage or narrowing of the bowel, the sphincter is intact and the bowels will not burst under the strain. Aim to reduce anxiety and create an expectation of positive change.
- Explain the treatment strategy in 'plumbing' terms to describe disimpaction ('clean them out') and maintenance ('keep them clear').

This is followed by treatment to achieve disimpaction and maintenance therapy.

Disimpaction
The availability of a palatable polyethylene glycol (PEG) laxative (Movicol) in the UK means that faecal disimpaction can be reliably achieved by the oral route rather than by enema or manual removal, which is now rarely required. A dosage schedule is recommended in which the number of sachets per day is gradually increased over 7 days.

Maintenance
This can be achieved using stool softeners, either PEG-based or lactulose. Lactulose usually requires the addition of a 'prokinetic' stimulant laxative, either senna, bisacodyl, or picosulphate. In addition, parents should be encouraged to:
- Increase fluid, fruit, and vegetable intake
- Use gastrocolic reflex in toilet training: encourage the child to sit on the toilet for 5 min after each meal
- Use a diary and star chart to monitor bowel habit and adherence to therapy.

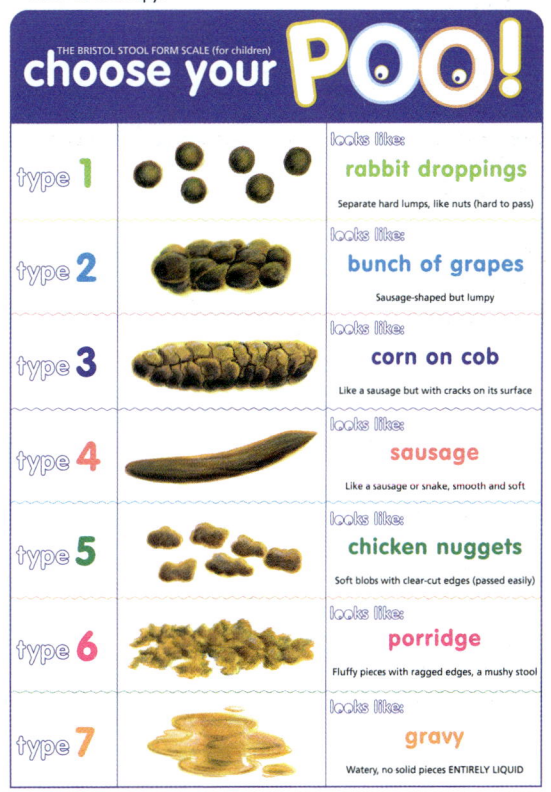

Fig 5.15 Bristol Stool Form Scale. Reproduced by kind permission of Dr KW Heaton, Reader in Medicine at the University of Bristol. © 2000 Norgine Ltd.

5.10 Pancreatic and gallbladder disease

Pancreatitis

Inflammation of the pancreas is rare in childhood. It may be local or diffuse and is classified as acute, recurrent, or chronic.

Aetiology

Abdominal trauma, infection, or drug reactions are the most common cause of an episode of acute pancreatitis. Release of activated digestive enzymes from pancreatic acinar cells leads to autodigestion of pancreatic parenchyma with necrosis and inflammation.

Recurrent episodes of acute pancreatitis are caused by congenital abnormalities of the pancreatico-biliary system and a number of inherited, familial disorders (Table 5.13). Common adult causes such as alcohol and gallstones are rare in childhood. One third of patients with chronic pancreatitis have no identified aetiology.

Table 5.13. Causes of pancreatitis in childhood	
Trauma (30% of cases)	Abdominal trauma from bicycle handlebars, seat belts
Viral infection	Mumps, rubella, coxsackie virus B, cytomegalovirus, HIV
Drugs	Valproic acid, azathioprine, tetracycline, L-asparagine, steroids
Gallstones	
Congenital anomalies	Choledochal cyst, pancreas division, duplication cysts
Hereditary pancreatitis	Mutations in *PRSS1*, *SPINK1*, *CFTR*
Metabolic disorders	Hypercalcaemia, hyperlipidaemia

Pathophysiology

Acute pancreatitis is a reversible process with sudden onset of abdominal pain, a rise in pancreatic digestive enzymes in the serum and the potential for complete recovery with no lasting effects on pancreatic structure or function.

Autoactivation of trypsinogen to trypsin is a key early acinar cell event in acute pancreatitis. Evidence for this has come from the analysis of hereditary pancreatitis. This is caused by mutations in the gene encoding cationic trypsinogen, *PRSS1*. The mutations increase autoactivation and render the protein resistant to inactivation through autolysis. Mutations in *SPINK1*, which encodes a serine protease inhibitor that normally inhibits trypsin, also cause pancreatitis.

Chronic pancreatitis is a progressive inflammatory disease of the pancreas characterized by irreversible morphological changes such as acinar cell loss, islet cell loss, inflammatory infiltration, and gradual fibrotic replacement. Recurrent acute pancreatitis progresses to chronic pancreatitis.

Cystic fibrosis is the most common cause of chronic pancreatitis in childhood. *CFTR* mutations that specifically block bicarbonate conductance selectively target the pancreas.

Clinical features

Abdominal pain is the hallmark. Pancreatic pain is dull or boring and worsens after eating. It is located in the epigastrium and often radiates to the back. There may be associated nausea and vomiting and examination may reveal abdominal distension, tenderness, guarding, and reduced bowel sounds. Fever, jaundice, and shock may be present.

Chronic pancreatitis with fibrosis leads to steatorrhea and weight loss. Endocrine insufficiency does not occur until late in the disease. Complications such as a chronic pseudocyst cause worsening abdominal pain and may be associated with biliary or gastric outlet obstruction.

Management

Diagnostic investigations

Blood tests

In >80% of cases serum amylase and lipase are elevated by >3 times the upper limit of normal, but these findings alone are not reliable as a screening tool. Serum lipase is more specific than amylase and remains elevated for 1–2 weeks longer. Either enzyme can be elevated in other conditions (e.g. mumps, burns, cholecystitis) and both can be normal when there is imaging evidence of acute pancreatitis. Markedly elevated LDH reliably predicts severe pancreatic disease.

Imaging

Plain films and transabdominal ultrasound are specific and non-invasive as initial screening tests but lack sensitivity for early or moderate disease. Ultrasound is useful for excluding other causes of abdominal pain such as gallstones. However, several imaging tests are of use in the diagnostic work-up, especially of CP.

- *Ultrasound (US):* is the primary screening tool for evaluation of the paediatric pancreas. It will demonstrate enlargement, altered echogenicity, dilated duct, calcification, cysts and fluid collections. Endoscopic ultrasound (EUS) gives increased sensitivity.
- *CT:* is useful for evaluation of CP and its complications.
- *Magnetic resonance cholangiopancreatography (MRCP):* method of choice for evaluating anatomy of ductal system.
- *Endoscopic retrograde cholangiopancreatography (ERCP):* invasive, but provides higher-resolution images than MRCP. Reserved for patients in whom a structural defect or duct disruption is suspected. Can be used therapeutically for stone removal or sphincterotomy.

Genetic testing

In patients with idiopathic recurrent or chronic pancreatitis or a family history of pancreatitis early identification of a *PRSS1* mutation can avoid prolonged and invasive evaluation. Genetic testing for *SPINK1* mutations is not advocated as heterozygous *SPINK1* mutations alone are usually not disease causing (<1% develop pancreatitis). If a sweat test and family history suggest atypical CF consideration of testing *CFTR* is appropriate, but available panels do not test for pancreatitis-associated mutations.

Management

Medical

Acute pancreatitis

The mainstays of treatment are intravenous fluids, analgesia, and pancreatic rest. Volume expansion is important to prevent development of pancreatic necrosis. Enteral nutrition via a jejunal tube is preferable to parenteral nutrition and nasogastric suction is used to eliminate gastric secretions from the duodenum. Antibiotics are unnecessary except in severe cases. Acute pancreatic pseudocysts are managed conservatively for 4–6 weeks as most resolve spontaneously. Acute pancreatitis can be life threatening if infected pancreatic necrosis and multisystem organ failure supervene.

Chronic pancreatitis
Pancreatic insufficiency may necessitate enzyme supplementation in conjunction with elemental or low-fat diets. Insulin-dependent diabetes is uncommon.

Surgical
Surgical intervention in acute pancreatitis is rarely required, but indications include:
- Congenital anatomical defects (e.g. pancreatic divisum)
- *Complications:*
  - pancreatic ascites
  - intra-abdominal abscess
  - chronic pancreatic pseudocyst (<3 months).

Indications for surgical intervention in chronic pancreatitis include intractable pain, malnutrition, and failed medical therapy. Options include:
- Distal pancreatectomy with Roux-en-Y
- Pancreaticojejunostomy (Duval procedure)
- Lateral pancreaticojejunostomy (Puestow procedure)
- ERCP sphincteroplasty.

Pancreatic insufficiency

Aetiology
Pancreatic insufficiency (without pancreatitis) may be primary or secondary.
- *Primary causes* include congenital agenesis or hypoplasia and genetic disorders of which CF is the most common. Shwachman–Diamond syndrome and Johnson–Blizzard syndrome are uncommon causes.
- *Secondary causes* include small bowel disease (e.g. coeliac disease), protein-energy malnutrition, and pancreatic resection.

Shwachman–Diamond Syndrome (SDS)
SDS is an autosomal recessive disorder caused by mutations in the *SBDS* (for Shwachman–Bodian–Diamond syndrome) gene on chromosome 7q11 which may have a role in RNA metabolism. It is characterized by:
- Exocrine pancreatic insufficiency
- Marrow hypoplasia with neutropaenia, anaemia, and thrombocytopaenia
- Skeletal abnormalities: metaphysical dysostosis, rib cage abnormalities.

Initial clinical presentation is similar to CF but the sweat test is normal. Diagnosis is generally based on evidence of exocrine pancreatic dysfunction and neutropaenia together with skeletal abnormalities and short stature.

Management includes pancreatic enzyme supplementation and consideration of granulocyte-colony stimulating factor (GCSF) or even bone marrow transplantation (BMT) for marrow failure.

Management
Tests of exocrine pancreatic function
- *Indirect tests* suitable for screening include measurement of faecal elastase and chymotrypsin levels.
- *Direct tests* require placement of double-lumen gastroduodenal tubes for pancreatic fluid collection after IV CCK or secretion stimulation. The fluid is analysed for enzyme and bicarbonate production.

Treatment
Supplements of pancreatin are given by mouth to compensate for reduced or absent pancreatic exocrine secretion. Pancreatin contains a mixture of protease, lipase and amylase in various proportions. Enteric-coated preparations are designed to deliver a higher enzyme concentration in the duodenum to avoid inactivation by gastric acid.

The dose is adjusted according to size, number and consistency of stools and the nutritional status of the child. Higher strength preparations have been associated with the development of large-bowel strictures (fibrosing colonopathy) in children with cystic fibrosis between 2 and 13 years.

Gallstones: cholelithiasis
Gallstone formation may be secondary to:
- Haemolytic anaemia (sickle cell disease, hereditary spherocytosis)
- Total parenteral nutrition
- Short bowel syndrome
- CF
- Liver disease.

Most gallstones are asymptomatic, but about 6% may occlude the cystic duct or common bile duct. This may lead to biliary obstruction, cholecystitis and cholangitis, intrahepatic abscesses, and biliary fibrosis or pancreatitis.
- *Clinical features* include abdominal pain and tenderness in the right hypochondrium. Gallstones are a differential diagnosis of vaso-occlusive crisis in sickle cell disease.
- *Investigations* reveal abnormal LFTs. Abdominal ultrasound is the imaging modality of choice.
- *Treatment options* include cholecystectomy.

5.11 Neonatal liver disease

Physiological jaundice is common in normal newborn infants but jaundice is also the most common manifestation of a wide variety of hepatic disorders which are individually rare and often have a genetic basis. Neonatal jaundice is usefully classified according to whether the hyperbilirubinaemia is unconjugated or conjugated and is considered in Chapter 1.11. Hepatic causes are discussed in more detail in this section

Unconjugated hyperbilirubinaemia

Inherited defects of bilirubin metabolism

Gilbert syndrome (GS)
This is the most common inherited cause of unconjugated hyperbilirubinaemia, affecting up to 5% of the population with a male preponderance.

GS is an autosomal recessive disorder caused by mutations in the promoter region of *UGT1A1*, encoding the uridine-diphosphate-glucurosyl transferase isoform IA1. A common mutation affects the promoter, reducing enzyme activity by 30–50%.

Neonates with GS may have an exacerbation of physiological jaundice in the first 48 h, but jaundice is usually first noted incidentally during adolescence. Patients may experience bouts of abdominal pain, anorexia, fatigue, and weakness during episodes of high bilirubin.

Diagnosis is by exclusion with unconjugated hyperbilirubinaemia in the range 30–90 mmol/L and otherwise normal LFTs. It is a benign condition and no treatment is required.

Crigler–Najjar syndrome
This very rare disorder is caused by mutations in the coding region of the same gene involved in Gilbert syndrome, *UGT1A1*. There is nearly complete absence of the enzyme. It is classified into type I and type II.

- *Crigler–Najjar syndrome type I:* severe unconjugated hyperbilirubinaemia presents soon after birth and rapidly progresses to levels associated with bilirubin encephalopathy. Diagnosis is by estimation of hepatic UDP glucuronyl transferase activity on a needle liver biopsy specimen. Repeated exchange transfusions and phototherapy aid short-term survival, but the only long term option is liver transplantation.
- *Crigler–Najjar syndrome type II (Avias syndrome):* less severe with detectable levels of enzyme. Kernicterus is rare and treatment with phenobarbital is effective.

Conjugated hyperbilirubinaemia

This is less common and has many causes, including biliary atresia for which treatment is critically dependant on early diagnosis. Definitions vary, but a conjugated (direct) bilirubin level >25 micromol/L is a valid cut-off point. Table 5.14 lists the causes. A mixture of raised unconjugated and conjugated bilirubin is often present.

No cause is identified in up to one third of cases, so called 'idiopathic neonatal hepatitis'. The emphasis is on early diagnosis of biliary atresia. It is vital to test for any liver-related coagulation defect which should be treated with parenteral vitamin K.

Table 5.14. Causes of conjugated hyperbilirubinaemia

Obstruction	Biliary atresia
	Choledochal cyst
Infection	Septicaemia, UTI
Congenital infections	TORCH
	Viral hepatitis (Hep A, B, C)
Genetic	Alagille syndrome
	α_1-antitrypsin deficiency
	Cystic fibrosis
Metabolic disorders	Galactosaemia
	Tyrosinaemia
	Progressive familial intrahepatic cholestasis
	Dubin–Johnson syndrome
	Rotor syndrome
Endocrine	Hypopituitarism
	Hypothyroidism
Toxic	Prolonged parental nutrition (TPN)
Idiopathic neonatal hepatitis	

Biliary atresia

Biliary atresia is a disease of unknown aetiology with an incidence of 1/14 000 live births. There is gradual fibrosis and destruction of the extrahepatic and intrahepatic biliary ducts.

It presents as neonatal cholestasis with jaundice apparent by the 2nd day and hepatomegaly apparent by 4 weeks. Not all patients fail to thrive, and normally pigmented rather than acholic stools may be present in the first weeks of life. Physical examination usually reveals jaundice, hepatomegaly, acholic (pale) stools, and dark urine.

LFTs reveal conjugated hyperbilirubinaemia, elevated alkaline phosphatase, elevated gamma-glutamyl transpeptidase, and mildly elevated transaminases.

Early consultation and referral to specialist paediatric hepatology services is required as severe intrahepatic cholestasis has various aetiologies which mimic biliary atresia and investigation is complex. Further investigations may include:

- *Ultrasound:* the gallbladder is absent or atretic and choledochal cyst (see below) is excluded.
- *TEBIDA scan:* radio-isotope hepatobiliary excretion studies using an imino-diacetic acid derivative are most useful in confirming bile duct patency in equivocal cases. False positive/false negative error rates are 10%.
- *Liver biopsy:* percutaneous liver biopsy is most valuable for evaluating neonatal cholestasis and differentiating hepatocellular from obstructive causes. Bile duct proliferation, inflammation and fibrosis is seen. The histopathology evolves and serial samples may be required.
- *Intraoperative cholangiography:* this definitively demonstrates the anatomy and patency of the extrahepatic biliary tract.
- *Endoscopic retrograde cholangiopancreatography (ERCP):* this is now available for neonates and may be useful.

Treatment is surgical using the Kasai porto-enterostomy procedure (Fig 5.16), which is more likely to be successful if performed <2 months of age. Postoperative cholangitis occurs in 50%. The majority of children will require liver transplantation at some stage.

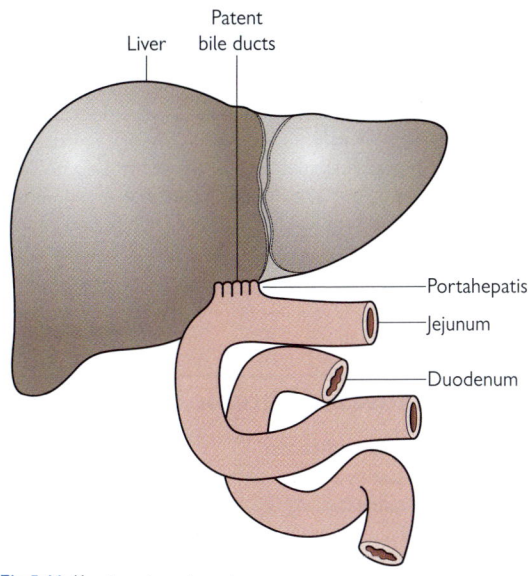

Fig 5.16 Kasai porto-enterostomy.

Alagille syndrome
This is an autosomal dominant disorder with variable expression and an incidence of 1/100 000 live births. It is caused by deletions of or mutations in the *JAG1* gene which encodes a ligand for the notch-1 receptor. Clinical features include:
- *Characteristic facial appearance:* prominent forehead, pointed chin, widely placed deep set eyes—and involvement of the liver, heart, skeleton, eye, and kidneys:
- *liver:* paucity of intrahepatic bile ducts causes cholestatic jaundice, hepatosplenomegaly and severe pruritus due to elevated serum bile acids. Deficiency of the fat-soluble vitamins K and D may cause coagulopathy and rickets
- *cardiovascular:* peripheral pulmonary stenosis
- *skeletal:* butterfly hemivertebrae in 50% and other abnormalities of vertebrae, ribs, forearm, and hands
- *eye:* posterior embryotoxon occurs in 70%
- *renal:* renal artery stenosis may cause hypertension
- *Neurologic:* developmental delay, learning difficulties.

Most patients present with neonatal cholestatic jaundice or a cardiac murmur, but expression is variable and some may only be diagnosed by examination after an index case is identified in the family.

Vitamin supplementation (A, D, E, K) is required, pruritus may respond to cholestyramine or rifampicin. Liver transplantation may be necessary.

α_1-Antitrypsin deficiency
This inherited disorder is caused by mutations in the *PI* (for protease inhibitor) gene which encodes α_1-antitrypsin, a serpin synthesized in the liver.

α_1-Antitrypsin (A1AT) has a major role in inhibition of several neutrophil-derived proteases (e.g. elastase, cathepsin G) providing an important protective screen that prevents alveolar wall destruction in the lung.

Over 80 mutations in the *PI* gene have been identified. The most common normal or wild-type allele is designated M, and homozygous individuals (PI MM) have normal serum levels of A1AT. Common mutant alleles are PI Z, PI S. Alleles causing absence of the protein are called Null.

A1AT levels depend on the phenotype:
- *PI MM:* 100% (normal)
- *PI MZ:* 60%
- *PI ZZ:* 10–15% (severe deficiency)
- *PI null null:* 0%

A1AT deficiency usually presents as lung disease in adults, but 10% of children with the PI ZZ, PI null null, or PI Z null phenotypes develop liver disease.

Clinical features include intrauterine growth retardation, cholestatic jaundice, and hepatomegaly. Serum A1AT levels are an initial screening test but definitive diagnosis requires determination of the phenotype by isoelectric focusing.

Prognosis is variable, with progressive liver disease in 50%.

Metabolic and transport disorders
Over a dozen AR inherited disorders can be associated with neonatal cholestasis: galactosaemia, tyrosinaemia type 1, Niemann–Pick type C disease, Zellweger syndrome, and disorders of bile acid synthesis.

Dubin–Johnson syndrome and progressive familial intrahepatic cholestasis (PFIC) are caused by mutations in transporter genes.
- *Tyrosinaemia type 1:* caused by defects in fumarylacetoacetase. Patients may present with acute infantile liver failure or chronic liver disease. Treatment with dietary restriction and nitisinone is effective and reduces the long-term risk of hepatocellular carcinoma. Liver transplantation is the definitive treatment.
- *Niemann-Pick type C disease:* neurovisceral accumulation of unesterified cholesterol. Expression is variable but about 50% present with neonatal cholestasis. Most have splenomegaly and vertical ophthalmoplegia is a pathognomonic neurological sign. Sea-blue histiocytes are found on bone-marrow biopsy.
- *Bile acid synthetic disorders:* defects in synthesis of cholic and chenodeoxycholic acid lead to cholestasis and accumulation of hepatotoxic metabolites. Presentation is with cholestasis, low gamma-GT levels and fat-soluble vitamin deficiency. Treatment is with cholic acid substitution.
- *Transporter defects:*
  - *Dubin–Johnson syndrome (DJS)* is a benign cause of conjugated hyperbilirubinaemia caused by defects in a canalicular membrane transporter for certain organic anions. Life expectancy is normal but jaundice may be exacerbated by alcohol, infection, and pregnancy. There is black pigmentation in the liver on biopsy.
  - *Progressive familial intrahepatic cholestasis (PFIC)* is a group of disorders caused by mutations in genes involved in transport of bile acids, *ATP8B1*, *ABCB11* or phospholipids, *ABCB4*.

Cholestatic jaundice and prolonged TPN
Cholestatic jaundice is common in preterm infants who have received prolonged parental nutrition, especially if accompanied by recurrent sepsis and gut resection.

In these circumstances a search for dual pathology is indicated if there is a progressive deterioration in liver function.

5.12 Childhood liver disease

Chronic liver disease

The causes of chronic liver disease in childhood include some of the inherited metabolic disorders which may also be present in the neonate (A1AT deficiency, tyrosinaemia type 1) together with additional inherited diseases, chronic hepatitis due to viral infection or autoimmune disease, and non-alcoholic fatty liver disease (Table 5.15).

Table 5.15. Chronic liver disease in childhood	
Chronic viral hepatitis	
Autoimmune hepatitis	
Metabolic disease:	A1AT deficiency Tyrosinaemia type 1 Wilson disease Cystic fibrosis Glycogen storage disease (types 3 and 4) Cholesterol ester storage disease Gaucher disease type 1
Primary sclerosing cholangitis	
Congenital hepatic fibrosis	
Hepatic tumour	
Non-alcoholic fatty liver disease (NAFLD)	

Pathophysiology

The final common histological pathway is cirrhosis, characterized by collapse of the normal lobule architecture and formation of islands of hepatocytes surrounded by dense connective tissue.

Hepatocellular failure leads to hypoalbuminaemia and a coagulopathy. Intrahepatic encroachment on the portal veins leads to portal hypertension and the development of splenomegaly and oesophageal varices.

Several factors may lead to ascites: hypoproteinaemia, hyperaldosteronism, and intrahepatic and lymphatic congestion.

Clinical features

These are highly variable at presentation. There may be a past history of neonatal cholestasis or infective hepatitis or an episode of apparent acute hepatitis which relapses or persists. The family history may be relevant. Uncommonly presentation may be with complications of portal hypertension such as bleeding from oesophageal varices.

Physical signs of chronic liver disease include:
- Jaundice
- Growth failure/muscle wasting
- *Cutaneous stigmata*: facial telangiectasia, spider naevi, palmar erythema, clubbing
- *Hepatomegaly*: hard or nodular liver
- Small liver (cirrhosis) with enlarged left lobe
- Splenomegaly
- Ascites, peripheral oedema.

Laboratory investigations

Blood tests to evaluate liver function (serum albumin, ALT, AST, coagulation screen) and test for specific diseases are done according to clinical context:
- *Chronic viral hepatitis*: HBsAg
- *Autoimmune hepatitis*: specific autoantibodies
- *A1AT*: PI phenotype

- *Cystic fibrosis*: sweat test.

Imaging modalities include:
- *Ultrasound*: allows assessment of liver parenchyma e.g. nodules and blood flow in portal veins and hepatic artery and veins.
- *CT and MRI*: allow high-resolution imaging of hepatic anatomy and circulation.

Percutaneous liver biopsy is essential in most cases for definitive diagnosis, but obviously requires prior correction of any coagulopathy.

Specific causes of chronic liver disease

Autoimmune liver disease

Autoimmune hepatitis is more common in girls and may present insidiously. Transaminases and IgG levels are raised with positive auto-antibodies:
- *Type 1*: antinuclear and/or anti-smooth muscle antibodies may be associated with auto-immune sclerosing cholangitis.
- *Type 2*: anti-liver and kidney microsomal antibodies. Liver biopsy shows interface hepatitis and multilobar collapse.

Wilson disease

Wilson disease is an autosomal recessive disorder caused by mutations in the *ATP7B* gene which encodes a copper transporting adenosine triphosphatase. The incidence is 1/30 000.

Defective copper transport leads to impairment of its incorporation in caeruloplasmin and biliary excretion with accumulation of copper in hepatocytes and hepatocellular injury. As liver copper levels increase it is released into the circulation and deposited in other organs, the iris, and basal ganglia.

About 50% of patients present with hepatic disease at 10–15 years of age. Neuropsychiatric presentation is rare before 10 years. Kayser–Fleischer rings (copper deposition in Descemet's membrane) are present in 50% of patients presenting with hepatic disease. Hepatic disease may manifest as chronic active hepatitis, cirrhosis, or fulminant hepatic failure.

Investigations indicated include:
- Serum caeruloplasmin (<20 mg/dL)
- Plasma copper (normal or raised)
- Urinary copper excretion (elevated >100 mg/dL) + after penicillamine
- *Liver biopsy*: for morphology (Mallory bodies) and copper content (raised)
- *Brain MRI*: basal ganglia lesions

Treatment is with chelating agents: D-penicillamine or trientine. Dietary management includes a low-copper diet, vitamin B6 and zinc which prevents intestinal copper absorption by inducing mucosal metallothionein synthesis. Liver transplantation is indicated for fulminant liver failure.

Non-alcoholic fatty liver disease (NAFLD)

Childhood NAFLD or non-alcoholic steatohepatitis (NASH) is an increasing problem in children and adolescents. The risk factors are obesity, insulin resistance, and hypertryglyceridaemia.

It is usually asymptomatic but vague recurrent abdominal pain may be a presenting feature. Liver enzymes (especially ALT) and triglycerides may be elevated.

Drug hepatotoxicity and genetic or metabolic disease associated with steatosis should be excluded. Liver biopsy is necessary for diagnosis and determination of disease severity. The mainstay of treatment is weight reduction. Progressive liver disease may occur in a minority.

Acute liver disease

Acute liver disease is usually associated with inflammation (hepatitis) and usually has an infectious viral aetiology. Non-infectious causes include toxins, autoimmune disorders, and various metabolic diseases. See Table 5.16.

Table 5.16 Aetiology of acute liver disease	
Infection	Viral hepatitis: hepatitis A, B, C, D, E; EBV, CMV, HLIV Measles
Drugs	Paracetamol Halothane Isoniazid Antiepileptics: valproate, carbamazepine
Metabolic	Wilson disease Galactosaemia Tyrosinaemia type 1 Mitochondrial disorders
Autoimmune hepatitis	

Acute hepatitis

This is an acute inflammation of the liver associated with hepatocyte degeneration and necrosis and by definition lasting <6 months. Table 5.16 includes the main causes. Viral infection accounts for around one half of all cases of acute hepatitis. Other infectious aetiologies include bacterial (leptospirosis), fungal, and parasitic agents (malaria, schistosoma).

Acute viral hepatitis

Five major hepatotropic viruses cause most cases: HAV, HBV, HCV, HDV, HEV. Other viruses which may be hepatotropic include herpesviruses (CMV, EBV, HHV), measles, and adenovirus. HDV and HEV are uncommon in the UK. Most childhood infections with hepatitis viruses are asymptomatic or result in anicteric illness.

- *Hepatitis A:* a picornavirus. Faecal–oral transmission, incubation 2–6 weeks, 80% of infections asymptomatic. Usually self-limiting (rarely fulminant). No carrier state and chronic liver disease does not occur.
- *Hepatitis B:* a hepadnavirus. 400 million carriers worldwide. Transmission parenteral, sexual or perinatal. Positivity for HBeAg increases transmission risk. Incubation period 30–180 days. Chronic infection develops in 90% of infected neonates, 5–10% older children. Fulminant hepatic failure in 0.5–10% and risk of cirrhosis and hepatocellular cancer in chronic infection.

Acute liver failure

Acute liver failure (ALF) is a rare but potentially fatal multisystem disorder in which severe impairment of liver function occurs in association with hepatocellular necrosis.

Aetiology varies with age. Infections and metabolic liver disease are most common in neonates or infants. In older children and adolescents paracetamol toxicity, autoimmune or viral hepatitis, Wilson disease, and infiltrative diseases (e.g. haemophagocytic lymphohistiocytosis) are more common but a substantial proportion are idiopathic.

Clinical features

Encephalopathy is often absent or difficult to recognize in younger patients. If present, it is a predictor of poor outcome. ALF should be considered if biochemical investigations reveal:

- Marked conjugated hyperbilirubinaemia
- Elevated aminotransferase levels (>10 000 iu/L)
- Raised plasma ammonia (>100 mmol/L)
- Coagulopathy (raised INR, prothrombin time >40 s) uncorrectable by IV vitamin K.

Complications include:

- *Neurological:* encephalopathy and cerebral oedema
- *Infection:* Sepsis; gram-positive or negative septicaemia; fungal infection (*Candida* spp.)
- *Metabolic:* hypoglycaemia in 40%
- Metabolic acidosis
- *Renal failure:* in 10–15%
- *Haematological:* coagulopathy, thrombocytopaenia
- *Haemodynamic:* hyperdynamic circulation with increased cardiac output and decreased peripheral vascular resistance
- GI haemorrhage.

Management

Children with ALF are best managed in a specialist centre but initial management while arranging transfer to ICU includes:

- Monitor BP and urine output
- Prevent hypoglycaemia: provide adequate calories (oral or NG feeding) or IV dextrose
- Restrict fluids to two thirds maintenance
- Broad spectrum prophylactic antibiotics
- Prophylactic ranitidine and proton pump inhibitors
- Correct coagulopathy with IV vitamin K.

Disease specific therapies include *N*-acetylcysteine infusion for paracetamol (acetaminophen) toxicity and high-dose steroids for autoimmune hepatitis. Liver transplantation has improved survival but certain conditions are not treatable by liver replacement (e.g. malignancies, mitochondrial disorders, giant cell hepatitis).

5.13 Case-based discussions

A child with an abdominal mass

A 9 year old white boy is seen in the hospital emergency department. He complains of feeling weak and exhausted for the last 3 months. He has slight diarrhoea and does not feel like eating, but there are no other specific symptoms, and no history of fever. There is no history of previous illness or recent travel and no family history of note. He takes no medications. Parents tell you that this has been a stressful few months because of the death of two of the child's grandparents.

On examination he is markedly cachectic (Fig 5.17).

His weight is on the 2nd centile for age, height 25th centile.

He is pale, with no lymphadenopathy. The only other abnormal finding is a smooth, non-tender mass in his right iliac fossa.

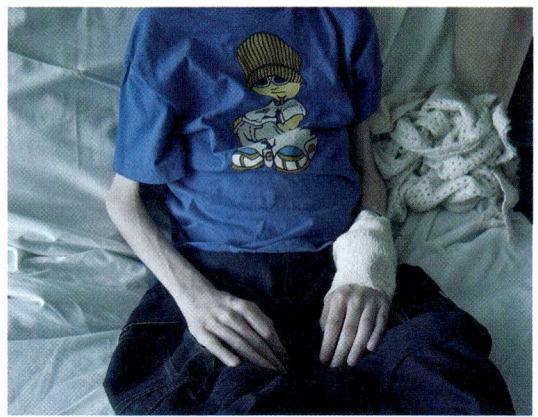

Fig 5.17 Cachectic body habitus.

What is your differential diagnosis?

Malignancy must be high on the list, with weight loss, systemic malaise, and an abdominal mass. Abdominal tuberculosis may account for his symptoms, although there is no history of contact or recent travel and he is not in a high-risk ethnic group.

Gastrointestinal pathology must also be considered in view of his diarrhoea and rapid weight loss. Possible diagnoses include coeliac disease (although this would not explain the mass), IBD, or CF, although this would be an unusual presentation of the latter. HIV should also be considered, although this child has no risk factors for this condition.

His blood results reveal:
Hb 8 g/dL, normocytic and normochromic.
WCC 12.1×10^9/L
Platelets 624×10^9/L
U&E and LFTs normal
CRP 63 mg/L
ESR 198 mm/h
Coagulation normal
Ferritin elevated
Tumour markers pending
Mantoux test negative at 48 h

What do these blood tests show?

The blood tests reveal evidence of inflammation (raised CRP, ESR, ferritin, and platelets). The anaemia is consistent with anaemia of chronic disease.

An urgent ultrasound scan is arranged. The report identifies a mass arising from the small bowel, but is otherwise inconclusive.

How would you proceed?

Further imaging, e.g. a CT scan, may be helpful. However, an endoscopy may yield more conclusive answers regarding possible gut pathology and will enable biopsies to be taken for histology.

An endoscopy was performed on this child the following day. It revealed extensive inflammation throughout the large and small bowel. Further information from biopsy samples showed that the inflammation was transmural, and demonstrated granuloma formation consistent with CD. The abdominal mass contained inflammatory tissue surrounded by adhesions.

How would you manage this patient?

A diagnosis of CD was made. Management was in consultation with the paediatric gastroenterologist.

The mass was removed at laparotomy. Re-anastamosis was possible. A temporary gastrostomy was inserted at the same operation to allow re-feeding, but an initial 3 week period of TPN was undertaken in the first instance to allow resting of the bowel.

An elemental diet was introduced, initially as a total exclusion diet, with gradual reintroduction of foods at 8 weeks. This induces remission in up to 90% of patients. Maintenance of remission was attempted with 5-ASA derivatives. Ongoing nutrition support and dietitian input is vital.

In the case of this child, remission was not maintained with 5-ASA derivatives, and courses of steroids were required, with return to elemental diet and later addition of azathioprine.

A vomiting infant

A 4 week old male infant presents for the second time to the hospital emergency department with a history of vomiting. He was seen there 1 week previously at which time a diagnosis of GOR was made and Gaviscon prescribed. The vomiting has worsened and now occurs after most feeds. It started at about 10 days of age. It is described as always being 'forceful' and consists just of milk with no blood or bile. He remains eager to feed but stool frequency is diminished. Birth history is unremarkable. He is the first child of young parents.

On examination he is afebrile and jaundiced with mild dehydration. He appears systemically well. There is no abdominal distension, but patient observation reveals visible peristaltic waves passing from left to right across the upper abdomen.

What is the diagnosis?

The clinical features strongly suggest infantile hypertrophic pyloric stenosis. The misdiagnosis of GOR indicates a failure to appreciate the difference between regurgitation and vomiting.

Investigations confirmed the diagnosis. He had a hypochloraemic, hypokalaemic metabolic alkalosis and pyloric hypertrophy visible on abdominal ultrasound examination. After rehydration >48 h he underwent Ramstedt's pyloromyotomy and made an uneventful recovery. This is not a surgical emergency.

Chapter 6
Nephrology and urology

- 6.1 The urinary system *120*
- 6.2 Clinical nephrology *122*
- 6.3 Urinary tract infection *124*
- 6.4 Glomerulonephritis *126*
- 6.5 Nephrotic syndrome *128*
- 6.6 Renal failure *130*
- 6.7 Congenital anomalies of the urinary tract *132*
- 6.8 Renal anomalies and inguinoscrotal disorders *134*
- 6.9 Cystic disease and tubulopathies *136*
- 6.10 Genetic syndromes and HUS *138*
- 6.11 Hypertension, urolithiasis, and nephrocalcinosis *140*
- 6.12 Case-based discussions *142*

6.1 The urinary system

Embryology
The urogenital system is divided into the urinary (excretory) system and genital (reproductive) system.

Development of the urinary system
Three sets of excretory organs develop sequentially: the pronephros, mesonephros, and metanephros.
- *Pronephros:* transitory structures appear early in the 4th week
- *Mesonephros:* caudal to the pronephros, appear late in 4th week and function as interim kidneys
- *Metanephros:* in the 5th week, ureteric buds arise from the distal portions of the mesonephric ducts and fuse with the metanephric mass to initiate nephrogenesis.

During weeks 6–10 the ureteric bud derivatives give rise to the renal pelvis, calyces and collecting tubules and the metanephric mesoderm gives rise to nephrons. Urine is produced from the 10th week. Nephrogenesis is completed by term and renal function continues to mature postnatally.

Renal anatomy
Each kidney has a pale outer cortex and darker inner medulla divided into conical renal pyramids (Fig 6.1). The apex of each pyramid ends in a renal papilla. These merge to form the renal pelvis which continues to form the ureter.

The nephron
The functional unit is the nephron (Fig 6.2), made up of a glomerulus, capsule, and tubule.

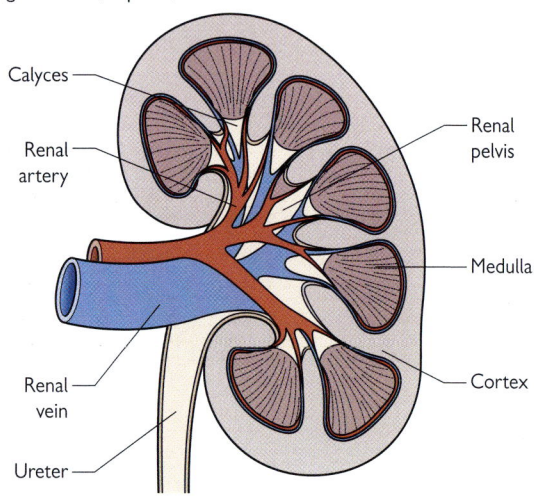

Fig 6.1 Renal anatomy.

- *Glomerulus and capsule:* the glomerulus is a tuft of capillaries interposed between the afferent and efferent arterioles. Each glomerulus is enclosed within an epithelial cell capsule (Bowman's capsule) which is continuous with the epithelial cells surrounding the glomerular capillaries and the cells of the proximal convoluted tubule.
- *Tubule:* each renal tubule is divided into several segments: the proximal convoluted tubule leads to the thin descending limb of the loop of Henle, followed by the thick ascending limb and finally the distal convoluted tubule which empties into the collecting duct.

Renal function
The primary function is the regulation of water and electrolyte balance and excretion of urea, but other functions include:
- Blood pressure regulation
- Regulation of haematopoiesis
- Metabolism of vitamin D.

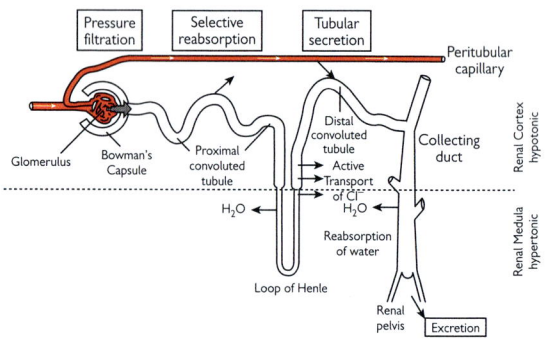

Fig 6.2 The nephron.

Glomerular function
The kidneys receive up to 25% of the cardiac output. A glomerular filtrate is formed which is then modified during passage through the renal tubule to form urine.

Glomerular ultrafiltration
The glomerular filtration rate (GFR) is mainly determined by the transcapillary hydrostatic pressure gradient which itself is influenced by the relative degree of constriction of the afferent and efferent arterioles. Angiotensin II causes preferential constriction of efferent arterioles and increases both glomerular capillary pressure and GFR.

GFR is expressed as a function of body surface area (BSA), and absolute values are corrected for surface area by the formula:

corrected GFR (mL/min per 1.73 m^2) = absolute GFR (mL/min) × 1.73/BSA

Measuring GFR
Plasma creatinine level provides an indirect estimate of GFR. The normal range increases with age.
GFR can be estimated from plasma creatinine concentration and height using the Schwartz formula:

GFR (mL/min per 1.73 m^2) = [height (cm)/plasma creatinine (μmol/L)] × K

where K is a constant that varies with age and sex.

GFR is overestimated in children with reduced muscle mass. GFR can be estimated from creatinine clearance, based on a timed urine collection and paired plasma samples using the formula:

[urine creatinine concentration (μmol/L)/plasma creatinine (μmol/L)] × urine flow (mL/min)

This overestimates true GFR, as creatinine undergoes tubular secretion.

Urea plasma concentration is influenced by dietary protein intake, catabolism, and hydration state as well as GFR and is therefore an unreliable marker of renal function.

The glomerular filtrate is a virtually protein-free solution of a similar composition to plasma. Tubular function converts the filtrate to urine.

Tubular function
The tubular epithelial cells express an array of transporters which confer distinct activities on individual segments. The proximal tubule and loop of Henle are the major site of reabsorption. The distal tubule and collecting duct are the site of 'fine tuning' of urine composition.

Proximal tubule
- 50% of filtered Na^+ is reabsorbed, via the Na^+–K^+ ATPase system with secondary transport by Na^+-coupled transport of various substrates (glucose, amino acids) and by the Na^+/H^+ exchanger NHE3.
- Glucose and amino acids are completely reabsorbed. Phosphate (80–90%) and calcium (60%) are reabsorbed. Creatinine, urate, and some drugs are secreted into the proximal tubule. 90% of bicarbonate and some Cl^- is reabsorbed by the Na^+/H^+ exchanger.

Loop of Henle (LoH)
- The water channel aquaporin-1 is expressed in the proximal tubules and descending thin limb of the LoH
- A further 40% of filtered Na^+ is reabsorbed via the Na^+–K^+–$2Cl^-$ co-transporter (NKCC2) in the thick ascending limb.
- Co-transported K^+ recycles into the lumen via the renal outer medullary K^+ channel (ROMK1). Na^+ is extruded across the basolateral cell membrane by the Na^+–K^+ ATPase and Cl^- exits via channels composed of the pore-forming unit CLC-Kb and the beta subunit barttin. The medullary concentration gradient is generated.

Distal tubule
- A further 5% of filtered Na^+ is reabsorbed by a luminal Na^+–Cl^- cotransporter (NCCT). Na^+ and Cl^- extrusion across the basolateral cell membrane is by the same channels as in the LoH.

Collecting duct
- 2% of filtered Na^+ is reabsorbed via aldosterone-sensitive Na^+ channels (ENaC), in exchange for K^+. ENaC is also expressed in the distal tubule. K^+ exits via the renal outer medullary K^+ channel (ROMK) and Na^+ exits via the Na^+-K^+ ATPase. Expression of all three proteins is stimulated by aldosterone via the mineralocorticoid receptor
- Aquaporin-2 (AQP2) is the arginine–vasopressin sensitive water channel of the principal cells of the collecting tubules/duct.

Water and electrolyte balance
Water and osmotic equilibrium
Total body water as a percentage of body weight decreases from 85% in preterm infants to 80% in term newborns and 65% in older children. The semipermeable cell membrane separates the intracellular and extracellular fluid compartments. Osmotic equilibrium is maintained between the compartments as fluid shifts from lower to higher osmolality.

Plasma (ECF) osmolality is calculated as:

$[(Na^+ + K^+) \times 2]$ + glucose + urea = osmolality in mOsmol/kg
- *Normal plasma osmolality* is 280–300 mOsmol/kg.
- *A small increase in ECF osmolality* stimulates thirst, water intake, and water retention by the kidneys via the release of antidiuretic hormone from the posterior pituitary. ECF depletion with hypovolaemia stimulates ADH release via carotid and atrial baroreceptors.
- *Urine osmolality:* neonates have reduced concentrating power, but infants >1 month of age should be able to concentrate urine >800 mOsmol/kg.

Renin–angiotensin–aldosterone system
A loss of blood pressure or hypovolaemia with decreased renal perfusion leads to release of renin from the juxtaglomerular apparatus.

Renin cleaves an inactive peptide called angiotensinogen, converting it to angiotensin I. Angiotensin I is converted to angiotensin II by angiotensin converting enzyme (ACE) which is found mainly in lung capillaries. Angiotensin II (AII) is the main bioactive molecule and causes vasoconstriction and release of aldosterone and ADH (Fig 6.3).

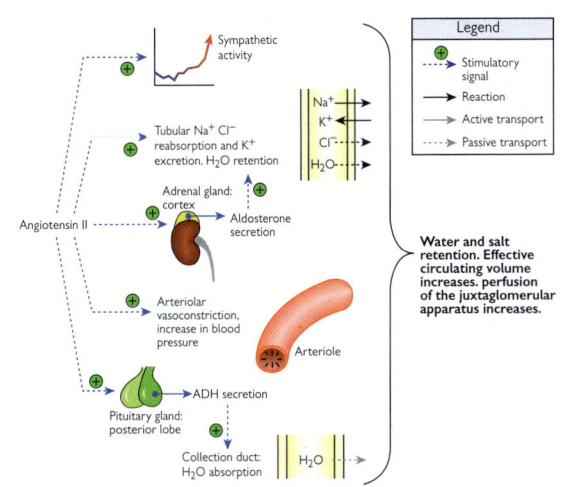

Fig 6.3 Actions of angiotension II.

Erythropoietin
Erythropoietin (EPO) is produced by peritubular fibroblasts of the renal cortex and stimulates erythropoiesis in the bone marrow. Deficiency of EPO is a major factor in the anaemia of renal disease.

Vitamin D metabolism
Cholecalciferol (Vitamin D3) is hydroxylated to 25 (OH)-D3 in the liver and to 1,25 $(OH)_2$-D3 or calcitriol in the kidney. Deficiency of calcitriol underlies the rickets associated with chronic kidney disease.

6.2 Clinical nephrology

History and examination
Presenting complaints may include:
- *Pain:* renal disease is an important cause of abdominal pain; acute pyelonephritis may cause flank pain in the older child.
- *Dysuria:* not all children with dysuria have a UTI. Other causes include local skin conditions such as vulvovaginitis or balanitis and the discomfort of passing concentrated urine.
- *Voiding problems:* enuresis which may be nocturnal or diurnal, frequency of micturition.
- Polyuria or polydipsia
- *Urinary abnormalities:* passage of cloudy urine or macroscopic haematuria may be reported.

A family history of renal disease or hearing impairment may be relevant.

Examination
Abnormalities of the genitourinary tract may be externally visible or palpable per abdomen. Blood pressure must be measured, and the acute or chronic effects of renal impairment may be evident on examination.

General
- *Fever:* a high fever is suggestive of upper UTI or pyelonephritis.
- *Anaemia:* is a feature of chronic kidney disease.
- *Failure to thrive:* kidney disease is an important cause of inadequate weight gain in the first year of life.
- *Short stature:* chronic kidney disease,
- *Oedema:* periorbital oedema may be apparent in both acute nephritis and nephrotic syndrome, but generalized oedema is generally only a feature of the latter.
- *Blood pressure (BP):* normally increases throughout childhood and must be compared with age, sex, and height centile. The cuff used should cover at least two thirds of the upper arm.
- *Abdominal examination:* bladder and/or kidneys may be palpable. Ascites and abdominal wall oedema occurs in severe nephrotic syndrome. An abdominal bruit may indicate renovascular disease.
- *Genitalia:* inguinoscrotal disorders are important particularly in boys including undescended testis, inguinal hernia or hydrocoele, the acute scrotum, or penile abnormalities.

Electrolytes: sodium (Na+)
The normal range of plasma Na^+ concentration is 135–145 mmol/L. Normonatraemia is consistent with salt depletion or overload if parallel changes in body water have occurred.

Hyponatraemia: plasma Na^+ <130 mmol/L
Hyponatraemia more often reflects gain or retention of water than Na^+ depletion. Causes include:

Excess water
Increase in body weight and inappropriately concentrated urine. The main treatment is fluid restriction.
- *Water overload:*
  - iatrogenic excess hypotonic oral or IV fluid
  - habitual drinkers
- *Water retention:*
  - syndrome of inappropriate ADH secretion (SIADH).
  - acute renal failure.

Na^+ depletion
- *Renal losses:* inappropriately high urine volume and Na^+ concentration (>20 mmol/l)
  - loop diuretics, e.g. furosemide
  - hypoaldosteronism, e.g. congenital adrenal hyperplasia
  - acute tubular necrosis: recovery phase
  - tubulopathies
- *Extrarenal losses:* appropriate oliguria and low urine Na^+ concentration (<10 mmol/l)
  - gastroenteritis
  - skin losses: severe sweating, cystic fibrosis.

Dehydration with reduced body weight is usually present and main treatment is rehydration with correction of Na^+ deficit, calculated as:

$$[140 - \text{plasma } [Na^+] \text{ (mmol)}] \times 0.65 \times \text{body weight (kg)}]$$

Both mechanisms may operate if dehydration and salt depletion is treated with inappropriately hypotonic fluid.

Artefactual hyponatraemia occurs in hyperlipidaemia states.

Hypernatraemia: plasma Na^+ >150 mmol/L
Hypernatraemia more commonly reflects loss of water, (in excess of Na^+) rather than a high load of Na^+ or solute. A shift of water from ICF to ECF makes hypernatraemic dehydration less obvious clinically.

Loss of water (dehydration)
- *Extrarenal losses:* urine is concentrated and reduced in volume
  - GI losses: diarrhoea
  - increased insensible water loss: pyrexia, radiant heater
- *Renal losses:* high volume of inappropriately dilute urine
  - diabetes insipidus: central or nephrogenic
  - diabetes mellitus: osmotic diuresis in DKA
  - reduced renal concentrating power: preterm babies.

Inadequate free water intake
- Iatrogenic: excess hypertonic oral or IV fluid
- Breast-fed neonate with inadequate maternal milk flow (compounded by high salt content of the milk).

Gain of Na^+
- *Iatrogenic:* excess hypertonic IV fluids
- Incorrect reconstitution of infant formula
- *Salt poisoning:* accidental or deliberate (in FII).

Rapid correction of hypernatraemia causes shift of water into the brain with encephalopathy and seizures. Standard oral rehydration solution is the safest approach. Intravenous treatment should be undertaken cautiously, avoiding falls in plasma Na^+ concentration >2 mmol/L per hour.

Electrolytes: potassium (K+)

K^+ is predominantly an intracellular electrolyte. Plasma K^+ does not necessarily reflect whole-body K^+ status as rapid shifts between the extracellular and intracellular compartments can occur.

Hypokalaemia
The causes include:

Excess renal losses
- Drugs including diuretics (loop and thiazide diuretics) and salbutamol.
- *Tubulopathies:* Bartter, Gitelman syndrome, distal RTA
- *Osmotic diuresis:* diabetic ketoacidosis
- Cushing syndrome.

Extrarenal losses
- GI losses.

Inadequate provision of K^+ intake
- Prolonged IV fluids without K^+ added.

Shift from ECF to ICF compartment
- During correction of metabolic acidosis and insulin treatment, classically during treatment of diabetic ketoacidosis.

Hyperkalaemia
The causes include:

Iatrogenic
- Excess administration in IV fluid. Accidental administration of K^+ concentrate solutions has fatal results.
- *Drugs:* spironolactone, ACE inhibitors.

Renal failure
- Acute or chronic.

Hypoadrenalism
- *Addison disease:* adrenal insufficiency
- Salt-wasting congenital adrenal hyperplasia
- pseudohypoaldosteronism (PHA).

Shift from ICF to ECF compartment
- Metabolic acidosis
- Tumour lysis syndrome
- Rhabdomyolysis (with acute renal failure).

Hyperkalaemia requires urgent treatment because of the risk of cardiac arrhythmia. ECG monitoring is essential to detect cardiac effects: peaked T waves, prolonged PR interval, QRS widening and ventricular arrhythmias.

Immediate measures include:
- Stop K^+ intake
- Calcium gluconate to stabilize myocardium
- Correct metabolic acidosis: shift K^+ into cells
- Salbutamol: nebulized or IV
- Administration of insulin and dextrose (caution as risk of hypoglycaemia)
- Calcium resonium or dialysis to reduce total body K^+.

Acid–base balance

(see Chapter 2.1)

The kidneys have a role in regulating pH by metabolic compensation. Primary or secondary disorders of tubular function may cause metabolic acidosis or alkalosis.

Bicarbonate ions are filtered at the glomerulus and virtually all are reabsorbed in the proximal and distal tubules. Channels in the distal tubule (controlled by aldosterone) exchange Na^+ for H^+ or K^+ ions.

Metabolic acidosis
Renal diseases associated with metabolic acidosis include:
- Acute or chronic renal failure
- Renal bicarbonate loss: proximal (type 2) renal tubular acidosis (RTA)
- Reduced renal H^+ ion excretion: distal (type 1) RTA.

There is hyperchloraemia with a normal anion gap.

Metabolic alkalosis
This is associated with:
- *Cl^- depletion:* Cl^- depletion leads to bicarbonate retention and alkalosis, and may occur in pyloric stenosis, congenital Cl^- diarrhoea, cystic fibrosis and furosemide therapy
- *Excess renal H^+ excretion:* occurs in hyperaldosteronism, Cushing syndrome, and Bartter syndrome.

Urinalysis

The kidneys are unique in producing an easily accessible fluid which reveals much about their function. Dipstick testing is used to detect blood, protein, glucose, pH, leukocyte esterase, and nitrite.

Urine microscopy followed by culture is commonly performed and measurements of urine osmolality and electrolyte concentrations are valuable in certain circumstances.

The use and interpretation of urinalysis is discussed in sections dealing with UTI, glomerulonephritis, and the nephrotic syndrome.

Renal biopsy

Common indications for renal biopsy include:
- *Nephrotic syndrome:* steroid resistant or atypical
- Macroscopic haematuria and/or proteinuria
- Acute nephritic syndrome
- Acute or chronic renal failure
- Post-transplant.

Procedure
Percutaneous renal biopsy is carried out after renal ultrasound to ensure two kidneys are present. It is performed using ultrasound guidance under sedation or brief general anaesthetic. Complications include subcapsular haematomas, macroscopic haematuria (in 10%, usually clears within hours), and infection.

6.3 Urinary tract infection

It is estimated that 1% of boys and 3% of girls have a UTI during the first decade. UTI is more common in boys than girls in the first 6 months, the sex incidence is equal during infancy, and by school age girls outnumber boys.

40% of girls have recurrent infection, one third of girls with a UTI having a further episode within a year.

UTI accounts for 5% of fevers in children <5 years.

Aetiology and pathogenesis

Aetiology
A UTI is infection (usually bacterial) in the normally sterile posterior urethra, bladder, ureters, renal pelvis, or renal parenchyma.

A continual and regular 'flushing' of the urinary tract normally ensures freedom from infection and most of the well-defined predisposing causes act via urinary stasis. Risk factors are usually classified as physiological or pathological:

Physiological
- *Female anatomy:* the short female urethra
- *Perineal hygiene:* forward wiping after defecation in girls
- *Poor fluid intake:* high urine flow protects against cystitis
- *Bladder dysfunction:* incomplete bladder emptying (may be associated with vesicoureteric reflux).

Pathological
- *Invasive bacteraemia:* acute infection of the kidneys may be bacteraemic in origin including translocation of bacteria
- *Urinary tract anomalies:* obstruction in pelvi-ureteric or vesi-coureteric junction obstruction, posterior urethral valves in males
- *Vesicoureteric reflux:* VUR is common among children with UTI and is assumed to be a causative factor
- *Neuropathic bladder:* e.g. in spina bifida
- *Renal calculi:* urothelial trauma predisposes to infection.

Pathogenesis
Pathogenic organisms differ from harmless bacterial flora in their ability to adhere to and invade the urothelium. 85% of infections are caused by *E. coli*, but other organisms are seen especially if there is underlying urinary tract pathology including *Klebsiella, Proteus, Pseudomonas, Strep. faecalis*.

UTIs are usually classified into:
- *Lower UTI:* cystitis
- *Upper UTI:* acute pyelonephritis.

Ascending infection may occur by reflux of infected urine or bacterial migration along the urothelium, or be blood borne. Upper UTI can cause renal parenchymal damage manifested as renal scarring. The risk is highest in young infants and appears to diminish with age. In a minority of cases hypertension and end-stage renal failure (ESRF) may occur although the extent to which this represents an association of congenitally small dysplastic kidneys with VUR remains unclear.

Clinical features
UTI can present in many ways. A high index of suspicion is especially necessary in infants who frequently present in a non-specific manner and in preverbal children unable to localize their symptoms. Differentiation between upper and lower UTI may be a challenge.

Presenting symptoms and signs in UTI by age
<3 months
• *Most common:* fever, vomiting, lethargy, irritability
• *Common:* poor feeding, failure to thrive
• *Less common:* jaundice, haematuria, offensive urine
>3 months (pre-verbal)
• *Most common:* fever, poor feeding
• *Common:* abdominal pain, loin tenderness, vomiting
• *Less common:* lethargy, haematuria, offensive urine
>3 months (verbal)
• *Most common:* frequency, dysuria
• *Common:* abnormal voiding, enuresis, abdominal pain
• *Less common:* fever, malaise, haematuria, offensive urine

Newborns and infants are susceptible to severe blood-borne infection, and urine culture is an essential component of the septic screen.

The history should include enquiry about:
- Previous history of possible or confirmed UTI
- Antenatal diagnosis of renal tract anomaly
- Family history of VUR or renal disease
- Constipation or dysfunctional voiding
- Loin pain
- Dysuria and urinary stream.

Examination
- *Fever:* >38 °C is consistent with upper UTI
- Signs of bacterial sepsis: circulatory compromise, prolonged capillary refill
- Palpable bladder or kidneys
- Inspection of external genitalia and spine
- Blood pressure
- Lower limb sensation and reflexes
- Growth.

Clinical features usually allow distinction between upper and lower UTI:
- *Upper UTI/acute pyelonephritis:* bacteriuria and fever >38 °C or loin pain and tenderness
- *Lower UTI/cystitis:* bacteriuria without systemic features.

Diagnostic investigations
Urine collection and testing
A urine sample should be tested in any infant or child with unexplained fever of 38 °C or higher, symptoms or signs of UTI, or persistent unexplained illness.

- *Urine collection:* a clean catch sample is the recommended method. Alternative non-invasive methods include use of a pad or bag. If non-invasive methods are not possible then consider a catheter sample or suprapubic aspiration (SPA).
- *Urine testing:* urgent microscopy and culture is optimal for diagnosis. If culture is delayed >4 h the sample should be refrigerated or inoculated on to a dipslide.

Bacteriuria on microscopy confirms the diagnosis, but pyuria without bacteriuria should not deter treatment if clinical features suggest a UTI. Absence of bacteria and white cells effectively exclude UTI if the observations are reliable.

Diagnosis is confirmed by culture of a pure growth of >10^5/mL organisms. Sensitivity of urine culture is high but specificity is low and varies with urine collection technique. Positive results should be interpreted in the clinical context.

Dipstick testing: used in children >3 years
Dipsticks test for nitrites and leukocyte esterase and haematuria. Uropathogens metabolize nitrate to nitrite but it takes several hours for detectable quantities to accumulate and children with UTI void frequently.

Nitrite testing has low sensitivity and false negatives are common. Pyuria is common in febrile children without UTI so detection of white cells is an unreliable guide to infection. If both nitrites and leukocyte esterase are positive infection is likely and if both are negative UTI is unlikely, but the tests must be interpreted in the clinical context. In a child >3 years, with a first UTI, dipstick testing is as useful as microscopy and culture.

Management
Acute management
Antibiotic treatment is commenced as soon as a suitable urine sample has been collected. Initial choice is based on local sensitivity patterns. Treatment is given intravenously in infants <3 months, in systemically unwell children or if acute pyelonephritis is suspected. Examples of suitable antibiotics:

- *Oral:* trimethoprim, nitrofurantoin, cefalexin, amoxicillin, co-amoxiclav
- *Parenteral:* cefuroxime, cefotaxime, ceftriaxone.

The child should be kept well hydrated. If the child is receiving prophylactic medication a different antibiotic should be used. A renal ultrasound should be performed during the acute infection in infants or children with 'atypical' UTI who are at greater risk of having an abnormal urinary tract. See Box.

Useful conservative measures include: treatment of constipation, frequent and double voiding and adequate fluid intake.

An 'atypical' UTI is defined by:
- Serious systemic illness or septicaemia
- Palpable bladder, kidneys, or poor urine flow
- Raised plasma creatinine
- Infection with organisms other than *E. coli*
- Failure to respond to suitable antibiotics in 48 h.

Investigation strategy
The imaging modalities available are:

- *Renal ultrasound:* can assess kidney size and shape, detect urinary tract dilatation, and identify calculi.
- *DMSA (99mTc-dimerruptosuccinic acid) scan:* the most sensitive test for detection of acute pyelonephritis and renal scarring. It is best delayed for 4–6 months after acute infection to distinguish acute parenchymal defects from renal scars.
- *MCUG (micturating cysto-urethrogram):* the definitive investigation for detection and grading of vesicoureteric reflux, but a very invasive procedure. Prophylactic antibiotics should be given for 3 days (with MCUG on day 2).
- *MAG3 (99mTc-mercaptoacetyltriglycine) scan:* with an indirect radionuclide cystogram may be performed in toilet-trained children. It provides functional imaging of the kidneys and by continuing during voiding it is possible to detect VUR.

Imaging recommendations
The UK NICE guidelines published in August 2007 recommend imaging schedules according to:

- *Age:* <6 months, 6 months–3 years, 3 years or older
- *Atypical UTI:* as defined above (see Box)
- *Recurrence of UTI:* defined as two or more UTIs (one or both of which is an upper UTI) or three or more lower UTIs.

Ultrasound during the acute infection is recommended at all ages if the UTI is atypical, except if a non-*E. coli* UTI is the only 'atypical' feature, and there is a good response, the ultrasound can be performed non-urgently within 6 weeks. A first infection responding well to treatment within 48 h and with no atypical features requires no further imaging in infants or children aged >6 months.

Recommended imaging schedule by age
- *Age <6 months:*
  - A renal ultrasound either acutely or within 6 weeks for atypical or recurrent UTI. If ultrasound abnormal consider MCUG even for a first UTI with no atypical features.
  - DMSA at 4–6 months and MCUG for all infants with atypical or recurrent UTI. This group of young infants is most likely to have an underlying abnormality and is most at risk.
- *Age 6 months–3 years:*
  - An ultrasound within 6 weeks for recurrent UTI and atypical UTI (if not performed acutely).
  - DMSA at 4–6 months for atypical or recurrent UTI.
  - MCUG considered if there is: dilatation on ultrasound, poor urine flow, non-*E. coli* infection, family history of VUR.
- *Age 3 years and older:*
  - Ultrasound within 6 weeks and DMSA at 4–6 months is recommended for recurrent UTI.
  - Antibiotic prophylaxis is not routinely used for a first UTI, but may be considered after recurrent UTI.

6.4 Glomerulonephritis

Glomerulonephritis (GN) is the term used for a group of primary or secondary immune-mediated renal diseases characterized by inflammation of the glomeruli or small blood vessels in the kidneys.

GN has many different causes ranging from post-infectious glomerulonephritis to systemic diseases such as Henoch–Schönlein purpura and systemic lupus erythematosus.

Glomerulonephritis may present as asymptomatic haematuria or proteinuria, acute nephritis, rapidly progressive glomerulonephritis (RPGN), a mixed nephritic/nephrotic syndrome, or nephrotic syndrome (see Section 6.5).

Aetiology and pathogenesis of GN

Aetiology
The cause may be post-infectious or non-infectious.

Post-infectious glomerulonephritis
Streptococcal
Post-streptococcal GN usually develops 1–6 weeks after infection with nephritogenic strains of Group A β-haemolytic streptococcus (GAS). The incidence is 5–10% in patients with pharyngitis and 25% after skin infection. Deposits of IgG and C3 are found in glomeruli and serum C3 is low.

Non-streptococcal
- *Bacterial:* infective endocarditis, typhoid, pneumonococcal pneumonia, meningococcaemia
- *Viral:* hepatitis B, Epstein–Barr virus, varicella, coxsackie virus
- *Parasitic:* malaria, toxoplasmosis.

Non-infectious
Primary glomerular diseases
- Membranoproliferative GN (MPGN)
- IgA nephropathy (Berger disease)
- Mesangial proliferative GN
- Focal and segmental glomerulosclerosis (FSGS).

Secondary to multisystem systemic disease
- Systemic lupus erythematosus
- Henoch–Schönlein purpura
- Goodpasture syndrome
- *Drugs:* penicillamine.

Renal histopathology
The histology may be non-proliferative or proliferative.

Non-proliferative GN
There is no cellular proliferation in the glomeruli and nephrotic syndrome is the usual clinical manifestation.
- *Minimal change GN:* accounts for 80% of nephrotic syndrome in children. There is no change visible on light microscopy but fusion of foot processes of podocytes on EM.
- *Focal and segmental glomerulosclerosis (FSGS):* presents as atypical nephrotic syndrome with microscopic haematuria and hypertension. Foci of glomeruli are affected with segmental sclerosis (fibrosis) and hyalinization of feeding arterioles. Aetiology includes mutations in *NPHS2* (podocin).
- *Membranous glomerulonephritis:* leading cause of nephrotic syndrome in adults. The basement membrane is thickened with diffuse granular uptake of IgG forming a 'spike and dome' pattern. Aetiology may be idiopathic, post-infectious (malaria, hepatitis), drug-related (penicillamine).

Proliferative GN
Nephritic syndrome is the usual clinical manifestation and progression to ESRF can occur. The glomerulus is hypercellular. Causes include:
- *Post-infectious glomerulonephritis:* deposits of IgG and C3 within glomeruli.
- *IgA nephropathy (Berger disease):* presents as macroscopic haematuria or the nephritic syndrome, incidentally or days after an URTI or GI tract infection. There is mesangial proliferation and IgA deposits within the matrix.
- *Henoch–Schönlein purpura nephritis:* a systemic variant of IgA nephropathy.
- *Membranoproliferative glomerulonephritis (MPGN):* there is proliferation of cells and matrix within the mesangium (Fig 6.4), with hypocomplementaemia (C3 and sometimes C4). Usually presents with nephrotic syndrome but may be nephritic. Aetiology may be primary or secondary to SLE, sickle cell disease, complement deficiencies, cryoglobulinaemia, and viral hepatitis.
- *Crescentic glomerulonephritis:* associated with rapidly progressive glomerulonephritis (RPGN). Passage of fibrin into Bowman's capsule and an influx of monocytes. Aetiology may include Goodpasture syndrome and vasculitides associated with anti-neutrophil cytoplasmic antibodies (ANCA) such as Wegener granulomatosis.

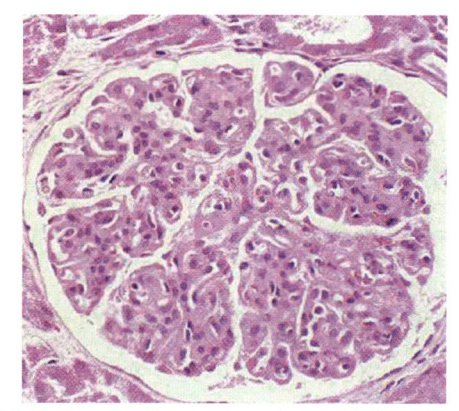

Fig 6.4 Membranoproliferative glomerulonephritis. Reproduced courtesy of Charles Jennette, MD.

Pathogenesis
Glomerulonephritis leads to:
- *Haematuria and proteinuria:* haematuria may be macroscopic or microscopic and is primarily of diagnostic value. Heavy proteinuria leads to hypoalbuminaemia and manifests clinically as nephrotic syndrome.
- *Decreased GFR:* may be associated with acute or rapidly progressive renal failure.
- *Salt and water retention:* salt and water retention leads to oedema, expansion of intravascular volume and systemic hypertension: the hallmarks of acute nephritis.

Clinical evaluation
Glomerulonephritis may present as asymptomatic haematuria or proteinuria, acute nephritis, rapidly progressive glomerulonephritis, nephrotic syndrome, or a mixed nephritic/nephrotic syndrome. Haematuria and acute nephritis are discussed here. Proteinuria and the nephrotic syndrome are discussed in Section 6.5.

Acute nephritis (AN)

Acute nephritis is twice as common in boys as in girls.

Clinical features

Presentation is often with a history of dark-coloured urine indicating macroscopic haematuria. Periorbital or peripheral oedema may be reported. Additional symptoms may include: recent throat or skin infection, personal or family history of GN, systemic disease symptoms (rash, arthritis), lethargy, breathlessness, decreased volume and frequency of urination.

Examination

Signs include hypertension and evidence of fluid retention with periorbital and peripheral oedema. If severe there may be pulmonary oedema (crackles and decreased oxygen saturation), ascites, and pleural effusion.

Signs of systemic disease associated with AN may be present such as a skin rash and arthropathy in HSP and SLE.

Management

Investigations

- Urine tests:
  - dipstick test for blood and protein
  - microscopy: red cells, white cells, granular casts. Red cell casts are pathognomonic of glomerulonephritis.
  - protein: creatinine ratio, urine electrolytes: Na^+ concentration and fractional excretion of Na^+ (FENa).
- Blood tests:
  - renal function: creatinine, urea and electrolytes
  - FBC, CRP, ESR
  - antistreptolysin-O titre, complement C3, C4 and C3 nephritic factor, immunoglobulins (including IgA)
  - ANA, dsDNA, ENA, ANCA
- *Cardiovascular status:* ECG, echocardiogram
- *Imaging:* CXR, renal ultrasound
- *Renal biopsy:* indications include impaired renal function, atypical presentation or delayed recovery. Histological diagnosis guides therapy and prognosis.

Treatment

General measures:

- *Monitor:* twice daily weight, fluid balance, BP
- Fluid restrict to urine output plus insensible losses
- *Diet:*
  - Na^+ restriction for fluid retention
  - increased carbohydrate intake in acute renal impairment
- *Loop diuretics:* furosemide for oedema and volume-related hypertension
- *Antihypertensive agents:* e.g. nifedipine.

Specific measures and prognosis

- *Henoch–Schönlein purpura nephritis:* 70% of patients with HSP have renal involvement ranging from microscopic haematuria/proteinuria to florid nephritic/nephrotic syndrome.
- *IgA nephropathy (Berger disease):* in severe cases ACE inhibitors may be necessary to control hypertension and immunosuppression to prevent progression.
- *Lupus nephritis:* SLE may present with acute nephritis. ANA and ds-DNA antibodies are positive.

Haematuria and proteinuria

Haematuria

Dipstick testing detects red blood cells, myoglobin, and haemoglobin but haematuria is confirmed by finding >5 RBCs per high power field on microscopy of fresh spun urine. Macroscopic haematuria should be distinguished from other causes of red urine: haemoglobinuria, ingestion of beetroot, treatment with rifampicin, and urate crystals.

Clinical evaluation

History and examination will usually identify the cause. Wilms tumour can cause painless macroscopic haematuria. Benign, transient haematuria may be idiopathic, familial, or exercise induced.

> **Pathological causes of haematuria**
>
> - *Renal disease:*
>   - *acute:* acute nephritis, trauma (abdominal or perineal) haemolytic uraemic syndrome, urinary tract infection, renal venous thrombosis
>   - *chronic:* Berger disease (IgA nephropathy), chronic glomerulonephritis, Alport syndrome, haemangioma/A-V malformation, Wilms tumour, hypercalciuria, renal stones
> - *Systemic disease:*
>   - Henoch–Schönlein purpura, SLE
>   - bleeding diatheses, drugs:sulphonamides, cyclophosphamide
> - *Fabricated or induced illness (FII).*

Proteinuria

Proteinuria may indicate significant renal disease or be a transient finding in a healthy child. Evaluation of the degree of proteinuria and its persistent or transitory nature, together with clinical examination, allows diagnosis.

Normal urine protein excretion is less than 60 mg/m^2 per day and increases with activity and upright posture.

Benign proteinuria

Benign proteinuria may be transient (fever, post-exercise) or orthostatic.

In the asymptomatic child with proteinuria detected on routine urine dipstick testing and normal clinical examination, repeat testing will establish whether proteinuria is transient or persistent.

If persistent, orthostatic proteinuria should be excluded by measuring the albumin or protein: creatinine ratio in urine samples voided on arising and in the evening. If there is no significant proteinuria on the early morning sample the proteinuria is orthostatic. Reassurance is appropriate.

Pathological causes of proteinuria

If significant, persistent, non-orthostatic proteinuria is present, history and clinical examination (especially BP) must be reviewed and further investigations considered including renal imaging and renal biochemistry. Concomitant haematuria and hypertension or impaired renal function should prompt a glomerulonephritis screen. IgA nephropathy can cause persistent asymptomatic proteinuria. Causes include:

- *Glomerular disease:* nephrotic syndrome, nephritis, CKD
- *Tubular disease:* tubulo-interstitial nephritis, poisoning (vitamin D, NSAIDs), inherited tubulopathies
- *Overload proteinuria:* myeloproliferative conditions (rare), rhabdomyolysis.

6.5 Nephrotic syndrome

Nephrotic syndrome is defined by
- Heavy proteinuria: >1 g/m² per day
- Hypoalbuminaemia: <25 g/L
- Generalized oedema.

In childhood, 80% of cases are idiopathic or minimal change nephrotic syndrome, MCNS with a UK incidence of 2–4/100 000 in white children and a male to female ratio of 3:2. The incidence is ~6 times higher in Asian children.

Aetiology and pathogenesis
Aetiology
Primary
Minimal change nephrotic syndrome (MCNS)
MCNS accounts for 70% of cases up to age 5 years and 20% in adolescents. There is no significant abnormality on light microscopy but electron microscopy shows effacement of podocyte foot processes. Most cases are steroid sensitive. Atopy is present in up to 50% of children with MCNS.

Miscellaneous glomerular diseases
- *IgM mesangial nephropathy*
- *Focal and segmental glomerulosclerosis (FSGS):* the second most common subtype. Some patients have *NPHS2* mutations.
- *Membranoproliferative glomerulonephritis (MPGN):* accounts for <1% of cases of NS in childhood
- *Congenital nephrotic syndrome:* mutations in *NPHSI* (nephrin), *NPHS2* (podocin) and *WT1* cause congenital nephrotic syndrome (see Section 6.10)

Secondary
Nephrotic syndrome may complicate Henoch–Schönlein purpura, SLE, diabetes mellitus, sickle cell disease, and hepatitis.

Pathogenesis
The glomerular filtration barrier (Fig 6.5) is made up of:
- *Glomerular basement membrane:* a very thick membrane rich in negatively charged glycosaminoglycans which repels negatively charged proteins.

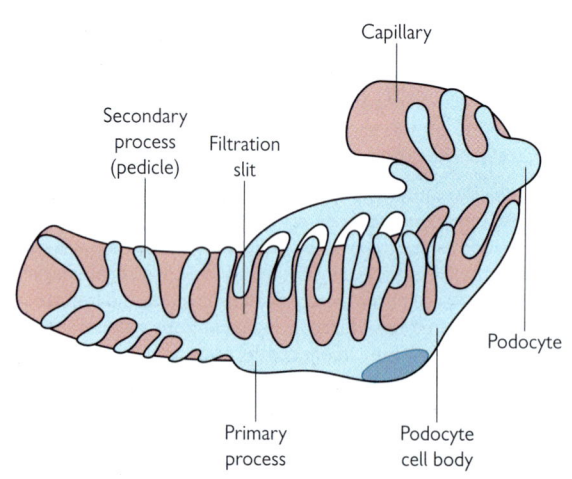

Fig 6.5 Glomerular filtration barrier. Adapted from Nilius, Owsianik, Voets, and Peters, Transient Receptor Potential Cation Channels in Disease. Physiol. Rev. 87: 165–217. 2007. Used with permission.

- *Podocyte slit diaphragm:* podocytes line the other side of the basement membrane and form an interdigitating network of foot processes. Neighbouring foot processes are connected by a continuous membrane-like structure called the slit diaphragm. The permeability-selectivity (permselectivity) allows small ions to pass freely but bars large proteins such as haemoglobin and albumin.

Altered permeability of the glomerular filtration barrier leads to:

- *Oedema and hypovolaemia:* hypoalbuminaemia reduces the plasma oncotic pressure causing passage of fluid into the interstitial space and contraction in plasma volume. This stimulates the renin–angiotensin system and secretion of vasopressin (ADH) leading to retention of Na^+ and water.
- *Blood pressure:* Children with MCNS are usually normotensive. Hypotension is a sign of severe hypovolaemia. Paradoxically, hypovolaemia may also cause hypertension because of excessive vasoconstriction.
- *Infection:* urinary losses of immunoglobulins and complement causes immunodeficiency in the acute phase. Pneumococcal peritonitis is a specific risk.
- *Thrombosis:* urinary losses of antithrombin III, raised plasma fibrinogen concentration and haemoconcentration all increase risk of vascular thrombosis, most commonly venous.

Clinical features
History and presentation
In 95% of cases, the presenting feature is oedema, initially mild and localized. Periorbital oedema usually appears first, particularly noticeable in the morning. Oedema then develops in dependent regions such as lower limbs and scrotum. Pleural effusions and ascites may then develop.

There may be a history of recent infection (viral URTI), 'foamy' urine, and general malaise and irritability.

A misdiagnosis of an allergic reaction as a cause for periorbital oedema is common. Once generalized oedema is present diagnosis is easy as other conditions causing this are rare.

Examination
Examination is focused on diagnostic features, presence or absence of 'atypical' features and complications.
- *Oedema:* periorbital, lower limb, abdominal wall, sacral, scrotal. Pleural effusions, ascites
- *CVS:* intravascular volume status: heart rate, blood pressure, capillary refill time
- *Fever:* sepsis, peritonitis
- *Abdominal examination:* abdominal pain and tenderness may be a sign of hypovolaemia, ascites or peritonitis.

Management
Diagnostic investigations
Urinalysis
Dipstick testing provides a semi-quantitative measure of urine protein concentration. The scale is not linear:

+	300 mg/L
++	1000 mg/L
+++	3000 mg/L
++++	20000 mg/L

Laboratory quantification is indicated for significant proteinuria. The simplest test is the albumin or protein: creatinine ratio on a spot sample. Normal ranges are age specific:

Age	Protein: creatinine ratio
0–2 years	<50 mg/mmol
>2 years	<25 mg/mmol

- *Haematuria:* haematuria + on dipstick is not uncommon
- *Microscopy:* microscopic haematuria is present at onset in 20–30% of MCNS patients but 80–100% of patients with MPGN. Macroscopic haematuria is uncommon in MCNS.

Blood tests
- *Plasma albumin:* <25 g/L in nephrotic syndrome
- *Plasma creatinine, urea and electrolytes.:* renal function is normal in most patients with MCNS, but a moderate rise in creatinine is found in 30%. Reversible acute renal failure can accompany hypovolaemia in MCNS but persistent high creatinine is an 'atypical' feature. Hyponatraemia is usually artefactual due to hyperlipidaemia.
- *Full blood count:* high Hb and PCV with hypovolaemia.

Additional first line investigations include:
- Complement C3 and C4 levels
- Varicella IgG antibody
- Hepatitis serology (B and C)
- Serum cholesterol and triglycerides
- CXR and renal ultrasound.

Second line investigations may include:
- Antistreptolysin O titre
- Antinuclear and anti-ds DNA antibodies.

Clinical evaluation and first-line investigations allow the patient to be diagnosed as:
- 'Typical' likely to be MCNS steroid-sensitive nephrotic syndrome (SSNS)
- 'Atypical' requiring referral and possible renal biopsy.

The main 'atypical' features are shown in the Box.

> **Features of atypical nephrotic syndrome**
> - Age: <12 months or >12 years
> - Macroscopic haematuria
> - Persistent hypertension (not due to hypovolaemia)
> - Persistent high creatinine (not due to hypovolaemia)
> - Low C3 concentration
> - *Systemic features:* rash, arthropathy (HSP or SLE)
> - Family history of FSGS
> - No response to corticosteroids by 28 days

Acute treatment
Observations and general measures
Monitoring of temperature, heart rate, BP, capillary refill time, respiratory rate and oxygen saturation, fluid balance and urine output, daily weight.
A salt-restricted diet is recommended (no added salt). In the absence of hypovolaemia fluid intake may be modestly restricted. Oral penicillin V is given until oedema has resolved.

Treatment of oedema
Moderate oedema will resolve spontaneously when steroid induced remission and diuresis occurs. Diuretics may be cautiously used to control oedema in the initial phase provided there is no hypovolaemia, renal impairment, or hypotension. Severe, diuretic resistant oedema may be treated using IV 20% albumin with furosemide. There is a risk of circulatory volume expansion and acute cardiac failure. Caution is required in renal failure.

Steroids
In typical SSNS, oral prednisolone is started with a single daily dose of 2 mg/kg per day (60 mg/m^2 per day) up to a maximum of 80 mg/day and continued for 4 weeks. Use 'ideal' weight for height if oedema is severe.

Remission is defined as resolution of proteinuria (trace on dipstick, <4 mg/m^2 per hour) for 3 consecutive days. Remission within 4 weeks indicates steroid-sensitive nephrotic syndrome (SSNS). Failure to remit within 4 weeks is defined as steroid-resistance and requires renal biopsy.

For patients with SSNS, prednisolone is then given in a tapering dose on alternate days for 12 weeks. The dose is reduced by 10 mg/m^2 each alternate day every 2 weeks, i.e. in six steps from 60 mg/m^2 per alternate day to discontinuation.

Acute complications
- *Hypovolaemia:* symptoms include nausea and abdominal pain and signs of circulatory compromise. Blood pressure may be normal or elevated due to compensatory vasoconstriction. Hypotension is an ominous sign. There is oliguria with low Na$^+$ content and haemoconcentration. Treatment is 10–20 mL/kg of 4.5% albumin solution.
- *Infection:* fever and evidence of sepsis or peritonitis is an emergency requiring broad-spectrum antibiotics.
- *Thrombosis:* prompt treatment of hypovolaemia and mobilization reduces risk of venous thrombosis.

Maintenance therapy
Immunisation
Children with SSNS should receive both pneumococcal and influenza vaccine. Non-immune immunosuppressed patients exposed to infectious varicella should receive varicella zoster immunoglobulin and aciclovir if clinical chickenpox develops. Human normal immunoglobulin is given if exposed to an infectious measles contact.

Relapsing SSNS
70% of SSNS patients relapse, the pattern of illness in the first 6 months being predictive of the future clinical course. Useful definitions in monitoring treatment are:
- *Relapse:* Albustix >2+ for 3 consecutive days
- *Remission:* Albustix 0 or trace for 3 consecutive days
- *Frequent relapsing nephrotic syndrome:* 2 or more relapses within 6 months of diagnosis or >4 relapses in any 12 months
- *Steroid-dependent nephrotic syndrome:* 2 consecutive relapses during steroid treatment or within 2 weeks of stopping.

Up to 25% of relapses resolve spontaneously, but treatment is usually given after 3–5 days of >2+ proteinuria. The standard regimen is 2 mg/kg/ per day (60 mg/m^2 per day) to a maximum of 60 mg/day on alternative days over a 28 day period.
Referral to a paediatric nephrologist is appropriate for frequent relapsing or SSNS.
Further management options include alternative-day maintenance prednisolone. If this fails alternative therapy options are levamisole, cyclophosphamide, and ciclosporin.

Prognosis of SSNS
Most children have a decrease in relapse rate and enter long-term remission, but up to 20% continue to relapse through adolescence and into adulthood. A minority develop 'secondary' steroid resistance and a small subset of these (mainly with FSGS histology) develop chronic kidney disease.

6.6 Renal failure

Acute kidney injury (AKI)

AKI is an acute but potentially reversible decline in glomerular filtration rate, with or without oliguria and associated with retention of nitrogenous waste products.

Aetiology

The common pathologic pathway for AKI is a reduction in renal blood flow which decreases the glomerular filtration rate (GFR). Causes are classified as:

- *Pre-renal:* GFR is depressed by reduced renal perfusion with normal glomerular and tubular function. Prerenal aetiology is most common in childhood AKI
- *Instrinsic:* diseases of the glomerulus or tubule
- *Post-renal:* obstructive uropathy causes an increase in tubular pressure which reduces the filtration driving force and is associated with renal afferent vasoconstriction.

Insults associated with prerenal AKI due to reduced renal blood flow may also impair cortical perfusion and progress to intrinsic renal failure due to acute tubular necrosis.
Causes in each category include:

Pre-renal
Circulatory failure ('shock') due to:

- *Hypovolaemia:* haemorrhage, burns, diarrhoea, sepsis
- *Cardiogenic:* congenital heart disease (hypoplastic left heart), myocarditis, sepsis.

Intrinsic

- *Acute tubular necrosis:* circulatory failure, toxins (myoglobinuria, gentamicin), acute nephritis
- *Vascular pathology:* haemolytic uraemic syndrome, renal venous thrombosis or asphyxia
- *Tubulo-interstitial nephritis:* furosemide, NSAIDs.

Post-renal

- *Congenital anomalies:* posterior urethral valves, bladder ureterocoele prolapse.
- *Obstruction:* tumour, stones, or blocked urethral catheter
- Neuropathic bladder.

Pathogenesis

Impaired renal blood flow eventually leads to ischaemia and cell death. When renal blood flow is restored, GFR recovery depends on the size of the surviving pool of nephrons. Complications include fluid retention and overload with congestive heart failure and hypertension, hyperkalaemia, metabolic acidosis, hypocalcaemia, and uraemia.

Clinical evaluation

Diagnosis usually rests on documentation of elevated plasma creatinine levels (×2–3 of normal) and oliguria, defined as a urine output of <0.5 mL/kg per hour (<1 ml/kg per hour in a neonate). Non-oliguric renal failure can occur in drug-induced nephrotoxicity.

Examination includes a careful assessment of circulatory status and fluid balance to identify circulatory failure or hypovolaemia consistent with prerenal failure or fluid overload. Important signs include:

- *General:* dehydration (hypovolaemia) or fluid overload (GN). Anaemia, jaundice or petechiae in haemolytic uraemic syndrome
- *CVS:* shock: tachycardia, hypotension, prolonged CRT, fluid overload: hypertension and gallop rhythm
- *Respiratory system:* crackles in pulmonary oedema
- *Abdomen:* palpable bladder or kidneys in obstruction.

Management: investigations

Urine tests

Dipstick test for blood and protein and microscopy (casts).

Urine osmolality and Na^+ concentration provides useful indicators of whether renal failure is prerenal or intrinsic.

- *Prerenal failure:* urine osmolality >500 mOsm/kg, urine Na^+ <10 mmol/L due to avid Na^+ and water retention
- *Acute tubular necrosis:* urine osmolality <300 mOsm/kg, urine Na^+ >40 mmol/L: dilute, Na^+-rich urine.

The fractional excretion of Na^+ (FENa) is a useful index of tubular function:

FENa = [(urine Na × plasma Cr)/ (plasma Na × urine Cr)] × 100%

FENa is

- <1% in prerenal failure (acute nephritis, obstruction)
- >1% in acute tubular necrosis.

Blood tests

- Changes in plasma creatinine (Cr) reflect changes in GFR, a doubling of plasma Cr corresponding to a 50% reduction in GFR
- Hyperkalaemia and hypocalcaemia are common
- *FBC and film:* leukopaenia and thrombocytopaenia suggest SLE or TTP. Microangiopathic anaemia suggests TTP or HUS.

Imaging and renal biopsy

- *Renal ultrasound* identifies obstructive uropathy, intrinsic renal disease, stones, renal venous thrombosis
- *Renal biopsy* is indicated in prolonged, unexplained acute renal failure.

Treatment

- *Fluid management:* in prerenal failure hypovolaemia should be corrected with a rapid fluid infusion (fluid challenge). In intrinsic renal failure, fluid intake is restricted to insensible loses and urine output. In a fluid overloaded, oliguric patient administration of a loop diuretic (furosemide) is indicated to prevent or treat pulmonary oedema. A urinary catheter is placed to allow accurate measurement of urine output (and relief of any lower tract obstruction).
- *Electrolytes:* plasma K^+ is monitored and hyperkalaemia treated. Hyponatraemia secondary to water excess requires fluid restriction and hypocalcaemia is treated with calcium supplementation.
- *Renal replacement therapy (dialysis):* indications for dialysis include failure of medical treatment to alleviate severe fluid overload, hyperkalaemia, symptomatic uraemia, or metabolic acidosis, and to remove dialysable intoxicants (low molecular weight and not highly protein bound: gentamicin, ethylene glycol).

Chronic kidney disease

Staging of chronic kidney disease (CKD) according to GFR as in Table 6.1 has been proposed.

Table 6.1. Staging of chronic kidney disease

Stage of CKD	Description	GFR mL/min/1.73 m²
0	Risk factors: diabetes, BP+	>90
1	Renal damage (proteinuria) normal GFR	>90
2	Mild ↓GFR	60–89
3	Moderate ↓GFR	30–59
4	Severe GFR	15–29
5	ESRF	<15

Aetiology and pathogenesis

The cause of chronic kidney disease varies with age:
- *Infants <2 years*: structural abnormalities including renal dysplasia and obstructive uropathy account for 50% of cases
- *Children 2–5 years*: in addition to renal dysplasia and obstructive uropathy, neonatal vascular accidents and haemolytic uraemic syndrome
- *Older children and adolescents*: glomerular disease (FSGS, crescentic GN, lupus nephritis), reflux nephropathy and genetic disorders (Alport syndrome).

Less common causes include rare genetic diseases such as cystic kidney disease, congenital nephrotic syndrome, cystinosis, hyperoxaluria, drug-induced nephrotoxicity, malignancy, tubular and interstitial disorders.

Pathogenesis

Chronic kidney disease generates a host of sequelae:
- *Failure to thrive*: anorexia and inadequate calorie intake
- *Short stature and delayed puberty*: multifactorial aetiology including poor nutrition
- *Anaemia*: caused by decreased erythropoietin production, iron and folate deficiency, reduced red cell survival (uraemia)
- *Osteodystrophy*: diminished hydroxylation by 1-α-hydroxylase reduces calcitriol synthesis and phosphate retention causes secondary hyperparathyroidism and bone resorption
- *Cardiovascular*: hypertension mediated by the angiotensin–renin pathway. Pro-atherogenic state with hyperlipidaemia and elevated calcium/phosphate product
- *Metabolic acidosis*: contributes to bone disease, growth failure, and hyperkalaemia.

Clinical evaluation

Presenting symptoms may include failure to thrive or growth failure, lethargy and malaise, anorexia and vomiting, polyuria, bone pain, or headaches. Clues to aetiology may exist in the past history (perinatal complications, oligohydramnios, recurrent UTI) or family history (renal disease, deafness).

Examination may be normal but can reveal causal factors or sequelae of renal impairment such as growth failure, anaemia, stigmata of osteodystrophy, hypertension, palpable bladder or kidneys.

Management: investigations

Urine tests
Dipstick testing for proteinuria, haematuria, osmolality, microscopy, and culture.

Blood tests
- *Renal function*: creatinine, U&E, capillary blood gases.
- Total corrected and ionized calcium, phosphate, alkaline phosphatase, PTH, and vitamin D
- FBC, ferritin.

Imaging
- *Renal ultrasound*: identifies small echogenic kidneys, cystic kidneys, obstructive uropathy.

Treatment

Preservation of renal function
The aim is to delay progression to ESRF. Strategies include prevention of recurrent upper UTI, relief of obstruction, control of hypertension and proteinuria.

Treatment of complications
- *Nutrition*: aim to promote growth by optimizing calorie and protein intake. Gastrostomy or nasogastric feeding may be necessary in infants.
- *Growth*: recombinant human growth hormone (rhGH) may be effective in increasing height velocity and final adult height.
- *Anaemia*: iron and folate deficiency should be addressed before initiation of erythropoietin therapy.
- *Renal osteodystrophy*: the key is adequate control of plasma phosphate by limiting dietary intake and the use of phosphate binders. Supplementation with 1-alfacalcidol may also be required for secondary hyperparathyroidism.
- *Hypertension*: an ACEi is used if there is proteinuria. Additional agents may be necessary such as furosemide, β-blockers, or calcium antagonists.
- *Fluid, electrolyte and acid–base abnormalities*: infants are often polyuric with renal Na^+ and bicarbonate wasting. Na^+ supplementation is given to the amount tolerated without hypertension, oedema, or hypernatraemia. Sodium bicarbonate supplementation is given for acidosis.
- *Psychosocial issues*: support from clinical psychologists may help with needle phobias and poor adherence to medication and diet. School attendance may falter and in-hospital education, home tuition, and participation of teachers in the multidisciplinary team are all of value.

Renal replacement therapy
- *Renal transplantation*: the ideal is a preemptive live-related transplant. This has the best outcome. Minimum weight for transplantation is 7.5 kg. Complications include early surgical problems, rejection, and the side effects of immunosuppressive drugs.
- *Dialysis*: if transplantation is not feasible or fails peritoneal dialysis (PD) is usually performed at home either overnight or using ambulatory PD in adolescents. Haemodialysis is also an option.

6.7 Congenital anomalies of the urinary tract

Congenital anomalies of the kidney and urinary tract (CAKUT) are now commonly identified on antenatal ultrasound scans. Problems may arise during fetal life or postnatally.

Fetal oliguria or obstructed urine flow is associated with oligohydramnios, pulmonary hypoplasia and positional deformities such as talipes equinovarus.

Postnatal presentation may include recurrent urinary tract infection or sepsis, oligoanuria, urinary retention, or silent, progressive renal disease. Evaluation requires biochemical assessment of renal function and imaging of the urinary tract with ultrasound initially.

Management is discussed in relation to each condition. Urinary tract obstruction requires early relief and may be followed by significant polyuria. Prevention and management of UTI and hypertension is discussed elsewhere.

Urinary tract anomalies

Outflow obstruction is the common feature and is associated with hydronephrosis (dilatation of the proximal collecting system), hydroureter (dilatation of the ureters), bladder enlargement, and oligohydramnios.

Hydronephrosis
- *Unilateral hydronephrosis:* may be caused by pelvi-ureteric junction (PUJ) obstruction or vesicoureteric junction (VUJ) obstruction in which case the ureter is also dilated. In PUJ obstruction MAG3 renogram shows poor drainage despite furosemide and reduced function (<40%) on the hydronephrotic side. Treatment is Anderson–Hynes pyeloplasty or nephrectomy if kidney function is poor. VUJ obstruction may require re-implantation, often with temporary stenting.
- *Bilateral hydronephrosis:* less common but more likely to be serious (e.g. posterior urethral valves in a boy).

Renal pelvis dilation (RPD)
RPD is a commonly detected abnormality on antenatal ultrasound with a prevalence of 1–2%. Postnatal management is controversial.

It is generally agreed that in the 2nd trimester a renal pelvis AP diameter of <5 mm is normal and >10 mm is probably significant. Obviously RPD with an abnormal lower urinary tract is significant and calyceal dilation is probably significant.

Postnatal ultrasound in the 1st week and again at 6–8 weeks is recommended. A ≤15 mm AP renal pelvis diameter without calyceal dilatation stable on follow-up is likely to be benign. Any suggestion of VUR requires further investigation and consideration of antibiotic prophylaxis.

Posterior urethral valves
The incidence is 1/5000–8000 male births. Mucosal folds or a membrane obstruct urine flow from the bladder with bilateral hydronephrosis and hydroureter and a thickened bladder wall.

Most are diagnosed on antenatal ultrasound in which case antenatal interventions are an option including vesico-amniotic shunt placement, bladder aspiration, and drainage of severe hydronephrosis. Postnatal management is by catheterization and later valve ablation.

Ureterocoele and megaureter
Cystic dilation of the terminal ureter may be intravesical (often asymptomatic) or extravesical (located at the bladder neck) which is often associated with duplex kidney. Severe hydroureter, or megaureter, may be primary or secondary to distal obstruction.

Vesicoureteric reflux (VUR)

Vesicoureteric reflux is the retrograde passage of urine from the bladder into the upper urinary tract.

VUR is found in up to 30% of children with UTI. In newborns the incidence is higher in boys than girls, but in later childhood it is 4–6 times more common in girls. About 30–50% of children with symptomatic VUR have evidence of reflux nephropathy which may be due either to congenital dysplasia or acquired scarring from recurrent pyelonephritis. Management of VUR remains controversial.

Aetiology
Primary VUR is a congenital anomaly of the vesicoureteric junction with a genetic basis. VUR may also be secondary to a number of disorders affecting the structure or function of the urinary tract, such as bladder outlet obstruction.

Primary VUR
A flap-valve mechanism at the junction of ureter and bladder normally ensures anterograde flow of urine and prevents retrograde flow during voiding. This depends on oblique insertion of the intramural ureter, adequate length of the intramural ureter (tunnel length to ureteric diameter ratio of 5:1) and strong detrusor muscle support. The valve operates by both passive and active mechanisms, either of which may be defective.
- *Passive:* bladder filling compresses the root of the intravesical ureter against underlying detrusor muscle. A lateral ureteral opening with short transmural and submucosal sections is associated with VUR.
- *Active:* the trigonal muscle and intrinsic muscles in the ureter terminus function as an active valve mechanism. Dysplasia and atrophy of the intravesical ureter is seen in VUR.

Primary VUR is a familial disorder which segregates as an autosomal dominant (AD) disorder with reduced penetrance and variable expression. The incidence of VUR in siblings of index cases is about 30%, and 1st degree relatives overall have a 20–50% risk of reflux.

Secondary VUR
Conditions associated with high intravesical pressures cause secondary VUR and include:
- *Bladder outlet obstruction:* posterior urethral valves
- *Neurogenic bladder:* myelomeningocele, spinal cord injury.
- *Bladder dysfunction:* it remains uncertain whether 'dysfunctional voiding' is more common in children with VUR.

Pathogenesis: reflux nephropathy (RN)
Reflux nephropathy is now known to represent both acquired kidney damage (chronic pyelonephritis) and congenital kidney malformation (renal dysplasia). The former is more common in girls and the latter in boys.

VUR and UTI
Up to 40% of children with symptomatic UTI investigated with cystourethrography have VUR, and VUR, UTI, and parenchymal kidney disease have long been linked. A plausible causal pathway exists in which recurrent intrarenal reflux of infected urine causes pyelonephritis and renal parenchymal damage with

subsequent scarring. Renal lesions are associated with higher grades of reflux. In a minority of children there is progression to renal impairment, hypertension, and ESRF. The risk of new scar formation appears to diminish with age and is low after age 5 years.

VUR and renal dysplasia
With increasing use of prenatal ultrasound it has become clear that renal abnormalities in patients with VUR may be present before birth, especially in boys. In these cases, VUR and reflux nephropathy are both developmental aberrations. The kidneys are dysplastic and small.

Clinical features
Vesicoureteric reflux itself is clinically silent and definitive diagnosis requires micturating cystourethrography. VUR may therefore present in:
- *Asymptomatic individuals:* investigation of renal pelvis dilation found on prenatal ultrasound or screening of relatives of affected individuals.
- *Children with symptomatic UTI:* a family history should be sought and examination should include BP measurement.

Imaging strategies for the investigation of infants and children with UTI or antenatal ultrasound abnormalities are set out in Section 6.3.

Grading of VUR
VUR is graded I–V according to the extent of retrograde filling and dilation of the ureter, renal pelvis, and calyces on a MCUG (Fig 6.6).
- *Grade I:* reflux into ureter only: varying degrees of ureteral dilatation
- *Grade II:* reflux reaches renal pelvis and calyces, no dilation of collecting system, normal fornices
- *Grade III:* reflux reaches renal pelvis and calyces: mild dilation of collecting system, mild blunting of fornices
- *Grade IV:* moderate dilation of ureter and collecting system with blunt fornices
- *Grade V:* intrarenal reflux with gross dilation of ureter and collecting system, tortuous ureter and blunted calyces

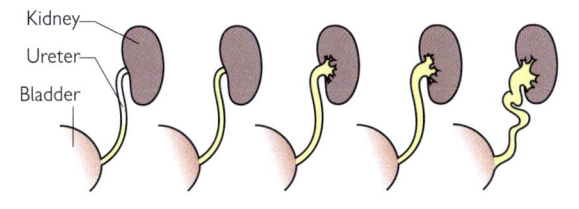

Fig 6.6 Grades of reflux.

Additional investigations in the diagnostic workup may include: urinalysis, urine culture and plasma creatinine and urodynamic studies for suspected dysfunctional voiding in patients with suspected secondary reflux.

Management
The management of VUR depends on:
- Grade of reflux, I–V
- Age and sex of the child
- Presence or absence of reflux nephropathy or renal impairment
- Occurrence of UTI.

The main aims are to prevent or rapidly treat acute UTI to preserve renal function. Medical options include antibiotic prophylaxis or watchful waiting. Surgical interventions remain controversial and are generally reserved for more severe cases.

Active treatment of childhood VUR using either antibiotic prophylaxis or antireflux surgery was introduced several decades ago but there is a surprising lack of robust evidence of long-term benefit.

Medical treatment
Spontaneous resolution of VUR grade I or II occurs in up to 90% within 5 years. Some advocate using antibiotic prophylaxis (trimethoprim, nitrofurantoin, or cefalexin) until VUR has resolved. However, evidence from two small studies showed no significant difference in risk for UTI or renal damage between antibiotic prophylaxis and no treatment. Watchful waiting with rapid diagnosis and treatment of acute UTIs appears an acceptable alternative.

Surgical treatment
Bilateral grade IV and V reflux (Fig 6.7) resolves spontaneously in less than 20% of patients after 5 years. Surgical treatment may be considered in severe reflux if there are frequent breakthrough febrile infections or a deteriorating DMSA appearance. However, large multicentre prospective trials of medical (antibiotic prophylaxis), surgical, or combined treatment did not show a clear difference between medical and surgical groups. Surgical interventions include:
- *Circumcision:* consider in boys with breakthrough infections despite prophylaxis
- *Transtrigonal reimplantation:* submucosal embedding of the ureter to lengthen the intramural part has a success rate in stopping reflux of 95% but it remains unclear whether outcome is superior to conservative management.

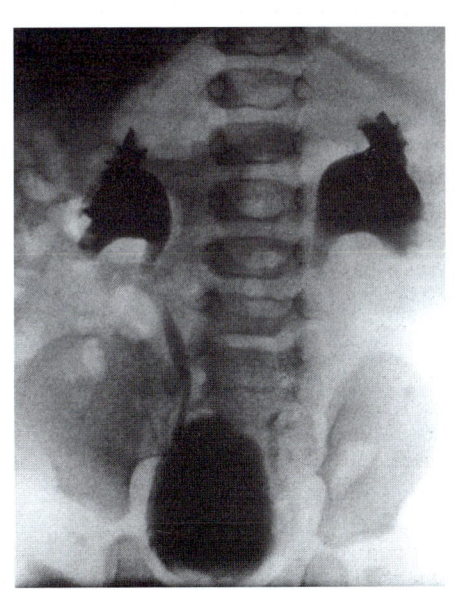

Fig 6.7 MCUG: bilateral severe (grade V) VUR.

6.8 Renal anomalies and inguinoscrotal disorders

Primary renal anomalies

Polycystic kidney disease and multicystic dysplastic kidneys (MCDK) are discussed in Section 6.9.

- *Renal agenesis:* unilateral agenesis is present in 1/1000 and may represent involuted MCDK. Bilateral agenesis results in Potter syndrome with stillbirth or lethal pulmonary hypoplasia causing neonatal death.
- *Ectopic kidney:* pelvic location most common.
- *Fused kidneys:* fusion of lower poles (95%) with horseshoe kidney (Fig 6.8A) may cause obstructive uropathy. Association with Turner and Bardet–Biedl syndromes (Fig 6.9). It may be asymptomatic or associated with VUR and recurrent UTIs.
- *Duplex kidney (Fig 6.8B):* usually two separate pelvicalyceal systems with ureters entering the bladder separately (upper pole ureter entering below that of lower pole) and lower pole at risk from reflux and scarring. The upper pole ureter may insert ectopically into urethra or vagina causing dribbling incontinence. There may be an associated bladder ureterocoele causing obstruction and hydronephrosis of the upper pole.

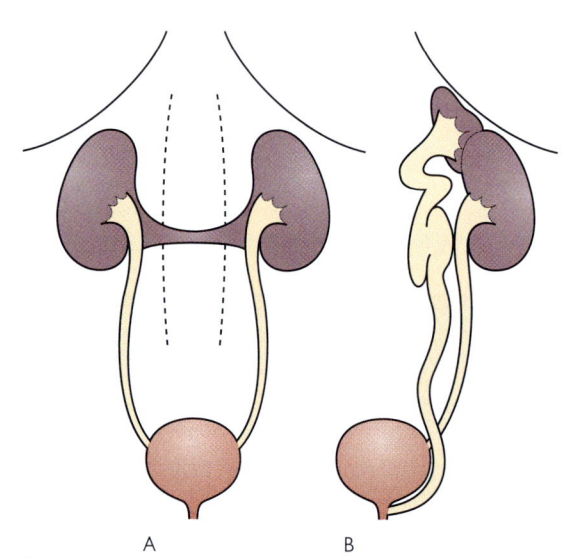

Fig 6.8 A. Horseshoe kidney. B. Duplex kidney.

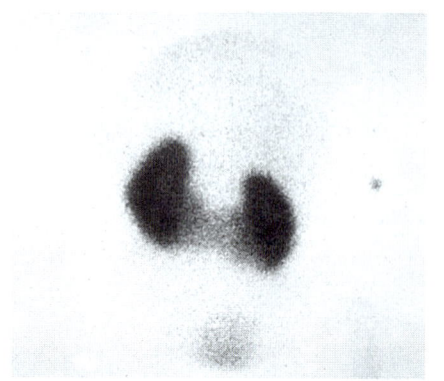

Fig 6.9 Horseshoe kidney in a girl with Turner syndrome (karyotype 46 XO): DMSA scan.

Inguinoscrotal disorders

Bladder exstrophy and epispadias

The incidence is 1/10 000–50 000. It is more common in boys. Disordered development of the cloacal membrane is associated with:

- Defect of lower abdominal wall and anterior bladder wall with outward herniation of posterior bladder wall mucosa.
- Genital abnormalities:
  - *males:* epispadias (dorsal-opening urethra) with dorsal chordee (upturned penis) often with bilateral undescended testes
  - *females:* epispadias with bifid clitoris
- Anteriorly displaced anus and separation of pubic symphysis.

Surgical reconstruction is required. Long-term complications include urinary incontinence and increased risk of bladder mucosa malignancy.

Cryptorchidism

The normal testis passes from an intra-abdominal position through the inguinal canal to lie in the scrotum between the 7th and 9th months of intrauterine life.

Cryptorchidism refers to absence of one or both testes from the scrotum.

This is the most common congenital anomaly of the male genitalia, affecting 7% of boys at birth, rising to 25% in preterm infants. Unilateral cryptorchidism is 4 times more common than bilateral and is more common on the right.

Aetiology

Cryptorchidism may be due to:

- *Maldescent:* the testis may be undescended or ectopic. Usually unilateral and due to an anatomical or hormonal abnormality. Descent may be arrested in the normal path with the testis near the pubic tubercle, in the inguinal canal (80%) or in the abdomen. The testis is usually small with a short spermatic cord and an associated inguinal hernia is common. Descent may deviate from the normal path to give an ectopic testis, usually in the superficial inguinal pouch.
- *Retractile testis:* prepubertal boys can have an exaggerated cremasteric reflex.
- *Ascending testis:* a previously normal or retractile testis becomes high with a shortened spermatic cord that prevents the testis from staying in the scrotum.
- *Anorchidism* (testicular agenesis, anorchia; rare): caused by ischaemic necrosis during descent.

Syndromes associated with cryptorchidism (usually bilateral) include Prader–Willi, Kallman, Bardet–Biedl, prune belly syndrome, and intersex syndromes.

Diagnosis: physical examination

Screening for cryptorchidism should be part of the newborn examination and 6 week check. Careful inspection of the femoral, perineal, and penile region is important. The important management issue is whether or not the testis is palpable.

Management

Treatment should be completed by age 12–18 months. Spontaneous descent is unlikely after age 1 year and there is a potential loss of testicular quality after 1 year which can affect fertility. Options include:

Medical treatment

Treatment with hCG or GnRH can be used with maximum success rates of 20%, success being more likely the lower the undescended testis is.

Surgical treatment

- *Testis palpable:* orchidopexy via inguinal approach. Success rate 92%.
- *Testis non-palpable:* examination under anaesthetic followed by inguinal exploration ± laparoscopy to find the testis. Orchidopexy, orchidolysis, or removal is then performed.
  - In children ≥10 years with a normal contralateral testis the intra-abdominal testis should be removed because of the risk of malignancy, torsion, and trauma.
  - In children ≤10 years with bilateral intra-abdominal testes an attempt is made to move them into the scrotum.

Penile abnormalities

Hypospadias

Hypospadias is second only to cryptorchidism as a common birth defect of the male genitalia with a reported incidence varying from 1/4000 to as high as 1/250 newborn males. The incidence may be increasing.

The urethral meatus is abnormally placed on the ventral surface of the penis and may open along a line (the urethral groove) from just below the normal position to junction of penis and scrotum or perineum. A hooded foreskin is common and more severe degrees are associated with chordee, in which the phallus is tethered downwards, and cryptorchidism (Fig 6.10).

Vesico-ureteric reflux is associated in 30–40% of cases.

Aetiology

Most cases are sporadic, and environmental agents interfering with androgen effects may contribute (e.g. fertilizers, pesticides). There is an association with vegetarian diet in pregnancy. Familial clustering suggests a genetic contribution.

Management

Severe hypospadias with cryptorchidism may be part of an intersex syndrome and requires further investigation (karyotype, abdominal ultrasound).

Circumcision is contraindicated, as the foreskin may be required for reconstructive surgery.

Mild hypospadias is primarily a cosmetic defect with little effect on function and does not need correction. Surgical repair of moderate hypospadias is usually successful in one procedure carried out in the first year of life but severe hypospadias may require multiple procedures and mucosal grafting.

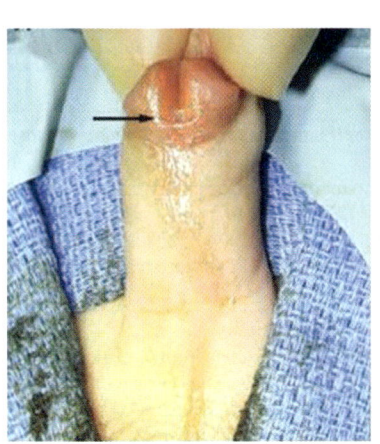

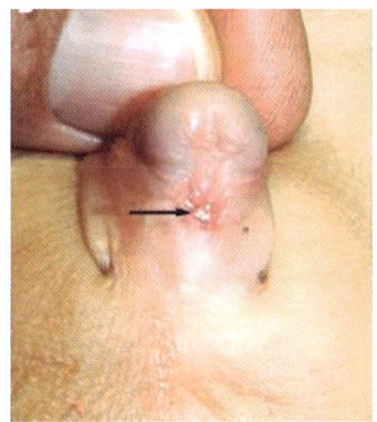

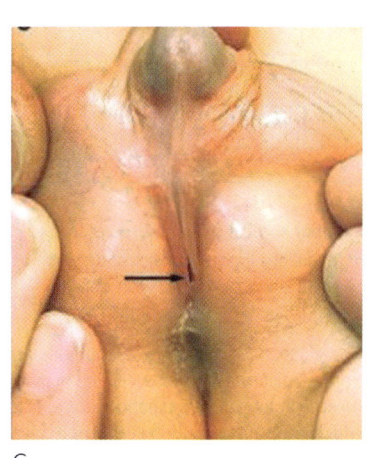

Fig 6.10 Hypospadias: A, glandular; B subcoronal; C, scrotal. Reprinted by permission from Macmillan Publishers Ltd: Nature Clinical Practice Urology, Willingham and Baskin, Candidate genes and their response to environmental agents in the etiology of hypospadias 4 (5) pp. 270–279, © 2007.

6.9 Cystic disease and tubulopathies

Cystic diseases of the kidney

Renal cystic disorders are a heterogeneous group of genetic, developmental, and acquired conditions. They are increasingly diagnosed by antenatal ultrasound and represent the most common genetic cause of ESRF in children and young adults.

Aetiology and pathogenesis
Genetic cystic diseases

Genetic cystic renal disease is non-syndromic or syndromic. Syndromic forms are shown in Table 6.2. Non-syndromic disorders include:
- Polycystic kidney disease: ARPKD and ADPKD
- Nephronophthisis (NPHP)
- Medullary cystic kidney disease (MCKD)

Table 6.2. Genetic cystic renal disease: syndromic		
Syndrome	Gene	Protein
Tuberous sclerosis (TSC)	TSC2/PKD1	Polycystin-1
Bardet–Biedl (BBS)	BBS1–12	Ciliary proteins
Meckel–Gruber (MKS)	MKS1, MKS2–4	Ciliary proteins
Von Hippel–Lindau (VHL)	VHL	pVHL
Orofaciodigital (OFD)	OFD1	CXORF5

Additional renal cystic disorders are:
- *Medullary sponge kidney (MSK):* with renal calculi and urinary calcification or acidification defects
- Multicystic dysplastic kidney *(MCDK)*.

The genes for many of these conditions encode proteins of the primary cilium. The primary cilium protrudes into tubular structures in kidney, liver and pancreas and acts as a mechano-sensor which transmits signals in response to flow that regulate proliferation of tubular cells. This explains why hepatic and pancreatic disease occurs in PKD.

Acquired cystic disease

The exact cause of the cyst formation in patients with ESRF remains uncertain. The prevalence increases with duration of dialysis. Complications include haemorrhage and renal cell carcinoma.

Clinical features and management
Cystic disease of the kidney presents in many different ways:
- Antenatal ultrasound screening
- Complications of bleeding, infection, or nephrolithiasis
- Hypertension
- Chronic kidney disease
- *Abdominal mass:* MCDK is a cause of a palpable abdominal mass in the newborn.

Autosomal recessive polycystic kidney disease (ARPKD)

Incidence 1/10 000. Up to 60% of cases are diagnosed on antenatal ultrasound: large echogenic kidneys with loss of corticomedullary differentiation (Fig 6.11). The neonate presents with massive bilateral nephromegaly and respiratory distress due to pulmonary hypoplasia. Liver involvement is variable and progresses to hepatic fibrosis. Progression to ESRF occurs requiring renal or combined liver–renal transplantation.

Autosomal dominant polycystic kidney disease (ADPKD)

ADPKD is common with a prevalence of 1/1000. Mutations in *PKD1* account for 85%. Presentation is usually in middle age but can occur in the second decade with recurrent UTI, hypertension, or haematuria. Treatment is symptomatic.

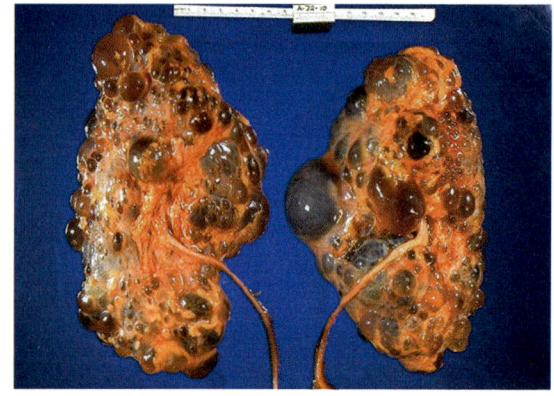

Fig 6.11 Polycystic kidneys. Source: CDC, Dr Edwin P Ewing Jr.

Nephronophthisis (NPHP) and medullary cystic kidney disease (MCKD)

Nephronophthisis and medullary cystic kidney disease are clinically similar with normal-sized kidneys and cysts mainly at the corticomedullary border. Juvenile NPHP (*NHP1*) has insidious onset with polydipsia and polyuria and progression to ESRF within the first 3 decades.

Multicystic dysplastic kidney (MCDK)

MCDK is a sporadic condition resulting from failure of union of the ureteric bud with the nephrogenic mesenchyme. It is a non-functioning structure with large cysts and no renal tissue. Most unilateral affected kidneys involute and disappear. Indications for nephrectomy include significant enlargement, suspicion of malignancy or hypertension.

Disorders of the renal tubule
Proximal tubulopathies
Cystinuria

This AR disorder is caused by defects in the renal dibasic amino acid transporter which causes excessive excretion of cystine and dibasic amino-acids.

Cystine is poorly soluble at normal urine pH and recurrent radio-opaque urinary stones are formed. Treatment is high fluid intake and alkalinization of urine with oral potassium citrate or D-penicillamine if that fails.

X-linked hypophosphataemic rickets

This X-linked dominant disorder is caused by mutations in the phosphate-regulating endopeptidase gene *PHEX* which causes a reduction of phosphate reabsorption and hypophosphataemia.

Presentation is in infancy with delayed dentition, rickets, and poor growth. There is hypophosphataemia, increased alkaline phosphatase, normal PTH and calcitriol levels. Treatment involves phosphate and vitamin D supplementation but nephrocalcinosis can be a complication.

Proximal (type 2) renal tubular acidosis
Proximal RTA results from a failure of bicarbonate reabsorption. Distal acidification mechanisms are intact.

Inherited proximal RTA is a rare AR disease caused by mutations in the gene for the sodium bicarbonate transporter. It usually occurs with ocular abnormalities. Proximal RTA is more common as part of the generalized tubular defect, Fanconi syndrome.

Clinical features include failure to thrive and vomiting. Urine pH may be <5.3 and ammonium chloride loading leads to acidification of urine. Nephrocalcinosis is not a feature.

Treatment is with sodium bicarbonate supplementation.

Fanconi syndrome
Fanconi syndrome is a generalized proximal tubular dysfunction leading to excessive loss of glucose, phosphate, amino acids, K^+, bicarbonate, Na^+, and water in the urine.

The causes include inherited metabolic disorders such as cystinosis, tyrosinaemia type I, Lowe syndrome, galactosaemia, glycogen storage disease, and Wilson disease. Acquired causes include heavy metal toxicity and drugs (expired tetracyclines).

Clinical features are failure to thrive, polyuria, polydipsia and dehydration, rickets (hypophosphataemia), acidosis (proximal type II), and hypokalaemia.

Loop of Henle and distal tubule
Bartter syndrome
Bartter syndrome is a group of AR disorders caused by mutations in any of three genes: *SLC12A1* encoding the Na^+-K^+-Cl^- co-transporter NKCC2, *KCNJ1* encoding ROMK, or *CLCNKB* encoding ClC-Kb (Fig 6.12)

There is increased urinary Cl^- and K^+ loss with a hypokalaemic alkalosis, and elevated plasma renin and angiotensin but normal blood pressure. Hypercalciuria and nephrocalcinosis may be a feature.

Presentation varies from the severe infantile form with polyhydramnios and life-threatening neonatal electrolyte disturbance to incidental asymptomatic abnormal biochemistry in later life.

The biochemical hallmark is hypokalaemic alkalosis with inappropriately high urine Na^+ and Cl^- and hypercalciuria. Therapy includes K^+ supplements and a prostaglandin synthetase inhibitor such as indomethacin.

Gitelman syndrome
Gitelman syndrome is caused by a defect in the thiazide-sensitive Na–Cl co-transporter in the distal tubule. There is hypocalaemic metabolic alkalosis with hypomagnasaemia and hypocalciuria. It is often asymptomatic but may present with episodic weakness, vertigo, or arrhythmias.

Distal (type 1) renal tubular acidosis
In distal type I RTA there is impaired excretion of acid into the distal tubule.

Inherited forms are caused by AD mutations in the gene for the anion exchanger AE1. An AR childhood-onset form associated with sensorineural deafness is caused by defects in a subunit of the renal tubule apical proton pump. This pump functions in inner ear epithelia as well as the renal distal tubule. Acquired forms occur in obstructive uropathy and drug toxicity (amphotericin, ciclosporin).

Clinical features are hypokalaemic acidosis and hypercalciuria with nephrocalcinosis. The urine fails to acidify in response to an ammonium chloride load. Treatment is sodium bicarbonate supplementation.

Collecting duct
Nephrogenic diabetes insipidus
Nephrogenic DI is caused by a failure of the kidney to respond to arginine vasopressin (AVP). Inheritance is:

- X-linked in 90%, caused by mutations in *AVPR2*, encoding the vasopressin V2 receptor.
- AR in 10%, caused by mutations in *AQP2*, encoding the aquaporin-2 water channel.

Affected males present in the newborn period with polyuria and polydipsia, vomiting, and constipation. There is hypernatraemia and increased plasma osmolality with inappropriately dilute urine and a low urinary Na^+. Plasma AVP levels are raised. Treatment is high water intake and low-solute feeds. (See Chapter 10.3 for a discussion of cranial diabetes insipidus)

Pseudohypoaldosteronism (PHAI) type I and Liddle syndrome
These rare disorders are caused by mutations in genes encoding any of the three subunits of the amiloride-sensitive epithelial Na^+ channel (ENaC).

PHAI is an AR disorder caused by *loss-of-function* mutations in *SCNN1A*, *SCNN1B*, or *SCNN1G*. End organ insensitivity to aldosterone causes severe salt wasting, hyponatraemia, and hyperkalaemia.

In contrast, AD *gain-of-function* mutations cause activation of ENaC and pseudoaldosteronism (Liddle syndrome). There is hypokalaemia and hypertension but normal aldosterone levels

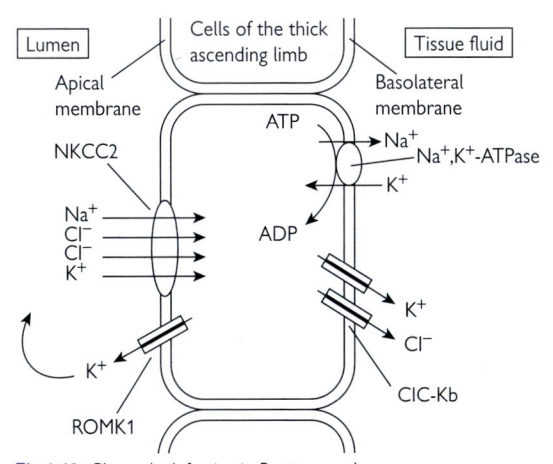

Fig 6.12 Channels defective in Bartter syndrome.

6.10 Genetic syndromes and HUS

Genetic syndromes

Alport syndrome
Alport syndrome (AS) is caused by mutations in any of three genes encoding subunits of type IV collagen, the major constituent of the glomerular basement membrane (GBM). Mutations in *COL4A5* on the X-chromosome account for 85% of cases (XLAS). These collagen chains are also important in basement membranes in the cochlea and eye.

The renal manifestations of XLAS are haematuria, usually macroscopic in males. Proteinuria is usually absent in childhood. Sensorineural deafness may only be detectable by audiometry in the early stages. Absence of α_5 (IV) chains of type IV collagen in the epidermal basement membrane on skin biopsy is diagnostic. Treatment with ACE inhibitors is used in patients with proteinuria, with or without hypertension, and renal transplantation is offered to patients who develop ESRD.

Cystinosis
Cystinosis is a rare AR disorder caused by mutations in the *CTNS* gene which encodes cystinosin, the lysosomal cystine transporter. Massive intralysosomal accumulation of cystine generates damage in renal tubular cells, manifested as Fanconi syndrome initially, and accumulation of crystals in the cornea causes photophobia.

Three clinical types exist: infantile (nephropathic), intermediate (juvenile), and non-nephropathic or ocular.

Infantile nephropathic cystinosis presents in infancy with features of Fanconi syndrome: failure to thrive, poor growth, excessive thirst and polyuria, acidosis, and hypophosphataemic rickets. Crystals in the cornea lead to photophobia. ESRF occurs by age 10 years (if untreated). Diagnosis is based on slit-lamp examination for cystine crystals in the cornea and raised white cell cystine levels.

Treatment is supportive with high fluid intake and supplements of phosphate, sodium chloride, potassium and sodium bicarbonate. Patients require alfacalcidol for rickets and thyroxine for hypothyroidism.

Specific treatment with mercaptamine reduces cystine accumulation and may prevent or delay renal failure and improve growth. Indomethacin ameliorates polyuria and electrolyte wasting by reducing GFR.

Intermediate cystinosis has the same clinical manifestations occurring with late onset (12–15 years). In non-nephropathic, benign cystinosis the only symptom is photophobia due to crystals in the cornea. The retina is not affected.

Congenital nephrotic syndrome
This is a rare but devastating inherited form of nephrotic syndrome caused by mutations in any of several genes encoding protein components of the podocyte slit diaphragm (Fig 6.13).

The Finnish type is usually caused by mutations in *NPHS1* which encodes nephrin. Mutations in *NPHS2*, encoding podocin, account for patients with congenital nephrotic syndrome and patients with early onset, steroid resistant nephrotic syndrome with focal and segmental glomerulosclerosis (FSGS) on histology.

The Finnish type presents early with oedema, proteinuria, and high mortality from malnutrition and sepsis. Treatment is supportive with albumin infusions, nutritional support, and ACE inhibitors and indomethacin to reduce GFR and protein loss in the remaining kidney. Progression to ESRF occurs necessitating bilateral native nephrectomies, dialysis, and transplantation.

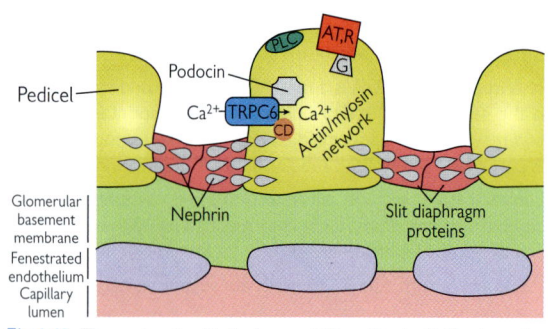

Fig 6.13 The podocyte slit-diaphragm. Nilius, Owsianik, Voets, and Peters, Transient Receptor Potential Cation Channels in Disease, Physiol. Rev. 87: 165–217, 2007. Used with permission.

Haemolytic uraemic syndrome (HUS)
Haemolytic uraemic syndrome (HUS) is a disease of infancy and early childhood characterized by the triad of:
- Microangiopathic haemolytic anaemia
- Thrombocytopaenia
- Acute renal failure.

The incidence of HUS <5 years is 3 cases/100 000 and the mortality rate is 5–15%.

Thrombotic thrombocytopenic purpura (TTP) has a similar underlying pathophysiology, but CNS rather than renal involvement predominates.

Aetiology and pathogenesis
HUS is classified into two forms depending on whether the patient has had diarrhoea: D+HUS (typical) and D–HUS (atypical). The causes of HUS are usefully classified as infectious or non-infectious:

HUS: infectious agents
- **Bacteria:** Shiga toxin producing *E. coli* 0157:H7 (STEC), *Shigella, Salmonella, Citrobacter*, and *Campylobacter* account for 70% of D+HUS. *Clostridium difficile, Strep. pneumoniae* (neuraminidase producing).
- **Viruses:** varicella, echovirus, coxsackie A and B, HIV.

HUS: non-infectious
- *Inherited:* complement factor H deficiency
- *Drugs:* mitomycin C, quinine, interferon alpha, tacrolimus
- *Malignancy:* gastric and pancreatic
- *Post-transplantation*
- *Autoimmune:* SLE.

Thrombotic thrombocytopenic purpura (TTP) is caused by deficiency of the von Willebrand factor-cleaving protease ADAMTS13 which may be inherited or acquired due to autoantibodies to this protein.

Pathogenesis
Endothelial cell injury appears to be the primary insult that triggers a cascade of events resulting in microvascular platelet-fibrin hyaline microthrombi. These occlude arterioles and capillaries causing a microangiopathic haemolytic anaemia and consumptive thrombocytopaenia. In HUS, microthrombi are essentially

confined to the kidneys whereas in TTP they occur throughout the circulation, especially the CNS.

Mechanisms of endothelial cell damage by toxins, drugs, or inherited predisposition vary. Verotoxins bind to glycosphingolipid receptors in kidney endothelial cells. *Strep. pneumoniae* produce neuraminidase capable of unmasking the Thomsen–Friedenreich antigen on erythrocytes and endothelial cells. Complement factor H has a role in protecting endothelial cells.

Clinical features

Children usually present following an acute diarrhoeal illness with grossly bloody stools. Risk factors include eating uncooked hamburgers, drinking unpasteurized apple juice, and visits to a petting zoo.

In D+ HUS, patients develop pallor, petechiae, or bleeding, and reduced or absent urine output within 2–14 (mean 6) days of onset of intestinal symptoms. Examination findings reflect the pathology and may include:

- Fever (low grade)
- *Pallor ± jaundice*: haemolytic anaemia
- *Petechiae and bleeding*: thrombocytopaenia
- *Oligo/anuria, hypertension*: acute renal failure
- *CNS signs*: encephalopathy due to uraemia.

In atypical, D−HUS there may be no history of preceding infection and HUS features may develop insidiously.

TTP usually presents insidiously with neurological symptoms such as headache, altered consciousness or behaviour, seizures, or coma. Fever is usual together with pallor, jaundice, and purpura or mucous membrane bleeding. Renal or cardiac involvement may occur.

Management: investigations

Diagnosis is clinical but confirmed by consistent laboratory investigations:

Blood tests

- *FBC and film*: anaemia (Hb <8 g/dL) with fragmented red cells on film (Fig 6.14). Thrombocytopaenia (usually <60 × 10^9/L), raised reticulocytes. Leucocytosis
- *Coagulation screen*: usually normal
- Low haptoglobin, elevated LDH and bilirubin: haemolysis
- Raised creatinine, urea concentrations. Hyponatraemia and hyperkalaemia. Hyperglycaemia
- Serum amylase, lipase (pancreatic involvement)
- *LFTs*: abnormal with low albumin.

Urine tests

Dipstick for proteinuria, haematuria, microscopy: red cells, white cells ± casts

Stool and blood culture

- Culture on sorbitol-MacConkey plates identifies *E. coli*. 0.157: H7 (most lack sorbitol fermentation)
- PCR for STEC virulence gene *stc*
- Typical HUS is not associated with bacteraemia but sepsis may be present in HUS associated with *Strep. pneumoniae* infection.

Imaging

- CXR, renal ultrasound
- In atypical HUS or possible TTP additional investigations include Thomson–Friedenrich antigen, complement C3, C4, ANA, anti-ds DNA antibodies (SLE), factor H and I levels, vWF cleaving protease activity.

Treatment

Treatment is supportive and specific depending on aetiology.

Supportive

Fluid balance

Patients with typical HUS are often dehydrated at presentation and require fluid resuscitation initially with subsequent maintenance to balance insensible losses and urine output. Diuretics are indicated for fluid overload or oligo/anuria.

Acute renal failure

- Hyponatraemia, hyperkalaemia, acidosis, and hypertension require medical treatment. 50% of typical HUS patients need dialysis.
- Blood transfusion to maintain Hb >7.0 g/dL. Platelets avoided except in active bleeding.
- Nutrition with high calorie intake.
- Antibiotics are not indicated in the first instance.

Specific

- No specific treatment is available for typical HUS. Atypical HUS or TTP may benefit from administration of fresh frozen plasma (FFP) to replace vWF-cleaving protease or plasmapheresis to remove antibodies to this protein.
- Long-term sequelae with proteinuria and hypertension occur in 15% of patients. Patients with atypical HUS have a worse prognosis. High neutrophil count and neurological complications in the acute phase are poor prognostic factors.

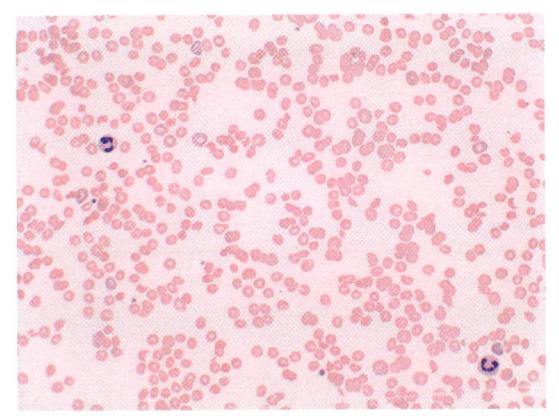

Fig 6.14 D+HUS: blood film with RBC fragments and few platelets.

6.11 Hypertension, urolithiasis, and nephrocalcinosis

Hypertension

Childhood hypertension is defined as an average systolic or diastolic blood pressure above the 95th percentile for age, gender, and height based on at least three measurements on separate occasions using a mercury sphygmomanometer with an appropriate-sized cuff. BP measurements between 90th–95th percentile are now designated 'pre-hypertension' rather than 'high-normal'.

Aetiology

Essential (primary) hypertension is common in adolescents, but in infants and children hypertension is usually secondary.

Secondary hypertension

Renal disease
- Renal parenchymal disease:
  - chronic disorders: cystic disease, reflux nephropathy, urinary tract obstruction, glomerulonephritis, FSGS
  - acute disorders: acute nephritis, acute tubular necrosis, haemolytic uraemic syndrome
- Renovascular disease:
  - renal artery or vein thrombosis
  - fibromuscular dysplasia
  - renal artery stenosis
  - mid-aortic syndrome (NF1, William syndrome)

Endocrine disorders
- *Aldosteronism:* congenital adrenal hyperplasia, glucocorticoid-remediable aldosteronism, Liddle syndrome
- Cushing syndrome: steroid therapy, tumour
- Catecholamine excess: phaeochromocytoma
- Hyperthyroidism

Coarctation of the aorta
- *Autonomic dysfunction:* Guillain-Barré syndrome

Primary (essential) hypertension

The pathogenesis of essential hypertension is multifactorial. Familial clustering indicates a genetic contribution which is polygenic. Hypertension is associated with the epidemic of obesity and metabolic syndrome, 20–30% of obese children have essential hypertension.

Pathogenesis: end-organ damage

Hypertension is an important risk factor for both cardiovascular disease and chronic kidney disease. Severe hypertension may be associated with congestive cardiac failure, left ventricular hypertrophy, renal failure, hypertensive encephalopathy, and retinopathy.

Clinical evaluation

Diagnosis

Blood pressure measurement

Blood pressure increases with age, is higher in males than females and is slightly higher in tall individuals. Short-term variation occurs with emotional state and there is a normal diurnal pattern with a fall during sleep.

Measurement

Centile charts are based on mercury sphygmomanometry and there are few other validated instruments in use. The cuff must cover at least two thirds of the upper arm and bladder length should be at least 80% of limb circumference.

Ambulatory blood pressure monitoring (ABPM)

ABPM is a useful adjunct to diagnosis and monitoring of hypertension in older children. Advantages include avoidance of observer error and documentation of circadian variability: normal night-time drop may be blunted in renal hypertension. Disadvantages are limited normal ranges (small cohorts, no young children) and lack of validation and comparability between devices.

History

Hypertension may be detected incidentally or during the course of an acute illness or chronic disease. It is often asymptomatic but if severe may present with symptoms such as headache, epistaxes, blurred vision or shortness of breath. Acute illnesses complicated by hypertension include acute nephritis, acute renal failure, Guillain–Barré syndrome.

In hypertension of uncertain aetiology the previous history may provide important clues to the presence of a renal cause. A family history may be revealed in rare cases of genetic hypertension or neurofibromatosis type I.

Examination

Careful examination may identify a cause and document end-organ damage.
- *General:* body habitus, obese, thin, short stature
- *Syndromic features:* neurofibromatosis Type I, Turner syndrome, Cushing syndrome
- *Cardiovascular system:* palpation of femoral pulses and four-limb BP measurement, left ventricular hypertrophy
- *Abdomen:* renal bruit
- *Genitalia:* ambiguous or virilized
- *CNS:* papilloedema, retinopathy, VII (facial) nerve palsy, encephalopathy.

Management

Investigations are guided by clinical features and proceed in a stepwise fashion:

Baseline investigations
- *Urinalysis:* dipstick, microscopy and culture
- *Biochemistry:* U&Es, creatinine, acid–base status
- TFTs, urate, fasting cholesterol and triglycerides
- Renal ultrasound, ECG.

Second line investigations: based on likely cause
- *Reflux nephropathy:* renal imaging: MCUG, DMSA/MAG3
- *Glomerulonephritis:* nephritis screen, renal biopsy:
- *Renovascular disease:* doppler ultrasonography
- *Phaeochromocytoma:* urine and plasma catecholamines, MIBG scan
- *Renal artery stenosis:* plasma renin activity and aldosterone levels
- *Cushing syndrome:* cortisol levels, abdominal ultrasound scan or CT scan
- *Coarctation of aorta:* echocardiogram.

Treatment

Acute hypertension: emergency treatment

The child should be on a high-dependency unit and management guided by a experienced team. The aim is safe reduction in BP whilst preventing end-organ damage and avoiding treatment side effects.

- *General measures:* children with intravascular depletion may be hypertensive due to renin production and respond to saline infusion. More usually there is salt and water retention as in acute nephritis, which responds to a loop diuretic such as furosemide plus a vasodilator such as nifedipine.
- *Drugs:* options include labetalol, sodium nitroprusside, nicardipine, or hydralazine. An infusion is given aiming at a controlled reduction, no more than one third of the desired reduction in the first 12 h. Too rapid reduction may cause stroke or cortical blindness.

Long term management

- *General measures:* mild primary hypertension is managed by weight reduction (in obesity), increased physical activity, and moderation of salt intake.
- *Drug therapy:* The evidence for when medication should be initiated is unclear. The aim is to maintain BP below the 95th centile. A long-acting, once-daily, single agent is optimal. Options include: calcium blocker, e.g. amlodipine; β-blocker, e.g. atenolol; ACE inhibitor, e.g. enalapril (contraindicated in renovascular disease, but logical choice in chronic kidney disease with proteinuria as there is an antiproteinuric effect).
- *Radiological intervention and surgery:* percutaneous transluminal angioplasty is used for renal artery stenosis. Surgical interventions may include nephrectomy, revascularization surgery for renovascular disease, removal of a phaeochromocytoma, and repair of coarctation of the aorta.

Urolithiasis and nephrocalcinosis

Urolithiasis is the formation of calculi (stones) within the urinary tract. Nephrocalcinosis is the presence of microscopic calcification within the renal parenchyma. Depending on aetiology, the two may coexist. Urinary tract calculi are more common in boys with a mean age presentation 3 years.

Aetiology and pathogenesis

Formation of renal calculi is promoted by several factors:
- Urine concentration of stone-forming substances: calcium, cystine, oxalate, and urate
- Urine pH: acid urine encourages calcium precipitation
- Urinary stasis and infection.

Metabolic

Metabolic abnormalities account for 50% of cases, with an infective aetiology in one third and no aetiology identified in about 25%. Inherited and acquired conditions predispose to formation of calcium, oxalate, cystine, or uric acid stones.

- *Calcium stones:* hypercalciuria is the most common metabolic abnormality identified, and is often associated with nephrocalcinosis. Causes include:
  - furosemide use in preterm infants and cardiac patients
  - distal renal tubular acidosis and Bartter syndrome.
  - Dent disease: X-linked disorder (mutations in *CLCN5*) causing LMW proteinuria, hypercalciuria, and nephrocalcinosis.
  - idiopathic hypercalciuria: immobility may be a factor.
  - hypercalcaemia: uncommon.
- *Oxalate stones:* these may be associated with primary hyperoxaluria (PH) or enteric hyperoxaluria. Enteric hyperoxaluria is due to small-bowel pathology such as bowel resection leading to increased dietary oxalate absorption.
- *Cystine stone:* cystinuria (see Section 6.8) is an inherited disorder of amino acid transport in the proximal tubule.
- *Uric acid:* uric acid gravel in both kidneys leading to acute renal failure as part of the 'tumour lysis syndrome' is now less common with the use of rasburicase and allopurinol pre-treatment. Lesch–Nyhan syndrome is associated with uric acid stones.

Infection

Infection-related stones are often located in the upper tract and are composed of magnesium ammonium calcium phosphate or 'triple phosphate' stones. *Proteus* infection is particularly associated with calculi.

Clinical features

Less than half present with the classic symptoms of abdominal or flank pain and macroscopic haematuria. Infants often have feeding and growth problems A stone may be detected fortuitously. Bilateral disease is more likely to have a metabolic aetiology. Most calculi (85%) are in the upper tract.

Management

Renal ultrasound to exclude urolithiasis is indicated in children presenting with a UTI or haematuria. Ultrasound is more sensitive in detecting nephrocalcinosis and may detect radiolucent stones. A very small stone may be detected on plain abdominal radiograph but missed by ultrasound.

Immediate management includes relief of any urinary obstruction, hyperhydration, and analgesia. Options for stone removal include:

- *Extracorporeal shock wave lithotripsy (ESWL):* for symptomatic stones >8 mm in the renal pelvis or upper ureter.
- *Nephrolithotomy:* stones >3 cm are removed either percutaneously or by open surgery.

Further investigations

Urine microscopy and culture is mandatory but presence of infection does not exclude an underlying metabolic abnormality which should be sought in all cases:

- *Blood tests:* plasma Ca, PO_4, creatinine, bicarbonate, Cl^-, Mg, PTH, urate.
- *Urinalysis:* 24 h urine collections are ideal but difficult. A spot urine sample can be used to infer excretion rate by comparing concentration with that of creatinine. Measure calcium, oxalate, urate, and cystine levels.

Medical treatment

Renal hypercalciuria may respond to a thiazide diuretic and a low Na^+ diet. Distal RTA responds to alkali supplementation. Cystinuria is treated with high fluid intake and oral potassium citrate. Alkalinization of urine with calcium citrate is indicated in primary hyperoxaluria and urate stones. Secondary (enteric) hyperoxaluria is treated with a low-oxalate diet.

6.12 Case-based discussions

A child with bloody diarrhoea

A 4 year old child presents to the hospital emergency deaprtment. Her mother tells you she has been miserable and listless all week, since she recovered from a bout of gastroenteritis a fortnight ago after eating some uncooked chicken. Further questioning elicits that she had been unwell for several days with bloody diarrhoea and vomiting, and had also been febrile. Stool cultures from the GP have gone missing. She is normally well, has no family history of note, nor any medications.

On examination, she is clinically anaemic and unhappy, with three small bruises. She is afebrile and is neither tachycardic nor hypotensive. She has no lymphadenopathy, but her spleen is palpable 1 cm below the costal margin. Her cardiovascular and respiratory systems are unremarkable. She has not passed urine since yesterday.

What is your differential diagnosis at this point?

This is a child presenting with lethargy, bruising, and a palpable spleen. Malignancy must be considered, and acute leukaemia excluded.

However, the history also mentions bloody diarrhoea, and this, associated with anaemia and thrombocytopaenia, should raise the possibility of haemolytic uraemic syndrome (HUS). This is the commonest cause of acute renal failure in young children, and occurs most commonly following infection with verotoxin-producing *E. coli* (0157:H7), which later grew from this child's stool culture. HUS refers to the triad of microangiopathic haemolytic anaemia, thrombocytopaenia, and acute renal failure, which in this child was suggested by the poor urine output and raised creatinine level.

Her investigations showed:
Hb 8 g/dL Plts 30 ×10^9/L WCC 6.13 × 10^9/L
Na 137 mmol/L K 7.1 mmol/L Urea 27 mmol/L
Creatinine 143 μmol/L.
Bicarbonate 12 mmol/L
Coagulation studies were normal
Urine dipstick +blood + protein
Urine culture negative

What might you expect the blood film to show? Should a renal biopsy be performed?

Typically the film will show helmet and burr cells and fragments of red blood cells. A biopsy should not be performed in the presence of thrombocytopaenia, and is not in any case necessary in a case of HUS which presents typically.

The child is admitted to PICU, and her acute renal failure is treated supportively, initially with fluid restriction, and later, in view of persistent anuria, with peritoneal dialysis. She required treatment for hyperkalaemia (calcium resonium and salbutamol nebulizers), and a bicarbonate infusion to treat her metabolic acidosis. She did not suffer active bleeding so did not require a platelet transfusion, though a blood transfusion was given in view of her symptomatic anaemia. While an inpatient, she developed severe headaches, and after several hours had a brief tonic-clonic seizure, which resolved without treatment, leaving no neurological deficit.

Why might this have occurred?

It important to exclude hypertensive encephalopathy and electrolyte abnormalities as a cause of headache and seizures in a child with renal pathology. However, this child's blood pressure was within normal limits for age. Children with HUS are prone to several complications believed to be related to intravascular thrombosis, and her CNS involvement may have been related to this. Other possible complications of intravascular thrombosis include colitis, diabetes mellitus, and rhabdomyolysis.

In addition to the supportive management which this child received, are there any other treatments for HUS?

No other treatment is of proven benefit. Anticoagulants have shown little effect. Fibrinolytics for intrarenal thrombi should, in theory, be useful, but risks appear to outweigh benefits. Supportive treatment of acute renal failure, anaemia, and thrombocytopaenia remains the mainstay of treatment, and peritoneal dialysis, as part of this supportive treatment, also promotes recovery by removal of an inhibitor of fibrinolysis. Plasmapherisis may have a role in the treatment of neurological complications of HUS and TTP.

Chapter 7
Neurology and neurodisability

- 7.1 The nervous system *144*
- 7.2 Clinical paediatric neurology *146*
- 7.3 Neural tube defects and hydrocephalus *148*
- 7.4 Cortical and cranial vault malformations *150*
- 7.5 Neurodegenerative disorders *152*
- 7.6 The cerebral palsies *154*
- 7.7 Childhood epilepsies: diagnosis and management *156*
- 7.8 Childhood epilepsies: causes and classification *158*
- 7.9 Movement disorders *160*
- 7.10 Headache *162*
- 7.11 Neuromuscular disorders: overview *164*
- 7.12 Specific neuromuscular disorders *166*
- 7.13 Muscular dystrophies *168*
- 7.14 Infection and injury *170*
- 7.15 Inflammatory disorders and stroke *172*
- 7.16 Case-based discussions *174*

7.1 The nervous system

Development of the nervous system

The nervous system consists of three parts:
- *Central nervous system:* brain and spinal column
- *Peripheral nervous system:* neurons outside CNS
- *Autonomic nervous system:* neurons that innervate smooth muscle, cardiac muscle, or glandular epithelium.

The nervous system develops from the neural plate, a dorsal thickening of ectoderm, which appears on the dorsal surface of the early embryo in the 3rd week of gestation. The neural plate is induced by signals from the notochord.

This strip of neuroectoderm folds in to form the neural groove with neural folds on either side which roll up and fuse to form the neural tube during the 4th week. Some neuroectodermal cells remain between the neural tube and surface ectoderm as the neural crest. Neural crest cells form the peripheral nervous system.

The subsequent main phases of CNS development involve cell proliferation, migration, and differentiation together with synaptogenesis and apoptosis and finally myelination. The principal stages are as follows.

CNS development
Primordial brain and spinal cord
The rostral (front) part of the neural tube develops into the brain and the rest develops into the spinal cord. The three brain primordia are the prosencephalon or forebrain, mesencephalon or midbrain, and rhombencephalon or hindbrain (Fig 7.1). These go on to form:
- *Prosencephalon*: telencephalon: cerebral cortex, basal nuclei
- *Diencephalon*: thalamus, hypothalamus, pineal, pituitary gland
- *Mesencephalon*: tectum, cerebral aqueduct, tegmentum, cerebral peduncles
- *Rhombencephalon*: metencephalon: pons, cerebellum.
- *Myelencephalon:* medulla oblongata.

Cranial neural tube closure occurs between 3 and 7 weeks. The neural canal becomes the ventricles of the brain and central canal of the spinal cord.

Cell proliferation
The single layer of primitive ectoderm begins to divide very rapidly and will in time form virtually all of the CNS. The walls of the neural tube thicken and the vesicles at the anterior end enlarge. Proliferating cells arise from zones adjacent to the ventricular system, the *ventricular* and *subventricular* zones.

Cell migration, differentiation, and synaptogenesis
Primitive nerve cells (neuroblasts) migrate using radial glial cells as a guiding scaffold. This process forms the six-cell-layered cortex in the area of the developing hemispheres. An 'inside-out' sequence of development occurs: deepest layers are formed first, each successive migration passing through earlier layers to form more superficial layers, so that the youngest neurons are closest to the surface.

Once neurons have reached their final location further differentiation occurs, dendrites form, and synaptic connections are made when growth cones contact their postsynaptic targets.

Apoptosis (programmed cell death)
Some neurons act as temporary targets for incoming fibres and form transient connections before being eliminated by apoptosis when a more appropriate and permanent set of target cells is in place.

Maturation and myelination
Neuronal maturation involves the development of dendrites axons and synaptic connections. Synaptic formation starts in the 2nd trimester and continues during postnatal life.

Oligodendrocytes begin to lay down myelin sheaths from 26 weeks gestation. Myelin acts as an insulating sheath which increases conduction velocity and prevents collateral spread. Myelination occurs sequentially into the 2nd decade. Fibres serving primary sensory and motor areas are myelinated shortly after birth while those associated with more complex cognitive functions are myelinated later.

Neuronal function: ion channels

The function of neurons and other excitable tissues depends on the action of ion channels which mediate changes in membrane potential by allowing the passage of charged ions through the lipid cell membrane.

Ion channels are membrane proteins, usually composed of one or more pore-forming subunits and a number of accessory subunits.

Ion channels are classified according to whether they are voltage-gated or ligand-gated by neurotransmitters and by the ion for which they are selectively permeable: sodium, potassium, calcium, or chloride. The neuronal action-potential is generated by sequential opening and closing of voltage-gated sodium and potassium channels. Glutamate receptors and GABA receptors are the most important excitatory and inhibitory neurotransmitter-gated ion channels in the CNS.

Mutations in >60 ion channel genes have now been associated with human diseases, the so-called *channelopathies*.

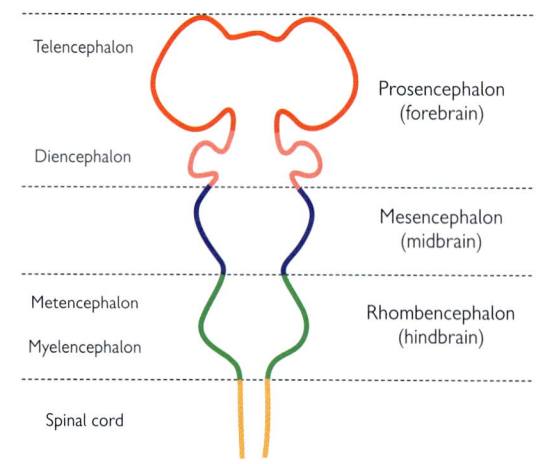

Fig 7.1 The primordial brain structures.

Cerebral blood flow and metabolism

Cerebral blood flow (CBF) is determined by cerebral perfusion pressure (CPP) and blood viscosity. The CPP is the difference between the mean arterial blood pressure (MABP) and the intracranial pressure (ICP). Cerebral blood flow is of critical importance in view of the high metabolic rate of brain tissue and its dependence on oxygen and glucose delivered by the circulation.

CBF is regulated by four main mechanisms:
- *Metabolic activity*: local flow is closely coupled to local metabolic demand.
- *Chemical control*: $PaCO_2$ has the most potent effect, hypercarbia causing vasodilatation and hypocapnia vasoconstriction.
- *Pressure autoregulation*: in normal adults CPP is maintained constant in the range of MABP 60–160 mmHg through autoregulatory dilatation or vasoconstriction of resistance vessels.
- *Neural control*: intense sympathetic activity causes vasoconstriction and a shift of the autoregulatory curve to the right.

Cerebral metabolic rate is influenced by neuronal activity. It increases during generalized seizures and is reduced in barbiturate-induced coma or hypothermia.

Blood–brain barrier

The capillaries of the cerebral circulation are unique in having endothelial cells joined by tight junctions rather than fenestrations. This forms the physical basis of the blood–brain barrier (BBB) which excludes water-soluble molecules with a molecular weight >500 Da. Lipid-soluble molecules able to cross cell membranes, such as oxygen, carbon dioxide, ethanol, and steroid hormones, penetrate the BBB. Specific endothelial transporters exist to allow passage of important hydrophilic molecules including glucose (GLUT1, insulin independent glucose transporter) and amino acids.

At certain sites, including the circumventricular organs, the capillaries are fenestrated and allow the neurons to 'sample' the circulating blood.

Inflammation of the meninges disrupts the BBB and may enhance the penetration of antibiotics into the brain.

The blood–CSF barrier is anatomically distinct and composed of the choroid plexus and arachnoid membrane. There is no major barrier between CSF and brain extracellular space, so drugs introduced intrathecally bypass the BBB.

Cerebrospinal fluid (CSF)

The CSF is produced by modified ependymal cells in the choroid plexus within the lateral ventricles. It circulates through the foramen of Monro into the 3rd ventricle and through the aqueduct into the 4th ventricle from where it exits through two lateral apertures, the foramina of Luschka and one midline aperture, the foramen of Magendie. Bulk flow then continues through the cerebromedullary cistern down the spinal cord and over the cerebral hemispheres. CSF returns to the vascular system by entering the dural venous sinuses via the arachnoid granulations (Fig 7.2).

The rate of CSF production is ~30 mL/h and the total volume at age >2 years is 150 mL of which 35 mL is in the ventricular system.

CSF functions include mechanical protection and distribution of neuroendocrine factors.

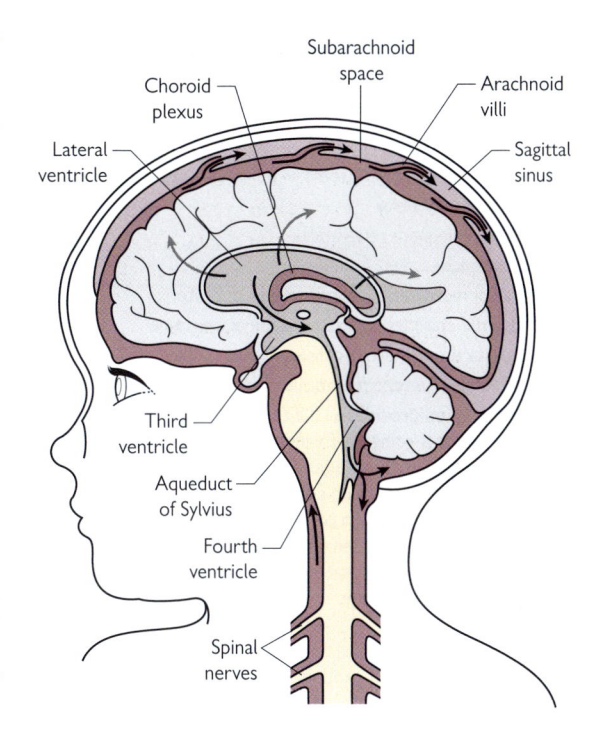

Fig 7.2 CSF circulation.

7.2 Clinical paediatric neurology

History
Common presenting symptoms of nervous system disorders:
- Developmental delay
- *Regression*: neurodegeneration
- *Pain*: headache
- *Abnormal movements or posture*: ataxia, dystonia
- *Paroxysmal episodes*: epileptic seizures, migraine
- *Weakness*: neuromuscular disease
- *Altered consciousness*: metabolic disorder, infection.

The history often provides a clue to the nature of the pathology. It tells you *what* is going on. Examination often reveals the localization of pathology. It tells you *where* the problem is.

The time course over which symptoms have evolved is particularly informative in relation to the probable pathology. Vascular events often have a sudden onset, whereas expanding lesions usually progress over several weeks. History is central to evaluation of certain conditions such as paroxysmal disorders and headaches.

The distinction between delayed development and actual regression with loss of skills becomes apparent from careful history taking and is crucial in distinguishing a neurodegenerative process from a static condition.

Examination
The aim is to assess the integrity of the nervous system and to localize any abnormality. Developmental examination may often overlap and is complementary but its primary aim is to assess the acquisition of learned skills.

Neurological examination is highly age dependent for obvious reasons, including extent of cooperation.

General examination is important and should include:
- *Skin*: cutaneous stigmata may provide important and subtle diagnostic clues such as hypopigmented macules in tuberous sclerosis
- *Dysmorphic features and organomegaly*: may be observed in neurometabolic disorders.

Important aspects of non-acute neurological examination at different ages include the following.

Infant
- *General inspection:* note dysmorphic features or cutaneous stigmata. Inspect sacrum and spine.
- *Head:* abnormalities of cranial vault size (measure occipitofrontal circumference, OFC) or shape. Palpate the cranial sutures and fontanelles.
- *Eyes:* eyeball size and protrusion, ptosis, strabismus or abnormal ocular movements, hyper- or hypotelorism, pupil size and pupillary reflexes.
- *Posture:* abnormal or asymmetric posture usually reflects abnormalities of tone. A hypotonic, floppy infant may show the 'frog's leg' posture when supine. Asymmetrical posture of freely hanging legs may be a sign of unilateral weakness or spasticity. Asymmetric upper limb posture occurs in brachial plexus injury.
- *Tone:* handling provides a general ideal of tone, i.e. resistance to passive movement. Hypertonia may reflect either corticospinal or extrapyramidal dysfunction. Hypotonia is indicated by floppiness on handling and may be due to a lower motor neuron lesion, muscle weakness or, on occasion, upper motor neuron lesions. Clonus, a rhythmic series of involuntary contractions elicited by stretching the muscle, is most easily tested at the ankle joint. Sustained clonus >5 beats is a sign of an upper motor neuron lesion.
- *Movements:* the quantity and quality of gross and fine movements is observed.
- *Reflexes:* test for persistence of primitive reflexes including Moro (to 6 months), stepping reflex (to 4 months), asymmetric tonic neck reflex (to 6 months).

Toddler/uncooperative child
- *Posture:* Abnormal postures at this age include:
    - *torticollis:* may be associated with a squint, sternomatoid tumour, posterior fossa or cervical tumour, or hemianopia.
    - *spinal curvature:* scoliosis or kyphosis
    - *opisthotonus:* extension of the neck and arching of back due to spasm of erector spinae.
    - *arms:* shoulder adducted, elbow flexed, wrist flexed, and hand clenched in upper motor neuron lesion.
    - *legs:* scissoring due to adductor spasm.
- *Tone:* lightly lift each leg and assess degree of resistance to flexing at knee and hip. Test tendon reflexes.
- *Movements:* assessment of handedness and gait. A clear hand preference in a child <18 months may indicate hemiplegia. Abnormal gaits are seen in hemiplegia, spastic diplegia, and cerebellar ataxia. Intermittent toe-walking is a normal variant but may indicate mild diplegia.

Older/cooperative child
Important points include the following:

Cranial nerves
A rapid screen of the cranial nerves is achieved by:
- *II:* pupillary reflexes and fundi
- *III, IV, VI:* eye movements
- *V:* motor: bite and waggle jaw from side to side.
  motor and sensory: jaw jerk.
  corneal reflex: sensory V, motor VII.
- *VII:* motor: raise eyebrows, screw up eyes, smile
- *IX, X:* motor: say 'aaah' to test pharyngeal movement.
- *XI:* shrug shoulders
- *XII:* put out tongue: it deviates to weak side.

Motor system
The pattern of movement is observed to distinguish peripheral, neuromuscular from central problems and to categorize CNS problems as pyramidal, extrapyramidal, or cerebellar. Screening manoeuvres include:
- Hold arms outstretched with eyes closed watching for drift, finger-nose touching, alternating movements, touching fingers in turn.
- Observe gait; observation is aided by age-dependent additional tasks:
    >3 years: walk on heels or toes, run, stand on one leg
    >4 years: hop
    >5 years: walk in straight line for 20 steps
    >7 years: heel-toe walking

- Gait may be abnormally narrow in mild diplegia or wide based (cerebellar dysfunction, weakness of legs or pelvic girdle), or asymmetrical (hemiplegia).
- Gowers' sign and Fogs' test.

If indicated, further examination includes:
- *Cerebellar function*: test for: scanning dysarthria, nystagmus, ataxia (heel-toe walking, Romberg's sign), tremor, dysmetria: 'finger-nose' touching, hand tapping alternate palm and back.
- *Sensation*: test for sensory modalities light touch, vibration, and proprioception if history has sensory component or there are motor signs.

Cranial imaging

Cranial ultrasound scanning

Ultrasound scanning (USS) of the brain is well suited to the study of the brain in the perinatal period. It is operator dependent and requires the anterior fontanelle to be at least 1 cm across.

Cranial USS is useful in the diagnosis of:
- Hypoxic-ischaemic encephalopathy
- Intracranial haemorrhage or ischaemic injury
- Ventricular enlargement
- *Malformations*: gross malformations can be recognized but MRI is the definitive procedure for delineation of developmental abnormalities.

Neuroradiology: cranial CT

CT scanning is readily accessible and has the advantage that images can be generated in seconds. It is useful in:
- Unstable patients
- Acute head injury
- Detection of intracranial calcification.

Cranial CT scan provides useful information on haemorrhage, infarction, gross malformations, hydrocephalus, cerebral abscess, and vascular malformations. CT has poor resolution for lesions causing focal epilepsy. In particular, it has poor resolution in the posterior and temporal fossae and is unable to detect mesial temporal sclerosis.

Magnetic resonance imaging (MRI)

MRI avoids the use of ionizing radiation, provides improved soft tissue contrast and high anatomical resolution, and has multiplanar imaging capability including the sagittal plane.

A major disadvantage is that scanners are noisy and claustrophobic and a complete study may require immobility for >30 min, necessitating general anaesthesia or sedation in children <8 years. Developmental changes in myelination are important in the interpretation of images at different ages.

Changes in the acquisition parameters can 'weight' the signals and generate different image contrasts (Figure 7.3).

Commonly used MRI protocols
- *Axial T2 weighted*: CSF appears bright (high signal); optimal for detecting most brain pathology (Fig 7.3B)
- *Axial T1 weighted*: CSF appears dark (low signal); optimal for defining normal soft-tissue anatomy (Fig 7.3A)
- *FLAIR (fluid attenuated inversion recovery)*: T2 weighted with suppression of CSF signal. Free water, e.g. CSF, appears dark; optimal for imaging periventricular white matter and for white matter inflammation.

Special MRI protocols
- *Diffusion weighted imaging (DWI)*: detects cytotoxic oedema as seen in acute cerebral infarction
- *Contrast enhancement*: gadolinium enhanced tissues and fluids appear bright on T1 weighted images' optimal for detection of vascular lesions such as tumours and assessment of brain perfusion
- *MRA/V*: angiography/venography to evaluate blood flow and blood vessel abnormalities
- *T2**: used in functional MRI (fMRI) and to detect iron-breakdown products (haem sequence) for ageing of intracranial haemorrhage.

Scans in the axial, coronal, and sagittal planes are all viewed to characterize and locate lesions.

CT vs MRI
- CT is fast and better in trauma and emergencies. Better bone detail and high sensitivity for acute haemorrhage. Detects intracranial calcification.
- MRI best as elective procedure but may require anaesthesia or sedation. Excellent high resolution anatomical detail and multiplanar views. High sensitivity for brain water allows early detection of changes in white matter, infarction and infection (e.g. encephalitis). Best for defining congenital malformations and for posterior fossa disease.

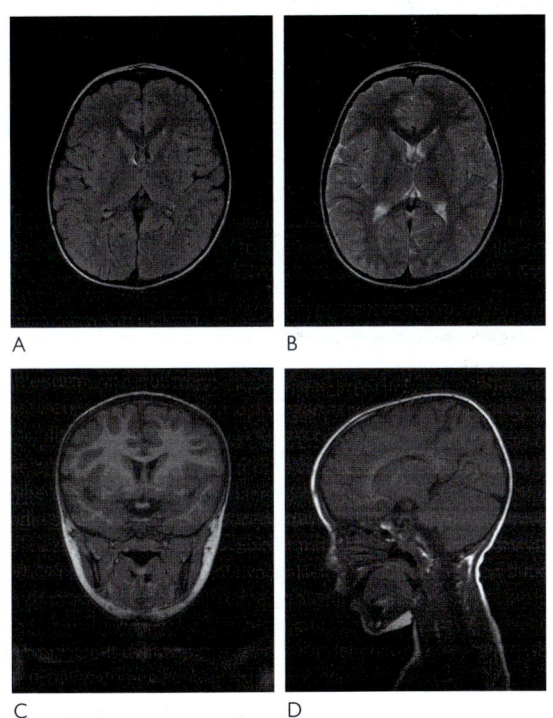

Fig 7.3 Cranial MRI: normal images.
A. Axial, T1 weighted.
B. Axial, T2 weighted.
C. Coronal, T1 weighted.
D. Sagittal, T1 weighted.

7.3 Neural tube defects and hydrocephalus

Neural tube defects (NTDs)

NTDs arise from failure of closure of the neural tube on or before 28 days gestation and encompass a range of malformations involving the brain or spinal cord and adjacent meninges, bones, and skin.

NTDs are amongst the most common birth defects causing death or serious disability. However, periconceptual folic acid supplementation and prenatal diagnosis reduced the incidence of NTDs in live births in the UK from 3.2 to 0.1/1000 between 1970 and 1997.

Aetiology and pathogenesis

Fusion of the edges of the neural groove starts cranially and progresses caudally, the anterior neuropore closing at about 25 days and the posterior neuropore closing at 27 days.

The causes of NTDs are multifactorial and include both genetic and environmental factors. Risk factors include:

- *Folic acid deficiency:* it is established that periconceptual folic acid supplementation can prevent some NTDs
- *Antiepilepsy drugs:* increased risk in pregnant women taking AEDs, sodium valproate, phenytoin or carbamazepine
- Maternal diabetes
- *Genetic factors:* a family history of NTDs increases risk.

Classification

Dysraphism is a synonym for NTD.

- *Cranial dysraphism*: anencephaly and encephalocele
- *Spinal dysraphism*:
  - spina bifida cystica: meningocele, myelomeningocele ± Chiari II malformation
  - spina bifida occulta
  - dorsal dermal sinus
  - diastematomyelia.

Anencephaly and encephalocele

The incidence is 1–3/10 000 live births. In anencephaly the cranial vault and cerebral hemispheres are absent. In encephalocele brain herniates through a defect in the skull.

Spina bifida cystica

- *Meningocele (5%)*: skin covered protrusion of meninges only.
- *Myelomeningoceles (90%)*: usually lumbosacral. In > 90% of cases there is an associated Chiari type II malformation: cerebellar hypoplasia, and displacement of hindbrain into cervical canal which causes hydrocephalus.

Spina bifida occulta

A defect of the posterior arch of one or more lumbar or sacral vertebrae, often L5 and S1. It may be associated with a naevus, hairy patch, dimple, sinus, or lipomyelomeningocole, and tethering of the spinal cord. Diastematomyelia refers to a complete or partial clefting of the spinal cord.

Antenatal screening

Antenatal screening detects 85% of NTDs. Maternal serum α-fetoprotein levels at 16–18 weeks are raised in anencephaly or spina bifida but may not detect closed defects and are less sensitive for women taking valproate.

USS is recommended for all at-risk women: positive serum α-fetoprotein, or previously affected child.

USS detects anencephaly from 12th week and spina bifida from 16–20 weeks. The 20 week anomaly scan will show ventriculomegaly, vertebral arch defects, and talipes. Amniocentesis to measure amniotic fluid α-fetoprotein and acetylcholinesterase (AChE) levels provides additional confirmation and MRI is increasingly used to define the lesion.

Postnatal management

Myelomeningocele

At birth, a midline defect in the posterior vertebrae with protrusion of the meninges and cord elements through an external sac is noted.

80% are lumbosacral. The neurological level is best determined by upper limit of sensory loss and may be higher than the anatomical level defined by MRI. At all levels there is a disturbance of bowel and bladder control. Hydrocephalus occurs in 90% of cases. It is usually associated with Chiari II malformation, but may also be due to aqueduct stenosis.

Management

MRI identifies contents of the defect and associated cranial malformations. CT scan allows visualization of the bony defect and anatomy.

The newborn with an open myelomeningocele should be positioned prone and the defect covered with a sterile saline dressing. Closure of the defect is usually done together with placement of a ventriculo-peritoneal shunt and administration of antibiotics.

Long-term management is multidisciplinary and requires attention to the many complications which occur as these patients survive into adult life:

- *Hydrocephalus*: VP shunt infections or blockage
- Cord tethering syndrome
- *Kyphoscoliosis*: may require spinal stabilization
- Trophic skin lesions
- Renal compromise secondary to neurogenic bladder is a leading cause of death after the 1st year of life
- Neuropathic bowel
- Cognitive impairment is common. Seizures in 10–30%.

Spina bifida occulta

Bony spiny bifida occulta at L5–S1 is a common incidental finding on radiographs and not usually associated with symptoms or signs. No action is necessary.

Cutaneous abnormalities such as dermal dimple, hairy patch, dermal sinus, or palpable lipoma may provide a clue to underlying spinal dysraphism. Newborns rarely exhibit neurological signs but symptoms and signs occur with growth as tension is put on the tethered cord.

Signs and symptoms may include lower limb pain and paraesthesia, bowel and bladder dysfunction, extended toilet training, recurrent UTIs, muscle weakness and gait disturbance, claw toes, pes cavus, and ankle rigidity. Early recognition is important as surgical intervention can prevent an irreversible neurological deficit and urological damage. Spinal MRI and urodynamic studies may be helpful.

Hydrocephalus

Hydrocephalus is a condition in which a disturbance of flow, absorption or formation of CSF leads to an increase in CSF pressure. The incidence of congenital hydrocephalus is about 3/1000 live births.

Classification and pathophysiology

Hydrocephalus is classified as:
- *Non-communicating/obstructive*: CSF flow is obstructed within the ventricular system or in its outlets to the arachnoid space. There is no communication between ventricular and subarachnoid space.
- *Communicating/non-obstructive*: full communication exists between ventricles and subarachnoid space. It is usually caused by defective absorption of CSF from arachnoid villi, rarely by overproduction of CSF from a choroid plexus papilloma or by foramen magnum and skull base malformations as occurs in Chiari II and achondroplasia.

Conditions such as cerebral atrophy lead to a vacant space which is filled passively by CSF. This is quite different, as CSF pressure is normal. Large subarachnoid spaces may be a normal appearance in infancy, or may occur in 'benign external hydrocephalus'.

Aetiology

Causes of hydrocephalus are congenital or acquired.

Congenital hydrocephalus
- *Malformations*:
  - *Aqueduct stenosis*: 10% neonatal cases
  - *Dandy–Walker malformation*: 2–4% neonatal cases with vermis hypoplasia and cystic dilatation of 4th ventricle
  - *Arnold–Chiari malformations I and II*: associated with NTDs
- *X-linked hydrocephalus*: including Bickers–Adams syndrome of aqueduct stenosis, mental retardation, thumb deformity
- Congenital toxoplasmosis.

Acquired hydrocephalus
- Intraventricular haemorrhage in preterm infants
- *Mass lesions*: posterior fossa tumours, cysts, abscesses
- *Infections*: bacterial meningitis
- Increased venous sinus pressure in achondroplasia, craniosynostosis, venous thrombosis
- *Iatrogenic*: hypervitaminosis A.

Clinical features

Infants
Symptoms include poor feeding, irritability, reduced activity, and vomiting. Examination reveals:
- *Progressive head enlargement*: the OFC crosses centile lines and may increase to >98th centile
- Tense anterior fontanelle, wide cranial sutures, and prominent scalp veins
- 'Setting sun' sign: caused by pressure on the mesencephalic tegmentum which paralyses upward gaze causing the eyes to deviate downwards and the upper lids to retract
- Increased limb tone: if stretching of pyramidal tract fibres causes lower limb spasticity.

The differential includes chronic subdural haemorrhage.

Children
Presentation is usually more acute and symptoms of raised intracranial pressure are dominant including headaches, initially in morning, vomiting, somnolence, and blurred or double vision. Spasticity may lead to difficulty in walking.
Examination may reveal a large head, papilloedema, failure of upward gaze, and unsteady gait due to ataxia or lower limb spasticity. Bradycardia, hypertension, and VI nerve palsies indicate severely raised ICP.

Management

Brain imaging options include cranial USS if fontanelle is open, cranial CT for acute assessment of ventricular size, and cranial MRI. MRI allows better definition of posterior fossa contents and evaluation of cerebral malformations.

Medical treatment
Medical treatment with diuretics and repeated lumbar puncture is used in preterm infants with posthaemorrhagic hydrocephalus. Normal CSF reabsorption may resume spontaneously.

Surgical treatment
Surgical intervention is required in most cases. Ventriculo-peritoneal shunting is the most common procedure. A silastic tube is placed into the ventricles to drain the CSF into the peritoneal cavity. Shunts may become blocked, infected, or outgrown. In addition, over drainage can cause problems from low-pressure symptoms including headaches and listlessness with slit-like ventricles on CT. Endoscopic 3rd ventriculostomy is an option in selected patients and avoids risks of infection and over-drainage.

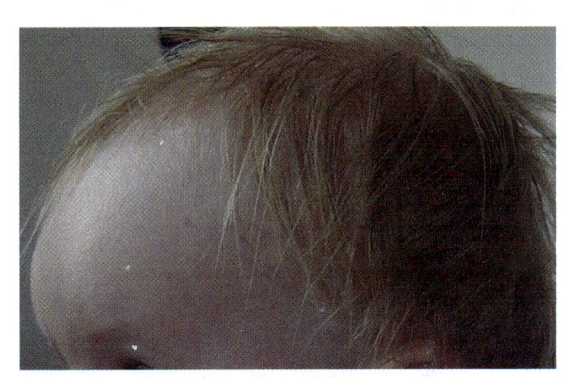

Fig 7.4 Enlarged skull vault in hydrocephalus.

7.4 Cortical and cranial vault malformations

Cortical malformations

Brain MRI and molecular genetic analysis have revolutionised understanding of this group of uncommon genetic disorders which cause developmental delay, cognitive impairment, and epilepsy.

A simple classification is based on the stage at which cortical development is first affected:

- Cell proliferation or survival
- Neuronal migration
- Cortical organization.

Disorders of neuronal proliferation or survival

Microcephaly

- A condition in which the brain fails to grow normally. The occipitofrontal circumference is less than 2 SD below the mean
- At least six genes (*MCPH1–6*) for autosomal recessive microcephaly have been identified
- Disorders of apoptosis are implicated in some cases of microcephaly and megalencephaly.

Disorders of neuronal migration

These include the lissencephalies (literally 'smooth brain') and heterotopias. Three main groups exist:

Lissencephaly/subcortical band heterotopia spectrum

Classical Type I lissencephaly is caused by two genes:

- *LIS1*: on chromosome 17p; large deletions cause Miller–Dieker syndrome (MDS) whereas small deletions or mutations cause isolated lissencephaly sequence (ILS)
- *DCX*: on chromosome Xq, encoding doublecortin. Inheritance is X-linked dominant. Females have subcortical band heterotopia or double cortex associated with epilepsy and cognitive defect. Hemizygous males have severe lissencephaly (Fig 7.5).

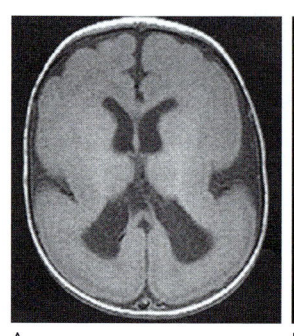

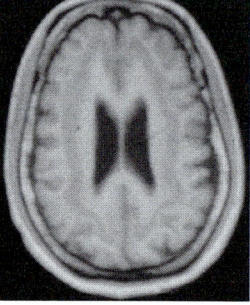

Fig 7.5 Cortical malformations: T1 weighted axial MRI.
A. Male: lissencephaly. B. Female: double cortex.

Periventricular nodular heterotopia (PNH)

Clusters of neurons fail to migrate out of the ventricular regions and form neuronal nodules along the walls of the lateral ventricles (Fig 7.6). Caused by defects in the filamin A gene, *FLNA*. Inheritance is X-linked dominant. Females have epilepsy with normal cognitive function, whereas hemizygous males almost invariably die in utero.

LIS1, *DLX*, and *FLNA* all encode proteins which are part of the cytoskeleton important in regulation of cell motility.

Cobblestone dysplasia (type II lissencephaly)

Over-migration of neurons occurs through the pial surface onto the outside of the brain causing a nodular ('cobblestone') appearance. Three rare autosomal recessive (AR) disorders in which muscular dystrophy and eye abnormalities also occur are:

- Fukuyama-type congenital muscular dystrophy (FCMD)
- Muscle–eye–brain disease (MEB)
- Walker–Warburg syndrome (WWS).

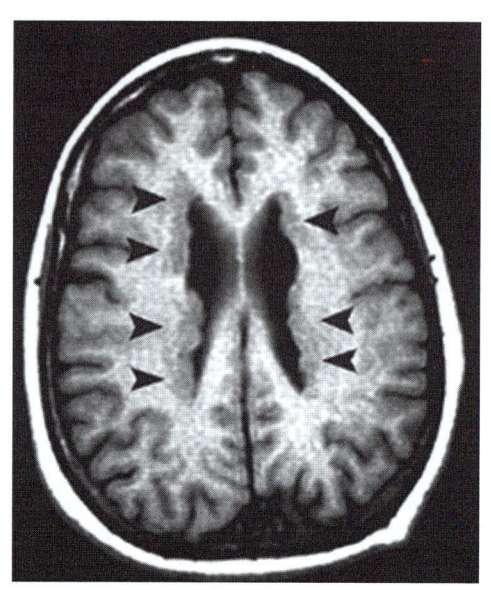

Fig 7.6 Periventricular nodular heterotopia.

The underlying genes all have a role in dystroglycan metabolism, disruption of which disturbs the integrity of the pial surface and the function of skeletal muscle.

Disorders of cortical organization

These include polymicrogyria, schizencephaly, and cortical dysplasias.

- *Polymicrogyria* is characterized by small, irregular and crowded gyri. It may be caused by cytomegalovirus infection or ischaemia as well as 22q11 deletions.
- *Cortical dysplasias* may be focal or widespread and may include giant neurons and glial cells together with embryonic cells and structures.

Cranial vault abnormalities

Normal skull development

At birth the human skull is made up of 45 separate bony elements. The bones of the cranial vault are separated by regions of dense connective tissue, the cranial sutures and fontanelles (Fig 7.7). Ossification of the cranial vault starts in the central region of each bone and extends outwards toward the sutures. The posterior fontanelle closes by 8 weeks and the anterior fontanelle by 12–18 months.

Fig 7.7 Normal newborn skull.

Craniosynostosis

The incidence is about 0.5/1000 live births. In craniosynostosis there is premature fusion of one or more cranial sutures causing problems with brain and skull growth and leading to an abnormal head size and shape.

A quite different and more common cause of abnormal head shape is deformational plagiocephaly (Fig 7.8B). This has become more common since the supine sleeping position ('back to sleep') has been recommended.

Classification
Craniosynostosis is classified as:
- *Primary craniosynostosis*: primary defect of ossification
- *Secondary craniosynostosis*: secondary to failure of brain growth. In microcephaly there is premature fusion of all sutures with normal ICP.

Primary craniosynostosis
Primary genetic craniosynostosis may be syndromic (in 20%) or non-syndromic.

Over 100 syndromes are associated with craniosynostosis, the most common of which are those caused by mutations in fibroblast growth factor receptor (*FGFR*) genes: Crouzon, Apert, and Pfeiffer syndromes.

Multiple suture fusion generates characteristic facial features, and there may be associated limb, ear, or cardiovascular abnormalities.

Premature fusion of specific sutures creates characteristic alterations in head shape (Fig 7.8) as skull growth is restricted in the plane perpendicular to the fused suture and enhanced in the parallel plane.
- *Metopic*: Trigonocephaly, narrow pointed forehead
- *Sagittal*: Scaphocephaly, elongated, narrow skull
- *Bicoronal*: Brachycephaly, short, broad skull
- *Unicoronal*: Plagiocephaly-anterior, unilateral flattening
- *Unilambdoid*: Plagiocephaly-posterior, unilateral flattening
- *Multiple*: Acrocephaly, high pointed head, syndromic.

In primary multiple craniosynostosis, ICP may be elevated.

Clinical features
Abnormal head shapes in babies are common and deformational plagiocephaly caused by repetitive sleep positioning is much more common than craniosynostosis. Craniosynostosis may be evident from birth or may present later on account of abnormal head size or shape, symptoms of raised ICP, or neurodevelopmental delay.
Examination should include:
- Measurement of OFC
- Palpation for tense fontanelle or suture ridges
- Evaluation of ICP
- *Syndrome recognition*: syndactyly, extra digits.

The differential diagnosis includes rickets. Vitamin D deficiency may cause frontal bossing and hypocalcaemia with raised ICP.

Management
Skull radiograph with AP and lateral views identifies premature suture fusion as increased density. Cranial CT with 3D reconstruction may be performed if surgery is considered.

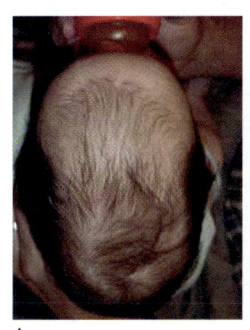

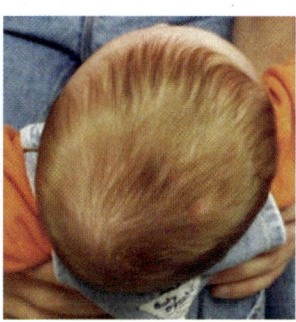

Fig 7.8 Abnormal head shapes: A. Scaphocephaly (or dolichocephaly). B. Plagiocephaly (positional). Image reprinted with permission from eMedicine.com. 2008. Available at: www.emedicine.com.

Treatment
Surgery may be recommended for increased ICP or cosmetic reasons. Optimal timing depends on severity but is usually performed before age 1 year. Positional plagiocephaly does not require surgery and is treated with repositioning manoeuvres.

Abnormal head size

Microcephaly
A small head may be caused by:

Failure of brain growth
- *Genetic*:
  - autosomal recessive microcephaly
  - *syndromic*: trisomy 21, 13, 18
- *Acquired*:
  - *prenatal insults*: congenital infection, maternal alcohol ingestion, maternal PKU, maternal iodine deficiency
  - *postnatal insults*: hypoxic-ischaemic insults, meningitis.

Craniosynostosis
Useful investigations include karyotype, TORCH screen, cranial MRI, and metabolic screen.

Macrocephaly
Causes of a large head include:
- Hydrocephalus
- Chronic subdural haematomas
- *Megalencephaly*: a big brain
  - benign familial macrocephaly
  - *neurocutaneous syndromes*: tuberous sclerosis, neurofibromatosis type 1
  - *neurometabolic disorders*: mucopolysaccharidosis, glutaric aciduria type I, Canavan disease
  - *overgrowth syndromes*: Sotos, Weaver
- *Thick skull bones*:
  - achondroplasia
  - *haemolytic anaemia*: thalassaemia.

7.5 Neurodegenerative disorders

Global developmental delay may be the result of a static condition of the CNS or a progressive neurodegenerative disorder. The recognition of a progressive disorder may be difficult, especially in the young child <4 years. In early-onset neurodegenerative disease the progressive pathology manifests as developmental delay rather than loss of acquired skills and a period of normal development may be difficult to demonstrate. In later-onset conditions a progressive neurodegenerative disorder is easier to identify.

Aetiology and pathogenesis

A definitive aetiology is more likely to become apparent in moderate to severe global delay or clear-cut progressive neurodegeneration with specific neurological abnormalities. Acquired causes are usually static. Genetic disorders may cause developmental delay or neurodegeneration.

The neurodegenerative disorders encompass a large group of genetic disorders with an overall incidence of 0.6/1000 live births. Inheritance is usually autosomal recessive so risk is greatly increased by consanguinity. Many therefore are inborn errors of metabolism (see Chapter 11) which affect the nervous system. Clinically, these disorders are usefully classified into:

- *Grey matter disorders*: affecting the cortex, with cognitive decline and seizures
- *White matter disorders*: the leucodystrophies, with prominent motor signs and according to age of onset.

Grey matter disorders

- Neuronal ceroid lipofuscinoses, Batten disease
- Mucopolysaccharidoses, e.g. MPSIII, San Filippo
- Sphingolipodoses
  - GM2 gangliosidoses: Tay–Sachs, Sandhoff
  - GM1 gangliosidosis
- Leigh disease (see Chapter 11.5)
- Mitochondrial disorders
- Rett syndrome (Chapter 12.9)

White matter disorders

Genetic leukodystrophies

A diverse group including lysosomal storage, peroxisomal, and organic acid disorders. Features of the more important are:

- *Krabbe disease*: AR defect in galactocerebrosidase. Globoid cells (macrophages with undegraded galactolipids) are found. Early onset with severe spasticity, irritability, and delay.
- *Metachromatic leukodystrophy (MLD)*: a defect in arylsulfatase. Presents in the 2nd year with regression, peripheral neuropathy, and then later hypotonia.
- *Adrenoleukodystrophy (X-ALD)*: (see Chapter 11.5) Mutations in *ABCD1* gene leads to accumulation of very long chain fatty acids (VLCFAs) in all tissues. Cerebral form has onset age 5–10 years with behavioural and cognitive decline followed by abnormal gait. Measurement of VLCFAs is diagnostic. Bone marrow transplantation is beneficial in early, presymptomatic patients.

Rarer forms include:

- *Alexander disease*: sporadic mutations in *GFAP* gene encoding glial fibrillary acidic protein, component of astrocyte intermediary filament. Presents in 1st year with megalencephaly and hypotonia.
- *Pelizaeus–Merzbacher syndrome*: X-linked recessive. Mutations in *PLP1* gene encoding proteolipid protein. Early onset hypotonia, spasticity, and nystagmus with diffuse, symmetrical demyelination.
- *Canavan disease*: AR mutations in gene encoding aspartoacylase. N-Acetylaspartate accumulates and is found in urine. Hypotonia and megalencephaly with 'spongy degeneration' of brain.

Acquired white matter disease

- *Toxic*: lead poisoning, drugs
- *Nutritional*: thiamine deficiency, B12 deficiency
- *Infective*:
  - AIDS encephalopathy
  - subacute sclerosing panencephalitis
  - Creutzfeld–Jacob disease
- *Inflammatory*: acute disseminated encephalomyelitis.

Clinical evaluation

History

The history should establish:

- *Age of onset*: infantile, late infantile or juvenile
- *Development*: static or regressive
- Global or specific developmental delay
- *Family history*: consanguinity, unexplained death
- *Previous history*: acquired brain insults such as perinatal hypoxia, intracranial infection
- *Seizures*: suggests grey matter disorder.

Examination

Developmental assessment is considered in Chapter 18. General examination may identify:

- *Dysmorphic features*: specific syndromes
- *Cutaneous stigmata*: neurocutaneous syndromes
- *Hepatosplenomegaly*: storage disorders.

Neurological examination is focused on:

- *Head size*: microcephaly or macrocephaly in Alexander and Canavan disease
- *Fundi*: cherry red spot (Fig 7.9), retinitis pigmentosa, optic atrophy
- *Pyramidal tract signs/spasticity*: white matter disorder
- *Cognitive impairment/seizures*: grey matter disorder.

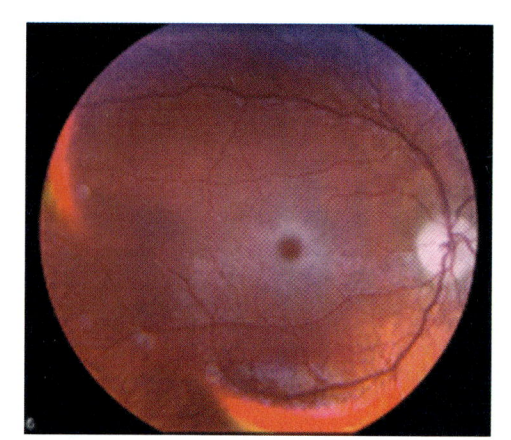

Fig 7.9 Tay–Sachs disease: cherry red spot. National Eye Institute, National Institutes of Health (NEI/NIH).

Management
Investigations
A diagnosis is made in about 75% of children with a neurodegenerative disorder. Investigations are guided by clinical suspicion. Useful investigations include:
- *Cranial MRI*: identifies cortical malformations and leucodystrophies
- *Neurophysiology*: EEG, ERG, and VEP. Useful in diagnosis of neuronal ceroid lipofuscinoses
- *White cell enzymes*: lysosomal enzymes can be measured in peripheral blood white cells (MLD, Krabbe disease)
- *Genetic analysis*: karyotype, FISH, DNA analysis, mitochondrial DNA deletions and mutations
- *Biochemistry*: plasma amino acids, lactate, ammonia, urine amino acids, organic acids, glycosaminoglycans
- Vacuolated lymphocytes are a hallmark of Batten disease (juvenile neuronal ceroid lipofuscinosis)
- *Muscle biopsy*: respiratory chain enzyme analysis for mitochondrial disorders, VLCFA; peroxisomal disorders.

A specific diagnosis is important even if no specific treatment is available for what may be a severe, debilitating, and fatal disorder. The benefits of diagnosis include:
- *Genetic counselling*: risk of recurrence and prenatal diagnosis
- *Prognosis*: improved accuracy
- *Contact with support groups:* in the UK, Contact a Family, CLIMB
- *Specific treatment*: available for some disorders including enzyme replacement therapy, bone marrow transplant, and substrate reduction therapy.

Management of the child with global delay or neurodegeneration associated with severe neurodisability is multidisciplinary.

7.6 The cerebral palsies

The cerebral palsies (CP) are disorders of movement or posture caused by a non-progressive defect or injury to the developing brain. The CPs are the most common cause of neurodisability in childhood with a prevalence of 2–3/1000 live births.

The term cerebral palsy emphasizes the motor deficit, but associated problems of vision, hearing, and cognitive function are common. Although the cerebral lesion is static, the manifestations evolve with age.

Aetiology and pathogenesis

Aetiology

Cerebral palsies are not only caused by problems arising during birth. In infants born at term the cause is prenatal in 75%. However, about 20% of children with CP were born preterm and perinatal factors are important in 90% of these.

Causal mechanisms by which the developing brain may be damaged are well recognized and include hypoxia–ischaemia, bilirubin toxicity, infection, and inflammation. In addition, a host of risk factors are recognized such as socio-economic disadvantage and multiple pregnancy which may exert their effect through multiple causal pathways.

It is useful to categorize causes of the CPs into prenatal, intrapartum, postnatal, and postneonatal.

Prenatal
- *Brain malformations*: chromosomal and genetic disorders of neuronal proliferation or migration
- *Intrauterine infections*: TORCH infections
- *Maternal factors*: e.g. iodine deficiency
- *Multiple pregnancy*: as a risk factor this increases likelihood of low birthweight and preterm birth. A co-twin fetal death increases likelihood of CP in the survivor, especially if monozygotic
- *Chorio-amnionitis*: ascending infection may trigger a fetal immune response causing inflammation which damages the fetal brain and initiates premature labour
- Placental insufficiency
- *Idiopathic*: e.g. cerebral vascular infarction.

Intrapartum
- *Birth asphyxia*: perinatal hypoxic–ischaemic brain damage accounts for 15% of cases of CP in infants born at term, although it is often difficult to exclude a contribution from prenatal factors. Intrapartum insults sufficient to compromise cerebral perfusion and oxygen delivery cause severe fetal acidosis, and bradycardia requiring postnatal resuscitation and subsequent hypoxic–ischaemic encephalopathy.

Postnatal
- *Preterm birth*: 20% of children with CP were born at <32 weeks gestation and 4–8% of survivors of ≤32 weeks delivery develop a CP. At 26–34 weeks gestation the periventricular white matter is most vulnerable to injury either from hypoperfusion or secondary to intraventricular haemorrhage
- Bilirubin encephalopathy
- Hypoglycaemia.

Postneonatal
- Intracranial infection (meningitis, encephalitis), traumatic brain injury (accidental and inflicted), post cardiopulmonary arrest, arterial ischaemic or haemorrhagic stroke.

Pathogenesis: patterns of brain injury

Specific aetiological insults result in recognizable patterns of brain injury which may determine the clinical category of CP that subsequently develops. The following classification is commonly used, but mixed varieties are common.

Spastic CP

Spastic diplegia (44%)
Lower limbs predominantly affected with variable but lesser involvement of upper limbs. 65% occur in preterm infants caused by damage to periventricular white matter which carries the fibres for motor control of lower limbs.

Spastic quadriplegia (7%)
Severe spasticity of all four limbs, usually worse in upper limbs and associated with severe cognitive defect. Associated with severe, prolonged intrapartum asphyxia in term infants.

Spastic hemiplegia (34%)
Upper limb predominant. 20% preterm and 80% term. Unilateral infarction of middle cerebral artery territory.

Dyskinetic CP

Selective damage to basal ganglia may occur in term infants with severe, short-lived asphyxia, leading to athetoid CP. Choreoathetosis associated with bilirubin encephalopathy and kernicterus is now rare. Cognition is often preserved in athetoid CP.

Ataxic CP

Most of these infants are born at term and have genetic disorders, often associated with cerebellar hypoplasia.

Multi-axial classification

This facilitates communication, guides investigations, and aids prognosis.

Axes of classification
- *Types of movement disorder*: record presence of spasticity, dystonia, dyskinesia, athetosis, hyperkinesia, ataxia, hypotonia
- *Pattern of anatomical involvement*: identify involvement of head, trunk, limbs; degree of symmetry. Classical patterns are simple but limited: monoplegia, hemiplegia, diplegia, quadriparesis/total body involvement, orobuccopharyngeal palsy (Worster–Drought)
- *Severity of motor impairment*: spasticity, strength, fixed contractures, and coordination
- *Co-morbidities*: neurological and systemic problem list: learning disability; epilepsy; visual impairment; chest infections
- *Functional abilities of daily living*: standard measurement tools are available
- *Known aetiologies and risk factors*: nature and timing; prenatal, perinatal, or postnatal/neonatal
- *Known neuroimaging findings*: white matter injury, cerebral malformations, etc.

Clinical features

About 50% of these children are diagnosed during follow-up of at-risk infants from the neonatal unit. The remainder may present on account of parental concern or be detected from routine developmental surveillance.

History
Presenting features depend on the nature and severity of the CP but may include:
- Delayed motor milestones
- *Early hand preference*: before 18 months.
- *Feeding problems*: may be first sign of severe CP
- Undue lethargy (the 'good' baby) or irritability
- Toe walking, speech delay, seizures.

If a CP is suspected, a detailed perinatal and family history should be taken to identify any risk factors.

Examination
Diagnosis is based on persistent motor abnormalities and often cannot be confirmed until 1 or 2 years of age. Many infants show transient abnormalities, such as hypertonia and brisk reflexes, which later resolve.

Examination is directed towards detecting any motor abnormalities and to evaluating their pattern and severity together with that of any associated deficits.
- *General examination*: dysmorphic features, length and weight, head circumference.
- *Neurological examination of motor system*:
  - *tone*: hypotonia or hypertonia with increased reflexes and sustained clonus may be apparent. Dystonia may be associated with rigidity (velocity-independent resistance) and increased resistance
  - *movements*: abnormal involuntary movements such as spasm or athetosis may only be evident in 2nd year. Lack of movement in lower limbs is an early sign of diplegia. Asymmetry may indicate hemiplegia
  - *posture*: poor head control is evident in severe CP. Persistent thumb adduction, fisting, or leg scissoring may be apparent. Trunk control is poor in severe CP causing delay in sitting alone and standing
  - *gait*: in ambulant children. asymmetry in hemiplegia, toe walking in spastic diplegia
  - *primitive reflexes*: persistence of grasp reflex beyond 4 months and Moro beyond 6 months.
- *Developmental assessment*: this depends on age but should encompass assessment of social interaction, language, vision, and hearing.

Management

Investigations
To determine aetiology and exclude alternative diagnoses, investigations may include:
- *Karyotyping*: to identify chromosomal abnormalities
- *TORCH screen*: congenital infections
- *Metabolic*: plasma amino acids, urine amino and organic acids
- *Brain imaging*:
  - *cranial USS*: helpful in early neonatal period, especially in unstable infants; can identify haemorrhage, hypoxic-ischaemic injury, or major structural abnormalities
  - *cranial CT*: identifies some congenital malformations, haemorrhage, periventricular leucomalacia
  - *cranial MRI*: optimal modality for older infants as it defines cortical and white matter abnormalities and myelination at high resolution
- Normal brain imaging does not exclude CP but suggests pursuit of a metabolic or genetic aetiology.
- EEG if seizures are suspected.

Treatment
There is no cure for CP as brain damage cannot be repaired. A multidisciplinary approach is implemented to reduce the impact, relieve symptoms, and improve prognosis: physiotherapy, speech and language therapy, medication, surgery, nutritional and respiratory support, and learning support.

Physiotherapy
An interdisciplinary assessment of motor impairment and function is made involving physiotherapists, occupational therapists and orthopaedic surgeons.
Analysis of video recordings may aid decision-making. Measurement scales are available to quantify motor impairment (Ashworth and Tardieu scales), dystonia (Barry–Albright scale) and mobility. The aim of physiotherapy is to retain and improve function and preserve muscle length.

Speech and language therapy
Oromotor dysfunction may limit feeding in infants and subsequently affect development of speech and language.

Medication
- *Spasticity*: baclofen, benzodiazepines, dantrolene. Botulinum toxin has a temporary effect for 3–6 months by weakening specific muscles and can reduce contractures and aid physiotherapy
- *Seizures*: antiepileptic drugs
- *Athetosis/dystonia*: antiparkinsonian drugs
- *Anticholinergics*: excessive salivation
- *Melatonin*: sleep disturbance

Surgery
- *Orthopaedic surgery* may be necessary in the management of hip dislocation, scoliosis, and contractures (e.g. tenotomy, tendon transfers)
- *Neurosurgery* is required for treatment of hydrocephalus, administration of intrathecal baclofen, or selective dorsal rhizotomy in severe spastic diplegia.

Nutritional and respiratory support
In severe CP feeding via a gastrostomy tube may be necessary and respiratory sequelae are common.

Learning support
A team specializing in children with special needs provides focused support. Many patients with CP have normal or above normal intelligence, but full expression of intellectual capacity is limited by severe motor impairment.

7.7 Childhood epilepsies: diagnosis and management

Paroxysmal disorders

A paroxysmal disorder is one in which normal good health is punctuated by episodes of illness. The most common neurological paroxysmal disorder is epilepsy, but in children there are a number of *non-epileptic* paroxysmal disorders from which epilepsy must be distinguished.

Paroxysmal disorders are sometimes grouped together as *'fits, faints, and funny turns'*. The important point is that not all paroxysmal episodes are epileptic seizures.

Definitions: seizures and epilepsy

Epileptic seizure

An epileptic seizure is a transient episode of abnormal, excessive neuronal activity in the cerebral cortex apparent to the subject or an observer. Synonyms include 'fit' and 'ictus'.

Note that an epileptic seizure does not necessarily involve either altered consciousness or abnormal motor activity.

Epilepsy

Epilepsy is a chronic brain disorder characterized by recurrent, usually unprovoked, epileptic seizures.

A single epileptic seizure does **not** make a diagnosis of epilepsy. Epileptic seizures may be provoked in young children by a host of different cerebral insults such as hypoxia, hypoglycaemia, electrolyte imbalance, fever, and meningitis. Provoked epileptic seizures can occur in any child and their occurrence does not make a diagnosis of epilepsy.

Of course, a patient with epilepsy may *on occasion* have epileptic seizures which are provoked for example by sleep deprivation or photic stimuli.

Clinical evaluation

Most children present with a history of one or more paroxysmal episodes, the nature of which must be judged from often incomplete reports of witnesses. A minority present during an actual episode which can be directly observed. A careful history is therefore often the most important component of clinical evaluation and seeks to answer the following questions:

- Are the paroxysmal episodes 'epileptic seizures'?
- If so, are they unprovoked and what seizure type are they?
- Does the child have epilepsy, i.e. recurrent, unprovoked epileptic seizures?
- If so, can the epilepsy or epilepsy syndrome be defined?

A patient may experience several different seizure types at different times but have a single epilepsy syndrome diagnosis.

History

A description of the paroxysmal episodes is obtained from witnesses and sometimes from the child. It should include:

- *Features of the episode*: loss of awareness, colour change, abnormal movements, duration
- *Preceding events*: time of day or night, relationship to sleep, provoking factors such as sleep deprivation, photic stimulation, warning prodrome, or aura
- *Post-episode events*: rate of recovery, period of reduced consciousness, so called postictal drowsiness, focal weakness
- *Frequency and variation*: several seizure types may occur.

Knowledge of the range of epilepsy seizure types (see below) and non-epileptic paroxysmal disorders which occur at different ages should allow a judgement as to whether the episodes are epileptic seizures or not and if so, which type.

The alternative diagnosis of a non-epileptic paroxysmal disorder includes the following conditions at different ages. Some of these conditions are considered elsewhere.

Infancy

- *Benign myoclonus*: brief bursts of jerks not involving the face may occur when the infant is awake or only during sleep. Development and the EEG are normal
- *Jitteriness*: a tremor with alternating movements of equal rate and amplitude observed in newborns and easily stopped by passive flexing
- *Gastro-oesophageal reflux disease (GORD):* writhing movements and opisthotonic posturing may occur.

Toddlers

- *Blue breath-holding attacks*: provoked by pain or frustration the angry child cries vigorously, remains in end-expiratory apnoea, turns blue, becomes limp, and loses consciousness for several seconds. Brief stiffening and clonic jerking occur followed by rapid recovery. No investigation or treatment is required.
- *Reflex anoxic seizures or pallid syncope*: provoked by fright or injury, there may be a brief cry followed by pallor and loss of consciousness caused by bradycardia or asystole. Stiffening or clonic jerks may occur followed by rapid recovery. Drug treatment with atropine to reduce vagal responsiveness is rarely required for very frequent or severe episodes.
- Benign paroxysmal torticollis/vertigo.

Childhood

- *Daydreaming*: inattentiveness and staring in tired or bored children are often mistaken for absence seizures
- *Night terrors*: the child screams and appears terrified but is not awake and cannot recall the episode
- *Sleepwalking*: with semi-purposeful behaviour.

Adolescence

- *Vasovagal syncope or faint*: common, especially in females. Simple faints are usually provoked by prolonged standing or heat and preceded by a feeling of dizziness or faintness. Pallor and clamminess is followed by sudden loss of posture and consciousness. Stiffness, urinary incontinence in 10%, and tonic-clonic movements in 75% may all occur. Syncope on exercise raises suspicion of a cardiac cause.
- *Pseudo-epileptic seizures or non-epileptic attack disorder*: briefer and less stereotyped than epileptic seizures, the patient may mimic unconsciousness by holding eyes tight shut. Movements are sometimes bizarre, such as pelvic thrusting and flailing, and wax and wane before suddenly stopping. There is no tongue biting, postictal drowsiness, or rise in prolactin levels. More common in females and may coexist with epileptic seizures.

Examination

The majority of children with epilepsy have an idiopathic generalized epilepsy and physical examination is normal. In a minority physical examination provides important clues to diagnosis. Important signs may include:

General examination
Cutaneous stigmata of neurocutaneous syndromes associated with epilepsy: hypopigmented macules in tuberous sclerosis, café-au-lait spots in neurofibromatosis, and port wine stain in Sturge–Weber syndrome. Dysmorphic features of syndromes associated with epilepsy, e.g. Fragile X.

Neurological examination
Focal neurological signs, signs of raised ICP, and examination of the fundi for signs associated with neurogenetic disorders such as retinitis pigmentosa, optic atrophy or 'cherry red' spot may provide clues to an underlying diagnosis. Developmental assessment is important, as delay is a common feature of the symptomatic epilepsies.

Management

Investigations
Special investigations including EEG and brain imaging may be necessary in some children in order to define the epilepsy syndrome and identify any underlying aetiology. Epilepsy remains a clinical diagnosis.

Electroencephalogram (EEG)
Routine EEG recordings are made from about 20 electrodes placed at standard positions on the head and identified by letters and numbers.

The normal EEG pattern evolves and matures from birth to adulthood. A posterior dominant rhythm appears at age 3 months. Theta activity at 4–8 Hz and delta activity at <4 Hz occur in the 1st month of life, and delta activity is dominant by 1 year. By 8 years of age this increases to reach α rhythm frequency at 8–12 Hz during wakefulness.

Electroencephalography is not a 'diagnostic' test for epilepsy. The routine EEG rarely captures ictal episodes. Methods of activation to enhance paroxysmal features include hyperventilation and intermittent photic stimulation. Video-EEG recording is useful for characterization of seizures and ambulatory EEG monitoring for 24 h periods may be useful in differentiating epileptic from non-epileptic episodes.

The EEG is useful for:
- *Aiding clinical diagnosis:* but note that 15% of normal children show non-specific EEG abnormalities and up to 2% have 'epileptiform' activity. Up to 50% of children with epilepsy have a normal routine, interictal EEG
- *Identification of epilepsy type or syndrome:* certain syndromes include EEG features in their diagnostic criteria, e.g. infantile spasms, absence epilepsy
- *Identification of structural brain lesion or neurodegenerative disorder.:* focal abnormalities may indicate a structural lesion such as a tumour. Some neurodegenerative disorders have characteristic EEG changes
- *Monitoring response to treatment:* in absence epilepsy, non-convulsive status, and West syndrome
- *Presurgical evaluation:* depth or brain surface recordings may be useful to define an epileptogenic focus.

Neuroimaging
Brain imaging is not indicated in children with a diagnosis of idiopathic generalized epilepsy, simple febrile seizures, or benign focal childhood epilepsy. It is indicated in children with neurocutaneous syndromes, focal seizures or focal neurological signs, neurodevelopmental regression and in infants < 12 months with infantile spasms, complicated febrile seizures, or intractable seizures of unknown aetiology.

MRI is preferred. It is more sensitive in the detection of subtle malformations and can detect mesial temporal sclerosis with high sensitivity (97%).
Single photon emission computed tomography (SPECT), positron emission tomography (PET), and fMRI are used in evaluation for epilepsy surgery.
Genetic/metabolic investigations may be indicated, especially in infants with epilepsy.

Treatment
Standard antiepilepsy drugs are the mainstay of treatment but education is also important. Additional treatment options in selected patients include surgery, steroids, a ketogenic diet, and vagal nerve stimulation.

Antiepilepsy drugs (AEDs)
AED medication is not indicated after a single, brief generalized tonic-clonic seizure or for infrequent minor seizures.

Monotherapy is the ideal. The dose is increased gradually until seizures are controlled or adverse effects become unacceptable. It is usually preferable to try alternative monotherapy before combination treatment. Withdrawal of first drug is done slowly when the new drug is at full dosage.

AEDs are categorized as first line, second line, and new AEDs.
- *First line*:
    - *sodium valproate:* first line therapy for generalized epilepsies including those with generalized tonic-clonic, absence and myoclonic seizures. Side effects include increased appetite and transitory hair loss. It is best avoided in women of childbearing age because of the risk in pregnancy
    - *carbamazepine:* is effective against focal seizures. It is also effective in treatment of generalized tonic-clonic seizures (GTCS) but may exacerbate myoclonic and typical absence seizures
    - *phenobarbital:* most commonly used drug for short-term control of neonatal seizures
    - *phenytoin:* used IV in convulsive status epilepticus and in neonatal seizures.
- *Second line*: ethosuximide is useful in intractable absence seizures, clobazam in partial or generalized seizures.
- *Newer AEDs*: lamotrigine, topiramate, levetiracetam, and vigabatrin. Lamotrigine is an alternative for generalized and partial seizures but may cause serious skin rashes. Vigabatrin is used as monotherapy in West syndrome but use is limited by visual field defects. Topiramate and levetiracetam may be used as adjunctive treatment.

When to stop: generally after seizure-free period of 2–3 years depending on epilepsy syndrome.

Education
Child and family need an explanation of epilepsy in lay terms and need to understand the prognosis and the importance of regular medication. Minimal restriction is the aim, but for the patient with generalised tonic clonic seizures (GTCS) it is wise to avoid unsupervised swimming or domestic baths, horse riding, and cycling.

7.8 Childhood epilepsies: causes and classification

Aetiology and pathogenesis

Epileptic seizures arise from an imbalance between excitatory and inhibitory influences causing neuronal hyperexcitability. Epilepsy may be associated with almost any cerebral pathology in which the normal pattern of neuronal connections is disturbed, or in which neuronal function is abnormal.

A genetic aetiology is present in ~50% of children with epilepsy, including those with 'idiopathic' epilepsy. In the rest, epilepsy is acquired and caused by:

- *Infections:* 10% of children develop epilepsy after meningitis, 20% after encephalitis
- *Head injury:* overall risk is 5% and is higher with focal damage
- *Hypoxic–ischaemic injury:* epilepsy complicates cerebral palsy due to HIE in a minority of about 20%
- *Brain tumours:* 10% present with seizures
- *Prolonged seizures:* there is an association between prolonged febrile seizures and hippocampal atrophy/mesial temporal sclerosis with temporal lobe epilepsy.

Genetics of epilepsy

Three genetic mechanisms can cause epilepsy:

- *Chromosomal anomalies:* ring chromosomes 14 and 20, trisomy 21, fragile X syndrome
- *Single-gene disorders:* over 200 monogenic disorders include epilepsy as part of the phenotype. Some rare monogenic epilepsies are caused by mutations in ion channel genes encoding voltage-gated or ligand-gated ion channels
- *'Complex' multifactorial traits:* the majority of patients with genetic epilepsy have a familial epilepsy syndrome which segregates as a complex polygenic trait.

Classification

Epileptic seizures and epilepsies are classified separately. Classification systems are evolving under the auspices of the International League against Epilepsy.

Epileptic seizures

The first division is into generalized or focal.

Generalized epileptic seizures

A generalized epileptic seizure is one in which abnormal activity occurs in both cerebral hemispheres from the onset of the seizure. Different subtypes include:

- *Tonic-clonic seizures (GTCS):* involuntary muscle contractions occur which may be sustained (tonic) or interrupted (clonic). Synonyms include 'convulsion' and 'grand-mal seizure' (a term best avoided). Tonic or clonic seizures may occur, as well as tonic-clonic.
- *Absence seizures:* a brief, 10–30 s loss of consciousness with staring and unresponsiveness but no loss of posture.
- *Myoclonic seizures:* brief, muscular contractions that occur singly or are repeated a few times. Consciousness is not altered.
- *Astatic (atonic) seizures, 'drop attacks':* a sudden brief reduction in muscle tone causing loss of posture.

Focal epileptic seizures

A focal seizure is one in which abnormal activity is initially confined to one part of the brain. 'Partial', 'local', or 'localized' are synonyms. Classification is into *simple*, in which consciousness is preserved, and *complex*, in which consciousness is impaired:

- *Simple focal seizures:*
  - *with motor activity:* 'Jacksonian' seizures
  - *with sensory symptoms:* somatosensory, numbness
  - *with autonomic features:* pupillary or skin colour changes
  - *with psychic symptoms:* feelings of fear, rage, déjà vu. There may be visual, auditory or olfactory hallucinations.
- *Complex focal seizures:*
  - *impaired consciousness:* may occur alone and may be present from onset or supervene in an initially simple focal seizure
  - *automatisms:* semi-purposeful activities during which the patient is vague and unresponsive, may occur.

Seizures occur which do not fit neatly into the above categories. It may be difficult to determine whether a seizure type is truly focal or generalized. Examples include:

- Focal seizures with rapid secondary generalization
- *Infantile spasms:* widespread muscular contractions.

Epilepsies and epilepsy syndromes

Epilepsies are classified by the type of epileptic seizure occurring into generalized epilepsies and focal epilepsies. A further subdivision is made according to aetiology into:

- *Idiopathic (primary):* no identifiable cause apart from genetic
- *Symptomatic:* in which the cause is identifiable or presumed.

Epilepsy syndromes are also defined by age of onset, EEG findings, and additional clinical or pathological features.

The classification continues to evolve in the light of new research, but a simplified version is as follows:

Generalized epilepsies and syndromes

- *Idiopathic generalized epilepsy (IGE):*
  - juvenile myoclonic epilepsy (JME)
  - childhood absence epilepsy (CAE)
  - juvenile absence epilepsy (JAE)
  - generalized epilepsy with febrile seizures+ (GEFS+)
  - benign familial neonatal seizures (BFNS)
  - benign familial infantile seizures (BFIS)
  - benign myoclonic epilepsy of infancy
  - epilepsy with GTCS on awakening
- *Symptomatic generalized epilepsy:*
  - cerebral malformations
  - inborn errors of metabolism.

Focal epilepsies and syndromes

- *Idiopathic focal epilepsy:*
  - benign childhood epilepsy with centrotemporal spikes
  - autosomal dominant nocturnal frontal lobe epilepsy
- *Symptomatic focal epilepsy:*
  - temporal lobe epilepsy with hippocampal sclerosis
  - Rasmussen's encephalitis
  - hemiconvulsion–hemiplegia syndrome.

In addition to the above, there are three further categories which do not fit easily into the above classification:
- *Reflex epilepsies:*
  - idiopathic photosensitive occipital lobe epilepsy
- *Epileptic encephalopathies:*
  - myoclonic-astatic epilepsy
  - West syndrome
  - *Dravet syndrome:* severe myoclonic epilepsy of infancy
  - Lennox–Gastaut syndrome
- *Progressive myoclonic epilepsies:*
  - Unverricht–Lundborg disease or Baltic myoclonus
  - neuronal ceroid lipofuscinosis
  - myoclonic epilepsy with ragged red fibres (MERRF).

Febrile seizures occurring alone are not classified as epilepsy but also occur, together with afebrile seizures in several epilepsy syndromes such as childhood absence epilepsy and generalized epilepsy with febrile seizures plus (GEFS+).

Epilepsy syndromes

The features of some common and important epilepsy syndromes are considered for each age group.

Infantile spasms (West syndrome)
An uncommon and severe epileptic encephalopathy with a peak onset at 5–9 months characterized by clusters of 'infantile spasms' in which neck and arms flex and legs extend ('salaam attacks'). A characteristic EEG pattern, hypsarrhythmia, is observed (Fig 7.10). The condition may be idiopathic or symptomatic. Tuberous sclerosis is an important cause. Initial treatment includes vigabatrin or steroids. Prognosis is poor, especially in symptomatic cases.

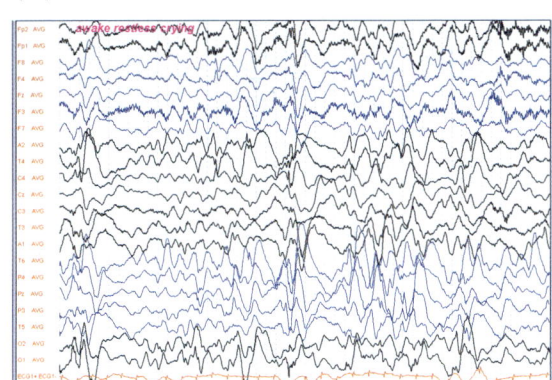

Fig 7.10 Hypsarrhythmia: high-amplitude slowing and multifocal spikes. Characteristics of infantile spasms.

Pyridoxine-dependent seizures
This AR disorder is a rare cause of intractable seizures with onset usually in the neonatal period. Multifocal or generalized seizures occur with a markedly abnormal EEG. Mutations in the antiquitin-1 gene, *ALDH7A1*, account for most cases. A diagnostic trial of pyridoxine or pyridoxal-5-phosphate should be considered in infants up to age 3 years with intractable seizures of unknown cause.

Dravet syndrome
Severe myoclonic epilepsy of infancy (SMEI) is a rare early-onset epileptic encephalopathy caused by sporadic severe mutations in *SCN1A*, the gene for a voltage-gated sodium channel. Prolonged febrile seizures evolve into frequent myoclonic, partial, and generalized seizures which are intractable.

Lennox–Gastaut syndrome
This is an uncommon severe epilepsy with onset between 1 and 7 years characterized by multiple seizure types: tonic, atonic, myoclonic, and atypical absences. The interictal EEG when awake shows diffuse slow <2.5 Hz spike-wave complexes and during sleep runs of fast 10 Hz rhythms. Episodes of convulsive and non-convulsive status are common.

Childhood absence epilepsy (CAE)
This is a benign epilepsy with peak onset at 6–7 years, more common in girls. Typical absence seizures occur and may be very frequent. The hallmark is an ictal EEG with generalized, symmetrical 3 Hz spike-wave discharges (Fig 7.11). Juvenile absence epilepsy (JAE) has a later onset (peak 9–12 years) and patients often have tonic-clonic seizures as well as absences. Sodium valproate is the first line treatment.

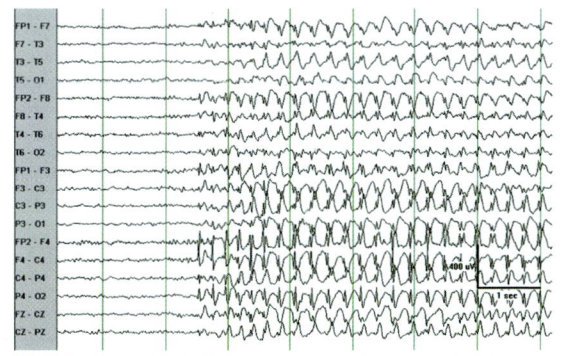

Fig 7.11 Generalized 3 Hz spike-wave complexes typical of absence epilepsy.

Benign childhood epilepsy with centrotemporal spikes
Previously called benign rolandic epilepsy, this is the most common idiopathic partial epilepsy of childhood. A sensory aura is followed by motor seizures involving tongue, lips, pharynx, and arm. 75% of seizures occur during sleep. Prognosis is good. Infrequent seizures do not require treatment.

Landau–Kleffner syndrome
This syndrome of acquired epileptic aphasia has an age of onset between 2 and 10 years. Insidious onset of a severe receptive and expressive language disorder leading to aphasia is accompanied by GCTS. EEG in sleep may demonstrate continuous spike and wave during slow sleep (CSWS).

Juvenile myoclonic epilepsy
The most common idiopathic generalized epilepsy syndrome of adolescence, characterized by myoclonic seizures often in upper limbs, GCTS in 90%, and absence seizures in 30%. Photosensitivity is common, as is a family history of epilepsy. Response to sodium valproate is good, but the condition is lifelong.

7.9 Movement disorders

The most important cause of motor deficit and disordered movement in childhood is CP, considered in Section 7.6. Genetic, inflammatory, neoplastic, and toxic pathological processes may present as movement disorders and manifest as ataxia, dystonia, paroxysmal dyskinesia or tics.

Ataxia

Ataxia is the inability to coordinate muscular movements and posture. It may be caused by cerebellar dysfunction, sensory impairment, or vestibular disease. Childhood ataxia may be acute, recurrent and episodic, chronic and static, or progressive.

Pathophysiology

Ataxia may be cerebellar, sensory, or vestibular. The three types have overlapping causes and may coexist or occur in isolation. Spinocerebellar dysfunction is common. Sensory ataxia occurs due to large-fibre neuropathy or dorsal column disease causing impaired proprioception and vibration sense. Vestibular ataxia is associated with prominent vertigo, nausea, and vomiting.

Aetiology

The causes are classified according to the time course.

Acute ataxia

- *Hours:* intoxication; drugs e.g. carbamazepine, antihistamines, alcohol
- *Days:* inflammation; postinfectious cerebellitis, acute disseminating encephalomyelitis
- *Weeks:* space-occupying lesion; posterior fossa tumour.

Episodic, recurrent

- *Genetic:*
  - *episodic ataxias:* a group of rare autosomal dominant disorders caused by mutations in at least six different genes (EA1–EA6), mostly encoding ion channels
  - urea cycle disorders, maple syrup urine disease
  - *mitochondrial disease:* neuropathy, ataxia and retinitis pigmentosa (NARP)
- *Paraneoplastic:* opsoclonus-myoclonus in neuroblastoma
- *Basilar migraine:* benign paroxysmal vertigo.

Chronic static

Cerebellar hypoplasia: trisomy 13, 18, Smith–Lemli–Opitz syndrome, Dandy–Walker malformation, Joubert syndrome, fetal alcohol syndrome.

Progressive ataxia

- *Genetic*:
  - *AD:* spinocerebellar ataxias SCA1–7, 10, 11
  - *AR:* Friedreich ataxia, ataxia telangiectasia, metabolic disorders: Menkes disease, phenylketonuria, Tay–Sachs disease, carbohydrate-deficient glycoprotein syndrome
  - *X-linked:* Rett syndrome
- *Brain tumours:* cerebellar astrocytomas, ependymomas
- *Demyelination:* multiple sclerosis.

Clinical evaluation

History

The time course is the most important guide to aetiology as described above. The history should aim to establish whether onset has occurred over hours, days, or weeks and whether the ataxia is episodic and recurrent or progressive.

Examination

General examination may reveal signs of syndromes associated with ataxia or recent infection such as chickenpox.
Neurological examination is directed towards identification of:

- *Cerebellar signs:* nystagmus, dysarthria, dysmetria
- *Sensory function:* Romberg's test (unsteadiness worse with eyes closed) is positive in sensory ataxia
- *Spinocerebellar degeneration:* absent tendon reflexes and upgoing plantar responses
- *Raised ICP:* papilloedema.

Clinical syndromes

Friedreich ataxia

Friedreich ataxia is the most common of the hereditary recessive ataxias with a prevalence of 1–2/50 000. Most patients have Friedreich ataxia type 1 (FRDA1) and are homozygous for expansion of a GAA triplet repeat sequence in the *FXN* gene on chromosome 9q.

Onset is usually at puberty with ataxia and clumsiness. Examination reveals reduced or absent deep tendon reflexes, reduced joint position and vibration sensation, and extensor plantar responses with pes cavus (Fig 7.12). Complications include cardiomyopathy, optic atrophy, diabetes, and deafness. Genetic testing is available for diagnosis.

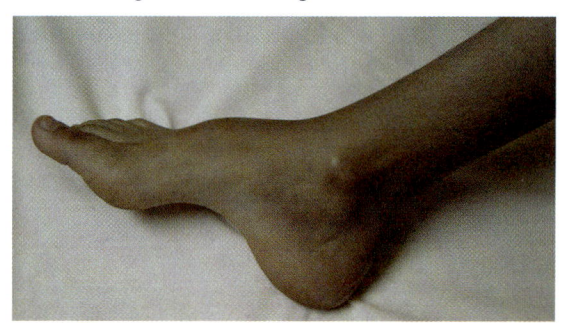

Fig 7.12 Friedreich ataxia: pes cavus.

Ataxia telangiectasia

This is the most common cause of inherited progressive cerebellar ataxia in early childhood. The incidence is 1/40 000.

It is an AR disorder caused by a defect in DNA repair associated with immune deficiency, predisposition to malignancy, especially after exposure to ionizing radiation, and telangiectasia.

Dystonia and choreoathetosis are prominent early features and oculomotor apraxia is a hallmark. Telangiectasia usually develops in sun-exposed areas such as bulbar conjunctiva behind the pinnae and the shoulders.

Diagnostic investigations include serum α-fetoprotein which is raised in 95%, chromosome fragility tests, immunoglobulin levels, and MRI.

Spinocerebellar ataxias (SCA)

This is a group of at least 10 AD cerebellar ataxias associated with progressive atrophy of cerebellum, spinal cord, and peripheral nerves. The mutation in several involves expansion of a CAG polyglutamine repeat which may be associated with *anticipation* or increasing severity and earlier onset in successive generations.

Clinical features include progressive incoordination and abnormal eye movements. Examples include SCA1, olivopontocerebellar atrophy and SCA3, Machado–Joseph disease.

Dystonia

The dystonias are movement disorders in which sustained muscular contractions cause twisting and repetitive movements or abnormal posture. The movements are involuntary, sometimes painful, and may affect a single muscle, a group of muscles, or the entire body.

Aetiology and pathogenesis

Pathology affecting the basal ganglia causes dystonia and is classified by aetiology into primary and secondary.

Primary dystonias (genetic 50%)
- Dystonia 1 (dystonia muscularis deformans, primary torsion dystonia)
- Dopa-responsive dystonia, Segawa syndrome
- Wilson disease
- Huntington disease.

Secondary dystonias
- *Perinatal hypoxia–ischaemia*: cerebral palsy
- *Drugs*: tardive dyskinesia
- Carbon monoxide poisoning, trauma, stroke.

Clinical classification

Dystonias are classified according to the muscles affected into
- *Generalized dystonia*
- *Segmental dystonia*: affecting two adjoining parts
- *Hemidystonia and focal dystonia*: spasmodic torticollis, blepharospasm, writer's cramp.

Clinical features

Muscle spasms lead to abnormal posturing and discomfort.

Dystonia 1, dystonia muscularis deformans

AD with onset in childhood or adolescence of involuntary posturing of trunk, neck, or limbs. Caused by defect in an ATP binding protein.

Dopa responsive dystonia, Segawa syndrome

AD with onset in 1st 5 years. Caused by defect in an enzyme in the pathway for dopamine synthesis.

Management

- *Medication*: antimuscarinics, GABA-ergic muscle relaxants (benzodiazepines, baclofen), levodopa, antiepilepsy drugs, botulinum toxin in focal dystonia
- *Surgery*: selective denervation, deep brain stimulation.

Paroxysmal dyskinesias

The paroxysmal dyskinesias are a group of conditions characterized by sudden episodes of involuntary movements. The movements may include any combination of:
- *Chorea*: irregular jerky movements
- *Athetosis*: slow, writhing motions
- *Dystonia*: twisting, patterned movements with distorted posturing
- *Ballismus*: uncontrollable flinging movements of an arm or leg, or both.

Classification and aetiology

Paroxysmal dyskinesias are often classified according to the factors that trigger the episodes of abnormal involuntary movement into:
- *Paroxysmal kinesogenic dyskinesia*: provoked by sudden movement or startle
- *Paroxysmal non-kinesogenic dyskinesia*: attacks occur spontaneously or provoked by stress, fatigue, alcohol, or caffeine
- *Paroxysmal exertion-induced dyskinesia*: prolonged exertion, cold, or stress
- *Paroxysmal hypnogenic dyskinesia*: induced by REM sleep.

They are further divided into short-lasting (<5 min) and long-lasting (>5 min). Age of onset may be from infancy to adulthood.

The cause may be genetic and familial or sporadic, or secondary to traumatic brain injury, hypoxic–ischaemic encephalopathy, metabolic abnormalities such as hypocalcaemia, AIDs, and drugs.

Management

There is no definitive diagnostic test. Many patients benefit from treatment with AEDs including valproate, carbamazepine, and clonazepam. Levodopa is also used.

Tics

A tic is an involuntary, rapid, recurrent, non-rhythmic motor or vocal action. Tic disorders are not uncommon in children.

Classification

Tics are classified into motor and vocal, simple and complex:
- *Motor tics*:
  - *simple*: eye blinking, grimacing, shrugging, frowning
  - *complex*: hopping, kissing, touching objects, clapping, squatting, echopraxia (imitating movements), copropraxia (rude gestures)
- *Vocal tics*:
  - *simple*: coughing, clearing throat, sniffing, whistling
  - *complex*: repeating words or phrases, unusual rhythms, tone or volume, coprolalia (rude or socially unacceptable words or phrases).

Tic disorders

These are classified into:
- *Transient tics*: onset 3–10 years, excess of boys, mostly motor ticks of neck and face. Duration <1 year
- *Chronic motor/vocal tics*: tics for >1 year
- *Tourette syndrome (TS)*: see Chapter 17.

7.10 Headache

Recurrent headache is a common childhood symptom. The prevalence of headache increases with age to become comparable to that in the adult population in the early teens. 50% of children age <10 years experience recurrent headache in the course of a year and this rises to 70%, with a female preponderance, by age 15 years.

In the majority, these are primary 'tension-type' headaches. Migraine affects 1–3% of children by age 7 years and 4–11% by age 15 years.

Secondary headaches are rare, and brain tumour as a cause of headache very rare: only 1/5000 children with recurrent headache has a brain tumour. Neuralgia, eye pain, and facial pain are distinct from headache.

Aetiology and pathogenesis

The causes of isolated acute, severe headache are different from those of recurrent headaches.

Acute isolated headache

Causes of a recent-onset headache with no previous history of similar episodes are:
- Viral illness with fever
- Sinusitis, dental caries
- *Intracranial infection*: meningitis, encephalitis
- Traumatic head injury
- *Rarities*: intracranial haemorrhage, substance use or withdrawal, post-seizure.

Recurrent headache

Causes of recurrent headache are usefully classified into primary and secondary:
- *Primary headache*:
  - migraine
  - tension-type headache
  - cluster headache
- *Secondary headache*:
  - *raised ICP*: tumour, hydrocephalus, idiopathic intracranial hypertension (IIH)
  - hypertension.

The brain parenchyma has no sensory innervation and the pain of headache is subserved by innervation of the vasculature and meninges. The pathophysiological basis of tension-type headaches remains uncertain. Migraine has a genetic component and in monogenic, dominant forms mutations in calcium and sodium channel genes have been identified.

Clinical evaluation

A thorough history and clinical examination is the key to diagnosis. Special investigations including brain imaging are rarely necessary and should not be used to allay unfounded fears of a brain tumour. In an acute, severe headache key features on examination include fever, signs of meningism, papilloedema, or focal neurological signs.

History

In recurrent headache, a careful history from child and parent should allow diagnosis although it must be remembered that there is significant overlap of features between tension-type and migraine headaches, and mixed types are common.
Clinically, it is useful to divide recurrent headache according to temporal pattern into:

- *Episodic acute recurrent:* headache separated by symptom-free intervals. Typical of tension-type headache and migraine.
- *Chronic progressive:* increasing frequency and severity. Commonly correlates with increasing ICP.
- *Chronic non-progressive headache*: includes chronic tension-type and chronic daily headache.

Important points to establish in the history include:
- *Pattern of headaches:*
  - how long have headaches been a problem?
  - frequency
  - timing during day, morning, evenings
  - getting better, worse or staying the same
- *Nature of headache:*
  - *onset*: sudden or gradual
  - *duration*: minutes, hours, days
  - *severity,* throbbing or constant
  - *location*: unilateral or generalized
  - *associated features*: prodrome, aura, visual symptoms, weakness, nausea, vomiting
  - variable or constant in nature
- *Provoking or relieving factors:*
  - *precipitants*: foods, light, stress, activity
  - *relieving factors:* including analgesia, rest
- *Effects:* school absence, academic progress
- Family history of migraine
- *Medication:* effect of analgesics.

Examination

In chronic, recurrent headache it is important to look for indicators of secondary headache:
- *Measure blood pressure*: hypertension
- *Fundi*: papilloedema in raised ICP
- *Focal neurological signs*: VI nerve palsy, cerebellar signs.

Specific headache syndromes

The features and diagnostic criteria for migraine and tension-type headache and the features suggesting a sinister secondary headache with raised ICP are considered in turn.

Tension-type headache (TTH)

The headache is usually bilateral, pressing/tightening, non-pulsating in quality, mild to moderate intensity, not aggravated by routine physical activity, not associated with nausea or vomiting, and associated with either phonophobia or photophobia but not both.

Episodic types last from minutes to days and may be infrequent, <1 day per month or frequent, >1 but <15 days per month. Chronic TTH lasts hours but may be continuous and occurs on ≥15 days per month. Chronic daily headache occurs in children, usually with a pattern of migraines superimposed on frequent TTH.

Examination is normal apart from pericranial tenderness in some cases.

Migraine

Typical migraine headaches are frontal, pulsating in quality, duration 2–48 h, moderate or severe intensity, aggravated by physical activity, exercise, noise, or bright lights, and relieved by resting in dark.

There may be a relationship between fatigue/stress, particular foods, or lack of sleep. A family history of migraine is present in 70%. In the teenage years migraine is more common in girls and symptoms may relate to menstruation.

Migraine is further classified into:
- *Common migraine*: migraine without aura
- *Classical migraine*: migraine with aura
- *Complicated migraine*: hemiplegic, ophthalmoplegic, basilar artery.

Migraine without aura is the usual pattern. Migraine with aura is more common in older children. A prodromal aura is usually visual, unilateral and does not last >1 h. The headache may begin before, during, or up to 1 h after the aura.

Complicated migraine, a type of migraine with aura, is uncommon and associated with focal, transient neurological signs or symptoms:
- *Hemiplegic migraine*: abrupt onset of hemiparesis followed by headache; strong family history
- *Ophthalmoplegic migraine*: periorbital pain with III, IV, VI nerve palsies which may persist for days
- *Basilar migraine*: dizziness, weakness, ataxia, and severe occipital headache.

Cluster headaches

Uncommon in children, characterized by severe unilateral headache with ipsilateral streaming of eye and nose and last up to 3 h.

Secondary headache

Features which should raise suspicion of a secondary headache include:
- *Recent onset of headache*:
- Severe headaches with progressive increase in frequency and duration
- Worse in recumbency, coughing, or bending
- Change in behaviour or educational performances
- Associated seizures or vomiting.

Signs of raised ICP or focal neurological signs on examination are to be expected.

Idiopathic intracranial hypertension (IIH)

Previously known as pseudotumour cerebri or benign intracranial hypertension, this rare disorder presents with headache and symptoms of raised ICP with visual symptoms: diplopia, blurred vision, transient visual loss. Papilloedema is found on examination but brain imaging is normal.

Diagnosis is confirmed by a raised opening CSF pressure, >20 cmH$_2$O, on lumbar puncture. It is a self-limiting condition lasting several months but the main concern is that raised ICP can cause severe optic nerve damage with irreversible visual loss. Visual field testing is essential.

Management

Routine investigations are not necessary in evaluation of the child with recurrent headaches. ENT examination and sinus radiographs are useful if sinus infection is suspected.

Indications for neuroimaging, cranial CT or MRI, include features suggestive of intracranial pathology, in particular progressive features and neurological signs. Headaches in very young children (<5 years) need careful evaluation.

Treatment

Education is most important. A simple explanation of headaches as a common and harmless biological fact of life may alter family expectations and help child and family understand management as an aid to minimizing rather than abolishing the problem. This reassurance should not be undermined by unnecessary investigations.

Tension-type headaches

Reassurance, simple analgesics such as paracetamol or ibuprofen, head massage, and relaxation techniques are all effective to some extent.

Migraine

Prognosis is good, especially in boys, with up to 90% of children headache free within 5 years. Measures include:

General measures
- *Self-help:* keep a diary to identify precipitants such as food or exercise and ensure regular food and sleep
- *Behavioural interventions:* thermal biofeedback and progressive muscle relaxation appear effective.

Drug treatment
- Acute attacks:
  - simple analgesics (paracetamol, ibuprofen) are first line combined with domperidone if vomiting is prominent. Analgesics combined with antiemetics can be used in children >12 years, e.g. paracetamol with metoclopramide, paracetamol, codeine, and buclizine. Analgesics at onset are most effective.
  - triptans (5HT$_1$ agonists) can be considered in older children. Sumatriptan nasal spray 10 mg is licensed for children aged 12–18 years for acute relief of migraine with or without aura.
  - treatment for acute attacks should not be used for more than 2 days a week because of the risk of medication overuse headache.
- *Prophylaxis* is considered for frequent, one every 1–2 weeks or severe attacks, duration >4 h and missing school. Options include:
  - *Propanolol:* contraindicated in asthma. Side effects depression, postural hypotension.
  - *Pizotifen:* side effects include drowsiness and weight gain.
  - *AEDs:* valproate and topiramate appear effective.
  - *Calcium channel blockers:* flunarizine

Idiopathic intracranial hypertension

Management options include:
- *Weight loss:* there is an association with obesity
- *Lumbar puncture:* to reduce and monitor CSF pressure
- *Acetazolamide:* reduces CSF production
- *Surgery:* optic nerve sheath fenestration or lumboperitoneal shunting.

7.11 Neuromuscular disorders: overview

Neuromuscular disorders affect any part of the pathway from anterior horn cell to skeletal muscle fibre:
- Anterior horn cell
- Peripheral nerve
- Neuromuscular junction
- Skeletal muscle.

The hallmark is hypotonia and weakness, but pathology may also be present outside the motor unit, affecting parts of the CNS or sensory system. Many pathologic mechanisms underlie these diseases including genetic defects, inflammation or autoimmunity affecting nerve or muscle, and mechanical injury.

Classification

The important neuromuscular disorders according to anatomic location and pathology are shown in Table 7.1

Table 7.1 Neuromuscular disorders of infancy and childhood		
	Genetic	**Acquired**
Anterior horn cell	Spinal muscular atrophy (SMA)	Poliomyelitis
		Cervical cord injury
Peripheral nerve	Hereditary sensory motor neuropathy (HSMN)	Guillain–Barré Syndrome (GBS)
		Brachial plexus injury
Neuromuscular junction	Congenital myasthenia syndrome	Myasthenia gravis
		Transient neonatal myasthenia Botulism
Muscle	Congenital myopathies	Inflammatory myopathy
	Metabolic myopathies	Viral myositis
	Muscular dystrophies (see section 7.13)	Endocrine myopathy

Clinical features

Presentation depends on age of onset, which varies from prenatal to late childhood:

Perinatal period
- Reduced fetal movement, polyhydramnios
- Arthrogryposis
- A 'floppy infant'.

Infancy/early childhood
- Delayed motor milestones
- Global developmental delay, if CNS involved
- *Episodic weakness*: metabolic myopathy, myasthenia.

Later childhood
- Difficulty with running
- Fatiguability
- Muscle pain or cramp on exertion
- Toe walking, foot deformity.

The 'floppy' infant

The term 'floppy' may refer to:
- *Hypotonia*: decrease in muscle tone
- *Weakness*: decrease in muscle power
- *Ligamentous laxity*: with increased joint mobility.

Strictly speaking, 'floppy' denotes hypotonia. Clinical signs of hypotonia include:
- 'Frog leg' posture when supine
- Head lag on traction
- *Ventral suspension*: 'rag-doll' posture
- *Vertical suspension*: slips through hands (Fig 7.13)

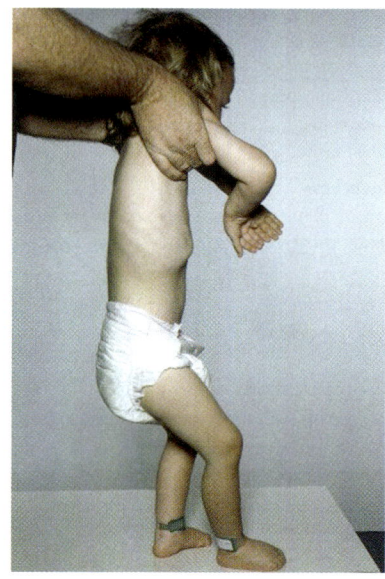

Fig 7.13 Vertical suspension: slips through hands.

Clinical evaluation

This is directed towards distinguishing floppiness:
- *Without weakness* (non-paralytic): central cause
- *With weakness* (paralytic): peripheral cause.

The following indicators help to distinguish central from peripheral causes of hypotonia in a 'floppy infant'.

Associations of central hypotonia
- *History of cerebral insult*: hypoxic-ischaemic encephalopathy or symptomatic hypoglycaemia,
- *Evidence of cortical dysfunction*: cognitive impairment, seizures, visual inattention, reduced awareness
- *Upper motor-neuron signs*: pseudo-bulbar palsy, scissoring, fisting of hands, brisk tendon reflexes.
- Dysmorphic features or multiple malformations.

Associations of peripheral hypotonia
- Family history of neuromuscular disorder
- 'Frog-leg' posture and paucity of spontaneous movement
- Delay in motor milestones/cognitive development normal
- Reduced or absent spontaneous anti-gravity movements, areflexia
- *Myopathic facies*: open mouth, tented upper lip, lack of facial expression, ptosis, restricted ocular movements.

Aetiology

Central (non-paralytic) hypotonia

- *Cerebral palsy*: HIE, hypoglycaemia
- *Cortical malformations*
- *Chromosomal disorders*: Prader–Willi syndrome, Down syndrome
- *Neurometabolic disorders*: Menkes syndrome, Zellweger syndrome
- *Endocrine*: hypothyroidism
- *Metabolic*: rickets, RTA
- *Connective tissue disorders*: Ehlers–Danlos syndrome
- Benign familial hypotonia.

Peripheral (paralytic) hypotonia

- *Anterior horn cell*: spinal muscular atrophy, paralytic poliomyelitis
- *Nerve*: congenital hypomyelinating neuropathy
- *Neuromuscular junction*: congenital myasthenia, transient neonatal myasthenia, botulism
- *Muscle*: congenital muscular dystrophies, congenital myotonic dystrophy, congenital myopathies.

The older child

Examination may reveal

- Muscle fasciculation, atrophy, or hypertrophy
- Hypotonia, reduced tendon reflexes
- Weakness reduced power
- Myopathic facies (Fig 7.14)
- *Abnormal gait*: 'waddling' gait, exaggerated lateral flexion of trunk towards weight bearing hip
- *Positive Gowers sign*: need to turn prone to rise due to proximal weakness (see Fig 7.15).

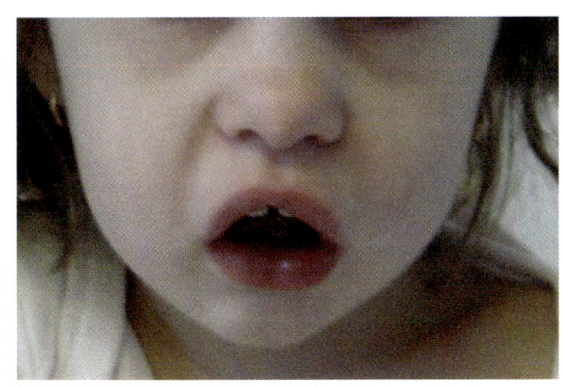

Fig 7.14 Myotonic dystrophy: myopathic facies.

Investigations

Investigations are guided by whether central or peripheral (neuromuscular) disease is suspected on clinical grounds.

Investigation of central hypotonia

- *Karyotype*: trisomy 21, Prader–Willi syndrome (15q)
- *Neuroimaging*: cranial MRI. Several congenital muscular dystrophy syndromes show brain or eye abnormalities.
- *Biochemistry*: Ca, PO_4, alkaline phosphatase, TFTs, plasma and urine amino acids, VLCFAs, Cu, caeruloplasmin
- Clinical genetics and ophthalmology review.

Investigation of peripheral hypotonia

- *Serum creatine kinase (CK)*: elevated in most but not all muscle diseases and should be measured in all late walkers or boys with speech or language delay
- *Neurophysiology*: nerve conduction studies and electromyography, EMG may distinguish between neurogenic, myopathic, myotonic, and myasthenic aetiologies
- *Muscle imaging*: ultrasound shows increased echogenicity in muscular dystrophy or myopathy and MRI to identify pattern of involvement
- *Muscle biopsy*: via needle or open biopsy, this allows histology, respiratory chain enzyme analysis, MtDNA analysis and immunohistochemistry for laminin α_2, collagen VI, and alpha dystroglycan
- *DNA analysis*: specific tests are available for some disorders, including spinal muscular atrophy, congenital myotonic dystrophy, dystrophinopathies, dystroglycanopathies, and facioscapulohumeral dystrophies.

Management

Specific treatment is not yet available for most of these disorders and supportive management is tailored to each individual. The main aims are family support and education together with prevention and management of complications.

- *Genetic counselling*: prenatal diagnosis may be feasible.
- *Nutrition*: nasogastric or gastrostomy feeding may be necessary but obesity from inactivity must be avoided. Gastro-esophageal reflux is common.
- *Respiratory sequelae*: risks arise from aspiration, bulbar palsy, weak cough and hypoventilation due to muscle weakness. Infection prevention includes vaccination (pneumococcus, influenza virus) and physiotherapy. Respiratory failure is a risk when FVC <30% predicted. Nocturnal hypoventilation occurs first and is managed by non-invasive positive pressure ventilation. This may progress to daytime respiratory failure and cor pulmonale.
- *Orthopaedic complications*: physiotherapy and passive stretching to avoid contractures and promote mobility. Scoliosis may be helped by bracing or spinal fusion.
- *Mobility*: knee–ankle–foot orthoses (KAFO) are used to prolong ambulation and independent mobility is prolonged with electrically powered indoor–outdoor chairs
- Cardiac failure or arrhythmias may require treatment.
- Ethical issues may arise around the appropriateness of cardiopulmonary resuscitation in the event of cardiac arrest or acute respiratory failure.

7.12 Specific neuromuscular disorders

Spinal muscular atrophy (SMA)

SMA is a group of AR disorders characterized by degeneration of anterior horn cells. The overall incidence is 1/6000 live births.

Genetics

The most common form is proximal SMA caused by mutations (usually deletions) of the survival motor neuron gene *SMN1* on chromosome 5q.

Rarer forms include spinal muscular atrophy with respiratory distress (SMARD1), X-linked SMA, and pontocerebellar hypoplasia with SMA.

Clinical features

Proximal SMA is classified into four types according to functional severity (Table 7.2).

Table 7.2. Classification of proximal SMA

Type		Onset	
I	Severe Werdnig–Hoffmann disease	0–6 m	Never sits
II	Intermediate	6–18 m	Never stands
III	Mild Kugelberg–Welander disease	>18 m	Stands and walks
IV	Adults	10–30 y	

Features include:
- Proximal, symmetrical wasting and weakness of muscles of trunk and limbs, more prominent in legs than arms
- Tongue fasciculation and absent tendon reflexes
- Weak intercostal muscles with sparing of the diaphragm
- Facial muscles are spared giving an alert, normal expression.

Type 1 SMA do not survive beyond 12–18 months, survival depending on bulbar and respiratory function.

Type II SMA have onset of weakness at 6–18 months, are able to sit but not stand or walk. Early scoliosis occurs and survival depends on degree of respiratory muscle involvement.

Type III SMA have onset >18 months and walk unsupported at some stage. Variation in severity depends in part on compensatory activity of a duplicate gene, *SMN2*.

Management

Prenatal diagnosis is available. Supportive care as described in Section 7.11.

Hereditary motor and sensory neuropathies (HMSN)

These are a heterogeneous group of degenerative disorders of the peripheral nervous system. Previously classified by clinical phenotype into Charcot–Marie–Tooth (CMT) disease, peroneal muscular atrophy, etc. elucidation of their molecular genetic basis has allowed a new classification (Table 7.3).

Table 7.3 Classification of HMSN

Type	Chromosome	Gene	Inheritance
HMSN1 demyelinating			
CMT1A	17p	PMP22	AD
CMT1B	1q	MPZ	AD
CMT1C	16p	LITAF	AD
CMT1C	8q	GDAP1	AR
HMSN2 axonal			
CMT2A1	1p36	KIF1B	AD
CMT2A2	1p3	MFNZ	AD
CMT2B	3q13-q22	RAB7	AD
HMSN3 hypertrophic			
Dejerine–Sotas syndrome	17p	PMP22	AD
	1q	MPZ	AD
	19q	PRX	AR
	10q	EGR2	AD
X-linked			
CMTX1	Xq13	GJB1	X-linked dominant

Pathogenesis

Two of the genes encode important structural components of peripheral myelin: peripheral myelin protein 22 and myelin protein zero. There is marked genetic heterogeneity: different alleles of the same gene cause different phenotypes, and the same phenotype can be caused by different genes.

Clinical features

Charcot–Marie–Tooth (CMT) type 1

AD CMT disease type 1 (CMT1A–C) has typical onset in school age with toe-walking, clumsiness, and falls. This progresses to foot drop, distal weakness, and wasting and later to weakness of intrinsic hand muscles, peroneal muscular atrophy, foot deformity (pes cavus, high arch, hammer toes), and mild distal sensory loss. Knee and ankle jerks are lost.

Neurophysiology demonstrates low motor nerve conduction velocity of 10–30 m/s, no conduction block. and absent sensory action potentials. DNA testing is available.

Charcot–Marie–Tooth (CMT) disease type 2

AD CMT disease type 2 (CMT2A) has later onset in the second and third decade and slower course. Weakness is less marked. Motor nerve conduction velocity is normal or slightly reduced. Autosomal recessive form has early onset <5 years and rapid progression.

The differential diagnosis includes Freidreich Ataxia (FA). In FA there is ataxia and marked sensory neuropathy with loss of proprioception and sensory neuropathy on nerve conduction studies. In CMT there is areflexia, distal weakness, and abnormal motor nerve conduction.

Myasthenic syndromes

Disorders of neuromuscular transmission characterized by fluctuating muscle weakness and fatiguability on exercise are classified into three main types: myasthenia gravis, transient neonatal myasthenia, and congenital myasthenia syndromes.

Myasthenia gravis (MG)
MG has an incidence of 2/100 000 and can occur at any age. It is most common in females between 18 and 25 years. It is an autoimmune disease in which antibodies are formed to either the acetylcholine receptor (AChR) or muscle specific kinase (MusK).

There is a genetic predisposition (HLAB8, DR3) and clustering in families with other autoimmune diseases such as rheumatoid arthritis, systemic lupus erythematosus, and thyroid disease. A thymoma is found in 25%. Penicillamine can induce MG.

Clinical features
Onset may be insidious with fluctuating subtle and variable symptoms, or sudden. The first symptom is often weakness of the eye muscles with asymmetrical ptosis and diplopia, or difficulty in swallowing and slurred speech. Involvement may be localized to eye muscles as ocular myasthenia or generalized affecting the trunk, arms and legs.

Examination reveals fatiguable weakness (e.g. poor sustained shoulder abduction with arms outstretched), proximal weakness, and normal or brisk tendon jerks.

A myasthenic crisis, with paralysis of respiratory muscles, may be triggered by infection, fever, emotional stress, surgery, pregnancy, or overexertion.

Management
Diagnostic investigations
- *Ice pack test:* for evaluation of ptosis
- *Serum antibodies:* anti-AChR, +ve in 80%; anti-MUSK, +ve in 14%
- *Neurophysiology:* repetitive nerve stimulation causes a decrement in the compound muscle action potential. Single fibre EMG shows increased 'jitter'. Edrophonium can be given to demonstrate a response
- *CXR ± CT or MRI:* to identify thymoma
- *Edrophonium test:* IV edrophonium (Tensilon) is given in HDU and improves muscle weakness within 1 min in MG. Used if other investigations inconclusive and easily observed weakness such as ocular is present.

Treatment
Options include:
- *Anticholinesterases:* neostigmine (Prostigmine) and pyridostigmine (Mestinon)
- *Steroids:* prednisolone may be used in conjunction with anticholinesterase but can cause initial deterioration
- *Thymectomy:* essential in cases of thymoma and may be of benefit in others especially those with AChR antibody positive generalised MG within 2 years of onset
- *Plasmapheresis and IVIG:* used for myasthenic crisis and pre-op thymectomy
- *Immunosuppressants:* azathioprine or cyclophosphamide are used for generalized MG if other medications fail.

Transient neonatal myasthenia
A temporary condition caused by transfer of maternal antibodies. Sucking, swallowing, and respiratory difficulties present on the first day of life. Anti-AChR antibodies are present and there is a response to anticholinesterases.

Congenital myasthenic syndromes (CMS)
These are AR genetic diseases of the neuromuscular junction and may be classified by site of defect: presynaptic, synaptic, or postsynaptic.

75% are postsynaptic and associated with AChR deficiency caused by mutations in genes encoding receptor subunits or genes essential for synapse formation. These rare disorders can also present beyond the neonatal period at any age.

Myopathies
Congenital myopathies
A group of at least six genetic disorders associated with hypotonia, muscle weakness, and motor delay in infancy. Classification is according to muscle histology:
- Central core disease
- Nemaline (rod) myopathies
- Myotubular (centronuclear) myopathy
- Minicore (multicore) myopathy
- Congenital fibre type disproportion
- Non-specific myopathy.

Central core disease
AD disorder caused by mutations in *RYR1* encoding the ryanodine receptor. Risk of malignant hyperthermia with general anaesthetics or muscle relaxants.

Nemaline (rod) myopathies
A group of rare disorders with a wide spectrum of onset from birth to adulthood defining six subgroups. Inheritance may be AD or AR. Five genes have been identified which encode muscle proteins. Mutations in *ACTA1* encoding α-actin account for 25%.

Myotubular (centronuclear) myopathy
Inheritance may be AD, AR, or X-linked recessive. X-linked myotubular myopathy is caused by defects in myotubularin. Most affected males fail to breathe at birth and do not survive beyond the first few months. Prenatal diagnosis is available.

Metabolic myopathies
Muscle tissue is involved in a number of inherited inborn errors of metabolism which may present in infancy with hypotonia or later in life with exercise-related weakness. Examples include glycogen storage diseases and mitochondrial myopathies.

Acquired myopathies
- *Inflammatory myopathies:* juvenile dermatomyositis is a rare systemic vasculopathy with median age of onset 7 years (it is more common in girls). Presentation is with slowly increasing proximal muscular weakness, heliotrope skin rash, fever, arthropathy, iritis. CK is high. Biopsy shows perivascular infiltrates and fibre necrosis.
- *Viral myositis:* a common, self-limiting disease, characterized by tender, aching calves or thighs and elevated CK, caused by coxsackie, echo, or influenza virus.

7.13 Muscular dystrophies

The muscular dystrophies are a group of genetic disorders characterized by defects in muscle proteins and changes in muscle tissue including variation in fibre size, necrosis, and excess of fatty and fibrous tissue.

The genes responsible encode proteins with a wide range of roles in the muscle fibre. Many of the proteins, including dystrophin, sarcoglycans, and laminins are components of the cytoskeleton which anchor muscle fibres to the extra-cellular matrix and normally ensure preservation of muscle integrity during contraction.

Classification

Classification by clinical phenotype is being supplemented by DNA mutation analysis and immunohistochemical demonstration of specific protein deficiencies. The main groups are:
- *Congenital muscular dystrophies (CMD)*
- *Dystrophinopathies:*
  - Duchenne muscular dystrophy (DMD)
  - Becker muscular dystrophy (BMD)
- *Muscular dystrophies of later childhood:*
  - Emery–Dreifuss muscular dystrophy (EDMD)
  - limb girdle muscular dystrophy (LGMD)
  - facioscapulohumeral muscular dystrophy (FSHMD)
- *Myotonic dystrophy (MD).*

Congenital muscular dystrophies

This is a group of AR disorders presenting with hypotonia as a 'floppy' infant, weakness and contractures at birth or during infancy. At least six different disorders exist. The conditions are mostly static or slowly progressive. The key diagnostic points are:

Is there also brain or eye involvement?
Defects in genes encoding proteins important in D-glycosylation are responsible for three disorders with abnormal α-dystroglycan in muscle and brain/eye malformations: Fukuyama CMD, muscle–eye–brain disease, and Walker–Warburg syndrome.

How high is the creatine kinase?
CMD with high CK is found in defects of D-glycosylation and defects of laminin. CMD with mild elevation or normal CK is found in Ullrich CMD and Bethlem myopathy caused by mutations in genes for the three α subunits of collagen VIA.

Immunolabelling
What are the results of immunolabelling of muscle tissue with antibody to laminin $α_2$ or merosin, and dystroglycan or collagen VI?

Dystrophinopathies

Mutations in the *DMD* gene on chromosome Xp21 encoding dystrophin cause a range of phenotypes from severe Duchenne muscular dystrophy (DMD) to mild Becker muscular dystrophy (BMD) depending on the level of residual functioning dystrophin.

Duchenne muscular dystrophy (DMD)
DMD is the most common form of muscular dystrophy, affecting 1/3500 liveborn males. A minority of female carriers are symptomatic.

Aetiology and pathogenesis
DMD is the largest known human gene, 2.4 Mb in size with 79 exons. It encodes dystrophin, a large cytoskeletal protein. Distinct isoforms are synthesized in muscle, brain, and heart. Dystrophin plays an important role in anchoring the cytoskeleton to the plasma membrane and protects the sarcolemma during contractions.

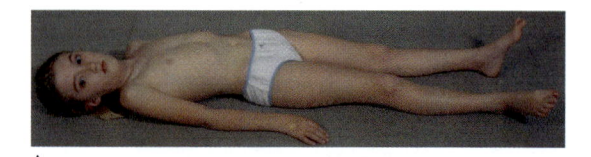

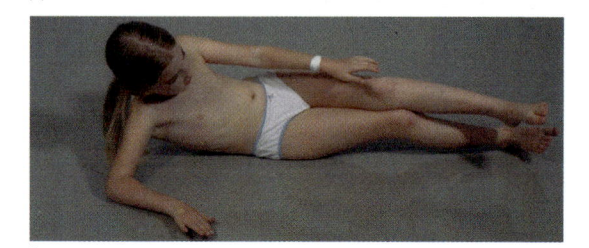

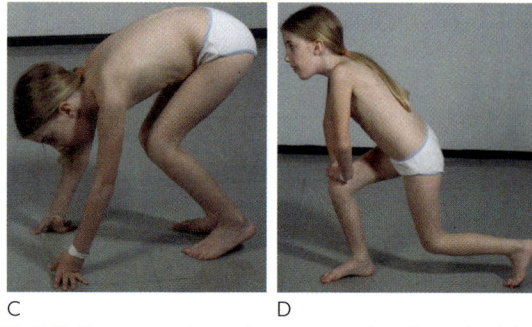

Fig 7.15 Gowers sign: the need to turn prone in order to rise. It is non-specific and indicates poor hip-girdle flexion and/or proximal weakness (it is not just a sign found in DMD).

An intragenic deletion in *DMD* is present in 70% of patients. Deletions, duplications, or point mutations cause complete absence of dystrophin. Mutations resulting in a shortened, partially functional dystrophin cause the milder Becker phenotype (see below). One third of cases are sporadic and caused by new mutations. Inheritance is X-linked recessive.

Increased oxidative stress damages the sarcolemma resulting in necrosis of muscle fibres, and their replacement with apidose and connective tissue. Humoral and cellular immune responses contribute to the pathological processes.

Clinical features
DMD mainly affects boys who present with delayed motor milestones, abnormal gait, inability to run, and difficulty in rising from the floor in the 1st 5 years of life. Examination reveals symmetrical, proximal muscle weakness, and pseudohypertrophy of some muscles especially the calves (see Fig 7.16). The Gowers sign may be positive (Fig 7.15).

Muscle weakness is progressive with loss of ambulation in classical cases at 8–12 years or 13–16 years in 'intermediate' forms.

Survival is limited and death occurs in the 3rd or 4th decade from respiratory failure or cardiomyopathy. Associations and complications include:
- *Learning difficulties, language delay:* in 60%
- *Cardiomyopathy:* in 100%, symptomatic in 20%
- Scoliosis, respiratory failure.

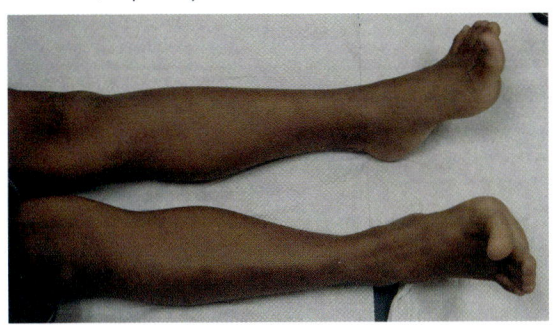

Fig 7.16 Pseudohypertrophy of calves in DMD.

Diagnostic investigations
Diagnosis is suspected on clinical presentation and elevated serum CK. **CK must be measured on any boy with delayed walking.** Confirmation requires:
- *Genetic testing:* routine testing is available for intragenic deletions and duplications, present in 70%
- *Muscle biopsy:* immunohistochemistry with monoclonal antibody to dystrophin reveals absence of dystrophin.

Management
There is as yet no cure for DMD but optimal multidisciplinary care can do much to help and prolong life.
- *General measures:* family support with modifications of housing, transport and schooling, and input from family care officers.
- *Supportive and symptomatic treatment:* physiotherapy for prevention of contractures, prolongation of walking by use of knee–ankle–foot orthoses (KAFO).
- *Medical treatment:* steroids hold the most promise. Evidence-based guidelines remain difficult to formulate but a consensus is that prednisolone may be considered in boys aged 7–10 years with impending loss of ambulation.
- *Management of complications:*
  - *respiratory:* a FVC of 40% predicts sleep hypoventilation, the first sign of impending problems. Nocturnal nasal mask IPPV is indicated when the patient is hypercapnic or has sleep hypoventilation
  - *cardiac:* echocardiography is performed at time of loss of ambulation and 2 yearly thereafter or if symptoms occur. ACE inhibitors may slow progress of cardiomyopathy
  - *nutritional:* obesity and undernutrition both occur.
- *Genetic counselling:* female relatives of affected males with an intragenic deletion or duplication can be offered carrier testing. The mother of a sporadic case is a carrier in two thirds of cases or may have somatic or gonadal mosaicism. Female carriers should have cardiac surveillance.

Becker muscular dystrophy (BMD)
BMD is a milder variant caused by production of a truncated, partially functional form of dystrophin. Presentation is later onset at 5–15 years with loss of ambulation >16 years and variable life expectancy. Diagnosis by DNA analysis and muscle biopsy (patchy dystrophin).

EDMD, FSHMD, and LGMD
These disorders tend to present later in childhood and are genetically heterogeneous. 17 disease genes have been identified for muscle proteins including subunits of sarcoglycan.

Emery–Dreifuss muscular dystrophy (EDMD)
- May be X-linked or ADt
- Clinical phenotype is mild with proximal weakness and prominent contractures of achilles tendon, neck, spine, and elbows. Cardiac surveillance is indicated as there is a risk of sudden death from arrhythmias or cardiac failure

Facioscapulohumeral muscular dystrophy (FSHMD)
- AD with an incidence of 1/20 000. Age of onset is variable with initial facial weakness followed by descending involvement with shoulder weakness causing scapular winging, proximal arm and peroneal weakness, and later pelvic and tibial weakness.
- Most patients have a deletion on chromosome 4q35, which forms the basis of a diagnostic molecular genetic test.

Limb-girdle muscular dystrophies (LGMD)
- A heterogeneous group of disorders, with a combined incidence of 1/10–20 000. Inheritance is AR in 90%. At least 14 different causal genes are known which encode muscle proteins such as lamin A/C and dysferlin.
- Phenotypes are diverse but classically manifest as proximal weakness of upper and lower limbs. Diagnosis may be difficult and relies on clinical features, immunohistochemistry on muscle biopsy, and genetic testing.

Myotonic dystrophy (MD1)
The common form of myotonic dystrophy, MD1, has an incidence of 1/8000 live births. MD1 is AD and caused by expansion of a CTG triplet repeat in the 3′-untranslated region of the last exon of *DMPK*.
Disease severity is determined by the number of CTG repeats, giving rise to different clinical phenotypes:
- *50–100 repeats:* mild MD, onset in middle age or later
- *100–500 repeats:* classical MD, variable age of onset
- *500–1500 repeats:* congenital myotonic dystrophy.

MD1 shows anticipation, increasing repeat length causing earlier onset and more severe phenotype in successive generations. Maternal transmission can be associated with a large expansion in the CTG repeat number, whereas paternal transmission is associated with a modest increase, or even a decrease. Congenital MD is therefore almost always inherited from the mother.

Clinical features
- *Mild form: form* presents with presenile cataracts.
- *Classical form:* adolescents and young adults with muscle weakness and wasting, grip and percussion myotonia, cataracts, testicular atrophy, cardiac arrhythmias, characteristic facial features: ptosis, facial weakness, male pattern baldness.
- *Congenital MD:* can present antenatally with reduced fetal movements and polyhydramnios or in the neonatal period with severe hypotonia, respiratory distress, feeding difficulties, talipes, facial weakness, and arthrogryposis. Cardiac features include cardiomyopathy and arrhythmias. The affected mother may be asymptomatic.

Genetic testing for MD1 is widely available.

7.14 Infection and injury

Intracranial infections

Infections of the CNS are classified as meningitis or encephalitis according to whether the pathology predominantly affects the meninges and CSF or the brain parenchyma. In *meningitis* the brain surface is usually involved and meningo-encephalitis would be a better term. In contrast, *encephalitis* may exist with little or no evidence of inflammation in the CSF.

The term *encephalomyelitis* is used for brain inflammation caused by a post-infectious autoimmune response rather than direct invasion by pathogens. Non-infectious causes of meningitis and encephalitis include drugs, vasculitides, and malignancy.

Meningitis

Acute meningitis is most commonly bacterial, but acute viral aseptic meningitis also occurs.

Chronic meningitis may be caused by infection with bacteria, especially *Mycobacterium tuberculosis*, but also by rickettsiae, fungi, and parasites in the immunocompromised host. Acute bacterial and tuberculous meningitis are considered in Chapter 15.

Encephalitis

Encephalitis is most commonly viral, but many non-viral causes exist: bacterial, rickettsial, fungal, and parasitic.

Viral encephalitis

Most CNS viral infections cause aseptic meningitis or meningo-encephalitis rather than encephalitis. Viral encephalitis is classified into:

- Acute viral encephalitis
- Post-infectious encephalomyelitis
- Slow viral infections of the CNS: subacute sclerosing panencephalitis.

Acute viral encephalitis

Acute viral encephalitis is uncommon with an incidence of ~4/100 000 per year. Herpes simplex virus (HSV1 and HSV2) is the most common cause in infants and children but other viruses which can cause encephalitis include:

- *Herpes viruses*: varicella zoster virus (VZV), cytomegalovirus (CMV), Epstein–Barr virus (EBV), human herpesvirus 6 (HHV6).
- Measles, mumps, and rubella virus
- Rabies
- *Arboviruses*: Japanese B encephalitis, West Nile encephalitis, tick-borne encephalitis viruses.

Herpes simplex encephalitis is the most common cause of sporadic encephalitis in children in Western countries and is considered further.

Herpes simplex encephalitis (HSE)

Herpesviruses cause a fulminant haemorrhagic and necrotizing encephalitis with severe oedema and massive tissue necrosis especially involving the temporal lobes.

HSV1 infection is the cause in infants and children. Neonatal herpes simplex encephalitis, typically HSV2, is a different entity. One third of HSE cases occur between age 6 months and 20 years.

HSV1 infection in childhood is almost universal and asymptomatic unless gingivo-stomatitis occurs and it remains unknown why encephalitis only occurs in a tiny minority.

Clinical features

Onset may be insidious with abnormal behaviour and memory problems or acute with headache, fever, reduced consciousness, and focal neurological signs.

The differential diagnosis is wide and includes:

- *Non-infectious encephalopathy*: inflicted TBI, metabolic disorders
- *Intracranial infections*: meningitis, brain abscess
- Acute disseminated encephalomyelitis.

Management

Diagnostic investigations, which may be normal in the early stage when treatment is most effective, include:

- *Neuroimaging*: cranial CT scan may not reveal abnormalities until 3–5 days after symptom onset. CT scans initially show low-density areas with mass effect localized to the temporal lobes, either unilaterally or bilaterally. T2 weighted MRI shows changes earlier, typically affecting temporal lobes.
- *Lumbar puncture*: CSF may be normal in the 1st 48 h and thereafter similar to viral meningitis: lymphocytic pleocytosis and elevated protein up to 6 g/L. PCR detection of HSV is the diagnostic method of choice and has specificity and sensitivity >95%.
- *EEG*: reveals diffuse background slowing and focal temporal abnormalities in 80%: a normal EEG renders the diagnosis unlikely. Later, periodic lateralizing epileptic discharges (PLEDs) may appear and support the diagnosis.

Treatment

Aciclovir 500 mg/m^2 BSA or 10 mg/kg IV 8 hourly is indicated if HSE is a diagnostic possibility. Aciclovir inhibits viral replication and is therefore only effective if started early in the illness. If HSV infection is confirmed treatment should continue for 21 days to avoid relapse. Rapid infusion can cause crystalluria so monitor renal function.

In severe cases neurointensive care is required with attention to seizure control, control of ICP, and steroids (methylprednisolone or dexamethasone).

Two thirds of survivors have significant sequelae.

Injury

The brain or spinal cord may be injured by mechanical trauma or a variety of other mechanisms including in particular hypoxia–ischaemia of the brain and compression or infarction of the spinal cord.

Traumatic brain injury (TBI)

TBI, either accidental or inflicted, is the commonest cause of death and acquired disability in children. Non-traumatic injury may be caused by infection (meningitis, encephalitis), tumours, or stroke. The diagnosis and acute management of TBI is considered in Chapter 2, hypoxic–ischaemic encephalopathy in the newborn in Chapter 1, and non-accidental head injury in Chapter 18.

Rehabilitation and outcomes

Outcome after TBI is highly variable and determined by:
- Mechanism and severity of injury
- *Age at injury*: late outcome is better for functions that were established at the time of injury. Developmental sequence is gross motor, language, and then cognition so there is particular concern for late cognitive outcomes in children injured at a young age
- *Time since injury*: some deficits may not manifest for many years. The consequences of frontal lobe injury in early childhood may not be apparent until frontal lobe skills are expressed in adolescence.

Recognition of 'low-level' states

Consciousness has two components:
- *Arousal*: a function of the reticular activating system and assessed by eye-opening scale of GCS
- *Awareness*: can only be assessed by observation of voluntary movement including eye movements and speech and is difficult to demonstrate if voluntary control of movement is limited.

Arousal without awareness is the 'vegetative state'. Hypoxic–ischaemic injury has a worse prognosis than TBI of apparently similar initial severity.

Rehabilitation

Rehabilitation requires cross-disciplinary, forward-looking setting of specific, relevant, and measurable goals involving both child and family.

Spinal cord injury

Traumatic injury to the spinal cord is most common in males aged 16–30 years.

Aetiology and pathogenesis

Injury may be traumatic or non-traumatic:
- *Traumatic*: a sudden blow to the spine fractures, dislocates, or crushes one or more vertebrae with damage to the spinal cord tissue. Common causes include road traffic accidents; sports and recreation injuries such as diving; falls; acts of violence.
- *Non-traumatic*: injury may be inflammatory (transverse myelitis, ADEM, abscess, tuberculoma), vascular (anterior spinal artery infarction), compression (tumours, syringomyelia) or secondary to disease of the spinal column (arthritis, discitis).

Spinal cord injuries are classified by the level (e.g. cervical, lumbar) and according to whether injury is complete or incomplete. Complete transection is rare.

Clinical features

A complete injury is indicated by a total lack of sensory and motor function below the level of the injury. A thoracic or lumbar level injury causes paraplegia and loss of bowel and bladder control. A cervical injury affects breathing in addition.

Spinal cord injury is not always obvious. Numbness or paralysis may have rapid or gradual onset after injury.

Management

Acute management

It is safest to assume that trauma victims have a spinal cord injury until proved otherwise. Key initial steps are:
- *Immobilizing the spine*: handle patient without moving neck or back, place rigid collar around neck, placed injured person on rigid board
- *Primary assessment*: neurological examination to test for a sensory or motor level if possible.

Diagnostic investigations include:
- *Spinal radiographs*: Spinal cord injury without radiological abnormalities (SCIWORA) is a well-described entity
- *CT scan or MRI*: MRI is the imaging modality of choice for the spinal cord but may not be feasible in patients on life support or cervical traction.

Immediate further management encompasses:
- Neurosurgical evaluation
- IV methylprednisolone to minimize secondary injury from oedema
- Ventilatory support for high lesions
- Urinary catheterization
- Autonomic dysreflexia management.

Complete lesions above T6 may cause this syndrome in which noxious stimuli below the level such as full bladder or constipation cause reflex vasoconstriction and hypertension leading to increased vagal tone and bradycardia. Relieving the cause and sitting upright provides emergency treatment.

Long-term management

Many issues are shared by children with neural tube defects. Attention is paid to:
- *Motor deficits*: management of spasticity and contractions, postural abnormalities, pathological fractures
- *Sensory deficits*: avoidance of skin breakdown
- *Sphincter control*: bladder dysfunction and constipation
- *Emotional and psychological support*: lack of independence and sexual dysfunction are important issues. Coping strategies, education and new technologies such as computer devices and functional electrical stimulation systems have all enhanced prospects for children with spinal cord injury.

7.15 Inflammatory disorders and stroke

Acute disseminated encephalomyelitis (ADEM)

ADEM is an uncommon but treatable inflammatory demyelinating disorder which typically affects the subcortical white matter. Synonyms include post-infectious encephalomyelitis and immune-mediated encephalomyelitis. Typically it is a disease of young children (age 5–8 years).

Aetiology and pathogenesis

ADEM is an autoimmune disorder probably caused by cross-reacting antibodies to myelin autoantigens such as myelin basic protein which share antigenic determinants with infecting pathogens.

It often occurs 7–14 days after a viral infection or, less commonly, vaccinations. It has been associated with many pathogens including:

- *Viruses*: HHV1, HHV6, HIV, measles, mumps, rubella, VZV, EBV, CMV, influenza, coxsackie
- *Bacteria*: Group A β-haemolytic streptococci, *Campylobacter*, *Mycoplasma*, *Borrelia burgdorferi*
- Rickettsiae

Clinical features

A prodromal phase with fever, malaise, and headache is often followed by meningism and drowsiness. Multifocal neurological signs may include cerebellar signs, hemiparesis, cranial nerve palsies, and optic neuritis.

Significant grey matter involvement is indicated by seizures and coma. Atypical cases may present with irritability and apparent psychiatric illness.

ADEM and multiple sclerosis (MS)

ADEM is typically monophasic but may show a multiphasic or recurrent course and must include a degree of encephalopathy. An episode of demyelination without encephalopathy is termed a clinically isolated syndrome (CIS) and is more likely to be MS. In the absence of a biological marker the distinction between ADEM, CIS, and MS cannot be made with certainty, especially at the first presentation.

In older children who relapse >6 months later MS may subsequently develop in 10%. MS is more frequently monosymptomatic without prodromal viral illness. MRI may show widespread CNS disturbance with thalamic involvement, and smaller periventricular lesions.

Diagnostic investigations

- *Neuroimaging*: cranial MRI, T2 weighted or FLAIR images is the investigation of choice and typically shows asymmetrical demyelination of hemispheric subcortical white matter, and symmetrical involvement of thalami and basal ganglia. Spinal cord involvement is common. Cranial CT is often normal.
- *Neurophysiology*: EEG may show excess background slow wave activity. VEPs may be attenuated if there is bilateral optic neuritis.
- *Serology*: rarely positive.
- *CSF*: a lymphocytosis and raised protein level (0.4–0.6 g/L) is common

Treatment

Children presenting with meningism, fever, and acute encephalopathy are often initially treated with cefotaxime and aciclovir until the diagnosis of ADEM is established.

Treatment starts with IV methylprednisolone 25 mg/kg per day (up to 1 G) for 3–5 days followed by oral prednisolone 2 mg/kg per day, tapered over 4–6 weeks depending on resolution of clinical signs. Other treatment options if steroids fail include plasmapheresis or IV immunoglobulins.

Steroids appear to hasten the rate but not the ultimate extent of recovery and a minority of children are left with neurological impairment that ranges from mild to severe.

Paediatric autoimmune neuropsychiatric disorders associated with streptococcal infections (PANDAS)

This name is given to an uncommon group of dyskinesias and associated psychiatric disorders which may occur after infection with β-haemolytic streptococci. Sydenham's chorea is the classical example. The aetiology is thought to be autoimmune reactivity targeting the basal ganglia, but this remains controversial.

The clinical spectrum of post-streptococcal dyskinesias has been expanded beyond chorea to encompass motor and vocal tics, dystonia, and myoclonus. Significant and disabling psychiatric co-morbidity occurs including obsessive–compulsive disorder, anxiety or depression, conduct disorders, and hyperkinetic disorders. Prevalence of movement and emotional disorders in close relatives suggests a genetic predisposition.

Treatment options include antibiotic treatment for tonsillitis in PANDAS and immunomodulation strategies such as plasma exchange and IV immunoglobulin, but the evidence base for this is very limited. Carbamazepine and sodium valproate are useful in Sydenham's chorea.

Guillain–Barré syndrome (GBS)

GBS is an acute inflammatory immune-mediated polyneuropathy with an incidence of 1–2/100 000 per year. The mortality is 3–8% and up to 15% of patients are left with permanent neurological sequelae.

Aetiology and pathogenesis

GBS is believed to result from an autoimmune response to recent infection or vaccination. Implicated infections include bacterial (*Campylobacter*, *Mycoplasma pneumoniae*, *Borrelia burgdorferi*) and viral (CMV, EBV, HIV).

Four different subtypes are now recognized:

- *Acute inflammatory demyelinating polyradiculoneuropathy (AIDP)*: 90% of cases are in this category
- *Acute motor axonal neuropathy (AMAN)*: 5–10%, more prevalent in paediatric age groups. A purely motor type. 70% seropositive for campylobacter
- *Acute motor-sensory axonal neuropathy (AMSAN)*: 5–10%. Typically in adults
- *Miller–Fisher syndrome (MFS)*: a rare variant with ataxia, ophthalmoplegia, and areflexia.

Clinical features

The classical presentation of GBS, AIDP type is with an ascending flaccid paralysis 2–4 weeks after a respiratory or gastrointestinal illness. Back or lower limb pain may be present with or without paraesthesia. Weakness progresses over hours or days to involve arms, trunk, muscles of respiration, and cranial nerves. A plateau phase ensues with a recovery phase lasting several months.

Examination may reveal:
- *Motor dysfunction:* symmetrical ascending limb weakness with inability to stand or walk., hypotonia and areflexia
- *Cranial nerve palsies:* facial weakness, dysarthria, ophthalmoplegia
- *Sensory dysfunction:* distal loss of vibration, proprioception and touch
- *Autonomic dysfunction:* cardiovascular instability, tachycardia, arrhythmias, hypotension, urinary retention, constipation.

Differential diagnosis
- *Spinal cord disease:* tumour, transverse myelitis
- *Brainstem disease:* infarction, tumour
- *Neuromuscular block:* myasthenia, botulism
- *Irritable hip, discitis:* pain with difficulty in ambulation
- *Poisoning:* heavy metals (lead, arsenic) botulinum toxin.

Management

Investigations

Diagnosis is clinical but useful investigations include:
- *Lumbar puncture:* Not always necessary in clear-cut cases. Elevated CSF protein without pleocytosis is supportive but CSF may be normal within 7 days of symptom onset
- *MRI scan:* Indicated if any suspicion of spinal cord pathology such as haemorrhage or tumour suggested by acute onset, distinct sensory/motor level, sphincter disturbance
- *Nerve conduction studies:* 80% slowing or increased distal latencies is consistent with GBS but may be normal early on.

To identify an underlying cause, acute and convalescent serum for viral and mycoplasma titres, a throat swab, and stool culture are indicated.

Monitoring and treatment
- *Supportive measures:* respiratory and cardiac complications can be life threatening. All patients require careful monitoring of ECG, blood pressure, and respiratory function. Vital capacity or FEV1 should be monitored every 1–2 h initially to identify incipient respiratory failure. Analgesics are given for pain which is often present.
- *Specific treatment: immunotherapy:* treatment options include intravenous immunoglobulin, IVIG, and plasmapheresis. IVIG is given at a dose of 2g/kg per day as a single dose or divided over 2–5 days if the child is deteriorating rapidly.
- Admission to PICU is indicated for rapid progression, flaccid tetraparesis, FVC <30% predicted, bulbar palsy, or cardiovascular instability. Despite paralysis the child is fully aware and careful communication is important.
- Prolonged multidisciplinary rehabilitation may be required.

Stroke in childhood

Stroke is a rare disorder in childhood with an incidence of about 3/100 000. A stroke is defined as a focal neurological deficit lasting >24 h, of vascular origin. Congenital stroke may be asymptomatic.

Aetiology and pathogenesis

Arterial ischaemic stroke (AIS) and haemorrhagic stroke occur with equal frequency but have different causes.

Conditions predisposing to arterial ischaemic stroke include:
- *Heart disease:* congenital or acquired, patent foramen ovale (PFO)
- Sickle cell disease
- Trauma
- *Infections:* meningitis, varicella
- Genetic thrombophilias
- Moya moya disease
- Down, Williams syndromes.

Haemorrhagic stroke may occur in thrombocytopaenia or coagulation defects.

Clinical features

Acute hemiparesis is most common, sometimes accompanied by hemisensory signs or visual field defects.

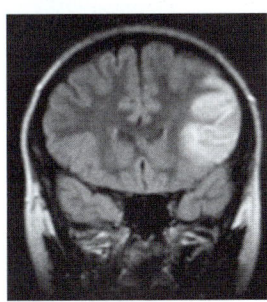

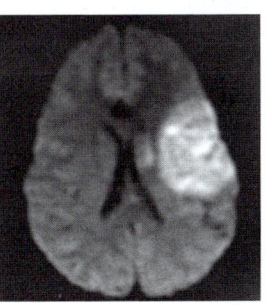

Fig 7.17 MRI: left middle cerebral artery infarct in a teenage girl presenting with acute hemiparesis and aphasia. Echo revealed PFO and aneurysm of atrial septum.

Management

Investigations

Brain MRI should be undertaken as soon as possible to image the cervical and proximal intracranial arterial vasculature (Fig 7.17). CT is an acceptable initial alternative to identify haemorrhage but cannot exclude arterial dissection. Cardiac echocardiography should also be done within 48 h if imaging indicates an embolic cause.

Investigations for a prothrombotic tendency are indicated including homocysteine levels, protein C and S deficiency. Viral studies may be appropriate.

Acute management

Avoid fever and treat acute seizures. Neurosurgical referral for haemorrhagic stroke or raised ICP. Urgent exchange transfusion for ischaemic stroke in sickle cell disease. Consider aspirin 5 mg/kg per day for arterial ischaemic stroke unless there is evidence of haemorrhage or sickle cell disease. Anticoagulation may be indicated in selected patients.

Secondary prevention

Recurrence rate is high at 6–20% and 60% in sickle cell disease. Measures depend on cause and include regular transfusion in sickle cell disease, low-dose aspirin, and rarely anticoagulation. A patent foramen ovale may be closed.

7.16 Case-based discussions

A teenage girl with headache

A 15 year old girl presents with a history of headaches. The headaches have been present for about 4 weeks and are getting worse. They are bilateral, throbbing, and worse in the mornings and on lying down. In the preceding week she has vomited twice and in the last few days has complained of blurred vision. There is a family history of migraine.

On examination she is obese and normotensive. She is afebrile, alert, and orientated. General neurological examination is normal with no cranial nerve palsies and no cerebellar signs. Examination of the fundi reveals bilateral papilloedema (Fig 7.18).

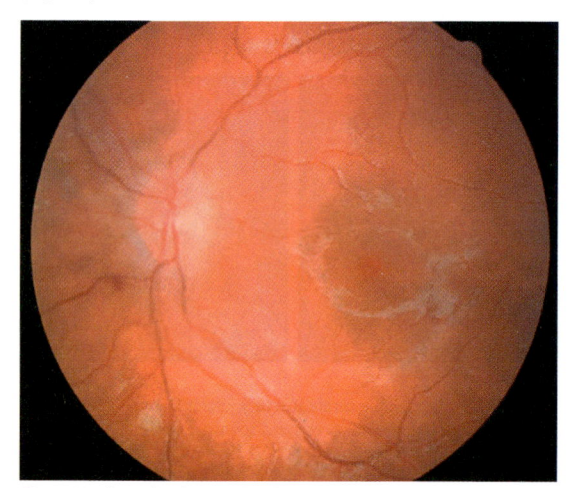

Fig. 7.18 Optic fundus: papilloedema.

What is the differential diagnosis?
The features of the headache suggest raised ICP which is confirmed by the finding of papilloedema. A posterior fossa tumour must be excluded but the lack of cerebellar signs raises the possibility of idiopathic intracranial hypertension (IIH). Obesity is a risk factor.

An urgent cranial CT is normal.

What further investigations are indicated?
A lumbar puncture to exclude IIH, an ophthalmological review to detect any visual field defect and cranial MRI.

A lumbar puncture was performed under sedation. An opening pressure of 40 cmH$_2$O was documented and 10 mL of CSF was drained off. Ophthalmic review found significantly constricted visual fields, right worse than left. Visual acuity was normal. Cranial MRI showed no mass lesion and patent dural sinuses. The optic nerve sheaths were distended with fluid and the optic nerve heads were protruding into the globes.

What is the diagnosis and management?
The CSF pressure >25 cmH$_2$O and neuroimaging confirm a diagnosis of IIH. 'Diagnostic' lumbar puncture can provide long-term relief of symptoms, and relief of severe headaches can be achieved by reducing CSF pressure through repeat lumbar punctures. Medication with acetazolamide is started in those whose headaches persist after initial lumbar puncture or who have visual compromise.

Surgical intervention is considered if medical measures fail and there is a progressive visual deficit.

Despite treatment with acetazolamide and a further lumbar puncture, headaches persisted and a progressive visual field deficit developed. She underwent optic nerve fenestrations and subsequently required a lumboperitoneal shunt insertion.

A boy with facial paralysis

A 12 year old boy presents with a history of a lopsided facial appearance developing over a few hours 1 week previously. He is now unable to close the right eye and is having difficulty drinking. There was no history of recent infection but he had recently been on a school camp in the New Forest region of the UK, home to a population of wild deer.

On examination, the only abnormality is a right-sided facial paralysis involving all the muscles. Taste sensation and examination of cranial nerves other than VII was normal. Blood pressure was normal. Figure 7.19 shows the response to a request to smile.

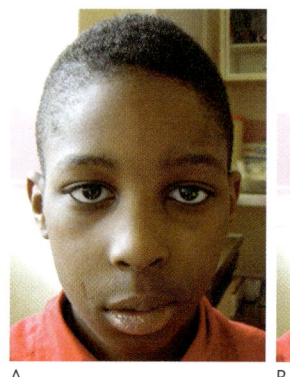

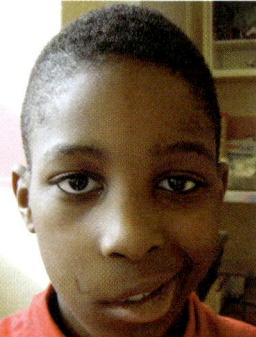

A   B

Fig 7.19 Facial paralysis: right side.

What is the most likely diagnosis?
The history and physical signs suggest a diagnosis of Bell's palsy. Bell's palsy is an acute idiopathic lower motor neuron VII nerve palsy which manifests as unilateral paralysis of all the facial muscles. There may be impaired taste and hyperacusis. A central *upper* motor neuron deficit causes weakness of the *lower* face only.

What are the possible causes?
Idiopathic Bell's palsy is believed to be an autoimmune reaction to infection. Recognized secondary causes include acute otitis media, hypertension, and Lyme disease. He has recently visited an endemic Lyme disease region. In Lyme disease facial involvement frequently becomes bilateral after a few days.

What is the management?
Cranial imaging is not necessary in the absence of additional cranial nerve palsies. If appropriate, Lyme disease should be investigated by serology for *Borrelia burgdorferi*.

Management of idiopathic Bell's palsy in children is symptomatic. An exposed cornea should be protected by lubrication and patching. A recent systematic review found no evidence of benefit from the routine use of corticosteroids for the treatment of Bell's palsy in children. Antivirals such as aciclovir are not recommended.

Complete recovery after 2–4 weeks is the rule in children. However, if denervation is complete improvement may be delayed and recovery may not be total.

Chapter 8
Ophthalmology

8.1 Eye anatomy and clinical ophthalmology *176*
8.2 Eye symptoms and signs *178*
8.3 Developmental anomalies and visual impairment *180*
8.4 Strabismus and nystagmus *182*
8.5 Eye infections and inflammations *184*
8.6 Childhood cataract and glaucoma *186*
8.7 Retinal and optic nerve disorders *188*
8.8 Genetic eye disease *190*
8.9 Case-based discussions *192*

8.1 Eye anatomy and clinical ophthalmology

Eye anatomy

The structure of the mammalian eye (Fig 8.1) consists of three main layers or *tunics*: fibrous, vascular (uveal tract), and nervous.
- *Tunica fibrosa oculi*: sclera and cornea
- *Tunica vasculosa oculi*: iris, ciliary body, and choroid
- *Tunica nervosa oculi*: inner sensory layer (retina).

The eye is also conveniently divided into the anterior and posterior segments:
- *Anterior segment*: cornea, iris, ciliary body, and lens
- *Posterior segment*: hyaline membrane and all structures behind it: vitreous humour, retina, choroid, and optic nerve.

Considering some important structures individually:
- *Sclera*: tough, fibrous outer protective coating, translucent with a bluish tinge in infants
- *Cornea*: transparent avascular tissue replacing the sclera anteriorly and inserted into the sclera at the limbus
- *Conjunctiva*: transparent mucous membrane that covers the posterior surface of the lids (palpebral conjunctiva) and anterior surface of the sclera (bulbar conjunctiva)
- *Lens*: consists of layers of tissue in a tough capsule; suspended from the ciliary body by the zonule fibres of Zinn
- *Uveal tract*: the iris, ciliary body, and choroid, each of which is pigmented and highly vascularized. The transparent innermost layer of the choroid is called Bruch's membrane
- *Hyaloid membrane*: a transparent membrane that encloses the vitreous humour, separating it from the retina. In front of the ora serrata (the area in which the retina terminates as it approaches the ciliary body) the hyaloid membrane is thickened by radial fibres to become the zonules of Zinn
- *Retina*: contains the rods and cones. The fovea centralis is the centre of the macula and has the highest visual acuity. The optic disc (optic papilla, blind spot) is located at the position from which the optic nerve leaves the retina.

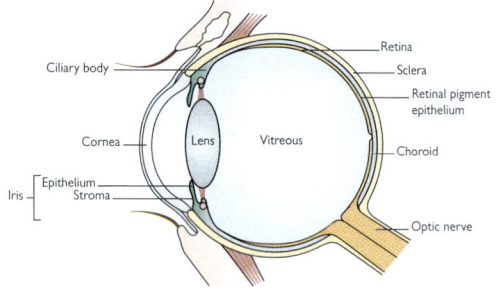

Fig 8.1 Cross-section of the human eye. Uveal tract boxed in red.

Extraocular anatomy
The orbits house the eyeballs, extraocular muscles, lacrimal glands, arteries, veins, and nerves. They are related to the frontal, maxillary, ethmoid, and sphenoid sinuses.

Clinical ophthalmology

History
This usually comprises an account of parental observations concerning some striking physical sign or concerns about the infant or child's visual function. Always listen to the parents.

Clues that visual function is impaired vary with age (see Chapter 18.7). However, visual impairment in the young may pass unnoticed. Any family history of eye disorders should be elicited.

Examination
Examination of the eyes should include:
- *External examination*: lids, conjunctiva, sclera, cornea, and iris together with the nasolacrymal gland
- *Pupils*: equal, round and reactive to light?
- *Red reflex*: detects opacities in the visual axis (cataract, corneal clouding) or abnormalities of the back of the eye (e.g. retinoblastoma)
- *Examination of the fundus*: by direct ophthalmoscopy
- Assessment of vision
- Assessment of ocular alignment and movements.

Of course, an ophthalmologist, optometrist, or orthoptist will undertake a much more detailed examination. The former has a host of additional instruments to hand including the slit-lamp (biomicroscope), the gonioscope (to view the iridocorneal angle), and indirect ophthalmoscope.

Examination under anaesthetic (EUA) may be necessary in young infants and pupillary dilatation is essential for fundoscopy.

Assessment of vision
This encompasses assessment of visual acuity, of contrast and colour vision, and of the visual fields.

Testing visual acuity
Visual acuity (VA) refers to the spatial resolving capacity of the visual system, the acuteness or clarity of vision as revealed by the ability to see fine detail. It depends on the quality of the image focused on the fovea (determined by the tissues of the visual axis including the lens), photoreceptor function in the fovea, and processing by the visual cortex. Measurement of VA is useful as it corresponds most closely with the visual capacity which permits normal daily activity.

In school-age children and adults VA is measured by assessing ability to identify or match black symbols on a white background (Snellen's optotype letters or numbers) at a standardized distance (6 m or 20 ft for distance VA) as the size of the letters is varied.

Reference VA, expressed as the ratio 6/6 (in UK) or 20/20 (in USA) corresponds to the ability to recognize a letter the individual parts of which subtend an angle of 1′ of arc at a distance of 6 m/20 ft. Each size letter has a corresponding distance at which its parts subtend this angle, the largest corresponding to 60 m/200 ft and the smallest to 3 m/10 ft. The larger the denominator, the worse the VA. For an eye with a VA of 6/60 the smallest letter recognized at 6 m would be seen by a 'normal' eye at 60 m. Near VA is done with a corresponding chart held at 40 cm/16 in.

The measurement of VA in infants and young children has to take account of their normal visual development and cognitive ability (e.g. verbal or preverbal).

Normal visual development
Vision develops from a very low level after birth to near adult levels by 12–18 months of age. By 4–6 months retinal maturation, myelination of visual pathways, and accommodation development is completed. This is known as the 'critical period'.

Maturation of the visual cortex occurs more gradually, over a 6–8 year period, with the most rapid phase being in the first 2 years of life. The development of vision and visual responses follows regular milestones (Table 8.1).

Table 8.1. Normal visual development		
Age	Visual Acuity	Other
Birth	6/60	Horizontal gaze in place Intermittent strabismus Limited visual fields
2 months	6/60	Vertical gaze in place Colour developing Central steady gaze Early binocularity
3–4 months		Good fixing and following Accommodation begins Good alignment
6 months	6/18–6/48	Normal ocular alignment
1 year	6/18	Visual fields fully developed
3 years	6/6	

Strategies for VA testing in infants and young children include behavioural testing, preferential looking, and recognition testing (Table 8.2).

Table 8.2. Visual acuity testing by age	
Age	Test
Newborn	Face fixation and following Preference for patterned objects
6–8 weeks	Smiles responsively Fixes and follows an object through 90°
3 months	Follows objects through 180°
10 months	Picks up small objects, e.g. raisin
2 years	Identify specific pictures of reducing size, e.g. Cardiff acuity cards
>3 years	Letter matching using single letter charts, e.g. Sheridan Gardiner test
>5 years	Identify a line of letters on a Snellen chart by naming or matching

Contrast and colour vision
Contrast sensitivity may be reduced in the presence of normal Snellen acuity which tests high contrast.

The most common form of colour blindness is failure of red–green discrimination which is X-linked and affects ~8% of boys and 0.5% of girls. It may be detected by Ishihara colour plates (Fig 8.2) or by colour matching in young children.

Visual fields
These can be assessed by simple confrontation techniques or formal Goldmann testing in older children.

Ocular alignment and motility
Alignment of the eyes must be checked to determine the presence of any abnormality (strabismus). This is done by simple observation, the corneal reflex test, and cover tests. These tests are considered in detail in Section 8.4.

The full range of eye movements should be tested and any abnormal supplementary movements such as nystagmus or saccadic movements noted.

Investigations
Imaging
CT is useful for visualization of the bony orbit and globe and indicated in suspected orbital cellulitis, trauma or other orbital pathology. MRI is indicated for suspected optic nerve disease such as glioma or suspected compressive optic neuropathy. Ultrasonography is useful for location of intraocular foreign bodies.

Electrodiagnostic tests
These objective tests of the integrity of the visual pathway are useful in infants who are not fixing and following or have supplementary abnormal eye movements and older children who are unable to communicate.

- *Electroretinography (ERG):* ERG is a record of the mass electrical activity from the retina when stimulated by an intense flash of light. It is useful in the diagnosis of generalized retinal degenerations such as retinitis pigmentosa.
- *Electro-oculography (EOG):* this indirectly measures the standing potential of the eye and reflects the activity of the RPE and photoreceptors of the entire retina. It is useful in diagnosing or screening for hereditary macular diseases (e.g. Best disease).
- *Visual evoked potential (VEP):* this is a gross electrical response recorded from the visual cortex in response to a changing visual stimulus e.g. multiple flashes. The visual pathway delay and amplitude of response is measured. It can document visual development in infants and reveal dysfunction of the optic nerve or chiasm. It can detect non-organic 'functional' visual loss.

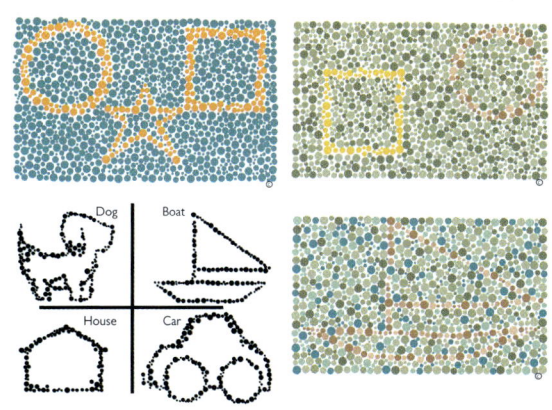

Fig 8.2 Ishihara test for colour blindness adapted for children age 3–6 years. Test plates located at www.colorvisiontesting.com and reproduced from 'Color Vision Testing Made Easy' by Dr Terrace L Waggoner (waggonert@aol.com).

8.2 Eye symptoms and signs

Red eye, watering, and photophobia

These common presentations, often in combination, are usually benign, but the presence of visual symptoms or photophobia suggests consideration of more serious causes.

Conjunctivitis or blepharoconjunctivitis and foreign bodies cause red eyes with watering or discharge but no photophobia.

Superficial conditions causing all three symptoms include corneal abrasions/erosions and keratitis. Look for circumlimbal injection.

Acute anterior uveitis, acute glaucoma, or endophthalmitis require slit-lamp examination to identify additional signs such as corneal oedema, keratic precipitates, anterior chamber activity, and chorioretinitis.

Watering

A watering eye may be caused by excessive secretion of tears (lacrimation) or overflow due to inadequate drainage (epiphora). A newborn infant does not shed tears when crying for the first 4–6 weeks. Nasolacrimal duct obstruction is the most common cause of chronic watering, without other ocular signs. There may be a sticky discharge and nasolacrimal sac swelling.

Photophobia

Photophobia (light sensitivity) is a symptom of excessive sensitivity to light or an aversion to sunlight or well-lit places. In folklore and mythology many creatures (e.g. vampires) suffer from photophobia. In paediatric practice the most common cause is intracranial infection (meningitis, encephalitis) or migraine but there are several important ophthalmic causes (see Box).

Ophthalmic causes of photophobia

- *Anterior segment disease:*
  - corneal abrasion or erosion
  - keratitis
  - anterior uveitis
  - glaucoma
  - aniridia
- *Posterior segment disease:*
  - endophthalmitis
  - retinal dystrophies

Dry eye

A dry eye is an uncommon problem. The actual complaint is usually of a burning sensation. Causes include:
- *Vitamin A deficiency:* xerophthalmia
- *Ectodermal dysplasia:* anhydrotic type
- Familial dysautonomia
- Sjögren's syndrome
- Congenital alacrima
- Facial nerve palsy.

Treatment is by the use of lubricant drops or gels.

Proptosis and globe size

Proptosis

Abnormal protrusion of the eyeball (proptosis) is uncommon, but usually signifies severe orbital disease when combined with reduced vision and restriction of ocular movements (Fig 8.3). Congenital proptosis is rare. Acquired proptosis occurs due to abnormal material (tumour, blood, or inflammatory exudate) within the orbit or oedema or infiltration of the extraocular muscles in thyroid eye disease.

The age of onset, whether unilateral or bilateral, and the rate of onset are important features bearing on the likely aetiology (Table 8.3).

Assessment of pupillary reactions, visual acuity, and ocular movements is essential together with systemic examination. The latter may provide clues to the diagnosis e.g. café au lait spots, an abdominal mass, or signs of hyperthyroidism.

Pseudo-proptosis may be caused by shallow orbits, ipsilateral large globe, contralateral enophthalmos or ptosis.

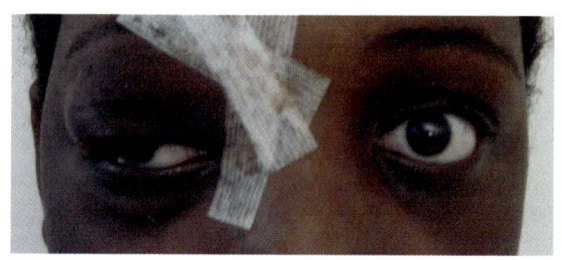

Fig 8.3 Right side proptosis due to orbital cellulitis.

Table 8.3. Causes of proptosis	
Orbital cellulitis	Acute unilateral proptosis with fever pain and lid swelling. Cavernous sinus thrombosis may be a complication
Thyroid eye disease	Bilateral with lid retraction and systemic signs. Rare in children

Tumours	Congenital dermoid cysts
	Metastatic:
	    neuroblastoma
	    retinoblastoma
	    leukaemic deposits
	Rhabdomyosarcoma
	Optic nerve glioma
	Langerhans cell histiocytosis
	Haemangioma
	Lymphangioma

Vascular anomalies	Congenital orbital varices Carotid-cavernous fistula
Bony anomalies	Craniofacial abnormalities

Abnormal eye (globe) size

Microphthalmia (small eyes) is usually developmental. An abnormally large eye is seen in glaucoma (bupthalmos) and axial myopia.

Pupil abnormalities

Leukocoria

Important causes of a white pupillary reflex include:
- *Lens:* cataract
- *Vitreous:*
  - persistent fetal vasculature
  - vitreous haemorrhage
- *Retina:*
  - retinoblastoma (Fig 8.4)
  - retinopathy of prematurity
  - coloboma
- *Infection:* toxocariasis.

Urgent investigation to exclude retinoblastoma is indicated.

Anisocoria

Inequality of the pupils may be physiological or due to a neurological disorder. It can be difficult to decide which is the abnormal pupil. Examination in bright or dim light can help to distinguish parasympathetic from sympathetic lesions. In Horner's syndrome (sympathetic lesion) anisocoria is more marked in dim light. The reverse is true for a parasympathetic lesion.

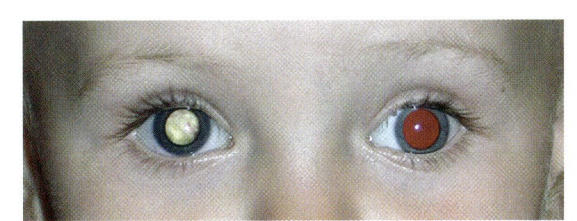

Fig 8.4 Right leukocoria due to retinoblastoma. Reproduced courtesy of John Ainsworth.

Causes of a small pupil
- Horner's syndrome
- Congenital miosis
- Uveitis
- Drugs.

Causes of a large pupil
- Third nerve lesion
- Coloboma
- *Drugs:* mydriatics, e.g. atropine.

Ptosis

*Blepharo*ptosis is a unilateral or bilateral abnormally low position of the upper eyelid. It is categorized by age of onset (congenital or acquired) or by aetiology (Table 8.4). Most cases of congenital ptosis are unilateral (Fig 8.5) and due to dysgenesis of the levator palpebrae muscle It may be severe enough to cause deprivational amblyopia.

Clinical evaluation

In congenital ptosis there will be some lid-lag on downward gaze. If acquired, the lid remains ptotic in all gaze positions.

Management

If severe, congenital ptosis requires early correction to avoid amblyopia. Otherwise patients should be monitored for signs of amblyopia or the development of ocular torticollis (abnormal head posture).

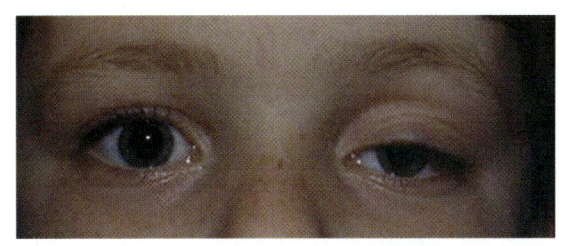

Fig 8.5 Left congenital ptosis.

Table 8.4. Causes of ptosis

Congenital	
Isolated congenital ptosis	Developmental dysgenesis of the levator muscle. Unilateral in 70%. May be familial (AD)
Blepharophimosis syndrome	AD condition with short palpebral fissures, epicanthus inversus, and telecanthus
Marcus Gunn jaw-winking syndrome	The motor nerve to the external pterygoid muscle is misdirected to the ipsilateral levator. Elevation of the ptotic lid occurs during chewing or movement of the jaw to the opposite side
Acquired	
Neurogenic ptosis	Horner's syndrome IIIrd nerve palsy
Myogenic ptosis	Myasthenia gravis, myotonic dystrophy, Kearns Sayre syndrome (chronic progressive external ophthalmoplegia), ocular myopathy
Mechanical	Tumours, infiltration or oedema of the upper lid

Horner's syndrome

A syndrome caused by interruption of the ocular sympathetic supply. The clinical features (Fig 8.6) include:
- Ptosis (partial)
- *Miosis:* small pupil with normal light and near reaction
- Enophthalmos (apparent)
- Anhidrosis (ipsilateral)
- Heterochromia iridis (in congenital type).

Congenital causes include obstetric trauma (to the brachial plexus), varicella syndrome, and cervical vertebra anomalies. Acquired causes include tumours such as neuroblastoma, surgery, and trauma; urgent neurological evaluation is indicated.

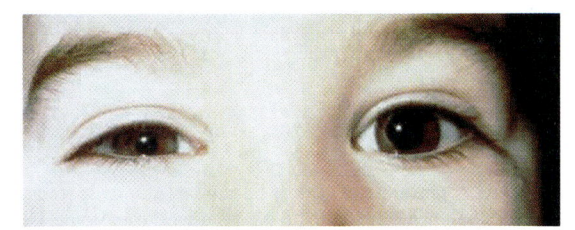

Fig 8.6 Right Horner's syndrome. Arch Soc Esp. Oftalmol 1998; 237–40.

8.3 Developmental anomalies and visual impairment

Developmental anomalies
Developmental anomalies affecting the eye are mostly rare and may have a genetic or acquired aetiology. Two important diseases with a developmental basis are discussed elsewhere: congenital cataract and congenital glaucoma.

A coloboma is a gap or cleft in any part of the eye caused by incomplete closure of an embryological fissure. The term dysgenesis is used for stable anomalies and dystrophy for those which progress.

Some of the more common and important anomalies affecting different parts of the eye's anatomy are the following.

Eyelids
A coloboma (clefting defect) of the eyelid may occur in isolation or in association with other clefting abnormalities or 1st arch syndromes. Bilateral lower lid clefts occur in Goldenhar syndrome.

Epicanthal folds are common, particularly in trisomy 21, and may give rise to a false appearance of squint (pseudostrabismus).

Globe and orbits
Microphthalmia occurs on a continuum with anophthalmia (absence of both eyes) which is very rare. Cyclopia, a single centrally placed eye, usually occurs as a component of severe holoprosencephaly.

Nasolacrimal duct
Stenosis or obstruction of the nasolacrimal duct is present in 30% of newborns and 90% resolve by age 1 year.

The anterior segment
Cornea
In sclerocornea the cornea is white and resembles sclera.
A corneal dermoid is a benign choristoma, which may be cystic the most common site being the inferotemporal limbus (Fig 8.7).

Abnormalities of size and shape include microcornea and keratoconus (thin, cone-shaped cornea).

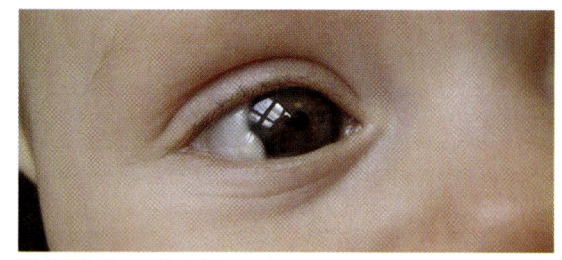

Fig 8.7 Epibulbar limbal dermoid.

Iris
Aniridia
Complete absence of the iris may be familial (AD) or sporadic and is caused by defects in the *PAX6* gene on chromosome 11. The sporadic form is more commonly found as a component of WAGR syndrome (**W**ilms' tumour, **A**niridia, **G**enitourinary abnormalities, and **R**etardation) associated with deletions of chromosome 11p. Associated eye findings include poor vision, cataract and glaucoma, nystagmus, foveal hypoplasia, and ectopia lentis.

Iris colobomas
Often in the inferonasal quadrant appearing as a notch or keyhole. If complete, these are often associated with other ocular and systemic disorders: trisomy 13 and 18, Aicardi syndrome and, rarely, as a component of the CHARGE syndrome (see below). See Fig 8.8.

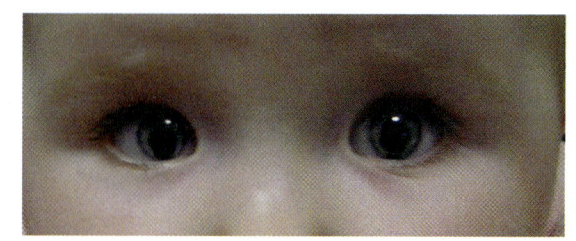

Fig 8.8 Bilateral iris colobomata.

Iris heterochromia
A difference in iris colour may be congenital or acquired from infiltrative processes such as naevi and melanomatous tumours.

Anterior segment dysgenesis
This comprises a spectrum of disorders involving the cornea, trabeculum, iris, and lens all with the potential consequences of glaucoma and opacity of the visual axis. They include the Axenfeld–Rieger group and Peter anomaly.

Lens
Aphakia (absent lens) and microphakia (small lens) are rare.

Ectopia lentis
The lens may be partially subluxed (displaced) or completely luxed (dislocated) and moved from its normal position. Ectopia lentis presents with blurred vision and may be associated with cataract (partial) or glaucoma (complete).
Inherited causes include Marfan syndrome, homocystinuria, and Ehlers–Danlos syndrome.

Optic nerve
Anomalies include optic disc pits, hypoplasia, and coloboma. Coloboma of the posterior segment may occur as part of the CHARGE syndrome: **C**oloboma, **H**eart defects, **A**tresia of the choanae, **R**estricted growth and development, **G**enitourinary abnormalities, **E**ar abnormalities and deafness.
This may be AD or sporadic and most cases are due to mutation of the *CHD7* gene on chromosome 8q.

Vitreoretinal
Persistent hyperplastic primary vitreous (PHPV) is a congenital ocular malformation caused by incomplete regression of the primary vitreous.
Retinal dyplasia is usually part of a syndrome such as trisomy 13 or 18, Warburg syndrome, or Incontinentia Pigmenti.

Visual impairment

Visual impairment is defined in a variety of different ways for epidemiological, legal, and clinical purposes, but the two main groups correspond to low vision (sight impaired/partially sighted) and blind (severely sight impaired).

The WHO definitions are:
- *Low vision:* VA less than 6/18 but equal to or better than 3/60 in the better eye with best correction or a visual field less than 20°.
- *Blind:* VA less than 3/60 or visual field loss to less than 10° in the better eye with best correction.

The causes of visual impairment vary markedly with age and geography. The global burden is about 160 million of whom 40 million (25%) are blind. 80% of blind people are aged 50 years or more, reflecting the increasing preponderance of age-related cataract, glaucoma, and macular degeneration. 90% of the world's visually impaired live in developing countries and impairment is caused by avoidable factors in 50%.

Causes in infants and children

Childhood blindness results from a group of conditions the prevalence of which varies widely by region, being largely determined by socio-economic development and availability of primary health and eyecare services.

Prevention of childhood blindness is high on the agenda of Vision 2020, the global initiative for the elimination of avoidable blindness.

Primary causes according to level of income are:

Low-income countries
- Corneal scarring due to vitamin A deficiency, measles, ophthalmia neonatorum, harmful traditional eye remedies, trachoma
- Cataract caused by congenital rubella
- Onchocerciasis (river blindness).

Middle-income countries
- Retinopathy of prematurity (ROP)
- Congenital cataract and glaucoma.

High-income countries
- Retinopathy of prematurity (ROP)
- Optic nerve hypoplasia
- Cortical visual impairment (CVI)
- Genetic diseases, e.g. albinism.

The leading cause of preventable visual loss in children worldwide is amblyopia, the most common cause of monocular visual impairment.

Amblyopia

This is a developmental defect of central visual processing resulting from anything less than perfect, balanced foveal image formation from both eyes during the first decade of life. The term is from the Greek for dullness of vision and the lay term is 'lazy eye'. Normal and equal visual input is necessary for proper development of the postchiasmal visual pathways which is finished by ~9 years of age. The younger the cortical visual system, the more sensitive it is to abnormal input, the first 18 weeks of life being a critical period. A clinical rule of thumb is that a week of abnormal visual input per week of life is amblyogenic.

Causes of amblyopia
- *Abnormal binocular interaction:* strabismus
- *No/reduced image:* ocular occlusion by cataract, ptosis
- *Image blurring:* refractive errors including
  - anisometropia: significant refractive difference between the two eyes
  - ametropia: severe bilateral refractive error from astigmatism or hypermetropia.

Treatment is directed towards reversing or decreasing the amblyogenic stimulus and forcing the use of the amblyopic eye by occlusion or penalization of the sound eye.

Refractive errors

Errors in the refractive power of the eye may lead to subnormal visual acuity. This may result from variations in the cornea or lens curvature, or changes in the axial length of the eye. The commonest forms of refractive error are:

- *Myopia (short-sightedness):* common in older children. It is usually due to an increase in axial length of the eye so distant objects are blurred. It is inherited as a multifactorial trait, which may also be associated with systemic conditions such as Stickler syndrome. Concave lenses correct.
- *Hypermetropia (far-sightedness):* the most common refractive error in young children. As the visual axis is reduced the optical image formed is focused behind the retina. Early correction with convex lenses indicated.
- *Astigmatism:* the cornea, lens, or retinal surface has a slightly varied curvature rather than a spherical one. This produces a blurred retinal image of an object at any distance. Astigmatism can be corrected by special lenses.
- *Anisometropia:* a condition where the eyes have different refractive errors, with one worse than the other. It may occur with myopia, astigmatism, absent lens, or a combination of these refractive errors.

Visual impairment support

Visual impairment commonly occurs in the context of multiple disabilities. It is essential to have a multidisciplinary approach to address the following areas:

- *Safe and independent mobility:* mobility aids and techniques, and specific orientation skills
- *Social interaction:* understanding body language
- Personal management and independent living.
- *Literacy:* reading and writing through large print, optical devices, powered magnifiers, and for those with severe visual impairment, the use of Braille
- Technology and computer proficiency.
- *Schooling:* although there are special schools for children with severely visual impairment, most partially sighted children remain in mainstream schools with special assistance
- *Disability:* assessment for associated systemic and neurological abnormalities
- *Genetic counselling:* when indicated
- Emotional support.

8.4 Strabismus and nystagmus

Control of eye movement
Six extraocular muscles control eye movement. The nerve supply and primary actions are as listed in Table 8.5.

Table 8.5. Nerve supply and action of extraocular muscles	
Lateral rectus VI nerve (abducens)	Abduction
Medial rectus III nerve (oculomotor)	Adduction
Superior rectus III nerve	Elevation
Inferior oblique III nerve	Elevation
Inferior rectus III nerve	Depression
Superior oblique IV nerve (trochlear)	Intorsion and depression

A simple formula to remember the innervation of the extraocular muscles is **LR6 SO4 R3** (LR, lateral rectus; SO, superior oblique; R, rest).

Strabismus (squint)
This is the term used to describe a misalignment of the eyes or visual axes. It interferes with binocular single vision which depends on correct alignment and similar image clarity of both eyes from the newborn period.

Binocular single vision
Two eyes in front, as found in hunting animals, sacrifices the peripheral vision provided by the lateral eye placement found in herbivorous or hunted animals such as rabbits.

Frontal placement favours the development of accurate depth perception (stereopsis) which is allowed by visual cues arising from the fusion of two images received by the brain from eyes with slightly different vantage points.

Eye movements
- *Monocular movements:* ductions (abduction, adduction)
- *Binocular movements:*
  - versions (conjugate): eyes move in same direction; include left gaze, right gaze
  - vergences (disconjugate): eyes move in opposite directions; include convergence (inward, *eso-*), divergence (outward, *exo-*).

Classification of strabismus (squint)
A squint may be manifest spontaneously, called a *tropia*, or only present with disruption of binocular vision, called a *phoria* or latent squint. It may be constant or intermittent. It is then classified as:
- *Concomitant:* angle of deviation constant regardless of the position of gaze
- *Incomitant:* angle of deviation changes according to the direction of gaze. This includes paralytic squint and may be associated with abnormal head postures (e.g. torticollis) which maintain binocular visual input.

Most childhood strabismus is concomitant and manifest (tropia), with either esotropic (inward deviating) or exotropic (outward deviating) misalignment. Hypertropia (upward deviation) or hypotropia (downward deviation) is uncommon.

Aetiology
Concomitant strabismus: esotropic
Many normal newborns show exotropic deviations and up to 3 months of age a normal infant's alignment may be esotropic or exotropic. Acquired accommodative esotropia is most common, presenting between 1 and 5 years of age. This is often due to refractive errors in which accommodation tries to compensate for hypermetropia and is accompanied by excessive convergence. Non-accomodative esotropias include essential or infantile esotropia presenting before 6 months. Secondary esotropias arise from a variety of diseases which reduce VA such as cataracts, retinoblastoma, corneal scars, and retinopathy of prematurity.

Incomitant strabismus (paralytic squint)
These are less common and reflect pathology in the cranial nuclei or nerves (III, IV, or VI), the neuromuscular junction, extraocular muscles or orbit. Cranial nerve palsies cause divergent squint (III), vertical squint (IV), or convergent squint (VI). A VIth nerve palsy may be associated with raised intracranial pressure. Myasthenia and myopathies may cause incomitant squints.

Restriction syndromes
Syndromic patterns of mechanical restriction due to developmental anomalies cause incomitant strabismus including:
- *Duane syndrome:* absence of the abducens (VI) nerve nucleus with aberrant innervation of the lateral rectus by the III nerve. There is deficient abduction with retraction of globe and narrowing of palpebral fissure on attempted adduction. It may be AD or sporadic, unilateral or bilateral and may be associated with deafness.
- *Mobius syndrome:* congenital facial diplegia (VII nerve) and failure of abduction (VI nerve) often with other neurological findings and systemic abnormalities (e.g. Poland anomaly—absent pectoralis major and minor).
- *Brown syndrome:* restriction of the superior oblique tendon as it traverses the trochlea causes inability to elevate the affected eye in the adducted field.

Clinical evaluation
History
Parents may describe an intermittent squint. Strabismus is more common in preterm infants or those with cerebral palsy. There may be a family history. Diplopia is rarely present, as vision is suppressed from the deviating eye.

Examination
Abnormal head posture should be noted. Various structural abnormalities may simulate strabismus (pseudostrabismus). These include epicanthic folds, asymmetrical facies, narrow or wide inter-pupillary distances. A full examination of the eye including tests of visual acuity and eye movements should be done followed by specific screening tests for strabismus:
- *Corneal light reflexes (Hirschberg test):* A penlight is shone in the child's eyes from 30 cm (12 in). If there is misalignment the reflection is not in the same spot in each eye.
- *Cover tests:* There are two types:
  - *cover/uncover test*: one eye is covered and the other is observed. If the uncovered eye moves to fix on the object there is a squint which is spontaneously present—a *manifest*

squint (heterotropia). Each eye should be covered in turn. As the cover is removed from the eye, the eye emerging from the cover is observed. If the position of this eye changes, interruption of binocular vision has allowed it to deviate, and a *latent squint* (heterophoria) is present (Fig 8.9).

- *alternate cover test*: used if the cover/uncover test is normal. The cover is alternately placed in front of one eye and then the other. This breaks up the control of heterophoria which may last through a single cover/uncover cycle. If the eye which has been uncovered moves, a latent squint is present.

Management

Amblyopia is the most common and important complication: suppression of vision in a structurally and functionally normal eye. Poor depth perception may occur due to monofixation and the cosmetic defect may cause bullying and teasing.

Early referral to an ophthalmologist is required for any constant or intermittent deviation present beyond the age of 3 months. Management strategies include:

- Correction of any refractive errors
- Occlusion (patching) or penalization (e.g. atropinization) of the good eye to prevent and treat amblyopia
- Surgery: only after full assessment and treatment of causative factors if significant stable deviation persists and further improvement is not anticipated. Extraocular muscles may be weakened, strengthened, or transposed. The benefits include relief of diplopia and possible restoration of binocular vision.

Cranial nerve palsies

- *III nerve*: ptosis, eye turned 'down and out', fixed and dilated pupil. A rare congenital form exists. Acquired causes include head trauma, intracranial infection (meningitis), tumours, intracranial aneurysms, and migraine.
- *IV nerve*: hypertropia occurs (vertical strabismus). The more common congenital form is usually unilateral. The most common acquired cause is head trauma.
- *VI nerve*: esotropia occurs: congenital as part of Duane syndrome; acquired due to hydrocephalus, tumours, head injury and infection (meningitis).

Nystagmus

An involuntary abnormality of fixation in which there are rhythmic oscillations of one or both eyes. These may be of equal amplitude and velocity (pendular nystagmus) or more usually with a slow initial phase and a fast corrective phase (jerk nystagmus). The direction is defined by the direction of the rapid phase. It may occur in a horizontal, vertical or rotary direction.

- *Congenital*: early-onset nystagmus is usually pendular and may be associated with decreased VA as in macular lesions, albinism, congenital cataract. Idiopathic congenital jerk nystagmus may be familial.
- *Acquired*: late-onset nystagmus has a variety of causes including cerebellar dysfunction, spinocerebellar degeneration, vestibular disorders and seizures.

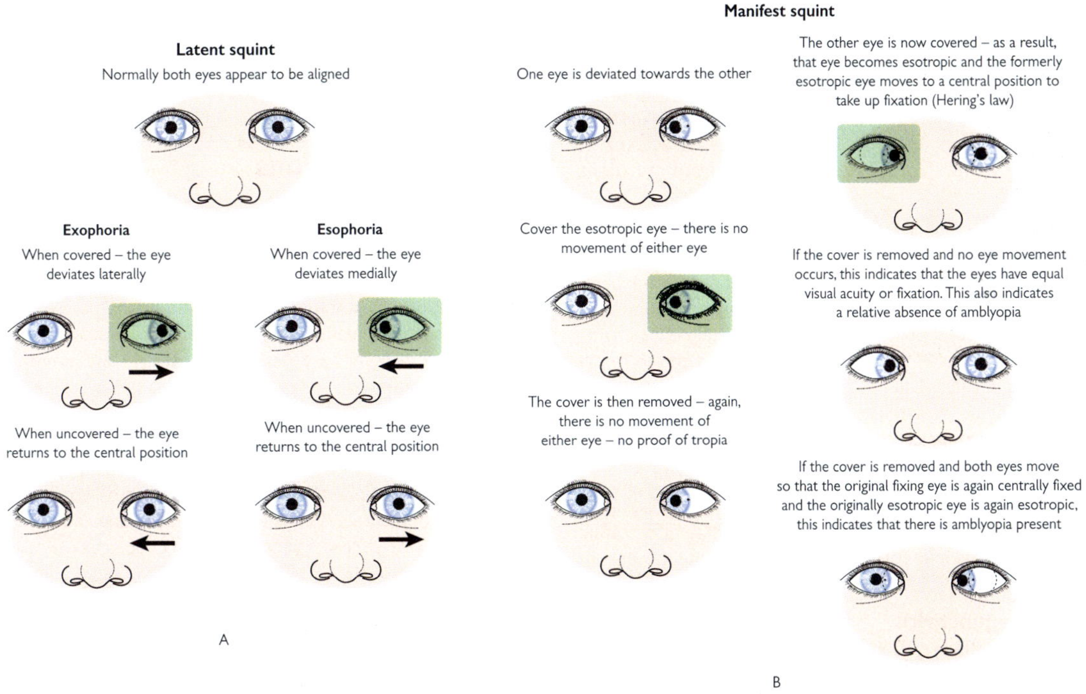

Fig 8.9 Cover/uncover tests: A. Phoria (latent). B. Tropia (manifest).

8.5 Eye infections and inflammations

These are classified by their anatomical location, infectious or inflammatory origin and age of occurrence.

Anatomical sites
Ocular
- *Eyelids:* blepharitis
- *Conjunctiva:* conjunctivitis
- *Cornea:* keratitis
- *Uveal tract:* uveitis
- *Globe:* endophthalmitis.

Periocular
- Periorbital (preseptal)
- Orbital.

Anatomical boundaries are not respected by pathogens and contiguous regions are often involved to give kerato-conjunctivitis or blepharo-conjunctivitis.

Pathogens include bacteria, viruses, fungi, protozoa (toxoplasma), and roundworms (toxocara). Inflammation may be allergic or part of a systemic autoimmune process.

Conjunctivitis

This may be bacterial, viral, chemical, or allergic. Clinical features are a mucopurulent discharge and injection of the palpebral and bulbar conjunctiva.

Bacterial conjunctivitis
This is nearly always unilateral. Pathogens vary with age. Neonatal conjunctivitis (ophthalmia neonatorum) is caused by *Chlamydia trachomatis, Pseudomonas aeruginosa,* and *Neisseria gonorrhoea.* In older children *S. pneumoniae, H. influenzae, Staphylococci,* and *Moraxella catarrhalis* cause purulent conjunctivitis.

Treatment depends on age and pathogen. Gonococcal conjunctivitis requires urgent treatment with systemic antibiotics (e.g. ceftriaxone) for 7 days, saline irrigation and chloramphenicol eye drops to avoid corneal perforation and blindness. *Chlamydia* is the most common cause of neonatal conjunctivitis and requires oral macrolides (e.g. azithromycin) and erythromycin ointment. *Pseudomonas* and *Haemophilus* require systemic antibiotics and topical gentamicin. Staphylococci and streptococci usually respond to topical antibiotics such as chloramphenicol.

Viral conjunctivitis
Adenovirus most common, presenting with a watery discharge. It is self-limiting and resolves over 1–2 weeks. May be systemic flu-like symptoms and sore throat. Conjunctivitis is seen in measles.

Allergic conjunctivitis
May be an acute hypersensitivity reaction to airborne allergens or a more chronic and seasonal disorder as one component of atopy. There is tearing and itching with conjunctival oedema. Vernal conjunctivitis is a chronic form which results in a cobblestone appearance of the palpebral conjunctiva. Topical sodium cromoglicate or steroids are used with systemic antihistamines.

Autoimmune systemic disease
Conjunctivitis occurs as a component of Stevens–Johnson syndrome, Kawasaki disease, juvenile chronic arthritis, and Lyme disease.

Keratitis

Corneal inflammation may be bacterial or viral. Bacterial infection can cause ulcers and abscesses with corneal perforation and was an important cause of blindness in pre-antibiotic days.

Human herpesvirus keratitis, which may be congenital, is potentially severe and sight threatening. Dendritic ulcers visible on fluorescein staining are typical. Recurrent disease may lead to severe corneal scarring. Treatment is with topical and systemic aciclovir. Topical steroids can be used under the direction of an ophthalmologist only when the corneal epithelium has healed and with aciclovir cover.

Blepharitis

This is commonly seen as part of a viral or bacterial blepharo-conjunctivitis as discussed above. Seborrhoeic dermatitis and lice may affect the eyelid margins.

A *hordoleum or stye* is an acute, painful localized bacterial infection arising either in a gland of the lid's tarsal plate or in one located around a lash follicle. Treatment is with warm compresses. A *chalazion* is a chronic lipogranulomatous inflammation caused by a blocked Meibomian gland which may resolve with moist heat and eyelid massage but sometimes has to be incised surgically.

Congenital infections

Eye morbidity is common in the congenital infections caused by the organisms referred to as TORCH syndromes (**TO**xoplasmosis, **R**ubella, **C**ytomegalovirus, and **H**erpes simplex virus). It also occurs in infections caused by syphilis, varicella, and HIV. Choroidoretinitis is commonly found. The impact is greatest with transplacental infection early in pregnancy. These infections are considered in more detail in Chapter 1, but essential features are as follows:

- *Congenital toxoplasmosis:* caused by the parasitic protozoa *Toxoplasma gondii,* usually acquired from contact with faeces from an infected cat. The spectrum ranges from an asymptomatic patch of peripheral choroidoretinitis to a blinding endophthalmitis. Treatment is with pyrimethamine and sulfadiazine (with folinic acid to prevent leucopaenia).
- *Congenital rubella:* typical ocular findings include microphthalmia, microcornea, nuclear cataract, anterior uveitis, corneal opacification, glaucoma, and diffuse retinitis.
- *Congenital CMV:* ocular manifestations can include microphthalmia, cataracts, keratitis, choroiditis, optic atrophy.
- *Congenital HSV:* usually acquired at birth. There may be involvement in disseminated herpes or a local blepharo-conjunctivitis and keratitis.

Periocular infections

Periorbital (preseptal) cellulitis

A common bacterial infection anterior to the orbital septum occurring usually in children <5 years.

It is usually caused by respiratory tract pathogens *Strep. pneumoniae*, *H. influenzae*, or *Staph. aureus*. It may be secondary to an URTI, stye, chickenpox, or impetigo. Fever is accompanied by generalized upper and lower lid erythema and oedema with possible extension beyond the lids (Fig 8.10). It is important to distinguish from orbital cellulitis, if necessary by CT.

Treatment is with intravenous antibiotics, e.g. co-amoxiclav, as there is a risk of progression to orbital cellulitis.

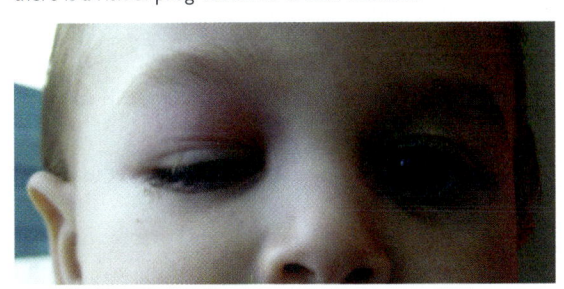

Fig 8.10 Right-sided periorbital cellulitis.

Orbital cellulitis

This uncommon infection is an ophthalmological emergency. It tends to occur in older children. Risk factors include ethmoid sinusitis, septal perforation from trauma, and orbital surgery. The cardinal signs in addition to those seen in periorbital cellulitis are:
- Proptosis
- Pain on eye movement
- Ophthalmoplegia and diplopia
- Afferent papillary defect.

Management

Investigations include blood cultures and eye swabs together with a CT of the orbits, sinuses, and brain. IV antibiotics (e.g. co-amoxiclav or a broad-spectrum cephalosporin and metronidazole) are indicated. The choice depends on age and advice of a microbiologist should be sought. Urgent ENT and ophthalmological consultation is mandatory as sinus drainage is often required. Complications include cerebral, orbital, or periorbital abscess formation, cavernous sinus thrombosis, meningitis, and visual loss from optic neuropathy

Dacryocystitis

This is a consequence of complete or partial nasolacrimal duct obstruction and may be acute or chronic. Respiratory pathogens are usually responsible. There is worsening epiphora (eye watering) and a tender erythematous lump just medial to the inferior canthus (Fig 8.11).

Pus may be expressed from the punctum on palpation and there may be a preseptal cellulitis. Treatment is with systemic (co-amoxiclav) and topical (chloramphenicol) antibiotics.

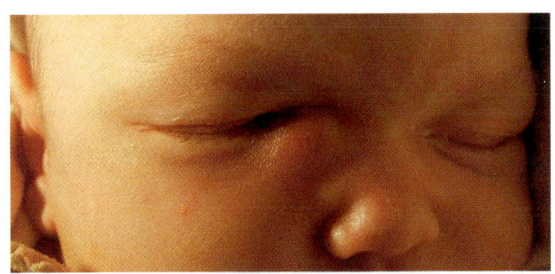

Fig 8.11 Dacryocystitis.

Uveitis

Inflammation of the uveal tract, which includes the iris, ciliary body and choroid, is classified by anatomic location into:
- *Anterior:* iris (iritis) and/or ciliary body (iridocyclitis)
- *Intermediate:* the posterior ciliary body, the pars plana (pars planitis) and/or peripheral retina
- *Posterior:* the choroid (choroiditis) or overlying retina
- Pan-uveitis: inflammation involving the entire uveal tract.

Retinal vasculitis refers to a predominant finding of retinal vascular inflammation.

Aetiology

Inflammation of the uveal tract in children is most commonly non-infectious but it may be caused by a variety of infections.

The 'silent' anterior uveitis of juvenile idiopathic arthritis accounts for 80%. Other non-infectious causes include ankylosing spondylitis, Kawasaki disease, inflammatory bowel disease, and idiopathic.

Infectious agents include toxocara, toxoplasma, tuberculosis, Lyme disease, and a host of viruses (herpes simplex and zoster, CMV in association with HIV and EBV).

Retinal vasculitis is seen in leukaemia, cat scratch disease, herpesvirus infections, and systemic vasculitis, e.g. SLE.

Clinical features

Uveitis in juvenile arthritis may be silent and screening is therefore required in this at-risk group to prevent irreversible visual loss.

Acute anterior uveitis is associated with pain, redness, photophobia, tearing, and blurred vision. Examination may reveal perilimbal injection, decreased visual acuity, photophobia and pupillary miosis. There may be pain on eye convergence (Talbot's test). Slit-lamp examination is necessary to see the keratitic precipitates (white blood cells on the endothelium, a hallmark of iritis) and flare due to raised protein content or cells in the anterior chamber in anterior uveitis.

Laboratory evaluation may include FBC, ESR, ANA, tuberculin test and CXR.

Complications of this vision threatening condition include band keratopathy, cataract (anterior uveitis), optic neuritis, retinal detachment, and glaucoma (posterior uveitis).

Management

Any underlying cause or infection may need specific treatment but the mainstay of treating the ocular inflammation is mydriasis and corticosteroids.

Cycloplegic agents decrease formation of adhesions of the iris to the anterior capsule of the lens (posterior synechiae). Steroid treatment may be topical or by injection, and systemic steroid treatment and/or immunosuppressant treatment may be necessary.

8.6 Childhood cataract and glaucoma

Lens anatomy and physiology

The crystalline lens is composed of a central nucleus surrounded by a lamellar cortex. Individual lens fibres meet at so-called 'sutures'. A layer of epithelial cells cover the anterior surface.

The entire lens is encased in a proteinaceous capsule (rich in type IV collagen) and suspended by the zonular fibres of Zinn, composed of fibrillin (the protein mutated in Marfan syndrome). The main lens proteins are crystallins. Most energy production is anaerobic.

Cataract

Cataract refers to any opacity of the crystalline lens and is the most common preventable cause of blindness in children worldwide, accounting for 40% of cases or 200 000 in total.

It may be bilateral or unilateral, complete or partial, and may occur in isolation or in association with other ocular developmental abnormalities or systemic diseases and syndromes.

Early diagnosis and treatment of dense or visually significant cataract is essential to avoid irreversible sensory deprivational amblyopia.

Cataracts are classified according to:
- *Density*
- *Shape:* punctuate or pulvurulent (dust like)
- *Location:* nuclear, lamellar, subcapsular, anterior, posterior
- *Aetiology*.

Causes of childhood cataract

In the UK about one third of bilateral congenital cataracts are idiopathic, one third are familial (genetic, non-syndromic) and one third are associated with systemic diseases including a large number of syndromes and metabolic disorders (see Box). Unilateral congenital cataract is idiopathic in 90%.

Maternal infections, especially rubella, are an important cause worldwide.

Clinical features

Cataracts may be asymptomatic and discovered on routine examination or may present with reduced visual acuity or its consequences: strabismus or nystagmus.

A pregnancy history should be elicited to identify maternal infection, drug use, or toxin exposure. There may be a family history but family members may have unrecognized partial cataracts.

Examination

Cataract is an important cause of leucocoria (white pupil) and of an abnormal red reflex (Fig 8.12). Age-appropriate assessment of VA is essential. Risk to vision is worse if the cataract is dense, posterior, axial and >3 mm in diameter. Nystagmus is an ominous sign. A full ophthalmological and systemic examination is required and ophthalmological review of parents and siblings.

Causes of childhood cataract

Congenital cataracts
- **Idiopathic:** 30% of bilateral, 90% of unilateral
- **Maternal factors:** intrauterine infections (TORCH), diabetes mellitus, drugs e.g. corticosteroids
- Transient cataract of prematurity
- **Genetic:**
  - non-syndromic (isolated): majority are autosomal dominant. 15 genes for inherited cataract are known and fall into 5 main groups including crystallins, *CRYAA, CRYAB*
  - syndromic:
    chromosomal disorders: trisomy 21, 18, 13, Cri-du-chat
    metabolic disorders: galactosaemia, galactokinase (GPUT1) deficiency, Lowe syndrome
    cranio-mandibulo-facial: Crouzon, Treacher Collins syndrome
    congenital ichthyosis
    anterior segment dysgenesis: aniridia, coloboma

Juvenile early-onset cataracts
- Acquired:
  - drugs (steroids), trauma, radiation
  - skin disorders: eczema, Cockayne syndrome
  - infections: herpes, toxoplasmosis, measles
- Genetic (syndromic):
  Down, Turner, Rubinstein–Taybi syndromes
  myotonic dystrophy
  abetalipoproteinaemia, homocysteinuria hypocalcaemia.

Investigations

Laboratory evaluation of congenital bilateral cataracts:
- Urine for amino acids and reducing substances
- *Serology:* TORCH screen
- *Enzyme assays:* galactokinase, GPUT1
- *Biochemical profile:* amino acids
- Glucose, calcium, phosphate
- Karyotype (if dysmorphic).

Management

Visually significant cataracts should be removed as soon as possible (before 6 weeks for congenital cataracts) to prevent irreversible visual loss from amblyopia. Partial cataracts may not need surgery.

Surgical techniques include lens aspiration and also anterior vitrectomy if the child is <5 years.

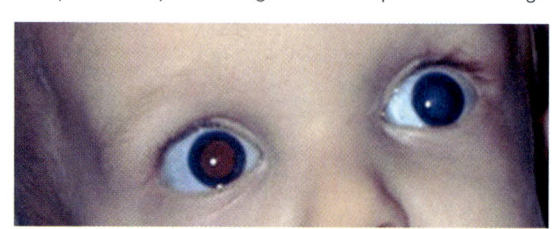

Fig 8.12 Left side unilateral cataract.

Childhood glaucoma

Glaucoma is a condition in which there is damage to the optic nerve caused by or related to a rise in intraocular pressure (IOP).

Pathophysiology

Aqueous humour is produced by the a tiny gland, the ciliary body and provides nutrients to the lens and cornea. Most aqueous humour exits the anterior chamber by a passive, pressure sensitive route through the trabecular meshwork and Schlemm's canal at the angle of the eye where iris and cornea meet (Fig 8.13) from which it drains into the venous system. Normal IOP in infants and young children is <20 mmHg.

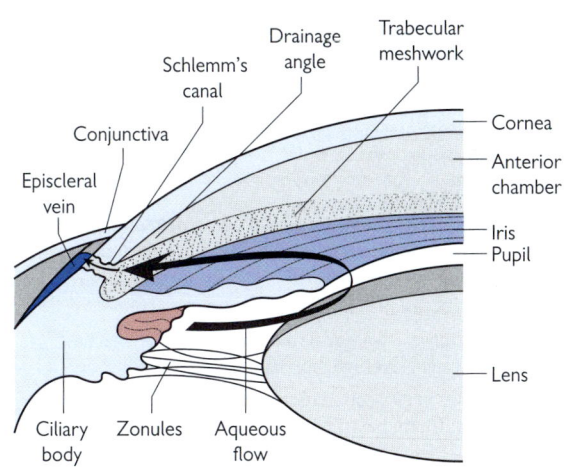

Fig 8.13 Angle anatomy. The angle is the recess formed by the iridocorneal juncture.

Causes of childhood glaucoma

Developmental glaucoma

- *Primary congenital glaucoma:* incidence 1/10 000 live births. Accounts for 50% childhood glaucoma. Bilateral in 70%. Most are sporadic but AR and polygenic inheritance recognized. One gene identified: *CYP1B1* which encodes P4501B1, and 2 loci mapped.
- *Systemic disease associated:*
  - Sturge–Weber syndrome
  - Neurofibromatosis (NF1)
  - Alagille syndrome
  - Rubinstein–Taybi syndrome
  - Wolf-Hirschorn syndrome
  - Down syndrome
- *Ocular anomaly associated:* aniridia and iris coloboma, Peter anomaly

Acquired (secondary) glaucoma

- Trauma
- *Drugs:* e.g. steroids
- *Intraocular neoplasm:* e.g. retinoblastoma
- *Ocular inflammation:* maternal rubella, uveitis
- *Lens-related:* ectopia lentis (Marfan), post cataract surgery.

Aetiology

Glaucoma occurs when a blockage of outflow of the aqueous fluid causes the IOP to rise. It may be developmental or acquired.

Developmental glaucomas include primary congenital glaucoma caused by a developmental abnormality of the trabecular meshwork, and those associated with systemic diseases (>30) or ocular anomalies (>10).

Causes of acquired, secondary glaucoma are numerous and include intraocular neoplasms, trauma, cataract surgery, lens dislocation, and drugs (e.g. steroids). See Box.

Clinical features

In infants and young children a rise in IOP leads to diffuse oedema and enlargement of the cornea with splits in Descemet's membrane (Haab's striae) and damage to corneal epithelial cells. The globe itself may enlarge causing 'bupthalmos' (ox-eye). See Fig 8.14.

The classical triad of presenting symptoms, due to corneal oedema and irritation, is present in only 30% of affected infants: epiphora (watering eye), photophobia, and blepharospasm (eyelid squeezing). Rhinorrhea may also be present. Physical signs on examination may include:

- Corneal enlargement (>11 mm at age <1 year)
- Corneal haze from oedema (Fig 8.15)
- Myopia, often extreme
- Optic nerve cupping.

Detailed ophthalmological and systemic examination may reveal a cause.

Investigations

Include tonometry (may require EUA) and gonioscopy to examine the anterior chamber angle.

Management

Untreated glaucoma leads to visual loss due to corneal scarring, optic nerve damage and, most importantly, sensory deprivation amblyopia. In most cases treatment is surgical, but medical treatment may also be required.

- *Surgical procedures:* goniotomy, trabeculotomy or trabeculectomy to open portions of Schlemm's canal and improve drainage
- *Cyclodestructive procedures:* destruction of the ciliary body by cryotherapy or photocoagulation to reduce aqueous fluid production. Long-term medical treatment may be necessary with β-blockers or carbonic anhydrase inhibitors.

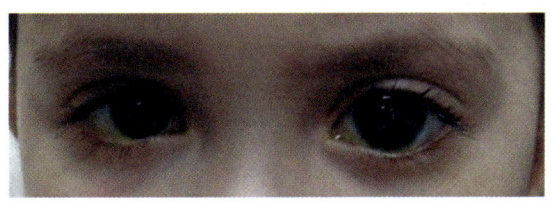

Fig 8.14 Glaucoma: corneal and globe enlargement on left. Source: www.medrounds.com, reproduced by permission of Medrounds Publications.

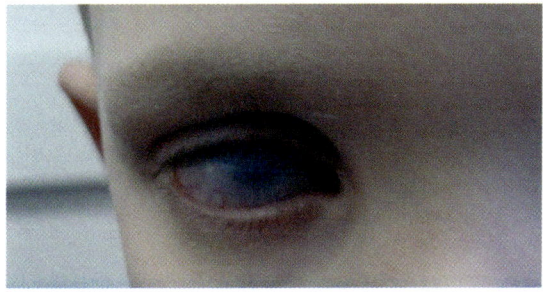

Fig 8.15 Advanced glaucoma with corneal clouding.

8.7 Retinal and optic nerve disorders

Retinal disorders

Retina
The retina is a transparent laminated structure comprising photoreceptors, interneurons, and ganglion cells overlying the retinal pigment epithelium. Superficial vessels form four arcades over its surface and collagen fibrils attach its internal limiting membrane to the vitreous, a transparent gel consisting of hyaluronic acid and collagen.

The retina may be affected by developmental disorders, tumours (retinoblastoma), congenital infections (Section 8.5) genetic diseases (Section 8.9), and acquired retinopathies including retinopathy of prematurity, diabetic retinopathy, and trauma.

Developmental disorders
These include:
- *Coloboma:* a defect of closure of the optic fissure may involve the retina
- *Albinism:* there is foveal hypoplasia and prominent choroidal vasculature with a pale fundus.
- *Retinal dysplasia:* usually part of a syndrome (Edwards, Patau, Norrie). Presents as bilateral leucocoria.

Acquired retinopathies
Retinopathy of prematurity (ROP)
This is a disorder of the retinal vasculature affecting premature newborn infants and remains a leading cause of blindness in children in the developing world. The manifestations range from mild, transitory changes in the periphery to severe vasoproliferative changes with scarring, retinal detachment, and blindness.

Aetiology and pathogenesis
Risk factors are low gestational age (<32 weeks) or birthweight (<1500 g), male sex, white ethnicity, and supplemental oxygen therapy. Genetic polymorphism in genes controlling normal retinal vascularization may contribute.

Retinal vessels grow out from the optic disc under the control of VEGF and other growth factors. Premature infants therefore have large areas of avascular retina, and the more premature the more posterior (closer to the optic nerve) the blood supply ends at the time of birth. It is possible that hyperoxia causes retinal vasoconstriction in peripheral vessels with resulting up-regulation of angiogenic factors and abnormal neovascularization.

International Classification of ROP (ICROP)
This consists of four basic elements: the stage (0–5), location by zone (1–3), extent (in clock hours), and presence or absence of 'plus disease'. The stages represent the phases through which the disease progresses:
- *Stage 0:* incomplete vascularization of the retina
- *Stage 1:* a white demarcation line between vascular and avascular zones
- *Stage 2:* elevation and thickening of the demarcation line to form a broad, thick ridge
- *Stage 3:* extraretinal fibrovascular proliferation into the vitreous
- *Stage 4:* contraction of the neovascular ridge pulls the retina up with subtotal detachment
  - *4A:* does not involve fovea
  - *4B:* involves fovea
- *Stage 5:* retinal detachment (retrolental fibroplasia).

'Plus disease' indicates engorged and tortuous vessels around the optic nerve (i.e. posterior pole) and indicates a more advanced and aggressive form of retinopathy.

Screening and treatment
Screening is recommended for all infants born <31 weeks gestation or weighing <1501 g at birth. Examination is carried out at postnatal age 6–7 weeks or at 31 weeks corrected gestational age whichever is later.

No treatment is necessary for stages 1 and 2. Stage 3 is treated by laser ablation of the avascular retina anterior to the ridge in eyes with sight-threatening ROP, usually under general anaesthesia. Stages 4 and 5 are rare and treatment is complex.

Prognosis: >90% of infants with stage 3 retinopathy do well and have good vision.

Diabetic retinopathy
Diabetic children >12 years should be screened annually. The risk increases with disease duration. The stages include:
- *Background:* microaneurysms, small haemorrhages, hard exudates, occasional cotton wool spots
- *Pre-proliferative:* intraretinal microvascular abnormalities, venous beading, blot haemorrhages, cotton wool spots
- *Proliferative:* neovascularization and fibrovascular tissue on the retina. Treated with laser photocoagulation.

Retinal haemorrhages
A common cause of retinal haemorrhage in infants is inflicted traumatic brain injury. However, a number of other causes should be considered:
- *Birth:* a normal finding after birth. Clear by 6 weeks
- *Accidental trauma:* very rare in minor domestic falls
- *Bleeding diatheses:* vitamin K deficiency
- *Intracranial infection:* meningitis, HSV, CMV
- *Metabolic disorders:* glutaric aciduria type 1
- Hypertension and raised ICP.

Optic nerve disorders
The optic nerve head or disc in infants is paler than in the adult and the vascular pattern more tortuous.

Developmental anomalies
Bilateral anomalies present with decreased vision and nystagmus, unilateral with strabismus. They include:
- *Optic nerve coloboma:* see Section 8.3
- *Myelinated nerve fibres:* appear as feathery white striated patches obscuring the retinal vessels and usually continuous with the optic disc
- *Optic nerve hypoplasia and dysplasia:* a small grey disc with poor vision. It may be syndromic as part of septo-optic dysplasia (de Morsier syndrome) in combination with short stature and growth hormone deficiency.

Optic disc swelling
Papilloedema refers specifically to swelling of the optic disc in association with raised ICP but optic disc swelling also occurs in a number of other conditions. See Box.

The fundoscopic appearances of papilloedema (Fig 8.16) progress from blurring of disc margins and elevation of disc to dilated capillary plexus and retinal veins and ultimately engorgement and tortuosity of retinal and disc capillaries with widespread haemorrhages.

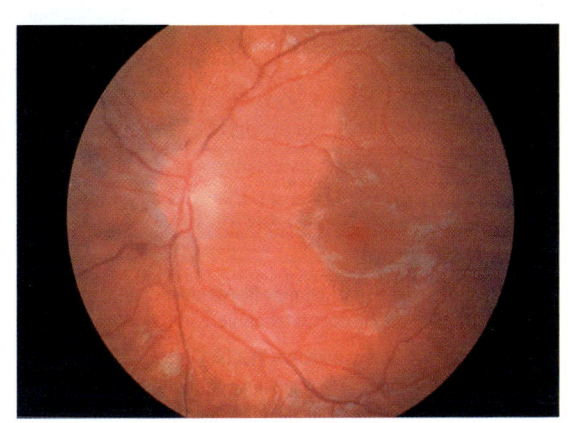

Fig 8.16 Optic disc swelling: advanced papilloedema.

Causes of a swollen optic disc
- *Papilloedema:* hydrocephalus, brain tumour, idiopathic intracranial hypertension
- Severe hypertension
- *Optic neuritis:* demyelinating or infectious
- *Tumours:* retinoblastoma, hamartoma, optic nerve glioma
- Ischaemic optic neuropathy
- Uveitis
- *Pseudopapilloedema:* disc colloid bodies (drusen), hypermetropia, myopia, angled or small optic disc.

Optic neuropathy (optic nerve atrophy)
The term neuropathy is preferred to atrophy as retinal ganglion cell axons have no capacity for regeneration. Irreversible loss of some or most of the fibres of the optic nerve causes the disc to become a pale yellow-white colour and appear sharply demarcated in association with reduced visual acuity and subsequent visual field defects (Fig 8.17). If bilateral it presents in infancy with blindness and roving eye movements. Unilateral cases may present with strabismus.

Many pathogenic mechanisms can lead to optic neuropathy ranging from inherited defects in mitochondrial function to the secondary effects of birth injury, trauma, toxins, compression and inflammation or oedema of the optic nerve (see Box).

Causes of childhood optic neuropathy
- *Perinatal:*
  - prematurity (IVH and hydrocephalus)
  - birth asphyxia
- *Tumours:*
  - astrocytoma, craniopharyngioma
  - optic nerve glioma
- Hydrocephalus
- *Trauma:* accidental and inflicted
- Genetic:
  - Kjer syndrome: (AD OA): mutations in *OPA1*, a gene involved in mitochondrial function
  - Leber hereditary optic neuropathy: mutations in MtDNA typically presenting in young adult males
  - Behr syndrome: AR with ataxia and spasticity
  - Wolfram syndrome: OA with early onset diabetes (DIDMOAD: **D**iabetes **I**nsipidus, **D**iabetes **M**ellitus, **O**ptic **A**trophy and **D**eafness)
- *Inflammation:* optic neuritis
- *Infections:* meningitis, measles
- *Toxins:* e.g. lead
- *Ocular:* glaucoma

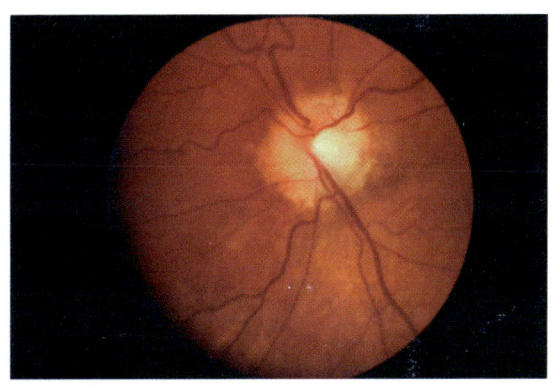

Fig 8.17 Optic atrophy.

8.8 Genetic eye disease

Mutations in several hundred genes can affect all parts of the visual system causing defects in development or progressive degeneration of the retina.

Disease may be confined to the eye, or the eye may be involved in genetic syndromes in which other features dominate the clinical phenotype. Genes also contribute to common problems such as refractive errors and retinopathy of prematurity.

Developmental defects

Anophthalmia
Complete failure of primary optic vesicle outgrowth with bilateral anophthalmia is a rare severe form of structural eye malformation associated with abnormalities of chromosome 3q27 involving the *SOX2* gene, a transcription factor expressed in the developing eye.

Anterior segment dysgenesis (ASD)
A spectrum of AD diseases ranging from iris hypoplasia (IH) to posterior embryotoxon (a ring-like opacity at Schwalbe's ring) and the more severe AR Axenfeld–Reiger malformations in which secondary glaucoma occurs in 50% of patients. Mutations in *PITX2* or *FOXC1* account for one third of patients with ASD.

Aniridia
See Section 8.3. Commonly due to submicroscopic deletions of chromosome 11p13 encompassing the aniridia-associated *PAX6* gene. FISH screening of this region is indicated in sporadic isolated aniridia.

Retina
See Section 8.7.

Retinal degenerations

The inherited retinal degenerations include stationary (non-progressive) and progressive disorders of photoreceptors, retinal pigment epithelium, choroid, and retinal vasculature. They include retinitis pigmentosa, Leber amaurosis, and albinism.

Retinitis pigmentosa (RP)
This heterogeneous group of disorders caused by >100 different genes is the most common of the retinal dystrophies with an incidence of 1/4000.

There is a progressive loss of rod and cone photoreceptor cells. It may be sporadic or inherited in AD (30%), AR (60%), or X-linked (10%) fashion. It may occur in isolation or as part of a syndrome (Table 8.6).

The causal genes identified account for about 50% of all patients and involve a very wide range of biological functions including:
- Components of the phototransduction cascade (*RHO*: rhodopsin)
- Synaptic interaction in Usher syndrome (*USH2A*)
- Maintenance of sensory cilia (Bardet–Biedl syndrome, *BBS* genes and *RPGR*).

Clinical features
Very variable, but the classic pattern is difficulties with dark adaptation and night blindness in adolescence followed by development of tunnel vision and eventual loss of central vision. Diagnosis depends on fundal findings together with documentation of progressive loss of photoreceptor function by visual field testing and electroretinography (ERG).

Table 8.6. Syndromes associated with retinitis pigmentosa

Usher syndrome	Types 1–3; associated with deafness
Bardet–Biedl syndrome	Obesity, polydactyly, hypogenitalism, and renal disease. 10 genes account for 70% cases
Batten disease	Neuronal ceroid lipofuscinosis (*CLN3*)
Bassen–Kornzweig syndrome	Abetalipoproteinaemia
Refsum disease	Phytanic oxidase deficiency

Management
There is some evidence of benefit from nutritional supplementation with vitamin A or docosatexanoic acid (DHA).

Leber congenital amaurosis (LCA)
This group of AR retinal dystrophies that is the most common genetic cause of congenital visual impairment.

LCA is characterized by profound visual impairment in early infancy presenting with searching nystagmus, sluggish papillary responses, and absent or attenuated ERG responses.

Additional features may include midfacial hypoplasia and hypermetropia. It is genetically heterogeneous with 11 loci mapped and mutations identified in 9 genes including *CEP290*.

Albinism
A group of inherited abnormalities of melanin synthesis resulting in pigment deficiency of the eye alone (ocular albinism, OA) or of the eye, skin, and hair (oculocutaneous albinism, OCA).

There is associated macular hypoplasia and smaller optic nerves with abnormal decussation of optic nerve fibres at the optic chiasm.

Clinical eye features include photophobia, nystagmus, hypopigmentation of the uveal tract and retinal pigment epithelium, and foveal hypoplasia.
- *Ocular albinism:* X-linked. *OAI* gene encodes a melanosome membrane glycoprotein
- *Oculocutaneous albinism*: AR
  - type 1 *OCA1*: mutations in *TYR*, encoding tyrosinase
  - type 2 *OCA2*: mutations in *P*, encoding substance P.

Syndromic forms occur (Hermansky–Pudlak, Chediak–Higaski, Griscelli syndromes).

Treatment involves lens tinting and correction of refraction, and treatment of any associated strabismus or amblyopia.

Ocular signs in genetic syndromes

Chromosomal syndromes
The eye is involved in several aneuploidy and chromosomal deletion syndromes:
- *Down syndrome:* mongoloid palpebral fissures and epicanthic folds, myopia, astigmatism, strabismus, nystagmus, keratoconus, Brushfield spots, cataract
- *Edwards syndrome:* epicanthal folds, ptosis, microphthalmia, corneal opacities, congenital glaucoma and cataracts, uveal colobomata
- *Patau syndrome:* cyclopia, microphthalmia, colobomata, corneal opacities, cataracts, retinal and optic nerve dysplasia
- *Turner syndrome:* antimongoloid palpebral fissures, epicanthal folds, ptosis, strabismus, cataracts, male levels of X-linked recessive disease, e.g. red–green colour blindness.

Craniofacial syndromes
A group of genetic disorders with cranial vault and facial malformations and systemic manifestations affecting the skeleton and CNS. They can be classified as clefting and synostotic (premature closure of the cranial sutures) syndromes.
- *Clefting syndromes:* Treacher–Collins, Goldenhar
- *Craniosynostoses:* Crouzon, Apert, Pfeiffer, Saethre–Chotzen, Carpenter.

The serious ophthalmic consequences include: orbital disease (proptosis), exposure keratitis, cataracts, glaucoma, colobomata, and optic nerve disease (hypoplasia, compression atrophy).

Neurocutaneous disorders (phakomatoses)
Ocular features of the phakomatoses are:
- *Neurofibromatosis type 1:* optic nerve glioma (in 5–10%), Lisch nodules (pigmented hamartomas of the iris), choroidal naevi, retinal astrocytoma, lid neurofibroma
- *Neurofibromatosis type 2:* early onset cataracts, combined hamartoma of retina and retinal pigment epithelium, bilateral acoustic neuromas
- *Tuberous sclerosis complex:* retinal hamartomas, eyelid angiofibromas
- *Von Hippel–Lindau syndrome:* retinal capillary haemangiomas (haemangioblastomas of cerebellum and spinal cord).

Neurocutaneous angiomatoses
- *Sturge–Weber syndrome:* haemangiomas of the choroid and episclera with glaucoma
- *Ataxia-telangiectasia:* an AR DNA repair defect with progressive ataxia and cutaneous and conjunctival telangiectasia occurring as a response to natural UV irradiation
- *Incontinentia pigmenti:* microphthalmia, corneal opacities, cataract and retinal dysplasia which may lead to blindness.

Connective tissue disorders
Marfan syndrome
Mutations in *FBN1* encoding fibrillin, a protein component of the zonule fibres which suspend the lens. Lens dislocation (ectopia lentis) is the most common ocular abnormality (up to 80% of patients). Dislocation is usually upwards.

Other problems include refractive errors (myopia), retinal detachment (up to 10%), and glaucoma. All children with Marfan syndrome should be examined by an ophthalmologist by age 10 years at the latest.

Osteogenesis imperfecta (OI)
OI is a heterogeneous collection of disorders with bone fragility caused by mutations in several genes: *COL1A1*, *COL1A2*. Blue sclerae may be present but are not invariable. Abnormal thinness or transparency allows the underlying blue-grey uveal pigment to show. Blue sclerae can also be seen in:
- Normal neonates: especially preterm infants
- Ehlers–Danlos syndrome, pseudoxanthoma elasticum
- Marfan syndrome
- Long-term corticosteroid treatment
- Iron-deficiency anaemia.

Ehlers–Danlos syndrome
Myopia, blue sclerae, and epicanthic folds are common and people with EDS VI (the ocular form) are at risk of more serious problems such as retinal detachment and glaucoma.

Metabolic and storage disorders
Over 30 inherited diseases affecting metabolism or characterised by abnormal storage have ocular manifestations. These most often affect the cornea, lens, iris, retina, or optic nerve. Causes of the most important abnormalities include:
- *Cloudy cornea:* mucopolysaccharidoses (MPS), GM1 gangliosidosis
- *Crystalline keratopathy:* cystinosis
- *Ectopia lentis:* Homocystinuria, Marfan syndrome
- *Kayser–Fleischer ring:* Wilson disease
- *Cherry-red spot:* Tay–Sachs disease, Sandhoff disease, Nieman–Pick disease type 1A
- *Retinitis pigmentosa:* see Table 8.6
- *Cataracts:* see Box, p. 186.

8.9 Case-based discussions

An infant with periorbital swelling

A 6 month old female infant presented with a 2 day history of coryza followed by swelling and redness around the left eye. There was no significant previous history except that her parents had declined immunisations because they believed that it was wrong to 'overload' the immune system

On examination she was miserable but systemically well. Temperature 38.4 °C. Periorbital swelling and redness as shown in Fig 8.18. Eye movements full.

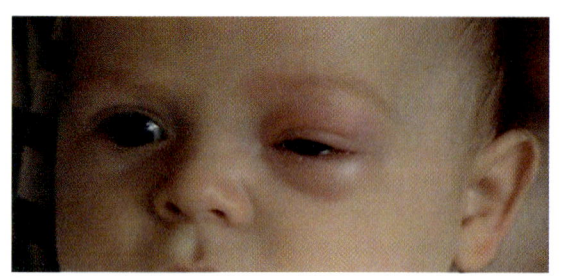

Fig 8.18 Periorbital oedema and inflammation.

What is the likely diagnosis?
The appearance and history is typical of periorbital (preseptal) cellulitis. Orbital cellulitis is a less common but more serious condition which must be considered. It is usually associated with a degree of proptosis and pain on eye movement and tends to occur in an older age group.

What is the management?
Blood culture and full blood count should be done. The usual pathogens are respiratory such as the pneumococcus or staphylococci. *Haemophilus influenzae* type B (Hib) was a common pathogen before immunisation was introduced but this infant has not been immunized against Hib.

If there is any suspicion of orbital cellulitis an ophthalmological and ENT opinion should be sought. A CT scan of the orbits is the definitive investigation. Surgical drainage may be required.

She was treated initially with an intravenous broad spectrum cephalosporin. Blood cultures grew Haemophilus after 48 h. She made a rapid recovery and was changed to oral antibiotics after 72 h.

An infant with a watering eye

A 4 month old male infant presented with an increasingly 'tearful' right eye. This problem was first noted at age 8 weeks, and the health visitor diagnosed a blocked nasolacrimal duct and recommended regular saline washes.

The parents had become concerned because they had observed his right eye to be looking cloudy and thought it was becoming bigger than the left eye.

On examination there was right-sided bupthalmos (Fig 8.19). There was right-sided epiphora (watering eye).

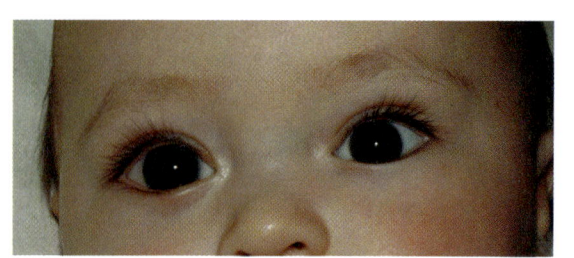

Fig 8.19

What is the most likely diagnosis?
The most common cause of a watering eye in a young infant, without other ocular signs, is a blocked nasolacrimal duct. However, in this case the corneal clouding and globe enlargement are strongly suggestive of congenital glaucoma.

Primary congenital glaucoma accounts for 50% of childhood glaucoma and is unilateral in 30%. Most are sporadic.

What is the management?
Urgent ophthalmological referral is required. Untreated glaucoma can lead to visual loss from corneal scarring, optic nerve damage, and sensory deprivation amblyopia.

Tonometry and gonioscopy confirmed a diagnosis of congenital glaucoma which required surgical intervention and long-term medical treatment.

Chapter 9

Dermatology

9.1 Skin: anatomy, development, and function *194*
9.2 Clinical dermatology *196*
9.3 Neonatal dermatology *198*
9.4 Eczema *200*
9.5 Skin infections and infestations *202*
9.6 Inflammatory dermatoses *204*
9.7 Hair, nails, mouth, and pigmentation *206*
9.8 Case-based discussions *208*

9.1 Skin: anatomy, development, and function

Skin anatomy
Human skin is composed of a superficial non-vascular epidermis and a deeper vascularized dermis. Beneath the skin lies a layer of subcutaneous fat and within the dermis are the adnexal structures: hair, sweat glands, and sebaceous glands (Fig 9.1).

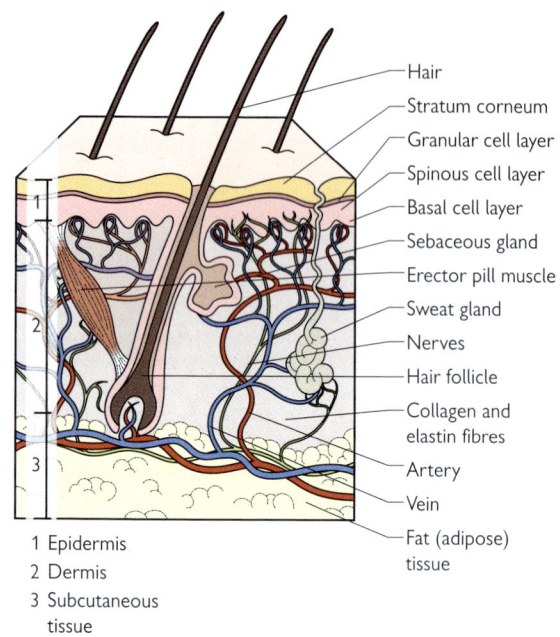

1 Epidermis
2 Dermis
3 Subcutaneous tissue

Fig 9.1 Skin anatomy.

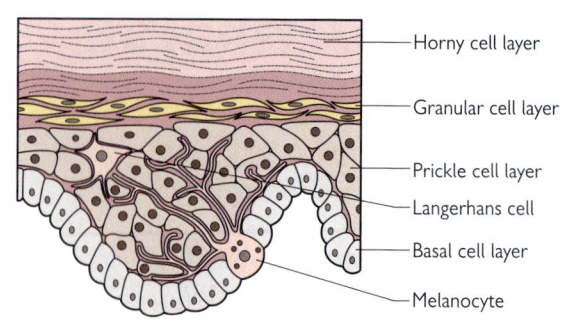

Fig 9.2 Structure of epidermis.

Epidermis
The main function is as a defensive barrier. There are four layers (Fig 9.2) which are, from deepest to most superficial:
- *Stratum basale:* the deepest, basal cell layer where mitotic division of keratinocytes occurs. Keratinocytes, the major cell type in the epidermis, are rectangular in this layer and tethered to the basement membrane by the hemi-desmosome. Melanocytes (10% of cells) produce melanin pigment in melanosomes which are passed to basal keratinocytes. The basal layer also contains oval, clear specialized sensory Merkel cells.
- *Stratum spinulosum:* after cell division, keratinocytes move into this prickle cell layer. Terminal differentiation begins leading to production of intracellular tonofilaments which attach to external desmosomes, providing firm intercellular connections which maintain structural integrity. Dendritic Langerhans cells, specialized antigen presenting cells, are also present.
- *Stratum granulosum:* here the cells begin to flatten and die and synthesize keratohyalin granules, filaggrin, and lipid before moving into the outer layer.
- *Stratum corneum:* in this outer horny layer the corneocyte cells are squamous and dead, forming a tightly compacted barrier layer. Outer corneocytes are continually shed as scale. The stratum corneum is thinnest over eyelids and thickest over palms and soles.

Dermis
The dermis provides fibrous strength, nutrient support, and elasticity to the epidermis. It compromises ~15% of body weight and varies in thickness. Fibroblasts are the most abundant cells and manufacture a supporting ground substance (proteoglycans, mucopolysaccharides) and fibrils composed of collagen I and III and elastin. Other cell types include mast cells and macrophages.

There is a rich blood supply, specialized nerve endings, and lymphatics. The deeper 9/10 is called the reticular dermis and the upper 1/10 the papillary dermis. Adnexal structures are considered below.

Subcutaneous layer (subcutis, hypodermis, panniculus)
Beneath the skin is a layer of fatty tissue divided into lobules by fibrous septae which contain blood vessels. The layer of fat provides insulation, physical cushioning, and protection of overlying skin.

Adnexal structures
Hair and sebaceous glands
Hair follicles are specialized invaginations of the epidermis and occur all over the body except for the palms, soles, and lips. A layer of cells at the base of each hair follicle, the hair matrix, continually divides pushing overlying cells upwards into the follicle.

There are three types of hair:
- *Lanugo hair:* fine and downy. Develops *in utero* and is shed before birth. Can develop in diseases such as anorexia nervosa
- *Vellus hair:* short, soft hairs present over most of the body
- *Terminal hair:* on the scalp and at secondary sexual sites after puberty.

Hair growth cycles through three phases:
- Anagen (~90%): active growth
- Catagen (<1%): hair bulb atrophies
- Telogen (~10%): resting state prior to shedding.

Anagen duration varies at different sites. Usually ~3 years on scalp. Sebaceous glands secrete sebum, a lipid-rich substance of uncertain function, into hair follicles.

Sweat glands
Two types exist. Eccrine glands are coiled ductal structures which open directly on to the skin surface and receive cholinergic innervation. Apocrine glands are found in axillae and groins, receive adrenergic innervation, and may have a vestigial role in scent communication.

Nails

Nails are plates of keratin that develop from specialized epidermal invaginations. Development begins at ~10 weeks gestation, fingernails preceding toenails by 2 weeks.

Skin development

Keratinization of the epidermis occurs from 22–24 weeks gestation and all layers of the epidermis are present from 24 weeks. Preterm infants have a thin stratum corneum and poor epidermal barrier with increased transepidermal water loss. Lack of subcutaneous fat compromises temperature regulation. There is a marked acceleration of the barrier when exposed to the extrauterine environment, with rapid formation of the stratum corneum. Within 2 weeks the skin resembles that of the term infant.

Vernix caseosa is unique to humans and made up of hydrated fetal corneocytes in a rich lipid matrix. It is synthesized during the 3rd trimester. At birth the skin surface is relatively neutral, pH 6.5, and an 'acid mantle' forms after birth which is beneficial for antimicrobial defence.

Skin function

Normal function

The integumentary system, which includes skin, hair, nails, and adnexal structures, is the largest organ system of the body. In humans it has seven main functions:
- *Barrier function:* provides a protective barrier against water and protein loss, pathogens, toxins, UV irradiation, and mechanical and thermal insults
- *Sensation:* provides sensory information about touch, pressure, pain, heat, and cold
- *Body temperature regulation:* there is significant heat loss through the skin which can be regulated by blood flow alterations and sweating. By sensing temperature it can mediate behavioural adaptive responses
- *Communication:* healthy skin is of fundamental importance to social interaction. Skin disease often causes significant psychological and social dysfunction
- *Immune:* skin has intrinsic immune functions, both innate (e.g. Toll-like receptors on keratinocytes) and acquired (Langerhans antigen-presenting cells)
- *Excretion:* waste products and excess salt are lost through insensible sweating
- *Metabolic:* the skin is the most important source of vitamin D3 and a site of steroid metabolism.

Skin failure

Acute skin failure is a medical emergency which requires a multidisciplinary intensive care approach. It has been defined as a loss of normal temperature control; inability to prevent percutaneous loss of fluid, electrolytes, and protein; and failure of the mechanical barrier. Patients with large areas of inflamed, peeling, or denuded skin will have some degree of skin failure.

Causes

Any condition causing extensive structural disruption and functional impairment of large areas of skin may cause skin failure. Important paediatric conditions include:
- *Erythroderma:* extensive and severe inflammation of the skin with >90% BSA involved. May occur in:
  - atopic dermatitis
  - extensive psoriasis
  - drug reactions
- Thermal burns
- Toxic epidermal necrolysis
- Erythema multiforme major (Stevens–Johnson syndrome, SJS)
- Epidermolysis bullosa
- *Infections:* staphylococcal scalded skin syndrome, toxic shock syndrome, eczema herpeticum.

Management

In the acute phase, intensive supportive care is the priority. Specific treatment depends on cause. The main hazards are hypothermia and dehydration. Attention is paid to:
- *Body temperature:* hypothermia is common. Fever (damaged keratinocytes produce interleukin-1) may occur even in the absence of infection. Sudden onset hypothermia may be a premonitory sign of septic shock. Environmental temperature should be 30–32 °C
- *Fluid and electrolyte balance:* percutaneous losses are increased and careful monitoring of fluid balance (e.g. by daily weight) is essential
- *Cardiovascular system:* increased cutaneous blood flow can cause high-output cardiac failure
- *Nutrition:* the hypercatabolic state and excessive loss of protein through the skin is associated with increased protein and energy requirements
- *Infection:* damaged barrier function and altered immune function increase the colonization of skin and facilitates systemic infection
- *Complications:* these include stress-induced gastrointestinal ulceration, pulmonary involvement (by the same process that caused the skin failure, e.g. in SJS), venous thrombosis
- *Specific measures:* depend on the aetiology, e.g. systemic steroids for erythrodermic eczema, IV immunoglobulins for pemphigus.

9.2 Clinical dermatology

Clinical evaluation
Assessment should always rely first on an appropriate history and then on examination of as much of the skin as possible. Laboratory investigations may be useful including blood tests, skin biopsy, and swabs for culture of viruses, bacteria, or fungi.

History
Key features of the presenting skin complaint include:
- Duration
- Distribution
- Pattern of evolution
- Associated symptoms, pruritus (itch), or pain.

Previous medical history and history of topical or systemic drug use including alternative therapies such as Chinese herbal medicine is important.

A family history of skin disease such as atopic dermatitis or pruritus in the case of scabies is often helpful.

A holistic approach exploring the psychological and functional effects of the problem on sleep patterns, social interactions, school attendance, and performance is essential.

Examination
General examination
- Is the child well or unwell?
- Any systemic upset such as fever, malaise
- Signs of systemic disease: organomegaly, lymphadenopathy.

Visual inspection of the skin should almost always be combined with palpation. Palpation provides vital diagnostic information and informs about the extent of dermal or subcutaneous involvement.

Examination of the whole skin as well as mucous membranes such as oral mucosa and conjunctivae and the adnexae (hair, teeth, and nails) will often yield important diagnostic clues.
Description of a skin abnormality should encompass:
- Location and distribution
- Colour
- *Morphology:* structure, shape
- Configuration
- Skin surface characteristics
- Active signs.

Location and distribution
Skin lesions may be single or multiple, generalized or local, symmetrical or asymmetrical, and on sun-exposed or protected skin. Locations include:
- *Acral:* distal portions of limbs and head (ears, nose)
- *Dermatomal:* distribution of a dermatome
- Extensor surface of a limb
- Flexural surface of a limb
- *Intertriginous:* under folds of skin
- *Follicular:* arising from hair follicles
- *Photosensitive regions:* head and neck, typically sparing eyelids, neck beneath earlobes and under the chin.

Colour
Erythema is redness and is usually due to increased blood flow. Black skin lesions may indicate the presence of melanin, haemorrhagic crust, or tissue necrosis. Hypo- or hyperpigmentation indicates alteration of melanin production (Fig 9.3). Orange skin may be seen in carotenaemia.

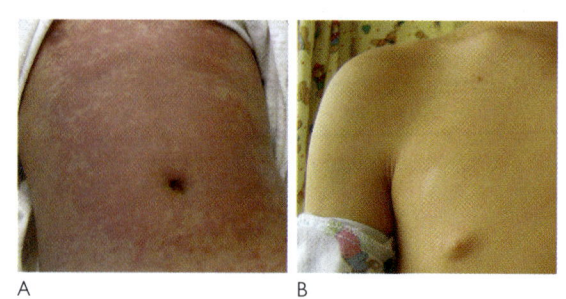

Fig 9.3 A. Confluent erythema. B. Hypopigmented macule.

Morphology
Morphology is the form and structure of a lesion: whether it is flat, elevated or depressed, the consistency, and the shape.

The following morphological lesions are recognized:
- *Macule:* a localized, flat non-palpable change in appearance
- *Papule:* a small raised palpable lesion (<5–10 mm diameter)
- *Nodule:* a larger, raised palpable solid lesion (>10 mm diameter)
- *Cyst:* a nodule or papule containing fluid
- *Vesicle:* a small, clear, fluid filled blister
- *Bulla:* a large, clear, fluid filled blister
- *Pustule:* an elevated yellow-white lesion containing pus (Fig 9.4)
- *Plaque:* a palpable, elevated flat topped lesion
- *Wheal:* a localized area of dermal inflammation seen in urticaria (hives). No visible epidermal change such as scale
- *Purpura:* a non-blanching lesion due to haemorrhage into the skin or mucous membranes which may be palpable (Fig 9.5A). Small pinpoint lesions are called *petechiae* (Fig 9.5B) and larger bruise-like areas *ecchymoses*
- *Telangiectasia:* a small area of visible arterioles.

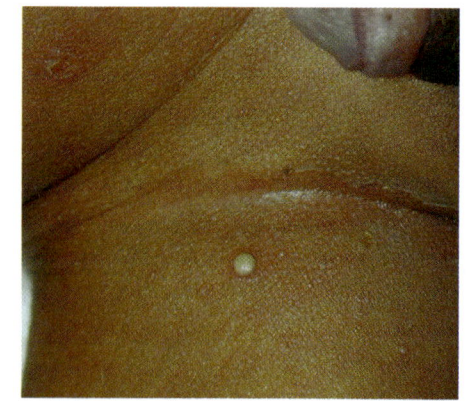

Fig 9.4 Pustule.

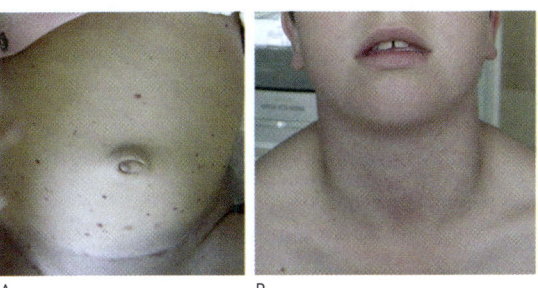

Fig 9.5 A. Purpura. B. Petechiae.

Configuration
Configuration refers to the shape of a lesion or the arrangement of clusters of lesions:
- *Linear:* a straight line (synonym: striate) (Fig 9.6B)
- *Nummular or discoid:* round (coin-shaped) lesions
- *Target:* concentric rings of erythema and pallor seen in erythema multiforme (Fig 9.6A)
- *Guttate:* multiple small scattered 'rain-drop' like lesions
- *Gyrate:* that appears to be whirling in a circle
- *Annular:* a ring with central clearing, e.g. tinea corporis
- *Reticular:* a lacy chicken-wire like pattern.

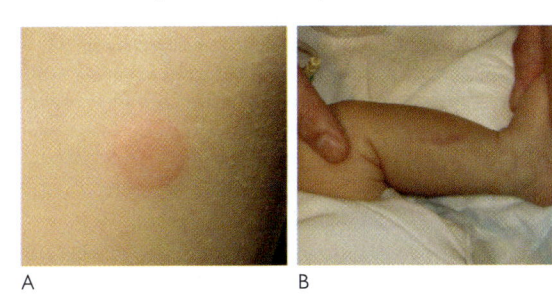

Fig 9.6 A. Target lesion. B. Linear bruise: inflicted.

Skin surface characteristics
Scaling (hyperkeratosis) is an increase in the stratum corneum. Descriptive terms for scale include:
- *Desquamation:* skin coming off in scales
- *Exfoliation:* skin peeling off in sheets (Fig 9.7)
- *Maceration:* moist peeling skin
- *Keratotic:* horny scale
- *Psoriasiform:* large white or silver flakes.

A host of secondary changes affect the skin surface:

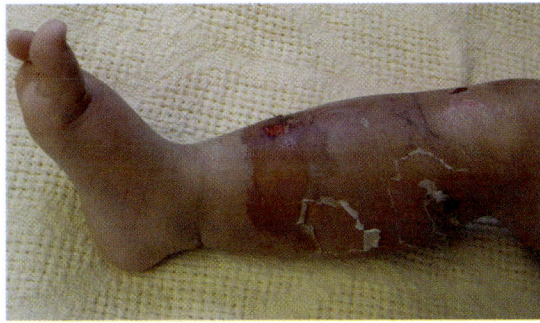

Fig 9.7 Exfoliation post cellulitis.

- *Lichenification:* palpably thickened skin with increased markings resembling tree bark, e.g. chronic eczema
- *Crusting:* yellow red or brown dried exudate (fibrinogen and plasma proteins), e.g. impetigo
- *Excoriation:* loss of the epidermal surface (partial or complete) due to scratching
- *Ulceration:* a large area of epidermal and dermal loss
- *Erosion:* a small area loss of the epidermis
- *Fissure:* a thin, narrow ulcer, e.g. in perianal region
- *Granulation:* a mass of new capillaries and fibrous tissue in a healing wound
- *Atrophy:* a sunken area of tissue loss and thinning of skin or subcutaneous tissue.

Active signs:
- *Dermatographism:* gentle scratching of normal skin produces a wheal
- *Darier's sign:* formation of a wheal when a pre-existing lesion is rubbed, e.g. in urticaria pigmentosa
- *Nikolsky's sign:* gentle pressure causes epidermal slippage and shearing
- *Koebner's phenomenon:* localization of lesions within areas of trauma.

Aids to examination
Dermoscopy
Usually is used to reveal the structure of pigmented lesions not discernible with the naked eye. Fluids (e.g. alcohol hand gel) are applied to the surface to eliminate surface reflection and make the epidermis more transparent. Examination is then performed with a magnifying 'dermatoscope'. It is useful for distinguishing between benign and malignant lesions.

Ultraviolet (Wood's) light
Examining the skin using a handheld UV (Wood's) light in a darkened room is useful in diagnosis of some infections: green fluorescence of tinea capitis, coral pink fluorescence of erythrasma. It also shows up hypopigmented ash-leaf macules in tuberous sclerosis.

Investigations
Culture
Skin scrapings or nail clippings are useful in diagnosis of fungal infection and swabs for bacterial infections.

Patch testing
Used to identify allergens responsible for contact dermatitis. Test materials are applied to the skin under patches for 48 h when the sites are inspected for signs of eczema. Inspection is repeated after a further 48 h.

Skin biopsy
Skin biopsy is an important diagnostic tool. Histology may help if a clinical diagnosis is elusive. Usually done under local anaesthetic. There are three main types:
- *Punch biopsy:* a core of tissue is removed using a circular punch biopsy blade which is rotated into the skin until it reaches the subcutaneous fat
- *Elliptical biopsy:* an ellipse incision can be used to remove an entire lesion or an incisional ellipse, e.g. across the edge of an ulcer or blister can be performed for diagnosis
- *Shave biopsy:* a thin slice is taken off a superficial lesion using a scalpel; not generally useful for diagnosis of inflammatory skin disorders.

9.3 Neonatal dermatology

Newborn skin: normal changes
Normal physiological appearances include:
- *Scaling:* desquamation often occurs on the 2nd day of life and may continue until the 3rd week. The post-term infant has thicker, dry, and cracked skin.
- *Cutis marmorata:* a reticulate bluish mottling on the trunk and extremities as a response to cold.
- *Acrocyanosis:* many normal babies have blue extremities in the first 24 h, especially if cold.
- *Harlequin colour change:* a transitory erythematous flush of the lower body with pallor of the upper half. Observed more commonly in preterm infants.

A number of transient vesiculopustular rashes occur:
- *Milia (milk spots):* due to blockage of sebaceous glands. Tiny white/yellow papules, usually on face. May persist for 1 month or longer.
- *Miliaria:* due to blockage of sweat ducts. May be tiny clear vesicles (miliaria crystallina) or surrounded by erythema (miliaria rubra, prickly heat). The latter occur in flexural areas (neck, groins, axillae) after excessive sweating. Avoid excessive heat and humidity.
- *Sebaceous gland hyperplasia:* multiple yellow tiny papules over the nose and cheeks.
- *Erythema toxicum neonatorum:* tiny yellow or white papules with generalized blotchy macular erythema. Unknown aetiology. Clear in 1–2 days.
- *Transient neonatal pustular melanosis:* superficial vesiculopustular lesions disappear leaving pinhead sized pigmented macules which last for 2–3 months.
- *Acropustulosis of infancy:* sterile pustules appear in crops on scalp, hands, and feet.

Infections
Candida infections are common, especially in the napkin area. Impetigo neonatorum due to *Staph. aureus* infection may present as:
- Superficial pustules
- *Bullous impetigo:* bullous, pus-containing lesions (Fig 9.8)
- *Staphylococcal scalded skin syndrome* caused by epidermolytic toxin from phage group 2 staphylococci. Widespread, tender erythema is followed by large flaccid bullae which peel away leaving scald-like areas.

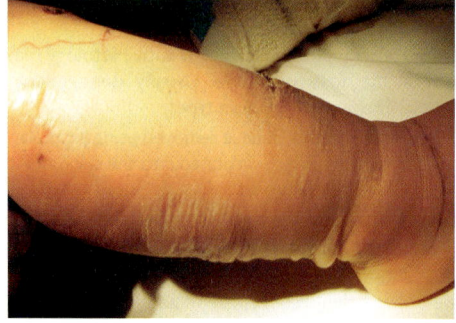

Fig 9.8 Bullous impetigo.

Staphylococcal skin infections in the newborn require treatment with systemic antibiotics, e.g. flucloxacillin.

Birthmarks (naevi)
A naevus is a circumscribed growth or mark on the skin which is either congenital (a birthmark) or an acquired stable hamartomatous malformation.

Vascular, pigmented and epidermal naevi occur.

Vascular naevi
- *Salmon patch (stork bite):* a flat, pink lesion on nape of neck, upper eyelids, or glabella. Most disappear, but 10–20% in occipital region persist.
- *Port wine stain:* a vascular malformation involving mature capillaries, usually large, irregular, deep red or purple, and unilateral. The face is a common site. These do not involute, and camouflage or laser treatment is often required. Associations include Sturge–Weber syndrome
- *Infantile haemangioma (strawberry naevus, capillary, cavernous, or mixed haemangioma):*
  - A proliferative lesion usually not present at birth but appearing in the first few weeks, more commonly in pre-term infants.
  - An erythematous lesion increases in size during the first year to form a vascular nodule (Fig 9.9B). The proliferative phase lasts 8–18 months. Involution usually follows.
  - Reassurance is usually sufficient, but active treatment with systemic steroids is indicated if vital functions are impaired such as airway, feeding or vision.
- *Diffuse neonatal haemangiomatosis:* multiple large cutaneous and visceral haemangiomas. Poor prognosis.

Sebaceous naevus (organoid naevus)
A slightly raised warty lesion containing high numbers of adnexal structures often seen on the scalp. Present at birth. Surgical excision in late childhood may be indicated because of a long-term risk of malignancy.

Pigmented naevi
- *Congenital melanocytic naevi:* present at birth in 1–2%.
- *Giant congenital melanocytic naevus (bathing trunk naevus):* an extensive (>20 cm diameter) hairy lesion usually of bathing trunk area. Increased risk of cutaneous melanoma or meningeal melanosis/melanoma.
- *Blue spots:* bluish-black macules usually in lumbosacral and buttock region of infants with pigmented skin (Fig 9.9A). Melanocytes are deep in dermis.

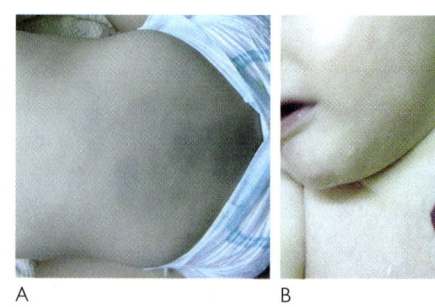

Fig 9.9 A. Blue spot. B. Strawberry naevus.

Icthyoses

The icthyoses are a heterogeneous group of disorders of keratinization. Ichthyosis vulgaris (IV) accounts for 95%.

Ichthyosis vulgaris (IV)

Inheritance is autosomal semidominant with a prevalence of 1/250. Heterozygotes are mildly affected and homozygotes severely affected.

Caused by mutations in *FLG*, the gene for profilaggrin, a high-molecular-weight precursor of filaggrin, a major component of keratohyalin granules. Loss of filaggrin disrupts the protective barrier which normally keeps water in and foreign proteins out.

Fine white scales appear in the first few months, typically sparing the flexures and face. In 25–50% of patients atopic eczema coexists and a significant association between *FLG* mutations and both eczema and asthma has been found.

Treatment is with hydrating agents such as copious emollients perhaps containing urea or salicylic acid. Topical retinoids may also be useful.

X-linked ichthyosis

This is caused by a defect in steroid sulfatase and affects 1/8000 males. Onset is in early childhood with scalp, ears, neck, and flexures developing polygonal dark scales.

Lamellar ichthyosis

This is a group of severe autosomal recessive (AR) disorders caused by mutations in at least four genes, including *TGM1*, encoding transglutaminase-1.

At birth the baby may be encased in a tough, film-like 'collodion membrane' (Fig 9.10) which is shed by 10–14 days revealing erythroderma and scaling.

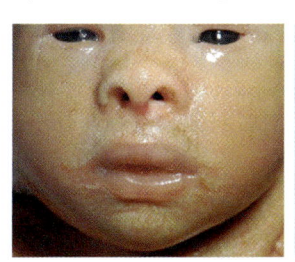

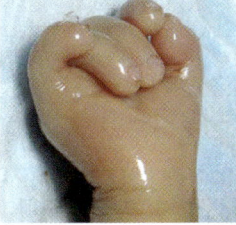

Fig 9.10 Collodion baby: face and hand. © Aukland District Health Board. For copyright information see. http://www.adhb.govt.nz/copyright.htm

Epidermolysis bullosa (EB)

EB is a group of inherited disorders characterized by formation of blisters (bullae) in response to mechanical trauma. It is caused by mutations in genes encoding proteins involved in the basement membrane zone (BMZ).

Basement membrane zone (BMZ)

The BMZ is a thin, sheet-like extracellular matrix structure which connects the basal cell cytoskeletal network with interstitial collagen fibrils in the dermis.

Three major forms of EB are recognized according to the depth of the split which is determined by the proteins involved. A deeper split causes more severe disease:

- *EB simplex (EBS):* superficial intraepidermal split
- *Junctional EB (JEB):* skin separation in lamina lucida
- *Dystrophic EB (DEB):* separation in sublamina densa.

Epidermolysis bullosa simplex (EBS)

Mutations in the genes for epidermal keratins mainly account for this autosomal dominant disease. Weber–Cockayne subtype is mild. Blistering usually confined to palms and soles. Superficial split so no scarring.

Junctional epidermolysis bullosa (JEB)

Mutations in genes encoding hemidesmosome proteins, including laminin 5 subunits and integrin β4, cause this severe group of AR diseases.

Separation is in the superficial part of the BM, the lamina lucida. Severe blisters occur at birth with involvement of larynx, gastrointestinal tract, bones, and teeth. Lethal and non-lethal forms occur.

Dystrophic epidermolysis (DEB)

Mutations in the gene for type VII collagen disrupt anchoring fibrils, causing separation beneath the basement membrane. AR and AD forms occur.

Extensive blistering and scars lead to fusion of digits, joint contractures, dysphagia, anal strictures, and teeth and nail abnormalities. Lifespan is reduced.

Incontinentia pigmenti (IP): Bloch–Sulzberger syndrome

IP is a rare ectodermal dysplasia caused by mutations in the *IKBKG (NEMO)* gene on Xq28. It is almost always lethal prenatally in males. It affects the skin, hair, teeth, and CNS.

In affected females skin manifestations evolve through four stages:

I: erythematous vesicobullous eruption from birth (Fig 9.11A)
II: verrucous hypertrophic wart-like rash in first few months
III: hyperpigmentation stage, swirled or linear pattern (Fig 9.11B).
IV: hypopigmentation stage

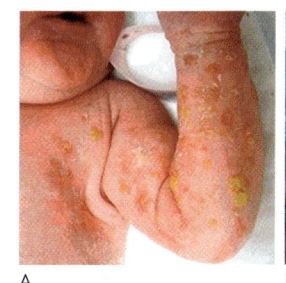

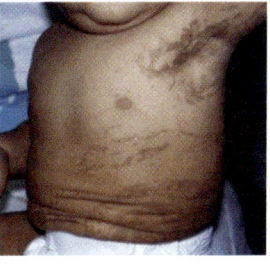

Fig 9.11 IP: A. Stage I, blisters. B. Stage III, pigmented. Source: www.genetests.org. © University of Washington, Seattle.

Acrodermatitis enteropathica

A rare AR disorder caused by defects in an intestinal zinc-specific transporter.

Infants develop diarrhoea and an eczematous eruption around orifices and on the extremities. It starts soon after birth in bottle-fed babies and at weaning in breast-fed babies, as breast milk is protective.

This potentially fatal disorder is important to recognize as it is reversed by oral zinc supplements.

9.4 Eczema

The terms *eczema* (Greek *ekzein*, 'to boil out') and *dermatitis* are both used for a distinct pattern of skin inflammation.

Atopic dermatitis (atopic eczema)

This is a chronic inflammatory skin disease which has a prevalence of 15% in children in developed countries. Atopy is defined as a genetic propensity for developing IgE-mediated (type 1) responses to environmental allergens and is manifested clinically as eczema, asthma, or hay fever.

Aetiology and pathophysiology

It is caused by strong genetic and environmental interactions. 70% of affected children have a positive history of atopy. Concordance in monozygotic twins is 86% and in dizygotic twins 21%. Mutations in *FLG* (R501X, 2282del4), the gene for fillagrin, are strongly associated with atopic eczema. The pathophysiology of atopic dermatitis is not fully understood. Factors include:

- *Skin barrier function*: identification of filaggrin mutations indicates that a failure of skin barrier function predisposes to dry skin, abnormal access of antigens and local infection.
- *Immune function*: immunological abnormalities may be primary (genetic predisposition), and secondary. An eosinophilia and raised IgE is common. Langerhans cells capture and present antigens to T cells causing production of TH2 cytokines which stimulate B cell IgE production, mast cell activation, and increased vascular permeability.
- *Environmental exposures*: environmental allergens provoke the immune response and may gain access via the gut, lungs, and skin. Food allergy is more common in atopic children, but food allergens exacerbate eczema in <10%.

All eczemas share a pattern of inflammation with epidermal oedema, thickening, scale, and perivascular inflammation.

Clinical features

Onset is in the 1st year of life in >50% of cases, and <5 years in 90%. Intense pruritus, or parental reports of rubbing in an infant, is the key feature in the history. A family history of atopy is significant.

Examination

The location of lesions and their morphology changes with age, chronicity, and complications such as infection (Fig 9.12).

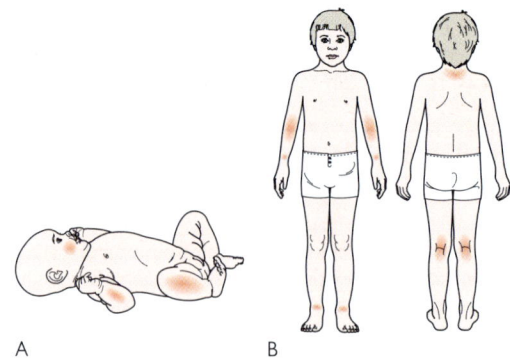

Fig 9.12 Atopic eczema: localization. A. Infant: face, flexural and extensor surfaces. B. Child: flexural surfaces. Adapted from the Illustrated Textbook of Paediatrics (Lissauer, Clayden) 2001, by permission of Elsevier.

- *Infancy*: onset usually after 2 months on the face and scalp. May occur anywhere with a predilection for the flexural regions. Extensor aspects of limbs often affected when crawling starts.
- *Childhood*: from 18–24 months elbows and knee flexures are most commonly involved. Lichenification (thickening with accentuation of skin creases) over bony protuberances may be seen (Fig 9.13). Asian or black children may develop a more papular form over the extensor surfaces.

Dennie–Morgan folds (prominent infraocular creases), loss of lateral eyebrows, and hypopigmentation of the face (pityriasis alba) may occur.

Acute and subacute eczema is characterized by erythema, dryness (xerosis), and weeping or vesiculation. Chronic eczema is characterized by lichenification and papules.

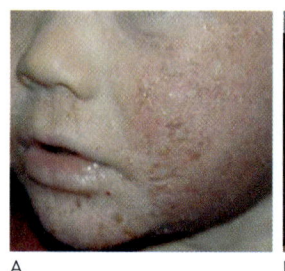

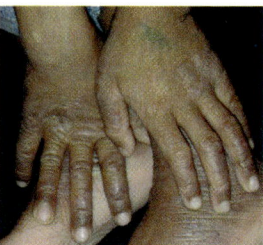

Fig 9.13 Atopic eczema: A. Facial. B. Lichenification of hands.

Atopic eczema is diagnosed when a child has an itchy skin condition plus three or more of the following:

- Dermatitis on flexures or cheeks/extensor areas in infants
- History of dermatitis as above
- History of dry skin in last 12 months
- Personal history or first degree relative with atopy.

An assessment of severity should place the child into one of the following three categories:

- *Mild*: areas of dry skin, infrequent itch, little impact on activity and no impact on sleep
- *Moderate*: frequent itching, redness, excoriation and localized thickening, impact on everyday activities and disturbed sleep
- *Severe*: widespread xerosis, incessant itching, extensive (or localized severe) redness, excoriation, cracking, weeping, flaking, hyperpigmentation, preventing sleep and everyday activities.

Management: first line

Investigations

No diagnostic tests exist, although high IgE level is supportive. Skin swabs should be taken if secondary infection is suspected. Allergy testing is generally not indicated.

A stepped approach to management is used which depends on the severity. This includes general and specific measures.

General measures

- *Avoidance of trigger factors*: clothing: cool, loose cotton clothing is preferable to synthetic or woollen fabrics. Rinse clothes well after washing. Avoid of excessive heat. Keep nails short and rub itchy skin with palm of hand, rather than scratch.
- *Diet*: exclusive breast-feeding during the first 3 months of life is associated with a lower incidence of eczema during

childhood in children with a strong family history of atopy. Food allergy exacerbates eczema in <10% of children.
- In bottle-fed infants aged <6 months with widespread eczema, a 6–8 week trial of a hydrolysed or amino acid formula could be considered.

- *Emollients (moisturizers):* these should be used regularly and copiously, even when the eczema is clear, and increased at any sign of dry skin. They should be prescribed in large quantities and application by smoothing on, not rubbing, should be demonstrated. Emollients should be used in the bath and soaps completely avoided. Useful emollients include:
  - *bath emollients:* oilatum junior, balneum bath oils. Diprobase cream or Epaderm ointment for washing
  - *after bathing and regularly through the day:*
    creams (oil in water suspension): Diprobase cream, Doublebase cream, Oilatum cream
    ointments (oil based): emulsifying ointment, Epaderm ointment, white soft paraffin (50/50).

Specific measures
Topical steroids (cream or ointment)

These are the mainstay of treatment. The lowest strength effective should be used, but only mild potency is used on face and neck and very potent preparations should not be used in children <12 years without specialist supervision. Use a preparation strong enough to settle the eczema in 3–7 days and then switch to a less potent preparation. Application is once or twice daily only to active areas.
- *Mild:* hydrocortisone 0.5–1.0%. for mild eczema or on face/neck.
- *Moderate:* betamethasone 0.025% (Betnovate RD), clobetasone 0.05% (Eumovate)
- *Potent:* betamethasone 0.1% (Betnovate) for chronic, severe, or lichenified eczema in school-age children.

Overall, steroids are underused because of excessive concern about side effects. Maintenance treatment with topical steroids for 2 days/week is useful for frequent flares.

Management: second line
Step up management for moderate to severe eczema. Second line treatment measures include:
- *Antihistamines:* itching is often worse at night so a nocturnal dose of sedating antihistamine such as hydroxyzine >6 months or trimeprazine or promethazine >2 years should be offered if there is significant sleep disturbance.
- *Topical calcineurin inhibitors:* topical tacrolimus and pimecrolimus are options as second line treatment for moderate or severe eczema in older children not controlled by topical steroid treatment. The long-term effects of these agents are not yet known.
- *Bandaging:* This is useful for extensively excoriated eczema particularly on the limbs. It is not indicated for infected eczema. Options include:
  - *occlusive bandages:* topical steroid is applied, followed by a zinc paste impregnated bandage and dry bandaging as the outer layer.
  - *wet wraps:* a moistened tubular bandage on the limbs after application of an emollient or emollient steroid combination. Dry tubular bandaged applied as a top layer. Parents can apply them.
- *Anti-infective chemotherapy:*
  - *Bacterial infection:* this is manifested by weeping, pustules or vesicles, crust, fever, malaise and failure to respond to therapy. *Staphylococcus aureus* is cultured from 90% of swabs from eczema patients, but swabs may identify bacterial resistance or β-haemolytic streptococcal infection.
  - *Minor, local infection* can be treated with topical antibiotics such as fusidic acid or topical antibiotic combined with steroid. Long-term use should be avoided. Extensive infection requires systemic antibiotic therapy with flucloxacillin or clarithromycin if there is a penicillin allergy. Chlorhexidine is effective in reducing bacterial skin flora but can be an irritant and is not suitable for infants.
  - *Herpes infection:* infection with HHV1 or 2, eczema herpeticum, is characterized by a very rapid development of clustered, painful vesicles, umbilicated blisters and punched out erosions 1–3 mm in diameter. Immunofluorescence or EM of blister fluid may give rapid confirmation, but treatment with systemic aciclovir should be initiated without delay if there is clinical suspicion as this is potentially life threatening.
- *Phototherapy or systemic treatment:* These options are considered in severe eczema when all others have been exhausted. UV light treatment is given two or three times weekly for 6–8 weeks. Long-term use confers a risk of skin cancer. Oral prednisolone may be used to obtain rapid control of severe eczema. Immunosuppressants (e.g. ciclosporin) may be very effective.
- *Complementary therapy:* Effectiveness and safety of many complementary therapies has not been assessed. Liver toxicity has been associated with Chinese herbal medicines, and some topical preparations contain potent steroids.

Infantile seborrheic eczema

This condition affects infants <3 months old. It starts in the scalp ('cradle cap') as thick yellow scales and goes on to spread to behind the ears, the folds of the neck, axillae, and nappy area. The flexural folds in the groin may be involved (in contrast to napkin dermatitis). Treatment options, if required, include emollients (aqueous cream), 0.5–1% hydrocortisone alone or with an imidazole (Daktacort).

Napkin dermatitis (nappy rash)

An irritant contact dermatitis which affects the nappy area as a result of occlusive contact of urine and faeces with the skin. The flexures are spared, giving a W-shaped pattern involving inner thighs and genitalia.

Differential diagnosis includes candidiasis (red, scaly, skin folds involved, satellite lesions) and infantile seborrhoeic eczema. Preventative measures include disposable nappies, frequent nappy changes, and protective creams (Epaderm, petroleum jelly). Treat with greasy emollients, exposure, and topical corticosteroid preparations.

9.5 Skin infections and infestations

Bacterial infections

Impetigo
Impetigo is a superficial skin infection with a golden crust on moist erythema, caused by *Staphylococcus aureus* or occasionally *Strep. pyogenes*. The face (around the nose and mouth) and hands are sites of predilection. Bullous impetigo is common in the newborn.

Impetigo is contagious and spreads rapidly. Topical antibiotics are suitable for early minor infections (e.g. fusidic acid) but most require a course of oral flucloxacillin. Nasal carriers of staphylococci in the family may need to be treated with cream containing chlorhexidine and neomycin.

Staphylococcal scalded skin syndrome
Specific phage types of staphylococci produce an exfoliative exotoxin. More common in infants and children <6 years.

A local upper respiratory tract infection, otitis externa, or conjunctivitis is followed by malaise, irritability, and fever. Tender erythema is a key feature. Wrinkled bullae form followed by sloughing (Fig 9.14). Treatment is with systemic flucloxacillin or fusidic acid.

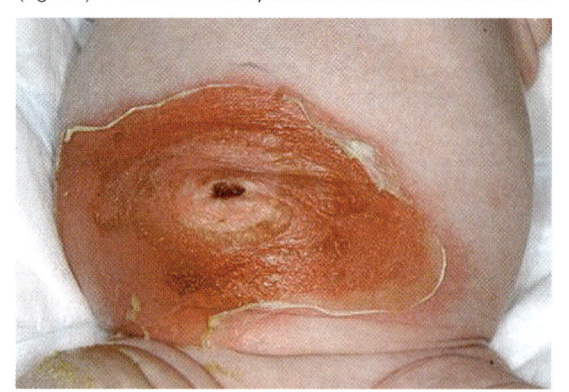

Fig 9.14 Staphylococcal scalded skin syndrome. Paediatrics & child health, 17(10) Oct 2007, by permission of Elsevier.

Streptococcal infections
- *Scarlet fever:* an erythematous exanthem caused by erythrogenic toxins produced by Group A streptococcus (GAS).
- *Erysipelas:* infection of the superficial dermis by GAS producing a well-demarcated red, tender, oedematous area with malaise and fever.
- *Cellulitis:* a deeper streptococcal (occasionally staphylococcal) infection involving subcutaneous tissue. There is erythema with ill-defined, non-palpable borders. Bullae and necrosis may occur, and there is fever. Antibiotic therapy should be prolonged (3–4 weeks).
- *Necrotizing fasciitis:* a life-threatening soft-tissue infection characterized by necrosis of the fascia and associated with various organisms (GAS, *Clostridium*.) It can complicate chickenpox, surgical wounds, and insect bites. Fever is accompanied by rapidly advancing erythema with severe pain and tenderness which reflect widespread tissue necrosis underlying apparently viable skin. Blistering necrosis may develop.
- ☛ This is an emergency requiring immediate intensive treatment and surgical referral. Broad-spectrum antibiotics are given IV (e.g. ampicillin, clindamycin, gentamicin). MRI or CT can delineate the extent of NF prior to immediate and extensive surgical debridement.

Viral infections

Viral warts
Warts are caused by the human papilloma virus (HPV). There are several varieties:
- *Common:* firm papules often on hands, knees, or face
- *Plantar:* verrucae occur on the soles
- *Plane:* multiple, flat-topped warts on hands or face
- *Filiform:* small frond like skin tags
- *Genital:* condylomata acuminata.

Virtually all warts in children disappear spontaneously within 3 years. Reassurance is the best treatment, but options for painful or unsightly lesions include wart paints (salicylic acid), podophyllin, or cryotherapy with liquid nitrogen.

Molluscum contagiosum
Hemispherical, domed, smooth, pearly papules with central umbilication caused by a pox virus (Fig 9.15). They occur in crops and seed by autoinoculation. Spontaneous resolution in 1 year is usual and no treatment is required initially. In the immunosuppressed, options include cryotherapy and curettage.

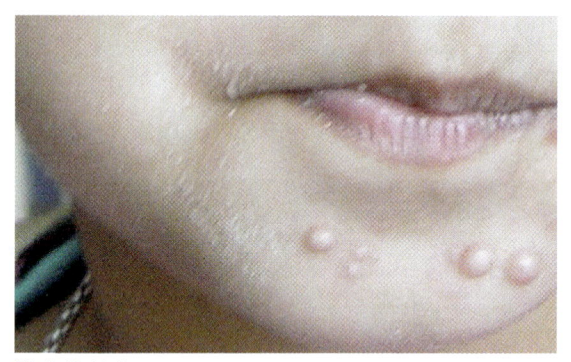

Fig 9.15 Molluscum contagiosum.

Herpesvirus infections

Herpes simplex virus 1 and 2 (HSV 1/2, HHV 1/2)
Infection is common and usually asymptomatic. Primary HHV1 infection can cause a severe gingivostomatis. Reactivation of latent virus causes 'cold sores' most commonly on lips (herpes labialis). Direct inoculation into finger causes a herpetic whitlow. Neonatal herpes simplex is usually caused by direct transmission of genital herpes during labour (usually HHV2).

Herpes simplex virus 3 (HHV3, varicella zoster)
Primary infection causes chickenpox and reactivation causes herpes zoster (shingles) which is usually unilateral and in a dermatomal distribution (Fig 9.16).

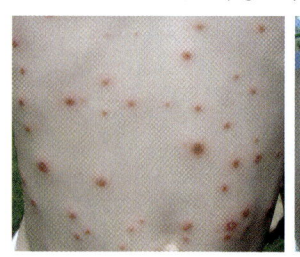

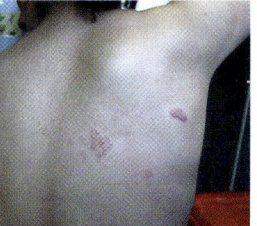

Fig 9.16 A. Chickenpox. B. Shingles.

Hand, foot, and mouth disease
Fever and malaise is followed by a painful stomatitis with superficial small blisters and similar vesicles over the hands and feet. It is caused by coxsackievirus A16 or enterovirus 71. Usually mild and self-limiting.

Fungal infections
Dermatophytosis (ringworm, tinea)
This is a fungal infection caused by dermatophytes, a group of fungi that invade the dead keratin of skin, hair, and nails. Infection is spread from person to person, animal to person, or rarely from the soil. Common organisms include species of *Trichophyton*, *Microsporum*, and *Epidermophyton*. Tinea infections are classified according to body region involved:
- *Tinea capitis*: scalp hair. Scalp ringworm is common. There is hair loss (alopecia) with a patch of scale and inflammation which may give rise to pustules (kerion). Occipital lymphadenopathy is very common and a useful diagnostic clue. The lesions may fluoresce under Wood's (UV) light, and skin scrapings and hair pulls should be sent to the mycology lab. It requires systemic treatment with oral griseofulvin for 8 weeks or terbinafine. An antifungal shampoo may be useful early on to reduce transmission risk.
- *Tinea corporis*: trunk or extremities. On the body, the lesion may clear centrally to form an annular patch (hence 'ringworm').
- *Tinea pedis*: athlete's foot. This affects the toe webs and is often unilateral affecting the lateral interspaces. Tinea corporis or pedis is treated with topical terbinafine cream.
- *Tinea unguium*: the nails (also called onychomycosis). Causes thickened, discoloured, dystrophic nails. Nail infections usually require systemic treatment with oral itraconazole or terbinafine.

Candidiasis
Candida albicans is a unicellular fungus or yeast and a normal gut commensal. Infections may cause oral candidiasis (thrush), cutaneous candidiasis (e.g. in napkin area), or systemic candidiasis (in the immunocompromised).

Oral thrush presents as white patches on the buccal mucosa and is treated with nystatin suspension or miconazole gel.

Skin infection, typically in the napkin area and superimposed on an infant dermatitis or seborrhoeic eczema, is treated with topical imidazole antifungals, e.g. clotrimazole (Canestan) or miconazole (Daktarin).

Pityriasis versicolor
This is commonest in young adults. It is caused by *Malassezia* yeast infection and manifests as scaly hypo- or hyperpigmented patches on the trunk. An imidazole cream (e.g. ketoconazole) twice daily for 10 days–3 weeks is effective.

Parasitic infestations
Scabies
Human scabies is caused by infestation with the mite *Sarcoptes scabies humanis*. After an incubation period of 2–6 weeks an intensely itchy (worse at night) skin eruption occurs which is an immune response to the mite. Features include:
- *Burrows*: the characteristic lesion, not always present (Fig 9.17)
- *Excoriations*
- *Rash*: widespread in infants with eczematization, papules, vesiculopustular lesions, urticaria, impetiginized lesions.

The distribution is typically over the soles of the feet in infants, but also on palms and sides of digits.

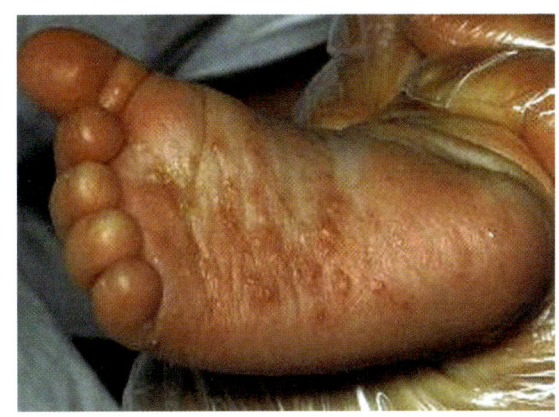

Fig 9.17 Scabies.

Treatment
Application of permethrin 5% cream to whole body including face if necessary (in infants). Particular attention to webs of fingers and toes and under nails. Wash off after 8–12 h. Two applications should be made, 1 week apart. Treat all family members even if asymptomatic. Itching and eczema of scabies may require treatment with topical steroid and sedating antihistamines. Secondary infection requires oral antibiotics. All clothing, bed linen, and towels should be washed at end of treatment.

Pediculosis (head lice, nits)
Head lice are most common, but lice may also reside on eyelashes and pubic hair. Presentation is with itching of the scalp. Nits (egg capsules) are visible on close inspection. Infestation is very common in children (prevalence 1–9%) and spreads by head to head contact.

Diagnosis is not always easy. Lice are small and well camouflaged, may be few in numbers, and hide when disturbed. Combing wet hair should detect infestation.

Treatment options include application of topical pediculocides and/or 'wet combing'. It is uncertain which is best.
- *Pediculocides*: carbaryl, malathion, or pyrethroids are all effective, although resistance is emerging. Lotion or liquid formulation should be applied with a contact time (e.g. overnight) of 12 h. Two applications 1 week apart.
- *Wet combing*: some parents prefer this to use of 'insecticides'. A 'Bug Buster kit' is prescribable but meticulous combing at 4 day intervals over 2 weeks is required and this is challenging for some families.

Papular urticaria
This is a hypersensitivity reaction to insect bites, e.g. cat fleas, bed bugs. Linear or closely grouped red papules occur over buttocks and limbs. Eradication of the cause is the best treatment. Pets should be treated for fleas; bed bugs often require professional control. Oral antihistamine and topical steroids may give symptomatic relief.

9.6 Inflammatory dermatoses

Psoriasis

Psoriasis is characterized by inflamed lesions covered by silvery-white scales of keratin It affects 2% of the population.

Aetiology and pathogenesis

Psoriasis is a multifactorial immune-mediated disease in which genetic predisposition interacts with environmental factors. Multiple susceptibility loci have been mapped. There is epidermal hyperproliferation with reduced keratinocyte transit time, endothelial proliferation, and inflammatory cell infiltration. Trigger factors include trauma (Koebner phenomenon), infection, emotional stress, drugs (systemic steroid withdrawal), alcohol, and HIV.

Clinical features

The hallmark is erythematous well-defined plaques with overlying silvery scales. Subtypes include:

- *Guttate psoriasis:* the commonest form in children. Sudden appearance of multiple small 'raindrop'-like red papules 0.5–2 cm diameter on trunk, face, and limbs. Sometimes occurs 1–4 weeks after streptococcal infection of throat or skin. Lesions typically persist for 3–4 months before resolving.
- *Plaque psoriasis:* larger, thick, scaly, erythematous plaques typically with predilection for extensor aspects of elbows, knees and scalp.
- *Flexural psoriasis:* macerated erythematous lesions with little scale. Often involve the napkin area first.
- *Nail psoriasis:* superficial pits, onycholysis, and subungual hyperkeratosis. May precede skin lesions.

Management

Topical treatment

- *Emollients and soap substitutes:* reduce scaling and pruritus
- *Coal tar:* has anti-inflammatory properties and is widely used, but strong odour limits acceptability
- *Dithranol:* useful for large thick plaques as a cream preparation; can irritate lesions and burn skin
- *Vitamin D analogues:* calcipotriol is licensed for children >6 years.
- *Topical steroids:* useful as monotherapy when itch is a major symptom; often combined with tar.

Systemic therapy

Ciclosporin, retinoids, and anti-TNF antibodies may be required for severe, resistant, or complicated psoriasis.

Phototherapy

Narrow-band UVB phototherapy or PUVA (psoralen +UVA), but long-term risk of skin cancer.

Acne

Acne is a chronic inflammatory disorder of the pilosebaccous unit affecting mainly the face and upper trunk. Acne vulgaris is an almost universal problem of adolescence.

Aetiology and pathogenesis

There is an increase in sebum production by pilosebaceous glands caused by an abnormal response of the glands to circulating androgens. Androgen levels peak in both sexes in early infancy and again at puberty.

In acne, increased sebum secretion is accompanied by hyperproliferation of keratinocytes at the orifice of the pilosebaceous duct forming the microcomedone, the precursor acne lesion.

Comedones are a later feature and may be closed (whiteheads) or open (blackheads). Colonization of the follicle by *Propionibacterium acnes* and an associated host inflammatory response leads to the development of papules and pustules.

Infantile acne, presenting between 3–6 months, is rare.

Association with underlying endocrine disease is not common and investigation is not warranted. Polycystic ovarian syndrome is a cause of acne (with hirsutism) in young women. Late-onset congenital adrenal hyperplasia and androgen-producing tumours are other rare causes.

Clinical features

Acne mainly affects the face and upper trunk. Lesions are polymorphic and include whiteheads, blackheads, papules, pustules and in severe cases deep nodules, cysts, and scars.

Treatment

Mild to moderate acne

Topical agents

- *Benzoyl peroxide 2.5–10%:* kills *P. acnes*
- *A retinoid (e.g. adapaline):* prevents micromedone formation
- *Topical antibiotics:* e.g. clindamycin, may be useful in inflammatory acne and is best used in combination with benzoyl peroxide to minimize development of drug resistance.

Moderate to severe acne, or failed topical treatment

Oral agents

- *Antibiotics:* >12 years: oxytetracycline or tetracycline 500 mg bd for 3–6 months. Doxycycline or lymecycline are once-daily alternatives. <12 years: erythromycin first choice. Trimethoprim is unlicensed for acne but often highly effective.
- *Isotretinoin:* an effective but toxic drug only for use under supervision of a dermatologist. It is a potent teratogen and females who are sexually active need contraception. May cause depression and hyperlipidaemia.
- *Co-cyprindiol:* a combination of cyproterone acetate (an antiandrogen) and ethinylestradiol (e.g. Dianette). Useful in polycystic ovarian syndrome. Increased risk of venous thromboembolism. Acts as an oral contraceptive.

Urticaria

Urticaria, also called hives, is a transient, itchy erythematous rash which forms raised oedematous wheals (Fig 9.18).

Aetiology and pathogenesis

Urticaria is caused by degranulation of mast cells which releases histamine and other vasoactive mediators causing vasodilatation and increased capillary permeability.

- *Ordinary urticaria*: idiopathic.
- *Allergic urticaria*: an IgE-mediated type 1 hypersensitivity reaction which may be precipitated by:
  - *infections*: viral, *Toxocara canis*, streptococcal infections, intestinal parasites
  - *drugs*: penicillins, NSAIDs, codeine
  - *Foods*: cow's milk, eggs, nuts, shellfish, exotic fruits, additives
  - *aeroallergens*: grass, moulds, feathers, house dust
  - *contact urticaria*: after exposure to latex.
- *Physical urticaria*: occurs following minimal trauma (dermographism) or after exposure to heat, cold, sun, or water.
- *Cholinergic urticaria*: precipitated by exercise, heat, or emotional stress; the wheals are small.

Clinical features

History is important as lesions are evanescent and may not be present when patients attend. Lesions usually appear within minutes to hours and resolve within 24 h. Urticaria may be associated with angio-oedema as part of an anaphylactic reaction in which there is swelling of lips, tongue, and larynx with risk of airway obstruction.

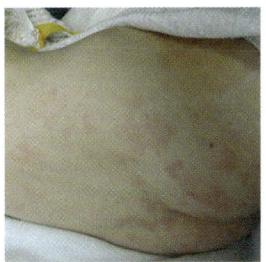

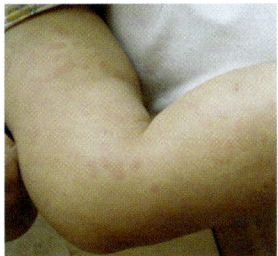

A   B

Fig 9.18 Urticaria or hives.

Management

Investigation is unrewarding in most cases and RAST/skin prick testing is rarely helpful. Non-sedating antihistamines (e.g. cetirizine) are the mainstay of treatment.

Erythema multiforme

Erythema multiforme (EM) is an immune-mediated acute symmetrical eruption, the hallmark of which is the target lesion: concentric rings of erythema, and pallor (Fig 9.6A).

Two main forms are distinguished:

- *Erythema multiforme minor*: no (or mild) mucosal lesions
- *Erythema multiforme major*: more severe with mucosal erosions, but <10% of body surface area involved. Some authorities regard EM major and Stevens–Johnson syndrome (SJS) as synonymous, others distinguish according to skin distribution and aetiology.

Aetiology and pathogenesis

EM minor is most commonly triggered by HSV infection and EM major by drugs. The list of precipitants includes:

- *Infections*:
  - *viral*: HSV, EBV, VZV, Orf
  - *bacterial*: *Mycoplasma*, *Chlamydia*, typhoid, TB
- *Drugs*: antibiotics: penicillins, cephalosporins, macrolides, antiepileptics, NSAIDs
- *Systemic disease*: SLE, malignancy (leukaemia, NHL).

Clinical features

In EM minor there is usually no prodrome, but a history of herpes labialis 3–14 days previously in 50%. In EM major a non-specific prodrome is present for 1–14 days in 50% including fever, discomfort, sore throat, vomiting, diarrhoea.

Target lesions develop abruptly on extensor surfaces of acral extremities and spread centrally. In the centre of target lesions a small papule, vesicle, or bulla may develop. Erosions of mucosal surfaces occur in EM major with haemorrhagic crusting of lips (Fig 9.19A) and involvement of eyes (conjunctivitis, corneal erosions) and genital areas.

In EM minor there may be mild involvement of one mucosal surface, usually the mouth, in 70%. More severe erosions of at least two mucosal surfaces occur in EM major.

Management

EM minor usually resolves within 2 weeks. Symptomatic treatment includes oral antihistamines and local skin care with soothing mouthwashes.

- EM major, and especially SJS, can evolve into a life-threatening condition requiring intensive supportive care in a burns unit or ITU.

Skin biopsy aids diagnosis by demonstrating epidermal necrosis. All drugs should be discontinued as soon as possible. Special attention is required to airway and haemodynamic stability, fluid status, pain control. No systemic treatment is of proven benefit. Eye care is required to prevent panophthalmitis.

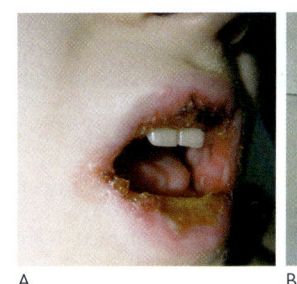

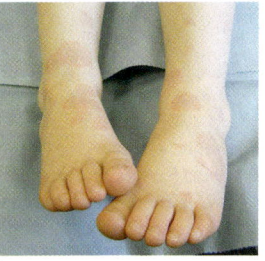

A   B

Fig 9.19 EM major: A. Mucous membrane lesions B. Skin rash.

Erythema nodosum

Tender erythematous nodules, on the shins thighs or forearms. Lesions start bright red but develop a bruise-like appearance. There may be fever, malaise, and arthralgia. It is usually idiopathic, but there is a long list of associations:

- *Infections*: streptococcal, TB, *Mycoplasma*, *Chlamydia*, *Campylobacter*, *Salmonella*, *Brucellosis*, *Yersinia*, cat-scratch fever, Epstein–Barr virus, hepatitis B
- *Drugs*: sulphonamides, penicillins, oral contraceptive pill
- *Systemic disease*: inflammatory bowel disease, sarcoid, malignancy (leukaemia, lymphoma).

Spontaneous resolution occurs in 3–6 weeks. A cause should be sought: streptococcal infection (throat swab, ASOT) and TB (CXR, Mantoux test).

9.7 Hair, nails, mouth, and pigmentation

Hair

Hair loss or absence
Alopecia (hair loss) may be diffuse or localized, scarring or non-scarring.
Causes of non-scarring alopecia include:

Alopecia areata
The most common form of alopecia with one or two well-circumscribed bald areas of scalp (Fig 9.20). Less common are alopecia totalis, whole scalp bald with loss of eyebrows and eyelashes, and alopecia universalis, loss of all body hair.

It is immune mediated and associated with vitiligo and autoimmune disorders. 'Exclamation-mark' hairs may be visible at the periphery of patches. The differential diagnosis is tinea capitis (scalp ringworm) and trichotillomania (see below). Most regrow in 12–18 months, but prognosis is worse if extensive, involving occiput, or associated with atopy.

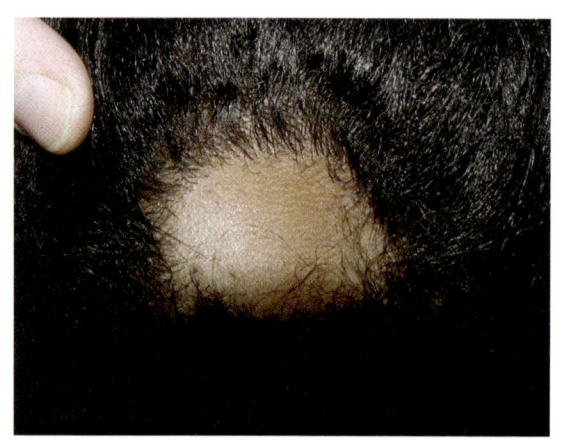

Fig 9.20 Alopecia areata.

Traumatic alopecia
Occipital hair loss is common in infants due to head rubbing on pillow. Trichotillomania is caused by pulling and twisting hair. Varying lengths of hair are found in the area of alopecia. There may be underlying emotional stress.

Traction alopecia
Patchy hair loss caused by hairstyles requiring tightly braided or tied hair, e.g. plaits, pony tails.

Loose anagen syndrome
Occurs in girls age 5–8 years with areas of hair loss and shedding which regrow. Examination reveals easily pluckable hair. Improves with age as hair becomes darker, thicker, and longer. Causes of localized absence of hair from birth include aplasia cutis congenita, naevus sebaceus, and xanthogranuloma.

Excessive hair growth
Hirsutism is the development of male pattern androgen-dependent hair growth in a female and occurs constitutionally in some girls and in polycystic ovarian syndrome.

Hypertrichosis is excess hair growth in either sex in a non-androgen-dependent distribution. Hypertrichosis is uncommon, but is seen in Cornelia de Lange and Rubinstein–Taybi syndromes and as a side effect of drugs (ciclosporin, diazoxide, phenytoin).

Nails

Congenital nail abnormalities
Nail patella syndrome (NPS) is an AD disorder characterized by dysplastic nails, small patellae, elbow deformities, iliac spurs, and nephropathy (in some cases).

Genetic disorders in which the nails may be affected include epidermolysis bullosa and incontinentia pigmenti (nail dystrophy in 40%).

Infections
Acute paronychia is a pyogenic bacterial infection of the nail fold requiring oral antibiotic therapy and on occasion incision and drainage. Herpetic whitlow is a primary infection with HHV1 or 2. Dermatophyte infection of the nail plate (tinea unguium) is relatively uncommon in childhood. Chronic paronychia (*Candida* infection) causes a tender boggy nail matrix with loss of the cuticle and nail dystrophy.

Trauma
Nail biting is common and best ignored.

Skin diseases
- *Psoriasis*: nail changes including pitting, onycholysis (separation of nail from nail bed) and nail dystrophy
- *Alopecia areata or lichen planus:* longitudinal ridges
- *Ectodermal dysplasia:* variable nail dystrophy.

Systemic diseases
- *Koilonychia:* spoon-shaped nails may be present with iron deficiency anaemia, but often occur as a normal finding in first few months due to a thin, soft nail
- *Beau's lines:* transverse depressions appear after onset of any severe illness or with chemotherapy
- *Leuconychia:* white nails can be associated with liver disease and hypoalbuminaemia.

Mouth

Oral mucosa
Causes of oral ulceration include:
- *Aphthous ulcers*: recurring, painful oval or round ulcers usually lasting 1–2 weeks. Affect 20% of population and of uncertain aetiology: trauma, allergy, stress, nutritional deficiency (iron, folate, B12, e.g. in coeliacs)
- *Herpes gingivostomatitis*: infection usually with HHV1
- *Erythema multiforme*: severe erosive lesions of oral mucosa and lips is a feature of the major form
- *Crohn disease*: associated with oral ulceration.

Teeth and gums
Gum hypertrophy may be a side effect of phenytoin and ciclosporin. Plumber's lines are a sign of lead poisoning (Fig 9.21). Discoloured teeth are found in severe neonatal jaundice, tetracycline staining, and congenital erythropoietic porphyria. Small, conical discoloured teeth in ectodermal dysplasia.

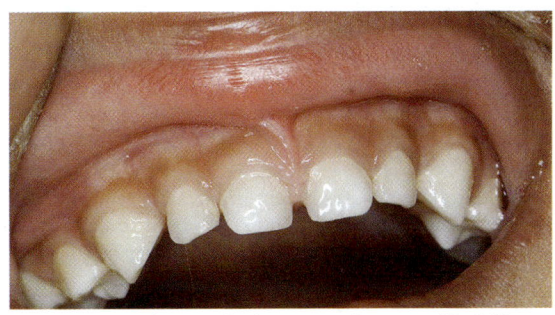

Fig 9.21 Plumber's lines in lead poisoning. Courtesy of Dr Ashley Reece and Dr Harriet Holme.

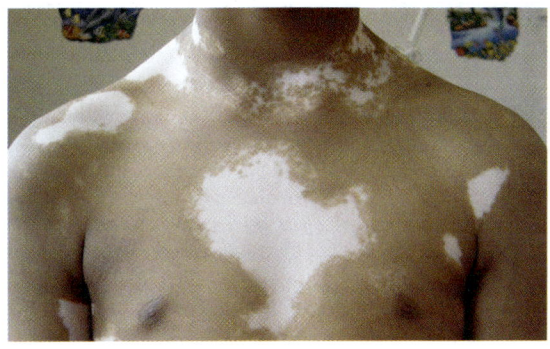

Fig 9.22 Vitiligo.

Disorders of pigmentation

Normal skin colour
Melanocytes in the epidermal basal layer synthesize melanin in organelles called melanosomes. Each pigment cell actively transfers melanosomes to multiple basal keratinocytes and skin colour (reflectance) is determined by number and distribution of melanosomes in keratinocytes.

Two types of melanin are synthesized from tyrosine:
- *Pheomelanin*: a cysteine rich red-yellow form
- *Eumelanin*: a less soluble black-brown form.

Human skin colour is a genetically determined multifactorial trait. Melanosomes of African skin are larger and more dispersed than those in Asian or European skin. Single-gene mutations can influence skin colour (see Albinism below). Loss-of-function alleles in the melanocortin 1 receptor, *MC1R*, are associated with red hair, fair skin, and freckling.

Hypopigmentation (hypomelanosis)
The most common cause of patches of pale or white skin is vitiligo. Genetic causes are numerous but individually rare (Table 9.1). Hypopigmentation can follow inflammation (eczema, psoriasis) and infection (pityriasis versicolor).

Table 9.1. Genetics of hypopigmentation	
Condition	**Gene**
Oculocutaneous albinism:	
Type 1 OCA1	*TYR*: tyrosinase
Type 2 OCA2	*OCA2 (P)*
Type 3 OCA3	*TYRP1*
Type 4 OCA4	*MATP (SLC45A2)*
Piebaldism	*KIT*
Waardenburg syndrome:	
Type 1 WS1	*PAX3*
Type 2 WS2	*WS2A-D*

Pigmentation disorders

Vitiligo
This presents as irregular patches which include areas of complete depigmentation (Fig 9.22). In most cases it is caused by an autoimmune loss of melanocytes; there is an association with autoimmune disorders such as thyroid disease, Addison's disease, and diabetes mellitus.

Lesions often progress to a static phase but spontaneous repigmentation is uncommon. Topical steroid or immunomodulator (tacrolimus) and UV phototherapy may help. Cosmetic camouflage and advice on protection from sunburn should be offered.

Albinism
A group of inherited diseases caused by a defect in the production of melanin. Two main categories are *oculocutaneous albinism* (OCA) involving colour of hair, skin, and eyes and *ocular albinism* in which only the eyes are affected.

OCA is caused by at least four different genes (see Table 9.1) and is AR. Hypopigmentation is present from birth. The main clinical problems are easy sunburn, increased incidence of skin cancer, and visual problems: photophobia, nystagmus, refractive errors, and impaired visual activity.

OCA also occurs in three rare syndromes in association with defects in CNS, platelets, or white cell function: Chediak–Higashi, Hermansky–Pudlak, and Griscelli syndromes.

Piebaldism and Waardenburg syndrome (WS)
Piebaldism is an AD condition characterized by a white forelock, a white patch in the central forehead, eyebrows, and chin and ventral chest, abdomen, and extremities.

In classical Waardenburg syndrome (WS1) the features include a wide bridge to the nose (dystopia canthorum), frontal white blaze of hair, white eyelashes, heterochromia iridis, and cochlear deafness.

Hyperpigmentation
A large number of conditions are associated with widespread or localized increased melanin pigmentation.

Other pigments can of course discolour the skin, including carotene in carotenaemia, haemosiderin in haemochromatosis, homogentisic acid in alkaptonuria, and copper in Wilson disease.

Important causes of hyperpigmentation include:

Acquired
UV light, postinflammatory after eczema, psoriasis, acne, drugs such as minocycline, psychotropics, oral contraceptives, chemotherapy, Addison's disease, Cushing's syndrome, primary biliary cirrhosis, porphyria, pellagra, kwashiorkor, ionizing radiation, pytiriasis versicolour.

Urticaria pigmentosa is a mastocytosis in which there is a naevoid accumulation of mast cells forming widespread small reddish-brown macules which urticate when rubbed.

Genetic
- *Peutz–Jäghers syndrome*: an AD disorder characterized by melanocytic macules of lips, buccal mucosa, and digits with multiple gastrointestinal polyps.
- *McCune–Albright syndrome*: features are pigment patches, polyostotic fibrous dysplasia, and endocrine abnormalities
- *Café-au-lait macules*: present in 2% of newborns and in numerous genetic syndromes, e.g. neurofibromatosis type 1.

9.8 Case-based discussions

A child with swollen lips

An 6 year old boy is seen in the hospital emergency department with a rash, which has developed over the course of the morning There is no pruritus. He has never had a rash like this before, and no one else in the family is affected. He takes no medications and has no allergies. He has had a troublesome cough for the last week, but has otherwise been well.

On examination he is afebrile and systemically well. There is a polymorphic erythematous rash affecting his face and trunk, with some small round lesions (Fig 9.23B). He also has swollen, painful erythematous lips (Fig 9.23A) and marked bilateral conjunctival involvement.

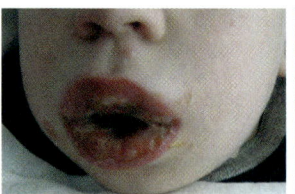

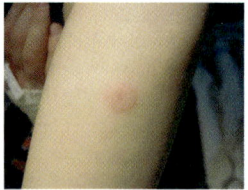

Fig 9.23 A. Lips with mucosal membrane involvement. B. Target lesion.

What is the likely diagnosis?
This child is presenting with classical target lesions of erythema multiforme. Involvement of two mucosal surfaces making the diagnosis of erythema multiforme major.

This is an immune complex-mediated hypersensitivity syndrome. Other mucosal surfaces which may be involved, or may become involved as the condition progresses, include the oral cavity, the upper airway, gastrointestinal tract. or anogenital mucosa.

The child is admitted to the ward. Investigations show only a mildly raised white cell count and a raised erythrocyte sedimentation rate.

What complications may occur in erythema multiforme major?
Possible complications may include corneal ulceration, anterior uveitis, panophthalmitis, bronchitis, pneumonitis, myocarditis, hepatitis, enterocolitis, polyarthritis, haematuria and acute tubular necrosis, and skin failure.

Ophthalmological review is essential as involvement of the eyes may require treatment with topical steroids. This can be a sight-threatening and life-threatening condition.

On day 2 of admission, this boy developed more extensive cutaneous lesions, which began to blister, leaving denuded areas of skin. The ulceration of his oral mucosa became more severe. He developed a temperature of 39 °C, and became tachycardic and hypotensive. He was tachypnoeic and developed an oxygen requirement. His urine output was poor.

What complications are likely to have occurred?
- *Severe dehydration* due to poor oral intake secondary to painful oral ulceration and cutaneous losses due to the extensive blistering.
- *Bacterial superinfection:* due to breakdown of local defences.
- Renal involvement
- Respiratory tract: pneumonitis.

His condition is serious and requires intensive care, best delivered in a burns unit as expert nursing and ventilatory support may be required.

IV fluids and broad-spectrum antibiotics must be commenced and careful skin toilet ensured, as bacterial infection is the leading cause of death in this condition.

Immunomodulatory treatment such as plasmapheresis and intravenous immunoglobulin has also been advocated as a treatment for this condition.

Chapter 10
Endocrinology

10.1 Hormones *210*
10.2 Hypothalamus and pituitary gland *212*
10.3 Hypopituitarism, diabetes insipidus, and SIADH *214*
10.4 Growth and its disorders *216*
10.5 Puberty and intersex *218*
10.6 Thyroid disorders *220*
10.7 Adrenal gland *222*
10.8 Adrenal disorders *224*
10.9 Calcium disorders *226*
10.10 Type 1 diabetes mellitus *228*
10.11 Type 2 diabetes mellitus and hypoglycaemia *230*
10.12 Case-based discussions *232*

10.1 Hormones

An endocrine hormone is a chemical messenger made by tissues or ductless glands and secreted into the blood.

In addition to the familiar glands of the endocrine system such as the pituitary, thyroid, adrenals, pancreas, and gonads several other organs and tissues are important sources of hormones: the gastrointestinal (GI) tract, kidney, heart, pineal gland, and adipose tissue.

Hormones

Types of hormone
Hormones can be classified according to their mode of transmission:
- *Autocrine:* act on the cells that synthesized them
- *Paracrine:* act on neighbouring cells in the same tissue
- *Endocrine:* act on distant cells to which they are carried by the circulation or lymphatic system
- *Pheromonal:* volatile hormones released into the atmosphere where they act on another individual.

Vertebrate hormones can also be categorized into three types according to their chemical nature:
- *Amines:* catecholamines, thyroxine (Fig 10.1)

Fig 10.1 Thyroxine (T4).

- *Peptides*: oxytocin (Fig 10.2), insulin, luteinizing hormone (LH)

Fig 10.2 Oxytocin: a nonapeptide

- *Lipid and phospholipid derived hormones:*
  - steroids: cortisol (Fig 10.3), testosterone
  - sterols: calcitriol
  - eicosanoids: prostaglandins.

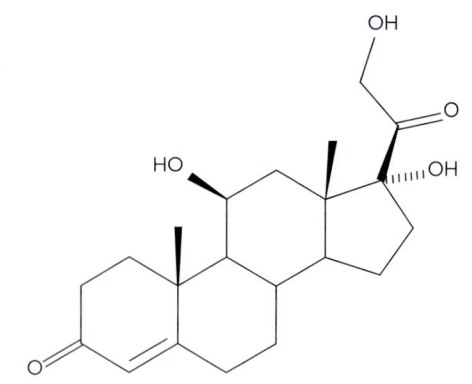

Fig 10.3 Cortisol.

Biosynthesis, transport, and metabolism
Biosynthesis
The classical hormones are synthesized in specialized cell types within a particular endocrine gland. The rate of biosynthesis and secretion is frequently controlled by homeostatic negative feedback and by mechanisms involving:
- Stimulating or releasing hormones
- Plasma concentrations of nutrients or binding globulins
- Nervous system signals
- Environmental effects such as light or temperature.

Secretion patterns
Patterns of hormone secretion vary and include:
- *Continuous:* e.g. thyroxine
- *Pulsatile:* e.g. follicle-stimulating hormone (FSH), LH, growth hormone (GH)
- *Circadian:* e.g. cortisol
- *Stress-related:* e.g. adrenocorticotropic hormone (ACTH)
- *Sleep-related:* e.g. GH.

Transport and metabolism
Most hormones are transported in the blood bound to carrier proteins in the plasma, which may be specific with high affinity for particular hormones or non-specific such as albumin which binds several hormones with low affinity. Examples include:
- *Thyroxine:* thyroid-binding globulin
- *IGF-1 :* IGF-binding proteins
- *Cortisol:* cortisol-binding protein.

Bound hormone is inactive and in equilibrium with a smaller, physiologically active free fraction. Hormones are most commonly measured in serum or plasma using immunoassays. Hormones are mostly metabolized in the liver or kidney but some are degraded in peripheral cells (thyroid hormones) or in the plasma (catecholamines).

Mechanisms of hormone action

Hormones stimulate or inhibit a range of biological processes and have effects on growth, development, the reproductive cycle, metabolism, immune function, and appetite.

Hormone receptors

Most hormones act by combining with a receptor protein. Hormone receptors are of two main types:

- *Cell surface membrane receptors:* water-soluble (polar) hormones such as amines and peptides act on membrane receptors
- *Intracellular receptors:* fat-soluble (non-polar) steroid and thyroid hormones, which easily penetrate the cell membrane, act on intracellular receptors.

Cell surface membrane receptors

Cell surface receptors are integral membrane proteins which react to hormone binding by interacting with other molecules to generate second messengers and complete signal transduction. There are two main types of cell surface membrane receptor:

G-protein coupled receptors (GPCRs)

The GPCRs are a large family of receptors with seven transmembrane (7TM) domains.

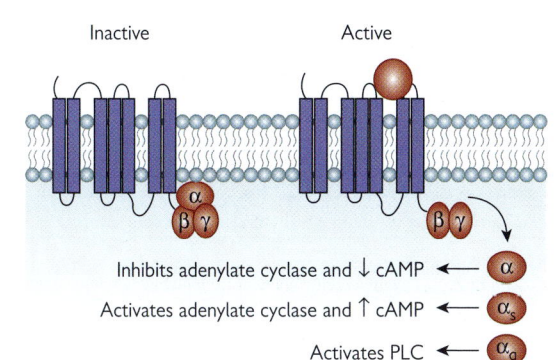

Fig 10.4 GPCR: mechanism of action via G proteins.

Binding of the hormone induces disassociation of an intracellular trimeric G protein (Fig 10.4), activating one of a variety of second-messenger systems:

- *Adenylate cyclase: cyclic AMP:* hormones which use this system include epinephrine, norepinephrine, FSH, LH, thyroid-stimulating hormone (TSH), calcitonin, parathyroid hormone (PTH).
- *Inositol triphosphate system:* e.g. epinephrine (adrenaline) and acetylcholine
- *Cyclic GMP:* used by peptide hormones such as atrial natriuretic factor (ANF) and nitric oxide (NO). Cyclic GMP regulates protein kinases and influences glycogenolysis, apoptosis, and smooth muscle relaxation. Its action is terminated by phosphodiesterases.

Receptor tyrosine kinase (RTK)

Ligand binding dimerizes and activates the receptor (Fig 10.5). Examples include the insulin receptor.

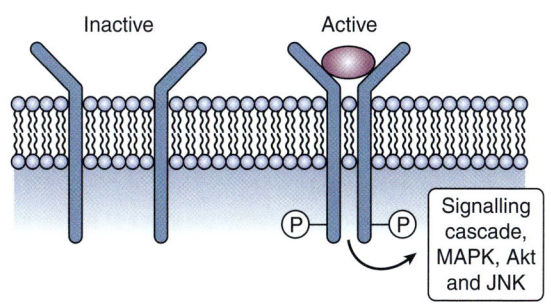

Fig 10.5 RTK mechanism: dimerization activates the receptor.

The receptor itself may be a tyrosine kinase which is activated by hormone binding. The receptor may phosphorylate itself, and other enzymes or interaction of hormone with receptor leads to activation of cytoplasmic tyrosine kinases.

Intracellular receptors

Receptors for lipophilic hormones, such as steroids and thyroxine are located in the cytoplasm or nucleus. These receptors function as ligand-dependent transcription factors: the hormone-receptor complex binds to the promoter region of specific genes and modulates their expression. They belong to the nuclear receptor super family.

Nuclear receptor superfamily

Nuclear receptors have a characteristic three-domain structure (Fig 10.6).

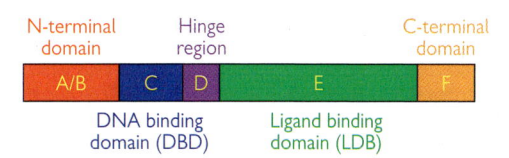

Fig 10.6 Nuclear receptor structure: three major domains.

The superfamily is divided into three classes:

- *Class I, steroid receptor family:* glucocorticoid receptor, progesterone receptor, oestrogen receptor, androgen receptor, and mineralocorticoid receptors. These receptors exist predominantly in cytoplasm bound to heat shock proteins (HSPs).
- *Class II, thyroid/retinoid family:* thyroid receptor, vitamin D receptor, retinoic acid receptor, and the peroxisome proliferator activated receptor. These receptors are typically located in the nucleus.
- *Class III, orphan receptor family:* share homology to known receptors but no ligands are yet identified.

Nuclear receptor signalling

All nuclear receptors modulate gene transcription.

- *Class I receptors:* bound to heat shock proteins (HSPs). Upon binding ligand the HSP complex is released, the receptor forms a homodimer and translocates to the nucleus where it binds to 'hormone response elements' at upstream promoter sites.
- *Class II receptors:* typically function as heterodimers and are bound to response elements regardless of whether ligands are present. However, gene activation is suppressed by a co-repressor which is displaced by ligand binding allowing activation of transcription.

Mutations in nuclear receptors

Inherited diseases, such as testicular feminization syndrome, vitamin D resistant rickets, pseudohypoparathyroidism, and some forms of pseudohypoaldosteronism arise from mutations in nuclear receptors which cause end-organ unresponsiveness. The clinical features of these 'pseudo-' diseases are those of hormone insufficiency, but hormone levels are raised.

10.2 Hypothalamus and pituitary gland

Hypothalamus

Anatomy
The hypothalamus occupies most of the ventral region of the diencephalon. It is divided into three regions, each with a medial and lateral area containing several nuclei. Major hypothalamic nuclei include: paraventricular (PVN), supraoptic (SON), arcuate (ARN), ventromedial (VMN), medial (MN), posterior hypothalamic (PHN), optic chiasm (OC), median eminence (ME), and lateral hypothalamic area (LHA). Two distinct cellular systems are recognized:

- *Magnocellular secretory system:* the PVN and SON contain large cells which produce and secrete oxytocin and vasopressin. Their axons project to the posterior pituitary as the hypothalamic-hypophyseal tract.
- *Parvocellular system:* the PVN has other smaller cells which contribute to a diffuse collection of neurons which send their axons to the median eminence where their terminals secrete the 'releasing hormones': corticotropin-releasing hormone (CRH), gonadotropin-releasing hormone (GnRH), and thyrotropin-releasing hormone (TRH) together with many other peptides including somatostatin and neurotensin. These are conveyed to the pituitary via a vascular link, the portal system.

The ARN are rich in prolactin (PRL) neurons and neurons which secrete galanin, growth hormone releasing hormone (GHRH), and somatostatin.

Functions
Via its neural projections and endocrine output the hypothalamus controls not only the 'endocrine orchestra' but also important bodily activities related to circadian rhythms, reproduction, body temperature, thirst, and hunger.

At the so-called circumventricular organs osmoreceptive and sodium-receptive neurons are in intimate contact with blood and cerebrospinal fluid (CSF) and control thirst, sodium appetite, vasopressin release, and sodium excretion. In addition, neurons with receptors for angiotensin and ANF regulate fluid and electrolyte balance, and interleukins act to elicit fever and ACTH secretion.

The hypothalamus receives many inputs from the brainstem which transmits information from cardiovascular stimuli and visceral stimuli carried by the vagus nerve. These inputs mediate secretion of oxytocin in response to suckling and vasopressin secretion.

Regulation of appetite and feeding behaviour
Neurons in the ARN project to the PVN and lateral hypothalamic area.

Neuropeptide Y (NPY) and Agouti-gene related peptide (AgRP) neurons stimulate feeding behaviour via Y1 and Y5 receptors.

Alpha melanocyte stimulating hormone (αMSH) and cocaine and amphetamine regulated transcript (CART) neurons inhibit appetite via MC3 and MC4 receptors. Pro-opiomelanocortin (POMC) is a precursor of αMSH. AgRP acts as an inhibitory antagonist at MC3 and MC4 receptors (Fig 5.2).

The LHA produces a set of appetite-stimulating (orexigenic) peptides called orexins (hypocretins). See Chapter 5.1. A variety of hormones released in the periphery influence this system (Fig 10.7). Ghrelin, the hunger hormone, stimulates appetite and leptin from adipocytes inhibits appetite. Eating releases a number of gut hormones including peptide YY (PYY3–36) and pancreatic polypeptide (PP) which inhibit appetite and inhibit release of ghrelin.

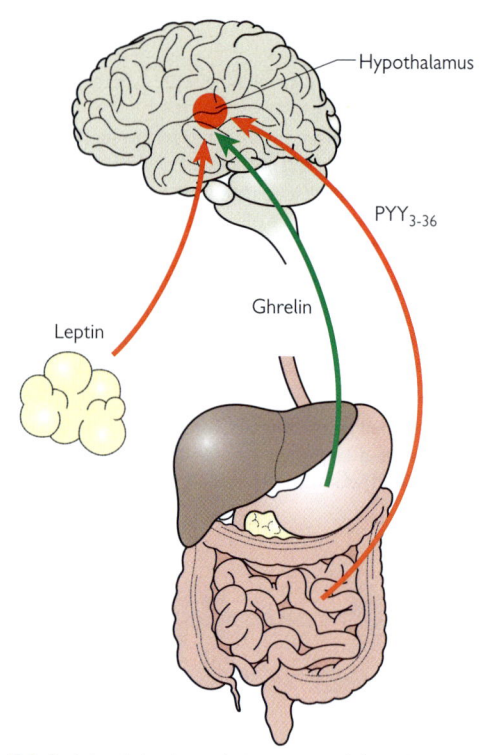

Fig 10.7 Peripheral signals regulating appetite. Adapted courtesy of the Physiological Society.

Anterior pituitary: adenohypophysis
The anterior pituitary arises from an invagination of the oral ectoderm (Rathke's pouch) and is divided into three regions:
- *Pars distalis*: majority of the gland
- *Pars tuberalis*: a sheath wrapped around the pituitary stalk
- *Pars intermedia*: often very small in humans.

It is functionally linked to the hypothalamus via the hypophyseal-portal vascular system in the pituitary stalk.

The anterior pituitary produces six hormones under the control of hormones from the hypothalamus, all but one of which stimulate release. The exception is PRL, which is inhibited by secretion of dopamine.

The nature and function of the individual hormones is considered in turn.

Adrenocorticotrophic hormone (ACTH)
ACTH is a 39 amino acid peptide cleaved from a larger glycosylated precursor, pro-opiomelanocortin. It stimulates production of cortisol by the adrenal cortex. ACTH release is stimulated by CRH and vasopressin.

Thyroid-stimulating hormone (TSH)
TSH is a glycoprotein which shares the same α subunit as LH and FSH. It binds to receptors on the thyroid follicular cell and stimulates release of thyroid hormones via activation of adenylate cyclase.

Gonadotropins (LH and FSH)
LH and FSH are glycoproteins composed of α and β subunits. LH stimulates Leydig cells to produce testosterone in the male, and stimulates ovarian steroidogenesis in the female. FSH acts

on sertoli cells in the male to increase the mass of seminiferous tubules and promote sperm development. In the female it acts on glomerulosa cells to stimulate oestrogen production from testosterone.

Synthesis and secretion of FSH and LH is stimulated by GnRH which is released in a pulsatile fashion. Production of FSH (but not LH) is suppresses by inhibin, a gonadal glycoprotein.

Growth hormone (GH)
GH is a 191 amino acid peptide secreted by somatotroph cells and circulating in bound and unbound forms. GH secretion is pulsatile, nocturnal release occurring shortly after onset of deep sleep.

Prolactin
Prolactin is a 199 amino acid polypeptide (24 kDa) with a high degree of homology to GH and placental lactogen. It is secreted and synthesized by lactotrope cells. Its main effects include the induction of lactation and cessation of menstruation during the puerperium. Secretion is regulated by neurosecretory dopamine neurons of the ARN which inhibit PRL secretion.

Posterior pituitary: neurohypophysis

The posterior pituitary consists mainly of neuronal projections from the hypothalamus extending via the infundibulum to terminate behind the anterior pituitary gland. Hormones are synthesized in cells of the hypothalamic nuclei and secreted into the capillaries of the hypophyseal circulation. There is also a specialized astrocytic cell called a pituicyte.

Two peptide hormones are synthesized in the hypothalamus and secreted into the circulation by the posterior pituitary: oxytocin and arginine vasopressin.

Oxytocin and arginine vasopressin (AVP)
These are both peptides consisting of nine amino acids with a sulfur bridge between two cysteines. Nearly all vertebrates have an oxytocin-like nonapeptide supporting reproductive functions and a vasopressin-like nonapeptide involved in water regulation. Their amino acid sequences differ at just two residues:

- *Oxytocin:* Cys-Tyr-**Ile**-Gln-Asn-Cys-Pro-**Leu**-Gly
- *AVP:*   Cys-Tyr-**Phe**-Gln-Asn-Cys-Pro-**Arg**-Gly

Both are synthesized in the magnocellular neurosecretory cells of the SON and PVN and released into the blood from the posterior pituitary.

Oxytocin
The actions of oxytocin are mediated by receptors expressed in the periphery and in many parts of the brain and spinal cord. The receptor is a Class I GPCR. Oxytocin's effects can be divided into peripheral and central (i.e. within the brain):

Peripheral actions

- *Letdown reflex*: oxytocin acts on the mammary glands causing milk to be 'let down'
- *Uterine contraction*: important during labour
- *Antidiuretic action*: weak antidiuretic action.

Central actions

- *Sexual behaviour and bonding*: oxytocin appears to have a role in arousal and is released during orgasm
- *Anti-stress functions*: there is evidence that oxytocin encourages 'tend and befriend' rather than 'fight or flight' activity
- *Fetal brain protection*: there is evidence that maternal oxytocin crosses the placenta and reduces the vulnerability of fetal cortical neurons to hypoxic damage.

Arginine vasopressin (AVP, ADH)
AVP acts on three different GPCRs (Table 10.1).

Table 10.1. AVP receptors: distribution and actions

Type	Second messenger	Location
AVPRIA	Phosphatidyl inositol /calcium	Liver, kidney, brain, vasculature, platelets
AVPRIB	Phosphatidyl inositol /calcium	Anterior pituitary, brain
AVPR2	Adenylate cyclase /cAMP	Kidney tubules

Reduced plasma volume, increased osmotic pressure, and angiotensin II stimulate release. Ethanol and caffeine suppress vasopressin secretion. Vasopressin is released into the brain in a circadian rhythm.

Peripheral actions

- *Antidiuretic effect:* acts on the AVPR2 receptor in the apical cells lining the collecting ducts of the renal tubules to cause insertion of aquaporin-2 channels, allowing water to be reabsorbed down an osmotic gradient
- *Vasoconstriction:* acting on AVPRIA receptors on vascular smooth muscle to cause vasoconstriction
- *Coagulation:* AVPRIA receptors are expressed on platelets and influence release of factor VIII and von Willibrand factor (VWF).

Central actions

- *ACTH secretion:* AVP acts on AVPRIB receptors in the anterior pituitary to promote secretion of ACTH
- *CNS effects:* AVP appears to be involved in regulation of blood pressure and temperature and social behaviour. Vasopressin released into the brain during sexual activity supports formation of pair bonds.

10.3 Hypopituitarism, diabetes insipidus, and SIADH

Hypopituitarism
Deficiency of one or multiple hormones of the anterior pituitary is termed *hypopituitarism*. Deficiency of all anterior pituitary hormones is *panhypopituitarism*. Onset can be at any time from the neonatal period through childhood. Underlying causes and clinical presentation varying with age.

Aetiology
Congenital hypopituaritism

Congenital hypopituitarism is caused by mutations in genes encoding transcription factors important in pituitary development. It may be syndromic and associated with developmental abnormalities and may cause isolated or combined hormone deficiencies. Examples include:

- *PIT1 (POU1F1)*: mutations cause deficiencies of GH, PRL, and TSH. ACTH and gonadotropin production is preserved. There is severe growth deficiency, midface hypoplasia, and a hypoplastic pituitary on MRI.
- *HESX1*: this is a homeobox gene important for the development of Rathke's pouch. Homozygous mutations may be associated with septo-optic dysplasia (agenesis of the corpus callosum, panhypopituitarism, optic nerve hypoplasia, absent septum pellucidum), and heterozygous mutations with milder phenotypes.
- *KAL1*: is mutated in X-linked forms of Kallman syndrome, characterized by hypogonadotrophic hypogonadism and anosmia. GnRH neurons and olfactory nerves fail to migrate normally from the olfactory bulb to the hypothalamus.

Acquired hypopituitarism

- *Perinatal insults*: birth asphyxia
- *Intracranial tumours*: craniopharyngioma
- Post-surgery
- Cranial irradiation
- Trauma.

Clinical features
Hypopituitarism in the newborn

Birthweight and length are typically within the reference range. There may be hypoglycaemia, hyperbilirubinaemia, or hyponatraemia. Signs may include microgenitalia, optic nerve hypoplasia, or dysmorphic signs of congenital syndromes such as septo-optic dysplasia or holoprosencephaly.

Hypopituitarism in older infants and children

- Growth failure with delayed skeletal maturation due to GH deficiency or hypothyroidism secondary to TSH deficiency
- Absent or delayed puberty or infertility due to gondadotropin deficiency
- Hypoglycaemia
- Weight gain with relative truncal obesity
- *Visual and neurologic abnormalities*: decreased visual acuity
- Anosmia in Kallmann syndrome with delayed puberty.

Investigations
Imaging

A lateral skull radiograph may show an abnormal pituitary fossa and calcification in a craniopharyngioma. Cranial MRI is best for evaluating the hypothalamic–pituitary axis.

Endocrine tests

Evaluation of the hypothalamic–pituitary axis is undertaken by a combination of random hormone level estimations and provocation tests.

Random hormone levels

- *Thyroid function*: FT4, TSH
- *Adrenal cortex*: glucose, urea and electrolytes, morning serum cortisol
- *Gonads*: in infants, random LH, FSH, oestradiol and testosterone are informative
- *Growth hormone*: a random serum GH level is useful in early infancy, or a 24 h profile.

Stimulation (provocation) tests

- *Synacthen stimulation test*: ACTH
- *Luteinizing hormone releasing hormone (LHRH) stimulation test*: FSH/LH response (up to 4 years)
- *TRH test*: TSH and PRL response
- *GH stimulation test*: a provocation test is usually required using GH secretagogues such as GHRH or glucagon. Other GH tests include the use of glucagon, arginine, clonidine, and exercise. Insulin tolerance tests are potentially hazardous and performed only in specialist centres.

A combined pituitary function test may be done with the injection of insulin or glucagon together with TRH and LHRH in the prepubertal child. Blood samples are taken before stimulation and at 20, 30, 60, 90, and 120 min after stimulation.
Evaluation of posterior pituitary function may be necessary.

Management
Direct treatment of the cause may be indicated. Craniopharyngioma is treated by surgical resection plus radiotherapy if initial resection is incomplete.

It is simpler for most purposes to replace target gland hormones:

- GH is replaced with synthetic somatropin
- TSH is replaced with thyroxine
- ACTH is replaced with hydrocortisone
- LH, FSH are replaced by testosterone or oestrogen and progesterone.

Diabetes insipidus

Hypofunction of the posterior pituitary gland causes cranial diabetes insipidus (DI).

Aetiology

Congenital diabetes insipidus
Wolfram syndrome (DIDMOAD)
WFS1 mutations cause Wolfram syndrome, characterized by **D**iabetes **I**nsipidus, **D**iabetes **M**ellitus, **O**ptic **A**trophy and **D**eafness. Most patients present with diabetes mellitus followed by optic atrophy in the 1st decade, DI and sensorineural deafness in the 2nd decade followed by variable neurological abnormalities including dementia and psychiatric disorders. A second locus, WFS2, exists. Some families harbour multiple deletions of mitochondrial DNA.

Mutations in the arginine vasopressin gene, *AVP*, cause autosomal recessive (AR) cranial diabetes insipidus.

Acquired
- Hypoxic-ischaemic brain damage
- *Intracranial tumours:* craniopharyngioma, leukaemia
- Post-surgery
- Head trauma
- *Infiltrations:* Langerhans cell histiocytosis, TB
- *Infections:* meningitis, encephalitis, TORCH infections.

Clinical features

Hypofunction of the posterior pituitary presents with polyuria and polydipsia. Polyuria is present if daily volumes of urine exceed:
- 1000 mL in preschool children
- 2000 mL in school-age children
- 3000 mL in adults.

This equates to volumes >2000 mL/m^2 body surface area. Children with DI are usually polyuric day and night.

The age of onset and pattern of fluid intake should be established. Children with DI are usually not fussy about fluid type or source and will drink from tap, toilet, or bath. The differential diagnosis of polyuria and polydipsia is shown in Table 10.2.

Table 10.2. Causes of polyuria and polydipsia	
Primary polydipsia	Behavioural/psychogenic
	Secondary to hypothalamic dysfunction
Diabetes mellitus	
Diabetes insipidus	Cranial diabetes insipidus
	Nephrogenic diabetes insipidus
	Genetic:
	X-linked: mutation in *AVPR2*, V$_2$ receptor gene
	Autosomal recessive: mutation in *AQP2*, aquaporin-2 gene
	Acquired: due to drugs, hypocalcaemia, or chronic renal disease

Investigations

First line
- *Blood:*
  - urea and electrolytes
  - creatinine
  - calcium, phosphate
  - plasma osmolality
  - glucose
- *Urine:* osmolality.

First line tests will detect diabetes mellitus, hypercalcaemia, and chronic renal failure. A relatively low plasma sodium concentration and osmolality suggests primary polydipsia.

Second line
- *Water deprivation test:* This tests the ability of the pituitary to make and the kidney to respond to AVP. Body weight is used to monitor short term changes in fluid states. A typical protocol would encompass:
1. Weigh patient at start and every 2 h
2. Restrict fluids for 8 h from early morning
3. Measure blood and urine sodium and osmolality, and urine volume at start and every 2 h
4. Stop test if weight loss exceeds 5%, thirst intolerable, or results confirm or exclude DI
- Urine osmolality >750 mOsm/kg with normal plasma osmolality suggests primary polydipsia.
- Urine osmolality <300 mOsm/kg suggests DI.
- Urine osmolality in the equivocal range 300–750 mOsm/kg is not uncommon, rendering a distinction between primary polydipsia (in which urine concentrating ability may be impaired) and partial DI difficult.

If DI is confirmed, renal responsiveness is assessed by administration of desmopressin (DDAVP). (See Chapter 6.9 for a discussion of nephrogenic diabetes insipidus).

Third line
Cranial MRI is undertaken in any child with evidence of cranial DI to look for loss of the posterior pituitary bright spot on T1 weighted images and evaluate evidence of inflammation or neoplasia. AVP levels are measured. Children with 'idiopathic' cranial DI may have a small tumour and tumour markers should be measured and the cranial MRI repeated at a later stage

Syndrome of inappropriate ADH secretion (SIADH)

Inappropriate secretion of vasopressin (ADH) leads to water retention, plasma hypo-osmolality with hyponatraemia, and inappropriately concentrated urine with high sodium content.

Causes include CNS pathology such as meningitis and hypoxic-ischaemic encephalopathy, surgery, and respiratory tract disease such as bronchiolitis and pneumonia.

The underlying cause is treated and fluid restriction is the mainstay of management.

10.4 Growth and its disorders

Normal growth
Four different growth phases are recognized:
- *Prenatal:* fetal
- *Postnatal:* infancy, childhood, and puberty.

The factors influencing growth are different during each phase and are considered in turn.

Fetal (intrauterine) phase
The very fast growth which occurs prenatally is regulated by several factors:
- *Maternal factors and placental function:* normal placental function is critical not only for fetal nutrition but also as a source of placental hormones and growth factors.
- *Genetic potential*
- *Hormones and growth factors:* GH is *not* the key hormone involved in regulating fetal growth, but insulin has a key role. Fetal hyperinsulinaemia is associated with macrosomia and organomegaly. IGF-2 and human placental lactogen are also important.

Failure of any of these factors may lead to intrauterine growth retardation (IUGR) and the birth of an infant who is 'small-for-dates'.

Infantile phase
Growth during infancy to 18 months is mainly determined by nutrition. Malnutrition is associated with a GH-resistant state with elevated serum GH but abnormal pulsatility and low IGF-1 levels and decreased GH receptors.

Childhood phase
During this phase of steady and prolonged growth GH secretion acting via IGF-1 at the epiphyses is the main determinant of growth rate. Thyroxine is also essential as an important regulator of GH secretion, and vitamin D and steroids influence cartilage and bone formation.

Pubertal growth spurt
Height velocity may double during the pubertal growth spurt. Increasing trunk length is predominant. The sex steroids testosterone and oestrogen appear to act both directly and indirectly by increasing GH secretion. The same sex steroids cause fusion of the epiphyseal growth plates and a cessation of growth, so final height is reduced if puberty is early.

Cellular mechanisms of growth
Growth hormone (GH)
GH (somatotropin), is synthesized in the somatotroph cells of the anterior pituitary. It is a single-chain 191 amino acid peptide, a member of a family of hormones including PRL and placental lactogen (PL). It circulates bound to GH binding protein.

Regulation of GH secretion
Secretion is pulsatile, increases during puberty, and is regulated by a host of factors.
- *GH stimulators:*
  - GHRH, ghrelin, arginine
  - sleep, exercise, hypoglycaemia
  - thyroxine, sex steroids
- *GH inhibitors:* somatostatin, GH and IGF-1, glucocorticoids.

Mechanism of GH action
GH acts directly on the GH receptor (GHR) and indirectly in the liver to promote synthesis of growth factors including insulin-like growth factors (IGFs).

The GHR is a membrane-bound tyrosine kinase receptor. Binding of GH causes dimerization and phosphorylation of GHR and JAK2, a tyrosine kinase.
- *Direct effects:* opposes insulin, being lipolytic in fat and causing gluconeogenesis in muscle. It stimulates division and multiplication of chondrocytes, promoting long bone growth
- *Indirect effects:* in the liver to stimulate synthesis and secretion of the peptide IGF-1. IGF-1 stimulates bone growth, protein synthesis in muscle and lipolysis in fat.

The major functions and effects of GH therefore include:
- *Bone:* growth and increased mineralization
- *Muscle:* increased muscle mass
- *Fat:* lipolysis with reduction of adipose tissue
- *Immunity:* stimulation
- *Internal organs:* growth stimulation.

Thyroxine
Thyroxine plays an important role in controlling growth after the prenatal period, in part by regulating GH secretion.

Sex steroids
Increasing levels of sex steroids at puberty stimulate growth by increasing endogenous GH secretion and may also have a direct effect on IFG-1 production.

Growth factors
These are proteins capable of stimulating cellular proliferation and differentiation. Some cytokines are growth factors, but others have an inhibiting effect. Examples include:
- *Insulin-like growth factors (IGF-1, IGF-2):* the IGFs have a high sequence similarity to insulin and form part of a system referred to as the GH/IGF axis.
- *Transforming growth factors (TGF):* TGF-α and TGF-β cause the growth of fibroblast cells
- *Fibroblast growth factor (FGF):* this family, also called heparin-binding growth factors (HBGF), promote angiogenesis and mitogenic action in several different cell types.

Auxology

Height is measured using a stadiometer: supine height at <2 years of age and standing at >2 years of age. The height is then compared to the population based centile charts and compared to mid-parental height to assess the child's genetic height potential. The height velocity in cm/year is determined from two measurements at least 4–6 months apart.

Centile charts
The UK growth chart (UK 1990) has nine centile lines: 0.4th, 2nd, 9th, 50th, 75th, 91st, 98th, and 99.6th. They are cross-sectional charts valid for all children living in the UK whatever their ethnic origin. Special charts are available for children with Down or Turner syndrome.

New UK-WHO Growth Charts
Key features of these charts (introduced from May 2009) include:
- Based on breast-fed infants.
- Separate section for preterm infants born at 32–37 wks.
- Term births plotted at age 0.
- No lines for 0–2 weeks of age.
- De-emphasised 50th centile.
- Length/height discontinuity at 2 years.

The new charts are used for age 0–4 years and should provide reassurance for parents of breast-fed infants, who are likely to gain weight more slowly.

A separate UK-WHO low birth weight chart is used for infants born at <32 weeks or low birth weight.

Mid-parental height
Mid-parental height is halfway between the corrected parental heights.
- Add 12.6 cm to mother's height to plot on a boy's chart.
- Subtract 12.6 cm from father's height to plot on a girl's chart.

Short stature

Clinical evaluation
The history should include information about birth size and weight gain during infancy and identify any chronic diseases or familial conditions.

Examination
General examination should encompass an assessment of pubertal status according to Tanner stages (see Fig 19.1) and identification of syndromes known to be associated with altered growth. The focus is then on measurement of height and growth velocity.

All children below the 0.4th centile height should be investigated for reversible causes of short stature. The majority (90%) of children track within one centile space (0.67 SD) for height. Many children diverge from their centile line during puberty, upwards if puberty is early or downwards if late.

The causes of short stature are listed in the Box below.

Familial short stature (short parents) and constitutional short stature in teenage boys with delayed puberty are most common. A syndrome diagnosis may be clinically apparent.

Causes of short stature
• Familial short stature and delayed puberty
• *Chronic illness:* cystic fibrosis, renal failure, IBD, coeliac disease
• *Endocrine:* GH insufficiency, hypothyroidism, Cushing's
• *Genetic syndromes:*
• Turner (45,X), Down, or Prader–Willi syndromes
• *skeletal dysplasias:* achondroplasia, mucopolysaccharoidosis (MPS).

Investigations
The following investigations may be considered:
- Full blood count, CRP, coeliac antibodies screen
- Karyotype
- *Bone age:* delayed in constitutional short stature, GH deficiency or hypothyroidism
- *Endocrine tests:* Thyroid function tests: fT4, TSH, GH provocation tests

Management
Synthetic human GH (somatropin) is available for treatment of proven GH deficiency. It is given by SC or IM injection, usually daily. Other indications for GH therapy include Turner/Noonan syndrome, chronic renal failure before puberty and Prader–Willi syndrome in which the main benefit is reduced body fat and increased muscle strength.

Hypothyroidism is treated with thyroxine.

Tall stature

Definition: a height >2 SD from the mean.

Clinical evaluation
Assessment of pubertal status and a search for clinical features indicating a pathological cause (see Box).

Causes of tall stature
• Familial (constitutional) tall stature
• Constitutional obesity
• *Endocrine causes:*
GH excess
hyperthyroidism
precocious puberty
androgen excess
• *Genetic syndromes:*
Marfan syndrome
Klinefelter syndrome (47,XXY)
Sotos syndrome
Beckwith–Wiedemann syndrome

If growth velocity is normal, the likely diagnosis is constitutional tall stature or obesity. Most obese children diagnosed <2 years are above the 50th centile for height and have an advanced bone age with a final height within the parental target height.

If growth velocity is accelerated, an endocrine cause is suspected. This may be in association with precocious puberty or due to a variety of rare causes such as: GH excess (pituitary adenoma), androgen excess (adrenal tumour), untreated congenital adrenal hyperplasia, or hyperthyroidism.

Investigations
- Karyotype
- *Bone age:* this can be used to predict final height
- *Endocrine tests:* as clinically indicated
- *Imaging:* cranial MRI, adrenal ultrasound.

Management
Indications for treatment are mainly psychological, although spinal and postural abnormalities occur. Tall children may be disadvantaged by being treated as older than their chronological age.

Induction of puberty using oestrogens accelerates skeletal maturity with early closure of epiphyses and limitation of adult height and has been used for excessive height in prepubertal or early adolescent females.

10.5 Puberty and intersex

Normal puberty
The hypothalamo–pituitary–gonadal axis is active during fetal life and early infancy, quiescent during childhood, and reactivated at onset of puberty. Quiescence is maintained by negative feedback by gonadal steroids and intrinsic CNS inhibition.

Within the hypothalamus, a neural mechanism drives the release of pulses of LHRH which stimulates pulsatile release of LH and FSH. Gonadal steroids inhibin and follistatin inhibit and activin stimulates FSH biosynthesis and secretion which leads to testicular testosterone production in boys and ovarian oestrogen in females.

Nutrition and puberty
The tempo of puberty is closely associated with changes in body composition. Under-nutrition delays the growth spurt and menarche whereas increasing food intake and moderate obesity is associated with earlier menarche. These effects may be mediated by leptin which stimulates the reproductive axis.

Normal changes at puberty
In boys puberty starts at an average age of 12 years. Growth of the testes and scrotum are the first sign. A testicular volume of 4 mL signifies onset of puberty and peak height velocity coincides with a volume of 10–12 mL. This is followed by reddening and rugosity of scrotal skin and the later development of pubic hair, penile growth, and axillary hair.

In girls, puberty starts at an average age of 10 years with the appearance of the breast bud and breast development as the first signs, followed by development of public and axillary hair. Peak height velocity coincides with breast stage 2–3 and menarche as late as breast stage 4.

See Figure 19.1 for Tanner stages 1–5.

Precocious puberty
This is defined as onset of puberty before 9 years in boys or 8 years in girls and is more common in girls. However, recent studies show that signs of early puberty (breasts and pubic hair) are frequent in girls (particularly black girls) aged 6–8 years.

The causes (see Box) are categorized into:
- *Central precocious puberty (CPP):* gonadotropin dependent
- *Precocious pseudo-puberty:* gonadotropin independent.

Clinical assessment
History and examination
A history of early puberty in a parent or sibling is relevant and increases the likelihood of idiopathic CPP. Headaches or visual disturbance suggests CNS pathology.

In girls, breast enlargement is usually the first sign of puberty and initially may be unilateral. Examination supine minimizes the chance of interpreting fat as true, glandular breast tissue. Enlargement of the clitoris indicates androgen excess.

In boys, the first sign is testicular enlargement (volume >4 mL) which depends on FSH and may go unnoticed. Signs of testosterone increase include penile growth and scrotal changes and in the presence of small testes suggest peripheral androgen production.

Causes of precocious puberty

Central precocious puberty (CPP)
- Idiopathic normal
- *Tumours*
  - *CNS:* astrocytoma, glioma
  - germ cell tumour, hypothalamic hamartoma
- *Congenital anomalies:* septo-optic dysplasia, arachnoid cyst, neurofibromatosis
- *CNS injury:* surgery, trauma, irradiation, inflammation

Precocious pseudo-puberty
- Mccune–Albright syndrome (95% female)
- *Tumours:* ovarian, testicular, or adrenal; ectopic hCG-secreting
- Congenital adrenal hyperplasia

Differential diagnosis
Precocious puberty must be differentiated from:
- *Premature pubarche:* early appearance of pubic and/or axillary hair with adult body odour caused by secretion of adrenal androgens, premature adrenarche, or exposure to exogenous androgens
- *Premature thelarche:* isolated appearance of breast development in young girls, usually age <3 years. In this benign condition there is no growth acceleration, no increase in breast tissue over time, and no changes in areola or nipples.

Investigations
Imaging
- *Bone age:* if bone age is within 1 year of chronological age puberty has not yet started.
- *Cranial MRI:* the younger the child with CPP (<6 years) the greater the chance of finding CNS pathology. For girls aged 6–8 years with no CNS signs the yield is 2%. Cranial MRI is **mandatory** in boys <9 years with CPP.
- *Pelvic ultrasound:* is indicated if precocious pseudopuberty is suspected in a girl to evaluate ovaries and uterus.
- *Abdominal MRI/CT:* for imaging the adrenal gland.

Endocrine tests
- *Sex steroid levels:* serum testosterone is useful in boys but oestradiol measurements are relatively unreliable in girls. Adrenal androgen production is measured by serum dehydroepiandrosterone sulfate (DHEA-S) levels.
- *Gonadotropins:* random LH level is the best screening test for central precocious puberty. A diagnosis of CPP is confirmed by measuring LH and FSH after infusion of GnRH.

Management
Active treatment is not necessarily required for idiopathic CPP in girls. It is important that all involved treat the child according to chronological rather than maturational age. Final adult height may be reduced due to premature closure of epiphyses, and therapy should be considered for girls with idiopathic CPP whose predicted height is unacceptable. Progress of puberty may be halted using a GnRH agonist such as triptorelin. CNS tumours may require resection and radiation therapy.

Delayed puberty

This is more common in boys. In most children changes occur within a span of 2 years before or after the mean. Delayed puberty is therefore considered if initial changes are not occurring in a girl aged 13 or a boy aged 14.

Constitutional delay of growth and puberty (CDGP) is the most common cause in boys, an organic pathology being more likely in a girl (see Box).

> *Causes of delayed puberty*
> - *Constitutional delay of growth and puberty*
> - *Systemic disease:*
>   - inflammatory bowel disease
>   - chronic renal failure
> - *Undernutrition:* anorexia nervosa
> - *Hypothalamic or pituitary disorders:*
>   - pituitary tumours
>   - post surgery, radiotherapy, chemotherapy
>   - Kallmann syndrome
> - *Gonadal dysgenesis:*
>   - Turner syndrome
>   - Klinefelter syndrome
> - *Hypothyroidism*

Clinical assessment
A complete history and examination will reveal most conditions associated with delayed puberty and provide clues to syndromic diagnoses. Investigations usually include a bone age and more complex endocrine investigations, karyotype, and cranial imaging as indicated.

Management
In constitutional delay reassurance may be sufficient, but if delay is extreme or causing distress a low dose of testosterone or oestrogen for a few months is often associated with onset of spontaneous puberty.

Intersex

Intersex usually manifests at birth as ambiguity of the external genitalia. The incidence is about 1/4500 live births

Normal sex determination
Genetic sex is determined at the time of conception. Possession of a Y chromosome normally determines development down the male pathway directed by the sex-related antigen encoded by the *SRY* gene. In the absence of a Y chromosome the ovary develops and the default female developmental pathway is followed

Intersex
An infant with ambiguous genitalia may be an inadequately masculinized XY infant, a masculinized XX infant, or a true hermaphrodite with both ovary and testis.

The most common cause of a masculinized 46,XX infant is congenital adrenal hyperplasia (CAH) due to 21-α hydroxylase deficiency or 11-β-hydroxylase deficiency. If 17-hydroxyprogesterone (17OHP) levels are normal (they may be falsely elevated at birth) and Mullerian structures are present, maternal androgens may be the problem.

The differential diagnosis is more complex in an undermasculinized 46,XY infant. If Mullerian structures are absent an HCG stimulation test will help to distinguish between defects in testosterone synthesis and androgen unresponsiveness

Clinical assessment

History and initial discussion
Enquire about the pregnancy, family history (consanguinity), and maternal drug use. Important points regarding the initial discussion with the parents are:
- Nursing staff should be present
- Refer to infant as 'your baby', not 'it', 'him', or 'her'
- Avoid sexually biased terms (penis, vagina) for genitalia.

Parents should be advised not to name the infant until sex of rearing is decided. This may require investigations over 10–14 days. Delay birth registration as long as possible.

Examination
- *Dysmorphic appearance:* Turner syndrome
- *Skin:* pigmentation in primary adrenocortical insufficiency
- *Systemic illness:* hypoglycaemia, vomiting, and salt depletion in congenital adrenal hyperplasia
- *External genitalia:* the genital appearance (phallus, position of urethral meatus, state of labioscrotal fusion) can be designated a Prader stage or given an external masculinization score (EMS) A maximum score of 12 represents normal external male genitalia
- *Gonads and uterus:* palpable bilateral gonads are usually testes.

Investigations
- *Karyotype:* an initial result is available in 48h by FISH
- *Biochemistry:* blood glucose, urea and electrolytes
- *Endocrine investigations:*
  - Serum 17OHP, gonadotropins, urine steroid profile
  - HCG stimulation test with pre- and post-testosterone, dihydrotestosterone, and androstenedione
- *Imaging:* to locate the uterus if present. Pelvic ultrasound urogenital sonogram or laparoscopy.

Management
Decisions about the sex of rearing are not easy. There are few long-term outcome studies, cultural factors are important, and the optimal timing of surgery may be when the patient is too young for informed consent. The aims include a contented childhood, a clear sexual identity, and the opportunity to enjoy a sexual relationship in adulthood.

10.6 Thyroid disorders

Thyroid gland

Anatomy
Thyroid tissue is composed of follicles containing colloid and lined by a single layer of follicular cells. Between the follicles are the parafollicular cells (c-cells) which are of neurogenic origin and secrete calcitonin. Thyroid hormone is produced by 12 weeks gestation.

Thyroid hormones
Synthesis
The follicle cells trap and take up iodine from the blood by an active uptake mechanism. Iodide is rapidly oxidized by a peroxidase system to iodine which reacts with tyrosine residues on thyroglobulin (organification) to form mono-iodotyrosine (MIT) and di-iodotyrosine (DIT). These then couple to form iodothyronines (T3, T4) stored in the colloid. Hydrolysis of thyroglobulin releases T3, T4, MIT, and DIT. T3 and T4 are released into the circulation whereas MIT and DIT are deiodinated and the liberated iodine recycled.

Regulation
TSH stimulates thyroid hormone synthesis and release at several points. Circulating free thyroid hormones feed back at both hypothalamic and pituitary level to suppress TRH and TSH synthesis. TSH receptor antibodies may inhibit or stimulate thyroid function.

Mechanisms and effects
Thyroid hormones act on nuclear receptors (THRs) which function as hormone-activated transcription factors and have tissue and developmental specific expression profiles.
The main actions of thyroid hormones are:
- *Calorigenesis:* increased mitochondrial oxygen consumption
- *Catabolic effects:* increased glycogenolysis, lipolysis, free fatty acid oxidation
- *Growth and development:* fetal thyroid hormones are essential for development of the brain *in utero*. Postnatally, thyroid hormones are essential for both the production and the normal action of GH.

Thyroid function tests
Thyroid hormones and TSH
About 1% of thyroid hormones are in the free state, the rest being tightly bound to transport proteins in the plasma. Assays of free thyroid hormones, fT4 and fT3, are most reliable.

In primary hypothyroidism, fT4 is low and TSH raised, but in secondary hypothyroidism both are low. A TRH rest will then distinguish patients with hypothalamic dysfunction in whom TSH continues to rise 60 min after injection.

Thyroid imaging
Thyroid ultrasonography can reveal nodules and cysts and aspiration, biopsy or drainage may be done under ultrasound guidance.

Thyroid scintigraphy or radionuclide imaging using radioiodine or technetium is useful for functional imaging. Uptake is uniformly increased in thyrotoxicosis and reduced in thyroiditis or in a 'cold' nodule which may be malignant.

Hypothyroidism
Hypothyroidism may be primary or secondary (central) and congenital or acquired. Iodine deficiency disorders (IDD) remain the most common cause of thyroid dysfunction and a major public health problem affecting almost 800 million people worldwide. Salt iodization is a proven cost-effective solution and is being progressively introduced.

Congenital hypothyroidism
Congenital hypothyroidism has an incidence of 1/4000 live births. The causes of primary hypothyroidism are:
- *Thyroid dysgenesis (85%):*
  - thyroid agenesis (30%)
  - ectopic thyroid (60%)
  - thyroid hypoplasia (10%)
- *Thyroid dyshormogenesis (10%):* goitre often present
- *Maternal thyroid diseases (5%):* autoimmune disease, drugs.

Thyroid dysgenesis
Most (98%) are sporadic. It is more common in females. Congenital non-goitrous hypothyroidism may be:
- *Non-syndromic:* mutations in *TSHR*, the TSH receptor gene
- *Syndromic:* mutations in *TTF1, TTF2, PAX8,* and *GNAS1*.

The TSH receptor is critical for gland development. Inactivating mutations may cause a spectrum of severity of hypothyroidism depending on compensation. Activating mutations in *GNAS1* (encoding $G_s\alpha$) cause Albright hereditary osteodystrophy.

Thyroid dyshormogenesis
Inheritance is AR and goitre is common. Mutations occur in:
- *TPO:* thyroid peroxidase
- *SLCA5:* the sodium-iodide symporter, NIS
- *TG:* thyroglobulin
- *DUOX1* and *DUOX2: NADPH* oxidases
- *SLC26A4 (pendrin):* causing Pendred syndrome.

Central hypothyroidism
Hypothalamic–pituitary disorders causing hypothyroidism are rare and may be isolated or as a component of a combined pituitary hormone defect.

Clinical features
Newborn screening identifies the majority of children with congenital hypothyroidism before the overt development of the clinical signs previously known as cretinism. Clinical features in the newborn classically include prolonged jaundice, macroglossia, hoarse cry, and umbilical hernia with or without a goitre. A goitre may be detected on antenatal ultrasound.

Newborn screening
TSH levels are the most specific and sensitive test and are used in programmes in the UK and Europe. Cut off levels are >10–20 mU/L depending on methodology. Cases of central hypothyroidism (rare) are detected by low TSH.

A physiological surge in TSH levels accompanies birth.

Investigations
Further investigations may include:
- *Thyroid function tests:* TSH, fT4, fT3, TGT, BG
- *Thyroid autoantibodies*: TPOAb, TgAb, TrAb

- *Imaging:*
  - thyroid ultrasound scan
  - *radionuclide scans:* ^{123}radioiodine, ^{99}technetium scans
  - *knee radiograph:* absence of distal femoral epiphysis in a term infant.

Management
Treatment with L-thyroxine should be started immediately the diagnosis is made and monitored by regular measurement of fT4 and TSH, initially fortnightly. An fT4 level in the upper range of normal and TSH 0.5–5 mU/L is the aim. Hearing should be screened in the neonatal period. Some detailed investigations can be delayed until 2–3 years of age when temporary cessation of treatment will not impair neurodevelopment.

Transient congenital hypothyroidism is a recognized entity with a wide variation in incidence. This may be due to maternal anti-TSHR antibodies or heterozygous *DUOX2* mutations.

Early diagnosis and treatment has improved prognosis, but although median IQ is normal some children have residual problems and 10% may have special educational needs.

Acquired hypothyroidism
Auto-immune mechanisms are the most common cause. It is a very important treatable cause of short stature and should be remembered as a treatable comorbid condition in Type I diabetes mellitus.

Hyperthyroidism
Thyrotoxicosis is uncommon in childhood. The incidence rises from around 0.1/100 000 in young children to 3/100 000 in adolescence, with a female to male ratio of 8:1.

Aetiology
95% of young people with thyrotoxicosis have Graves disease (GD) caused by stimulatory antibodies to the TSH receptor. Genetic factors account for 80% of the susceptibility. GD is a multisystem autoimmune disorder involving the skin, eyes, and thyroid gland.

Very rarely a monogenic genetic cause is found. Activating mutations occur in the TSH receptor gene and thyrotoxicosis may occur in McCune–Albright syndrome when mutations in *GNAS1* cause constitutive activation of the TSH receptor.

Neonatal thyrotoxicosis is a rare condition caused by the placental passage of thyroid-stimulating antibodies from a mother with either Graves disease or Hashimoto's thyroiditis. The condition is usually self-limiting in 4–12 weeks.

Clinical features
Manifestations of thyrotoxicosis may include:
- *Symptoms:* palpitations, fatigue, insomnia, heat intolerance, secondary amenorrhoea
- *Signs:* tachycardia, tremor, hyperactive precordium, exophthalmos.

A goitre is common. Other signs in GD may include vitiligo and ophthalmopathy due to retro-orbital inflammation. Thyroxine promotes growth, and tall stature may be evident in the prepubertal child.

Investigations
These may include:
- *Thyroid function tests:* TSH, fT3, fT4, TGT, BG
- *Thyroid autoantibodies:* TPOAb, TgAb, TrAb

- *Imaging:*
  - thyroid ultrasound scan
  - *radionuclide scans:* ^{131}I or ^{99}Tc.

TrAb are positive in 95% of patients with GD. Imaging may allow GD and Hashimoto's appearances to be distinguished.

Management
Short-term supportive therapy with β-blockers (propranolol, atenolol) may be necessary for symptomatic relief and control of tachycardia and hypertension in severe cases.

There are three long-term treatment options, each with advantages and disadvantages:
- *Antithyroid drug (ATD) therapy*
- *Surgery:* partial or total thyroidectomy
- Radio-iodine.

Antithyroid drugs (ATDs)
A course of carbimazole for 2–4 years is the standard approach to the management of thyrotoxicosis. It acts as a preferential substrate for thyroid peroxidase, inhibiting organification of iodine and coupling of iodotyrosine residues.
There are two alternative regimens:
- *Dose titration to achieve normal TFTs:* lower dose with fewer side effects
- *A blocking dose with thyroxine replacement:* less intensive monitoring and possible increased remission rate.

A major disadvantage is the side effect profile which includes urticaria, rash, transient reduction in granulocyte count or rarely, agranulocytosis. Patients are warned to discontinue ATDs and seek advice if fever and sore throat occur.

Unfortunately, relapse is common when ATD therapy is stopped and long-term remission rates are lower than in adults. Up to 95% of patients <16 with GD will relapse within 1 year when a 2–3 year ATD course is stopped.

Surgery
Most UK surgeons favour total thyroidectomy with long-term thyroxine replacement rather than subtotal thyroidectomy. The mortality rate is 1/1000 thyroidectomies. Morbidity includes recurrent laryngeal nerve damage and hypoparathyroidism.

Radio-iodine
This is an increasingly popular option in adolescents. A dose that will ablate the thyroid gland is given and subsequent monitoring and replacement therapy undertaken.

10.7 Adrenal gland

Adrenal gland

Anatomy
The adrenal glands lie adjacent to the upper poles of the kidneys and are composed of an outer cortex and inner medulla surrounded by an outer capsule. The cortex has three histologically distinct zones: zona glomerulosa, zona fasciculata, and zona reticularis (Fig 10.8).

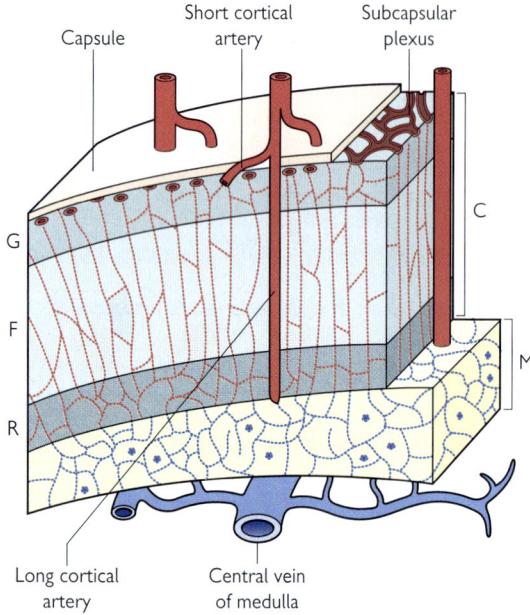

Fig 10.8 Adrenal gland structure. C, cortex; M, medulla; G, zona glomerulosa; F, zona fasciculata, R, zona reticularis.

Adrenocortical function

Corticosteroids
Adrenal steroids are synthesized in the cortex from cholesterol in a series of enzymatic steps (Fig 10.9). Three main types of steroid hormone are produced:
- *Mineralocorticoids:* aldosterone
- *Glucocorticoids:* cortisol
- *Sex steroids:*
  - androgens: testosterone, dehydroepiandrosterone, androstenedione
  - oestrogens: oestradiol.

Biosynthesis and regulation
Steroidogenic enzymes are cytochrome P450 oxidases or members of the hydroxysteroid dehydrogenase (HSD) group.

The glucocorticoid and androgen branch is under the control of ACTH via the hypothalamic–pituitary–adrenal axis. ACTH binds to the melanocortin-2 receptor causing increased uptake of cholesterol and up-regulation of enzyme activity. Cortisol is secreted in a pulsatile manner and follows a circadian rhythm (peak at 8 a.m.).

Aldosterone is influenced by salt and water balance via the renin–angiotensin axis.

Mechanisms and effects
The physiological actions of adrenal steroids are listed in Table 10.3.
- *Aldosterone* acts via the intracellular mineralocorticoid receptor (MR) which on activation translocates to the nucleus and stimulates expression of proteins including the epithelial sodium channel (ENaC). Glucocorticoids have some action on this receptor. Spironolactone blocks the action of aldosterone on the MR.
- *Glucocorticoids* act via the intracellular glucocorticoid receptor (GR) The GR protein is expressed in almost all cells and resides in the cytoplasm complexed to HSPs (hsp90, hsp70).

Ligand binding leads to two mechanisms of action:
- *Transactivation:* translocation into nucleus and activation of gene transcription
- *Transrepression:* activated GR complexes with other transcription factors and prevents them from activating their target genes.

Table 10.3. Physiological actions of adrenal steroids	
Steroid	**Effect**
Mineralocorticoids	Na$^+$ retention/K$^+$ excretion Proton (acid) excretion Raised BP

Glucocorticoids	*Intermediary metabolism*
	Anabolic: gluconeogenesis in liver
	Catabolic:
	   lipolysis in fat
	   proteolysis in muscle
	Immune system
	Suppression of immunity and anti-inflammatory
	Thymus regression
	Salt and water balance
	Salt and water retention
	↑BP
	Central nervous system
	Suppress ACTH and CRH release
	Neuroactive: psychosis and seizure suppression
	Stress response

Sex steroids	Adrenarche: pubic hair Virilization Muscle maintenance Sexual function

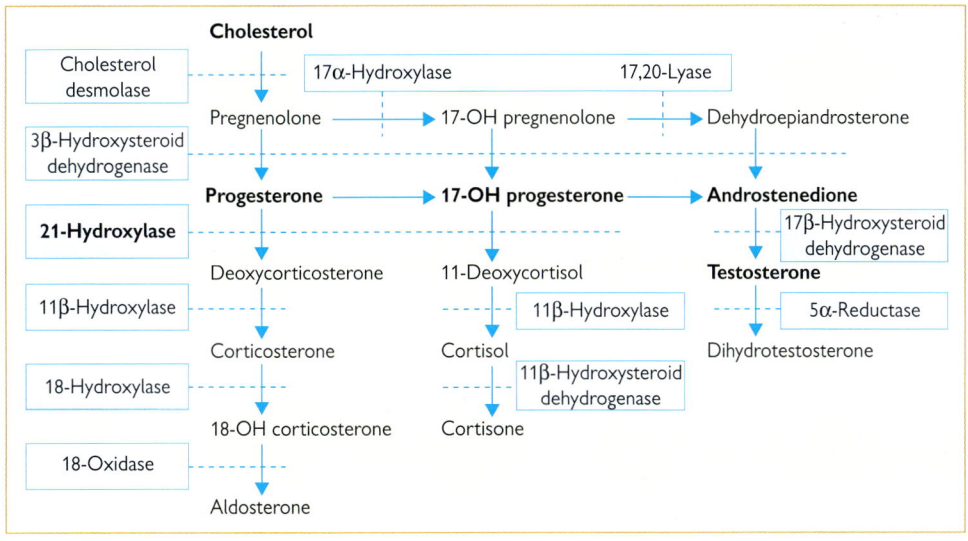

Fig 10.9 Biosynthesis of corticosteroids. Enzymes shown in boxes. Effects of 21-hydroxylase deficiency shown with increased androgen synthesis. Reproduced from the Oxford Textbook of Endocrinology, with permission from OUP.

Adrenal medullary function

Catecholamines

The medulla is essentially a large ganglion receiving preganglionic axons via the splanchnic nerve. Activation occurs mainly in response to stress. The catecholamines dopamine, noradrenaline, and adrenaline are synthesized from tyrosine in a pathway shared by melanin (Fig 10.10).

Mechanisms and effects

The physiological actions of catecholamines are listed in Table 10.4. Catecholamines act via adrenoreceptors which are G-protein coupled and mediate distinct effects. Overall the action is the response to stress ('fight and flight').

Table 10.4. Physiological actions of catecholamines

Receptor	Actions
α1	*Cardiovascular:* inotropic, vasoconstriction, ↑BP
α2	Sweating, Vasoconstriction, Inhibition of sympathetic outflow, insulin secretion
β1	*Cardiovascular:* inotropic, renin secretion
β2	Vasodilatation, Smooth muscle relaxation

Fig 10.10 Biosynthesis of catecholaminines.

10.8 Adrenal disorders

Cushing syndrome
Caused by excess corticosteroids.

Aetiology
The most common cause is administration of exogenous corticosteroids (Fig 10.11). Endogenous hypercortisolism may be:
- *ACTH dependent*: pituitary ACTH-secreting tumour (Cushing disease), ectopic ACTH production by tumours
- *ACTH independent*: adrenal tumour (adenoma or carcinoma) primary adrenal micronodular hyperplasia.

Clinical features
Presentation may be with weight gain, growth failure, lassitude, diabetes, hypertension. Classical signs include:
- *Obesity*: central and truncal
- 'Moon face' (Fig 10.11)
- Striae and easy bruising
- *Virilization*: acne, hirsutism
- Hypertension.

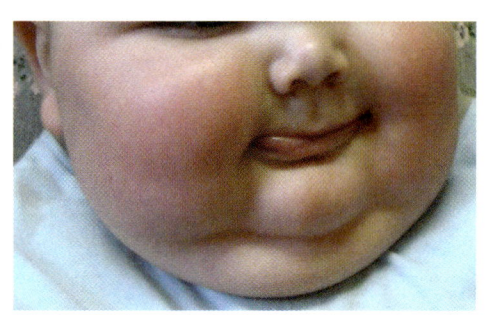

Fig 10.11 Iatrogenic Cushing syndrome facies.

Investigations
- *Urea and electrolytes*: hypokalaemia, alkalosis
- *Blood glucose*: hyperglycaemia
- *Endocrine investigations*:
  - midnight and 8 a.m. serum cortisol, ACTH levels
  - 24 h urine collections for urinary free cortisol
- *Dexamethasone suppression tests*: In Cushing syndrome, low-dose dexamethasone fails to suppress cortisol and ACTH. No suppression at low-dose, but high-dose suppression suggests an ACTH secreting pituitary tumour (Cushing disease)
- *Imaging*: Adrenal imaging by ultrasound and CT to identify an adrenal tumour if indicated. Benign non-functioning adrenal adenomas are common. Cranial MRI to identify a pituitary tumour.

Management
Surgical excision of pituitary adenoma by trans-sphenoidal hypophysectomy or adrenalectomy for a cortisol-secreting adrenal adenoma. Perioperative steroid therapy is required and subsequent hydrocortisone replacement may be needed. Iatrogenic Cushing syndrome is managed by withdrawing or reducing the dose of exogenous steroid.

Addison's disease
Primary adrenal insufficiency and secondary insufficiency due to deficiency of ACTH are both uncommon. Deficiency of both cortisol and aldosterone, leads to hypersecretion of ACTH and melanocytic stimulating hormone (MSH).

Aetiology
The most common cause of Addison's disease in childhood is autoimmune adrenalitis, but other rare causes exist (see Box).

> **Causes of Addison's disease**
> - Autoimmune adrenalitis (80%):
>   - HLA associated
>   - antibodies against 21-hydroxylase
> - Tuberculosis (calcification on XR or CT), HIV, haemorrhage
> - Genetic:
>   - X-linked adrenoleucodystrophy (*ABCD1*)
>   - X-linked congenital adrenal hypoplasia (*DAX1*)
>   - familial glucocorticoid deficiency (*MC2R*)
>   - autoimmune polyendocrinopathy syndrome (*AIRE*)

Clinical features
Presentation is usually insidious, but an acute Addisonian crisis precipitated by stress may be the presenting feature.
Chronic adrenal insufficiency presents with a variety of non-specific symptoms:
- Weakness, fatigue, weight loss
- Pigmentation, persistent tan
- Dizziness and syncope.

Signs may include:
- *Pigmentation*: skin and mucous membranes especially
- Hypotension
- Vitiligo, hypothyroidism, short stature
- Neurological signs in adrenoleucodystrophy.

Investigations
- *Urea and electrolytes*: hyperkalaemia, hyponatraemia
- *Blood glucose*: hypoglycaemia
- *Endocrine investigations*:
  - Low morning cortisol with high ACTH
  - Synacthen stimulation produces a minimal cortisol response
- Antiadrenal antibodies
- Very long chain fatty acids to exclude ALD in a male.

Management
An Addisonian crisis is treated with:
- *IV hydrocortisone*: bolus 4 mg/kg then 6 hourly or by infusion and IV normal saline volume replacement 20 mL/kg
- *IV dextrose 10%*: to correct hypoglycaemia.

Replacement treatment is with hydrocortisone and fludrocortisone.

Congenital adrenal hyperplasia (CAH)

This is an AR disorder caused by mutations in genes encoding enzymes in the steroid biosynthesis pathway (see Fig 10.9). 95% of cases are caused by 21α-hydroxylase deficiency due to mutations in CYP21. The incidence is 1/1000 live births.

Aetiology
In about 95% of cases 21-hydroxylation is impaired, blocking the conversion of progesterone to deoxycorticosterone (DOC) and 17-hydroxprogesterone to 11-deoxycortisol (see Fig 10.9). Low cortisol levels stimulate ACTH production which stimulates adrenal hyperplasia and precursors spill over to make adrenal androgens.

The CYP21 (CYP21A2) gene encoding 21α-hydroxylase is on chromosome 6p close to a pseudogene CYP21A. This arrangement predisposes the functional gene to mutations. Less commonly, mutations are found in:
- CYPIIB1, encoding 11β-hydroxylase: 11-deoxycortisol and 11-deoxycorticosterone accumulate, causing hypertension
- STAR, encoding the steroidogenic acute regulatory protein This causes a severe form, lipid congenital adrenal hyperplasia.

Clinical features
Three main types of 21α-hydroxylase deficiency CAH are recognized and correlate with severe, moderate, or mild degrees of enzyme deficiency:
- *SW 21-OHD:* classical salt-wasting
- *SV 21-OHD:* simple virilizing
- *NC 21-OHD:* non-classical (late onset).

Classical SW 21-OHD deficiency
Females present with ambiguous genitalia due to virilization by adrenal androgens. The clitoris is enlarged and labia majora fused. Males prevent with a salt-losing crisis usually within the first 2 weeks of life. Dehydration and circulatory collapse occur and hyperpigmentation may be apparent. Investigation reveals hyponatraemia, hypokalaemia, acidosis, and hypoglycaemia. Virilization of females continues after birth with early puberty and short stature.

Simple virilizing 21-OHD deficiency
There may be no or mild virilization initially, the effects of excess adrenal androgens manifesting later in childhood with phallic enlargement, public hair, greasy skin, and rapid growth with advanced bone age. The early exposure to sex hormones may also 'prime' the hypothalamic–pituitary axis to initiate a centrally mediated precocious puberty.

Non-classical 21-OHD deficiency
This presents in females post-puberty in adolescence or young adulthood with acne, hirsutism, and irregular menses, a clinical picture similar to that of polycystic ovary syndrome.

Investigations
These obviously depend on the clinical context:
- *Urea and electrolytes:* hyponatraemia, hypokalaemia
- *Blood glucose:* hypoglycemia
- *Endocrine investigations:*
  - serum cortisol and aldosterone low, ACTH high
  - classical SW 21-OHD: elevated 17OHP

In non-classical forms, unstimulated 17OHP may be normal with an exaggerated rise after Synacthen.
- *Genetic tests:* DNA analysis of CYP21 (CYP21A2) is not routinely used in diagnosis. It is useful for genetic counselling if prospective parents are either carriers or sufferers of CAH. This allows the option of prenatal treatment of the mother of a female fetus with a virilizing form of CAH with dexamethasone.

Management
This encompasses prenatal management, management of a salt-losing crisis, and long-term management in childhood.

Prenatal management
The virilizing effects of hyperandrogenism in the female fetus are potentially remediable to suppression by maternal dexamethasone therapy. The potential risks and benefits remain uncertain. Side effects in the mother may include weight gain and hypertension.

Postnatal salt-losing crisis
- This life-threatening illness requires urgent treatment with hydrocortisone, volume replacement with normal saline, and correction of hypoglycaemia with IV dextrose.

Infancy and childhood
Once the diagnosis is made, replacement therapy is required. Neonates are usually started on oral hydrocortisone, fludrocortisone, and salt supplements.

During childhood careful monitoring of treatment is necessary to avoid the ill effects of insufficient or excess glucocorticoids. Insufficient dosage permits androgen excess driving growth with early physeal fusion which limits adult height. Excess glucocorticoids results in cushingoid features with growth failure and impaired final height.

Intercurrent illness requires a doubling of the dose of hydrocortisone or IV hydrocortisone if there is vomiting. Virilized females may need corrective surgery.

Phaeochromocytoma

Catecholamine secreting tumours of chromatin cell origin are rare. The 'rule of 10s' is useful:
- 10% are malignant
- 10% are extra-adrenal (paragangliomas)
- 10% are bilateral
- 10% are familial.

Familial forms occur in neurofibromatosis type I, Von Hippel–Lindau disease, and multiple endocrine neoplasia.

The cardinal feature is labile hypertension but symptomatology may be non-specific and include sweating, palpitations, headaches, anxiety, and abdominal pain. If suspected a 24 h urine collection for free catecholamines, adrenaline and noradrenaline is done. CT or MRI scanning may localize the tumour and isotope imaging with ^{123}I-*meta*-iodo-benzyl-guanidine (MIBG) confirms its nature. Treatment is surgical after full adrenergic blockade to prevent an acute hypertensive crisis or cardiac dysrrhythmias.

Endocrine hypertension

Some rare genetic disorders cause hypertension by excess aldosterone or enhancement of its effects: see Chapter 6.11.

10.9 Calcium disorders

Calcium homeostasis

Calcium is essential for bone growth, blood clotting, and membrane function and is an intracellular signalling molecule.

Circulating calcium includes free ionized calcium (50%) and protein-bound calcium, most of which is bound to albumin. Binding to albumin is pH dependent: acidosis decreases binding and increases ionized calcium whereas alkalosis increases binding with a decrease in ionized calcium.

Calcium homeostasis is maintained by exchange between the blood and three organs: bone, kidney, and intestine. This is controlled by PTH, calcitonin, and 1,25 $(OH)_2D_3$, the circulating active form of vitamin D (Fig 10.12).

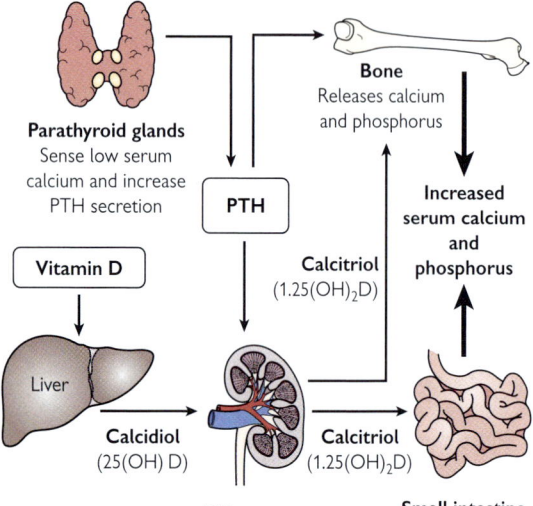

Fig 10.12 The calcium homeostatic system. A small decrease in serum-free calcium concentration results in the release of parathyroid hormone by the parathyroid cells. Parathyroid hormone acts on the kidney to increase calcium reabsorption and phosphate excretion and stimulates the synthesis of 1,25- $(OH)_2D_3$ or calcitriol, the active form of vitamin D.
In addition, parathyroid hormone acts on bone to mobilize calcium and phosphate. All these effects result in a return of the extracellular calcium to the normal range. Adapted from Jane Higdon © 2008 LPI, used with permission.

Parathyroid hormone (PTH)

PTH is synthesized by the chief cells of the parathyroid glands as a pre-pro-PTH peptide which is cleaved twice to form the circulating form. It has a short half-life of 90 s. Calcium sensing receptors (CaSR) on the parathyroid gland mediate secretion of hormone in response to hypocalcaemia or hyperphosphataemia.

Actions of PTH

PTH increases serum calcium by acting on the PTH receptor in three organs:
- *Bone:* stimulates osteoblasts to produce a factor which activates osteoclasts to increase calcium and phosphorus resorption from bone
- *Kidney:* promotes renal tubular phosphate and bicarbonate excretion and calcium reabsorption
- *Intestine:* enhances absorption of calcium in the intestine by increasing 1α hydroxylation of vitamin D in the kidney.

Calcitonin

Calcitonin (CT) is synthesized and secreted by the parafollicular (C) cells in the thyroid gland. CT acts to lower serum calcium by inhibiting bone resorption and increasing renal excretion of calcium.

Vitamin D

Vitamin D is a group of related steroid compounds:
- *Vitamin D1:* compound of ergocalciferol and lumisterol
- *Vitamin D2:* ergocalciferol (calciferol) from plants
- *Vitamin D3:* colecalciferol derived from animal sources and synthesised in skin from dehydrocholesterol under influence of UV irradiation.

Vitamin D3 is hydroxylated in the liver and kidney to its active forms:
- *Calcidiol:* 25-OH-D_3, 25-hydroxycolecalciferol (alfacalcidol)
- *Calcitriol:* 1,25- $(OH)_2D_3$, 1,25 dihydroxycolecalciferol.

The active, circulating form functions as a hormone, mediating its biological effects via the vitamin D receptor (VDR), a member of the nuclear receptor superfamily.

Actions of vitamin D
- Increased intestinal absorption of calcium and phosphate
- Increased osteoclastic resorption of calcium from bone
- Increased reabsorption of calcium from renal tubules and promotion of phosphate excretion.

Hypocalcaemia

Aetiology

In children, hypocalcaemia is more common than hypercalcaemia and outside the neonatal period is most commonly caused by rickets. There are many rare causes, mostly genetic, associated with hypoparathyroidism and with end organ resistance to PTH (see Table 10.5)

Clinical features

Important symptoms and signs include:
- Perioral tingling and paraesthesia, seizures, laryngospasm (stridor), raised intracranial pressure
- *Tetany:* manifested as carpo-pedal spasm. Latent tetany may be revealed by:
  - Trousseau's sign, eliciting carpo-pedal spasm by inflating BP cuff
  - Chvostek's sign, tapping zygoma to produce facial spasms.

Features of the syndromes associated with hypocalcaemia:
- *DiGeorge syndrome (DGS):* this and related syndromes arising from microdeletions of chromosome 22q are linked by failure of development of the 3rd and 4th branchial arches. There is hypoplasia of the thymus and parathyroids together with cardiac anomalies
- *Albright's hereditary osteodystrophy (pseudohypoparathyroidism):* mental retardation, short stature, dysmorphic facies, shortening of 4th and 5th metacarpals and soft tissue calcification (e.g. calcification of basal ganglia).

Investigations
- *Blood tests:* calcium, phosphate, alkaline phosphatase, magnesium
- *Imaging:*
  - wrist radiograph for rickets
  - chest radiograph for thymic hypoplasia (DGS)
  - bone mineral density scan (DEXA)
- *Hormone levels:* vitamin D, PTH
- Urine calcium, phosphate, creatinine, cAMP
- Genetic analyses
- Maternal serum calcium in neonatal hypocalcaemia.

Table 10.5. Causes of hypocalcaemia

Vitamin D deficiency	
Nutritional	Rickets
Genetic	Vitamin D-dependent rickets type 1 (defect of 25-α hydroxylase)
	Vitamin D-dependent rickets type 2 (defect of vitamin D receptor)
	Vitamin D-resistant, hypophosphataemic rickets (renal phosphate wasting)
Hypoparathyroidism	
Genetic	Microdeletions of chromosome 22q including DGS
	Familial isolated hypoparathyroidism caused by mutations in *CaSR*, *PTH*, and *GCM2*
Acquired	Maternal hypercalcaemia
	Thalassaemia: iron overload
	Autoimmune diseases
Hypomagnasaemia	
PTH resistance	Pseudohypoparathyroidism (PHP). End-organ resistance to PTH occurs in a heterogeneous group of rare genetic disorders: some are caused by mutations in the *GNAS1* gene encoding the GSα protein vital for PTH action. This gene is imprinted. The group includes PHP1a, 1c, Albright hereditary osteodystrophy

Treatment
Severe, symptomatic hypocalcaemia is treated with IV infusion of calcium gluconate. Mild, asymptomatic hypocalcaemia is treated with oral calcium supplements.

Nutritional deficiency of vitamin D is treated with ergocalciferol (D_2) or cholecalciferol (D_3), 3000–10 000 u/day.

Hypoparathyroidism is treated with the active metabolites of vitamin D_3: alfacalcidol (1α-hydroxycolecalciferol) or calcitriol which has a shorter half-life.

Hypomagnesaemia
Magnesium deficiency inhibits PTH release and causes secondary hypocalcaemia. The most common cause is malabsorption, but several cytotoxic drugs cause renal tubular magnesium loss. Primary genetic hypomagnesaemia is rare.

Hypercalcaemia

Aetiology
Hypercalcaemia is uncommon. Causes include Williams syndrome and iatrogenic hypercalcaemia (Table 10.6).

Clinical features
Hypercalcaemia is frequently asymptomatic, but can cause symptoms arising from the nervous system: irritability, malaise, headache, personality changes, proximal muscle weakness, or GI tract: anorexia, nausea, vomiting, constipation.

Renal stones may occur and ectopic calcification may cause pancreatitis and conjunctivitis.

Examination may reveal bradycardia, hypertension, altered sensorium, and weakness. Eye examination may reveal band keratopathy.

Table 10.6. Causes of hypercalcaemia

Hyperparathyroidism (PTH high)	
Genetic:	Multiple endocrine neoplasia (MEN)
	MEN1: AD. Parathyroid adenomas with tumours of endocrine pancreas and pituitary
	MEN2A,B: Parathyroid hyperplasia with tumours of the thyroid and adrenal medulla
	Familial hypocalciuric hypercalcaemia (FHH). AD and benign. In homozygous individuals it causes neonatal severe primary hyperparathyroidism
Miscellaneous (PTH low)	
Malignancy	Parathyroid carcinoma (rare)
	Tumours secreting PTH-related peptide
	Osteolytic bone lesions
Williams syndrome	Deletions of 7q11.23 (15%)
Thyroxicosis	
Granulomatous disease	Sarcoidosis, TB
Idiopathic infantile hypercalcaemia	
Renal failure	
Iatrogenic	Vitamin D or vitamin A excess
	Thiazides
	Excessive calcium supplements, TPN

Investigations
As for hypocalcaemia but include:
- *Renal US, radiograph:* nephrocalcinosis, renal stones
- *Parathyroid imaging:* ultrasonography
- *Radionuclide scanning:* 99mTc MIBI, 99mTc-tetrofosmin.

Treatment
Acute management of hypercalcaemia involves saline diuresis with isotonic NaCl in combination with furosemide to inhibit tubular reabsorption of calcium. Biphosphates (e.g. pamidronate) block bone resorption by inhibiting osteoclast activity and can be used orally or IV. Surgical intervention including subtotal or complete parathyroidectomy may be required.

10.10 Type 1 diabetes mellitus

Physiology of glucose homeostasis
Insulin is the key regulator of glucose uptake by muscle and liver in the fed state. Counter-regulatory hormones such as glucagon, cortisol, catecholamines, and GH maintain blood glucose levels during fasting by promoting glycogenolysis, gluconeogenesis, and lipolysis.

The endocrine pancreas
The human pancreas has 1–2 million islets composed of four cell types: α, β, δ and F. The β cells (60% of the islets) secrete insulin, α cells secrete glucagon, δ cells secrete somatostatin, and F cells pancreatic polypeptide.

Insulin
Insulin is synthesized from a proinsulin precursor molecule by the action of enzymes which remove the centre portion of the molecule, C-peptide, leaving a 51 amino acid peptide (A chain of 21 amino acids, B chain of 30 amino acids), bound together by disulfide bonds.

Insulin secretion
Glucose stimulates the β cell to secrete insulin via the mechanism shown in Fig 10.13.

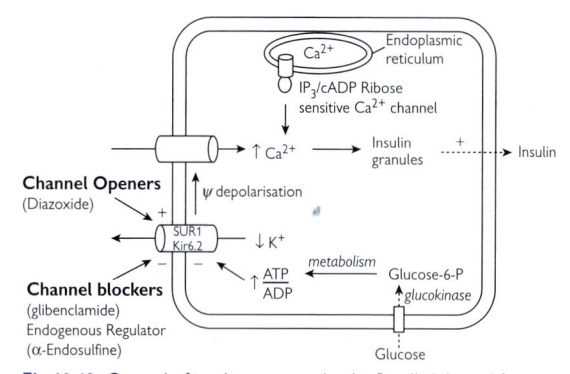

Fig 10.13 Control of insulin secretion by the B cell. Adapted from the Oxford Textbook of Medicine, with permission from OUP.

Glucose enters the β cell through the transporter GLUT2 and is metabolized with generation of ATP.

ATP-sensitive potassium channels (SUR1/Kir6.2) close, depolarizing the cell membrane which opens voltage-gated Ca^{2+} channels. Increased Ca^{2+} level causes exocytosis of stored insulin and activation of insulin gene expression. Channel openers and blockers affect the K channel.

Insulin secretion in response to a rise in blood glucose is therefore biphasic: an immediate release of stored insulin followed by a sustained release of both stored and newly synthesized insulin. It circulates as an unbound monomer with a half-life of 5 min. Insulin release is also under autonomic control.

Insulin action
The transmembrane insulin receptor is a tyrosine kinase receptor consisting of two α and two β subunits. After binding insulin the receptor is internalized by endocytosis. Activation triggers a cascade of phosphorylation which leads to an increase in the high-affinity glucose transporter (GLUT4) molecules in the outer membrane of insulin-responsive tissues.

Insulin effects
The main effects of insulin are to:
- Increase glucose uptake into muscle and fat cells
- Stimulate liver glycogen synthesis
- Stimulate lipogenesis and reduce ketogenesis.

Glucagon
Glucagon is a 29 amino acid peptide synthesized in and secreted by the α cells of the islets. It is cleaved from a larger precursor molecule, pre-pro-glucagon. Increased secretion of glucagon is caused by decreased plasma glucose, catecholamines, cholinergic and β-adrenergic stimulation and cholecystokinin. Secretion is inhibited by insulin and somatostatin.

Glucagon opposes insulin. It increases blood sugar by promoting glycogenolysis and gluconeogenesis from glycerol, lactate and amino acids.

Type 1 diabetes mellitus (T1DM)
The incidence of T1DM in children ≤14 years varies geographically from 0.1/100 000 per year in China up to 37/100 000 per year in Finland. Incidence is bimodal with peaks at 4–6 years and 10–14 years. T1DM accounts for 90% of diabetes mellitus in childhood.

Aetiology and pathogenesis
T1DM is caused by insulin deficiency from autoimmune destruction of the pancreatic β cells triggered by environmental factors in genetically predisposed individuals.

Other less common causes of insulin deficiency include:
- Congenital absence of pancreas or islet cells
- Pancreatectomy
- Pancreatic damage in cystic fibrosis, thalassaemia
- *Wolfram syndrome:* **d**iabetes **i**nsipidus, **d**iabetes **m**ellitus, **o**ptic **a**trophy, **d**eafness (DIDMOAD).

Genetics
There is clear evidence of a genetic component to T1DM:
- *Concordance in twins:* monozygotic 30–50%, dizygotic 8%.
- *Familial clustering:* offspring risk 2–3% if affected mother, 5–6% if affected father, 30% if both parents are affected.

At least six genes or chromosomal regions are implicated:
- *HLA class II genes on chromosome 6:* individuals who are HLA DR3 and DR4 have the highest risk.
- The insulin gene *INS, CTLA-4,* and *PTPN22.*

Environmental factors
Low concordance in MZ twins, wide geographical variations in incidence and incidence changes over short time spans all implicate a role for environmental factors such as viral infections and diet. Breast-fed infants have a lower risk.

Pathogenesis
Islet cells are progressively destroyed by an immune-mediated process. Various antibodies may be found, some of which predict risk.: islet cell antibodies (ICA), insulin antibodies (IAA), antibodies to glutamate decarboxylase (GAD). Children with T1DM are at risk of autoimmune thyroid disease and coeliac disease.

Pathophysiology
Lack of insulin causes failure of glucose uptake by tissues with concomitant hyperglycaemia. A profoundly catabolic state ensues with increased glycogenolysis, gluconeogenesis, and lipolysis. As hyperglycaemia exceeds the renal threshold an osmotic diuresis with dehydration and electrolyte losses ensues. Diabetic ketoacidosis supervenes as ketones are generated.

Clinical features

History
The classical history in the older child is of increasing thirst and polydipsia, polyuria which may lead to enuresis, and weight loss despite a good appetite. Non-specific malaise and irritability are common. The diagnosis is more easily overlooked in the very young. Diabetic ketoacidosis (DKA) is often accompanied by vomiting, abdominal pain, and altered consciousness.

Examination
Apart from wasting and mild dehydration there may be no specific clinical findings in the early stages. Signs of DKA include:
- *Severe dehydration:* hypovolaemia, poor perfusion
- *Ketoacidosis:* acidotic breathing (Kussmaul respiration), tachypnoea, smell of ketones on breath.

Diagnosis and investigations
T1DM is not usually difficult to diagnose although hyperglycaemia and impaired glucose tolerance have proved difficult to define. The WHO relies on fasting plasma glucose >7.8 mmol/L for the diagnosis of diabetes. Testing for impaired glucose tolerance is not usually necessary for diagnosis in childhood. Investigations for suspected T1DM include:
- Urine glucose and ketones
- *Blood (or plasma) glucose:* random whole-blood glucose >11 mmol/L
- *Glycosylated haemoglobin:* HbA1c
- Urea and electrolytes
- *Acid–base status:* capillary blood gas estimation.

T2DM and MODY may occasionally present with insulinopenia and DKA and definitive diagnosis may only be possible retrospectively.

Management
The treatment of DKA is considered elsewhere (see Chapter 2.10). For the majority of children in whom diagnosis is made prior to the onset of DKA, long-term management involves insulin therapy. All children with T1DM require insulin therapy which is given regularly by SC injection.

Insulins
A number of new insulin analogues are now available which may be rapid or long-acting: see Chapter 20.9.
- *Rapid-acting analogues*: Insulin Lispro (Eli Lilly), Insulin Aspart (Novo Nordisk). Onset of action is at 10 min, peak at 30 min, duration 3 h.
- *Long-acting analogues:* Insulin glargine precipitates in subcutaneous tissues and has delayed absorption. This provides a better profile of action than isophane (intermediate-acting) insulin with less risk of early hypoglycaemia and dawn hyperglycaemia when given at night. The flat profile lasts 18–26 h.

Insulin regimens
- Most children are treated with multiple injection regimens using pre-mixed formulations given twice daily or basal bolus injections of short-acting insulin with meals and a long-acting insulin in the evening.
- Insulin requirements may be low during the 'honeymoon period' but thereafter prepubertal children usually require 0.5–1.0 u/kg per day. Intensification is often required at puberty and some adolescents require up to 2 u/kg per day.
- Continuous subcutaneous insulin infusion (insulin pump therapy), using a short-acting insulin, may improve glycaemic control in highly motivated patients.

Dietary management
Management emphasizes a healthy, balanced diet containing adequate protein, small amounts of fat, and complex carbohydrates (e.g. cereal) that are digested slowly. Mealtimes and carbohydrate content need to be consistent on the twice-daily regimens, but the intensive regimes allow a more flexible eating pattern.

Monitoring control and complications
Daily monitoring of blood glucose using a finger-prick sampling device and monitor is optimal.

Measurement of HbA1C is useful for medium to long-term monitoring, and the level should be checked every 3 months. HbA1c levels <7.5% are optimal.

Microvascular complications (retinopathy, renal damage) are rare before puberty, at which time risk increases three-fold. The risk of complications is in part inherited but additional risk factors include poor glycaemic control, female sex, smoking, and duration of diabetes. Microalbuminuria (MA), is predictive of renal and cardiovascular disease, but 50% of teenagers with MA return to normoalbuminuria in young adulthood.

There should be regular review of cardiovascular risk factors including weight, blood pressure, dyslipidaemia, and discussion regarding smoking and exercise.

Education and the management of hypoglycaemia
Education is necessary concerning all aspects of diabetes, but the recognition and management of hypoglycaemia is of particular importance. In a patient receiving glucose-lowering treatment this is defined as a blood glucose <4 mmol/L.

Initial symptoms and signs reflect the effects of sympathetic stimulation: pallor, sweating, nausea, and vomiting. Neuroglycopenia causes altered behaviour, visual disturbance, headache, and seizures with eventual coma.

In the alert patient with intact airway protection oral carbohydrate in the form of a gel (e.g. Glucogel) or high-calorie drink is indicated. In the patient with altered consciousness IM glucagon or IV dextrose is used.

Management during intercurrent illness, surgery
Intercurrent illness creates a catabolic state requiring additional insulin, even if carbohydrate intake is reduced. This is managed by adjusting short-acting insulin dosage.

10.11 Type 2 diabetes mellitus and hypoglycaemia

Type 2 diabetes mellitus (T2DM)

Type 2 diabetes mellitus, previously called non-insulin dependent diabetes mellitus (NIDDM) or maturity-onset diabetes, is a metabolic disorder characterized by insulin resistance, relative insulin deficiency, and hyperglycaemia.

Incidence

T2DM accounts for 90% of cases of diabetes mellitus overall, but as its previous name suggests, onset is usually in late adult life. The first cases of T2DM were reported in UK children in 2000, reflecting a trend seen in North America for 20 years.

Aetiology

Affected children are usually overweight or obese, female, pubertal, and of ethnic minority (South Asian) origin. There may be a family history of T2DM or gestational diabetes.

There is a clear genetic contribution combined with environmental factors constituting the 'diabetogenic' lifestyle: excessive calories combined with reduced activity and calorie expenditure (Fig 10.14).

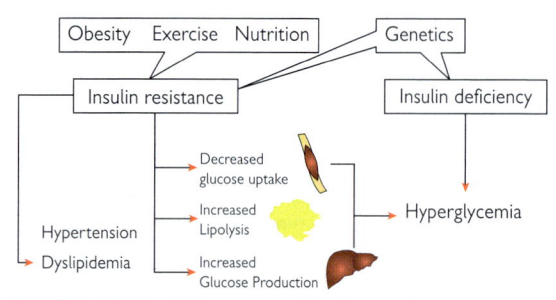

Fig 10.14 T2DM aetiology: genes and environment.

Genetics

In most patients with T2DM the genetic susceptibility is polygenic but at least six single-gene, AD forms of T2DM exist. Although these forms are called maturity-onset diabetes of the young (MODY), presentation may be in adult life.

Polygenic T2DM

Robust, replicated associations in non-isolate populations have been found for variants in *PPARG* and *KCNJ11*, genes which may influence β cell function.

Autosomal dominant T2DM (MODY 1–6)
Mutations in six genes including:
- *MODY 3 TCF1*: encoding a hepatic transcription factor-1 (also called *HNF1A*). Accounts for 87% of UK MODY patients.
- *MODY 2 GCK*: encoding glucokinase. Impaired phosphorylation of glucose impairs the β cell response to hyperglycaemia.

Pathogenesis

T2DM arises from a combination of β cell failure and peripheral insulin resistance. The cellular mechanisms are not fully understood but include:
- Loss of the early phase of insulin release
- Decreased insulin-mediated transport in muscle and adipose tissue
- Increased hepatic glucose production.

Clinical features

Most patients with T2DM are asymptomatic but occasionally T2DM may present with ketoacidosis. Onset is usually insidious. If they occur, symptoms may include lassitude, thirst, polyuria, and weight loss.

Examination is usually unrevealing but risk factors (obesity, hypertension) should be sought and rarely, acanthosis nigricans may be present: dark, thick, velvety skin around the neck or in the armpits.

Investigations

Diagnosis of diabetes mellitus rests on a fasting or random plasma glucose concentration of:
- *Fasting* >7.8 mmol/L
- *Random:* >11 mmol/L.

If there is uncertainty as to whether the diagnosis is type 1 or type 2 diabetes mellitus, additional investigations which may aid diagnosis include:
- *Islet cell GAD antibodies:* presence more likely in T1DM
- *Insulin or C-peptide concentrations:* high levels in T2DM
- Fasting lipids
- Genetic testing is indicated in MODY.

Management

Treatment for T2DM focuses on diet and exercise. Insulin is occasionally required at diagnosis and oral hypoglycaemia agents may be required.
- *Diet:* a healthy diet of protein, carbohydrate, and fat aiming at modest weight loss
- *Exercise:* aim at 30 min/day of exercise such as brisk walking, swimming, riding a bicycle, or team sports
- *Oral agents:* metformin is the oral antidiabetic agent of first choice in children in whom the above measures fail.

Self-monitoring of blood glucose is implemented, together with monitoring of:
- *HbA1C:* aim for range < 7%, unless hypoglycaemia is a problem
- *Blood pressure:* control with ACE inhibitors
- *Microalbuminuria (MA):* screen yearly using albumin/creatinine ratio (abnormal >30mg/g). MA is a good indicator of early renal damage and a risk factor for microvascular disease.

Hypoglycaemia

The normal range of circulating glucose concentration varies with age as does the level at which neuroglycopenia causes symptoms. Different methods measure the glucose concentration in whole blood (most glucometers and 'dextrostix') or plasma (most lab estimations). Red cells have a lower glucose concentration, so blood glucose measurements tends to be lower than plasma by 10–15%.

Accepted definitions of hypoglycaemia are:
- <2.6 mmol/L in the newborn
- <3.5 mmol/L in childhood
- <4.0 mmol/L in a child on a glucose-lowering agent.

Aetiology

Causes vary with age and can be classified into those with inadequate glucose production (ketotic or non-ketotic) or excess glucose consumption due to hyperinsulinism (non-ketotic). Neonatal hypoglycaemia is also usefully categorized into transient and persistent (see Tables 10.7 and 10.8. See also Chapter 1.12).

Table 10.7. Causes of neonatal hypoglycaemia

Transient	
↓Glucose production	Preterm or SGA infants
	Low glycogen stores, immature gluconeogenic enzymes
↑Glucose consumption	Hyperinsulinaemia:
	Infants of diabetic mother
Persistent	
↓Glucose production	Defective counter-regulatory hormones:
	Panhypopituarism, congenital adrenal hyperplasia (CAH)
	Inborn errors of metabolism
	Glycogen storage disorders
	Galactosaemia
	Organic acidaemias
↑Glucose consumption	Familial hyperinsulinaemia (HHF)
	Beckwith–Wiedemann Syndrome

Table 10.8. Causes of childhood hypoglycaemia

Ketotic
- Idiopathic ketotic hypoglycaemia: most common
- Addison's disease
- Inborn errors of metabolism:
    Glycogen storage diseases
    Organic acidaemias
- Hepatic failure

Non-ketotic
- Hyperinsulinaemia:
    Insulinoma
    Exogenous insulin
- Inborn errors of metabolism:
    Fatty acid oxidation defects: medium chain acyl CoA dehydrogenase (MCAD) deficiency
    Carnitine transport deficiency
- Poisoning: accidental or non-accidental

Idiopathic ketotic hypoglycaemia
This syndrome, of uncertain aetiology, is the most common cause of hypoglycaemia in the age range 1–5 years. Episodes of hypoglycaemia characteristically occur in the morning after an overnight fast, presenting with features of neuroglycopenia: lethargy and malaise. The children are usually underweight and it often resolves by 10 years.

Hyperinsulinaemic hypoglycaemia, familial (HHF)
Previously called persistent hyperinsulinaemic hypoglycaemia of infancy this may be caused by mutations in at least six different genes: *HHF1–6*.

Most cases are accounted for by mutations in *ABCC8* which encodes the sulfonylurea receptor (SUR) and *KCNJII* which encodes Kir 6.2, both subunits of the β cell ^{K}ATP-sensitive K channel. See Fig 10.13.

Focal or diffuse (nesidioblastosis) histopathologies occur.

Clinical features
The presenting features reflect the effects of adrenergic stimulation and counter-regulatory responses together with the effects of neuroglycopenia.

Infants may be asymptomatic or present with hypotonia, lethargy, poor feeding, jitteriness, apnoeic episodes, or seizures.

In children, manifestation of autonomic nervous system activation include anxiety, tremulousness, sweating, pallor, tachycardia, hunger, and nausea. Neuroglycopenia causes headache, confusion, behavioural changes, visual disturbances, altered consciousness, and seizures.

Investigations
Capillary blood glucose estimation and urine ketones are the baseline investigations. Venous blood samples should also be taken during hypoglycaemia for a diagnostic screen to identify the cause.
- Laboratory plasma glucose estimation
- Insulin and C-peptide levels
- Cortisol and GH
- Lactate
- Free fatty acids (FFA)
- Amino acids
- Ketones (β-hydroxybutyrate, acetoacetate)
- Urine organic acids.

In non-ketotic hypoglycaemia, FFA levels help to distinguish between hyperinsulinaemia (normal FFA) and fatty-acid oxidation defects (raised FFA).

Management
Prevention of hypoglycaemia is preferable and can be achieved in at-risk newborns and children with T1DM. MCAD deficiency is now part of UK neonatal screening.

Prompt recognition and correction of hypoglycaemia is vital to avoid the brain damage caused by neuroglycopenia, especially in the presence of seizures.

In an alert patient with intact airway protection oral liquids containing 10–20 g carbohydrate can be administered, e.g. non-diet Lucozade or Coca-Cola (50–90 mL) or Glucogel (glucose 9.2 g). This can be repeated in 10–15 min.

In the unconscious or fitting patient 2–5 mL/kg of 10% dextrose IV is indicated, or IM glucagon 1 mg if venous access is problematic.

Hyperinsulinaemia
Options in infants with HHF and chronic intractable hypoglycaemia include:
- *Glycaemic agents:* diazoxide, octreotide, nifedipine
- Pancreatic resection.

Idiopathic ketotic hypoglycaemia
Frequency and duration of episodes can be reduced by avoiding extended fasts: giving a bedtime snack and avoiding late breakfasts. An underweight child may benefit from nutritional supplements. If vomiting complicates acute episodes, hospitalization and IV saline and dextrose may be required.

10.12 Case-based discussions

An infant with ambiguous genitalia and vomiting

A 10 day old infant presents to the emergency department with a history of vomiting for 48 h. He had been born at term by a normal vaginal delivery. Bilateral undescended testes were diagnosed on the newborn examination at 24 h.

On examination there was severe dehydration with a sunken fontanelle, dry mucous membranes, and reduced skin turgor. His central capillary refill time was 5 s.

Urea and electrolyte and blood glucose results:
- Sodium 130 mmol/L
- Potassium 5.8 mmol/L
- Urea 11 mmol/L
- Blood glucose 1.9 mmol/L.

What is the most likely diagnosis?
A salt-losing crisis caused by classical congenital adrenal hyperplasia due to 21-hydroxylase deficiency. This is likely to be a virilized female. Hyponatraemia and hyperkalaemia is characteristic of mineralocorticoid deficiency. This is a life-threatening emergency.

What is the immediate management?
IV normal saline at 20 mL/kg initially with dextrose together with IV hydrocortisone 50 mg. Oral fludrocortisone can then be added. Oral salt supplementation may be necessary.

What diagnostic tests would you perform?
Measure serum 17OHP and 11-deoxycortisol (cortisol precursors) and ACTH.

A very high concentration of 17OHP (>240 nmol/L, normal <3 nmol/L at 3 days in a term infant) is diagnostic of classic 21-hydroxylase deficiency. In borderline cases a corticotropin stimulation test can be used with measurement of 17OHP at 60 min.

Investigation results
- The 17-OHP level was 300 nmol/L
- Abdominal ultrasound identified a normal uterus
- Karyotype 46,XX

What is the further management?
There are many challenges in the future management of a girl with classical salt-wasting CAH.
- *Surgery*: the management of a child with ambiguous genitalia remains complex and controversial. Early surgery may be technically easier but must be done at an age when the patient cannot participate full in an informed consent process.
- *Growth and development*: treatment during the first 2 years may influence final height outcome. Excess glucocorticoids suppress growth, but high concentrations of sex steroids will induce premature epiphyseal closure. A difficult path must be found between hypercortisolism (over-treatment) and hyperandrogenism (under-treatment).
- *Fertility*: reduced fertility is reported, especially in females with classical CAH. An increased incidence of polycystic ovaries is a common finding and may be contributory.

A case of short stature

A 5 year old boy presented with short stature. He was born at term, with a birthweight on the 50th centile. He fed well during infancy and had sustained his weight between the 50th and 75th centiles. During infancy his height had followed the 50th centile but from the age of about 18 months his parents had noticed that he appeared shorter than his peers. He was otherwise well.

On examination he appeared plump with immature facies, and small hands, feet, and genitalia.

His standing and sitting heights were on the 2nd centile and his weight on the 50th. The calculated midparental centile was the 50th. A height velocity over the preceding 6 months was calculated as 3 cm/year.

What is the most likely diagnosis?
The most likely diagnosis is GH deficiency (GHD). This is the most common endocrine disorder presenting with short stature, with a prevalence of 1/2000–4000. In most cases there is an isolated deficiency but it may occur as part of a multiple or combined anterior pituitary hormone deficiencies: TSH, ACTH, LH, FSH, PRL, and/or diabetes insipidus.

He grew normally in height and weight during the nutritional phase of growth in infancy. His height was then noted to fall away from his peers as he entered into the hormonal phase of growth. In severe GHD the height velocity may be <4 cm/year.

How would you confirm this diagnosis?
Random GH levels are of little or no diagnostic value. GH is secreted in a pulsatile fashion with peaks and troughs. A low GH measurement could therefore simply be a natural trough. The diagnosis of GHD is confirmed by a peak plasma GH level <20 mU/L (depending on assay method) on one or two provocation tests.

It is also important to demonstrate normal thyroid function tests.

What treatment is recommended?
The management of GHD is by daily subcutaneous injections of GH using r-hGH. With GH treatment final height is increased by about 8–11 cm (slightly more in boys than girls).

Regular assessment of response every 3 months for the 1st year is necessary. Bone age and thyroid function is assessed annually. Adverse effects include local discomfort, transient headache, and intracranial hypertension (rare).

Other licensed indications for GH treatment include Turner syndrome, chronic renal failure, Prader–Willi syndrome, and SGA children. The dose of GH depends upon the indication for use.

Chapter 11
Metabolic medicine

11.1 Metabolic pathways *234*
11.2 Inborn errors of metabolism *236*
11.3 Disorders of carbohydrate and fat metabolism *238*
11.4 Disorders of amino acid metabolism *240*
11.5 Mitochondrial and peroxisomal disorders *242*
11.6 Lysosomal storage diseases *244*
11.7 Case-based discussions *246*

11.1 Metabolic pathways

Carbohydrate metabolism

Glucose
Most dietary carbohydrate is in the form of polysaccharides, including the two disaccharides:
- *Lactose:* galactose + glucose.
- *Sucrose:* fructose + glucose.

Galactose and fructose are rapidly converted to glucose after absorption.

Circulating glucose is maintained by dietary absorption and from the breakdown of liver glycogen, a large glucose polymer that allows the body to store glucose molecules in a compact form. Glucose is used in most cells as a source of energy and metabolic intermediate. Only the D-isomer, D-glucose (dextrose) is biologically active. Control of glucose entry into cells and glycogen production and breakdown is under tight hormonal control, particularly the ratio between insulin and glucagon (see Chapter 10).

Glucose metabolism
The main metabolic fates of glucose are:
- Oxidation for energy
- Storage as glycogen
- Conversion to amino acids and triglycerides.

Oxidation of glucose
Glycolysis
Anaerobic glycolysis is the first stage of glucose breakdown and takes place in the cytoplasm. A six-carbon glucose molecule is broken down to two pyruvate molecules with the net gain of only two ATP molecules.

Pyruvate is converted to lactate under anaerobic conditions, or enters the tricarboxylic acid cycle in the mitochondrion under aerobic conditions. Pyruvate is then converted to oxaloacetate by pyruvate carboxylase or is decarboxylated to acetyl-CoA by the pyruvate dehydrogenase (PDH) enzyme complex.

Tricarboxylic acid (TCA) cycle
The TCA cycle (citric acid cycle, Krebs cycle) occurs in all cells with mitochondria and provides the final common pathway for glucose, fatty acids and amino acid oxidation (Fig 11.1).

The cycle provides reduced cofactors (NADH, FADH2) which donate electrons to the respiratory chain for ATP production in the process of 'oxidative phosphorylation'. Complete aerobic breakdown of one glucose molecule generates 36 ATP molecules.

Glycogen metabolism
Glycogen is a branched glucose polymer stored predominantly in the liver, but also in muscle and kidney.

Glycogenesis is stimulated by insulin and involves:
- Synthesis of UDP-glucose from glucose-1-phosphate
- Polymerization to form glycogen.

Glycogenolysis is promoted by adrenaline and glucagon. Liver glycogen releases glucose to the circulation for general use whereas muscle glycogen supports muscle glycolysis only.
- Monomers of glucose-1-phosphate are cleaved off by glycogen phosphorylase
- Glucose-1-phosphate is converted to glucose-6-phosphate (G6P). G6P can enter glycolysis via the pentose phosphate pathway or be dephosphorylated back to glucose
- A special debranching enzyme removes the α (1–6) branches

Gluconeogenesis
Gluconeogenesis, the generation of glucose from non-carbohydrate precursors, takes place mostly in the liver.

Substrates that can enter the gluconeogenesis pathway include:
- Lactate and pyruvate
- Citric acid cycle intermediates
- *Amino acids:* especially alanine, aspartate, and glutamate
- Glycerol.

Most fatty acids can not be converted to glucose because they are broken down into acetyl-CoA which enters the TCA cycle.

Protein metabolism

Proteins are composed of 20 different amino acids. There is a pool of amino acids in the body in dynamic equilibrium with tissue protein.

Breakdown of protein leads to a net daily loss of nitrogen (as urea) from the body which is compensated by dietary intake. Positive nitrogen balance occurs in growth, pregnancy and convalescence, and negative balance in malnutrition, starvation or in catabolic states, e.g. severe burns, sepsis.

Amino acids
Amino acids consist of a carbon skeleton and amino group (Fig 11.2).

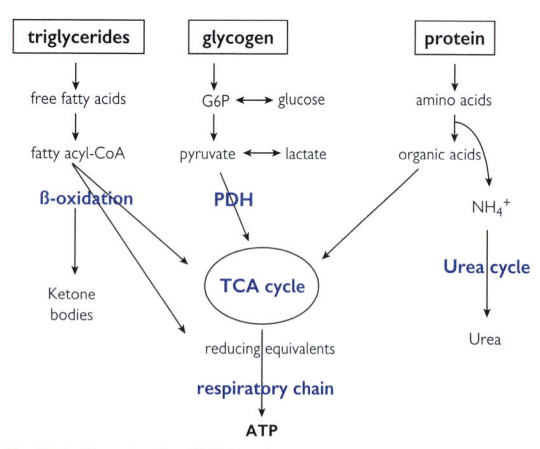

Fig 11.1 Central role of TCA cycle.

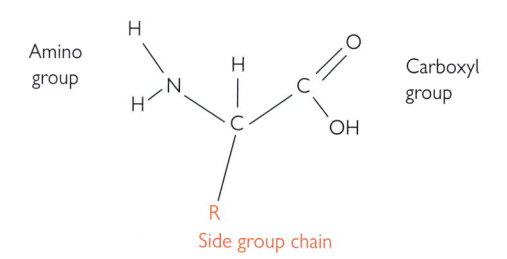

Fig 11.2 Amino acid structure.

The R-group side chain varies and determines the amino acid and its properties: polar or non-polar, basic or acidic.

There are 10 essential amino acids which have to be obtained from the diet and 10 non-essential ones which can be synthesized.

Amino acid metabolism

Catabolism

The two main reactions in amino acid catabolism are:

- *Transamination:* aminotransferases (transaminases) catalyse the transfer of the α-amino group (NH_3^+) to an α-keto-acid (pyruvate, oxaloacetate, or α-ketoglutarate). The most important enzymes are alanine aminotransferase (ALT) and aspartate aminotransferase (AST).
- *Oxidative deamination:* glutamate dehydrogenase (in the mitochondrion) removes the amino group from glutamate to form ammonia which enters the urea cycle and a carbon skeleton (α-ketoglutarate).

Amino acid carbon skeletons may be converted to acetyl-CoA which is oxidized, converted to ketone bodies or to pyruvate which is oxidized, or converted to glucose by gluconeogenesis.

Urea cycle: disposal of nitrogen

In the urea cycle, urea (NH_2-CO-NH_2) is synthesized from CO_2 and NH_4^+ in the liver (Fig 11.3).

Ammonia is extremely toxic and by converting it to urea, a small, non-toxic, water soluble molecule, 50% nitrogen by weight, nitrogen can be easily excreted in the urine.

The urea cycle has 5 reactions, the first two occurring in the mitochondrion, the last three in the cytosol. One nitrogen is supplied by ammonia and the other derives from aspartate. The cycle uses a carrier molecule, ornithine, which is regenerated. See Figure

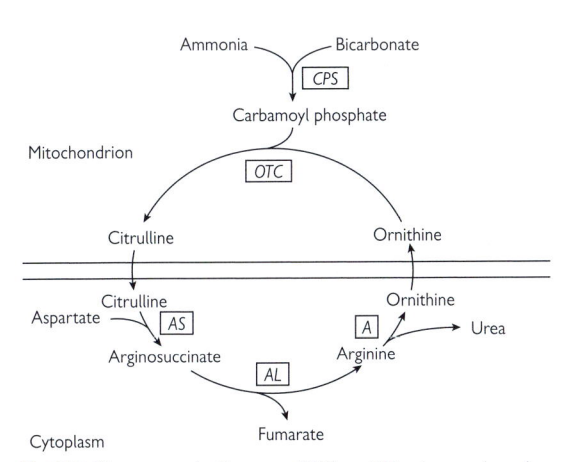

Fig 11.3 The urea cycle. Enzymes: OTC, ornithine transcarbamylase; CPS, carbamoyl phosphate synthase; AS, arginosuccinic acid synthetase; AL, arginosuccinic acid lyase; A, arginase.

Fat metabolism

Animal and plant fats are triesters of glycerol and fatty acids. Lipids are important for energy storage, as structural components of cell membranes and as signalling molecules. Fat stores 9 kcal/g of energy, compared to 4 kcal/g stored by carbohydrates and proteins.

Fatty acids

A fatty acid is a carboxylic acid with an unbranched aliphatic chain of 8–22 carbon atoms. The term 'saturated' refers to hydrogen. In a saturated fatty acid all carbons contain as many hydrogens as possible, with no double bonds. One or more double bonds renders the fatty acid mono- or poly*unsaturated*.

The human body can synthesize all but two fatty acids it needs from acetyl-CoA by sequential addition of two carbon atoms. The essential fatty acids in the diet are linoleic acid and the longer-chain omega-3 fatty acids present in fish oils.

Free fatty acids (FFAs)

FFAs come from the breakdown of triglyceride into its components (fatty acids and glycerol) by lipolysis. Lipolysis is stimulated by adrenaline and glucagon. FFAs are an important source of fuel for many tissues, in particular heart and skeletal muscle. FFAs are transported attached to albumin in the circulation and undergo β-oxidation to ketones in the mitochondrion.

Circulating lipids

Cholesterol and triglycerides are transported in the circulation bound to lipoproteins. The four main classes are:

- *Chylomicrons:* carry dietary lipids from gut to liver
- *Very low density lipoprotein (VLDL):* carries triglycerides and cholesterol synthesized in the liver to the periphery
- *Low density lipoprotein (LDL):* transports cholesterol and triglycerides. Uptake by cells via the LDL receptor
- *High density lipoprotein (HDL):* carries cholesterol from the periphery to the liver.

11.2 Inborn errors of metabolism

Inborn errors of metabolism (IEMs) are a group of genetic disorders of metabolism most of which are due to defects of single genes that code for enzymes.

Inheritance

IEMs are individually rare, but have an overall incidence of >1/4000 births. Certain diseases are enriched in specific populations. They are nearly all single-gene disorders, inherited in mendelian fashion. A specific disease phenotype may show:
- *Locus heterogeneity:* different genes in the same pathway give rise to a similar phenotype e.g. urea cycle disorders
- *Allelic heterogeneity:* different mutations (alleles) in the same gene may vary in their severity and influence the age of onset or expressivity of the phenotype.

The genes for most IEMs are located on autosomes, and as most encode enzymes the pattern of inheritance is usually autosomal recessive (AR). This is because most biochemical pathways function adequately with 50% of enzyme activity so heterozygotes (carriers) are normal. Consanguinity, e.g. when parents are first cousins, increases the risk of AR disorders.

There are exceptions. Some genes are on the X chromosome, some are caused by mutations in mitochondrial DNA which is maternally inherited, and mutations in some genes cause autosomal dominant (AD) disease. Genetic heterogeneity allows some disease phenotypes to have several different patterns of inheritance.

Pathophysiology

Pathogenetic mechanisms include:
- Intoxication due to upstream effects
- Deficit of normal products, e.g. glucose
- Energy failure
- Storage of macromolecules
- Defects in processing of complex molecules.

Intoxication

This occurs most commonly in disorders of protein metabolism and classically presents in the newborn with decompensation after a symptom free period of 2–3 days.

Ammonia is commonly the toxic metabolite. Decompensation is provoked by the stress of exogenous protein or the catabolic breakdown of endogenous protein that accompanies birth. Feeding is the essential stressor only in galactosaemia. Later presentation may occur after an unusual substrate load or catabolic stress during fasting or intercurrent illness. Intoxication may occur progressively over months or years (e.g. in phenylketonuria).
- *Examples:* galactosaemia, aminoacidopathies (tyrosinaemia, hyperphenylalaninaemia), urea cycle defects (hyperammonaemia), organic acidaemias.

Acid–base balance disturbances

Acid–base disturbances are common in IEMs with 'intoxication'. Metabolic acidosis arising from accumulation of organic acids or bicarbonate loss is most common. Calculation of the anion gap allows these two mechanisms to be distinguished:

$$\text{Anion gap} = [Na^+] + [K^+] - [Cl^-] - [HCO_3^-]$$

The normal anion gap is +12–16 mmol/L. An increased anion gap indicates the accumulation of acids giving an excess of unmeasured anions e.g. lactate, keto-acids. A normal level with metabolic acidosis indicates hyperchloraemic acidosis associated with bicarbonate loss via the kidney or gut. See Fig 11.4.

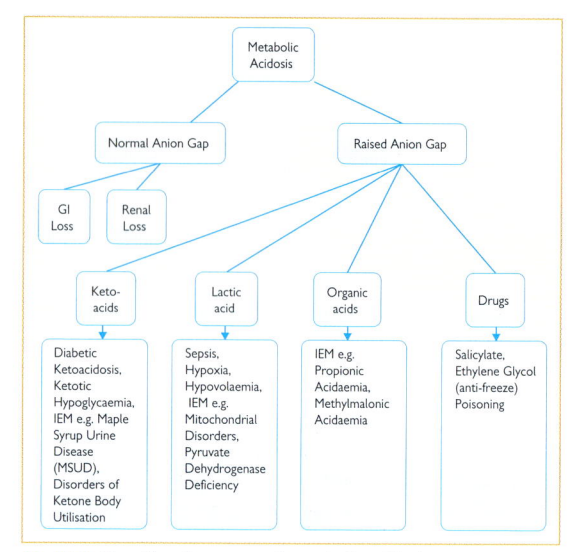

Fig 11.4 Algorithm for causes of metabolic acidosis.

Deficit of normal products

Hypoglycaemia is the most common problem and occurs in defects of carbohydrate metabolism (e.g. glycogen storage disorders), fatty acid oxidation defects (e.g. medium-chain acetyl-CoA dehydrogenase deficiency), and endocrine disorders (congenital adrenal hyperplasia).

Energy failure

Defects in energy production pathways present with dysfunction in multiple organs, especially those with high energy consumption. The deficit may be constant with early onset of symptoms, e.g. pyruvate dehydrogenase deficiency, or may only occur if there is a deficit in provision of a particular fuel.
- *Examples:* respiratory chain defects, fatty acid oxidation defects, glycogen storage disease.

Storage of macromolecules

Failure to metabolize macromolecules leads to their accumulation usually in the lysosomes. This commonly leads to a dysmorphic syndrome, which may be evident at birth or become progressively more obvious with time.
- *Examples:* mucopolysaccharidosis (MPS).

Defects in processing of complex molecules

Many proteins require post-translational modification for normal function. Defects in this process include the congenital disorders of glycosylation.

Clinical features

Presentation is highly variable and notoriously non-specific, the features depending on the pathophysiology. In acute presentations the most common differential is sepsis, which may mimic or accompany an IEM. An IEM should be suspected in children of any age with:
- Unexplained acute encephalopathy
- Acid–base disturbance, e.g. lactic acidaemia
- Unexplained multi- or single-organ disease
- Progressive neurological disease
- Dysmorphic features and organomegaly.

History

Important clues in the history include:
- *Consanguinity:* increases risk of AR disorders
- Previous multiple miscarriages (non-viable fetuses)
- Previous sudden unexplained death in infancy
- Ethnicity (for certain conditions).

Clinical presentations

- *Newborn presentation:* many disorders of intermediary metabolism present soon after birth. Clinical illness usually becomes apparent within the first 48–72 h. Encephalopathy is the most common presentation but onset may be subtle with poor feeding, vomiting, and lethargy followed by apnoea, fits, and coma. Similar features occur in sepsis and duct-dependent cardiac problems.
- *Infant or young child (1 month–5 years):* an IEM may present with poor feeding, failure to thrive, or developmental delay and/or regression. Episodes of vomiting, ataxia, seizures, lethargy, or coma may occur, or intercurrent illnesses may be severe or prolonged.
- *Older children, adolescents, and adults:* features may include mild to profound learning difficulties, behavioural disturbance, coma, exercise intolerance, or weakness.

Examination

The sick neonate will usually have non-specific signs such as temperature instability, tachypnoea or apnoea, circulatory compromise, and encephalopathy.

Useful signs are more common in older infants and children, especially in the storage disorders. There may be dysmorphic features, skeletal abnormalities, organomegaly or a variety of eye signs: cataracts, corneal clouding, pigmentary retinopathy, a cherry-red spot in the retina.

Investigations

In the acutely unwell infant the following investigations are a useful first line screen. Some abnormalities may be transient and present only during decompensation.

Blood tests

- *Blood gases:* venous, capillary or arterial
- Glucose, lactate, and ammonia
- LFTs, urea and electrolytes, creatinine
- Acylcarnitines (bloodspot on Guthrie card)
- Full blood count and coagulation screen.

Urine tests

- pH, ketones
- Organic acids (reducing substances and/or orotic acid)
- Amino acids.

Secondary lactic acidosis occurs in hypoxia, sepsis, shock, and liver failure and is more common than primary metabolic disease.

The degree of hyperammonaemia shows some correlation with aetiology. Fatty acid oxidation defects are associated with the range 40–250 μmol/L, organic acidaemia 40–450 μmol/L, and in urea cycle defects or liver failure levels can exceed 2000 μmol/L.

Second line investigations

These may include:
- Very long chain fatty acids, uric acid, plasma amino acids
- *CSF:* glucose, lactate, pyruvate, glycine, amino acids
- White cell or fibroblast lysosomal enzymes
- Biopsy of bone marrow, liver, skin, skeletal muscle
- DNA analysis.

Specimens are still important in a child who is dying or has died without a diagnosis, to facilitate evaluation of asymptomatic siblings and genetic counselling.

Newborn screening

This offers the opportunity for presymptomatic diagnosis and preventative measures in a number of IEMs. Mass spectrometry has extended the range of conditions for which screening is feasible. In the UK specific criteria are applied.

Treatment

Acute management using an 'emergency regimen' is aimed at correcting any life threatening metabolic abnormalities. Long-term management is based on several potential strategies (Table 11.1).

Acute management

- Stop feeds to eliminate protein, galactose, fructose.
- Give calories as IV 10% dextrose with appropriate electrolytes (sodium) to promote anabolism. Add insulin if hyperglycaemia develops and use 5% dextrose if primary lactic acidosis suspected.
- Treat severe acidosis and electrolyte abnormalities.
- Remove abnormal metabolites. Hyperammonaemia may respond to IV sodium benzoate or sodium phenylbutyrate and arginine in UCD and, if severe, haemofiltration.

Table 11.1. Long-term treatment strategies in IEMs

Strategy	Example
Substrate restriction	Dietary restriction in PKU
Diverting metabolic pathway	Urea cycle disorders
Correcting product deficiency	Glucose polymers in GSD
Co-factor therapy	Biotin for biotinidase deficiency
Transplantation (BMT)	X-linked adrenoleukodystrophy
Enzyme replacement therapy (ERT)	Lysosomal disorders, e.g. Gaucher disease, Fabry disease, Pompe disease

11.3 Disorders of carbohydrate and fat metabolism

Carbohydrate metabolism

Glycogen storage disorders (GSDs)

The GSDs are a group of diseases caused by deficiencies in enzymes involved in either the synthesis or breakdown of glycogen or in the transport of their substrates (Table 11.2).

Liver or muscle may be primarily involved. Eleven distinct enzyme defects have been described, five of the more important of which are shown in the table.

Liver glycogenoses
GSD I and III present with recurrent hypoglycaemia as their main symptom. As glycogen cannot be utilized, excessive storage with hepatomegaly develops. In the most severe form (GSD 1, Von Gierke) a low blood sugar can occur in less that 2 h after feeding. As the body is in a constant state of catabolism, trying to maintain an energy supply by gluconeogenesis, typical biochemical abnormalities develop which include lactic acidaemia, hypertriglyceridaemia and hyperuricaemia. Failure to thrive is typical.

In GSD Ib there is also a neutrophil dysfunction, leaving the child open to aphthous ulceration, recurrent infections, and inflammatory bowel disease. Type VI and type IX glycogenosis are usually mild disorders without hypoglycaemia.

Treatment of these GSDs is by frequent feeds during the daytime, overnight tube feeds, and the use of uncooked corn starch to prolong the fasting interval.

Muscle glycogenoses
Disorders such as muscle phosphorylase deficiency (GSDV, McArdle disease) present with localized muscle complaints, especially on exercise. Any anaerobic activity results in pain, cramps, and even rhabdomyolysis. Serum creatine kinase and uric acid are usually elevated.

These are rare disorders which usually present later in life except for Pompe disease (GSDII), which is a disorder of glycogen degradation within the lysosome.

Infantile Pompe disease presents with severe, early hypotonia with cardiomyopathy. There is a raised creatine kinase and aspartate aminotransferase, and diagnosis can be made by enzyme analysis of lymphocytes.

Early diagnosis is especially important as the early death associated with this condition can now be avoided with enzyme replacement therapy using a recombinant human enzyme.

Galactosaemia

A deficiency of enzymes involved in the conversion of galactose to glucose (usually galactose-1-phosphate uridyl transferase, Gal1-Put) results in galactosaemia. The incidence is 1/47 000 live births.

Galactose and its metabolites accumulate, and children present in the first few weeks with vomiting, failure to thrive, jaundice, and lethargy. If the diagnosis is not recognized, they may progress to liver and kidney impairment, nuclear cataracts, and episodes of *E. coli* sepsis.

Galactose (a reducing substance) is present in the urine but this test is not sensitive or specific enough for diagnosis. Diagnosis is confirmed by enzyme assay in red cells, but this is unreliable up to 3 months after a blood transfusion.

Treatment is with a non-lactose-containing formula (usually a soya milk) and later by a minimal-galactose diet. *Galactokinase deficiency* is a rarer form of galactosaemia that presents only with cataracts and is otherwise benign.

Hereditary fructose intolerance (HFI)

Patients with hereditary fructose intolerance have gastrointestinal symptoms and hypoglycaemia after ingesting fructose and this may lead to an aversion to fruits and sweets. Continued intake may cause liver and kidney disease.

HFI is caused by a deficiency in fructose 1,6-bisphosphate aldolase (aldolase B).

Three mutations in *ALDOB* account for >80% of HFI cases in the European population so that the diagnosis can most often be confirmed by DNA analysis from a blood specimen. Treatment is lifelong avoidance of fructose.

Fructose-1,6-bisphosphatase (F-1,6-BP) deficiency

This IEM does not present simply on ingestion of large amounts of fructose (a common sugar in fruit and vegetables, and a component of the disaccharide sucrose), as F-1,6-BP deficiency is primarily a disorder of gluconeogenesis.

Half present in the neonatal period with lactic acidosis and hypoglycaemia, and the remainder later, associated with intercurrent illnesses or following a fructose load.

Management is with intravenous dextrose and bicarbonate initially, followed by avoidance of fasting and frequent ingestion of starch-based foods.

Table 11.2. Glycogen storage disorders						
Number (Type)	Gene	Enzyme	Eponym	Liver	Muscle	Other
Ia	G6PC	Glucose-6-phosphatase	Von Gierke	+++		
Ib	G6PT1	Glucose-6-phosphatase translocase		+++		Neutrophil defect
II	GAA	Acid maltase (Glucosidase, α acid)	Pompe		++++	Cardiomyopathy
III	AGL	Debrancher enzyme	Cori	++	+	
V	PYGM	Muscle phosphorylase	McArdle		++	

Disorders of fat metabolism

Disorders of fatty acid oxidation

FFAs liberated from triglycerides are a major fuel source during fasting and are oxidized by most tissues except the brain. They are the preferred substrate for cardiac muscle and a vital energy source for skeletal muscle during exercise.

Fatty acid oxidation

Fatty acids are first activated in the cytoplasm by the action of fatty acyl-CoA synthetase to form the corresponding acyl-CoA. The fatty acyl-CoA is transported into the inner mitochondrial space via an acyl-carnitine intermediate where it undergoes β-oxidation. Entry into the β-oxidation cycle requires the action of acyl-CoA dehydrogenases of which there are three, each specific for different chain lengths:

- Short-chain acyl-CoA dehydrogenase: <C6
- Medium-chain acyl-CoA dehydrogenase: C6–C12
- Long-chain acyl-CoA dehydrogenase: >C12

Medium-chain acyl-CoA dehydrogenase deficiency (MCADD)

This is the most common of the acyl-CoA dehydrogenase deficiencies with an incidence similar to PKU in white people. During fasting or metabolic stress severe hypoglycaemia develops with no ketogenesis, but accumulation of dicarboxylic organic acids and mild hyperammonaemia.

Clinical features

Neonatal presentation can occur but most infants with MCADD present at 6–18 months with poor feeding during an intercurrent infection (particularly gastroenteritis). There is vomiting, lethargy, encephalopathy (hypoglycaemia), and tachypnoea. There may be an enlarged liver due to fatty infiltration. Mortality may be as high as 20% on first presentation and one third of survivors have neurological sequelae.

Diagnostic investigations

- Hypoketotic hypoglycaemia
- Mild to moderate hyperammonaemia
- ↓Bicarbonate
- ↑Octanoyl carnitine: tandem mass spectrometry
- Organic aciduria: dicarboxylic acids, hexanoylglycine.

Neonatal screening has been introduced in the UK.

Management

Episodes of decompensation are best prevented by using an emergency regimen of glucose polymer drinks during intercurrent illness or admission for IV 10% dextrose if drinks are not tolerated. In the at risk newborn feeds should be frequent, with intervals no longer than 3 h.

Long-chain deficiencies (LCHAD, VLCAD)

Deficiencies can occur in long-chain hydroxyl-acyl-CoA dehydrogenase (LCHAD) and very-long-chain acyl-CoA dehydrogenase (VLCAD). These are more severe.

The carrier mother may develop liver dysfunction in pregnancy either as acute fatty liver of pregnancy (AFLP) or HELLP syndrome (**H**aemolysis, **E**levated **L**iver enzymes, **L**ow **P**latelets), a severe form of pre-eclampsia/eclampsia. Treatment is dietary but prognosis is guarded.

Hyperlipidaemias.

Hypertriglyceridaemias

Familial hypertriglyceridaemia is rare and may be caused by mutations in *LIP1*, encoding lipoprotein lipase. Secondary causes include obesity, diabetes mellitus, glycogen storage disorders, liver disease, and chronic renal failure.

Clinical features include abdominal pain with eruptive xanthomas and organomegaly. There is an association with pancreatitis at triglyceride levels >20 mmol/L.

Diagnosis may be made incidentally by observation of a separated fat level in plasma. Management involves a very low fat diet.

Familial hypercholesterolaemia (FH)

Familial hypercholesterolaemia (FH) is an AD disorder caused by mutations in the LDL receptor gene, *LDLR*. It is the most common IEM in the UK with a heterozygote incidence of 1/500. Homozygotes are rare at 1/1 000 000.

Reduced LDL receptor numbers or function impairs endocytosis of cholesterol into hepatocytes. Negative feedback by repression of HMGCoA, the rate limiting step in cholesterol synthesis, is impaired and LDL cholesterol levels rise.

- Heterozygotes do not present in childhood but affected children may be identified by screening (see below)
- Homozygotes have cholesterol levels >15 mmol/L and develop tendon xanthomas by age 5 years and coronary artery disease in the 2nd decade.

Management

Screening

UK NICE guidelines published in 2008 recommend that children at risk of FH because of an affected parent are offered a DNA test by age 10 years if the family mutation is known. Otherwise, LDL cholesterol concentration should be measured and repeated after puberty if necessary.

Treatment

Treatment for heterozygous FH is initially with a low fat diet, but this may lower cholesterol by only ~10%. Treatment with HMG CoA reductase inhibitors (statins) is effective in children and should be initiated at 10 years. Initial studies have shown good tolerance and efficacy even in early childhood but as yet there are no long term published data on safety.

Homozygous FH is largely resistant to dietary and medical therapy and requires regular plasmapheresis or liver transplant.

11.4 Disorders of amino acid metabolism

Aminoacidopathies

The toxic effects usually arise from the accumulation of metabolites upstream of the defect.

A summary of the main conditions is shown in Table 11.3.

Phenylketonuria (PKU)

The incidence of classical PKU is about 1/12 000 live births in whites but is higher in certain populations (Turkey, Northern Ireland) and lower in others (African-Americans, Finns).

Aetiology

PKU is caused by mutations in *PHA* which encodes the hepatic enzyme phenylalanine hydroxylase responsible for converting phenylalanine to tyrosine. Inheritance is AR. Over 500 different mutations have been identified.

A much rarer form of hyperphenylalaninaemia is caused by disorders of the synthesis or recycling of biopterin, a cofactor for phenylalanine hydroxylase.

Pathophysiology and clinical features

Infants with PKU are clinically normal at birth. Deficiency of phenylalanine hydroxylase causes hyperphenylalaninaemia and low tyrosine levels which, in untreated patients, causes developmental delay, mental retardation, and seizures. There may be fair hair, mousy odour, and eczema.

Neonatal screening

In the UK the newborn blood spot sample is taken between days 5 and 7 of life. About one fifth of infants identified by screening have less severe mutations causing a mild increase in phenylalanine. This is designated *hyperphenylalaninaemia* (HPA). Positive screening tests must be confirmed with a quantitative measure of phenylalanine on a repeat specimen, and investigations done to exclude biopterin defects.

Management

Dietary treatment prevents the neurological impairment and should be initiated by day 21 at the latest.

The diet involves severe restriction of natural protein and supplementation of other amino acids, vitamins, and minerals. Infants can partially breast-feed.

Phenylalanine levels should be monitored weekly to age 6 months, fortnightly from 6 months to 4 years and thereafter monthly to ensure levels are kept within age-defined targets. Dietary compliance becomes more difficult after age 10 years and higher values can be accepted.

Maternal PKU

Untreated PKU often leads to miscarriage or severe fetal damage. Strict control of the diet prior to conception is necessary to prevent microcephaly and heart defects.

Maple syrup urine disease (MSUD)

This is caused by a deficiency of branched-chain keto-acid decarboxylase. Although it affects the catabolism of all three branched-chain amino acids (leucine, valine, and isoleucine), the primary neurotoxic agents are leucine and its keto-acid (2-ketoisocaproic acid).

The condition has acquired its name from the characteristic sweet maple-syrup-like odour that is present. Infants with MSUD usually present with a progressive encephalopathy towards the end of the first week. Although ketosis is characteristic there is generally no significant metabolic acidosis or hyperammonaemia.

The diagnosis can be made from urine organic acid or urine or blood amino acid analysis. Emergency treatment consists of reducing leucine levels as rapidly as possible, which usually necessitates extracorporeal dialysis. Subsequent management is similar to PKU except that branched-chain amino acids are restricted rather than phenylalanine. The long-term outcome can be good if irreversible damage has not occurred during the initial encephalopathy.

Tyrosinaemia type 1

This is caused by mutations in *FAH* encoding fumarylacetoacetase. Tyrosine metabolism is blocked with the accumulation of succinylacetone. Early-onset forms present with liver disease and coagulopathy and a proximal renal tubulopathy. Late-onset presentation is with faltering growth and rickets (secondary to renal Fanconi syndrome). Hepatocellular carcinoma is a risk during childhood.

Diagnosis is based on raised blood tyrosine levels and succinylacetone in urine. Enzyme assay requires liver biopsy. Nitisinone (NTBC) acts by blocking the catabolic pathway proximal to the production of toxic metabolites and reverses the acute complications. It is used together with a low tyrosine diet.

Homocystinuria

This is caused by defects in cystathionine B synthase which is involved in the breakdown of methionine and homocysteine. The clinical features are similar to Marfan syndrome: Marfanoid habitus, stiff joints, ectopia lentis, learning difficulties, intravascular thrombosis.

Table 11.3. Important aminoacidopathies			
Disorder	**Toxic metabolite**	**Presentation**	**Treatment**
Phenylketonuria (PKU)	Phenylalanine	Slowly progressive CNS damage	Diet: restrict phenylalanine
Maple syrup urine disease (MSUD)	Leucine and 2-ketoisocaproic acid	Rapidly progressive encephalopathy	Diet: restrict leucine, isoleucine, valine
Tyrosinaemia type 1	Tyrosine and succinylacetone	Severe and progressive hepatic failure, tubulopathy	Diet: restrict tyrosine and give nitisinone (NTBC)
Glycine encephalopathy	Glycine	Early onset seizures	None effective
Homocystinuria	Homocysteine	Venous thrombosis, ectopia lentis, joint stiffness	Diet: restrict methionine and/or give betaine

Investigation reveals raised plasma homocysteine levels together with raised plasma methionine and homocystinuria.

Protein restriction including a low-methionine diet is instigated in patients identified in screening. About 50% of patients respond to cofactor supplementation with vitamin B6 (pyridoxine). Betaine is used as an alternative methyl donor if the diet is not tolerated.

Glycine encephalopathy (GCE)
This term is preferred to non-ketotic hyperglycinaemia.

GCE is caused by mutations in any of several genes encoding proteins (P, T, or H) in the mitochondrial glycine cleavage system. The classical neonatal form presents with a history of increased fetal movements (in utero seizures), hypotonia, apnoeas, and encephalopathy with seizures. Diagnosis is by measuring the CSF/plasmaglycine ratio.

Treatment with sodium benzoate reduces glycine levels and dextromethorphan, a partial NMDA receptor antagonist, may control seizures in some patients. Prognosis is poor.

Organic acidaemias
Propionic, methylmalonic, and isovaleric acidaemias
These organic acidaemias are caused by enzyme deficiencies involved in the later stages of amino acid catabolism, after the amino group has been removed. Many affected children present with encephalopathy in the neonatal period after a symptom-free period, have a high anion gap, metabolic acidosis, and often a raised blood ammonia. Subsequent episodes can occur with intercurrent infection. Developmental delay is common.

The disorders are differentiated on the basis of the urine organic acid profile, but blood spot acylcarnitine analysis is often useful (and faster!).

Treatment of these disorders is in general by lowering the ammonia, managing the acidosis with bicarbonate, stopping feeds, giving high-calorie fluids (usually 10% dextrose IV) and l-carnitine (to aid excretion of the organic acid by conjugation). Dialysis may be required if these treatments do not control the acidosis and hyperammonaemia, especially in the neonate.

Long-term management is with a low-protein diet, carnitine and in propionic acidaemia and methylmalonic acidaemia, metronidazole (to eradicate propionate-producing bacteria from the gut). Outcome is variable and depends mainly on the presenting illness. Children treated from birth with these conditions (i.e. siblings of known cases) often have a relatively good outcome, although methylmalonic acidaemia is also associated with progressive kidney disease.

Glutaric aciduria type 1
This is caused by a defect in glutaryl CoA dehydrogenase.

There is normal development to about 1 year. Examination reveals macrocephaly, choreoathetosis, and dystonia. Cranial MRI shows bilateral frontotemporal atrophy, subdural haematomas, and white matter hypodensities. The occurrence of subdural haematomas make it important in the differential diagnosis of inflicted head injury.

Diagnosis is made on urine organic acids, acylcarnitine analysis, and enzyme estimation in fibroblasts.

Biotinidase deficiency
Biotinidase cleaves biotin from biocytin, preserving the pool of biotin which is a cofactor for the four human carboxylases. So biotinidase deficiency is associated with *multiple carboxylase deficiency*, the alternative name.

Clinical features may include developmental delay, intractable seizures, skin signs (alopecia, intractable eczematous, scaly rash), and chronic candidiasis.

Diagnosis relies on biotinidase levels, urine organic acid, and acylcarnitine profiles.

❶This condition is important not to miss as it responds to treatment with oral biotin.

Urea cycle disorders (UCDs)
Aetiology
Deficiencies in any of the six enzymes of the urea cycle (N-acetylglutamate synthase, carbamoyl phosphate synthetase, ornithine carbamoyl transferase, arginosuccinate synthetase, arginosuccinate lyase, arginase) result in a failure to excrete excess nitrogen and an accumulation of ammonia, a substance that is highly toxic to the CNS (See Fig 11.3).

The UCDs are AR except for ornithine carbamoyl transferase (OCT) deficiency which is X-linked.

Clinical features
Infants with these disorders typically present with hyperammonaemic encephalopathy some days after birth with lethargy, poor feeding, hyperventilation, vomiting, and coma. The blood ammonia is usually >500 µmol/L. An initial presentation later in life is rarer but can occur, particularly in females with OCT deficiency who may be affected on account of lyonization with inactivation of the non-mutated X-chromosome.

Arginase deficiency has a different presentation, with a progressive spastic diplegia without severe hyperammonaemia.

Diagnosis and management
Specific disorders are differentiated by the pattern of plasma amino acids (especially citrulline levels) and the presence of orotic aciduria in OCT deficiency. Citrulline is low in CPS, NAGS, and OCT deficiency, and high in AS and AL deficiency (see Fig 11.3). Definitive diagnosis requires enzyme estimation (on fibroblasts or liver biopsy) or DNA mutation analysis if available.

Initial treatment of the urea cycle disorders is by stopping protein feeds, promoting anabolism by giving calories as 10% dextrose intravenously, arginine and medications that remove nitrogen by alternative pathways (sodium benzoate and sodium phenylbutyrate). Neonatal hyperammonaemia is rapidly fatal if not recognised and treated aggressively. Even with such treatment the long term neurological prognosis is often poor. Severe hyperammonaemia will usually require requite extracorporeal dialysis.

Long-term management includes:
- Dietary protein restriction
- Arginine supplementation (except in arginase deficiency)
- *Use of alternative pathway substrates:* sodium benzoate, sodium phenylbutyrate
- Carbamylglutamate in NAGS deficiency.

11.5 Mitochondrial and peroxisomal disorders

Inborn errors of metabolism may affect the function of three important cellular organelles: mitochondria, peroxisomes, and lysosomes.

Mitochondrial disorders

Function of mitochondria
Mitochondria are intracellular organelles which produce cellular energy as ATP by oxidative phosphorylation.

They are also involved with most of the major metabolic pathways, housing enzymes responsible for pyrimidine biosynthesis, part of the urea cycle, cholesterol synthesis, and many other pathways.

The term 'mitochondrial disorder' is generally used for one in which the primary abnormality affects the respiratory chain.

Mitochondrial DNA
The mitochondrial genome (mtDNA) is 16 kb long and encodes 13 respiratory chain proteins, 22 tRNAs, and 2 ribosomal RNAs. (see Chapter 12.10). It is maternally inherited.

Mitochondrial respiratory chain disorders
The respiratory chain consists of four protein complexes (I–IV) interlinked within the mitochondrial inner membrane together with complex V (ATP synthase).

The many subunits of the respiratory chain have a dual genetic origin: most are encoded by nuclear DNA, but 13 are encoded by mtDNA. Over 200 mutations in mtDNA are now recognized as causing disease, and mutations in nuclear genes may cause depletion of mtDNA or render it prone to deletions or rearrangements.

Clinical features
Dysfunction of tissues with a high metabolic demand such as the brain, eye, and muscle is most common.

The highly variable and evolving clinical feature of mtDNA diseases arises in part from 'heteroplasmy': the proportion of mutant mtDNA molecules varies between tissues and must exceed a threshold level before dysfunction occurs.

The variety of symptoms and signs which occur and the various syndromes are listed in Tables 11.4–11.6.

Clinical syndromes
Mitochondrial encephalomyopathy, lactic acidosis, stroke-like episodes (MELAS)
Most patients (80%) are heteroplasmic for a point mutation in the *MTTL1* gene, encoding tRNA leucine, but mutations in at least eight other mitochondrial genes are known.

Recurrent migraine-like headaches evolve into stroke-like episodes with hemiparesis and cortical blindness associated with progressive cognitive impairment. Blood and CSF lactase are elevated. Inheritance is maternal.

Myoclonic epilepsy with ragged-red fibres (MERRF)
Most patients (80–90%) are heteroplasmic for a point mutation in the *MTTK* gene, encoding tRNA lysine but mutations in at least six other mitochondrial genes are known. Inheritance is maternal.

Table 11.4. Mitochondrial respiratory chain disease: features by system

Organ/system	Features
Muscular system	Myopathy, rhabdomyolysis
CNS	Seizures, migraine Stroke-like episodes Cerebellar dysfunction Neurodegeneration
Eyes	Ptosis/ophthalmoplegia Cataract, corneal opacities Retinitis pigmentosa
Ears	Sensorineural hearing loss
Cardiovascular	Cardiomyopathy, conduction defects
Kidneys	Proximal tubulopathy
Endocrine	Diabetes mellitus types 1 and 2 Growth hormone deficiency
Gastrointestinal	Intestinal pseudo-obstruction Exocrine pancreatic dysfunction
Bone marrow	Sideroblastic anaemia
Liver	Hepatomegaly, liver dysfunction

Table 11.5. Mitochondrial respiratory chain disease: clinical syndromes due to mtDNA mutations

Mitochondrial encephalomyopathy, lactic acidosis, stroke-like episodes	MELAS
Myoclonic epilepsy with ragged-red fibres	MERRF
Neurogenic muscle weakness, ataxia, retinitis pigmentosa	NARP
Leber hereditary optic neuropathy	LHON
Kearns–Sayre syndrome	KSS
Pearson syndrome	
Leigh syndrome (some cases)	
Aminoglycoside-associated deafness	mI555A→G
Diabetes with deafness	

Table 11.6. Mitochondrial respiratory chain disease: clinical syndromes due to nuclear DNA mutations

Syndrome	Gene
mtDNA depletion:	
Hepatocerebral variant	DGUOK
Myopathic variant	TK2
Alpers syndrome	POLG1
Leigh syndrome	SURFI, PDHA1
Barth syndrome	TAZ (X-linked)

Patients develop myoclonic epilepsy, progressive ataxia and cognitive decline, and muscle weakness. Deafness and optic atrophy also occur. Proliferation of the mitochondria render the muscle fibres 'red' on Gomori trichrome staining.

Leigh syndrome (subacute necrotizing encephalomyelopathy)
This is an early-onset progressive neurodegenerative disorder with characteristic neuropathology: bilateral necrotic lesions in thalamus, brain stem, and spinal cord.

Leigh syndrome shows genetic heterogeneity and is caused by mutations in >20 different genes encoding components of the mitochondrial respiratory chain (complexes I–V) and the pyruvate dehydrogenase complex.

Inheritance of Leigh syndrome may therefore be:
- *Maternal:* mtDNA mutations in nine different genes
- *Autosomal recessive:* mutations in *SURF1* (assembly of complex IV)
- *X-linked:* mutations in *PDHA1* (E1-α subunit of PDH).

Investigations
- *Blood and CSF lactate:* a persistently elevated blood lactate level in a child with multisystem disease should arouse suspicion of a mitochondrial respiratory chain disorder.
- *Investigation of specific organ systems:* cranial MRI, echocardiography and ECG, audiology, electroretinogram, visual evoked responses.
- *Tissue biopsy:* a muscle biopsy is usually preferred, although liver biopsy is sometimes useful. Histology may reveal ragged red fibres and COX-negative fibres. Enzyme assays can be done for complex I, II–III, and IV.
- *Genetic studies:* analysis of nuclear genes or mtDNA is guided by the clinical context and results of enzyme assays. Certain syndromes have a common underlying mtDNA mutation.

Management
The mainstay is supportive and preventative therapy. Oral ubiquinone (CoQ10) can be helpful in complex III deficiency. Bicarbonate is given during episodes of decompensation and acidosis. Genetic counselling is fraught with difficulties and unless a nuclear gene mutation has been identified empirical risks are usually given.

Peroxisomal disorders

Function of peroxisomes
Most mammalian cells contain several hundred peroxisomes, oval bodies bound by a lipid bilayer membrane containing membrane proteins (peroxins) which participate in import of proteins with a peroxisomal targeting signal. Peroxisomes in liver and kidney cells are most active. Catalase, involved in hydrogen peroxide metabolism, is the identifying marker, but >50 biochemical reactions involve the peroxisome.

Peroxisomal functions include:
- β-oxidation of VLCFAs
- Biosynthesis of ether phospholipids (plasmalogens), platelet activating factor, and cholesterol
- α-oxidation of fatty acids.

Peroxisomal disorders
There are two main groups.

Peroxisomal biogenesis disorders (PBDs)
PBDs are due to mutations in the *PEX* genes encoding peroxin proteins necessary for peroxisome biogenesis.
- *Examples:* Zellweger syndrome, infantile Refsum disease.

Zellweger syndrome (ZWS, cerebrohepatorenal syndrome)
ZWS is caused by mutations in any of eight *PEX* genes. Patients have decreased number of peroxisomes, impaired plasmalogen synthesis, and raised levels of VLCFA, bile acids, pipecolic, and phytanic acids.

Clinical features include multiple congenital anomalies, severe psychomotor retardation, seizures, cortical dysplasia, renal cysts, hepatic cirrhosis and cholestasis, and calcific stippling of epiphyses. Survival is limited.

Single-enzyme deficiencies with intact biogenesis
Examples:

Adrenoleucodystrophy (X-ALD)
X-linked adrenoleucodystrophy is caused by mutations in the *ABCD1* gene encoding a transporter molecule involved in the uptake of VLCFAs by peroxisomes.

Clinical phenotypes are diverse and include a cerebral childhood form which presents in mid-childhood with school failure, neurological regression, and progressive dementia, Diagnosis is assisted by measurement of VLCFAs in blood and DNA analysis. Oral administration of a mixture of glyceryl trioleate and trierucate oils (Lorenzo's oil) normalizes plasma VLCFA levels but clinical effects are uncertain. Bone marrow transplantation in the presymptomatic patient may be life-saving.

Refsum disease

There is a defect in the α-oxidation of phytanic acid. Clinical features include retinitis pigmentosa, sensorimotor polyneuropathy, hearing loss, and cerebellar ataxia. It is also known as hereditary sensorimotor neuropathy type IV (HSMNIV). Treatment is with a low-phytanate diet.

11.6 Lysosomal storage diseases

Lysosomal storage diseases (LSDs) are a group of inherited disorders characterized by the intralysosomal accumulation of macromolecules.

There are >50 different LSDs, including:
- Mucopolysaccharidoses (MPS)
- *Sphingolipidoses:*
  - Gaucher disease
  - Niemann–Pick disease
  - Tay–Sachs disease
  - Fabry disease
- Glycogen storage disease type II (Pompe disease)
- *Mucolipidoses:* I-cell disease.

Lysosomes

Lysosomes are subcellular organelles containing a set of catabolic enzymes, mostly hydrolases requiring a low optimum acidic pH (4.8) to function. Lysosomal enzymes are synthesized in the cytoplasm and endoplasmic reticulum and targeted to the lysosome by a mannose-6-phosphate tag.

Lysosomes have a role in the degradation of macromolecules derived from phagocytosis, endocytosis (in which receptor proteins are recycled from the cell surface), and autophagy (in which old organelles or microbes which have invaded the cytoplasm are delivered to the lysosome).

Mucopolysaccharidoses (MPS)

The MPS are a group of disorders caused by deficiency of lysosomal enzymes involved in the degradation of glycosaminoglycans (GAGs), previously called mucopolysaccharides.

The GAGs are sulfated polymers composed of a central protein moiety attached to repeating disaccharide branches. Examples include:

- *Dermatan sulfate:* in many connective tissues
- *Heparan sulfate:* in plasma membranes
- *Keratin sulfate:* in cartilage, cornea
- *Chondroitin sulfate:* in cartilage and cornea.

Stepwise degradation of GAGs requires four glycosidases, five sulfatases, and one non-hydrolytic transferase. The different forms and their corresponding eponyms and enzyme deficiencies are shown in Table 11.7.

Clinical features
Patients appear normal at birth and usually present with developmental delay in the 1st year. Coarse facial features (Fig 11.5), clouding of the cornea, hepatosplenomegaly, and learning difficulties are common. Diagnosis can be made by screening urine for GAGs followed by white cell enzyme assay.

MPS IH (Hurler syndrome)
Hurler syndrome is highly representative of the MPS and is caused by mutations in *IDUA*, encoding α-L-iduronidase. Dermatan and heparan sulfate are found in the urine. Clinical features emerge at 6–24 months:
- Coarse facial features and skeletal deformities (dysostosis multiplex, stiff joints)
- Cardiomyopathy, valvular disease
- Hernias (umbilical, inguinal, femoral) and hepatosplenomegaly
- Corneal clouding and glaucoma, developmental delay and retardation, communicating hydrocephalus
- *ENT problems:* secretory otitis media, deafness.

Early bone marrow transplantation significantly modifies the phenotype. Supportive care is provided for untransplanted patients with particular regard to airway/breathing difficulties. Life expectancy is reduced, with survival >10 years unusual. Enzyme replacement therapy (ERT) is now licensed for non-Hurler phenotypes.

Type		Disorder	Gene	Enzyme	Eye	Brain	Skeletal	Viscera
I	H	Hurler	IDUA	α-L-Iduronidase	√	√√	√	√
	H/S	Hurler/Scheie						
	S	Scheie						
II		Hunter	IDS (X-linked)	Iduronate-2-sulfatase	–	√√	√	√
III	A	Sanfillipo	SGSH	Heparan-N-sulfatase		√√		
	B		NAGLU	N-α-Acetylglucosaminidase				
	C		HGSNAT	α-Glucosaminidase acetyltransferase				
	D		GNS	N-acetylglucosamine-6-sulfatase				
IV	A	Morquio	GALNS	Galactosamine-6-sulfatase	√		√√	
	B		GLB1	β-Galactosidase				
VI		Maroteaux–Lamy	ARSB	Arylsulfatase B	√		√	√
VII		Sly	GUSB	β-Glucuronidase	√	√	√	√

Table 11.7. The mucopolysaccharidoses (MPS)

11.7 Case-based discussions

A neonate with a positive newborn blood spot

A newborn baby is found to have a positive newborn blood spot test for phenylketonuria. The child, now 10 days old, had a Phe of 1200 µmol/L (normal: 64–92) on day 6, with a normal tyrosine level. The parents and midwife are contacted and seen the next day. The child appears very well, and is bottle-feeding well.

What would you tell them and what tests would you do?

The repeat Phe is 1800 µmol/L and the urine shows the presence of phenylketones, confirming the diagnosis as phenylketonuria (PKU). Further blood and urine are taken to exclude the rare atypical forms of PKU (defects in biopterin).

The parents are told about PKU and the formula is stopped, the child now being given milk that contains no phenylalanine. Four days later the level is 300 µmol/L and so small amounts of term formula are introduced to provide sufficient phenylalanine for growth and repair.

The health visitor is requested to arrange to monitor Phe levels weekly to guide the quantities of term formula.

Mother says her sister is pregnant and is worried about the possibility of her baby having PKU.

What advice should be given to her sister?

The mother's sister is counselled about the AR nature of PKU and the 1:4 risks of recurrence with every pregnancy.

Her sister has a 2 in 3 risk of being a carrier for PKU (assuming she was screened at birth and does not have PKU), her partner (assuming non-consanguinity) has the population risk of ~1/50. If both were carriers, there is a 1/4 chance with each pregnancy of having a affected child. This equates to a risk of around 1/300.

What do you know about the newborn blood spot test?

The newborn blood spot test is performed at 5–7 days of age, usually by community midwives. A drop of blood is taken from a heelprick, and the test is used to screen for phenylketonuria (PKU), congenital hypothyroidism, and MCADD, in order to enable treatment to be started by 21 days of age. Sickle cell disease and thalassaemia have been tested for since 2005. In some regions of the UK, galactosaemia, cystic fibrosis, and homocystinuria are also tested for.

These conditions fulfil the criteria for screening of Wilson and Jungner (WHO 1968):

- The condition should be an important health problem for the individual and community
- There should be an accepted treatment or useful intervention for patients with the disease
- The natural history of the disease should be fully understood
- There should be a latent or early symptomatic stage
- There should be a suitable and acceptable screening test or examination
- Facilities for diagnosis and treatment should be available
- There should be an agreed policy on whom to treat as patients
- Treatment started at early stage should be of more benefit than treatment started later
- The cost should be economically balanced in relation to possible expenditure on medical care as a whole
- Case finding should be a continuing process.

The newborn bloodspot test has good sensitivity (high rate of true positives) and specificity (low rate of false positives) for the above conditions.

The introduction of a new screening programme, based on tandem mass spectroscopy, is currently under evaluation. This would test for many inborn errors of metabolism, providing a metabolic profile.

A boy with hypoglycaemia

A 18 month old boy presented to the hospital emergency department after 12 h of a diarrhoea and vomiting illness. The parents were unable to rouse him from sleep at breakfast time so called an ambulance. There is no significant previous medical history but a sibling died unexpectedly at 2 days of age. On examination he is afebrile and the only abnormality is a depressed level of consciousness (responding to pain only). His blood sugar on bedside testing was 1.1 mmol/L. A urine sample tested positive for a trace of ketones.

What is the differential diagnosis?

The most common cause of early morning hypoglycaemia at this age is idiopathic *hyper*ketotic hypoglycaemia (IKH), a condition of uncertain cause in which hypoglycaemia and ketosis occurs after a period of fasting, as occurs overnight. However, although fatty acid oxidation defects are classically *hypo*ketotic ketone production can occur and IKH should be regarded as a diagnosis of exclusion. Hormonal causes include Addison disease (plasma Na^+ usually low) and hyperinsulinism (non-ketotic).

The family history of unexplained death is a vital clue.

What is the immediate management?

A bolus of 10% dextrose (5 mL/kg) is given after appropriate investigations, and a dextrose infusion commenced. The child responds rapidly to the dextrose infusion.

The results of further investigations are as follows:

- Lactate, blood gases, renal and liver function tests normal. Cortisol, insulin, and C-peptide are all appropriate for the blood sugar.
- Urine organic acids show the presence of hexanoylglycine and bloodspot acylcarnitines show an increased level of C_8, octanoylcarnitine.

What is the likely diagnosis?

On the basis of these results a diagnosis of medium-chain acyl-Co dehydrogenase deficiency (MCADD) is made. His older sibling almost certainly died as a result of this condition. An emergency dietary regimen is taught to the parents and the child discharged to a specialist metabolic clinic.

MCADD is now screened for on newborn blood spot in the UK.

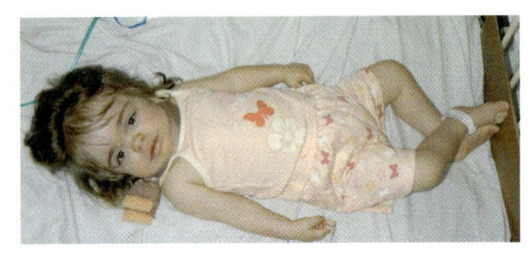

Fig 11.5 MPS 1H: Hurler syndrome.

MPS II (Hunter syndrome)
Hunter syndrome is caused by mutations in *IDS*, encoding iduronate-2-sulfate, and is the only X-linked MPS. Dermatan and heparan sulfate are found in the urine. Incidence is 1/100 000 live births.

The phenotype is variable, ranging from a severe form similar to *MPSIH* (Hurler syndrome), with coarse facial features, short stature, skeletal deformities, and progressive neurological involvement, to a mild variant with preserved intelligence. There is no corneal clouding. ERT is now licensed for Hunter syndrome patients.

Sphingolipidoses

Sphingolipids are a class of lipids derived from sphingosine. Their biological roles include forming a stable outer leaflet of the plasma membrane, cell recognition and signalling, and formation of 'lipid rafts' important in membrane transport. There are three main types:
- Ceramides
- Sphingomyelins
- *Glycosphingolipids*: cerebrosides, gangliosides.

The more important disease entities are listed in Table 11.8.

Table 11.8. Sphingolipidoses

Disorder	Gene	Enzyme
Gaucher disease	GBA	Glucocerebrosidase (acid β-glucosidase)
Niemann–Pick disease		
types A, B	SMPD1	Sphingomyelinase
types C1, D	NPC1	NPCI protein-cholesterol trafficking
Tay–Sachs disease	HEXA	Hexosaminidase A
Fabry disease	GLA	α-Galactosidase A

Gaucher disease
Gaucher disease is caused by mutations in the *GBA* gene encoding glucocerebrosidase. There is intracellular accumulation of glucosylcerebroside primarily within cells of mononuclear phagocyte origin.

It is characterized clinically into three main subtypes which differ in the extent of CNS involvement:
- *Type I: Non-neuronopathic (noncerebral juvenile)*: presents in childhood or later with splenomegaly, hepatomegaly, and pancytopaenia (anaemia, bleeding tendency) due to bone marrow infiltration by 'Gaucher cells'. Skeletal involvement may manifest as pain, deformities, and osteopaenia.
- *Type II: Acute neuronopathic*: early onset in infancy. Severe CNS involvement with bulbar palsy, convergent squint, spasticity, seizures, hepatosplenomegaly.
- *Type III: Subacute neuronopathic*: bulbar involvement with convergent squint and horizontal gaze palsy, hepatosplenomegaly, slow neurological deterioration.

Biochemical abnormalities include high alkaline phosphate, angiotensin-converting enzyme (ACE), and chitotriosidase levels. Bone marrow aspiration may reveal Gaucher cells. The enzyme glucocerebrosidase is assayed in white cells.

For type I and most type III patients, enzyme replacement therapy with mannose-terminated recombinant glucocerebrosidase (given IV) is effective for visceral disease. Bone-marrow transplantation has been useful for neurological manifestations in type III disease. Splenectomy can correct anaemia and thrombocytopaenia.

Niemann–Pick disease
The eponymous term for the sphingomyelinoses, a genetically heterogeneous group of disorders caused by mutations in two different genes: *SMPD1*, encoding acid sphingomyelinase (sphingomyelin phosphodiesterase-1) and *NPC1*, encoding a protein involved in intracellular cholesterol trafficking.

Niemann–Pick types A and B
Mutations in *SMPD1* cause types A and B. More common in Ashkenazi Jews (incidence 1/40 000).
- Niemann–Pick type A, the infantile form, is characterized by hepatosplenomegaly, feeding difficulties, and progressive neurodegeneration; survival is uncommon beyond age 3 years. A cherry-red spot is present in the fundus.
- Niemann–Pick type B occurs in all populations. There is hepatosplenomegaly and pulmonary infiltrates with hypercholesterolaemia. Survival into adulthood is usual.

Diagnostic investigations include bone marrow aspirate for Niemann–Pick cells and assay of acid sphingomyelinase in white cells. Treatment is supportive.

Niemann–Pick types C and D
Niemann–Pick types C1 and D (Nova Scotia variant) are caused by mutations in *NPC1* (95% of type C). The earliest sign is conjugated hyperbilirubinaemia with development of hepatosplenomegaly and progressive neurological deterioration of variable age of onset. A vertical supranuclear gaze palsy is the neurological hallmark of this disease.

Tay–Sachs disease
This disease, also called GM2-gangliosidosis type 1, is caused by mutations in *HEXA*, encoding the α subunit of hexosaminidase A. The classic infantile form presents with developmental regression in the 1st year, hyperacusis, and macrocephaly with a cherry-red spot at the fovea. Progressive spastic quadraplegia leads to death within 2–4 years. Diagnostic investigations include vacuolated lymphocytes and hexosaminidase A assay on white cells.

Fabry disease
This X-linked disorder, also called angiokeratoma corporis diffusum, has an incidence of at least 1/40 000 males and is caused by mutations in *GLA*, encoding α-galactosidase A. Accumulation of glycolipids occurs, especially in lysosomes of the vascular endothelium. Clinical features are more severe in males, but heterozygous female carriers show a variable phenotype depending on X-inactivation.

Presentation in childhood is with episodic pain in the extremities (acroparasthesia), hypohidrosis and angiokeratomas (tiny, painless papules), corneal and lens opacities, fever, fatigue, and exercise intolerance.

Birefringent lipid deposits are seen in urine. Diagnosis is by enzyme assay in leucocytes or mutation analysis in females.

ERT with IV recombinant human α-galactosidase A has been used successfully. Renal failure, cerebrovascular disease, and cardiomyopathy are the most serious long-term complications.

Chapter 12

Genetics

12.1 Genetics and genomics *248*
12.2 Human genetic disease *250*
12.3 Paediatric clinical genetics *252*
12.4 Trisomies: Down, Edwards, and Patau syndromes *254*
12.5 Turner and Klinefelter syndromes *256*
12.6 Microdeletion syndromes: DiGeorge, Williams *258*
12.7 Marfan, Crouzon, and other syndromes *260*
12.8 Neurofibromatosis type 1 and tuberous sclerosis *262*
12.9 X-linked disorders: Fragile X and Rett syndrome *264*
12.10 mtDNA and imprinted gene disorders *266*
12.11 Case-based discussions *268*

12.1 Genetics and genomics

Genetics is the study of heredity. *Genomics* is the study of genomes and their function and seeks to understand the structure and function of the entire genetic complement of an organism based on knowledge of the organism's entire DNA sequence.

Genetics

Chromosomes
In eukaryotes the nuclei of all cells contain a set of chromosomes, each of which is composed of a single long molecule of double-stranded DNA complexed with protein (histones) in the form of chromatin.

Structure of chromosomes
Chromatin allows the immensely long DNA molecules to be packaged in the confined space of the nucleus.

The structure of chromatin varies during the cell cycle:
- *Interphase:* during the period between cell divisions chromatin structure is relaxed to enable DNA to bind regulatory proteins and facilitate transcription. Euchromatin is active and heterochromatin inactive. The chromosomes are invisible.
- *Metaphase:* in the early stage of cell division the chromatin becomes condensed into a compact transportable form. Chromosomes become visible and form the classic four arm structure, a pair of sister chromatids attached at the centromere. The centromere is the site of attachment of the spindle fibres during division.

Chromosomes are classified according to centromere location:
- *Acrocentric:* centromere at one end (13, 14, 15, 21, 22, Y)
- *Metacentric:* centromere in the middle
- *Submetacentric:* intermediate position.

Each chromosome has a short arm labelled p and a long arm labelled q. The tip of each arm is the *telomere*.

The human karyotype
Modern banding techniques allow precise identification of each chromosome. Dyes used stain for A-T (G bands) or G-C (R bands), and a standardized numbering system is used for the G banding pattern (Fig 12.1). 550 bands are resolved routinely.

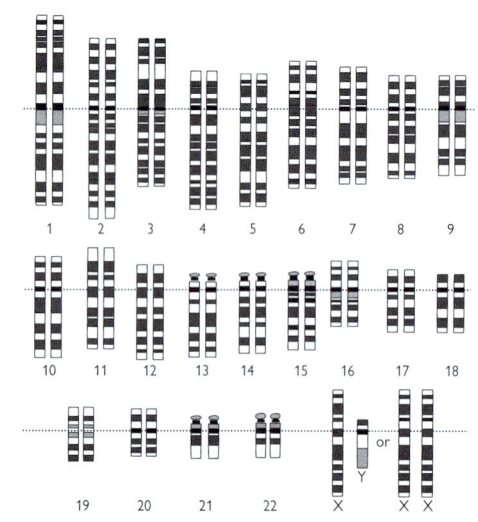

Fig 12.1 Ideogram (G banding) of human karyotype. Note acrocentric chromosomes 13, 14, 15, 21, 22, Y.

Each nucleated somatic cell contains 46 chromosomes: 22 pairs of autosomes (numbered 1–22 by size) and one pair of sex chromosomes: XY for males, XX for females. Humans are therefore diploid organisms with two copies of the nuclear genome in each somatic cell, one from each parent.

Cell division
- *Mitosis:* the process of cell division in somatic cells. It results in diploid daughter cells which are genetically identical to each other and to the original cell.

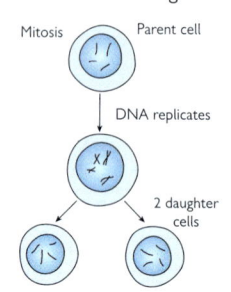

Fig 12.2 Mitosis: results in two diploid daughter cells.

- *Meiosis:* occurs in the germ cells of the gonads and is known as 'reduction division' because it results in four haploid cells each containing just one member (homologue) of each chromosome pair. Moreover, each germ cell is genetically distinct because of the phenomenon of *crossing over*. Meiosis consists of two successive divisions:
  - meiosis I: chromosomes condense, pair up, and exchange genetic material at cross-over points (chiasmata). Chromatids which have exchanged material are called *recombinants*. Homologous chromosomes move to opposite poles and the cell divides into two haploid cells.
  - meiosis II: this resembles a mitotic division resulting in four haploid cells (gametes) (Fig 12.3).

In males, onset of spermatogenesis is at puberty. In females, replication of chromosomes and crossing over begins during fetal life but the oocytes remain suspended before the first cell division until just before ovulation.

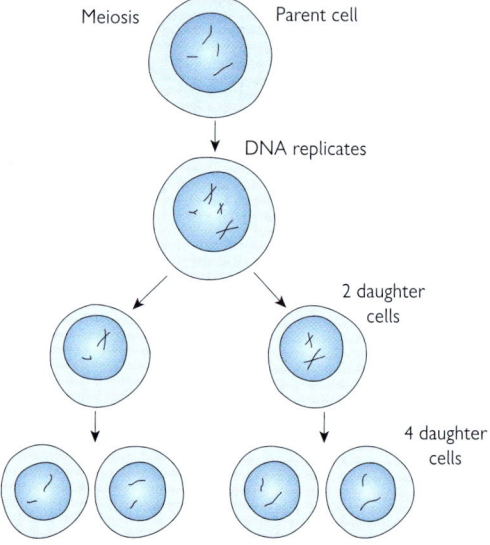

Fig 12.3 Meiosis: results in four haploid germ cells.

Gene to protein
DNA
Deoxyribonucleic acid (DNA) is the genetic material. DNA molecules are paired strands with a double-helical structure composed of four nucleotide bases: adenine (A), thymine (T), guanine (G), and cytosine (C). Bases on opposite strands pair specifically, A-T and G-C (Fig 12.4).

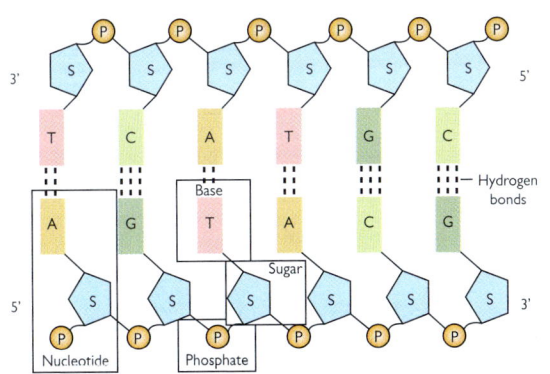

Fig 12.4 DNA: Each nucleotide is composed of a base (A, T, C, or G) a sugar and a phosphate group. Base pairing A-T and G-C occurs by hydrogen bonding.

RNA
Several different forms exist:
- *Messenger RNA (mRNA):* acts as messenger taking information to the ribosome for protein synthesis
- *Transfer RNA (tRNA):* transfers specific amino acids to the ribosome for protein synthesis
- *Ribosomal RNA (rRNA):* structural component of ribosomes
- *Micro RNA (miRNA):* controls expression of target genes.

Protein synthesis
This involves four steps:
- *Transcription:* the coding strand of DNA is transcribed into messenger RNA by the enzyme RNA polymerase.
- *Post-transcriptional processing:* the initial transcript is edited to remove introns and splice together exons. Multiple different transcripts may be produced (alternative splicing).
- *Translation:* at the ribosome the mRNA is translated into a polypeptide chain. A tRNA bound to a specific amino acid recognizes a sequence of three bases (termed a codon) in the mRNA. The correlation between codons and amino acids is the *genetic code*. Some codons are stop signals that terminate protein synthesis.
- *Post-translational modification:* many proteins undergo further modification such as cleavage of the polypeptide chain or the addition of sugar residues (glycosylation).

Genomics: the human genome
A genome is the complete DNA complement of an organism. The human genome is found in all cells except mature red blood cells and encompasses:
- *Nuclear genome:* the DNA in chromosomes in the nucleus
- *Mitochondrial genome:* mitochondrial DNA in the mitochondria in the cytoplasm.

Features of the human genome include:
- *Size:* the haploid human nuclear genome is 3200 million base pairs in length (3200 Mb). It is packaged into 23 chromosomes with DNA molecules ranging in length from 50 to 250 Mb.

The mitochondrial genome (mtDNA) is just 16 000 base pairs long (16 kb) and exists as a circular strand of naked DNA. Each mitochondrion may contain several molecules of mtDNA and a cell may contain several hundred mitochondria.

- *Gene number and size:* the human genome contains ~25 000 genes of which about 5000 are known to be associated with diseases. The average human gene occupies 3000 base pairs (3 kb) of genomic DNA. Enhancer and promoter regions control expression and coding exons are separated by introns. See Fig 12.5.

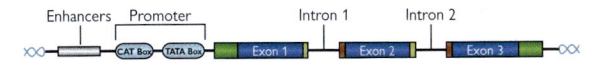

Fig 12.5 Gene structure.

- *Coding DNA:* genes occupy just 2% of the genome
- *Junk DNA:* repeat sequences of uncertain function occupy 50% or more of the genome.

Genetic variation: mutations
Mutations are rare spontaneous alterations in the base sequence of a gene which arise from errors in DNA replication or DNA damage and may alter the phenotype and cause disease. Variants of a gene are called *alleles*. Missense and nonsense mutations commonly cause disease (Fig 12.6)

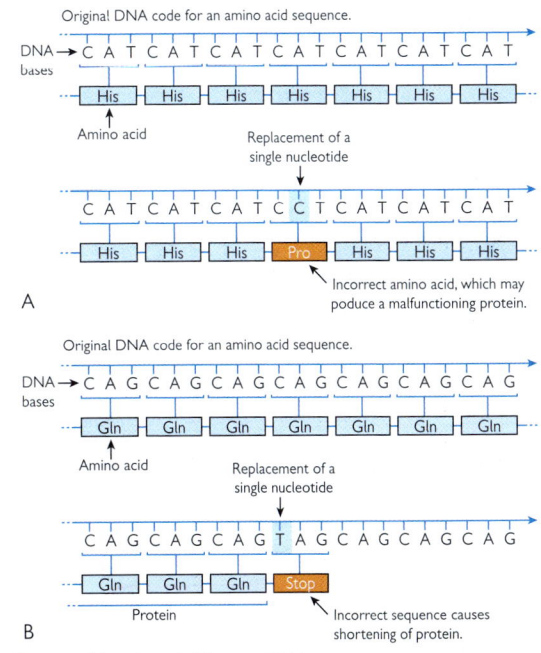

Fig 12.6 Mutations: A. Missense. B. Nonsense.

12.2 Human genetic disease

Phenotype and genotype

The observable characteristics of an individual are termed the *phenotype*. The phenotype is made up of individual traits, a trait being one form of a character. Eye colour is a character, blue or brown eye colour are traits. Phenotypes may be controlled by one or more genes, by the interaction of gene(s) and environment, or by the environment.

A *genotype* is the composition of that part of an individual's genome which contributes to determining a specific trait.

A genotype is determined by observing DNA; a phenotype is determined by observing or investigating a patient.

Genotype and phenotype may or may not be directly correlated (see below). Variable expressivity and penetrance and genetic heterogeneity all disturb the correlation between genotype and phenotype.

Mechanisms of disease

Human genetic diseases can be classified according to the genetic mechanisms into three main groups:
- *Chromosomal disorders:* caused by abnormalities of chromosome structure or number.
- *Single gene (monogenic) disorders:* caused by mutations in a single gene. Most display a mendelian pattern of inheritance, but the exceptions are mutations in mitochondrial DNA and imprinted genes.
- *Multifactorial disorders:* caused by sequence variation in several genes interacting with environmental factors.

A particular disease phenotype may arise from several different genetic mechanisms. For example, there are rare monogenic variants of many multifactorial disorders, and patients with mutations in single genes within chromosomal deletion regions can have a phenotype similar to those with deletions.

Chromosomal disorders

Aberrations of the chromosomes are common and probably affect at least 7.5% of all conceptions. Most are spontaneously miscarried so the live birth frequency is <1%. There may be abnormalities of chromosome number or structure.

Numerical abnormalities: aneuploidy

Aneuploidy may involve autosomes or the sex chromosomes and may include:
- *Trisomy:* an extra copy of a chromosome pair
- *Monosomy:* a missing copy of a chromosome pair.

Aneuploidy usually arises from failure of paired chromosomes to separate at anaphase: non-disjunction. Two cells are produced, one with an extra copy (trisomy) and one with a missing copy (monosomy) of that chromosome. Aneuploidy can arise during mitosis or meiosis. Increased maternal age increases the risk of chromosome aneuploidy. The most common autosomal aneuploidies seen in live births are Down syndrome (trisomy 21), Edwards syndrome (trisomy 18), and Patau syndrome (trisomy 13). Turner syndrome is the most common X chromosome aneuploidy.

Structural abnormalities

Gross changes visible at the microscopic level result from chromosome breakage and can take several forms including deletions, duplications, translocations, inversions, and ring forms.

It has recently emerged that structural variation in the genome including large but submicroscopic insertions and deletions of DNA causing variation in the copy number of genes (CNVs) is widespread and underlies a diverse group of so-called 'genomic disorders'.

- *Translocations:* this most common type of rearrangement may be balanced, containing the correct amount of genetic material or unbalanced, in which chromosomal material has been lost or gained overall. Translocations are further classified into:
  - *reciprocal:* segments distal to breaks in two chromosomes are exchanged. Any pair of chromosomes may be involved. A balanced carrier is usually healthy, unless the breakpoint disrupts a critical gene. There is a risk of unbalanced gametes resulting in miscarriage or liveborn abnormal child.
  - *Centric fusion (Robertsonian):* two acrocentric chromosomes fuse at their centromeres e.g. 13:14, 14:21 (Fig 12.7). Balanced carrier usually healthy, but risk of unbalanced gametes.

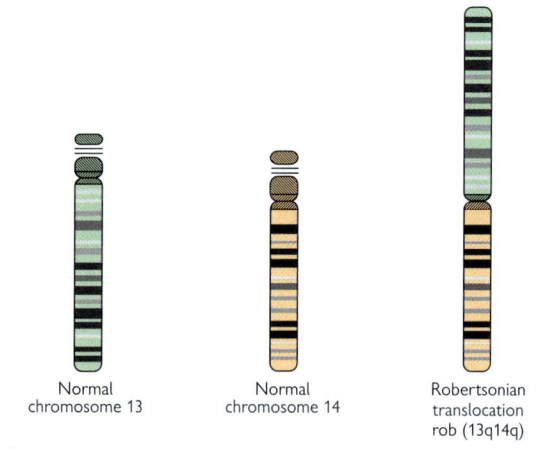

Fig 12.7 Robertsonian translocation 13:14.

- *Deletions:* a portion of the chromosome is missing or deleted. Microdeletions are too small to be seen under the light microscope.
- *Duplications:* a portion of the chromosome is duplicated.
- *Inversions:* a portion of the chromosome has broken off, turned upside down, and re-attached.
- *Rings:* terminal ends of both arms of a chromosome break off and the proximal ends fuse to form a ring.

Mosaicism

A mosaic is an individual with two or more distinct cell lines derived from a single zygote. Mosaicism may be somatic or gonadal. Gonadal mosaicism is a special form in which some gametes, either sperm or oocytes, carry the abnormal genotype and the rest are normal. About 1% of patients with trisomy 21 are somatic mosaics. This is usually due to a nondisjunction event in an early somatic mitosis.

Single-gene disorders: mendelian

If allelic variation at a single gene is necessary and sufficient to produce the disease phenotype, a mendelian pattern is usually seen. Non-mendelian patterns of inheritance occur in traits influenced by mtDNA or by genes subject to genomic imprinting (see below).

Mendelian single-gene disorders display patterns of inheritance consistent with Mendel's laws. It is the particular allele (mutation) which may determine whether a disease displays dominant or recessive inheritance and the gene's location determines whether the pattern is autosomal or X-linked.

Genetic heterogeneity is divided into locus and allelic heterogeneity:

- *Locus heterogeneity*: mutations at different genes cause the same phenotype. The genes may encode proteins involved in the same pathway or subunits of a multimeric protein assembly. One phenotype is caused by mutations in several different genes. Tuberous sclerosis, for example, is caused by mutations in *TSC1* or *TSC2*.
- *Allelic heterogeneity*: different alleles (mutations) at the same gene may cause different phenotypes or the same phenotype with different inheritance patterns (e.g. dominant or recessive). For example, inactivating mutations in *RET* cause Hirschsprung disease, but activating mutations cause multiple endocrine neoplasia (MEN) type 2.

The definitions of expression and penetrance are important:

- *Expression*: variable expression is variation in the severity of the phenotype between individuals within the same family i.e. individuals with the same mutant allele.
- *Penetrance*: is the proportion of heterozygotes or homozygotes who manifest the phenotype, however mildly.

Autosomal dominant (AD) diseases

Disease is manifest in heterozygotes: mutation in one copy of a gene on an autosome. See Box for examples

AD conditions presenting in childhood	
Achondroplasia	Myotonic dystrophy
Alagille syndrome	Neurofibromatosis I
Familial hypercholesterolaemia	Noonan syndrome
Huntington disease (rare)	Tuberous sclerosis
Marfan syndrome	von Willebrand disease

Autosomal recessive (AR) diseases

Disease is manifest in homozygotes: mutations in both copies of an autosomal gene. Most common pattern in diseases arising from mutations in genes encoding enzymes such as inborn errors of metabolism. See Box for examples. AR diseases are discussed in the relevant chapters.

AR conditions presenting in childhood	
Cystic fibrosis	Thalassaemia
Inborn errors of metabolism:	Sickle cell disease
Phenylketonuria	Fanconi anaemia
Congenital adrenal hyperplasia	Ataxia telangiectasia
Galactosaemia	Spinal muscular atrophy
Glycogen storage disorders	Xeroderma pigmentosa
Homocystinuria	Wilson disease

X-linked recessive (XLR) diseases

These arise from mutation in a gene on the X chromosome and affect males because they have just one copy. Females are usually unaffected but may have mild manifestations as a result of lyonization. Most X-linked disorders are recessive. See Box for examples.

XLR conditions presenting in childhood	
Becker muscular dystrophy	G6PD deficiency
Duchenne muscular dystrophy	Haemophilia A and B
X-linked agammaglobulinaemia	Hunter syndrome (MPS II)
Ocular albinism	Wiskott–Aldrich syndrome

X-linked dominant (XLD) diseases

Mutation in one copy of the X chromosome causes disease in females as well as males. Females are more mildly affected and the disorders are often lethal in males. Examples include Rett syndrome, vitamin D resistant rickets, incontinentia pigmenti, and periventricular nodular heterotopia.

Single-gene disorders: non-mendelian

Single-gene disorders may display a non-mendelian pattern if the gene is in the mitochondrial genome or imprinted.

Mitochondrial DNA disorders and genomic imprinting disorders are discussed in Section 12.10.

Multifactorial inheritance

Most common diseases with a genetic aetiology are caused by the interaction of sequence variants at more than one gene (oligogenic 2–5, polygenic >5) and the environment.

The hallmarks of a multifactorial trait include:

- Common in population
- Familial clustering is non-mendelian: frequency in 1st-degree relatives low (2–15%), but higher than population.
- Monozygote twin concordance <100% but higher than dizygote concordance.

Many important childhood onset diseases display multifactorial inheritance (see Table 12.1).

Table 12.1. Childhood multifactorial disorders	
Congenital abnormalities	Cleft lip and palate Neural tube defects Pyloric stenosis
Immune mediated disorders	Atopy Inflammatory bowel disease Diabetes mellitus type I Juvenile idiopathic arthritis
Metabolic disorders	Obesity Diabetes mellitus type 2
Neurological disorders	Epilepsy Autism Attention deficit disorder

12.3 Paediatric clinical genetics

The paediatric clinical geneticist is involved with the diagnosis and management of genetic disorders and has a role in providing information, risk assessment for future pregnancies, and counselling regarding future reproductive options.

Pedigrees and inheritance
When constructing a pedigree, ask about miscarriages, stillbirths, and consanguinity. Take details from both sides of the family and record dates of birth rather than current ages. The symbols in common use are shown in Fig 12.8.

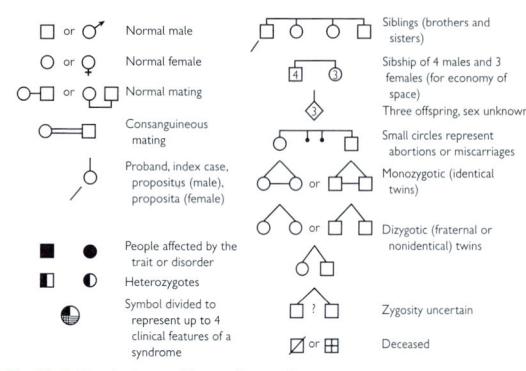

Fig 12.8 Symbols used in pedigree diagrams.

Genetic disorders determined by a single gene and inherited in a mendelian fashion display patterns of inheritance with the following features.

Autosomal dominant (AD)
An affected person usually has an affected parent but variable expression and reduced penetrance (heterozygous carriers who appear normal) may obscure the pattern and *de novo* mutations are common in some disorders.
- High recurrence rate in 1st-degree relatives with multigenerational pedigrees (Fig 12.9)
- Males and females affected equally
- Male to male transmission occurs
- 50% risk to offspring of affected parent.

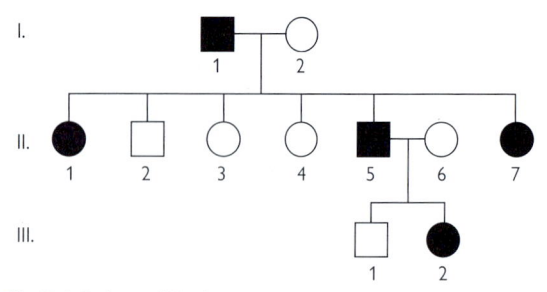

Fig 12.9 Pedigree: AD inheritance.

Autosomal recessive (AR)
Everyone carries some mutated AR genes but close relatives are more likely to carry *the same* mutated gene, so consanguinity increases the likelihood of having children with an AR disease (Fig 12.10). The risk for 1st-cousin parents is increased from 2% to 5%. The carrier rate for specific diseases is increased in certain population groups, e.g. cystic fibrosis in whites, sickle cell disease in Afro-Caribbeans, thalassaemia in Asians and those of Mediterranean origin.
- Parents are both unaffected 'carriers' (heterozygotes)
- 1 in 4 (25%) risk to offspring of two carriers
- Healthy sibling of affected individual has 2/3 risk of being a carrier.

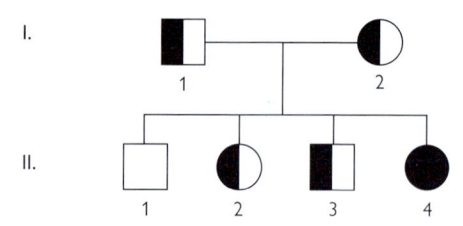

Fig 12.10 Pedigree: AR inheritance.

X-linked recessive
Nearly all affected individuals are male. New mutations are common so the mother of an affected boy with no preceding family history is not necessarily a carrier (Fig 12.11).
- Affected male never transmits the trait to his sons
- Carrier (heterozygous) females usually unaffected, depending on pattern of X-inactivation (lyonization).
- Sons of female carrier have 50% risk of being affected
- Daughters of female carrier have a 50% risk of being carriers
- All daughters of affected males are carriers.

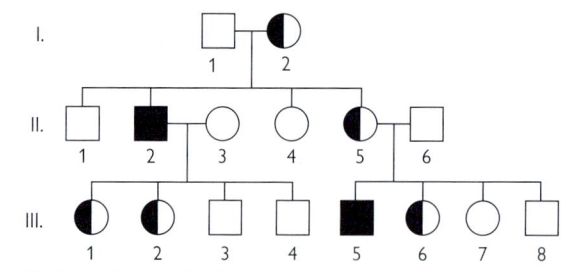

Fig 12.11 Pedigree: X-linked recessive inheritance.

X-linked dominant
Most are rare disorders. Males are so severely affected that there may be *in utero* or perinatal lethality with increase in spontaneous abortions. Heterozygous females manifest the disease but are less severely affected than surviving males (Fig 12.12).

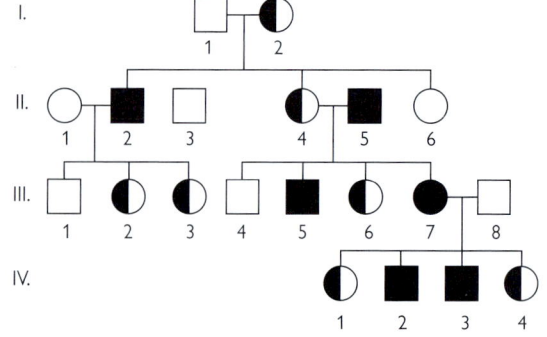

Fig 12.12 Pedigree: X-linked dominant inheritance.

- Affected males transmit the trait to all of their daughters but none of their sons
- Affected heterozygous females transmit the trait to 50% of their children of either sex

Genetic tests
Clinical testing
- *Screening tests:* the population may be screened for carrier detection or affected status. Some prenatal screening is undertaken in the entire population (e.g. ultrasound anomaly scan). Neonatal screening in the UK is for PKU, congenital hypothyroidism, sickle cell disease, cystic fibrosis, and MCADD.
- *Diagnostic tests:* useful for confirmation of a diagnosis suspected on clinical grounds.
- *Predictive tests:* undertaken in a clinically normal individual who is at risk for developing a familial disorder in the future. Special ethical considerations arise in children and adults.
- *Carrier tests:* undertaken to determine risk to offspring but the result usually has no implications for the health of the individual.
- *Preimplantation genetic diagnosis (PGD):* embryos are generated by *in vitro* fertilization. At the 8–16 cell stage a single cell is removed to test for a specific genetic disorder. Only unaffected embryos are re-implanted into the mother. This may be used for couples for whom termination of an affected fetus is unacceptable.

Techniques
Karyotyping
A karyotype is a photomicrograph of an individual's chromosomes arranged in a standard format showing the number, size, and shape of each chromosome. The karyotype can identify abnormalities of the number or structure of the chromosomes. A karyotype may be done on white blood cells, amniocytes or skin fibroblasts. The limit of resolution is 4 Mb. The chromosomes must be in metaphase, so cultured dividing cells are required.

Fluorescence in situ hybridization (FISH)
In situ hybridization is the annealing of specific single-stranded DNA probes to complementary sequences in immobilized chromosomes (i.e. in situ). If the probes are visualized by labelling the probes with a fluorescent dye, the procedure is termed FISH.

Probes may be locus specific, specific for centromeric repeats or cover an entire chromosome or the entire genome (CGH: comparative genome hybridization).

FISH is useful for detection of microdeletion syndromes, detailed characterization of chromosome structural abnormalities, trisomy detection and rapid sexing. It can be applied to interphase chromosomes (Fig 12.13).

Mutation analysis
Direct analysis of DNA for specific detection of disease mutations is increasingly available. Amplification of the DNA using the polymerase chain reaction (PCR) is frequently the first step. Specific probes bracket the target DNA sequence and repeat cycles lead to exponential amplification (Fig 12.14).

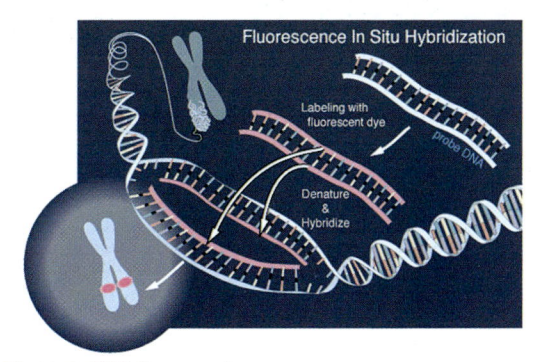

Fig 12.13 FISH. Courtesy of www.genome.gov.

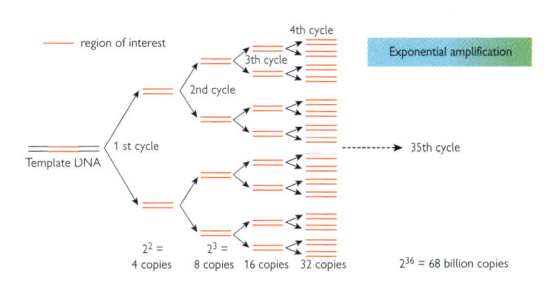

Fig 12.14 PCR amplification of specific DNA sequences.

Genetic counselling and ethics of testing
Genetic counselling involves giving advice or information on:
- Mechanisms of inheritance of a disease
- The recurrence risks of a disease within a family
- Advice on antenatal screening
- Advice on reproductive options
- Advice on predictive testing of children.

Counselling should be non-directive. The genetic testing of children raises special issues. A young child may be unable to give informed consent and testing for a late-onset disorder would not usually be considered in childhood. The decision to test for conditions that manifest in childhood lies with the parents. Specific issues arise in several contexts:

Predictive testing
Tests exist that may allow presymptomatic testing of a healthy child for a disease which may have onset in childhood or in adult life. Considerations include: existence or not of a presymptomatic medical treatment; performing the investigation deprives the child of the right to decide when they are older; potential psychological harm of a healthy child being labelled as 'sick'.

It is generally agreed that predictive testing for adult-onset conditions for which there is no presymptomatic medical treatment, e.g. Huntington disease (HD), should not be done. For childhood-onset conditions the situation is less clear and parents should have the right to make an informed choice.

Carrier testing
By definition, this usually has no implications for the health of an individual being treated but may have a larger effect on reproductive decisions. Ideally, children should be tested only when of an age to be involved with the decision. In most cases therefore, the issue of carrier status is best dealt with at puberty or when the child becomes sexually active.

12.4 Trisomies: Down, Edwards, and Patau syndromes

The most common autosomal aneuploidies seen in live births are:
- *Down syndrome:* trisomy 21
- *Edwards syndrome:* trisomy 18
- *Patau syndrome:* trisomy 13.

The gene-poor nature of these three chromosomes probably enhances survival to birth.

Down syndrome (DS)

This is the most common and best known human chromosomal disorder. It is named after John Langdon Down, a British doctor who first described it in 1866.

The overall incidence is approximately 1/1000 live births, but the incidence varies markedly with maternal age:
- *17 years:* 1 in 1550
- *35 years:* 1 in 385
- *40 years:* 1 in 106
- *45 years:* 1 in 30.

Aetiology

Down syndrome is caused by the presence of all or part of an extra chromosome 21. The exact genetic basis varies:
- *Trisomy 21 (95%):* caused by nondisjunction at meiosis; 90% are nondisjunction in the maternal gamete.
- *Robertsonian translocation (3%):* usually long arm of chromosome 21 attached to chromosome 14 or to itself. There is no maternal age effect and the translocation may be maternal or paternal in origin. 75% de novo, 25% familial.
- *Mosaicism (2%):* a nondisjunction event during early cell division in a normal embryo leads to a fraction of cells with trisomy 21. The fraction varies and influences phenotype severity.
- *Duplication (<1%):* rarely, a region of chromosome 21 is duplicated, e.g. dup 21 (q22.1–22.2) is sufficient to cause DS and is called the Down syndrome critical region (DSCR). Chromosome 21 contains about 350 genes but the DSCR is believed to harbour the major genes involved in DS.

Clinical features

There are phenotypic features which are characteristic together with common associated defects and common medical complications.

Phenotypic features
- *Dysmorphic facies:* epicanthic folds, upslanting palpebral fissures, Brushfield spots in the iris, short nose with depressed nasal bridge, protruding tongue, brachycephaly
- *Other features:* hypotonia (especially in newborn), single palmar crease (Fig 12.15), 5th finger clinodactyly, sandal gap (between hallux and 2nd toe).

Associated defects
- *Cardiac defects in 40–50%:* common defects include endocardial cushion defects (43%), VSD (32%), secundum ASD (10%), Fallot's tetralogy (6%), isolated PDA (4%). About 70% of all endocardial cushion defects are in DS patients.
- *GI system defects:* duodenal atresia or stenosis, Hirschsprung disease (<1%), tracheo-oesophageal fistula, imperforate anus
- *Eyes:* congenital cataracts
- *Genitourinary tract:* hypospadias, cryptorchidism.

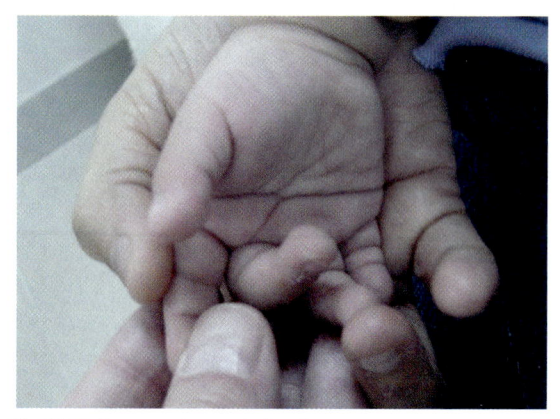

Fig 12.15 Down syndrome: single palmar crease.

Diagnostic investigations

A clinical diagnosis requires confirmation by cytogenetic studies, including karyotyping of the infant and parent if a translocation is present. Interphase FISH or quantitative fluorescence PCR (QF-PCR) may provide rapid diagnosis.

Prenatal screening

Screening is offered to women of all ages. Even the best non-invasive screens have a sensitivity of only 90–95% and false positive rates of 2–5%. A nuchal translucency scan is done at 11–13 weeks. Maternal serum markers (α-fetoprotein, unconjugated oestriol, total human chorionic gonadotropin (hCG)) can be measured between 10 and 18 weeks gestation.

If the screening test shows a risk of less than 1/250 (low risk) a diagnostic test is not offered. If the screening tests give a risk of greater than 1/250 (high risk) a diagnostic test is offered. About 1/20 (5%) of women screened have a high-risk result.

Diagnostic tests include chorionic villus sampling (CVS) or amniocentesis (after 15 weeks gestation) followed by QF-PCR and/or full karyotyping.

Management

Important aspects of management include:

Genetic counselling

Recurrence risk for trisomy 21 is 1% and for a *de novo* Robertsonian translocation is 2–3%. For a Robertsonian carrier parent the theoretical risk of affected liveborn is 1/3. Actual recurrence rate is 10–15% for carrier mothers and 2–3% for fathers.

Investigations: at diagnosis
- Cardiac echo, thyroid function tests, immunoglobulin levels
- Ophthalmological examination, hearing tests.

Medical follow up

This is designed to screen for and manage the many complications that occur.
- *Central nervous system:* moderate to severe learning difficulties occur, but cognitive development is quite variable. The prevalence of psychiatric disorders is 17% in children and 27% in adults. Increased risk of autism, ADHD, conduct disorder, and obsessive compulsive disorder. Epilepsy occurs in 5–10%. An Alzheimer-like dementia may develop early

with prevalence of up to 25% at 50 years, 50% at 60 years, 75% >60 years. Speech and language therapy.
- *Respiratory tract/ENT:* obstructive sleep apnoea, dental problems, chronic otitis media, hearing loss.
- *Eyes:* refractive errors, strabismus, blepharitis, cataracts
  - annual ophthalmic and audiological evaluation.
- *Endocrine:* short stature and obesity, hypothyroidism (16–20%), diabetes, decreased fertility (near complete in males)
  - *monitor growth:* Down syndrome charts available.
- *Skeletal:* atlantoaxial instability (14%) can lead to spinal cord compressions, acquired hip dislocation (6%)
  - cervical radiography to detect atlanto-axial instability at 3 years.
- *Haematological:* risk of acute leukaemia increased × 50. Acute myeloid leukaemia (AML) as common as acute lymphoblastic leukaemia (ALL). Transient neonatal leukaemoid reactions are common.
- *Immune function:* immunodeficiency, impaired cellular immunity, increases risk of infectious disease
  - screen for autoimmune disorders: hypothyroidism, coeliac disease, diabetes.
- *Skin problems:* hyperkeratotic lesions, alopecia areata, vitiligo, recurrent skin infections.

Prognosis
Outlook is much improved with better integration and increased longevity. Congenital heart disease is the main cause of early mortality. Many develop Alzheimer-like dementia by age 40 years.

Edwards syndrome: trisomy 18

Trisomy 18 has an incidence of 1/3000 conceptions and 1/6000 live births. 95% are trisomy 18 due to meiotic non-disjunction. 5% are translocations or mosaics.

Clinical features are variable but include:
- Intrauterine growth retardation
- *Dysmorphic facies:* micrognathia, narrow palpebral fissures, ptosis, ocular hypertelorism, microcephaly, cleft lip/palate, low-set or malformed ears
- *Skeletal abnormalities:* rocker-bottom feet, over-riding fingers, clenched fists, absent radius or thumbs
- Cardiac and renal anomalies.

Edwards syndrome is frequently diagnosed prenatally. The triple test may indicate increased risk and a targeted ultrasound may identify markers such as the rocker-bottom feet.

50% die *in utero*. Of liveborn infants 50% live to 2 months and 5–10% to 1 year.

Patau syndrome: trisomy 13

This is the least common of the autosomal trisomies. The incidence is 1/9500 live births. 90% are trisomy 13 due to meiotic non-disjunction; 5–10% are Robertsonian translocations, usually 13:14; <5% are mosaics.

Clinical features include:
- *Dysmorphic facies:* holoprosencephaly, microcephaly, low-set ears, structural eye defects, microphthalmia
- Cleft lip/palate
- *Skeletal abnormalities:* rocker-bottom feet, postaxial polydactyly

- Cardiac and renal anomalies
- Omphalocoele, cutis aplasia.

Screening tests in the 1st trimester may indicate high risk. Diagnosis may be suspected on the fetal anomaly scan at 20 weeks. Confirmatory diagnosis is by karyotype or QF-PCR.

Median survival is 7–10 days, 90% dying within the 1st year.

12.5 Turner and Klinefelter syndromes

Turner syndrome (45,X)

The classic karyotype of Turner syndrome is 45,X. The incidence is about 1/2500 live female births, but as many as 15% of spontaneous abortions have a 45,X karyotype.

Aetiology

The condition is usually sporadic. In 80% of cases the paternal X chromosome is missing. Variants of the karyotype include:
- *Mosaics:* 46,XX/45,X or 46,XY/45,X
- Structural abnormalities of the second X chromosome which may be inheritable or a ring X chromosome which may cause a more severe phenotype.

Patients with Y chromosome material have a high risk of gonadoblastoma.

Clinical features

The hallmarks, present in 95% of patients are short stature and ovarian failure. Diagnosis may be prenatal, neonatal, or during childhood and the presenting features are different at each age.

Prenatal diagnosis
- Elevation of hCG, oestradiol, or α-fetoprotein raises the possibility of Turner syndrome.
- Ultrasound features include: cystic hygroma or rasied nuchal translucency, non-immune fetal hydrops (Fig 12.16), horseshoe kidney and left-sided cardiac anomalies
- A karyotype by amniocentesis or CVS confirms the diagnosis.

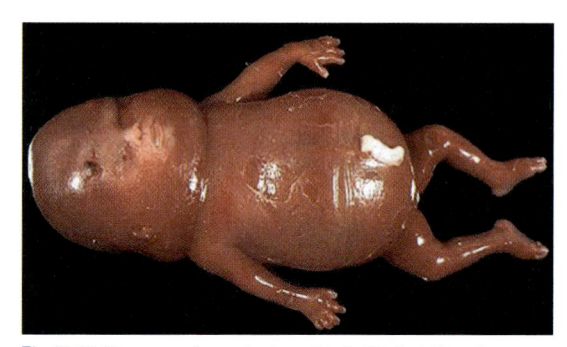

Fig 12.16 Turner syndrome: hydrops fetalis. Medical Genetics (Second Edition); Jorde, Carey, Bamshad, and White (2000) © Mosby.

Newborn
Phenotypic features may include neck webbing, lymphoedema, low posterior hairline, shield chest and widely spaced nipples, coarctation of the aorta, loose folds of skin particularly in neck and oedema of hands and feet.

Childhood
Turner syndrome is often diagnosed during investigation of short stature or delayed puberty. Important features (Fig 12.17) include:
- *Short stature:* <11 years some girls have normal growth but the adolescent growth spurt fails.
- *Ovarian failure:* no breast development by 12 years and no menarche by 14 years. LH and FSH levels are raised. Pubic hair development is normal. Ovarian dysgenesis is present.

- *Skeletal system:* cubitus valgus, short 4th metacarpal or metatarsal, shield chest. Hip dislocation (in infants), scoliosis (10% of adolescent girls).
- *Cardiovascular system:* left-sided lesions: coarctation of aorta, bicuspid aortic valve.
- *Renal system:* horseshoe kidney, collecting duct anomalies in 30%.
- *Webbing of neck:* broad neck and low or distinct hairline.
- *Skin and nail:* hypoplastic or hyperconvex nails and multiple pigmented naevi.
- *Eyes and ears:* ptosis, strabismus, amblyopia, and cataracts are more common.

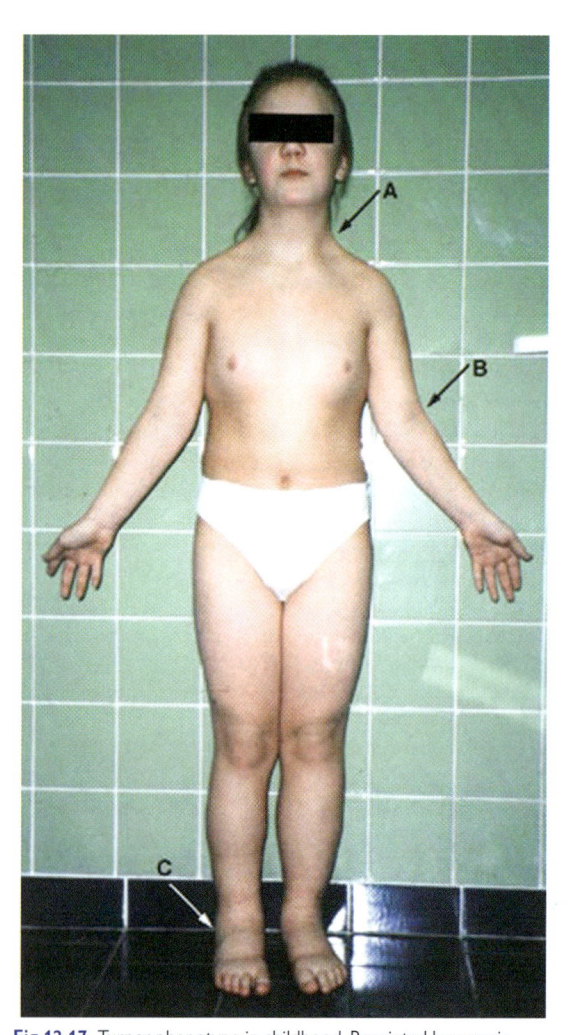

Fig 12.17 Turner phenotype in childhood. Reprinted by permission from Macmillan Publishers Ltd: Nature Clinical Practice Endocrinology & Metabolism: Gawlik and Malecka–Tendera; Hormonal theraphy in a patient with a delayed diagnosis of Turner's syndrome 4, 173–177, © 2008.

Management

Diagnosis is confirmed by karyotyping. Multidisciplinary management is designed to detect and treat the many complications to which these children are prone.

Genetic

- Test for Y chromosome material using a Y-centromeric probe. Monitor for gonadoblastoma and consider prophylactic gonadectomy.

Endocrine

- Growth hormone is given before the epiphyses are fused to increase adult height. Oestrogen replacement therapy is usually started from age 12–15 years
- Thyroid function tests at diagnosis and monitor 1–2 yearly
- Screen for diabetes mellitus and prevent obesity
- Measure bone density in adolescents as osteoporosis is common.

Cardiovascular

- Cardiac echocardiography and evaluation at diagnosis
- Significant cardiac anomalies may require surgical intervention. Cardiovascular evaluation should be repeated every 5 years to assess the risk of aortic dissection.

Renal

- Girls with horseshoe kidneys have an increased risk of Wilms tumour and should have regular renal ultrasound
- Yearly urine culture, creatinine, urea and electrolyte monitoring. Monitor blood pressure.

Psychological

- Intelligence and mental health is usually normal but counselling and support may be required concerning short stature and infertility.

Klinefelter syndrome (47,XXY)

Affects 1/600 liveborn males. The karyotype is 47,XXY. Phenotypic features become apparent at puberty (Fig 12.1 8).

- Tall stature due to delayed closure of epiphyses
- Secondary sexual characteristics show variable development and there is poor growth of facial and body hair
- Small testes, azoospermia, low testosterone levels
- Gynaecomastia, female fat distribution, high-pitched voice
- Mild developmental and behavioural problems with cognitive function normal or low normal (20%).

47, XXY is a leading cause of male infertility and testosterone deficiency, yet most reach adulthood without diagnosis. There is an increased risk of breast cancer and autoimmune disorders.

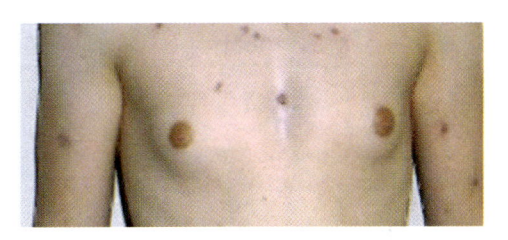

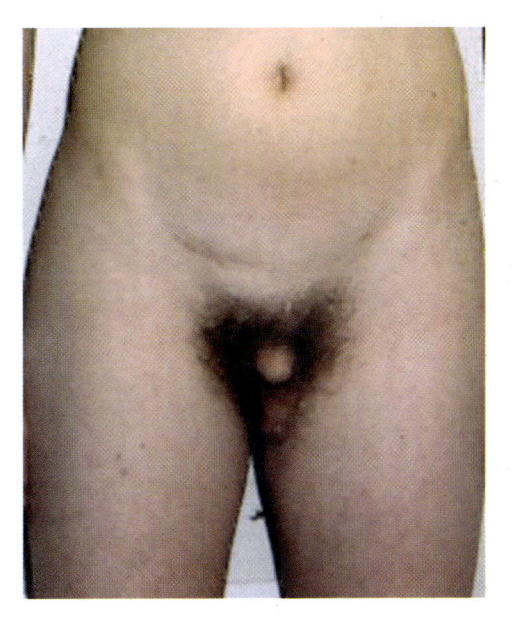

Fig 12.18 47, XXY: adolescent with small testes and gynaecomastia. Image reprinted with permission from eMedicine.com, 2008. Available at http://www. emedicine.com/ped/topic 1252.htm.

12.6 Microdeletion syndromes: DiGeorge, Williams

Microdeletion syndromes are caused by deletions too small to be seen under the microscope by conventional cytogenetic methods, i.e. <4 Mb. They arise because the chromosomal regions concerned contain low copy number repeats, which leads to unequal pairing of chromosomes at meiosis with formation of deletions or duplications. The most well known are:

- *DiGeorge syndrome:* del 22q11
- *Williams syndrome:* del 7q11.23
- *Smith–Magenis syndrome:* del 17p11.2
- *Wolf–Hirschhorn syndrome:* del 4p
- *Cri-du-chat syndrome:* del 5p15.2

22q11 deletion syndromes

Microdeletions of the chromosome 22q11 region cause a spectrum of developmental defects attributable to abnormal development of the 3rd and 4th branchial arches. The prevalence is 1 case per 3000 persons. The best known is DiGeorge syndrome.

The phenotype is variable, but the hallmarks are a combination of dysmorphic facies, congenital heart defects, immunodeficiency, and hypocalcaemia caused by hypoplasia of thymus and parathyroids.

Genetics

This is the most common contiguous gene deletion syndrome in humans. 90% of patients have a microdeletion of ~2 Mb at 22q11.21–22q11.23 including a 250 kb DiGeorge critical region (DGCR) (Fig 12.19).

The T-box transcription factor gene *TBX1* is implicated in the cardiac lesions and some patients have mutations in *TBX1* rather than a detectable genomic deletion.

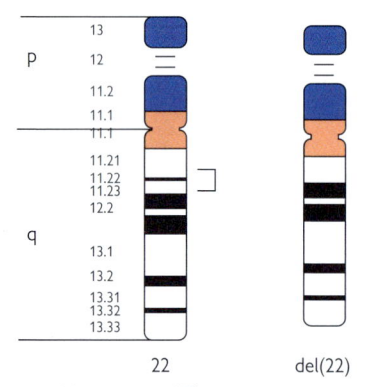

Fig 12.19 22q11 deletion region.

Phenotype

A number of distinct but overlapping phenotypes are recognized:
- DiGeorge syndrome (DGS)
- Velocardiofacial syndrome (VCFS, Schprintzen syndrome)
- Conotruncal anomaly face syndrome (CAFS).

The main features of DiGeorge syndrome are:
- *Facies:* prominent nose, wide nasal bridge, short philtrum, micrognathia, hypertelorism, short palpebral fissures (Fig 12.20).
- *Otolaryngic:* low-set ears, defective pinnae, cleft palate (9%), velopharyngeal insufficiency, fissures, hooding of upper eyelids, antimongoloid slant.

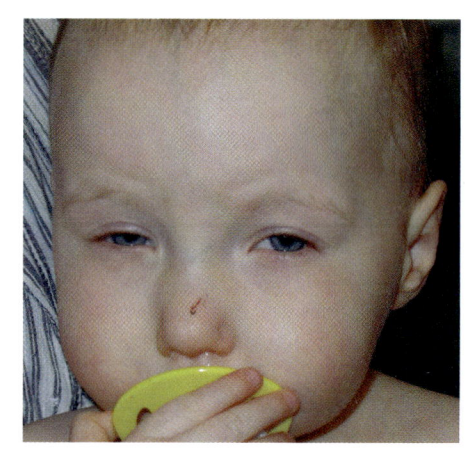

Fig 12.20 DiGeorge syndrome, 22q11 deletion: facies.

- *Cardiovascular defects:* in 75% of patients, especially conotruncal anomalies including tetralogy of Fallot (17%), VSD and interrupted aortic arch (14%), pulmonary atresia/VSD (10%), truncus arteriosus (9%). These are a major cause of mortality.
- *Immunodeficiency:* in 80% of patients. Thymic hypoplasia or aplasia leads to defective T-cell function (mitogen responsiveness) and numbers. Humoral defects may also be present. Immune function should be checked before giving live vaccines or non-irradiated blood transfusions. Increased susceptibility to systemic fungal infections and disseminated viral infections.
- *Hypoparathyroidism/hypocalcaemia:* parathyroid hypoplasia leads to hypocalcaemia in the neonatal period in 60% of patients. This may cause tetany or convulsions.
- *Renal anomalies:* in 30% of patients. Include renal agenesis and horseshoe kidney. A renal ultrasound should be performed at diagnosis.
- *Behavioural problems/learning difficulties:* behavioural problems present in many patients and psychiatric disorders including schizophrenia and bipolar disorder may develop. 60% have learning difficulties.

Skeletal abnormalities, hearing loss, growth hormone deficiency, and autoimmune conditions (e.g. eczema) may occur as complications.

Management

Diagnosis is confirmed by FISH or multiplex ligation-dependant probe amplification (MLPA). A parent is affected in about 12% of cases and testing should be offered.

Initial investigations in a newborn should include:
- *CXR:* to assess thymic shadow
- *Parathyroid evaluation:* parathyroid hormone (PTH) levels and plasma calcium levels
- Cardiac echocardiography
- *Immunological tests:* T-cell numbers and proliferative response to mitogens and antigens; immunoglobulin levels (B-cell development requires normal T-cell function).

Management may include:
- Surgical treatment of cardiac malformations
- Calcium supplements and vitamin D

- Prophylactic regimes for T- and B- cell deficiency
- Developmental surveillance
- Speech therapy and pharyngoplasty for velopharyngeal insufficiency.

Williams syndrome

The incidence is 1 /10 000 births and most cases are sporadic. The syndrome is also called Williams–Beuren syndrome (WBS) and is a contiguous gene deletion syndrome associated most usually with a hemizygous deletion of a 1.5 Mb region encompassing at least 17 genes at 7q11.23. Two genes known to be important are the elastin gene *(ELN)* and the LIM kinase-1 gene *(LIMK1)*.

Phenotype
Facies: small upturned nose, long philtrum, wide mouth, small chin, stellate (white-lacy pattern) iris in blue and green-eyed children (Fig 12.21).

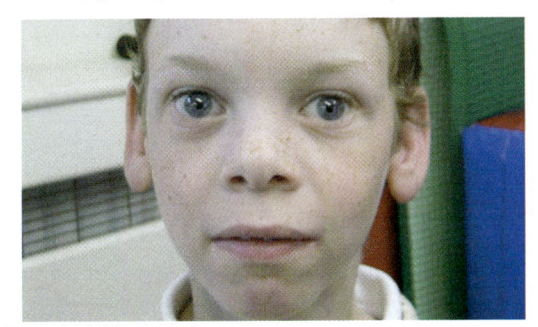

Fig 12.21 Williams syndrome.

- *Cardiovascular malformations:* supravalvular aortic stenosis (SVAS) is most common and ranges from trivial to severe. Pulmonary artery stenosis may also occur. The elastin gene is implicated.
- *Hypercalcaemia:* the exact frequency and cause of the hypercalcaemia which occurs in some patients is unknown. If present it may be associated with extreme irritability and usually resolves spontaneously.
- *Personality and cognitive function:* patients are sociable and endearing (very polite) with well-developed expressive language skills. Most have some developmental delay and learning difficulties. Older children display strengths (speech, social skills, long-term memory) and weaknesses (impaired fine motor and visuospatial cognition). *LIMK1* hemizygosity is implicated in the latter.
- *Miscellaneous:* hypertension due to generalized arteriopathy or renal artery stenosis, renal anomalies, hyperacusis, hernias; musculoskeletal problems: hypotonia, joint laxity, contractures. Intrauterine growth retardation/failure to thrive.

Management
Diagnosis is confirmed by FISH or MLPA (Fig 12.22). Routine karyotyping should be done and mutation analysis of *ELN* may be indicated. If one parent is affected the recurrence risk is 50% as the deletion behaves in an AD manner.

Initial investigations should include: cardiac echo, renal ultrasound, and baseline serum calcium and renal biochemistry.

Multidisciplinary management involves monitoring for hypertension and hypercalcaemia. Supravalvular aortic stenosis requires lifelong cardiac follow-up.

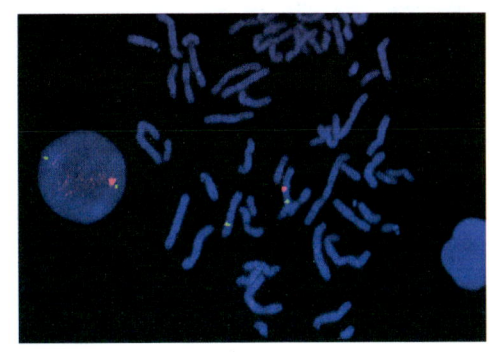

Fig 12.22 FISH analysis: green control probe identifies two copies of chromosome 15. Red probe hybridizes to only one copy of chromosome 7, indicating deletion in Williams region.

Smith–Magenis syndrome (SMS)

This is caused by a microdeletion at 17p11.2. The incidence is 1/25 000 live births.

Most cases are sporadic but occasionally one parent carries a 'balanced' rearrangement so parental chromosomes should be checked. Characteristic facies are associated with severe behavioural difficulties.

- *Facies:* flat broad head, heavy brows, depressed nasal bridge, wide mouth. Hoarse deep voice, short stature, and eye problems may be present.
- *Behavioural problems:* self-injurious behaviour, hyperactivity and severe sleep disturbance. Autistic features.

Wolf–Hirschhorn syndrome

This syndrome is caused by a deletion of the tip of the short arm of chromosome 4 (del4p). The incidence is 1/90 000 births.

There may be a parental 'balanced' rearrangement. The phenotype is variable but includes dysmorphic facies: broad nasal bridge, hypertelorism, small chin, 'Greek helmet' profile, epilepsy and learning difficulties, cleft lip and/or palate, heart defects, and hypospadias

Cri-du-chat syndrome

This syndrome is caused by deletion of the chromosome 5p15.2 region. Most are sporadic (deletions) but 10–15% are inherited (parental translocations). The incidence 1/37 000 births. High-pitched monochromatic cat-like cry at birth gives rise to the name. Facies are round with hypertelorism, low-set ears, and prominent epicanthal folds. The phenotype becomes less striking with age (Fig 12.23). Learning difficulties and self-injurious behaviour may emerge.

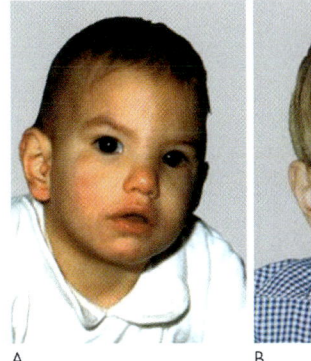

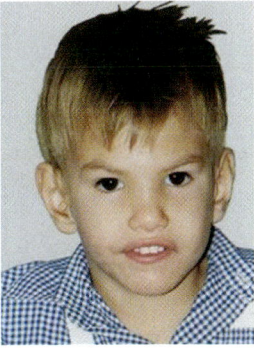

Fig 12.23 Cri-du-chat syndrome: A. At 8months. B. At 2 years.
Source: Orphanate Journal of Rare Diseases.

12.7 Marfan, Crouzon, and other syndromes

Marfan syndrome (MFS)
This is an AD disorder of connective tissue with an incidence of 1/5000 births.

Genetics
Classical Marfan syndrome (MFS1) is caused by mutations in the gene encoding fibrillin, *FBN1* on chromosome 15q.

Over 500 different mutations have been identified. MFS1 is fully penetrant but the clinical phenotype is variable. 25% of patients are sporadic with a *de novo* mutation.

A similar phenotype (MFS2) is caused by mutations in the *TGFBR2* gene on chromosome 3p. Beal congenital contractural arachnodactyly is caused by mutations in *FBN2*.

Pathogenesis
Fibrillin is a constituent of microfibrils which are the structural components of the suspensory ligament of the lens and act as substrates for elastin in the aorta and other connective tissues. Mutant fibrillin monomers disrupt multimerization necessary for microfibril formation: a dominant negative effect.

Deficient fibrillin deposition reduces the structural integrity of the aortic wall, lens zonules, ligaments, lung airways, and spinal dura.

Clinical phenotype and diagnosis
There is a severe neonatal form with aortic dilatation present from birth but diagnosis (in the absence of a family history) usually becomes apparent in mid childhood. However, clinical diagnosis is challenging due to phenotypic variability and the age-dependent nature of some features, and children may need to be kept under review.

Children may present with visual problems, cardiac signs, skeletal problems, delayed motor milestones, spontaneous pneumothorax, or back pain due to dural ectasia.

In difficult cases formal clinical diagnosis relies on the Ghent criteria. Features by system include:

Skeletal
- Pectus carinatum or pectus excavatum (Fig 12.24)

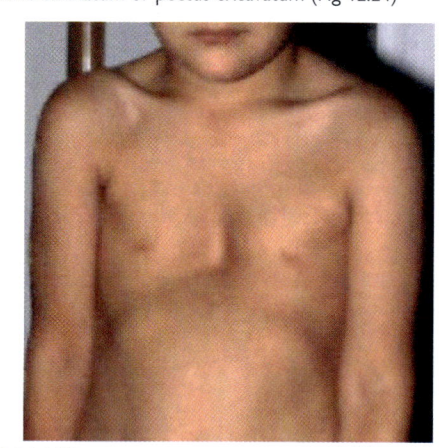

Fig 12.24 MFS: pectus excavatum.

- Upper to lower body segment ratio <0.85 or arm span to height ratio >1.05
- Arachnodactyly demonstrated by positive wrist or thumb signs (Fig 12.25). Thumb projects beyond ulnar border when

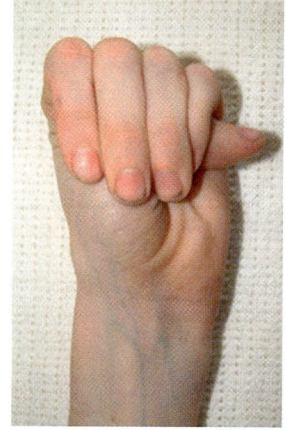

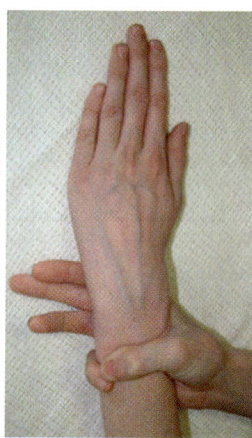

Fig 12.25 MFS: Positive thumb (A) and wrist (B) signs.

opposed in clenched hand. Wrist sign positive if distal phalanges of thumb and little finger overlap when wrapped round opposite wrist.
- Scoliosis and joint hypermobility
- *Typical facies:* dolichocephaly, high arched palate with dental crowding, malar hypoplasia, enophthalmos, retrognathia, down-slanting palpebral fissures
- *Ocular:* ectopia lentis (lens dislocation) present in 50%, flat cornea, increased axial length of globe, hypoplastic iris or ciliary muscle
- *Cardiovascular:* aortic root dilatation in 70–80%, dissection of ascending aorta, mitral valve prolapse, dilatation of main pulmonary artery
- *Dura:* dural ectasia (widening of the dural sac), usually in the lumbosacral region on CT or MRI
- *Pulmonary:* spontaneous pneumothorax or apical blebs on CXR
- *Skin and integuments:* stretch marks (striae atrophicae), recurrent or incisional hernia.

Management
Investigations
- CXR and cross-sectional echocardiography to determine aortic root diameter at the sinus valsalva and evaluate for mitral valve prolapse.
- Blood pressure measurement, ophthalmological review.

Medical care
Directed towards the prevention and treatment of complications: see Case-based discussions, p. 274.

Crouzon syndrome
Crouzon syndrome is an inherited craniofacial disorder. The incidence is 1/50 000 births. Inheritance is AD but up to 50% of cases result from *de novo* mutations in the paternal germ cells for which increased paternal age is a risk factor. Most cases are caused by mutations in the *FGFR2* gene for a fibroblast growth factor receptor.

Facial features are usually apparent by 1 year and include maxillary hypoplasia, shallow orbits, and proptosis arising from early fusion of coronal, lambdoid, and sagittal sutures (craniosynostosis).

Complications include feeding and breathing difficulties, hearing loss, and hydrocephalus. Intelligence is normal.

Multidisciplinary care includes input from plastic, craniofacial, and neurosurgeons.

Treacher–Collins and Goldenhar syndromes

Treacher–Collins syndrome or mandibulofacial dysostosis is an inherited craniofacial disorder resulting from defective 1st arch development. The incidence is 1/50 000. Inheritance is AD with over half due to *de novo* mutations. Mutations are found in *TCOF1* which encodes a protein called treacle expressed in developing branchial arches.

Clinical features are highly variable and are evident at birth. Maxillary and mandibular hypoplasia are associated with downsloping palpebral fissures, and there is a variable degree of malformed or absent ears. Bilateral conductive hearing loss and cleft palate each affect about one third of cases.

Hemifacial microsomia is a birth defect involving 1st and 2nd branchial arches. In addition to craniofacial anomalies there may be eye, cardiac, vertebral, and CNS defects which if present constitute *Goldenhar syndrome* (Fig 12.26). Most are sporadic and no gene defect has been identified. Features include unilateral deformity of the external ear and small ipsilateral half of the face. Intelligence is normal.

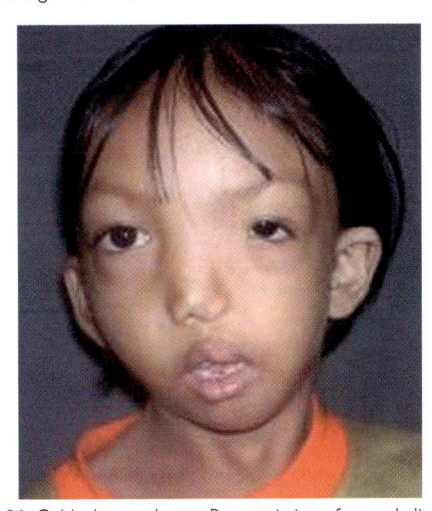

Fig 12.26 Goldenhar syndrome. By permission of seyumbali.org.

CHARGE syndrome

'CHARGE' are the initial letters of the most common features of this condition (promoted from association to syndrome with the discovery of a causative gene).
- **C**oloboma: eye defect affecting iris (keyhole appearance) retina or optic nerve head with visual impairment
- **H**eart defects: e.g. VSD, ASD
- **A**tresia of choanae: one or both nasal passages narrow or blocked
- **R**etardation: of growth and development
- **G**enital anomalies: hypogonadism, micropenis, undescended testes
- **E**ar anomalies: abnormal pinnae (Fig 12.27) and deafness.

The incidence is 1/10 000 births. 60% have mutations in the *CHD7* gene.

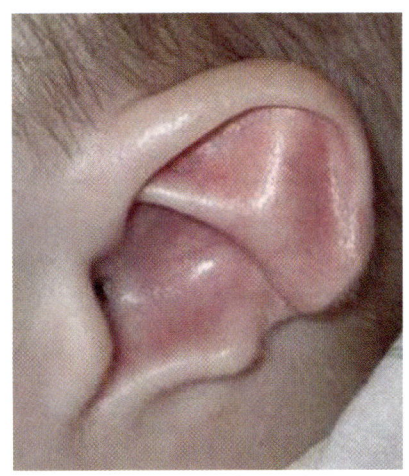

Fig 12.27 CHARGE syndrome: typical external ear.

Cornelia de Lange syndrome (CdLS)

CdLS (Amsterdam dwarfism) is characterized by low birthweight and characteristic facial appearance. The incidence is 1/50 000 births and nearly all cases are sporadic. Mutations in *NIPBL* account for 50% of cases.

There is microcephaly, thick eyebrows that meet in the middle, long eyelashes, an upturned nose, and long philtrum. Hands and feet are small and limb abnormalities common. Development including speech is severely delayed and most children have psychological and behavioural abnormalities: autistic features and self-injury.

Noonan syndrome (NS)

Noonan syndrome is an AD multiple anomaly syndrome with an incidence of 1/2500 live births. It shares phenotypic features with Turner syndrome: webbing of neck, cardiovascular anomalies.

Genetics

NS1 is caused by gain of function mutations in *PTPN11* (encoding a protein tyrosine phosphatase, SHP2) and accounts for about half the patients. Additional loci account for a minority: NS2, NS3 (*KRAS2,*) NS4 (*SOS1*). These genes all participate in the MAP kinase signalling cascade.

Clinical phenotype
- *Facies*: epicanthic folds, ptosis, antimongoloid slant, hypertelorism, strabismus, low-set ears, short neck with extra folds of skin (webbing), and low hairline
- *Cardiac anomalies (80%):* the most common are pulmonary stenosis, hypertrophic cardiomyopathy, ASD, VSD
- *Growth and development:* birthweight is average but subsequent growth in height and weight usually low normal
- *CNS:* developmental delay is common and 10% have learning difficulties requiring educational support
- *Lymphatic system:* nuchal oedema in utero and lymphoedema of hands and feet
- *Bleeding diathesis (50%):* easy bruising or a bleeding tendency is associated with thrombocytopaenia or partial deficiency of a variety of coagulation factors

Management

Diagnosis is clinical. The phenotype becomes more striking in early childhood. Cardiac and haematological are indicated at diagnosis. Prognosis depends on the cardiac lesion. Follow-up includes ophthalmological (refractive errors in 60%) and audiological (progressive sensorineural hearing loss) monitoring.

12.8 Neurofibromatosis type 1 and tuberous sclerosis

Neurofibromatosis type 1

Neurofibromatosis type 1 (NF1, Von Recklinghausen disease) has an incidence of 1/4000 live births. NF2 is a quite different disease with bilateral acoustic neuromas caused by mutations in *NF2* encoding schwannomin.

Genetics

NF1 is caused by mutations in the *NF1* gene on chromosome 17q. *NF1* encodes neurofibromin, a putative tumour suppressor. The gene is large, spanning 350 kb of genomic DNA with 60 exons. Over 500 different mutations have been identified, many of which are 'private' to a specific family. All types of mutation occur and the *NF1* gene is deleted in 5% of patients. NF1 results from haploinsufficiency. Inheritance is AD with highly variable expression. 50% of cases are new mutations.

Clinical features

Clinical diagnosis requires the presence of two or more of the following seven criteria (National Institutes of Health criteria):

- Six or more café-au-lait (CAL) patches (hyperpigmented macules) (Fig 12.28):
  - ≥5 mm in size in children <10 years (prepuberty)
  - ≥15 mm in size in adults (postpuberty)
- Axillary or inguinal freckles
- Two or more typical neurofibromas or one plexiform neurofibroma
- Optic nerve glioma
- Two or more Lisch nodules (iris hamartomata)
- Bone lesions: sphenoid dysplasia, pseudoarthrosis
- 1st-degree relative with NF1.

Many of these signs do not appear until later childhood or adolescence, so diagnosis may be delayed. Multiple CALs is usually the first sign and may be present at birth. Freckling appears during childhood.

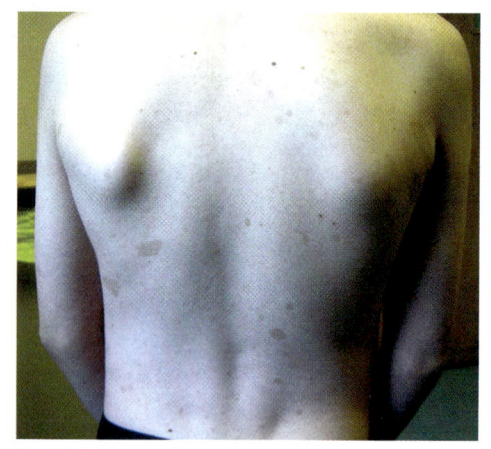

Fig 12.28 NF1: Café-au-lait spots.

Less common features include:

- *Plexiform neurofibromas:* these diffuse growths can be locally invasive and deep. They rarely develop on face and neck in children >1 year and on other parts after adolescence
- *Optic nerve gliomas:* these may be clinically silent and occur primarily in children <5 years. They occur in 12% of patients and are bilateral in 4%
- *Bony lesions:* sphenoid bone dysplasia, usually asymptomatic. Pseudoarthrosis usually causes bowing of the tibia.

Complications of NF1 include:

- *Increased risk of benign and malignant tumours:* malignant tumours include cerebral gliomas, peripheral nerve sheath tumours and neurosarcomas, small bowel leiomyoma/leiomyosarcoma, meningiomas, lymphoma, neuroblastoma, phaeochromocytoma
- *Hypertension:* caused by pheochromocytoma or renal artery stenosis from fibromuscular dysplasia
- *Macrocephaly:* common and benign unless head is rapidly expanding (hydrocephalus)
- *Learning difficulties:* some learning disability with or without ADHD is seen in 40% of patients
- *Scoliosis:* a subset of children develop a rapidly progressive form of scoliosis requiring intervention.

Management

Diagnosis is clinical. Mutation testing is limited because of the high proportion of new mutations. Prenatal diagnosis is possible by linkage analysis or mutation testing.

Parents of a new case require careful examination (including slit-lamp for Lisch nodules). If neither is affected there is a 1–2% recurrence risk (possible gonadal mosaicism). Initial evaluation should include slit-lamp examination; baseline cranial imaging is recommended by some authorities.

Medical care is directed towards detection of complications by annual surveillance for:

- Hypertension
- Symptomatic bony lesions or neurofibromata
- Ophthalmological evaluation: optic nerve tumours present with asymptomatic visual loss, optic nerve pallor, proptosis
- Scoliosis or long-bone modelling defects.
- Spinal cord neurofibroma which may cause paraesthesia, weakness and muscle atrophy.

Surgical care may be required for resection of neurofibromata, correction of rapidly progressive scoliosis or severe bony defects or renal artery stenosis.

Tuberous sclerosis (TSC)

Tuberous sclerosis complex (TSC) is a multisystem disorder associated with benign tumours (hamartomas) in the brain and many other organs including skin, eyes, kidneys, heart, and lungs. The incidence is 1/6000 live births.

Genetics

TSC is caused by mutations in either of two tumour suppressor genes:
- *TSC1*: encoding hamartin on chromosome 9q
- *TSC2*: encoding tuberin on chromosome 16p.

Inheritance is AD with high penetrance and variable expressivity. 60% of cases are new mutations. In familial cases, mutations in *TSC1* and *TSC2* are equally frequent, but *TSC2* accounts for 80% of sporadic cases. *TSC2* is contiguous with the gene for autosomal polycystic kidney disease and overall is associated with a more severe phenotype. Loss-of-function mutations in these genes results in constitutive mTOR signalling in multiple organs.

Clinical features

TSC may present at any age and physical signs are highly variable. Neurological manifestations are a common presentation in infancy.

Nervous system (80%)
- Epilepsy occurs in 65% of patients, often presenting in infancy with infantile spasms. Impaired cognition and learning difficulties are common (60–70%), as are behavioural problems (autistic features, ADHD).
- Tubers (glial proliferation) occur in the cerebral cortex and ventricular walls as subependymal nodules (SENs) but are uncommon elsewhere. The number, size, and location varies widely. Subependymal nodules can transform into subependymal giant cell astrocytomas (SEGAs) causing ventricular obstruction.

Eyes (50%)
- There may be retinal astrocytomas (phakomata) which appear as rounded areas, becoming whitish as they calcify, or hypopigmentation of iris or retina.

Skin (70–80%)
- *Hypomelanotic macules:* 'ash-leaf' shaped macules on the trunk or limbs offer an excellent opportunity for early diagnosis (Fig 12.29). May only be visible under UV (Woods) light.

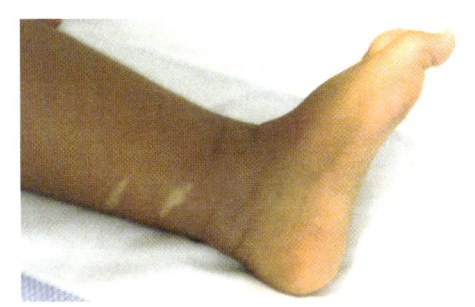

Fig 12.29 TSC: hypomelanotic macules (ash-leaf spots).

- *Angiofibromas:* previously misnamed 'adenoma sebaceum', papules in nasolabial folds and cheeks appear during childhood (Fig 12.30)

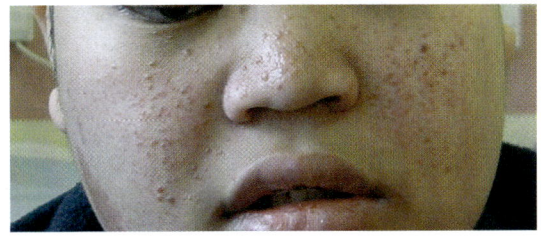

Fig 12.30 TSC: facial angiofibromas.

- *Shagreen patch:* a rough (shagreen is a term for untanned leather) plaque often found in lumbosacral area
- *Fibromas:* periungual fibromas are most common.

Cardiac and lungs
- Cardiac rhabdomyomas are present in 50% of infants and may be detected prenatally. Most are benign and asymptomatic. Spontaneous regression occurs. Rarely they cause mechanical obstruction or arrhythmias.
- Symptomatic pulmonary disease is rare and occurs mostly in adult women in the form of cysts or lymphangiomyomatosis (LAM).

Renal
- Angiomyolipomas (AMLS) are present in 80% of patients; these benign tumours are usually multiple and spontaneous retroperitoneal bleeding may occur
- Polycystic kidney disease: in 2–3% when a deletion affects *TSC2* and *PKD1*.
- Renal cysts (*not* polycystic kidney disease) in 10–20%; usually asymptomatic
- Renal cell carcinoma in increased in frequency.

Diagnosis is based on a set of major and minor criteria some of which require imaging investigations in addition to fundoscopy and examination of skin with UV light.

Management

Molecular genetic testing is available. Both parents of an affected child should be carefully examined for cutaneous and retinal manifestations and some advocate cranial CT or MRI and renal ultrasound scans in addition. If parents are unaffected the recurrence risk is 2–3% (gonadal mosaicism). Prenatal diagnosis can be offered to families in which a mutation has been identified in an index case.

Medical care is directed towards detection and treatment of complications with a multidisciplinary approach:

Complete remission of epilepsy can occur but multiple AEDs may be necessary. Urgent cranial imaging is indicated if raised intracranial pressure or focal neurological signs occur. Identify developmental disorders and learning difficulties early and provide remedial help.

Laser therapy is useful for facial angiofibromas and skin tags can be removed with cryotherapy.

Clinical trials for the treatment of angiomyolipomas are in progress.

Monitoring should include annual blood pressure measurement, renal function tests, and renal ultrasound. PKD (rare) may cause hypertension and renal failure. Angiomyolipomas (AMLs) may bleed with abdominal pain and haematuria.

12.9 X-linked disorders: Fragile X and Rett syndrome

The X chromosome

The X chromosome is 150 Mb in size and harbours >1400 genes including a large number that cause disease (Fig 12.31). X inactivation (or lyonization) is a process by which one of the two copies of the X chromosome in females is inactivated. Which of the two X chromosomes is inactivated in a cell is normally random in higher mammals.

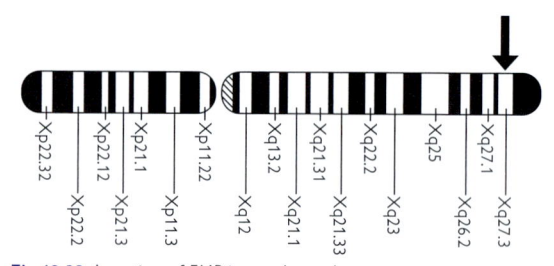

Fig 12.33 Location of *FMR1* gene (arrow).

Genetics

FXS is caused by mutations in the *FMR1* gene which encodes the FMR protein, FMRP (Fig 12.33). The mutation is a triplet CGG repeat expansion which gives rise to a complex pattern of inheritance:

- A normal *FMR1* gene has 30 (range 5–54) CGG triplet repeats in the first exon 5′ regulatory region of the gene. This small number is stable.
- A premutation with 56–200 repeats is unstable. Males carrying a premutation are normally unaffected and transmit the premutation to their daughters unchanged (a 'normal transmitting male'). However, a premutation can expand during oogenesis so offspring of a female with a premutation may inherit a longer full mutation (Fig 12.34).
- A full mutation is >200 repeats. Males with a full mutation are always affected. Up to 50% of females with a full mutation (carrier females) are affected with learning and behavioural difficulties. Older men and women with a premutation can develop fragile X-associated tremor/ataxia syndrome (FXTAS).

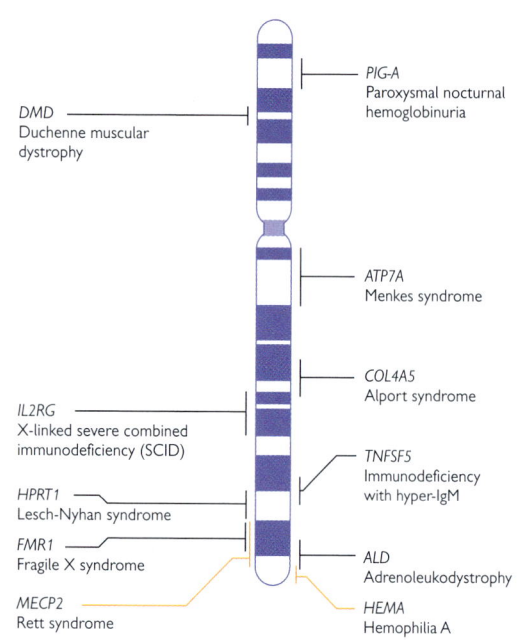

Fig 12.31 The X chromosome: location of some diseases.

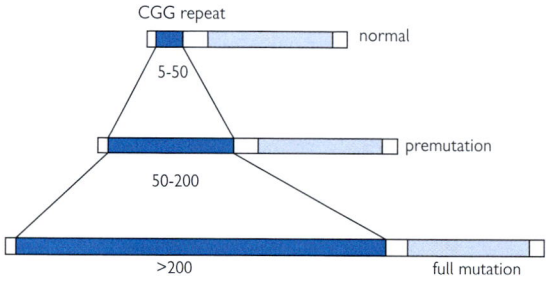

(DMD – Duchenne muscular dystrophy; IL2RG – X-linked severe combined immunodeficiency (SCID); HPRT1 – Lesch-Nyhan syndrome; FMR1 – Fragile X syndrome; MECP2 – Rett syndrome; PIG-A – Paroxysmal nocturnal hemoglobinuria; ATP7A – Menkes syndrome; COL4A5 – Alport syndrome; TNFSF5 – Immunodeficiency with hyper-IgM; ALD – Adrenoleukodystrophy; HEMA – Hemophilia A)

Fig 12.34 FXS: expansion of triplet repeat numbers.

The full mutation leads to hypermethylation and silencing of *FMR1* gene transcription, resulting in reduction or absence of FMRP.

Pathogenesis

FMRP is present in high levels in brain and testes and at synapses in neurons. It is an mRNA-binding protein and regulates synthesis of a set of proteins. The human FXS brain has some gross morphological abnormalities

Fragile X syndrome (FXS)

Fragile X syndrome is the most common form of inherited mental retardation and is associated with specific physical features, cognitive patterns, and behavioural problems. The name derives from the 'fragile' appearance of the long arm of the X chromosome in lymphocytes cultured in a folate-depleted medium (Fig 12.32).

Clinical features

Physical features

These are subtle and difficult to recognize before puberty.

- *Facies:* prominent ears, long thin face, prominent forehead and jaw, facial asymmetry, macrocephaly (Fig 12.35)
- *Extremities:* hyperextensible finger joints, hand calluses, soft skin over dorsum of hand, hallucal crease, pes planus or cavus

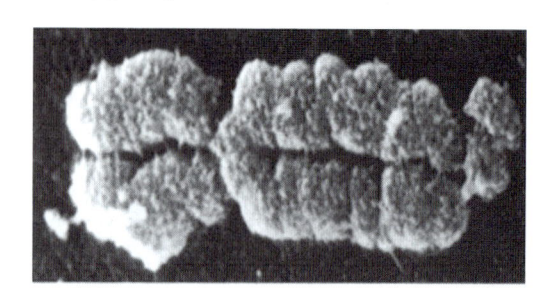

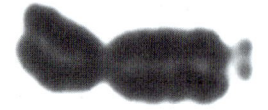

Fig 12.32 Fragile X chromosome appearance.

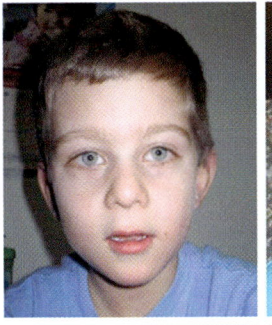

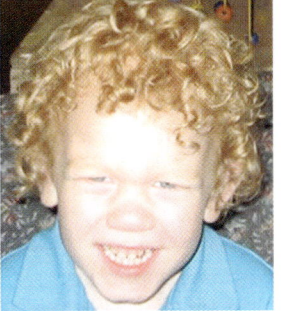

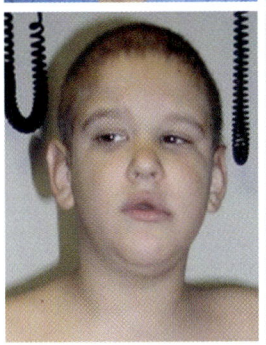

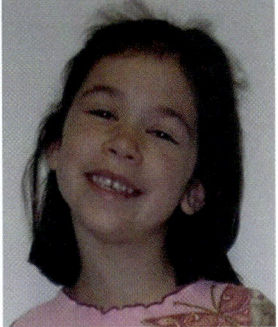

Fig 12.35 Fragile X syndrome: facies.

- *Genitals:* macro-orchidism postpuberty
- *Cardiac:* mitral valve prolapse.

Cognition and behaviour

- *Cognitive function:* the average adult IQ is 40 in males and 80 in females with the full mutation, but variability is wide. Males with intelligence in the normal range are mosaics with *FMR1* expression of >30% normal. In females intellect correlates with X-inactivation ratios. The cognitive profile includes strengths in vocabulary/verbal skills, impairment of expressive language, and weakness in spatial processing and numbers. Mild motor delay is common.
- *Behaviour:* autistic features: 15–40% of males meet criteria for autistic spectrum disorders with features such as poor eye contact, social anxiety, sterotypies, hand flapping.
- *ADHD:* poor concentration and impulsive behaviour is common.

Medical complications

- Gastro-oesophageal reflux (30%)
- Recurrent otitis media (60%)
- Strabismus (30%), hypermetropia (60%)
- Hypotonia and motor incoordination all occur
- Seizures occur in 20% of males
- Sleep problems are common.

Management

Genetic testing is by testing DNA for CGG repeat size by Southern blot or PCR. Fragile X testing is recommended for most children with developmental delays, mental retardation, or autistic spectrum disorder of unknown aetiology especially if a family history is present.

Rett syndrome (RS)

This X-linked dominant syndrome is an important cause of developmental arrest and regression in females with an incidence of 1/10 000 live female births.

Genetics

RS is caused by mutations in *MECP2*, encoding methyl-CpG-binding protein 2, located on Xq28. Over 170 mutations in *MECP2* have been described.

In females the phenotype severity is determined by both the mutation and pattern of X-inactivation. In males mutations are usually embryonic lethal but surviving males display a variety of mental retardation phenotypes or severe neonatal encephalopathy. Most cases are sporadic but recurrence may result from gonadal mosaicism or inheritance from a mother who is mildly affected on account of favourably skewed X-inactivation.

Pathogenesis

Mutations in *MECP2* allow unregulated expression of genes crucial for normal brain development.

Clinical features

Classical RS in a female is characterized by normal early development followed by deceleration of head growth, developmental stagnation followed by regression with autistic features and hand stereotypies (Fig 12.36).

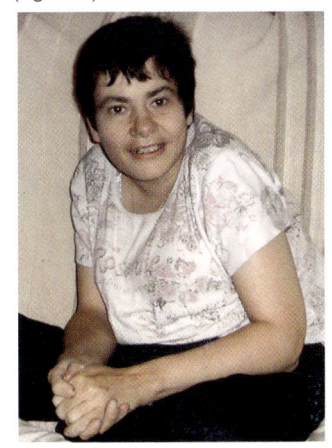

Fig 12.36 Rett syndrome: hand stereotypy.

Four stages are identified (see Chapter 7):
- *Stage I:* developmental arrest (age 6–18 months)
- *Stage II:* developmental regression (age 1–4 years)
- *Stage III:* pseudostationary (age 2–10 years)
- *Stage IV:* late motor deterioration (age>10 years).

Increasing motor problems occur, including hypertonia and dystonia. Some patients stop walking and scoliosis or kyposcoliosis develops.

Atypical or variant forms occur and *MECP2* mutations have been found in girls with autism or mild intellectual disability and healthy females (carriers).

Management

DNA analysis of *MECP2* is available and mutations are identified in 80% of females with classical RS.

Medical care is multidisciplinary and supportive. Antiepilepsy drugs for epilepsy, management of feeding disorders (consider gastrostomy), help with communication, and surgery for scoliosis may all be required.

12.10 mtDNA and imprinted gene disorders

Single gene disorders with patterns of inheritance which do not follow Mendel's rules occur in disease caused by mutations in mtDNA or imprinted genes.

mtDNA disorders

These are considered in detail in Chapter 11.5. Mitochondrial disorders arise from a dysfunction of the mitochondrial respiratory chain and may be caused by mutations in nuclear genes or mtDNA.

mtDNA: maternal inheritance

The mitochondrial genome is a 16 kb double-stranded circular DNA molecule encoding 13 respiratory chain proteins (out of a total of ~100), 22 tRNAs, and 2 rRNAs (Fig 12.37).

The mtDNA molecules in a cell are normally identical and this is called *homoplasmy*. Coexistence of normal and mutant mtDNA molecules is *heteroplasmy*. The mitochondrial genome is inherited maternally. An affected male does not transmit a mutation to any offspring whereas an affected female may transmit a mutation to all her offspring.

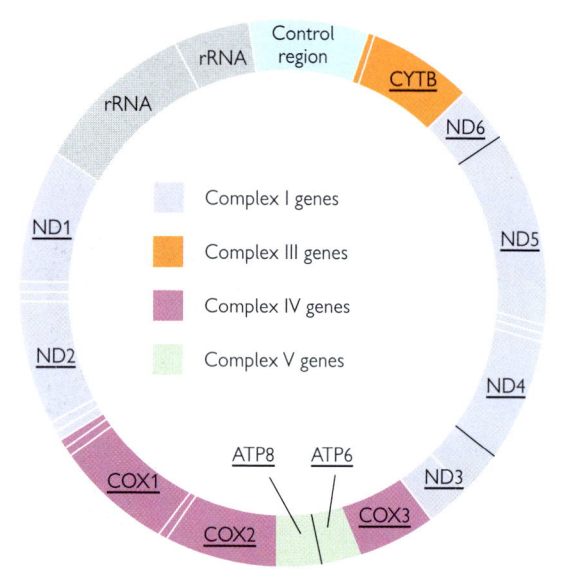

Fig 12.37 mtDNA encodes 13 respiratory chain proteins. Control region regulates transcription and replication. White lines represent tRNA genes.

Pathogenesis

Respiratory function is more critical in tissues with a high metabolic demand such as brain, eye, or muscle. A critical threshold level of mutant mtDNA is necessary before function is impaired. The variable and evolving level of mutant mtDNA (heteroplasmy) in tissues accounts for the highly variable and evolving phenotype.

Clinical features

The hallmark is a seemingly unrelated set of clinical symptoms and signs with multiple organ involvement. Neurological features tend to predominate. Most patients are sporadic but any familial clustering displays a maternal inheritance pattern. See Chapter 11.5.

Imprinted gene disorders

The best-known examples are Prader–Willi syndrome and Angelman syndrome, both of which involve imprinted genes on chromosome 15q, and Beckwith–Wiedemann syndrome on chromosome 11p. Imprinting is also involved in Silver–Russell syndrome (SRS).

Genomic imprinting

There are two copies of each autosomal gene, inherited from each parent at fertilization. For the vast majority expression of the paternal and maternal copy (allele) is equal. However, a small minority (<1%) are preferentially expressed from one allele dependent on the parent of origin. This phenomenon is known as *imprinting*.

Imprinting occurs in germline cells. The original imprint is erased and re-established according to the sex of the individual, e.g. a paternal imprint in developing sperm. Imprinting occurs by DNA methylation and histone modifications. 'Imprinted' usually refers to the silenced allele but, confusingly, is sometimes also used to denote the expressed allele.

Imprinted genes occur in clusters and may be under the control of an imprinting control region (ICR). Paternally expressed genes tend to promote growth and maternally expressed genes tend to limit growth.

Imprinting can cause disease if the active gene is deleted, mutated or silenced or if both copies of a chromosome are inherited from the same parent. This is known as uniparental disomy (UPD).

Prader–Willi and Angelman syndromes

These two genetic disorders arise from abnormalities in a region of imprinting at chromosome 15q11.

- **P**rader-Willi syndrome arises if neither chromosome has genes normally expressed on the **P**aternal chromosome. The relevant genes show 'maternal' imprinting.
- Angel**M**an syndrome arises if neither chromosome has genes normally expressed on the **M**aternal chromosome. The relevant genes show 'paternal' imprinting.

Prader–Willi syndrome (PWS)

PWS has an incidence of between 1/10 000 and 1/15 000.

Genetics

There are four different mechanisms:
- Microdeletion of *paternal* 15q11.2–13 (70%)
- *Maternal* uniparental disomy for chromsome 15 (25%)
- Unbalanced translocation with loss of *paternal* chromosome 15q11.2–13 (4%)
- Imprinting centre defect (1%).

Clinical features

These mainly reflect hypothalamic dysfunction. Newborns with PWS present with hypotonia and poor feeding. Major motor milestones are delayed and hyperphagia and progressive obesity develops at age 1–6 years.

- *Facies:* almond-shaped palpebral fissures, down-turned mouth, thin upper lip
- *Short stature:* most patients have GH insufficiency

- *Genital hypoplasia:* secondary to hypogonadotrophinism
- *Obesity* and moderate learning difficulties.

Management
Genetic DNA diagnosis is available using methylation analysis or FISH. The recurrence risk for the common *de novo* microdeletion is <1%.

Investigations to assess the GH and adrenal axis are undertaken.

Medical care is directed towards:
- Management of hypotonia and poor feeding in infancy
- Prevention of obesity: limitation of access to food, increased activity
- *Sleep disorders:* monitor for sleep apnoea
- Psychiatric/psychological input for behavioural problems.

Angelman syndrome (AS)
AS has an incidence of between 1/12 000 and 1/40 000 live births. An older term, 'happy puppet syndrome' alludes to the typical happy demeanour, and is no longer used.

Genetics
AS is caused by abnormal expression of *UBE3A*, encoding ubiquitin protein ligase E3A, a paternally imprinted gene in the PWS/AS critical region.

There are four different mechanisms:
- *Class I:* a deletion (or rearrangement) involving 15q11.2–13 in the *maternal* chromosome. (70%)
- *Class II: paternal* uniparental disomy (2%)
- *Class III:* imprinting centre defect (3%)
- *Class IV:* mutations in *UBE3A* (75%).

Clinical features
Severe developmental delay occurs from 6 months with hypotonia and poor feeding due to sucking problems.

There are subtle dysmorphic features with deep set eyes, a wide mouth, and prognathia; microcephaly (by age 2 years); hypopigmentation of skin and eyes (Fig 12.38). Motor delay is severe with an ataxia jerky gait and hand-flapping, and there is a happy demeanour with frequent laughter and smiling. Seizures occur by age 3 years with a characteristic EEG.

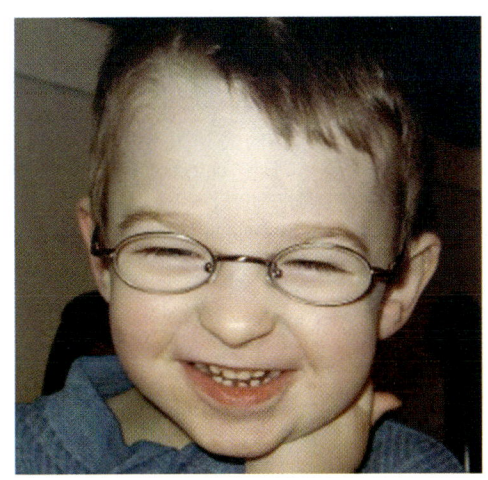

Fig 12.38 Angelman syndrome: facies.

Management
Genetic DNA diagnosis is available using methylation analysis or FISH. Recurrence risk for the common *de novo* microdeletions is <1%, attributable to maternal germ line mosaicism.

Medical care is directed towards: epilepsy treatment with antiepilepsy drugs, sleep problems (melatonin may assist in promoting satisfactory sleep patterns), and physiotherapy to encourage joint mobility

Beckwith–Wiedemann syndrome (BWS)
BWS, also known as exomphalos–macroglossia–gigantism (EMG) syndrome, has an incidence of 1/13 000.

The genetic mechanisms are complex and involve the expression of a cluster of genes in an imprinted region on chromosome 11p15. The BWS critical region has at least 2 imprinting centres and 12 genes. 85% of cases are sporadic, 15% familial. Most cases are caused by abnormal methylation of imprinted loci within 11p but some have uniparental disomy or mutations in *CDKN1C*.

The cardinal features, usually apparent at birth, include:
- *Overgrowth:* large size, macroglossia (Fig 12.39), visceromegaly (liver, kidneys), hemihypertrophy
- Anterior abdominal wall defects (exomphalos)
- Neonatal hypoglycaemia (50%)
- Embryonal tumours (5–20% by 4 years), most frequently Wilms tumour.

Hypoglycaemia is prevented by frequent feeds and diazoxide. Regular abdominal ultrasound (3–6 monthly) is indicated to screen for embryonal tumours.

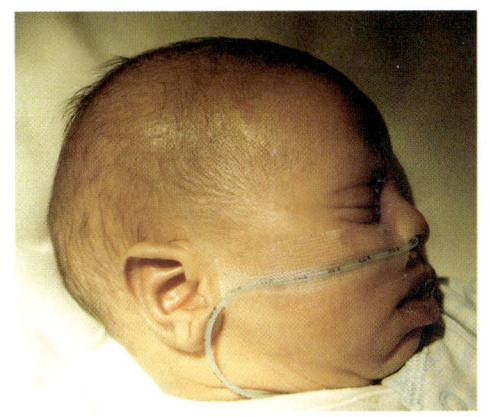

Fig 12.39 BWS: macroglossia and ear crease.

Silver–Russell syndrome (SRS)
Incidence estimates range from 1/3000 to 1/100 000.

There is clinical and genetic heterogeneity. 10% have maternal uniparental isodomy of chromosome 7. 30% have methylation defects of 11p15.

Clinical features include intrauterine growth retardation, poor postnatal growth, feeding difficulty, fasting hypoglycaemia, developmental delay. Classical dysmorphic features include triangular facies with high forehead and small jaw, prominent nasal bridge, and blue sclerae. Head size is normal although the body is small.

12.11 Case-based discussions

An infant with Down syndrome
You are called by the midwife to the delivery suite as she is concerned that a baby boy that has just been born has features of Down syndrome. On reviewing the notes you establish that the mother is 35 years old and that this is her first baby. The nuchal scan and 20 week anomaly scan were both normal. The mother did not have a CVS or an amniocentesis and her booking bloods were unremarkable. You introduce yourself to the parents and examine the baby.

Examination findings
The infant is lying in the frog-leg position and appears quite floppy. He is warm and well perfused. Looking at his face you note that he has up-slanting palpebral fissures and epicanthic folds. He also has a protruding tongue and a short nose with a flat nasal bridge. On examining his hands you notice single palmar creases and bilateral 5th finger clinodactyly. His feet reveal a wide sandal gap between his 1st and 2nd toes. Cardiovascular and abdominal examination are unremarkable.

What should you do next?
The suspicion of Down syndrome in a newborn requires prompt discussion with the parents by a senior paediatrician who should be alerted immediately.

Arrange for both parents and /or other family members to be present in a private quiet space without unnecessary observers or staff. The infant should be present and referred to by name. Balance concerns with positive observations and explain the process of confirming the diagnosis.

Provide immediate access to good information about Down syndrome. An open-ended opportunity to ask questions and clear information about next steps and follow up is given. Telling parents this news is not a single encounter but a process that may last weeks or months.

How is the diagnosis of Down syndrome made?
Take blood for rapid FISH, looking for trisomy 21. This will then be confirmed by a full karyotype which requires cell culture and takes several days.

What is your immediate management plan?
Monitor feeding closely: hypotonia can affect the ability to feed. There is an increased incidence of gastrointestinal abnormalities, e.g. duodenal atresia.

Organize an ECG, cardiac echo and renal ultrasound, ophthalmology review, and follow-up.

Plot head circumference, weight, and length on Down syndrome specific growth chart.

Inform the GP, health visitor, and community paediatric team.

A child with Marfan syndrome
You are asked to see a 12 year old girl with MFS for her annual review in the general paediatric clinic. She is 12 years old and has a clinical diagnosis of MFS according to the Ghent criteria. Her father has MFS and has been shown to have a mutation in FBN1. He recently underwent prophylactic surgery to correct dilatation of his aortic root. Her paternal grandfather died from aortic dissection before a diagnosis of MFS was made.

What test would you want to ensure has been done?
Annual echocardiogram, including measurement of aortic diameter at sinus of valsalva.

Cardiovascular complications of MFS include mitral valve prolapse and regurgitation, LV dilatation and cardiac failure, and dilatation of the pulmonary artery. Aortic root dilatation, often associated with aortic regurgitation, is the most common cause of morbidity and mortality in MFS. It is also the most common indication for cardiovascular surgery in childhood.

Advice is given to avoid competitive sports involving severe exertion. β-Blockers are used to prevent or delay aortic dilation and are initiated at the first sign of aortic expansion. Prophylactic aortic root surgery is indicated if the aortic diameter exceeds 5.0 cm in a child or 5.5 cm in an adult.

In addition to a cardiac examination, what other system should be examined in clinic?
The skeletal system.
The development of scoliosis is age dependent and commonly occurs following rapid growth. Even if no clinical scoliosis is present children should have an erect AP plain radiograph of the spine (with gonadal shielding) before puberty.

Scoliosis is likely to progress if it exceeds 20°. A child with clinical scoliosis or >40° curvature requires formal orthopaedic assessment and 6 monthly follow-up until growth is complete.

Severe pectus excavatum or carinatum may need surgical repair to prevent cardiac or pulmonary compromise. Children may also have concern over the appearance of these skeletal abnormalities. Surgery unless urgent is normally delayed until growth is completed.

What advice would you give regarding ocular manifestations of MFS?
For children, annual review by an optometrist until at least 12 years is recommended. Early detection and correction of refractive errors help prevent amblyopia.

Ocular manifestations are common in MFS. 60–80% develop ectopia lentis, 28% develop myopia, 36% retinal detachment, and 15% glaucoma.

Any deterioration in sight or visual symptoms should be taken seriously. Patients should be informed about the symptoms of retinal detachment such as, flashers, floaters, and visual field changes, so that they can seek urgent specialist attention.

Chapter 13

Haematology

- 13.1 Blood cells: formation and function *270*
- 13.2 Haemostasis *272*
- 13.3 Clinical haematology *274*
- 13.4 Investigations, transfusion, and transplantation *276*
- 13.5 Iron deficiency anaemia and aplastic anaemia *278*
- 13.6 Haemolytic anaemias *280*
- 13.7 Sickle cell disease and thalassaemia *282*
- 13.8 Haemophilia and von Willebrand disease *284*
- 13.9 Coagulation disorders and thrombophilia *286*
- 13.10 Platelet and white cell disorders *288*
- 13.11 Case-based discussions *290*

13.1 Blood cells: formation and function

Haemopoiesis

Location

Embryonic haemopoiesis

In developing embryos, blood formation occurs in blood islands in the yolk sac from the end of the 3rd week of gestation and declines to an insignificant level by the end of the 1st trimester. Hepatic haemopoiesis then predominates reaching a maximum at around the 3rd month and declining from the 3rd month until birth.

Bone marrow

Haemopoiesis in bone marrow begins at around the 5th month of gestation and this eventually becomes the main site. Bone marrow is a mesenchymal-derived tissue divided up into interconnected spaces by bone trabeculae. The haemopoietic component is supported by a microenvironment of stromal cells, extracellular matrix, and vascular structures.

Some lymphoid cells are produced in the spleen, thymus, or lymph nodes and extramedullary haemopoiesis may occur in liver, thymus, and spleen.

Cell lineages

All the cells originate from pluripotent haemopoietic stem cells (HSC). HSCs have an intrinsic capacity for self-renewal and comprise just <0.001% of total. The next stage of committed progenitor cells or colony-forming cells accounts for the massive cell proliferation which maintains blood cell production.

Common lymphoid progenitors develop into lymphoblasts and lymphoid dendritic cells, the former going on to form natural killer cells and T and B lymphocytes. Common myeloid progenitors develop into megakaryocytes, proerythroblasts, and myeloblasts (Fig 13.1).

Haemopoiesis is regulated and sustained by a network of cytokine growth factors including interleukins and colony stimulating factors (CSFs).

Red blood cells

Erythropoiesis is regulated by the hormone erythropoietin (EPO), synthesized in the kidney, liver and elsewhere. Immature red cells or reticulocytes comprise 1% of circulating red blood cells and mature in ~7 days. The normal erythrocyte lifespan is 120 days.

Red cell membrane

The red cell membrane has an external phospholipid bilayer and an internal protein cytoskeleton. which interact to maintain structural integrity and cation homeostasis within the cell. Cytoskeletal proteins include spectrin, the most abundant, and ankyrin.

Haemoglobin

Haemoglobin is the iron-containing oxygen-transport metalloprotein in the erythrocytes. In humans, the haemoglobin molecule is an assembly of four globular protein subunits each with a pocket containing a haem group. Each haem group contains an iron atom in a flat porphyrin ring and is the site of oxygen binding.

Haemoglobin synthesis

During development different globin chains are synthesized resulting in different types of haemoglobin: see Table 13.1.

Table 13.1. Embryonic, fetal and adult haemoglobins

Haemoglobin type	Globin chains	
	α-gene cluster	β-gene cluster
Embryonic		
Hb Gower 1	ξ2	ε2
Hb Gower 2	α2	ε2
Hb Portland	ξ2	γ2
Fetal		
HbF	α2	γ2
Adult		
HbA	α2	β2
HbA2	α2	δ2

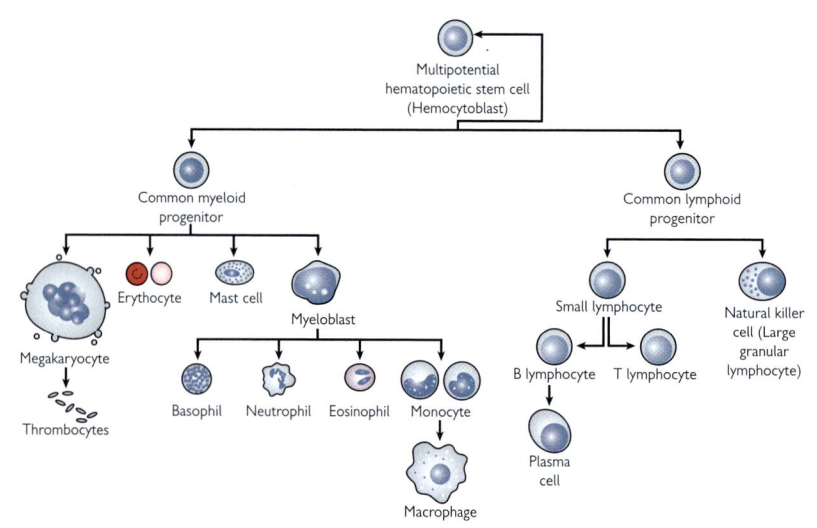

Fig 13.1 Haemopoiesis: cell lineages.

Haemoglobin function

The main function of haemoglobin is oxygen delivery to the tissues. As oxygen binds to the iron atom it causes a conformational change in the molecule which increases the affinity of the remaining haem groups for oxygen. This makes the oxygen dissociation curve sigmoid in shape.

Several factors alter the oxygen affinity of haemoglobin:

Right shift

↓O_2 affinity with increased release to tissues.

↓pH, ↑CO_2, ↑2,3-diphosphoglycerate (DPG), ↑temperature. Hb variants, e.g. HbS.

Left shift

↑O_2 affinity with increased uptake from lungs

↑pH, ↓CO_2, ↓2,3-Diphosphoglycerate (DPG), ↓temperature. Hb variants, e.g. HbF.

The effect of CO_2 and pH is called the Bohr effect (Fig 13.2).

Methaemoglobin is a derivative in which the iron is oxidized from the ferrous (Fe^{2+}) to the ferric (Fe^{3+}) state.

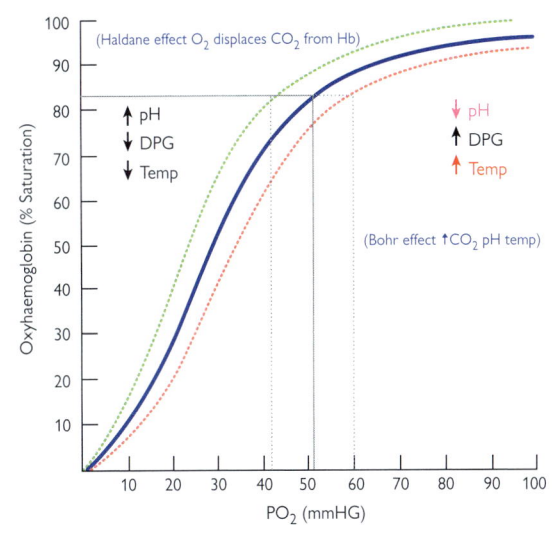

Fig 13.2 Bohr effect.

Red cell metabolism

Mature red cell metabolism is dependent on the enzymes of the Embden–Meyerhof and associated pathways (Fig 13.3). These:

- Generate reducing power as NADH and NADPH. This prevents oxidative injury to the cell and reduces oxidized methaemoglobin to active reduced Hb.
- Generate ATP which drives the cell membrane Na^+/K^+ pump to maintain osmotic equilibrium.

White blood cells

White cells or leucocytes are classified into:

- *Immunocytes:* T and B lymphocytes
- *Phagocytes:*
  - monocytes
  - granulocytes: neutrophils, eosinophils, basophils.

Production is controlled by growth factors from stromal cells (endothelial cells, fibroblasts, macrophages) and T cells. GM-CSF increases differentiation of stem cells into phagocytes.

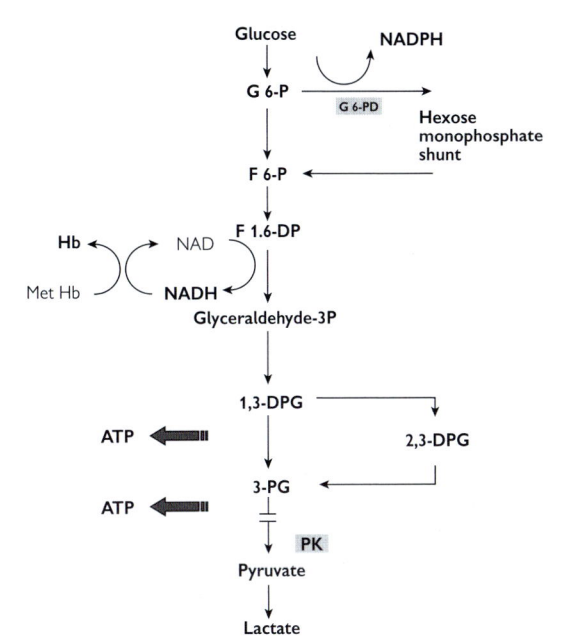

Fig 13.3 Red cell metabolism showing G6PD and PK.

A large reservoir of granulocytes is present in the marrow, up to 15 times the number in the circulation. Two pools of bloodstream granulocytes exist:

- The *circulating pool*, included in the blood count
- The *marginating pool*, which adheres to endothelium and is not included in the blood count.

The circulating lifespan of neutrophils is 6–10 h.

The lymphocyte lineage includes T and B lymphocytes, produced in the bone marrow and thymus and modified in secondary lymphoid tissue, lymph nodes, spleen, and respiratory and gastrointestinal (GI) tracts.

Platelets

Platelets or thrombocytes bud from megakaryocytes in the bone marrow and play an essential role in primary haemostasis.

Platelet production is controlled by thrombopoietin (TPO) and IL-6, and both GM-CSF and IL-3 stimulate megakaryocyte colonies. Platelet lifespan is 7–10 days.

Since they are cell fragments, platelets have no nucleus but they do have microfilaments which hold the unactivated platelet in a discoid shape, a canalicular system, and mitochondria. They also have two types of granule the contents of which differ:

- *Dense granules:* ADP, ATP, bioactive amines, Ca^{2+}, Mg^{2+}
- *Alpha granules*: von Willebrand factor (vWF), fibrinogen, factor V (FV), platelet derived growth factor (PDGF).

Numerous glycoprotein receptors are expressed on the platelet surface:

- *GP IIb/IIIa*: binds fibrinogen allowing platelet aggregation
- *GP Ib/IX*: binds vWF and co-links to collagen.

Pro-inflammation

In addition to being the chief cell involved in haemostasis, platelets are rapidly deployed to sites of injury or infection and potentially modulate inflammatory processes by interacting with leucocytes and secreting cytokines and other inflammatory mediators.

13.2 Haemostasis

Haemostasis: overview
Haemostasis is the cessation of blood loss from a damaged blood vessel and has three main components:
- Vasoconstriction
- *Primary haemostasis:* adhesion, activation, and aggregation of platelets to form a platelet plug
- *Secondary haemostasis:* a complex cascade of coagulation factors ultimately resulting in the transformation of fibrinogen into polymerized fibrin making a stable clot.

In all mammals, coagulation involves cellular and protein components which are also involved in inflammation, vasculogenesis, and tissue repair. Anticoagulant mechanisms keep the coagulation cascade in check.

Primary haemostasis
Following endothelial damage platelets undergo adhesion, activation, and aggregation (Fig 13.4) and also act as procoagulants.

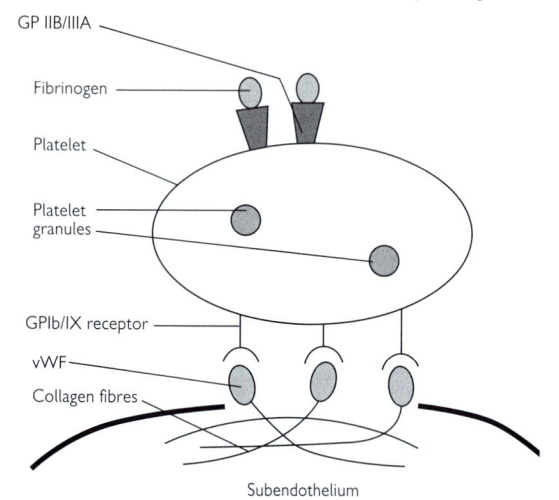

Fig 13.4 Platelet adherence and activation. Reproduced from the Journal of Paediatrics and Child Health, with permission from Elsevier.

- *Adhesion:* platelets adhere to the subendothelial lining of injured vessels via vWF which binds to GPIb/IX, a surface glycoprotein which is constantly expressed. vWF acts to cross-link platelets to collagen on the subendothelium.
- *Activation:* following adherence to collagen platelets are activated and change shape, forming pseudopodia and increasing surface area. Platelet activation releases granular contents including thromboxane A2, ADP, FV, and vWF which promote coagulation. Activated platelets express GP IIb/IIIa which binds to fibrinogen causing aggregation. Platelet factor 3 is a phospholipid which moves to the surface when activation occurs and catalyses conversion of FX to FXa and prothrombin to thrombin.
- *Aggregation:* activation initiates a cascade of mediators resulting in platelet aggregation to form a haemostatic plug in conjunction with fibrin. Aggregating platelets release arachidonic acid. This is converted to thromboxane A2 which is a powerful vasoconstrictor and stimulus for aggregation.

Secondary haemostasis

The coagulation cascade
This is classically divided into two pathways: the tissue factor (TF) extrinsic pathway, and the contact activation intrinsic pathway, both of which lead to the final common pathway of FX, thrombin, and fibrin.

The pathways are a series of reactions in which inactive precursors of serine proteases and their glycoprotein cofactors are activated and catalyse the next reaction, allowing amplification.

Extrinsic: tissue factor pathway
This is the pathway of primary importance. TF, a cell surface glycoprotein, is the principal biological initiator of coagulation. TF released from damaged endothelium forms a complex with and activates circulating plasma FVII to FVIIa. TF–FVIIa activates FIX and FX. FXa and cofactor FVa (the prothrombinase complex) activate prothrombin (FII) to thrombin (IIa), generating thrombin (Fig 13.5).

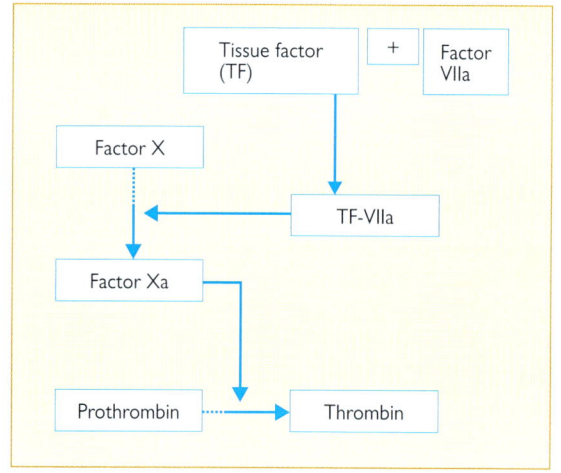

Fig 13.5 Extrinsic pathway: initiation of coagulation.

Intrinsic contact phase pathway
The precise *in vivo* mechanism of the intrinsic pathway is unclear. Thrombin feeds back to activate FXI, which activates FIX and FVIII. Activated FVIII, FIX, and FV forms a complex that activates larger amounts of FX, resulting in a huge 'thrombin burst'. A simplified scheme is shown in Fig 13.6.

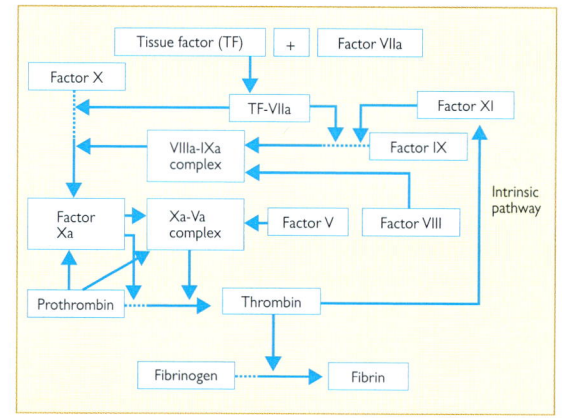

Fig 13.6 Amplification via the intrinsic pathway.

Final common pathway
Prothrombin is activated to thrombin in the *propagation* phase. Thrombin converts fibrinogen to fibrin and also activates FVIII and FV and their inhibitor protein C (in the presence of thrombomodulin). It also activates FXIII which cross-links fibrin polymers to form a stable, lysis-resistant clot.

Cofactors
Calcium and phospholipid platelet factor 3, a constituent of platelet membrane, are required for the tenase and prothrombinase complexes to function. Vitamin K is an essential cofactor for the hepatic gamma-glutamyl carboxylase that adds a carboxyl group to glutamate residues on FII, FVII, FIX and FX, as well as protein C and protein S.

Coagulation screening tests

A coagulation screen includes PT, APTT, TT and a fibrinogen level. A platelet count should be available as part of the FBC. These test different parts of the system (Fig 13.7).

- *Prothrombin time (PT)*: a prolonged PT reflects abnormalities of FII (prothrombin), FV, FVII, and FX. It tests extrinsic and common pathways. A prolonged PT is seen in liver disease, vitamin K deficiency, oral anticoagulant therapy, and disseminated intravascular coagulation (DIC).
- *Activated partial thromboplastin time (APTT)*: a prolonged APTT reflects deficiency of FVIII, FIX, FXI, or FXII. It tests the intrinsic and common pathways. A prolonged APTT is seen in FVIII or FIX deficiency due to haemophilia or von Willebrand disease and heparin treatment.
- *Thrombin time (TT)*: TT reflects the time taken to convert fibrinogen to fibrin. An isolated prolonged TT is likely to indicate an abnormality or deficiency of fibrinogen. TT is prolonged by heparin and DIC.

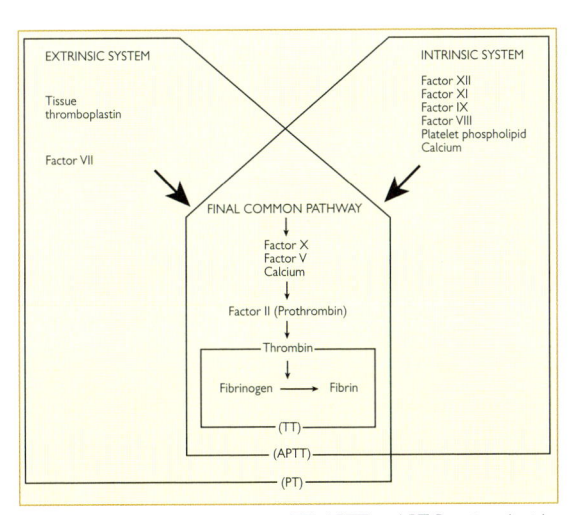

Fig 13.7 Coagulation screen tests: TT, APTT, and PT. Reprinted with permission of PasTest Ltd

A combination of abnormalities is common. A normal coagulation screen *in vitro* does not exclude a coagulation defect being present *in vivo*.

Anticoagulant mechanisms

Under physiological conditions, pro-and anticoagulant mechanisms are balanced in favour of anticoagulation, maintaining blood in its fluid phase. Three main anticoagulant mechanisms keep the coagulation cascade in check (Fig 13.8):

Tissue factor pathway inhibitor (TFPI)
This inhibits FVIIa-related activation of FIX and FX, controlling the initiation phase.

Protein C (PC)
The amplification phase is blocked by the protein C pathway. PC is activated to APC by a complex of thrombin, thrombomodulin (TM), and endothelial protein C receptor (EPCR). APC, with its coenzyme protein S, inactivates FVa and FVIIIa.

The Leiden variant of FV leads to APC resistance and thrombophilia.

Antithrombin (AT)
This serine protease inhibitor or serpin degrades the serine proteases thrombin, FXa, FXIIa, and FIXa. Heparin acts by increasing the affinity of AT for FXa and thrombin. It is constantly active.

The protein C pathway acts mainly in the microcirculation and TFPI and AT exert their effects primarily in the macrocirculation.

Eventually clots are reorganized and resolved by fibrinolysis mediated mainly by the enzyme plasmin and regulated by various activators and inhibitors.

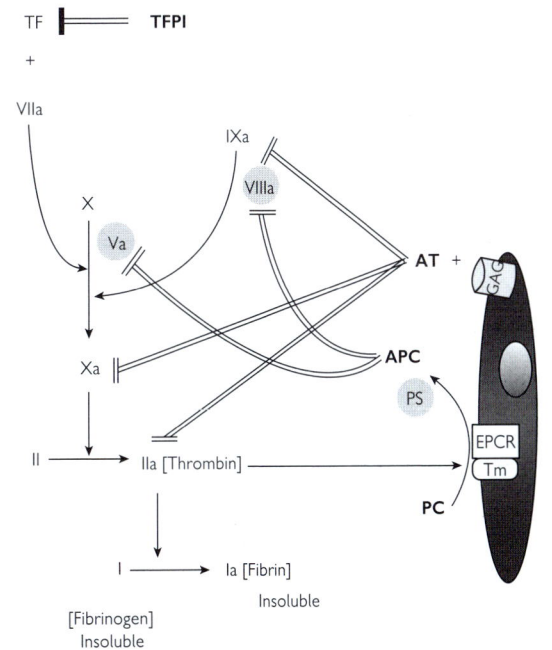

Fig 13.8 Anticoagulant mechanisms. GAG: glycose aminoglycan

13.3 Clinical haematology

Blood disorders often present with striking physical signs such as pallor caused by anaemia, bruising, or bleeding due to a failure of haemostasis or splenomegaly.

A diagnostic approach to these is considered in turn.

Anaemia

Anaemia in a child may be the presenting feature of a primary blood disorder such as leukaemia or secondary to other pathology such as malabsorption with haematinic deficiency or chronic renal failure.

The cause may be apparent clinically but investigation is usually necessary to confirm the aetiology.

Clinical assessment

History
Anaemia is remarkably well tolerated in children who may be asymptomatic until the Hb drops below 7 g/dL. Infants may feed more slowly and children tire more easily. Specific enquiry depends on suspected aetiology but may include:
- *Dietary history:* iron deficiency
- *Family history:* sickle cell disease, thalassaemia, spherocytosis, G6PD deficiency.

Examination
Pallor of the mucous membranes is the key sign of anaemia. Skin pallor is unreliable and anaemia is easy to miss in children with pigmented skin.

Important further signs to seek in an anaemic child are:
- *Excessive bruising:* thrombocytopaenia in marrow failure
- *Splenomegaly:* often present in haemolytic anaemia
- *Jaundice:* a sign of haemolysis.

Diagnostic investigations
Confirmation requires measurement of haemoglobin concentration in peripheral blood. Reference values vary with age and haemoglobin concentration is influenced by haemoconcentration or haemodilution.

A FBC with red cell indices and review of peripheral blood film allows the major causes to be identified.

The two key parameters are:
- Reticulocyte count
- Red cell parameters:
  - mean corpuscular volume (MCV)
  - mean corpuscular Hb (MCH).

Reticulocyte count
The reticulocyte count expressed as a percentage of the total RBC count is normally 0.5–1.5%, 2–5% in newborn infants. Anaemia with a low total RBC count falsely elevates the reticulocyte percentage. A reticulocyte production index allows for this.

Reticulocyte count distinguishes between anaemia due to reduced red cell production and anaemias in which red cells have been lost, sequestrated, or prematurely haemolysed.

Reticulocytes normal or high
- *Blood loss:* haemorrhage, sequestration
- *Haemolysis:* e.g. HS, G6PD deficiency
- *Sickle cell disease:* haemolytic crisis.

Reticulocytes low
- *Marrow failure:*
  - aplastic anaemia
  - bone marrow infiltration
  - parvovirus B19 infection
  - chemotherapy
- Haematinic deficiency
- *Ineffective erythropoiesis:* β-thalassaemia
- Reduced erythropoietin drive.

Blood film, MCV, and MCH
Red cell morphology may provide the diagnosis if spherocytes, sickle cells, or red cell fragments are seen and red cell size and Hb content may be visibly abnormal (Figs 13.9, 13.10).

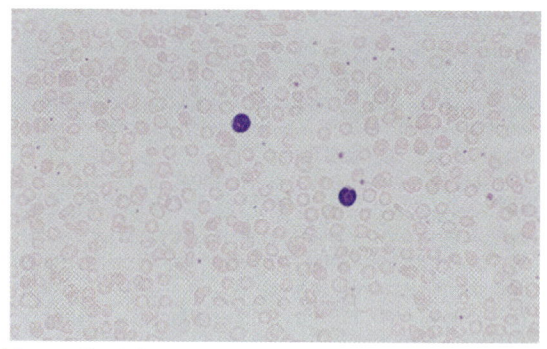

Fig 13.9 Blood film: hypochromic, microcytic anaemia

The blood film, the mean corpuscular volume and haemoglobin allow the anaemia to be classified as:
- *Normocytic and normochromic anaemia:* found in renal disease, acute blood loss, splenic pooling, and occasionally in bone marrow failure. A reticulocyte count and blood film usually resolves the aetiology.
- *Microcytic and hypochromic anaemia:* most commonly caused by iron deficiency anaemia (IDA), but less common possibilities include thalassemia trait in which anaemia is mild, Hb >9 g/dL, chronic lead poisoning, chronic infection, and sideroblastic anaemia.
- *Macrocytic anaemia:* uncommon in childhood. Aetiology is further resolved according to whether the marrow is:
  - megaloblastic: vitamin B12 or folate deficiency.
  - macronormoblastic: Fanconi anaemia, Diamond–Blackfan anaemia and other bone-marrow failure syndromes, haemolytic anaemias.

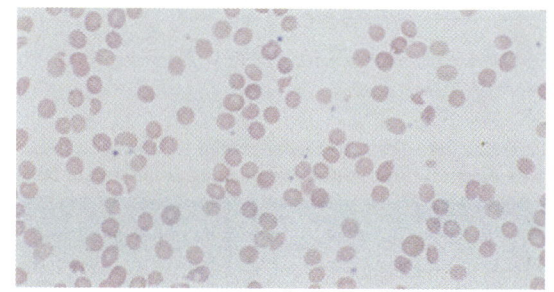

Fig 13.10 Schistocytes in microangiopathic haemolytic anaemia.

Bleeding disorders

A bleeding disorder is most commonly suspected because of spontaneous or excessive bruising or a petechial or purpuric rash. It is an important differential diagnosis of non-accidental injury.

The clinical pattern of bleeding differs according to the haemostatic mechanism involved:

- *Vessels:* Henoch–Schönlein purpura is associated with superficial bleeding in skin and mucosal surfaces.
- *Primary haemostasis:* thrombocytopaenia or impaired platelet function is associated with petechiae and purpura or bleeding from mucosal surfaces such as nose bleeds, GI, genitourinary (GU) tract, or retinal haemorrhage.
- *Secondary haemostasis:* inherited or acquired defects of coagulation cause excessive bruising and bleeding in deep structures such as joints, brain parenchyma and muscle. Bleeding often occurs after a delay as the primary haemostatic mechanisms function initially.

Clinical assessment

A careful family history and history of exposure to haemostatic challenges such as circumcision (Fig 13.11), tooth extraction, tonsillectomy, or other operative procedures is important.

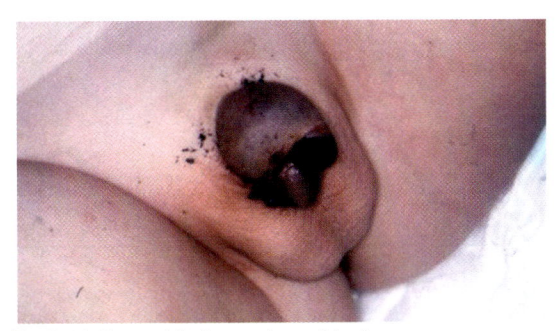

Fig 13.11 Haemophilia A: post-circumcision haematoma.

Investigations

- *FBC and film:* platelet count
- *Coagulation screen:* PT, APTT, TT, fibrinogen levels
- Fibrin degradation products, liver function tests.

Splenomegaly and asplenia

Functions of the spleen

These include:

- *Immune system:* filtering of blood by allowing macrophages to remove blood borne bacteria, especially encapsulated organisms. Exposure of antigen presenting cells to antigens, production and maturation of B and T cells
- *Red cell disposal:* senescent or abnormal red cells are removed from the circulation in the spleen
- *Haemopoiesis:* up until 5th month of gestation.

Splenomegaly

Splenic enlargement may occur in isolation or together with hepatomegaly. When palpable the spleen has usually reached twice its normal size. Features of an enlarged spleen include:

- Moves with respiration
- Upper margin lies under ribs; cannot palpate above it
- Palpable notch, dull to percussion.

Splenomegaly may be accompanied by pancytopaenia. Symptoms include pain in the left upper quadrant.

Splenomegaly may arise from increased function, infiltration or abnormal blood flow (Table 13.2).

Table 13.2. Causes of splenomegaly

Increased function	*Haemolytic anaemias* Thalassaemia, spherocytosis, HbSS (before infarction) *Infections* Viral: EBV, CMV, HIV Bacterial: infective endocarditis, typhoid, TB Protozoal: malaria, leishmaniasis *Systemic diseases* Sarcoidosis, SLE, juvenile chronic arthritis Immune thrombocytopaenia purpura
Infiltrations	*Malignancies:* leukaemia, lymphoma, Langerhans cell histiocytosis, neuroblastoma *Metabolic storage disorders:* Gaucher, Nieman-Pick
Abnormal blood flow	*Portal hypertension:* liver cirrhosis, Budd Chiari syndrome, portal or splenic vein obstruction

Hepatosplenomegaly is common in metabolic storage disorders and haematological malignancies. Massive splenomegaly may occur in tropical diseases such as chronic malaria and visceral leishmaniasis. Infarction abolishes the initial splenomegaly found in sickle cell disease. Massive splenomegaly in sickle cell disease suggests splenic sequestration.

Asplenia

Asplenia is most commonly a result of surgical splenectomy and functional asplenia caused by recurrent infarction is an important feature of sickle cell disease. The causes of asplenia are listed in Table 13.3.

Hyposplenism may be manifested by elevated platelet and white cells in peripheral blood, and Howell–Jolly bodies (nuclear fragments) or 'pits' in red cells visible on the blood film. Howell–Jolly bodies indicate significant hypo-splenism.

The most important consequences are the increased risk of overwhelming bacterial sepsis with capsulated organisms (*S. pneumoniae, H influenza,* or *N. meningitidis*) and of parasitic infection, malaria, and babesiosis.

Table 13.3. Causes of asplenia

Congenital asplenia	Associated with right-sided isomerism, cardiac anomalies
Surgical splenectomy	Post-traumatic removal Hereditary spherocytosis *SCD:* recurrent sequestration Thalassaemia: hypersplenism
Splenic infarction	Sickle cell disease
Splenic atrophy	Coeliac disease, SLE, IBD, JCA HIV/AIDS, chronic GvHD Post irradiation
Splenic infiltration	Malignancy

13.4 Investigations, transfusion, and transplantation

Bone marrow trephine and aspiration

Bone marrow trephine or biopsy removes a core of bone with the marrow. Aspiration removes a small amount of marrow through a needle.

Marrow is sampled from the posterior iliac crest in children and the medial tibia in infants. It is usually done under general anaesthetic, but local anaesthetic and sedation may be appropriate in an older child.

Indications

Indications for bone marrow examination include:
- Diagnosis of the cause of anaemia, thrombocytopaenia, pancytopaenia (Figures 13.12, 13.13)
- Diagnosis and monitoring of haematological malignancies such as acute leukaemia
- Staging of malignancies, e.g. lymphoma, neuroblastoma
- *Diagnosis of metabolic disease:* identification of storage cells, e.g. in Gaucher disease
- Diagnosis of infectious diseases: atypical TB, leishmaniasis.

Complications may include excessive bleeding and infection, especially if the child has a coagulopathy or is immunocompromised.

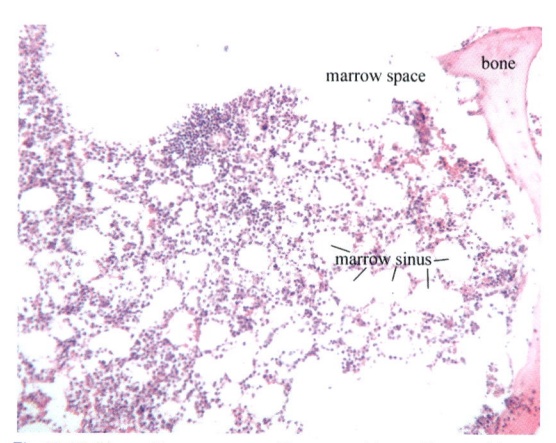

Fig 13.12 Normal bone marrow. Courtesy of Loren Evey and Ian Zagon.

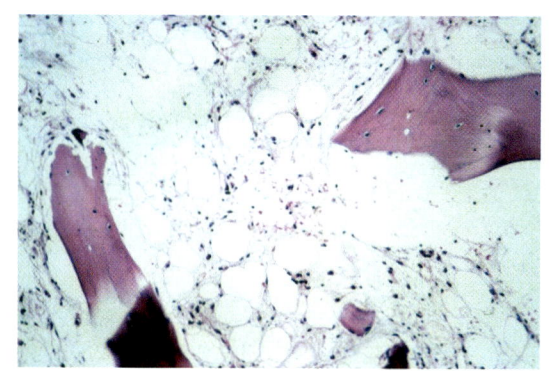

Fig 13.13 Bone marrow in aplastic anaemia: marked hypocellularity.

Blood transfusion

Red cell antigens: blood groups

Blood group or type is a classification based on inherited antigenic substances on the surface of red cells. These antigens may be proteins, carbohydrates, glycoproteins, or glycolipids and may also be present in other types of cells.

There are 26 blood group systems corresponding to red cell surface antigens, but few are of clinical significance.

ABO blood group

The antigens are oligosaccharide components of glycoproteins and glycolipids of unknown function. Antibodies against A and B antigens occur naturally in people without these antigens.

Rh blood group

The antigens are membrane proteins encoded by two genes: *RDH, RHCE*. There are many antigens of which D, C, E, c, and e are most significant. Other antigens are the Kell, Duffy, Kidd, MNS, Hh groups.

Antibodies to these antigens do not occur naturally but require exposure, either by blood product transfusion or feto-maternal exposure. The antibodies are mainly IgM immunoglobulins.

ABO system

This system is determined by a gene for an enzyme which modifies a common precursor, the H antigen (Fig 13.14).

	Group A	Group B	Group AB	Group O
Red blood cell type	A	B	AB	O
Antibodies present	Anti-B	Anti-A	None	Anti-A and Anti-B
Antigens present	A antigen	B antigen	A and B antigens	No antigens

Fig 13.14 ABO blood group system: antigen and antibody status.

Blood groups, corresponding genotypes and naturally occurring antibodies, with their corresponding worldwide frequencies are shown in Table 13.4.

Group O individuals are 'universal donors'. Group AB individuals are 'universal recipients'. Inheritance is codominant.

Table 13.4. ABO blood groups			
Blood group	Genotype	Antibodies	Frequency (%)
O	OO	Anti-A, Anti-B	46
A	AA or AO	Anti-B	42
B	BB or BO	Anti-A	9
AB	AB	–	3

Blood product transfusion
Cross-matching
The cross-match comprises:
- ABO and D grouping of the recipient
- Antibody screen of the recipient, or mother in the case of neonatal transfusion. Serum is tested against a panel of RBCs which carry all important antigens
- A comparison of these results with any previous record ('group and screen' finishes at this point)
- Testing of patient serum against the RBCs to be transfused.

Blood products
- Red cell concentrate:

Dose (mL) = desired rise in Hb × (3 × recipient wt [kg])
- *Platelets*: 'platelet concentrate' from whole blood donation or platelet apheresis. Dose =15 mL/kg
- *White cells*: granulocyte concentrates from whole blood donation or apheresis (rarely used)
- *Fresh frozen plasma (FFP)*: includes all coagulation factors (except FVII and fibrinogen) and complement. Dose=15 mL/kg.
- *Cryoprecipitate*: rich in FVIII, fibrinogen, vWF, and FXIII. Dose = 10–15 mL/kg. Used in DIC.

Red cells and platelets are leukodepleted to remove leucocytes which can cause immune reactions and harbour infections such as CMV.

Adverse transfusion reactions
Signs and symptoms of severe acute adverse reactions often begin within 15 min and may include fever, flushing, urticaria, hypotension, anxiety or restlessness, pain at the transfusion site and respiratory distress. Causes include:
- *Haemolytic reaction*: ABO incompatibility. Recipient's plasma antibodies attack donor red cell antigens causing life threatening intravascular haemolysis with dyspnoea, back pain and haemoglobinuria. DIC and renal failure may ensue.
- *Febrile non-haemolytic reaction*: usually after platelet transfusions. Non-specific reaction to foreign antigens.
- *Bacterial contamination*: severe reaction with rigors and hypotension. Usually seen with platelets.
- *Transfusion-related acute lung injury (TRALI)*: Donor antibodies react with recipient's leucocytes causing acute respiratory distress. Bilateral infiltrates on CXR.
- *Anaphylactic reaction*: increased risk with large volumes of plasma and in patients with IgA deficiency which is often asymptomatic and unrecognized. Rare but life-threatening.
- *Volume overload and air embolism*: uncommon.

Response to adverse reaction
- Stop transfusion and resuscitate if necessary
- Cross check patient and product identification
- Examine product appearance
- Order septic screen, CXR, indicators of haemolysis
- Repeat cross-match and antibody screen

Long-term adverse events include: transmission of pathogens, graft vs host (GVH) disease, iron overload.

Bone marrow transplantation (BMT)
Bone marrow transplantation is the collection and transfer of haemopoietic pluripotential stem cells from a donor to a recipient. Bone marrow is the usual source for these stem cells but other sources include the peripheral blood stem cells and umbilical cord blood.

Transplantation may be:
- *Autologous*: donor and recipient are the same
- *Allogeneic*: genetically non-identical donor:
  - matched (HLA-identical) family member
  - mismatched family member
  - matched unrelated donor (MUD)
  - mismatched unrelated donor (MMUD)
- *Syngeneic*: identical twin donor.

The key difference between a bone marrow and solid organ transplant is the significant component of *donor* lymphoid cells which proliferate to constitute a new immune system. These proliferating effector cells can have both beneficial effects such as graft versus leukaemia, and adverse effects such as GVH disease.

Indications for BMT
Stem cells have the potential for repopulating and reconstituting complete haemopoietic systems if a supportive stroma exists. The main indications for BMT include:
- *To restore bone marrow function*: following high-dose or bone marrow ablative chemotherapy
- *To treat or immunomodulate a disease process*:
  - graft vs leukaemia: leukaemias, lymphomas, haemophagocytosis, autoimmune disease
  - graft vs virus: EBV-induced lymphoproliferation
- *To correct inherited enzyme deficiency*: mucopolysaccharidosis, e.g. Hurler syndrome, adrenoleukodystrophy
- *To facilitate gene therapy*: stem cells harvested for *ex vivo* gene therapy protocols prior to autologous re-infusion, e.g. in SCID.

The transplant process
This is divided into five phases:
- *Conditioning*: chemotherapy and or irradiation eliminates malignancy, prevents rejection of new stem cells, and creates space for the new cells. Lasts 7–10 days.
- *Stem cell processing and infusion*: duration depends on volume and is done through a central venous catheter. Depletion of T cells may decrease GVH disease.
- *Neutropenic phase*: for 2–4 weeks there is severe myelosuppression and immunosuppression and a high risk from nosocomial infection, herpes, and fungal infection.
- *Engraftment phase*: during this period GVH disease and veno-occlusive disease may occur.
- *Postengraftment phase*: this lasts for months or years. Most patients need re-immunisation beginning 1 year after transplant.

Outcome of BMT
Mortality and morbidity of the procedure is balanced against that of the disease. Risks include toxicity related to the conditioning treatment, failure of marrow engraftment, infection, GVH disease, and later problems affecting growth and development, infertility, and second neoplasms.

13.5 Iron deficiency anaemia and aplastic anaemia

Iron deficiency anaemia (IDA)
IDA is the most common cause of isolated chronic substrate deficiency anaemia worldwide. In the UK, the prevalence of IDA between age 6 and 24 months varies between 25% and 40% in socio-economically deprived populations.

Iron metabolism and dietary sources
In healthy humans the body concentration of iron is regulated by absorptive cells in the small intestine. 70% of total body iron is in the blood.

Dietary iron in infants and young children is 10% haem and 90% non-haem iron. Numerous chelators in the diet such as bran, tannin in tea, phytates in high-fibre foods, calcium and phosphate in cow's milk may render non-haem iron unabsorbable.

The term newborn infant has iron stores sufficient for 4–6 months, from which time exogenous iron is required. During rapid growth from 4–12 months ~0.8 mg of iron per day from the diet is required. Breast milk has iron in low concentration (~0.08 mg/100 mL) but it is well absorbed.

Iron deficiency
Iron deficiency as a decreased total iron body content may precede the diminished erythropoiesis that causes anaemia. There is evidence that iron deficiency affects both growth and development in children.

Iron deficiency may arise from inadequate dietary intake, malabsorption, or excessive losses.

Diet
Risk factors vary with age:
- *Preterm infants*: stores are inadequate so iron supplements are given routinely.
- *Infants*: early introduction of unmodified cow's milk at 6–8 months is a risk factor. Cow's milk is low in iron, but additional factors include decreased ingestion of other iron sources, poor absorption and possibly increased losses from GI mucosal damage.
- *Children*: diets low in iron-rich foods such as meat, green vegetables.

Malabsorption
Coeliac disease may present as IDA, and iron deficiency may complicate short-bowel syndrome and inflammatory bowel disease.

Haemorrhage
Each mL of blood lost results in a loss of 0.5 mg of iron. Bleeding from most orifices is soon noticed but chronic GI tract bleeding may go unrecognized and excessive menstrual losses may be overlooked.

Worldwide, hookworm infestation is the most important cause of GI blood loss but in the developed world Meckel diverticulum and cow's milk protein intolerance are recognized causes.

Clinical features
A dietary history is essential in a child presenting with anaemia, and a family history of inherited anaemia should be sought.

Pallor may be apparent in the nail beds, conjunctivae, and oral mucosae. Koilonychia (spoon-shaped nails) is rare.

Investigations
First line: FBC, reticulocyte count and peripheral blood film.

Features consistent with IDA are:
- Hb <11.0 g/dL (in age range 6 months–4 years)
- Hypochromic, microcytic anaemia on film. Occasional target cells, anisocytosis
- Red cell indices: ↓MCV, ↓MCH.

The differential diagnosis of a hypochromic, microcytic anaemia includes
- *Thalassaemia trait:* MCHC normal, RBC count raised
- Anaemia of chronic disease (ACD)
- Lead poisoning, congenital sideroblastic anaemia (rare).

Supplementary investigations to confirm iron deficiency if necessary are:
- *Serum ferritin:* low serum ferritin confirms iron deficiency with a 99% positive predictive value. Normal ferritin does not exclude IDA as it is an acute phase protein and may be elevated by an inflammatory or infective process.
- *Serum iron:* low in IDA and ACD but normal in thalassaemia.
- *Total iron binding capacity (TIBC):* high in IDA, low in ACD and normal in thalassaemia.
- *HPLC or Hb electrophoresis (EP):* HPLC is more sensitive. In β-thalassaemia trait HbA2 is raised, but HbA2 may be within the normal range if there is coexistent iron deficiency. It should be checked again after iron therapy.

The anaemia of chronic disease, due to defective incorporation of iron into Hb and a blunted response to EPO, can coexist with iron deficiency, particularly in inflammatory bowel disease.

If occult blood loss or malabsorption is suspected additional investigations might be considered:
- Screening tests for coeliac disease by assay of anti-tissue transglutaminase antibodies, serum folate
- GI tract endoscopy.

Management
Prevention

In the UK, primary prevention of IDA is the aim, with advice to avoid unmodified cow's milk and the provision of iron-supplemented formula milk up to the age of 24 months in at risk groups. Low birthweight babies should receive 5 mg/day elemental iron from age 6 weeks until mixed feeding starts.

Treatment

If IDA is diagnosed in a clinical context strongly suggestive of dietary insufficiency, management requires dietary advice and oral iron supplementation using iron salts at a dose of 3–6 mg/kg per day elemental iron for at least 3 months after haemoglobin levels normalize. Haemoglobin concentration should increase by 2 g/dL over 4 weeks. Failure to respond would prompt a search for malabsorption or occult blood loss.

Transfusion should only be considered if there is significant acute bleeding or severe anaemia.

Folate or B12 deficiency

These substrate deficiencies may occur in isolation or in combination and are associated with megaloblastic anaemia, i.e. macrocytosis with large immature dysfunctional red cell precursors (megaloblasts) in the marrow. Folate deficiency is more common.

Folate deficiency
Folate deficiency may occur in periods of rapid growth, especially in the preterm infant, infection, or diarrhoea and is a risk in all patients with a chronic haemolytic anaemia such as sickle cell disease or spherocytosis. Folic acid supplements are given to all children with a haemolytic anaemia.

Vitamin B12 deficiency
Vitamin B12 deficiency is uncommon and is usually caused by deficiency of intrinsic factor caused by surgical blind loops or juvenile pernicious anaemia.

Aplastic anaemia

Aplastic anaemia is a condition characterized by marrow hypoplasia and peripheral pancytopaenia. In rare instances committed progenitor cell development is affected leading to isolated red cell aplasia.

Aetiology
About 80% of cases are acquired and 20% congenital or inherited (Table 13.5). Some of the rare inherited causes are considered individually below.

Table 13.5. Causes of aplastic anaemia	
Acquired (80%)	Idiopathic (autoimmune)
	Infections: EBV, parvovirus, hepatitis viruses, HIV
	Toxins: radiation and chemicals, e.g. benzene, DDT
	Drugs: acetazolamide, chloramphenicol
Inherited (20%)	Fanconi anaemia
	Diamond–Blackfan anaemia
	Shwachman–Diamond syndrome
	Familial aplastic anaemia

Clinical features
Onset is insidious with symptoms related to anaemia, thrombocytopaenia, or neutropaenia. Physical stigmata of inherited marrow failure syndromes may be present such as short stature, skin pigmentation, skeletal anomalies.

Cases are classified into severe or very severe aplastic anaemia (VSAA). The latter, with neutrophil count <0.2×10^9/L, is less likely to respond to immunotherapy.

Diagnostic investigations
- *FBC and blood film:* pancytopaenia with reduced reticulocyte count is usual. Leukoerythroblastic changes suggest an infiltrative process.
- *Bone marrow aspiration and biopsy:* biopsy is required to confidently establish hypocellularity.

Management
This is initially supportive with blood transfusion and prevention and treatment of infections. Bone marrow transplantation from an HLA-matched sibling donor is the treatment of choice for severe aplastic anaemia.

If no donor is available, immune suppression using antithymocyte globulin (ATG) and cyclosporin may be used with beneficial effect, but relapse is not uncommon.

Fanconi anaemia (FA)
FA is a rare autosomal recessive form of inherited aplastic anaemia characterized by multiple congenital abnormalities, bone marrow failure, and susceptibility to malignancy, including myeloid leukaemias and squamous cell carcinomas.

There are 11 different genes for FA. FA cells have a defect in cell cycle regulation and in the DNA damage repair pathway.

Clinical features

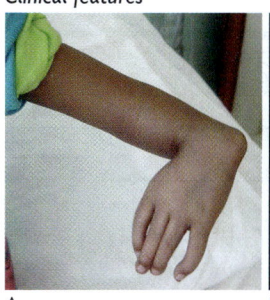

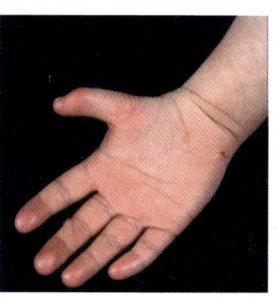

Fig 13.15 Fanconi anaemia: radial ray anomalies.

FA may present at birth with congenital anomalies or later with manifestations of bone marrow failure at any time from childhood to adulthood. Typically, presentation is with thrombocytopaenia between age 5 and 10 years.

About 75% have birth defects including upper limb radial ray anomalies (Fig 13.15), café-au-lait spots, short stature, GU abnormalities, microphthalmia, cataracts, cardiac defects. Malignancies may precede bone marrow failure in 25%.

Investigations

Thrombocytopaenia and leucopaenia may precede full-blown aplasia. Chromosome breakage: cultured lymphocytes show increased breaks, gaps, etc. in presence of DNA cross-linking agents. Gene mutation analysis is available.

Management

Supportive treatment with red cell and platelet transfusions. Aggressive iron chelation is initiated when ferritin level rises above 1000 microg/L. Bone marrow transplantation from an HLA identical donor is the treatment of choice. Androgens (e.g. danazol) should be considered if a suitable bone marrow donor is not available, as up to 75% respond.

Diamond–Blackfan anaemia (DBA)
This rare congenital erythroid aplasia has an incidence of 1/5 million live births. Up to 25% are familial and usually display autosomal dominant (AD) inheritance. One third have associated congenital abnormalities including craniofacial (snub nose, hyperteleorism), radial ray (triphalangeal thumbs), renal, and cardiac defects. Blood transfusion and oral prednisolone is the mainstay of treatment.

Shwachman–Diamond syndrome
A rare autosomal recessive (AR) disorder characterized by bone marrow failure, pancreatic exocrine failure, and skeletal abnormalities: short stature and metaphyseal dysostosis.

The most common haematological problem is isolated neutropaenia or mild pancytopaenia. There is an increase risk of malignancy. Clinical presentation may resemble cystic fibrosis. Mutational analysis of the *SBDS* gene is available.

13.6 Haemolytic anaemias

Haemolysis is the premature destruction of red cells and leads to haemolytic anaemia when the bone marrow cannot compensate for the shortened red cell lifespan. Red cell destruction may occur in the circulation as intravascular haemolysis or as extravascular haemolysis in the spleen.

The causes of haemolytic anaemia in childhood are shown in Table 13.6. Most acquired forms are immune mediated; inherited forms are caused by abnormalities of the red cell membrane or red cell enzyme defects. The haemoglobinopathies cause anaemia due to a combination of abnormal Hb molecule, ineffective erythropoiesis and reduced red cell lifespan.

Table 13.6.	Causes of haemolytic anaemia	
Inherited	Red cell membrane defects	Hereditary spherocytosis
		Hereditary elliptocytosis
	Red cell enzyme defects	Glucose-6-phosphate dehydrogenase (G6PD) deficiency
		Pyruvate kinase (PK) deficiency
	Haemoglobinopathies	Sickle cell disease, thalassaemia
Acquired	Immune-mediated	
	Alloimmune	Haemolytic disease of newborn (HDN)
		Transfusion mismatch
	Autoimmune	Evans syndrome
		Infection :EBV, mycoplasma
		Drugs: penicillin
	Non-immune mediated	Microangiopathic haemolytic anaemia : HUS, TTP
		Malaria, septicaemia
		Drug toxicity: dapsone, sulfasalazine
		Burns, animal venoms

Clinical features

Minimal or long-standing haemolytic anaemia may be asymptomatic. Features of haemolysis in addition to those attributable to anaemia may include:

- *Jaundice:* breakdown of haem may cause an unconjugated hyperbilirubinaemia. Haemolytic anaemia is an important cause of neonatal jaundice.
- *Gallstones:* bilirubin stones can develop in persistent haemolysis.
- *Haemoglobinuria:* acute intravascular haemolysis is usually associated with dark urine caused by haemoglobinuria.
- *Splenomegaly:* a variable finding.

Investigations

The hallmarks of a haemolytic anaemia include:
- *Reticulocytosis:* elevated count above 1%; associated macrocytosis (young red cells are larger)
- *Blood film:* polychromasia (reticulocytosis). Specific features related to aetiology may be seen such as spherocytes or red cell fragments in microangiopathy
- *Haptoglobin:* decreased in intravascular haemolysis
- *Bilirubin:* unconjugated hyperbilirubinaemia
- *Lactate dehydrogenase (LDH):* raised.

Hereditary spherocytosis (HS)

HS is the most common hereditary haemolytic anaemia in northern Europeans with a prevalence of about 1/2000.

Aetiology and pathophysiology

HS is usually an AD disorder caused by defects in proteins of the red cell cytoskeleton including spectrin, ankyrin, band 3, and band 4.2. Spectrin deficiency is the most common defect.

The spherical RBCs are rapidly destroyed by the spleen and have a lifespan of about 28 days. Haemolysis leads to jaundice and gallstones and is balanced by accelerated erythropoiesis. Anaemia worsens if there is increased splenic activity causing a haemolytic crisis or decreased erythropoiesis due to infection with parvovirus B19, causing an aplastic crisis.

Clinical features

There may be a family history of HS or history of a family member having had splenectomy or cholecystectomy. The wide variation in severity—mild (20–30%), moderate (60–75%), and severe (5%)—determines presentation.

Neonatal jaundice is common and may be severe enough to require exchange transfusion.

Mild HS may be asymptomatic until a haemolytic or aplastic crisis occurs. Moderate HS is characterized by mild anaemia, modest splenomegaly, and intermittent jaundice. Severe HS is usually the recessive form and characterized by severe haemolytic anaemia.

Diagnostic investigations

FBC and blood film

HS spherocytes, or microspherocytes are uniform in size and density, in contrast to spherocytes seen in thermal injury or immune haemolytic disease (Fig 13.16). RBC indices show increased MCHC. Reticulocytosis is apparent except in an aplastic crisis.

LDH is elevated and haptoglobin decreased.

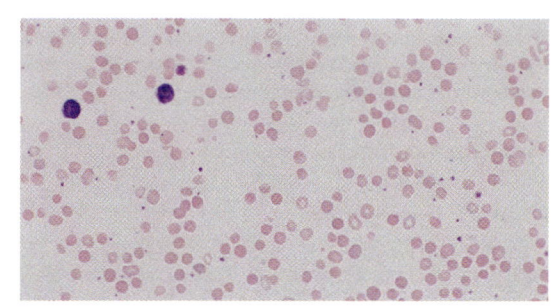

Fig 13.16 Hereditary spherocytosis: blood film.

EMA test

Eosin-5-maleimide is a fluorescent dye which binds to band 3 protein. Reduced binding has a sensitivity of 93% and specificity of 99% for HS.

Management

All patients should receive daily folic acid supplements. Blood transfusion may be required for severe anaemia in haemolytic or aplastic crises. The latter usually last 10–14 days and Hb values often fall by 50%.

Splenectomy
Splenectomy corrects the anaemia but not the underlying red cell defect. It should be considered in children with:
- Anaemia requiring repeat transfusions
- Pigment gallstones requiring cholecystectomy
- Poor growth and development, exercise intolerance.

Where possible it should be delayed until after the 6th birthday because of the risk of severe sepsis. Vaccination against *Pneumococcus*, *Haemophilus*, *Meningococcus* and hepatitis B, and lifelong prophylactic oral penicillin is recommended.

Glucose-6-phosphate dehydrogenase (G6PD) deficiency

G6PD deficiency is an X-linked red cell enzyme defect which affects 400 million people worldwide.

Aetiology and pathophysiology
Red cell enzymes support two important pathways:
- *Embden–Meyerhof pathway:* generates NADH and ATP
- Hexose monophosphate shunt: generates NADPH.

G6PD is important for generation of NADPH that is then utilized for glutathione reduction. Reduced glutathione is the main defence against oxidative damage to Hb.

Genetics of G6PD deficiency
The *G6PD* locus is at Xq28. Over 300 variants are known. Inheritance is X-linked recessive so males are predominantly affected, but incomplete lyonization can result in affected females.

The frequencies of allelic variants shows population specific variation. Variants have been divided into 4 classes according to severity of the enzyme deficiency from class 1 (severe) to class 4 (mild). In general, African variants are much less severe than those in Mediterranean populations.

The common variants are:
- Gd^B: normal activity; all world populations
- Gd^{A-}: 8–20% normal activity; African variant
- Gd^{Med}: <5% normal activity; Iraq, India, Greece, Sardinia.

Clinical features
This varies with severity of the enzyme deficiency. Severe class 1 variants causing chronic haemolytic anaemia are rare. Most common are the variants associated with acute intermittent haemolysis with oxidative stress.

Neonatal jaundice may occur, usually by age 1–4 days.

Most patients are asymptomatic with normal Hb levels and present with an acute haemolytic crisis characterized by anaemia, jaundice, splenomegaly, and haemoglobinuria. Precipitants may include:
- *Diet:* notably fava beans, hence the name favism, especially fresh and raw fava beans. *Vicia faba* are called broad beans in the UK.
- *Drugs:* risk is dose related and may be 'definite' or 'possible'.
  - *definite risk:* dapsone, primaquine, nitrofurantoin, quinolones, ciprofloxacin, nalidixic acids, sulphonamides: co-trimaxole
  - *possible risk:* aspirin, chloroquine + quinine
- *Infection:* oxidative metabolites produced by microbial pathogens, especially in viral hepatitis and typhoid fever.

Investigations
- *FBC and film:* during haemolytic episodes Heinz bodies may be seen either directly or after preincubation with oxidants.
- *G6PD enzyme assay:* a rapid fluorescent screening test or quantitative spectrophotometric analysis is available. An acute haemolytic episode selects for survival of young erythrocytes with higher enzymatic levels so the screening test may give a falsely high result during the acute episode.
- *DNA analysis:* useful for heterozygous females.

Management
Folate supplements for patients with chronic haemolytic anaemia. Education about precipitants of acute haemolysis and the importance of their avoidance.

Pyruvate kinase deficiency (PKD)

PKD is an AR disorder. It occurs worldwide but most cases are in the USA, northern Europe, and Japan. It is caused by defects in the isoenzymes PK-L and PK-R. Over 100 allelic variants are known, with a wide variation in severity.

PK catalyses glycolytic reactions which generate ATP.

Clinical features are highly variable, from a life-threatening anaemia to a mild haemolytic process. Management is folate, blood transfusions, and splenectomy for severe anaemia.

13.7 Sickle cell disease and thalassaemia

Sickle-cell disease (SCD)
SCD is a group of genetic disorders caused by the presence of sickle haemoglobin, HbS. It includes
- *Sickle cell anaemia:* HbSS
- *Haemoglobin SC disease:* HbSC
- *Sickle β-thalassaemia:* Hb S β-thal.

In the UK, up to 1 in 10 people of African or Caribbean descent have sickle cell trait and up to 1 in 60 have SCD giving a total of about 6000 adults and children with SCD.

Aetiology and pathogenesis
Genetics
Sickle cell haemoglobin results from a mutation in the β-globin gene which causes a single amino acid substitution, valine for glutamate, at position 6. Sickle cell anaemia is caused by homozygosity (HbSS) and sickle cell trait by heterozygosity. The other forms of SCD are compound heterozygous states in which one copy of the HbS gene is combined with another abnormal β-globin allele.

Pathogenesis
In the deoxy form, HbS polymerizes and precipitates causing red cell distortion with sickling and loss of elasticity in red cells (Fig 13.17). The RBCs are unstable with shortened survival, causing a chronic haemolytic anaemia. The rigid blood cells are unable to flow through narrow capillaries, causing vessel occlusion and ischaemia.

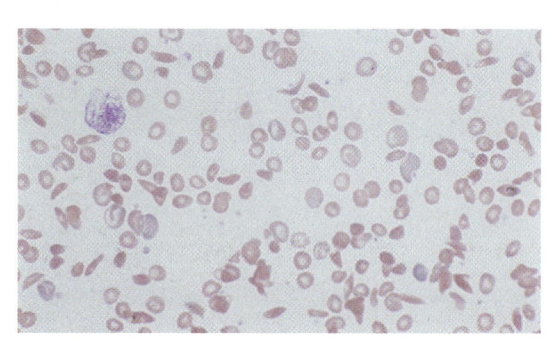

Fig 13.17 Sickle cell anaemia: blood film.

Clinical features
The features of different forms of SCD vary; this section describes sickle cell anaemia, HbSS.

The protective effect of high levels of circulating HbF can delay clinical presentation until 6–12 months. Antenatal or newborn screening is being introduced and will allow presymptomatic diagnosis.

There is a chronic haemolytic anaemia with haemoglobin levels in the range 5–9 g/dL. The clinical course is punctuated by four distinct types of 'crisis':
- *Vaso-occlusive crises:* dactylitis, painful crises, acute chest syndrome, stroke and priapism
- *Aplastic crises:* caused by parvovirus B19 infection
- *Haemolytic crises:* infection shortens red cell lifespan
- *Sequestration crises:* acute, painful splenic enlargement.

In addition, patients with HbSS disease are at risk of:
- Overwhelming infection due to functional hyposplenia
- Cholelithiasis and cholecystitis
- Osteomyelitis caused by *Salmonella* or *Staphylococci.*

Vaso-occlusive crisis
A painful crisis is the most common clinical manifestation of SCD. The usual site of vaso-occlusion is bone marrow causing bone pain. In infants, painful and usually symmetrical swelling of hands and feet, dactylitis, or hand–foot syndrome may be the initial manifestation (Fig 13.18). In older children pain affects joints, chest wall and long bones. Triggers include dehydration, infective episodes, acidosis, temperature extremes and sleep apnoea.

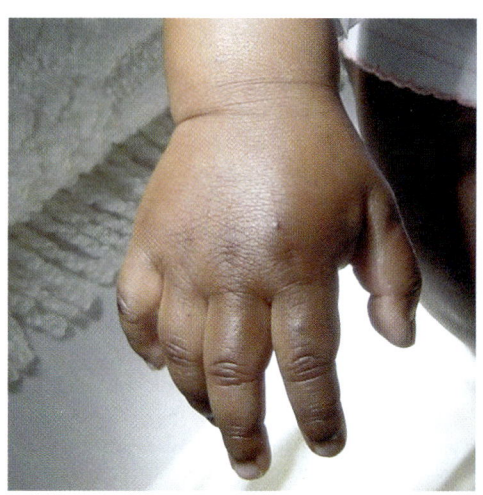

Fig 13.18 Sickle cell anaemia: dactylitis.

Vaso-occlusion at specific sites may cause:
- *Abdominal pain:* small infarcts of mesentery and viscera cause severe abdominal pain with diffuse tenderness.
- *Acute chest syndrome (ACS):* cough, chest pain, and tachypnoea. Aetiology is multifactorial and includes infection, fat embolism, and atelectasis as well as vaso-occlusion. CXR shows new infiltrates. ACS can be life-threatening.
- *Stroke:* cerebrovascular occlusion may occur in large or small vessels and manifest as transient ischaemic events, silent infarction, seizures, or stroke.
- *Priapism:* this may be acute or stuttering and is categorized as low flow (decreased outflow from penile veins) or high flow (unregulated arterial inflow).

Aplastic, sequestration, or haemolytic crises
These less common crises cause acute worsening of the anaemia. Aplastic crises are caused by infection with parvovirus B19 which causes transient red cell aplasia. The reticulocyte count is low. Splenic sequestration occurs in infants and young children before splenic infarction has occurred. Hepatic sequestration occurs in older children.

Chronic complications
- *Respiratory:* restrictive lung defects and asthma are common. Pulmonary hypertension in 30% of patients.
- *Renal:* tubular pathology commonly causes a concentrating defect which predisposes to dehydration.
- *CNS:* silent infarction may contribute to learning difficulties and a proliferative retinopathy may occur.
- *Orthopaedic:* chronic osteomyelitis, avascular necrosis of hip.

Sickle cell trait
Heterozygotes have RBCs with 30–40% HbS and have a benign clinical course. However, vaso-occlusive episodes can occur under hypoxic stress.

Investigations
Newborn screening for haemoglobinopathies is being introduced, using dried blood spots and high performance liquid chromatography (HPLC) or isoelectric focusing (IEF).

Diagnostic investigations include:
- *Solubility test, Sickledex:* detects HbS >10% and other abnormal HbS. Positive in sickle trait and disease but unreliable <6 months.
- Hb electrophoresis, HPLC, or IEF.

Management
Emergency measures are required during crises. All patients with HbSS anaemia should receive prophylactic oral penicillin V, folate supplements, and immunisation against *S. pneumoniae*. Additional long-term strategies include:
- *Hydroxyurea:* this increases fetal haemoglobin levels, and improves RBC hydration It reduces frequency of painful and chest crises. but is myelosuppressive.
- *Transfusion programme:* transfusion every 3–4 weeks is indicated following acute stroke.
- *Bone marrow (stem cell) transplantation:* this is potentially curative.

Management of crises
The mainstays of treatment of acute painful crises are:
- *Analgesia:* stepwise from paracetamol to opiates
- *Hydration:* IV fluids are usually required
- *Antibiotics:* IV cephalosporin if infection suspected.

Acute chest syndrome is responsible for 25% of deaths in children with SCD. In addition to analgesia, hydration, and antibiotics, oxygen is important. Top-up blood transfusion for significant anaemia of 1–2 g/dL less than baseline, and exchange transfusion may be life saving.

Red cell transfusion is usually required for aplastic or sequestration crises.

Thalassaemia

The thalassaemias are inherited disorders of haemoglobin synthesis caused by a decrease in production of one or more globin chains. The frequency is higher in populations from the Mediterranean basin, India, South-east Asia, North Africa. Worldwide, 15 million people have thalassaemia.

Aetiology and pathogenesis
The genes that control the production of globin chains lie within one of two clusters located on two chromosomes:
- *Chromosome 11:* five β-like globin genes: including β, γ, δ
- *Chromosome 16:* two α-like globin genes.

Each Hb molecule has four chains, two β-like and two α-like. HbF is $\alpha_2\gamma_2$, HbA is $\alpha_2\beta_2$, and HbA2 is $\alpha_2\delta_2$.

Thalassaemia genotypes and phenotypes
Thalassaemias are classified into β-thalassaemia and α-thalassaemia according to whether the mutation affects β-globin like or α-globin like genes.

The gene is designated + if synthesis is reduced, e.g. β+ The gene is designated 0 if synthesis is abolished, e.g. β0. Gene deletions abolish synthesis. The disorders are recessive and compound heterozygotes are common. This results in a spectrum of phenotypic severity from mild (minor) to moderate (intermedia) and severe (major).

Cellular pathophysiology
Imbalanced globin chain synthesis occurs, but the excess chains behave differently. In β-thalassaemia, excess α chains precipitate in RBC precursors causing intramedullary destruction, ineffective erythropoiesis, and premature destruction in the bone marrow, extramedullary sites, and circulation.

In α-thalassaemia, the excess chains change from γ to β and are able to form homotetramers, HbBarts (γ4) and HbH (β4) which are unstable but relatively soluble.

Chronic anaemia stimulates erythropoietin production, causing bone marrow expansion and bone deformity. Extramedullary haematopoiesis causes hepatosplenomegaly.

Clinical features
β-Thalassaemia
Several clinical forms are recognized, in order of severity:
- *Silent carrier:* heterozygous for a mild mutation.
- *Thalassaemia trait:* hypochromic, microcytic red cells, mild anaemia with abnormal Hb electrophoresis: elevated HbA2, HbF or both. Heterozygous for β0 or β+ mutation.
- *Thalassaemia intermedia:* compound heterozygosity causing anaemia of intermediate severity.
- *Thalassaemia major:* severe anaemia causing poor feeding from age 6 months when HbF levels decline.

α-Thalassaemia
Usually caused by gene deletions. The clinical phenotype depends on the number of genes deleted:
- *Silent carrier:* one gene inactivated (aa/ao). Subclinical with occasional low RBC indices
- *α-Thalassaemia trait:* two genes inactivated (aa/oo or ao/ao). Mild anaemia with low RBC indices.
- *HbH disease:* three genes inactivated (ao/oo). Usually a thalassaemia intermedia with mild to moderate anaemia, splenomegaly, and jaundice
- *Thalassaemia major:* loss of all four genes (oo/oo) is incompatible with life and results in death *in utero* from hydrops fetalis.

Investigations
Most children with β-thalassaemia in the UK are diagnosed antenatally or by newborn screening. If presentation is with anaemia, FBC and peripheral blood film is sufficient to indicate the diagnosis. Diagnosis is confirmed by HPLC.

Management
Patients with thalassaemia traits do not require medical care, but genetic counselling may be appropriate. β-Thalassaemia major requires regular blood transfusion with well-monitored chelation therapy.

- *Blood transfusion:* transfusion every 3–4 weeks to maintain Hb >9.5 g/dL. Iron overload occurs and if untreated toxic haemosiderin accumulates causing lethal cardiac disease, liver damage, and endocrine problems: hypothalamic and pituitary damage, diabetes mellitus, hypothyroidism.
- *Chelation therapy:* is started when the ferritin level reaches 1000 microg/L. Subcutaneous overnight infusion of desferrioxamine for 5–6 nights a week is the standard regimen. New oral agents are available. Monitoring iron status is critical. T2-weighted MRI is an indicator of cardiac iron status and annual echocardiography monitors function. Bone marrow (stem cell) transplantation is curative but limited by donor availability.

13.8 Haemophilia and von Willebrand disease

Disorders of coagulation

Disorders of coagulation may cause a bleeding diathesis or conversely, an increased tendency to intravascular coagulation, thrombophilia. Each category has inherited or acquired forms. The most important bleeding disorders are listed in Table 13.7.

Table 13.7. Disorders of coagulation: bleeding disorders	
Inherited	Haemophilia
	von Willebrand disease
	Rare factor deficiencies
	Fibrinogen disorders
Acquired	Vitamin K deficiency
	Liver disease
	Disseminated intravascular coagulation
	Drugs

Haemophilia

The haemophilias are a group of inherited disorders of coagulation and include:

- *Haemophilia A:* FVIII deficiency. Incidence 1: 10,000 male births, X-linked
- *Haemophilia B:* FIX deficiency. Incidence 1: 30,000 male births, X-linked.

Aetiology and pathogenesis
Genetics

Haemophilia A and B are X-linked recessive disorders. Up to one half of new cases are sporadic with no family history.

The FVIII gene, *F8*, is very large with 26 exons. A 'flip inversion' mutation in intron 22 of *F8* accounts for 45% of all serious cases of haemophilia A. Missense mutations are more common in patients with mild disease or who produce normal levels of a non-functional protein and are 'cross-reacting material' positive.

Molecular pathogenesis

Mutations interfere with the synthesis, stability, or function of the proteins generating a spectrum of severity in the phenotype determined by the level of activity.

The FVIII protein is very large, with three A domains, one B domain, and two C domains. The B domain is excised during activation. Most patients with severe disease do not produce a protein with either antigenic or coagulation activity and are at risk of developing antibodies to exogenous FVIII given as therapy.

Clinical features

Males are affected. Female carriers can have below-normal levels of coagulation factors, determined by random inactivation of the X chromosome (lyonization), and a mild bleeding diathesis. In the presence of a family history, antenatal diagnosis can be carried out by chorionic villous sampling (CVS) or diagnosis made on a cord blood sample at birth.

Haemophilia is classified clinically as:
- Mild: factor activity level >5%
- Moderate: factor activity level 2–5%
- Severe: factor activity level <1%.

Moderate to severe sporadic cases typically present with birth trauma related bleeding, bleeding post-circumcision, excessive toddler bruising, or soft-tissue, muscle, or joint bleeds at 6–18 months. Oral bleeds may occur as teeth erupt. Mild haemophilia typically presents in an older child with excessive bruising or bleeding following a traumatic or surgical event.

In an untreated case, repeated musculoskeletal bleeding occurs as physical activity increases with a high risk of crippling arthropathy from recurrent joint bleeds (Fig 13.19).

Other bleeding manifestations such as intracranial, iliopsoas, intra-abdominal, or GU tract bleeding are uncommon.

Diagnostic investigations

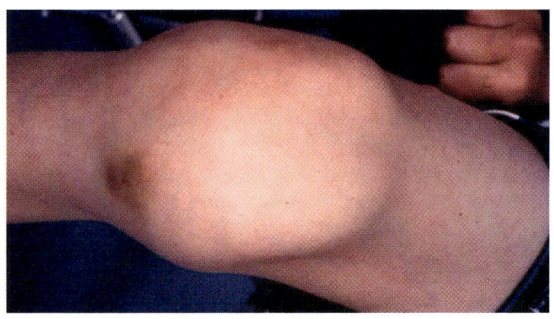

Fig 13.19 Severe haemophilia: arthropathy

The APTT is prolonged and factor assay levels reveal reduced FVIII or FIX levels. Bleeding time and PT are normal.

A DNA-based diagnosis is possible in 95% of cases. Diagnosis of the common flip inversion (seen in ~50% of patients with severe FVIII deficiency) and general mutation screening are widely offered. Carrier detection by molecular analysis is more reliable than methods based on assays of coagulation activity.

Management

The aims of modern management, which is provided in the UK by specialist centres, includes:
- Prevention of life-threatening bleeds and chronic joint damage
- Facilitation of social and physical well being
- Avoidance of harm by exposure to blood products.

Management involves prophylactic therapy to normalize haemostasis, treatment of bleeding episodes, and treatment of patients who develop factor inhibitors.

Maintaining haemostasis:primary prophylaxis

In severe haemophilia regular doses of FVIII or FIX may be given, three times weekly in haemophilia A and twice weekly in Haemophilia B.

Factor levels do not usually drop below 1% at any given time so the child is converted from a severe to a moderate or mild haemophiliac for most of the time. This allows participation in normal activities including non-contact sports. Younger boys may require a central venous catheter.

Products available for FVIII and FIX replacement therapy include plasma-derived products, monoclonal-antibody purified, and recombinant FVIII.

Treatment of bleeding episodes
Weight-bearing joints are most commonly affected. Prompt and adequate replacement therapy is essential to avoid long-term complications.

Deep intramuscular haematomas are difficult to detect. Intracranial haemorrhage is usually post-traumatic (beware the haemophiliac with a headache), and cranial imaging is indicated following factor infusion.

Oral bleeding is aggravated by fibrinolytic activity in saliva and helped by the antifibrinolytic agent tranexamic acid.

DDAVP is the treatment of choice in mild haemophilia as it stimulates a transient increase in FVIII levels sufficient to stop a bleeding episode or prepare patients for dental or minor surgical procedures.

Treatment in patients with factor inhibitors
Antibodies to infused factor concentrate develop in 25% of boys with haemophilia A and 5% of those with haemophilia B. This presents with poor response to treatment. Treatment options include use of agents that bypass the defect, such as recombinant FVIIa. Inhibition can be eradicated by inducing immune tolerance but this is expensive, time consuming, and difficult.

von Willebrand disease (vWD)
vWD is the most common inherited bleeding disorder with an incidence of up to 1% and is caused by quantitative or qualitative deficiency of vWF, a large multimeric protein.

Aetiology and pathogenesis
The gene for vWF is on chromosome 12p. Inheritance of the most common forms is AD but the molecular genetics remains complex and not fully resolved.

Quantitative or qualitative deficiency of vWF disrupts:
- Primary haemostasis due to failure of platelet adherence to vessel wall
- Secondary haemostasis due to destabilization of Factor VIII.

vWF is composed of complex multimers of low, intermediate, or high molecular weight. Small multimers function mainly as FVIII carriers.

Acquired forms of vWD due to autoantibodies have been described in Wilms tumour, SLE, congenital heart disease, and hypothyroidism.

Clinical features
There is considerable phenotypic variation even within the same family due to both genetic modifiers such as ABO blood group and environmental factors such as hormones and stress. Several types are recognized:

Type 1 vWD (70–80% of cases)
Quantitative deficiency of vWF and FVIII. Features include easy bruising, menorrhagia, epistaxis, gum bleeding after tooth brushing, post-traumatic or post-surgical bleeding. Usually mild and often asymptomatic.

Type 2 vWD (15–20% of cases)
Qualitative deficiency of vWF. Normal levels but multimers structurally abnormal.
There are four subtypes: 2A, 2B, 2M, and 2N. In 2A and 2B the clinical features are similar to type 1 with mucosal and skin bleeding and epistaxis. In type 2B the abnormal vWF has increased affinity for platelets and causes intermittent thrombocytopaenia.

Type 3 VWD (rare: 1–2 per million)
AR with complete absence of vWF. Frequent severe mucosal bleeding and haemarthroses may occur. FVIII levels can be as low as 2%.

Diagnostic investigations
Laboratory findings are variable. The following results are usually found:
- PT, TT normal
- Platelet count normal, but low in type 2B
- APTT prolonged or at upper end of normal range
- *FVIIIc:* reduced or low normal in types 1, 2B
- *vWF antigen:* reduced or low normal in type 2B
- *vWF activity:* measured by ristocetin-induced platelet aggregation, acts by causing vWF to bind to platelets. Impaired, but enhanced in type 2B.

Mutation analysis is possible at specialized centres and if antenatal diagnosis has been done for type 3 disease.

Management
Patients with vWD do not normally require regular treatment but should be advised against use of aspirin and NSAIDs. Treatment to correct the haemostatic defect is required for surgical procedures or bleeding episodes. Optimal therapy depends on the subtype and severity:
- *Mild disease:* DDAVP promotes release of vWF from storage pools in endothelial cells. The side effects of seizures and hyponatraemia limit use in young children. It is useful in most patients with a quantitative deficiency but efficacy needs to be assessed in each patient. It may be given IV, SC, or intranasally. Contraindicated in type 2B patients in whom it causes thrombocytopaenia.
- *Severe disease:* type 3 or type 2B: best treated with vWF and FVIII concentrates. Consider cryoprecipitate or platelet transfusion for severe uncontrolled bleeding.

13.9 Coagulation disorders and thrombophilia

Rare factor deficiencies and fibrinogen disorders

The rare factor deficiencies have a frequency between 1 and 2 per million. They include deficiencies of factors V, VII, X, XIII and prothrombin and fibrinogen. They are AR and more likely in consanguineous couples. A severe bleeding tendency is usually present from birth, and may cause bleeding from the umbilical stump.

All result in an abnormal coagulation screen except for FXIII deficiency.

Vitamin K deficiency: haemorrhagic disease of the new born (HDN)

The incidence of HDN in the UK is 8.6/100 000 live births (1987–1990) and has been reduced by prophylaxis.

Aetiology and pathogenesis
Vitamin K deficiency in newborns is caused by several factors including low amounts of vitamin K in breast milk, lack of gut synthesis of vitamin K, functional immaturity of the liver, and low levels of vitamin K dependent factors at birth.
Risk factors include:
- *Breast feeding*: the risk of HDN is increased 20-fold in breast-fed infants.
- *Maternal drugs*: isoniazid, rifampicin, anticoagulants, and anticonvulsants increase risk of early HDN.
- *Unsuspected liver disease*: α_1-antitrypsin deficiency or malabsorption in cystic fibrosis.

Vitamin K is a cofactor for the gamma-carboxylase enzyme which is vital for synthesis of factors II, VII, IX, and X and proteins C and S. Deficiency leads to failure of secondary haemostasis.

Clinical features
HDN is classified into:
- *Early*: 1st 24 h. Limited to infants of mothers receiving the drugs mentioned above and presents with bleeding related to birth trauma: cephalhaematoma, intracranial bleeding.
- *Classic*: days 1–7. Presents with bleeding from umbilical stump, GI tract, nose, or gums.
- *Late*: weeks 2–12. High morbidity and mortality due to CNS haemorrhage which may be intraventricular, subdural, or subarachnoid.

The differential diagnosis includes haemophilia in boys, thrombocytopaenia, DIC and trauma, accidental or non-accidental.

Diagnostic investigations
Both PT and APTT are prolonged.

Management
Prevention by routine administration of vitamin K to babies at birth has reduced the UK incidence. A single dose of 1.0 mg of intramuscular vitamin K after birth is effective in the prevention of classic HDN. Oral vitamin K has not been tested in randomized trials and there is a danger of late HDN if dosing is incomplete.

Treatment is with vitamin K together with solvent/detergent plasma if bleeding is severe.

Liver disease

The aetiology of coagulation disorders in children with liver disease is multifactorial:
- Malabsorption of fat-soluble vitamin K
- Impaired synthesis of coagulation factors
- Impaired clearance of activated clotting factors and increased fibrinolysis.

Management includes administration of vitamin K, solvent/detergent plasma, and administration of cryoprecipitate or fibrinogen concentrate.

Disseminated intravascular coagulation (DIC)

DIC is the uncontrolled activation of the coagulation and fibrinolytic pathways.

Aetiology and pathogenesis
The list of causes is long and includes:
- Severe infections, e.g. meningococcal septicaemia
- Intravascular haemolysis, e.g. ABO-incompatible transfusion
- Liver disease
- Malignancy.

DIC usually occurs in children who are critically ill.

There is consumption of coagulation factors and platelets, intravascular fibrin deposition, and accelerated degradation of fibrin and fibrinogen.

Clinical features
DIC can cause profuse bleeding into the skin, GI tract, and CNS.

Laboratory investigation shows prolonged APTT and PT, thrombocytopaenia, low fibrinogen, and elevated D-dimers.

Treatment of the underlying cause is a priority and options to control bleeding include fresh frozen plasma and platelets as first line treatment. Other forms of intervention include the use of concentrates such as cryoprecipitate, fibrinogen concentrate, and anticoagulant concentrates.

Thrombophilia

Thrombophilia is an increased tendency to develop clots in veins, arteries, or both. Thromboembolic disease is relatively uncommon in childhood.

Aetiology of thrombophilia in children.
Thrombophilia may be inherited or acquired. See Table 13.8.

Table 13.8. Causes of thrombophilia	
Inherited	Thrombotic thrombocytopenic purpura
	Congenital deficiencies of antithrombin, protein C, or protein S
	Homocysteinaemia
	Factor V Leiden (rarely causes problems pre-puberty)
	Prothrombin variant G20210A
	Dysfibrinogenaemia
Acquired	Indwelling vascular catheters
	Acquired natural anticoagulant deficiency
	Nephrotic syndrome: antithrombin deficiency
	Purpura fulminans:
	varicella may cause protein S deficiency
	meningococcaemia may cause protein C deficiency (Fig 13.20)
	Neonatal diseases: respiratory distress syndrome, necrotizing enterocolitis, birth asphyxia, maternal anticardiolipin antibodies
	Heparin-induced thrombocytopaenia/ thrombosis syndrome (HIT/HITTS)
	Extracorporeal membrane oxygenation
	Haemolytic uraemic syndrome/thrombotic thrombocytopaenic purpura.

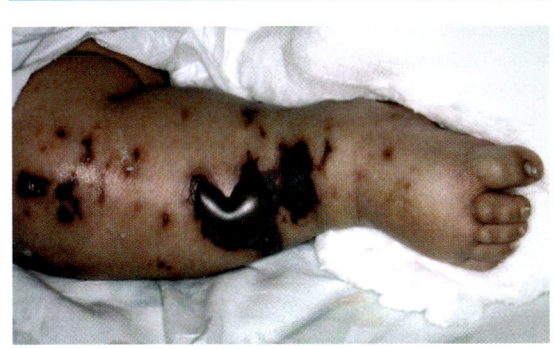

Fig 13.20 Purpura fulminans: secondary to acquired protein C deficiency in meningococcal septicaemia.

Venous thromboembolism (VTE)
The incidence is low at 5.3/10 000 hospital admissions in children and 0.5/10 000 live births in neonates. Idiopathic, primary VTE is rare and serious risk factors are usually present.

The most common risk factors are central venous lines, associated with VTEs in the upper venous system and extracorporeal circulation devices.

Clinical manifestations may be non-specific and diagnosis rests on venography, ultrasound, and echocardiography. Umbilical vein catheters may cause thrombi in the IVC or portal vein which may be clinically silent. Renal vein thrombosis is the most common non-catheter-related VTE in the 1st month of life. Cerebral sinovenous thrombosis may occur in neonates with dehydration and sepsis.

Antithrombotic prophylaxis may be considered in paediatric patients under certain circumstances such as Fontan operation, sick children with multiple risk factors, or the presence of congenital prothrombotic disorders.

Heparin is used acutely or oral anticoagulants such as warfarin or low-molecular-weight heparin for longer-term management. Screening for congenital thrombophilia is recommended in children with spontaneous or recurrent VTE.

Arterial thromboembolism
Arterial catherization is the most common risk factor. Non-catheter-related arterial thrombosis may occur in Kawasaki disease, familial hyperlipidaemia, congenital cardiac arterial abnormalities, and sickle cell disease.

Arterial ischemic strokes are rare. Predisposing conditions include sickle cell disease, moya moya disease, and congenital cardiac malformations especially ASD and PFO.

Thrombotic thrombocytopenic purpura (TTP)
This rare condition is caused by reduced activity of ADAMTS13, an enzyme responsible for cleaving large multimers of vWF protein into smaller fragments.

Aetiology and pathogenesis
- *Inherited (congenital) TTP:* mutations in *ADAMTS13*
- *Idiopathic:* autoimmune disorder caused by antibodies to ADAMTS13.
- *Secondary TTP:* complication of malignancy, BMT, HIV infection, drugs (immunosuppressants, platelet aggregation inhibitors).

Deficient ADAMTS13 function leads to the presence of ultra-large vWF which causes platelet aggregation and formation of microthrombi in the microcirculation. This leads to microangiopathic haemolytic anaemia and reduced blood flow and end-organ damage in brain and kidneys. Pathogenesis overlaps with that in haemolytic uraemic syndrome in which renal pathology predominates.

Clinical features
A 'pentad' of five key features is recognized:
- Fever
- *Fluctuating CNS dysfunction:* headache, stroke, fits
- *Thrombocytopaenia:* bruising and purpura
- Microangiopathic haemolytic anaemia
- Renal impairment.

Congenital TTP presents during infancy or early childhood with recurrent episodes of low platelets and haemolytic anaemia. Episodes may be precipitated by viral infections.

Management
Congenital TTP is treated with prophylactic plasma infusions every 2–3 weeks to maintain adequate functioning levels of ADAMTS13.

Acquired TTP is a life-threatening emergency requiring urgent plasmapheresis to remove antibodies and restore ADAMTS13 levels.

13.10 Platelet and white cell disorders

Thrombocytopaenia

Megakaryocytes develop into platelets by shedding cytoplasmic granules which have developed into platelets. Platelet production is under the control of growth factors including thrombopoietin and IL-6.

The normal circulating platelet count is $150-400 \times 10^9/L$ and does not vary with age. The average lifespan is 7–10 days. Platelets are disposed of in the spleen.

Absolute platelet counts do not correlate in a simple way with the haemostatic defect. Vascular factors are also important and with high turnover, an excess of new active platelets may exist.

Aetiology
Thombocytopaenia may be caused by impaired production or decreased survival (Table 13.9).

Table 13.9. Causes of thrombocytopaenia

Impaired production	
Inherited	Thrombocytopaenia absent radius (TAR) syndrome
	Fanconi anaemia
	Wiskott–Aldrich syndrome
	Aplastic anaemia
Acquired	Bone marrow infiltration
Decreased survival	
Immune-mediated	ITP
	Neonatal isoimmune, alloimmune or idiopathic thrombocytopaenic purpura
	Autoimmune disorders: SLE
	Infections, drugs, malignancy
Non-immune mediated	DIC
	Haemolytic uraemic syndrome
	TTP
	Kasabach–Merritt syndrome
	Liver disease
	vWD type 2B
	Drugs: valproate, rifampicin

Immune thrombocytopaenic purpura (ITP)

ITP is defined as an immune mediated thrombocytopaenia not associated with drugs or other evidence of disease. It is the most common cause of childhood thrombocytopaenia. Most cases are benign and self-limiting.

ITP is classified as acute or as chronic if it persists >6 months. Acute ITP has an equal sex incidence with ~500 new cases per year in the UK. A peak is seen in autumn and winter. Peak age of presentation is 2–5 years. Chronic ITP is more common in females. 72% of patients >10 years are female.

Aetiology and pathogenesis
Acute ITP usually follows a viral infection or immunisation. Pathogenesis involves a complex immune response combined with a relative failure of marrow compensation. Platelet antibodies coat the platelets which are then removed by the reticuloendothelial system, usually in the spleen.

Clinical features
Acute ITP usually manifests as an abrupt onset of purpura with excessive or spontaneous bruising. Less common is nose or mouth bleeding, known as 'wet purpura'. Bleeding from bowel or GU tract is rare. Intracranial haemorrhage is extremely rare (1/500). The prevalence of a palpable spleen (12%) is not different from that in the non-ITP paediatric population. The child is systemically well.

The differential diagnosis includes non-accidental injury, aplastic anaemia, and acute leukaemia. In older girls SLE may present with isolated thrombocytopaenia.

Diagnostic investigations
- Isolated thrombocytopaenia in the range $1-30 \times 10^9/L$ is characteristic.
- Purpura with a platelet count $>30 \times 10^9/L$ should prompt a search for an alternative diagnosis.
- Bone marrow biopsy is not usually required for diagnosis.

Management
Acute ITP
Most children recover quickly with no treatment, 80% within 6 weeks in one study. Severe haemorrhage from GI tract, GU tract, or nose occurs in 3–5% of patients and intracranial haemorrhage in <1/1500. This cannot be predicted and is not prevented by treatment.

If there is no severe haemorrhage admission is unnecessary. Information and advice should be provided on avoidance of contact sports, exposure to head injury, and antiplatelet medication such as NSAIDs. The plan of action should include a contact person to call in emergency.

The patient, rather than the platelet count, should be the focus of management. In ITP the few platelets circulating are more efficient. Air travel is not a risk.

Platelet transfusions are not indicated except in very severe bleeding as consumption is rapid. If severe haemorrhage is present, treatment options include:
- *Steroids*: steroids are first line treatment. Oral prednisolone 4 mg/kg per day for 4 days or 1–2 mg/kg daily for a maximum of 14 days.
- *Intravenous immunoglobulin (IVIG)*: this raises the platelet count within 48 h, but side effects are common such as headaches and chills. IVIG is reserved for emergency treatment of patients with active bleeding who do not respond to steroids.
- *Anti-D*: is effective in Rh D-positive non-splenectomized patients, given as a single IV dose but can cause severe intravascular haemolysis..

Chronic ITP
Management of chronic ITP is more challenging. Splenectomy may be considered but has a 25% failure rate. New therapies include a monoclonal antibody, anti-CD20.

Neonatal thrombocytopaenia

There are two types of neonatal thrombocytopaenia:
- *Neonatal isoimmune thrombocytopaenia*: occurs in infants of mothers with active or previous ITP due to transplacental passage of antiplatelet antibodies. Antenatal maternal steroid treatment may improve the fetal platelet count.
- *Neonatal alloimmune thrombocytopaenia*: this usually occurs if a HPA-1a negative mother has a HPA-1a positive fetus. However, only 6% of at-risk mothers are sensitized.

In contrast to haemolytic disease of the newborn it may occur in the first born. Treatment options include maternal infusions of IgG, steroids, or perinatal transfusions of immunologically compatible platelets. Maternal platelets can be used.

Platelet function disorders

Inherited
Inherited forms fall into several groups:

Defects of the platelet membrane:
- *Disorders of adhesion*: Bernard–Soulier syndrome is caused by deficiency of glycoprotein Ib. Bruising and mucosal bleeding occur. Platelets are giant and few and do not aggregate with ristocetin.
- *Disorders of aggregation*: Glanzmann thrombasthenia is due to abnormalities of glycoprotein IIb/IIIa. Episodic mucocutaneous bleeding and unprovoked bruising manifests soon after birth. Platelets fail to aggregate.

Storage pool disorders
- *Dense granules storage pool disease:* Hermansky–Pudlak, Chediak–Higashi, Wiskott–Aldrich, Thrombocytopaenia absent radii. May–Hegglin syndromes.
- α-*Granule storage pool disease:* grey platelet syndrome.

Release defects
- Deficiency of cyclo-oxygenase or thromboxane synthetase.

Acquired
Acquired disorders of platelet function occur with drugs—aspirin and NSAIDs, furosemide, nitrofurantoin, cephalosporins; renal and hepatic failure, leukaemia, and myeloproliferative disorders

Neutropaenia

The normal range of circulating white cells varies with age. Newborns have a high total count and relative neutrophilia. Africans and Afro-Caribbeans have lower counts than whites, Chinese, and Asians. About 25% of healthy black infants may have a neutrophil count $<1.0 \times 10^9$/L.

Neutropaenia is defined as a reduction in the absolute neutrophil count below the normal for age, sex, physiological status, and ethnic origin. It is classified as:
- *Mild*: $>1.0 \times 10^9$/L but < lower limit of normal
- *Moderate*: $0.5–1.0 \times 10^9$/L
- *Severe*: $0.2–0.5 \times 10^9$/L
- *Very severe*: $<0.2 \times 10^9$/L.

The risk of infection is higher when neutropaenia is due to reduced production rather than increased consumption. Neutropaenia persisting for >6 months is chronic.

Aetiology
The most common cause of neutropaenia is chemotherapy for malignant disease. However, there are many rare inherited disorders which cause neutropaenia and a variety of acquired disorders (Table 13.10).

Clinical features
Viral infection is the most common cause of transient neutropaenia in children, developing in the first 2 days of illness and persisting for 3–6 days.

Table 13.10. Causes of neutropaenia

Inherited defects	*Non-syndromic:* Severe congenital neutropaenia: Kostmann disease (SCN1–4) *Syndromic:* Shwachman–Diamond syndrome Fanconi anaemia Cartilage hair hypoplasia Glycogen storage disease type 1b Organic acidaemias.
Acquired defects Production failure:	Marrow infiltration: acute leukaemia, osteopetrosis Aplastic anaemia Drugs: chemotherapy, antibiotics, NSAIDs Nutrition: Vit B12, folate deficiency, copper deficiency Viral infection: parvovirus B19, EBV, varicella, HIV
Excess consumption:	Hypersplenism Severe bacterial sepsis. Neonatal alloimmune neutropaenia Chronic benign (autoimmune) neutropaenia

Chronic benign or autoimmune neutropaenia is the most common cause of chronic neutropaenia in infancy and childhood. Median age of presentation is 8–11 months with increased incidence of minor infections. Anti-neutrophil antibodies are detected. Spontaneous remission is the norm.

Clinical problems are uncommon with neutrophil counts $>0.5 \times 10^9$/L but are potentially severe and life threatening if below 0.5×10^9/L. Infections are commonly bacterial such as cellulitis, pneumonia, septicaemia, or abscess formation and prone to disseminate. There is an increased risk of fungal infection and infection with *Pneumocystis carinii*.

Management
- *Investigations:* in a well child, the first priority is to establish whether neutropaenia is transient or persistent, so repeat FBCs should be done over several weeks. Useful initial investigations for persistent neutropaenia include neutrophil antibodies, B12 and folate levels, immunoglobulin levels, T and B cell subsets, and a viral screen including antibodies to HIV.
- *Treatment:* in prolonged neutropaenia preventative measures are important and include: mouth care and dental hygiene and prophylactic medication: co-trimoxazole for pneumocystis, itraconazole for fungi, aciclovir for herpes simplex virus. Treatment options depend on cause but include G-CSF therapy and bone marrow transplantation. Fevers or severe infections require broad spectrum antibiotics.

13.11 Case-based discussions

A girl with pancytopaenia and organomegaly

A 4 year old girl presented to her GP with a 1 week history of recurrent mild nose bleeds. Nasal pressure and cotton wool plugs were advised. She returned 6 weeks later with increasingly frequent, heavy nose bleeds, pallor, tiredness on exertion, and mouth ulcers. Referral was made for a paediatric opinion.

Examination revealed anaemia, several oral ulcers, and hepatosplenomegaly. The liver was 3 cm below the costal margin and spleen 12 cm. Excessive bruising was apparent on the trunk and arms.

What is the likely diagnosis?
The clinical features of anaemia, easy bruising, and mouth ulcers suggest pancytopaenia. Organomegaly suggests an infiltrative process and acute leukaemia is the most likely diagnosis. The splenomegaly is unusually marked.

A FBC shows:

> Haemoglobin 5.2 g/dL
> WBC 2.9 × 10^9/L
> Neutrophils 0.09 × 10^9/L
> Lymphocytes 2.34 × 10^9/L
> Platelets 41 × 10^9/L

Examination of the blood film confirms pancytopaenia but identifies no other abnormality. A provisional diagnosis of acute leukaemia is made.

A more detailed history reveals recent foreign travel. The family have visited southern Spain on four occasions during the previous year. They had stayed with friends who lived in a forest area inhabited by many feral dogs.

What further investigation is required?
A bone marrow examination is essential. A diagnosis of leukaemia cannot be made on peripheral blood examination.

The bone marrow aspirate is shown in Fig 13.21.

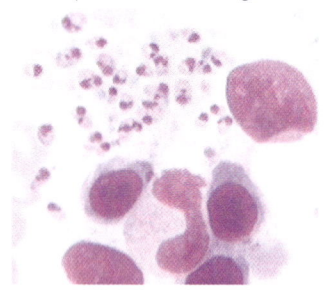

Fig 13.21 Bone marrow aspirate

What is the diagnosis?
Leishmania donovan bodies are seen, making a diagnosis of visceral leishmaniasis (kala-azar). This is a zoonosis transmitted by sandflies from mammals including dogs. Enquiry about recent foreign travel is often worthwhile. She responded well to treatment with IV liposomal amphotericin B.

A girl with excessive bruising

A 6 year old girl is referred for assessment by the social work department. A neighbour raised concern about her 'black eyes'. The family is known to social services on account of a history of domestic violence and alcohol misuse by the child's mother. No explanation for the black eyes has been offered by the child or her family.

On examination she appears systemically well. There is no fever or pallor. She has bilateral black eyes, a large bruise over the left loin, and multiple large bruises over both lower limbs (Fig 13.22). A spleen tip is just palpable.

What is the differential diagnosis?
Accidental bruises are common in mobile 6 year olds and usually occur over anterior bony prominences. The lower limb bruises could be accidental. Bruises to the face or back are more consistent with physical abuse but a bleeding diathesis must always be excluded. Finger-tip bruising can occur from normal interactions in a child with a bleeding diathesis. A spleen may be palpable in immune thrombocytopaenic purpura. Neuroblastoma may present with bilateral black eyes. The distribution is not typical of Henoch–Schönlein purpura.

A

B

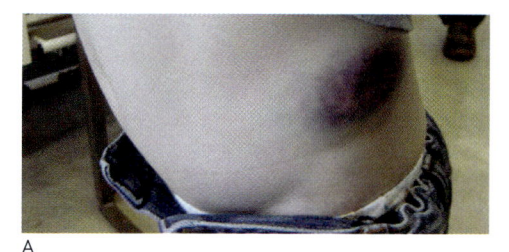

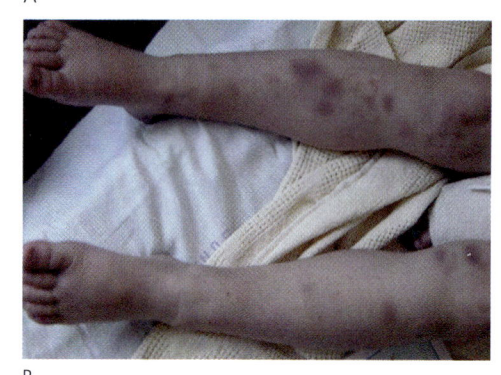

Fig 13.22

What investigations are indicated?
Initial tests should include:

Coagulation screen: PT, APTT, TT, and fibrinogen levels.

FBC: platelet count and film.

Second line tests may include FVIII and FIX levels and vWF antigen and activity (ristocetin cofactor). The initial screen may be normal in vWD, Henoch–Schönlein purpura, and rarities such as FXIII deficiency and platelet function disorders,

The only abnormality identified was isolated thrombocytopaenia: platelet count 5 × 10^9/L/

She made a spontaneous recovery without any intervention from her immune thrombocytopenic purpura (ITP).

Chapter 14

Oncology

14.1 Cancer in childhood *292*
14.2 Treatment of childhood cancer *294*
14.3 Acute leukaemias *296*
14.4 Lymphomas *298*
14.5 CNS tumours, retinoblastoma, and germ cell tumours *300*
14.6 Wilms tumour, neuroblastoma, and STS *302*
14.7 Bone tumours and LCH *304*
14.8 Case-based discussions *306*

14.1 Cancer in childhood

Epidemiology

Cancer in childhood is rare. The overall risk of developing cancer under 15 years of age is just 1/600. There are 1500 new cases of childhood cancer in the UK each year, accounting for 0.5% of all cancer. However, malignancy is the most common cause of death at age 5–14 years in the UK.

The frequency of particular cancers differs from that in adults. Leukaemia accounts for one third of cases followed by CNS tumours (brain and spinal cord) which account for one quarter. The most common extracranial solid tumours are Wilms tumour, lymphoma, neuroblastoma, and soft tissue sarcomas (Fig 14.1).

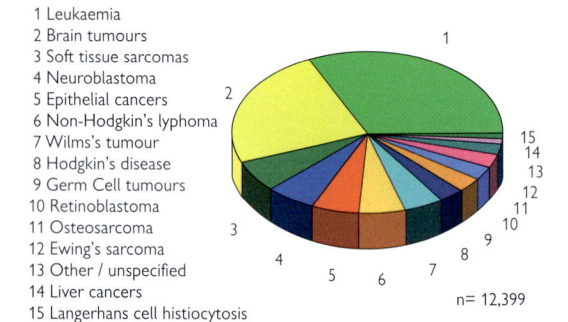

1 Leukaemia
2 Brain tumours
3 Soft tissue sarcomas
4 Neuroblastoma
5 Epithelial cancers
6 Non-Hodgkin's lyphoma
7 Wilms's tumour
8 Hodgkin's disease
9 Germ Cell tumours
10 Retinoblastoma
11 Osteosarcoma
12 Ewing's sarcoma
13 Other / unspecified
14 Liver cancers
15 Langerhans cell histiocytosis

n= 12,399

Fig 14.1 Frequency of childhood cancers.

Aetiology

The cause of most childhood cancers is unknown. Inherited predisposition accounts for a small minority of cases (<5%) and environmental factors play a minor role.

Environmental factors
Established factors include:
- *Ultraviolet radiation:* skin cancer
- *Ionizing radiation:* increased incidence of leukaemia
- *Cytotoxic drugs:* alkylating agents or topoisomerase II inhibitors may increase incidence of leukaemia
- *HIV infection:* increased risk of non-Hodgkin's lymphoma, Kaposi's sarcoma, and leiomyosarcoma.

Genetic predisposition
Cancer can be regarded as a genetic disorder of the somatic cells but an inherited genetic predisposition is found in only a minority of cases. Retinoblastoma is the most common example of a cancer with a clear genetic aetiology which may run in families, but several genetic syndromes have an increased risk of malignant disease (see Table 14.1).

Table 14.1. Genetic syndromes and susceptibility to cancer

Down syndrome	Acute leukaemia
Neurofibromatosis type 1	Optic glioma, phaeochromocytoma
Von Hippel–Lindau disease	Renal cell carcinoma, phaeochromocytoma
Familial adenomatous polyposis	Hepatoblastoma
Beckwith–Wiedemann syndrome	Wilms tumour
WAGR (**W**ilms tumour, **A**niridia, **G**enitourinary abnormalities, **R**etardation)	Wilms tumour
Xeroderma pigmentosum	Skin cancer
Ataxia telangiectasia	Leukaemia, lymphoma
Li–Fraumeni syndrome	Sarcoma, breast cancer, adrenocortical cancer

Molecular pathogenesis

The molecular mechanisms underlying malignancy relate to alterations in the structure and function of genes which regulate cell growth and differentiation. The majority of genetic alterations occur in the somatic cells and are manifested as major chromosomal rearrangements (translocations, deletions, insertions) as well as point mutations and gene amplifications.

The genes affected by these alterations fall into three groups: oncogenes, tumour-suppressor genes, and stability genes. These genes encode proteins which fall into several classes: transcription factors, growth factors and their receptors, kinase inhibitors, and signal transducers.

Oncogenes
Proto-oncogenes encode normal cellular proteins involved in growth signalling pathways, most commonly transcription factors. Mutated proto-oncogenes are called oncogenes.

Mutations usually cause a gain of function and act in a dominant way: only one mutant allele is sufficient to alter cell function. Examples include:
- *MYC:* in Burkitt lymphoma the translocation t (8;14) moves one allele of *CMYC* from chromosome 8 to the immunoglobulin heavy chain locus in chromosome 14 where enhancer elements lead to over-expression. *MYCN* is amplified in a subset (25%) of neuroblastoma patients and associated with poor outcome.
- Translocations fuse *PAX3* or *PAX7* with *FKHR* in alveolar rhabdomyosarcoma or *EWS* and *FL11* in Ewing sarcoma.

Tumour-suppressor genes
These genes encode products which normally regulate cell number by inhibiting progress through the cell cycle or promoting programmed cell death (apoptosis). See Fig 14.2.

Mutations usually cause inactivation and act in a recessive way: inactivation of both alleles is necessary. This mechanism underlies Knudson's 'two-hit' hypothesis in which individuals inherit a germline mutation in the gene (first hit) and subsequently acquire a somatic mutation in the second allele (second hit) (Fig 14.3). Loss of heterozygosity (LOH) is a marker of a putative tumour suppressor gene.

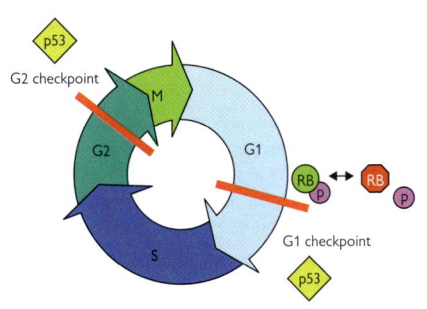

Fig 14.2 The cell cycle. G1 and G2 checkpoints control progression through the four phases. The RB protein controls progression through G1. Activation of p53 induces cell cycle arrest at G1 or G2 checkpoints.

Fig 14.3 Knudson's two-hit hypothesis illustrated for familial and sporadic retinoblastoma. Reprinted from Current Paediatrics, Strahm and Capra, © 2005, with permission from Elsevier.

Examples
- *RB1*: this is the classical tumour-suppressor gene. Familial retinoblastoma (RB) occurs in individuals who have inherited a germline mutation and subsequently acquire a somatic mutation. Sporadic RB is caused by two independently acquired somatic mutations. The retinoblastoma protein pRB acts as the molecular switch controlling passage through the G1 checkpoint.
- *TP53*: this gene encodes p53, sometimes called 'the guardian of the genome'. It is switched off in normal cells and activated by multiple stimuli such as DNA damage, viral infection, and oncogene activation. Activation causes expression of proteins that induce cell cycle arrest or apoptosis, preventing replication of damaged cells. The p53 protein is therefore a critical inhibitor of tumour development and loss of normal function allows tumours to grow.

Mutations of *TP53* are present in 50% of human tumours. Germline mutations occur in most families with Li–Fraumeni syndrome, a hereditary cancer syndrome.

Stability genes
These encode proteins involved in the control of processes such as DNA repair and chromosome segregation during mitosis. Loss of function results in a general increase in the rate of mutations. Mutations behave in a recessive way. An examples is:
- *ATM*: mutations in ATM are associated with ataxia telangiectasia. 20% of patients develop malignancy, especially leukaemia or lymphoma.

Cell physiology
At least six alterations in cell physiology are essential for malignant growth:
- Self-sufficiency in growth signals
- Insensitivity to growth inhibitory signals
- Evasion of programmed cell death
- Limitless replicative potential, achieved in part by telomere maintenance mechanisms which prevent the telomere shortening associated with cell senescence
- *Sustained angiogenesis:* solid tumour growth requires a vascular supply and many tumours express stimulators of angiogenesis (VEGF, FGF) or decreased expression of angiogenesis inhibitors
- *Tissue invasion and metastasis:* the molecular mechanisms allowing cells to migrate via the circulation to a new microenvironment remain uncertain.

Presentation of malignancy
All clinicians caring for children are concerned that seemingly innocuous symptoms may be a feature of malignancy, and early diagnosis does remain a challenge.

However, hindsight often ascribes undue significance to symptoms present in the months before a malignancy is diagnosed and the fact is that optimal early diagnosis is in many cases very difficult to achieve. Some 'red flags' are listed in the Box.

'Red flags' for childhood malignancy	
Pain	Bone pain that is persistent and present at night
	Persistent backache
	Headaches: becoming more severe and frequent
Lumps	Any enlarging mass in abdomen or elsewhere
	Enlarging, non-tender, rubbery lymph nodes
Vomiting	Persistent, worsening, worse in morning and associated with headache
General	Lethargy, anorexia, weight loss, pallor, easy bruising

Characteristic symptoms and signs of common childhood malignancy include:

Haematological malignancies
Leukaemias usually present with the clinical consequences of pancytopaenia due to marrow infiltration: pallor (anaemia), easy bruising (thrombocytopaenia), or recurrent infections (neutropaenia). Limb or back pain may be an early feature.

A lymphoma may present with persistent lymphadenopathy. Suspicious features include progressive enlargement of non-tender, rubbery glands in the supraclavicular or axillary location.

Solid tumours
Obviously this depends on anatomical region.
- *CNS tumours:* features of raised intracranial pressure (ICP) such as early morning headache and vomiting are the typical presentation. Papilloedema and focal neurological deficits (squint, ataxia, torticollis) are important signs. Persistent back pain may be a feature of spinal cord tumours and is rarely an innocent symptom in children.
- *Abdominal tumours:* Wilms tumour may be painless and present as an isolated finding.
- *Endocrine tumours:* may present with the consequences of hormone deficiency (e.g. short stature, diabetes insipidus) or excess (e.g. precocious puberty, Cushing syndrome).

14.2 Treatment of childhood cancer

Principles of cancer treatment

Therapeutic strategies include chemotherapy, radiotherapy, and surgery either in combination or alone. A multidisciplinary team approach is central with specialist nurses, dietitians, play therapists, teachers, and psychologists. In the UK, care is 'shared' between specialists in regional centres and local hospitals which provide supportive care, and most patients are entered into national and international studies. Palliative care is provided for those whose disease is no longer curable.

The prognosis for childhood cancer in the developed world is much improved with cure rates in the range 60–70%. It remains a challenge to maximize cure rates whilst minimizing the long-term side effects of treatment.

In patients with haematological malignancy the first step is to induce remission. This is followed by consolidation, intensification, and maintenance chemotherapy as required. In contrast, patients with solid tumours usually require sequential, multimodal treatment. Chemotherapy and/or radiotherapy may need to precede surgery if a localized primary tumour is large, or may follow surgery as adjuvant therapy.

Chemotherapy

The cell cycle involved in cell division is divided into four active phases, G_1, S, G_2, and M, and a resting phase, $G0$ (see Fig 14.2). Aggressive tumours with a high 'mitotic index' are more likely to respond to chemotherapeutic agents than slow-growing, indolent tumours in which many cells are in the G0 resting phase. The main categories of cytotoxic drugs are:

- *Alkylating drugs:* chlorambucil, cyclophosphamide
- *Cytotoxic antibiotics:* daunorubicin
- *Antimetabolites:* 6-mercaptopurine, methotrexate
- *Vinca alkaloids and etoposide:* vinblastine, vincristine, etoposide
- *Other drugs:* asparagine, carboplatin, cisplatin.

These act in a variety of ways including interference with DNA synthesis and disruption of mitosis. Agents may act throughout the cell cycle (e.g. alkylating agents and cytotoxic antibodies) or at specific phases (e.g. M-phase: vinca alkaloids; S-phase: anti-metabolites, etoposide).

Combination therapy is used to increase efficacy by exploiting additive or synergistic mechanisms of action, minimize development of resistance and limit single-organ toxicity.

Administration

Chemotherapy should only be given by individuals who have been trained in the potential risks and complications and are working in fully equipped and staffed centres.

Most agents are given IV, but oral and intrathecal administration is also used. Central venous access is optional to avoid the risk of extravasation from peripheral veins (highest with vinca alkaloids, anthracyclines). Concomitant IV fluids are given with cyclophosphamide and ifosfamide to protect against haemorrhagic cystitis.

Intrathecal methotrexate is used for treatment and prophylaxis of CNS disease in leukaemia and non-Hodgkin lymphoma (NHL). Arrangements are now in place in the UK to guard against the catastrophic consequences of administering vincristine intrathecally by mistake.

Side effects

The most common short-term side effects are vomiting, myelosuppression, mucositis, and alopecia. Less common side-effects include hepatitis, nephrotoxicity, and encephalopathy. Long-term side effects include:

- *Infertility:* cumulative doses of alkylating agents (e.g. procarbazine) diminish fertility
- *Second malignancies:* the most common second malignancies are leukaemia and lymphoma, especially following treatment with etoposide or alkylating agents
- *Cardiomyopathy:* with anthracycline treatment
- *Ototoxicity:* with platinum-containing agents
- *Nephropathy:* platinum containing agents cause a reduced GFR and many agents are associated with tubular damage causing a Fanconi like syndrome.

Radiotherapy

Ionizing radiation is effective in killing malignant cells. The aim is to deliver effective treatment to a 'target' volume while sparing surrounding tissues. A total dose is calculated and 'fractionated' into a number of individual treatments.

Radiotherapy is used in the management of Hodgkin lymphoma, neuroblastoma, Wilms tumour, soft tissue sarcoma, Ewing sarcoma, and most CNS tumours. In leukaemia it is used for treatment of the CNS, in testicular disease, and in preparation for bone-marrow transplantation.

Administration

The target volume is delineated by imaging (CT or MRI). Immobilization is necessary (by sedation or general anaesthesia) and if necessary surrounding tissues (e.g. gonads) are protected by lead shields. Play therapists have a key role in facilitating radiotherapy.

Side effects

Acute side effects include nausea and vomiting, skin erythema, diarrhoea, marrow suppression, and inflammation of lungs and liver. Toxicity may be potentiated by certain chemotherapeutic agents such as actinomycin D. When these agents are used after radiotherapy the phenomenon of 'radiation recall' may cause further damage.

Late effects in the developing child are a particular problem and may be delayed for months or years. They include:

- *Specific organ damage:* cardiac, lung, gastrointestinal
- *Endocrine problems:* hypopituitarism, hypothyroidism, infertility
- Musculoskeletal hypoplasia
- Spinal growth failure
- Neurocognitive sequelae
- Cataracts
- *Second malignancies:* e.g. lymphoma, sarcoma.

Surgery

Surgical intervention may be an option for solid tumours. This may involve biopsy only or resection. Resection may be primary or follow chemotherapy. The completeness of resection influences the need for subsequent treatment.

Bone marrow transplantation

Transplantation of stem cells harvested directly from the bone marrow (bone marrow transplantation, BMT) or from the peripheral blood (peripheral blood stem cell transplantation, PBSCT) is used in conjunction with myeloablative chemotherapy and/or total body irradiation. Cord blood stem cells are now becoming an option.

The stem cells may be autologous (derived from the patient) or allogeneic (from a donor who may be a sibling, a matched unrelated donor or a haplo-identical parent).
Indications include:
- Selected high-risk or relapsed leukaemias (allograft)
- High-risk solid tumours e.g. neuroblastoma, Ewing sarcoma (autologous).

PBSCT is favoured for autologous transplantation. Stem cells are harvested by leukopheresis after being mobilized by granulocyte colony stimulating factor. They are then re-infused after myeloablation. There is less risk of tumour contamination and more rapid engraftment.

Complications include graft failure, infection (secondary to immunosuppression), veno-occlusive disease of the liver and graft vs host disease (GVHD). The latter may affect any organ but most commonly skin or gastrointestinal tract. Conversely, the immune effects of donor cells may actually be a component of malignant disease control.

Supportive and emergency care

Supportive care

Increased survival in childhood cancer has been helped by the availability of supportive care for the inevitable and life-threatening complications of treatment. These include infection, anaemia, renal toxicity, malnutrition, and mucositis.

- *Infection*
  Febrile neutropaenia may signal sepsis which can be fatal within hours (but note that fever may be absent even in severe neutropenic sepsis). It is usually defined as fever >38 °C with a neutrophil count <1.0 × 10^9/L. Causative organisms include *Pseudomonas*, skin or gut flora, and gram-positive organisms (from a central venous catheter). Careful inspection of mouth, anus, and skin may reveal a focus.

Local protocols are usually in place for the investigation and management of febrile neutropaenia. These vary by institution but always include suitable cultures (blood, urine, stool, swabs of throat, nose, skin sites) and administration of broad-spectrum antibiotics. Fungal infection should be suspected in prolonged febrile neutropaenia.

Viral infections are potentially lethal in immunocompromised patients. Active chickenpox, shingles, or herpes stomatitis is treated with aciclovir. Pneumonitis has a high mortality and may be caused by adenoviruses, cytomegalovirus or respiratory syncytial virus, or *Pneumocystis jirovecii*.

- *Haematological support*: blood products are used to maintain Hb >8.0 g/dL and platelets >10–20 × 10^9/L. Irradiated products are used following bone marrow transplantation or in patients with Hodgkin disease.
- *Nausea and vomiting*: preventive treatment is usually implemented using domperidone or metoclopramide as first line agents. Second line options include ondansetron, dexamethasone, cyclizine, nabilone, and chlorpromazine.
- *Nutrition*: nasogastric or gastrostomy feeding, or TPN should be employed early to maintain nutritional status.
- *Mucositis*: this is associated with pain and diarrhoea. Treatment includes oral hygiene and antiseptic mouthwashes
- *Tumour lysis syndrome*: rapid lysis of malignant cells on initiating chemotherapy may be associated with this syndrome which is manifested by hyperkalaemia and hyperuricaemia together with metabolic acidosis and deranged calcium metabolism (hypocalcaemia, hyperphosphataemia). Acute renal failure may occur. It should be anticipated in 'bulky' disease (high count acute leukaemia, B-cell NHL) and prevented by hyperhydration, allopurinol or urate oxidase, and diuretics (furosemide) to ensure good urine output. In extreme cases haemofiltration may be necessary.

Emergency care

Malignancy in childhood may on occasion present with clinical features requiring urgent treatment. Syndromes include:
- *Hyperviscosity syndrome*: in leukaemia with white blood count >200 × 10^9/L venous stasis may occur in cerebral vessels. Prompt treatment of leukaemia with hydration and avoidance of transfusion (unless essential) is indicated. Severe cases may require leukopheresis.
- *CNS emergencies*: raised ICP is a neurosurgical emergency and requires treatment with high-dose dexamethasone. Spinal cord compression is manifested by back pain, abnormal gait, and bowel or bladder disturbance. Urgent MRI is indicated prior to surgical decompression.
- *Acute abdomen*: this may occur with neutropenic enterocolitis or typhlitis (inflammation of the cecum, appendix and/or ileum) which is associated with leukaemia, lymphoma, and aplastic anaemia. Management includes systemic antibiotics and surgical review.
- *SVC obstruction*: this may occur with a large mediastinal mass and presents with plethora, engorgement of chest wall veins, and dilatation of veins in the optic fundus.

Palliative care

This phase of treatment starts when it is recognized that cure is unattainable and prognosis is limited. The focus changes to quality of life and symptom control. A multidisciplinary team approach includes a specialist paediatrician, psychologists, nurses, play therapists, and social workers. Care offered should embrace the physical, emotional, spiritual, and social needs of the child and family.

Important strategies for symptom control include:
- *Dyspnoea*: opioids, steroids, and oxygen. Positioning and play therapy may help
- *Excess secretions*: hyoscine patch
- *Pruritus*: cimetidine or antihistamines if opioid induced
- *Anxiety/depression*: levomepromazine, diazepam, amitriptyline.

Most children prefer to die at home; some prefer a hospice.

14.3 Acute leukaemias

Acute leukaemia accounts for 95% of all childhood leukaemia and chronic myeloid leukaemia (CML) for the remaining 5%. Acute lymphoblastic leukaemia (ALL) accounts for 80% and acute myeloid leukaemia (AML) for 20% of childhood acute leukaemia.

Acute lymphoblastic leukaemia (ALL)

ALL is the most common childhood malignancy with an annual incidence of 1/25 000 children and peak age of presentation between 2–6 years of age.

Aetiology and pathogenesis

A lymphoid progenitor cell becomes genetically altered and undergoes dysregulated proliferation and clonal expansion. Immunophenotyping has allowed ALL to be classified broadly into B-cell or T-cell lineage

- *B-cell ALL:* >80% of childhood ALL are B-cell origin. These are further subdivided into pre-B cell (the majority) and common ALL.
- *T-cell ALL:* 15% of childhood ALL.

A minority (2%) have mixed lineage.

Cytogenetic and molecular genetic alterations
Specific genetic changes are found in leukaemia blast cells of 90% of ALL patients. These include changes in chromosome number (ploidy) and structure e.g. chromosomal translocations: *BCR-ABL* (t9:22), *E2A-PBX1*, *TEL-AML1* (t12:21), *MLL* gene rearrangements (translocations involving 11q23). These influence prognosis (see below).

No environmental factor has been definitively implicated. Although ALL arises in the bone marrow leukaemic blasts may be widespread at presentation and present in reticuloendothelial system, testes, and CNS.

Clinical features

The presenting symptoms and signs reflect the consequences of bone marrow infiltration (Fig 14.5) and occasionally those of extramedullary disease. There may be a history of fatigue, weight loss, malaise, bone pain, and recurrent infections.

Signs at presentation
- *Pallor:* anaemia
- *Petechiae, bruising or bleeding:* thrombocytopaenia
- *Fever, oral ulceration:* neutropaenia
- *Hepatosplenomegaly and lymphadenopathy:* RES infiltration.

CNS involvement is rarely manifested at presentation (raised ICP, cranial nerve lesions) and testicular involvement (painless, unilateral enlargement) is also rare.

Prognostic factors
A poor prognosis is indicated by high total WCC, $>50 \times 10^9$, bulky organomegaly, male sex, and CNS involvement. Cytogenetic analysis (see below) defines further prognostic features.

Investigations

The FBC usually demonstrates anaemia and thrombocytopaenia and blast cells may be apparent on the blood film. The total white cell count may be normal or elevated ($>10 \times 10^9$/L in 50%) and neutropaenia may be present. A high white cell count ($> 50 \times 10^9$/L) is a poor prognostic factor.
The complete work-up includes:
- *Biochemistry:* urea and electrolytes, LFTs, urate
- *CXR:* to identify a mediastinal mass
- *Lumbar puncture:* cytospin morphology on CSF
- Bone marrow aspiration and trephine.

Complete morphological, immunological and genetic examination of the bone marrow is required to confirm the diagnosis and establish prognostic factors.

Immunophenotyping allows classification of B/T cell lineage. Cytogenetic analysis using FISH and molecular techniques such as RT-PCR allows identification of translocations and genetic alterations not visible on routine karyotyping.
These identify changes of prognostic significance:
- *Favourable prognosis:* hyperdiploidy (chromosome number >50), *TEL-AML* gene rearrangement
- *Poor prognosis:* hypodiploidy (chromosome number <44), Philadelphia chromosome (Ph+), *ALL* gene rearrangement, T-cell ALL.

Management

Supportive care may be required at presentation including transfusion of blood products, treatment of infection, and prophylaxis of tumour lysis syndrome.

Treatment then follows protocols established from many years of clinical trials which encompass the following stages and are stratified by risk.

Remission induction
This lasts 4 weeks and involves administration of vincristine, dexamethasone, asparagine, and anthracyclines for high-risk patients. Bone marrow examined at day 28 defines the risk group.

Consolidation phase
This provides CNS prophylaxis and includes weekly doses of intrathecal methotrexate. Intensification blocks are included according to the risk group.

Maintenance phase
This involves oral daily 6-mercaptopurine (6-MP) and weekly methotrexate together with monthly IV vincristine with 5-day pulses of oral dexamethasone and 3-monthly intrathecal methotrexate. Doses are adjusted to achieve mild marrow suppression without prolonged neutropaenia. Duration is 2 years for girls, 3 years for boys.

Prognosis is improving with 80% overall survival for standard risk patients. Molecular techniques are being developed to detect minimal residual disease (MRD) which will allow patients to be allocated to more or less intensive chemotherapy regimens at 28 days. At present only 20% of children treated who are destined to relapse receive the most intensive treatment.

Relapse may be confined to bone marrow or be extramedullary (CNS, testes). Treatment involves intensive re-induction and consolidation with a further 2 years maintenance therapy. BMT is considered for high risk cases.

Acute myeloid leukaemia (AML)

AML is a rare form of childhood leukaemia affecting <100 children in the UK each year. The incidence increases with age and AML accounts for 90% of all acute leukaemias in adults.

Aetiology and pathogenesis

The most important risk factor in childhood is Down syndrome, which is associated with a 10–20-fold increase in risk of AML. Environmental risk factors include exposure to chemotherapy agents and ionizing radiation.

The malignant cell is the myeloblast. A single myeloblast accumulates genetic changes which prevent further differentiation and further mutations lead to uncontrolled growth of an immature clone. Marrow replacement interferes with development of normal blood cells.

Cytogenetic and molecular genetic alterations

Specific cytogenetic abnormalities are common and usually result in abnormal fusion proteins which cause the 'differentiation arrest'. These are of great prognostic significance. Examples include:

- *Favourable prognosis*: t (15,17); *PML-RARα* (acute promyelocytic leukaemia)
- *Unfavourable prognosis*: monosomy 5 or 7, del (5q), complex cytogenetics.

Classification

The French-American-British (FAB) system divides AML into eight subtypes, M0–M7, based on the type of cell and degree of maturity, each with a different behaviour and cytogenetics.

- M0: Myeloid leukaemia (*with minimal differentiation*)
- M1: Myeloblastic leukaemia
- M2: Myeloblastic leukaemia (*undifferentiated*)
- M3: Promyelocytic leukaemia (*favourable prognosis*)
- M4: Myelomonocytic leukaemia
- M5: Monocytic leukaemia
- M6: Erythroblastic leukaemia
- M7: Megakaryoblastic leukaemia (*unfavourable prognosis*).

Clinical features and investigations

These are similar to those of ALL. Extramedullary, including intrathoracic disease, is less common. A presumptive diagnosis may be made by examination of the peripheral blood film but definitive diagnosis requires bone marrow aspiration and biopsy. Diagnosis requires involvement of >20% of blood or bone marrow by leukaemia myeloblasts. 'Pre-leukaemic' conditions such as myelodysplastic or myeloproliferative syndromes must be differentiated.

Management

Treatment involves induction with intensive chemotherapy followed by consolidation. Prolonged maintenance is not given. Induction chemotherapy involves 4–5 courses of therapy using cytarabine (ara-c) and an anthracycline (e.g daunorubicin). The M3 subtype of AML (acute promyelocytic leukaemia) is treated in addition with the drug ATRA (all-trans-retinoic acid) to prevent disseminated intravascular coagulation (DIC). CNS prophylaxis is given. For patients at high risk of relapse allogeneic stem cell transplantation is usually recommended.

Overall survival in AML is only 50–60%.

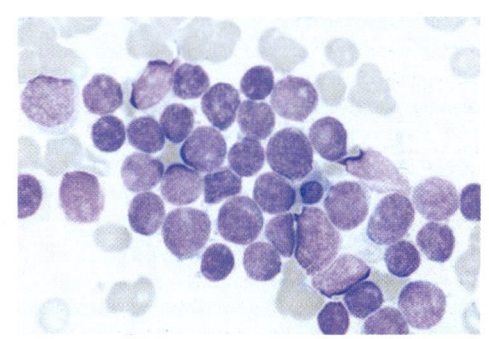

Fig 14.5 ALL: bone marrow replacement by blasts with round nuclei and scanty cytoplasm. Diagnostic Service, St James's.

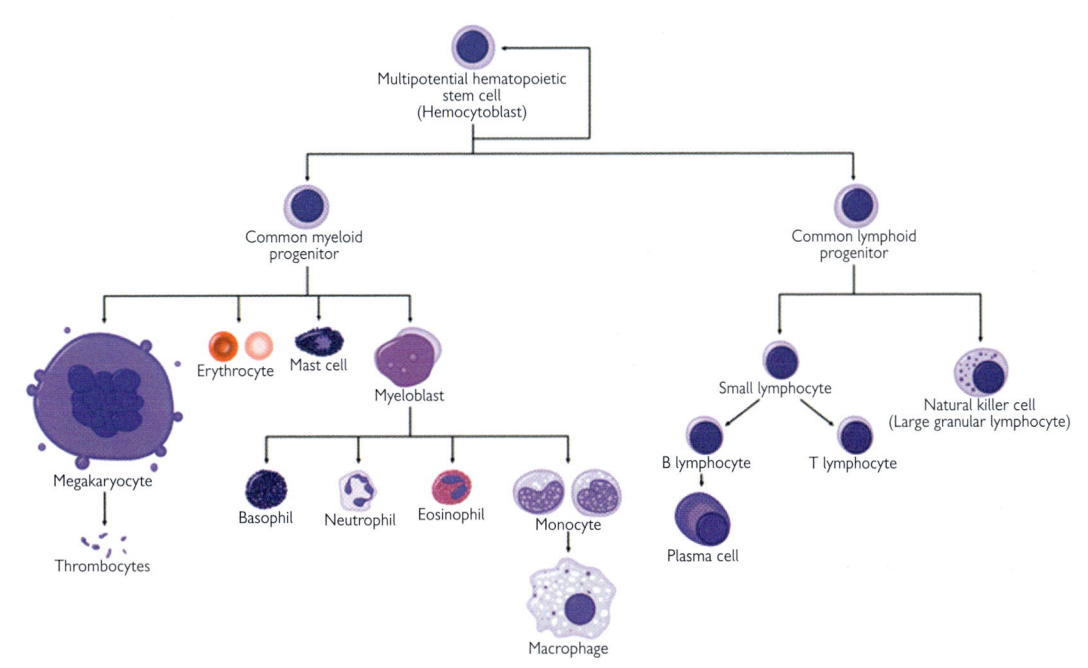

Fig 14.4 The lineage of blood cells.

14.4 Lymphomas

Lymphomas are malignant proliferations of lymphoid precursor cells. Two distinct disease entities are recognized: Hodgkin (HL) and non-Hodgkin lymphoma (NHL).

Hodgkin lymphoma (HL)

The incidence of HL in Western Europe increases from 5.5/million at <15 years to 12.1/million for individuals aged 15–20 years. A male to female preponderance of 3:1 is observed in children <10 years.

Aetiology and pathophysiology

The aetiology of HL is multifactorial and includes:
- *Genetic predisposition*: there is familial clustering with increased incidence in monozygotic twins and same-sex siblings. Familial cases account for 5% of total.
- *Infectious agents*: there is an association with Epstein–Barr virus infection (50% EBV positivity in HL in UK) but a causal link is yet to be established.
- *Immune dysregulation*: association with HIV infection, immunodeficiency syndromes.
- *Socioeconomic factors*: in the US, incidence is inversely related to parental income and education.

Malignant B cells proliferate in the reticuloendothelial and lymphatic systems and may invade lungs, bone, bone marrow, liver parenchyma, and CNS.

Clinical features

Persistent, painless lymphadenopathy is the most common presenting feature. Systemic 'B' symptoms (see below) include unexplained fever (>38 °C for 3 consecutive days), weight loss (>10% in 6 months), drenching night sweats, pruritus, urticaria, and fatigue. A mediastinal mass may cause dyspnoea, cough, chest pain, or SVC obstruction syndrome.

Physical examination commonly reveals firm, non-tender lymphadenopathy cervical in 70–80%, axillary in 25%. Splenomegaly and/or hepatomegaly may be found.

Investigations

The laboratory work-up confirms the diagnosis and allows both classification and staging of the disease. It includes:
- *FBC*: this may reveal anaemia (haemolytic, anaemia of chronic disease or from marrow replacement), leukocytosis and/or lymphopaenia, and thrombocytopaenia.
- *Biochemistry*: elevated lactate dehydrogenase levels reflects disease bulk and raised alkaline phosphatase indicates bony metastases.
- *Lymph node biopsy*: excision biopsy is preferred to needle-biopsy. The Reed–Sternberg (RS) cell is pathognomonic (Fig 14.6).

The WHO histological classification distinguishes:
- *Classic nodular sclerosing*: most common type overall
- *Classic mixed cellularity*: more common in younger children
- *Classic lymphocyte rich*: very rare
- *Classic lymphocyte depleted*: very rare
- Nodular lymphocyte predominant: 'popcorn' cells visible.

Immunophenotyping is undertaken.
- *Bone marrow aspiration*: in all patients with suspected bone marrow involvement or stage II a or higher.

Imaging
- *CXR*: to assess bulk of mediastinal mass. Mass with a thoracic ratio >33% is poor prognostic indicator
- CT or MRI imaging of neck, chest, abdomen, and/or pelvis to assess sites of disease
- *PET scan*: uptake of radioactive glucose analogue identifies tumour activity in bone and other locations.

Management

After a tissue diagnosis is made the disease is staged using imaging studies and treatment stratified according to stage.

The Ann Arbor staging system is used:
- *Stage I*: single lymph node region or extranodal site
- *Stage II*: two or more lymph node regions on same side of diaphragm
- *Stage III*: lymph node regions on both sides of diaphragm
- *Stage IV*: diffuse or disseminated involvement of one or more extralymphatic organs (liver, bone marrow, lung) with or without node involvement (spleen is counted as a nodal site).

A or B designations are added:
- *B*: presence of at least one of: drenching night sweats, unexplained fever, or loss of body weight.
- *A*: absence of B symptoms.

HL is one of the most curable of childhood malignancies. Radiation therapy and chemotherapy alone or in combination are used. Modern strategies focus on minimizing late effects of therapy, while maintaining cure rates.

Chemotherapy regimens include various combinations of steroids (prednisone), anthracyclines, alkylating agents, and etoposide. Radiation therapy is used for residual disease. Prognosis is excellent with 80–100% long-term survival. Problematic late effects of treatment include second malignancies in 20% (e.g. breast cancer), cardiomyopathy (anthracyclines and radiation), and reduced fertility (alkylating agents).

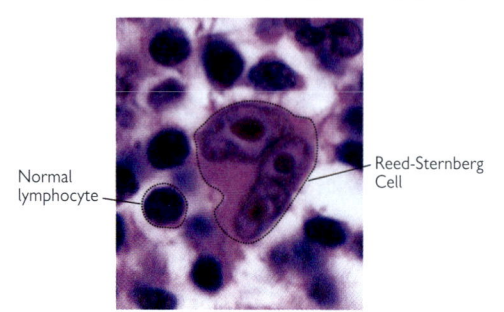

Fig 14.6 Hodgkin lymphoma: Reed–Sternberg cell.
Source: National Cancer Institute.

Non-Hodgkin lymphoma (NHL)

NHL encompasses a heterogeneous group of malignant proliferations of lymphoid tissue, and accounts for 7% of all childhood cancers. The annual incidence is about 10/million with 100 new cases each year in the UK. NHL is more common in white males with peak incidence in the 2nd decade. It is the most common malignancy in children associated with AIDS and often occurs in young children <4 years if HIV has been vertically transmitted.

Aetiology and pathogenesis
Genetic and environmental factors operate:
- *Chromosomal and molecular rearrangements:* The most common abnormality is the t (8;14) translocation which juxtaposes the *c-myc* (*bcl-2*) gene to immunoglobulin locus regulatory elements leading to overexpression of *c-myc*
- *Viral infection:* 25% of B-cell lymphomas contain EBV genomes
- *Immunodeficiency states:* congenital immunodeficiency (e.g. ataxia telangiectasia, Wiskott–Aldrich syndrome), HIV
- Cancer chemotherapy and/or radiation therapy.

Classification
This remains rather complex and controversial. 90% of childhood NHL are 'high-grade' tumours and can be classified into one of four main categories by histology, cytogenetics and immunophenotype:
- *Burkitt/Burkitt-like (45–50%):* a mature B-cell lymphoma
- *Lymphoblastic (25–30%):* T-cell (90%), pre B-cell (10%)
- *Large-cell diffuse (15–20%):* B-cell
- *Large-cell anaplastic (10–15%):* T-cell (70%), null cell (20%), B-cell (10%).

Clinical features
Presentation varies with the site affected, which differs between subtypes. Endemic (African) Burkitt lymphoma associated with early EBV infection frequently affects the jaw, and abdominal involvement is common in both endemic and sporadic Burkitt lymphoma.

T-cell lymphoblastic lymphoma typically presents in teenagers with a mediastinal mass which may cause dyspnoea, cough, chest pain, pleural effusions, and swelling of head and neck (if there are >25% blasts in marrow the patient is considered to have ALL).

Diffuse large B-cell lymphoma (DLBL) is often localized and involves the mediastinum. Anaplastic large-cell lymphoma (ALCL) has a variable presentation with involvement of nodes and various extranodal sites: skin, bone, lungs, muscle.

Two life threatening situations may occur: superior vena cava syndrome and acute tumour lysis syndrome.

Investigations
- *FBC:* assesses bone marrow function and identifies any abnormal circulating cells
- *Biochemistry:* U&E, LFTs, lactate dehydrogenase (LDH), β_2-microglobulin, protein electrophoresis
- *HIV serology:* if risk factors present (routine in some countries)
- *Diagnostic biopsy and bone marrow aspiration:* this may involve lymph node biopsy, pleural tap, or biopsy of other sites including bone marrow. Patients with a large mediastinal mass are at risk of cardiac or respiratory arrest during general anaesthetic or heavy sedation: the least invasive procedure is advisable. Biopsy material is analysed using immunohistochemistry, FISH, and other specific techniques.
- *Imaging:*
  - CXR
  - CT scans of thorax, abdomen, and pelvis
  - MRI is useful in revealing bone and CNS involvement.

Management
The St Jude staging scheme is used to guide treatment and inform prognosis:
- *Stage I:* single tumour or nodal area (except abdomen or mediastinum)
- *Stage II:*
  - single tumour plus regional nodes
  - two or more tumours/nodal areas on one side of diaphragm
  - primary gastrointestinal tract tumour (resected)
- *Stage III:*
  - involvement both sides of diaphragm
  - any primary intrathoracic, paraspinal, or epidural tumour
  - extensive intra-abdominal disease
- *Stage IV:* any above with bone marrow or CNS disease.

Chemotherapy is the mainstay of treatment. Lymphoblastic lymphoma is treated with regimens similar to those used in ALL (e.g. CHOP: cyclophosphamide, doxorubicin, vincristine, and prednisolone).

Burkitt lymphoma and anaplastic large cell lymphoma are treated with brief intensive courses (e.g. COMP: cyclophosphamide, vincristine, methotrexate, and prednisolone). CNS involvement necessitates intrathecal therapy and radiotherapy is used for residual disease.

The most important prognostic factor is the extent of disease at diagnosis. The cure rate is 70% overall and 90% for patients with very localized disease. However, children with extensive disease who relapse have a poor outcome despite attempts at salvage (e.g. high-dose therapy with stem cell rescue).

14.5 CNS tumours, retinoblastoma, and germ cell tumours

Brain tumours

Brain tumours are the most common solid tumours that occur in children and constitute 25% of childhood malignancies. In the UK each year about 350 children develop brain tumours. Boys are more often affected than girls. Only primary tumours are considered here as secondary brain metastases are extremely rare in children.

Aetiology and pathogenesis

Although grouped together on anatomical grounds, CNS tumours have diverse biological origins. In most cases the cause is unknown but certain genetic syndromes are associated with CNS malignancies including Li–Fraumeni syndrome, neurofibromatosis type 1 (optic pathway gliomas), and tuberous sclerosis complex (gliomas and ependymomas).

Grading and classification

Brain tumours are classified according to the cell of origin and how potentially slow-growing (low-grade, grade 1) or fast-growing (high-grade, grade 4) they are.

The main types are listed in the Box.

Main types of brain tumour

Gliomas
- *Astrocytomas (90%):*
  - low-grade glioma (30%)
  - moderate-grade glioma (astrocytoma) (45%)
  - high-grade glioma (glioblastoma multiforme) (10%)
  - brainstem glioma (<5%)
- *Ependymomas (10%)*

Primitive neuroectodermal tumours (PNET)
- *Infratentorial:* cerebellar medulloblastoma
- *Supratentorial:* pineoblastoma

Craniopharyngioma

Clinical features

Brain tumours may cause a wide variety of symptoms depending on their location, and late diagnosis is unfortunately common. The mean time from onset of symptoms to diagnosis is 5 months.

As infratentorial tumours are most common (>50%) and frequently obstruct CSF drainage, the most common presenting symptoms are those of raised ICP. These include early morning headache and vomiting, but it should be remembered that brain tumours are a very rare cause of childhood headache (1/5000). More subtle symptoms and signs depending on focal neurological deficits include:

- Changes in personality, behaviour, school performance
- Cerebellar ataxia
- Diplopia with squint, head tilting
- *Diencephalic syndrome:* weight loss, hypogonadism, nystagmus
- Seizures.

A careful search for signs of raised ICP (papilloedema), cerebellar dysfunction (ataxia, nystagmus, dysmetria), and cranial nerve deficits is important in any child with a headache or in whom a brain tumour is suspected.

Investigations

Cranial imaging is the key investigation. Cranial CT is useful initially to identify raised ICP, but MRI is definitive. Additional investigations include

- *Lumbar puncture:* to identify malignant cells in CSF
- *Tumour markers:* α-fetoprotein, B-hCG for midline, possible germ cell tumours
- *Tumour biopsy:* diagnostic biopsy may be indicated even in inoperable tumours.

Management

Raised ICP requires prompt management if it is of recent onset. This may involve dexamethasone to reduce oedema, CSF diversion by 3rd ventriculostomy or external ventricular drain or even intensive care and assisted ventilation in severe cases. Anticonvulsants may be used to prevent seizures.

For definitive treatment, surgery, radiotherapy, or chemotherapy may be used alone or in combination. Many children have treatment as part of a clinical research trial. The exact strategy depends on the size, position, and type of tumour as follows.

Low-grade glioma

Most cerebellar astrocytomas are cured by surgery alone Unresectable tumours (e.g. involving optic pathway or hypothalamus) are treated with chemotherapy or radiotherapy in older children (but not in those associated with NF1) as risks are increased of second tumours).

High-grade glioma

These occur in older children and are often supratentorial and incompletely resectable. Prognosis is poor.

Brainstem glioma

Intrinsic pontine gliomas have a characteristic MRI appearance. They are inoperable with variable response to radiotherapy and chemotherapy and median survival <1 year. Exophytic brainstem tumours may be low-grade and have a better prognosis.

Ependymomas

Complete surgical excision may be possible (>70% survival). If not, radiotherapy or chemotherapy is used in addition.

Primitive neuroectodermal tumours (PNETs)

These include cerebellar medulloblastomas and supratentorial PNETs. CSF-borne metastases may be present. Resection and craniospinal radiotherapy is the basis of treatment with additional chemotherapy. Localized medulloblastomas have an overall survival rate of 50% in <3 years and 80% in >3 years. There is, however, significant long-term morbidity from radiotherapy: neurocognitive impairment, endocrine deficiency, and second malignancies.

Craniopharyngioma

This midline benign epithelial tumour is completely resectable in most cases (80%). However, although most patients survive long term the complications of both the disease and its treatment remain significant and include hypothalamic dysfunction, vision defects, and behavioural problems.

Spinal cord tumours

Primary spinal cord tumours are uncommon but account for 10% of paediatric CNS tumours.

Aetiology and pathogenesis

The cause is unknown in most cases but there is an association with certain genetic syndromes. Astrocytomas and ependymomas are more common in neurofibromatosis type 2 and spinal haemangioblastomas occur in 30% of patients with Von Hippel–Lindau syndrome.

Anatomically a spinal cord tumour may be extradural or intradural. Intradural tumours may be intrinsic (intramedullary) or extrinsic (extramedullary).

Most intramedullary spinal cord tumours are histopathologically benign or slow growing. Compression of the spinal cord and its vascular supply is the principle pathological effect.

Clinical features

Chronic back pain referred from the level of the lesion is the most common symptom, followed by numbness or paraesthesia, weakness, and bladder dysfunction.

Examination reveals a mixture of upper and lower motor neuron signs in the lower limbs. The differential includes discitis and Guillain–Barré syndrome.

Investigations

Plain radiography lacks specificity and sensitivity. MRI with and without gadolinium is the definitive imaging modality. Lumbar puncture is not indicated as the initial investigation and may precipitate neurological deterioration.

Management

Surgical resection is the usual treatment of choice. Radiotherapy and/or chemotherapy may also be indicated, and postoperative physiotherapy is important.

Retinoblastoma

This rare tumour accounts for 3% of childhood cancer with 40 cases diagnosed in the UK each year. It may be inherited (40%) or sporadic (60%).

Aetiology and pathogenesis

In the inherited forms (40% of cases) a mutation in the *Rb* gene is inherited (first hit) followed by a second somatic mutation (second hit). Tumours are often bilateral. Sporadic retinoblastoma (60%) tend to be unilateral.

Clinical features

Children born into a family in which a member has retinoblastoma are screened from birth every few months for 5 years by ophthalmoscopy. Sporadic retinoblastoma is often asymptomatic and may present as leucocoria (white pupil) noted in pictures taken using flash photography (Fig 14.7). Alternatively a squint or painful red eye may develop.

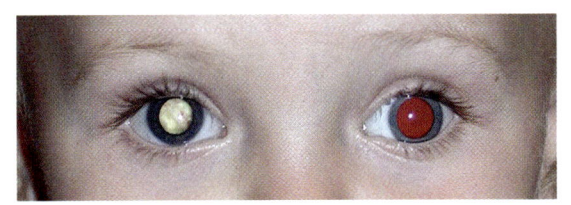

Fig 14.7 Retinoblastoma: abnormal red reflex. Reproduced courtesy of John Ainsworth.

Investigations

Examination under anaesthetic by an ophthalmologist may confirm the diagnosis. A biopsy is not usually required. Imaging modalities used include ultrasound, CT, and MRI. Lumbar puncture and bone marrow aspiration may be necessary to identify metastases. Genetic testing of Rb is available.

Staging

Retinoblastoma is staged according to whether or not it is intraocular (local tumour in one or both eyes) or extraocular (local spread or metastases).

Management

Small, local tumours may respond to cryotherapy, laser therapy, thermotherapy, or plaque therapy (application of a radioactive disc). Larger tumours with extraocular spread are treated with chemotherapy or radiotherapy. Enucleation may be necessary.

Germ cell tumours

A germ cell tumour (GCT) is a neoplasm derived from germ cells, and most therefore affect the ovaries or testes.
Fewer than 45 children develop malignant germ cell tumours in the UK each year.

Aetiology and classification

The aetiology is unknown. Extra gonadal germ cell tumours are congenital, the most notable being sacrococcygeal teratoma. Klinefelter syndrome increases the risk ×50.
Germ cell tumours may be benign or malignant and include:
- *Germinomas:* dysgerminoma and seminoma
- Embryonal carcinoma
- Yolk-sac tumours
- *Teratomas* : mature and immature
- Choriocarcinoma
- Gonadoblastoma

Clinical features and diagnosis

A lump is the usual presentation. Diagnostic investigations include imaging, biopsy and tumour markers such as α-fetoprotein (AFP) and human chorionic gonadotrophin (hCG).

Treatment

Treatment usually involves a combination of surgery and chemotherapy. Levels of AFP and hCG are monitored during follow-up.

14.6 Wilms tumour, neuroblastoma and STS

Wilms tumour
Wilms tumour (WT), or nephroblastoma, accounts for 6% of childhood malignancies with ~70 new cases per year in the UK. 75% occur in children <4 years of age.

Aetiology and pathogenesis
There is a clear genetic aetiology in some cases of WT which show both familial clustering and an association with certain genetic syndromes. Two Wilms tumour genes have been identified: *WT1* (chromosome 11p13) and *WT2* (11p15). In addition, loss of heterozygosity (LOH) at chromosome 1p and 16q confers a worse prognosis.

Genetic syndromes that are associated with WT include:
- Beckwith–Wiedemann syndrome (macroglossia, gigantism, umbilical hernia) (2%)
- Hemihypertrophy
- Congenital aniridia (1%)
- WAGR syndrome: Wilms tumour, aniridia, genitourinary malformations, retardation (5%)
- Denys–Drash syndrome (WT, pseudohermaphroditism, glomerulopathy)
- Trisomy 18.

Wilms tumour arises from metanephric blastema cells, primitive embryonic renal tissue. These cells have usually disappeared by birth but in many children with WT they may persist as 'nephrogenic rests'. It typically arises as an intrarenal solid or cystic mass which displaces the collecting system and extends into the renal vein (40% cases). It is bilateral in 6%. Tumour spread is usually via lymphatic and vascular routes to the lungs or liver.

Clinical features
The most common presenting symptom is swelling in the abdomen, usually painless. Haematuria, macroscopic or microscopic and often painless may occur. Hypertension may be caused by pressure on the renal artery. Fever, weight loss, and anorexia may occur. Stigmata of associated syndromes may be apparent on examination (e.g. aniridia, hemihypertrophy). Lung metastases are present in 10%.

Investigations
- Blood count, U&E, urinalysis
- Imaging:
  - *ultrasound:* allows initial evaluation of an abdominal mass and can identify renal vein or IVC and hepatic involvement.
  - *CXR:* pulmonary metastases
- CT or MRI of the chest and abdomen allows distinction of nephroblastoma from neuroblastoma, assessment of lymph nodes and other kidney, identification of liver metastases (Fig 14.7)
- *Biopsy:* Tissue from the tumour is examined histologically and using cytogenetic and molecular techniques. Histopathology may be:
  - *favourable, low risk (90%):* epithelial, stromal and blastemal elements present
  - *unfavourable, high risk (10%):* anaplastic and blastemal subtypes.

Staging
A commonly used surgical staging system is:
- *Stage I:* tumour limited to kidney and excised completely
- *Stage II:* tumour extends beyond kidney but is excised completely
- *Stage III:* residual intra-abdominal tumour (non-hematogenous) after surgery
- *Stage IV:* haematogenous or lymph node metastasis outside abdomen or pelvis
- *Stage V:* synchronous bilateral tumours.

Management
Treatment usually includes surgery, chemotherapy, and sometimes radiotherapy and is determined by tumour histology and stage. All children have surgery at some stage. Initially this may involve diagnostic tumour biopsy and tumour resection either then or following chemotherapy. Postoperative chemotherapy is determined by the extent of surgical resection (complete or incomplete) and histology. Radiotherapy may also be given to the area of the affected kidney or the whole abdomen and for lung metastases.

Chemotherapy may include vincristine or several months of an anthracycline-based regimen.

Bilateral disease (stage V) is usually treated with chemotherapy followed by bilateral partial nephrectomy to avoid the need for dialysis. Overall survival ranges from 95% in stage I to 70% in stage IV. Follow-up investigations include abdominal ultrasound (local recurrence) and CXR (pulmonary metastases). Late side affects include growth failure, infertility, cardiac and pulmonary damage, and second malignancies.

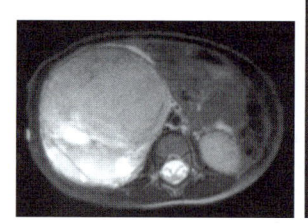

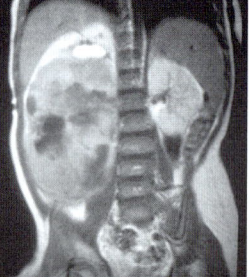

A   B

Fig 14.8 Wilms tumour: MRI.

Neuroblastoma

Neuroblastoma is an aggressive tumour originating from neural-crest-derived sympathetic nerve cells. It is one of the most common extracranial tumours of childhood with ~100 cases per year in the UK. The median age of onset is 2 years.

Aetiology and pathogenesis
The cause is unknown but genetic factors are important (see below). Tumours most commonly arise from the adrenal gland but may arise in the sympathetic chain anywhere in the neck, chest, abdomen, or pelvis. Secretion of catecholamines may cause hypertension.

Clinical features
Presenting symptoms are highly variable and often non-specific and vague. Depending on the primary site, the presence of metastases, and associated metabolic disturbances caused by catecholamine secretion, presenting features may include:
- *Local effects:* abdominal swelling, constipation, bladder dysfunction, dyspnoea or difficulty swallowing, visible cervical swelling, limping and pain from cord compression, Horner syndrome
- *Catecholamines:* pallor, sweating, diarrhoea, hypertension
- *Metastases:* proptosis and periorbital (superior) ecchymosis ('racoon eyes'), blueberry muffin skin (stage 4S: see below), pallor, bone pain
- *Nervous system:* opsoclonus–myoclonus ('dancing eyes' syndrome) with cerebellar ataxia.

Investigations
A wide range of investigations may be necessary:
- *Blood tumour markers:* neuron specific enolase (NSE), lactate dehydrogenase (LDH)
- *Urine catecholamines:* vanillylmandelic acid (VMA) and homovanillic acid (HVA) to creatinine ratios raised in 80%
- *Imaging:*
  - ^{131}I-mIBG (meta-iodobenzylguanidine) scan. This is taken up by neuroblastoma cells and is useful for identification of primary tumour and metastases (also used as treatment)
  - CXR
  - CT and/or MRI imaging for primary and metastases
- *Bone marrow aspiration and biopsy:* Bilateral marrow aspiration is necessary as disease infiltration may be patchy
- *Biopsy:* the lesion or a lymph node may be accessible for biopsy. Tissue (and bone marrow is subjected to histological, cytogenetic and molecular analysis). Unfavourable prognostic features include N-myc amplification, DNA diploidy (worse than hypo- or hyperdiploidy), 1p deletion, unbalanced chromosome rearrangement with partial gain of chromosome 17.

Staging
The international neuroblastoma staging system (INSS):
- *Stage 1:* localized disease, surgically excised
- *Stage 2A:* localized disease, incompletely excised. No lymph node involvement
- *Stage 2B:* localized disease, incompletely excised. Lymph nodes positive
- *Stage 3:* unresectable unilateral tumour extending across midline
- *Stage 4:* any primary tumour with dissemination (except 4S)
- *Stage 4S:* in child <1 year. Localized tumour (1–2B) with dissemination to liver, skin or bone marrow.

Management
Treatment and prognosis depends on staging and risk:
- *Low risk:* stage 1: surgery alone. Survival is >95%.
- *Intermediate risk:* stage 2 or 3, age >1 year, no N-myc amplification. Surgery combined with intensive chemotherapy. Survival is 75–85%
- *High risk:* stage 4 and N-myc amplification. A combination of surgery, high dose chemotherapy with stem-cell rescue and radiotherapy (either external or internal using radioactive mIBG). Survival is <40%.
- *Stage 4S:* neuroblastoma in infants <1 year can spontaneously regress or evolve into a ganglioneuroma. Chemotherapy is required only for life-threatening symptoms. Survival is >90%.

Late side-effects include cardiac or renal damage, ototoxicity, growth and fertility problems, and second malignancies.

Soft tissue sarcoma (STS)

These rare cancers develop in muscle, fat, cartilage, blood vessels, or other tissues that support or surround the organs of the body. Rhabdomyosarcoma (RMS) develops in muscle and is the most common variety and represents 6% of childhood malignancies. Fewer than 60 children develop RMS in the UK each year. Most are <10 years and it is more common in boys.

Aetiology and pathogenesis
Children with certain rare genetic disorders such as Li–Fraumeni syndrome have a higher risk of STS. Alveolar RMS is characterized by t (2;13) or t (1;13) which produce fusion products of *PAX* and *FKHR* genes (poor prognosis).

Clinical features
This depends on tumour location but the most common presentation is a swelling or lump. Common sites include bladder, pelvis, nasopharynx, orbit, parameningeal, or trunk. There may be a blockage and discharge in the nose or throat, proptosis, abdominal discomfort, or difficulty passing urine.

Investigations
The primary tumour size and extent is established by MRI or CT. Imaging to detect metastatic disease includes:
- ^{99}Tc bone scan
- CT or MRI of chest, abdomen, pelvis.

Bilateral bone marrow aspiration and trephines are required. Biopsy of the lesion allows histological and cytogentic/molecular characterization. Histology is classified as embryonal, ERMS (80%) or alveolar, ARMS (20%).

Management
This depends on size, location, dissemination, and risk stratification base on known prognostic indicators. Treatment usually includes surgery, radiotherapy, or chemotherapy or a combination of all three. Surgical resection is usually done post chemotherapy and radiotherapy is the primary treatment for unresectable tumours. Overall survival is 70%.

14.7 Bone tumours and LCH

Bone tumours

Osteosarcoma (osteogenic sarcoma) and Ewing sarcoma are both rare and account for only 4% of childhood malignancy. There are <30 cases of each per year in the UK but the former is more common.

Osteosarcoma

This has a peak incidence in the teenage years and is more common in boys.

Aetiology and pathogenesis

Children with hereditary retinoblastoma have a higher risk and it may occur as a second malignancy following chemotherapy or radiotherapy. Most are high-grade but there are rare subtypes such as periosteal, periosteal telangiectatic, and small-cell osteosarcoma.

Clinical features

Osteosarcoma has a predilection for the growing ends of long bones. 80% occur around the knee in the distal femur or proximal tibia. Pain in the affected bone is the most common symptom, initially intermittent but gradually becoming severe and constant. Overlying swelling and erythema may be evident and pathological fractures can occur. Metastases (in lung or bone) at diagnosis are uncommon (10%).

Investigations

A plain radiograph of the bony lesion usually identifies the tumour (Fig 14.9). MRI of the primary site defines the extent of the tumour and aids surgical planning. The whole bone must be included to identify 'skip' metastases.

Assessment for disseminated disease includes CXR, CT chest, ^{99}Tc bone scan. Biopsy of the lesion should be carried out at a specialist centre by an experienced orthopaedic oncology surgeon or musculoskeletal radiologist working within a sarcoma team.

Staging is carried out based on histology, the extent of local spread and the presence or absence of metastases.

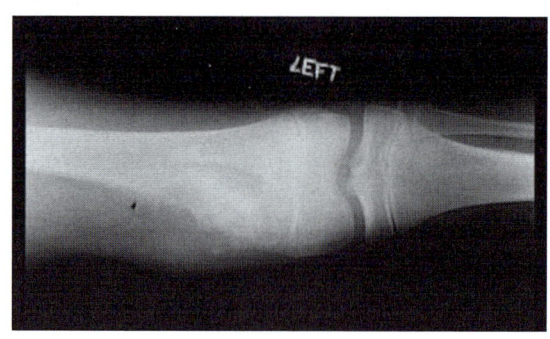

Fig 14.9 Osteosarcoma of the femur: radiograph.

Management

Treatment is surgical with pre- and postoperative chemotherapy. Neoadjuvant chemotherapy reduces tumour size to improve limb salvage options and decrease dissemination.

The type and extent of surgery depends on the tumour size and location, which is usually in a limb. Options are limb-sparing surgery and amputation, which is sometimes unavoidable. The need for complete resection is balanced against the requirement for a good functional result. Excised bone is replaced with either a metal prosthesis or bone from another part of the body. The prosthesis needs to be lengthened as the bone grows.

Radiotherapy is rarely an option as osteosarcoma is not radiosensitive, but may be used in palliation. Overall survival is 60–70%. The current trial is EURAMOS I.

Ewing sarcoma

The Ewing sarcoma family of tumours (ESFT) is a group of small round-cell tumours derived from cells of the neural crest. It includes Ewing sarcoma and various extraosseous tumours. Incidence peaks in the late teens.

Aetiology and pathogenesis

One of a series of related translocations (e.g. t (11;22)) occurs in 95% of the ESFTs which join the Ewing sarcoma gene (*EWS*) with a gene of the ETS family, *FLI1*. The *EWS–FLI1* fusion transcript encodes an aberrant transcription factor.

Histologically these are small, round blue cell tumours. They occur most commonly in flat bones of the axial skeleton, e.g. pelvis, ribs, vertebrae.

Clinical features

Pain is the most common symptom. A painful swelling may be apparent at the location. Metastases are present in 25% at diagnosis and bone marrow metastases occur. Pathological fractures may occur. Systemic symptoms of fever and weight loss suggest metastatic disease.

Investigations

Radiography of the painful bony area usually identifies the tumour (Fig 14.10). MRI delineates the extent of disease, and additional imaging is done to assess dissemination: CT chest, Tc99 bone scan. Bone marrow aspiration and trephine is done to detect bone marrow dissemination.

A biopsy of the lesion should be evaluated histologically and immunophenotyped to distinguish from rhabdomyosarcoma and lymphoma.

Management

Treatment depends on size and position and may include a combination of surgery, chemotherapy, and radiotherapy. Preoperative neo-adjuvant chemotherapy is often given to reduce tumour size and enhance limb salvage options, and continued postoperatively.

The aim of complete tumour excision is balanced against the need for a good functional result. Limb amputation may be unavoidable but limb-sparing surgery may be an option.

Ewing sarcoma responds well to radiotherapy which may be used pre- and postoperatively if resection is incomplete for lung metastases, and instead of surgery for inoperable (e.g. vertebral) tumours.

Overall survival is 70%.

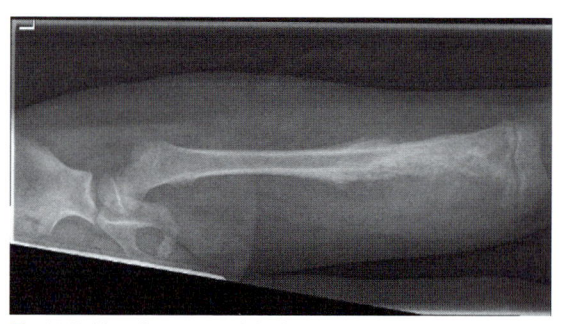

Fig 14.10 Ewing's sarcoma of the femur: radiograph.

Langerhans cell histiocytosis (LCH)

This is a group of disorders characterized by proliferation of Langerhans cells from bone marrow and mature eosinophils. LCH is rare, affecting 50–100 children in the UK each year, and is more common in boys than girls (2:1). Histiocytosis is divided into three different groups:

- Dendritic cell histiocytosis, e.g. LCH
- Erythrophagocytic macrophage disorders
- Malignant histiocytosis.

Aetiology and pathogenesis
The pathogenesis of LCH remains uncertain and debate exists as to whether it is a malignant neoplastic or reactive process. There is evidence that a permissive immunosurveillance system allows the proliferation of Langerhans cells, perhaps induced by viral infection. The clonal proliferation, infiltration of organs by aberrant cells and response to anticancer therapy are all consistent with neoplasia.

Clinical features
Several clinical subtypes exist:

- *Single-system LCH:* Eosinophilic granulomas. Age 5–15 years. Chronic indolent lesions of bones or skin. Unifocal eosinophilic granulomas usually present as a lytic bone lesion found incidentally (Fig 14.11).
- *Multisystem LCH:*
  - age 2–10 years: Hand–Schuller–Christian disease: Classical triad of diabetes insipidus, proptosis, lytic bone lesions. Often presents with recurrent episodes of otitis media and mastoiditis with polyuria and polydipsia.
  - age <2 years: Letterer–Siwe disease: acute, fulminant systemic disease of great malignancy. Letterer–Siwe disease presents with widespread skin eruption, anaemia and hepatosplenomegaly (Fig 14.12).

Investigations
These depend on the clinical subtype and presentation but may include:

- FBC, ESR, Ig levels, Coagulation studies, LFTs
- Bone marrow aspiration if anaemia, leucopaenia, or thrombocytopaenia is present
- Imaging:
  - *Skeletal survey:* single or multifocal osteolytic lesions may be found
  - *CXR:* LCH may show micronodular, interstitial infiltrate in mid zone and bases. Older lesions show a 'honeycomb' appearance.
  - *CT and/or MRI* of hypothalamic-pituitary region
- Water-deprivation test if diabetes insipidus suspected
- *Biopsy of skin lesions:* a pathological LCH cell resembles the normal skin Langerhans cell but is not dendritic. The ultrastructural hallmark is the Birkbeck granule, an intracytoplasmic membranous body with a tennis-racket shape.

Management
This is based on severity.

- *Single-system disease:* solitary lesion may resolve spontaneously. Bone lesions may be treated by curettage or excision and steroid injections if painful. Multiple bone lesions treated with indomethacin or systemic steroids. A lymph node may be excised. Localized skin lesions are treated with topical steroids or topical nitrogen mustard if severe.
- *Multisystem disease:* systemic chemotherapy is used for multisystem disease (or unresponsive single-system disease). Low to moderate doses of prednisone, methotrexate, and vinblastine are used. Bone marrow transplantation is considered in poor prognosis patients, if a suitable donor is found. Diabetes insipidus is treated with DDAVP.

Prognosis is excellent for a single focus. In multifocal disease 30% achieves remission, 60% have a chronic course and 10% die. Letterer–Siwe disease has a mortality of 50%. Long-term complications include growth retardation, liver cirrhosis, and neuropsychological defects.

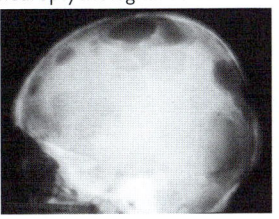

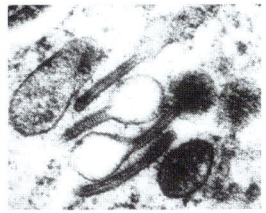

Fig 14.11 A. LCH: eosinophilic granuloma form. Discrete punched-out lesions affecting the skull (pepperpot skull). B. Electron microscopy of Langerhans cell showing tennis-racket-shaped Birkbeck granules. Image reprinted with permission from eMedicine.com 2008. Available at http://www.emedicine.com/derm/topic 216.htm

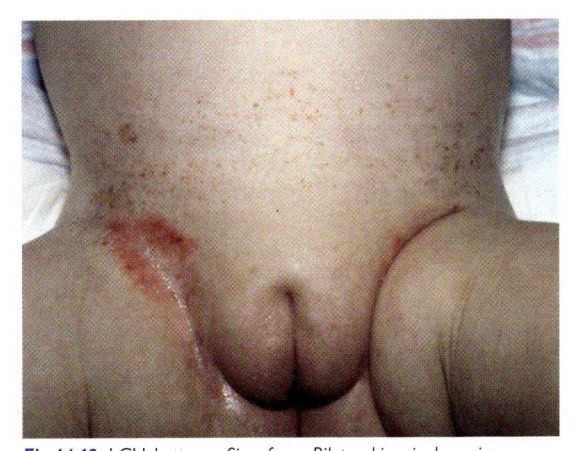

Fig 14.12 LCH: Letterer–Siwe form. Bilateral inguinal erosive plaques and erythematous papules. Image reprinted with permission from eMedicine.com 2008. Available at http://www.emedicine.com/derm/topic 216.htm

14.8 Case-based discussions

A child with an abdominal mass

A 3 year old girl was referred by her GP to an emergency clinic with a diagnosis of pneumonia. In the preceding week she had a productive cough, fever, and seemed quite tired. Six months previously she had been treated for a urinary tract infection following an episode of painless macroscopic haematuria. Microbiology records from that illness report red cells on urine microscopy and a mixed growth of uncertain significance. No further investigations were done.

On examination she looked pale and unwell.
T 38 °C, HR 120, BP 125/75 mmHg, capillary refill <2 s
RR 25/min, dull to percussion with crackles left base.

Abdominal examination revealed a 4 cm × 7 cm mass in the left upper quadrant. It was smooth, oval, non-mobile and did not appear to cross the midline. No organomegaly.

What is the most likely diagnosis?

Her acute symptoms are consistent with a community-acquired pneumonia which may have contributed to her anaemia, making her fatigued. Alongside this she also has an abdominal mass, a history of haematuria, and hypertension.

The most likely diagnosis is Wilms tumour. Most cases present at <4 years of age and painless haematuria is common. The UTI was a misdiagnosis. Hypertension may occur from pressure on the renal artery.

The differential includes a neuroblastoma or lymphoma. Neuroblastoma usually crosses the midline and has an irregular border. Hypertension and haematuria may occur. Hydronephrosis and polycystic kidney are also possibilities.

What is the immediate management?

Immediate supportive treatment requires IV antibiotics for her pneumonia. Full blood count, renal biochemistry, and blood cultures are indicated. Urgent antihypertensive therapy is not required.

Confirmation of the diagnosis will be most rapidly achieved by imaging: abdominal ultrasound scan and CXR followed by CT or MR imaging of chest and abdomen. A CT scan of the chest and abdomen identifies any involvement of lymph nodes, liver, or lung and enables differentiation from other abdominal masses.

In this case a mass arising from the right kidney was identified with the characteristics of a nephroblastoma (Wilms tumour). No lung metastases were detected on CT of the chest.

What is the further management?

Treatment includes surgery, chemotherapy, and sometimes radiotherapy depending on tumour histology and stage.

Surgical staging was at Stage III: there was residual intra-abdominal tumour after surgery. Histology of a tumour biopsy was favourable: mixed epithelial, stromal, and blastemal elements. Postoperative chemotherapy was with vincristine and actinomycin D.

A child with leg pain

A 3 year old girl presents to the emergency department with a painful limp. Her mother reports that she has been complaining of pain in her left leg for about 2 months. It has been getting steadily worse and over the last few days she has begun to limp. She took her to the GP 6 weeks previously and was told that it was 'growing pains'. She cannot recall her daughter being examined at that time. There is no history of trauma.

On examination she is afebrile and systemically well. She has an obvious limp. Examination using pGALS and pREM (see Chapter 16) identifies normal joints in all four limbs, but a localized tender region above the left knee with a suspicion of swelling.

What is the likely diagnosis?

The most common causes of a painful limp at this age include transverse synovitis, trauma, and infection. However, the length of history and clinical signs raise the possibility of a bone tumour. These are rare, but limb pain in a young child should always be treated with circumspection and examination is of course essential to identify a sinister cause.

Imaging (Fig 14.13) confirmed a Ewing sarcoma of the left femur.

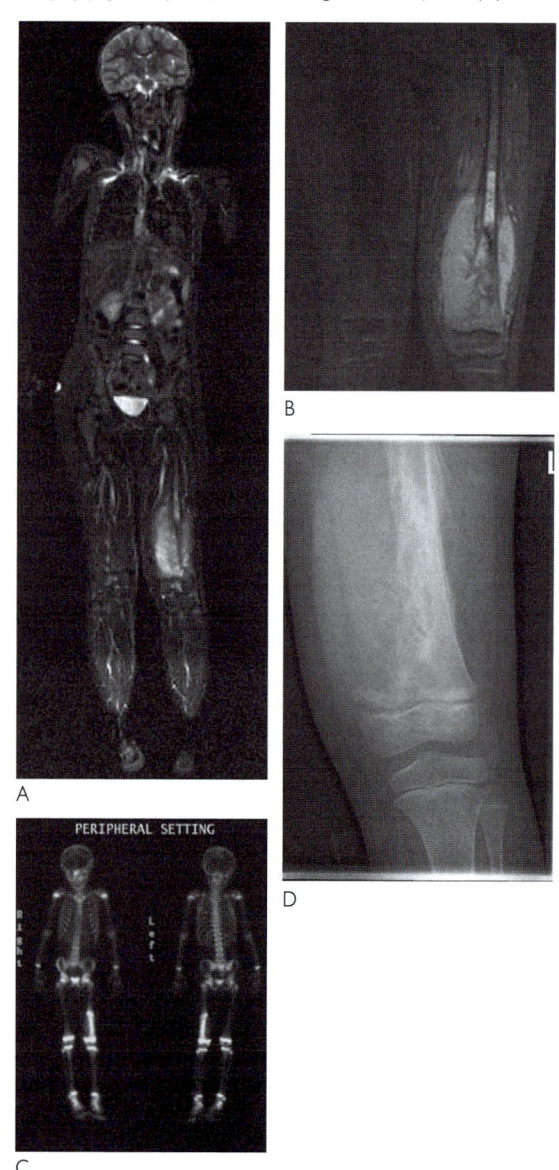

Fig 14.13 Imaging of Ewing sarcoma left femur. A, B. MRI. C. Isotope bone scan. D. Plain AP radiograph.

Chapter 15
Infection and immunity

15.1 Immune system *308*
15.2 Pathogens: infectious disease *310*
15.3 The feverish child: aetiology and assessment *312*
15.4 The feverish child: management *314*
15.5 Immunodeficiency *316*
15.6 Specific primary immunodeficiencies *318*
15.7 Measles, mumps, and rubella *320*
15.8 Enterovirus and parvovirus infection *322*
15.9 Herpesvirus infections: HSV and VZV *324*
15.10 Herpesviruses: EBV, CMV, and HHV-6, 7, and 8 *326*
15.11 Human immunodeficiency virus: HIV/AIDS *328*
15.12 Tuberculosis *330*
15.13 Staphylococcal and streptococcal infections *332*
15.14 Pneumococcal and meningococcal infections *334*
15.15 Zoonoses *336*
15.16 Malaria and typhoid *338*
15.17 Allergy *340*
15.18 Henoch–Schönlein purpura and Kawasaki disease *342*
15.19 Case-based discussions *344*

15.1 Immune system

Infectious disease arises from the interplay between pathogenic microbes and the defences of the host they infect. Host defence depends on the immune system.

The immune system is concerned with the recognition and disposal of 'non-self' material such as microbes, drugs, or food that enters the body. Immunity to infectious microbes is the chief desirable function, but undesirable consequences include allergy, autoimmune disease, and graft rejection.

External factors represent the first line of defence against microbes. These include:

- Intact skin and mucous membranes
- *Antimicrobial secretions:* lysozyme, lactoferrin, defensins, peroxidases
- Acidity of stomach
- Cilia of respiratory tract.

Immune mechanisms are usefully classified into 'innate' and 'adaptive' and in each case are mediated by both cellular and humoral elements. Adaptive mechanisms evolved most recently, in vertebrates, and perform many functions by interacting with older innate mechanisms.

Each system has a capacity for identifying non-self molecules based on soluble recognition molecules and cell-associated receptors. The latter include the antibody molecule, the T-cell receptor, and the major histocompatibility complex (MHC) which is part of the immunoglobulin (Ig) superfamily.

Innate immunity

Innate immunity is the first line of defence and plays a vital role in initiating the adaptive immune response. It is stimulated via receptors which recognize microorganisms and activate disposal mechanisms including some that produce inflammation.

Recognition systems

A limited number of pattern-recognition receptors recognize structures common to pathogens, called *pathogen-associated molecular patterns* (PAMPs). These may be soluble or cell-membrane associated and include:

- *Soluble recognition molecules:* complement, mannan-binding lectin (MBL), lipopolysaccharide (LPS)-binding protein (LBP), and C-reactive protein (CRP).
- *Cell-associated recognition:* Most pattern-recognition receptors are restricted to macrophages and dendritic cells. Examples include:
  - *mannose receptor:* recognizes mannan, a fungal cell wall component
  - *toll-like receptors:* recognize LPS, flagellin, haemagluttinin.

Cellular and humoral components

Cells of the innate system include:

- *Phagocytes:* neutrophils or polymorphonuclear cells (PMNs) and the mononuclear phagocyte system (monocytes in blood, macrophages in tissue). Neutrophils destroy ingested pathogens by superoxides and proteases. Macrophages also present antigens to T cells.
- *Dendritic cells:* rare cells in T-cell area of lymphoid tissues which present antigens to T-cells.
- *Natural killer (NK) cells:* a lymphocyte like cell capable of killing virus-infected and tumour cells.
- *Mast cells:* epithelial cells in skin, gut, and respiratory tract that release inflammatory mediators.

Humoral components include the complement system, acute phase proteins, interferon, and cytokines.

Complement system

The complement system consists of ~30 proteins including circulating serum proteins and cell membrane receptors.

Most components are part of a sequential activation pathway in which inactive proteases are converted into active proteases producing an amplifying cascade (comparable to the coagulation cascade).

Three pathways activate the system resulting in opsonization, chemotaxis, and cell lysis or the maladaptive response, anaphylaxis.

The three activation pathways are:

- *Classical pathway:* binding of antigen to antibody leads to activation of the C1 complex (C1q, C1r, and C1s).
- *Alternative pathways:* spontaneous conversion of C3 to C3b occurs continuously, C3b normally being spontaneously inactivated. Bacterial products or antibody aggregates allow C3b to bind Factor B and form a C3 convertase which activates the system.
- *Lectin pathway:* mannose-binding lectin, MBL binds to mannose residues on the pathogen surface which activates MBL-associated serine proteases which function similarly to C1r and C1s.

The three pathways all generate the protease C3 convertase which cleaves and activates C3 by creating the fragments C3a and C3b.

The subsequent effector mechanisms include:

- *Opsonization:* C3b binds to cell surface and receptors on macrophages and neutrophils, acting as an opsonin.
- *Chemotaxis:* C5a attracts phagocytic cells.
- *Anaphylatoxins:* C3a and C5a act as anaphylatoxins, binding to mast cells and causing release of vasoactive contents and promoting the inflammatory response.
- *Membrane attack complex:* C5b, C6, C7 and C8 guide polymerization of 18 molecules of C9 into the cell lipid membrane punching a hole which allows cell lysis.

Factors which regulate complement activity include Factors H and I and C1 inhibitor (C1INH) which shuts down the proteolytic activity of C1r and C1s.

Adaptive immunity

Adaptive immunity is based on the properties of lymphocytes which can respond selectively to thousands of different antigens, resulting in development or augmentation of defence mechanisms in response to a specific stimulus. The adaptive response acts as a 'memory' of the specific exposure and of course forms the basis of immunization.

Recognition systems

The adaptive immune system has four recognition systems:
- *Antibodies:* antibodies synthesized in B lymphocytes are exposed on the surface membrane and also secreted into the blood to act as a soluble recognition element. Antibody molecules represent millions of distinct and specific receptors. Some cells have Fc receptors which insert antibodies into their cell membrane.
- *T-cell receptor:* T lymphocytes carry receptors specialized to recognize small peptides bound to MHC molecules.
- *MHC molecules:* the MHC molecules present small antigenic peptides to the T-cell receptor. MHC class I molecules are found on all cells, MHC class II on B lymphocytes, macrophages, and dendritic cells.
- *NK cell receptors:* natural killer cells have activating and inhibitory receptors.

Cellular and humoral components

Lymphocytes

Lymphocytes have several unique features:
- *Specificity:* restricted receptors
- *Long lifespan and clonal proliferation:* memory
- *Body-wide distribution:* recirculation from tissues to bloodstream.

Lymphocytes may be immature, naive, memory, or effector cells. The two main subpopulations are T or thymus-dependent and B or bone-marrow dependent cells.

T cells

All T cells express the T-cell receptor (TCR) and further mature into effector cells including:
- *Helper T cells (Th):* CD4 T cells are essential for most antibody and cell-mediated responses. CD4 cells further divide into:
  - *Th1 cells:* pro-inflammatory, produce interferon-gamma (IFN-γ), tumour necrosis factor-alpha (TNF-α), and interleukin-2 (IL-2). They activate macrophages and help CD8 responses.
  - *Th2 cells:* produce IL-4, 5, and 6 cytokines necessary for helping B cells make IgA, IgE, and IgG2 and for eosinophil recruitment. Important for parasite eradication.
  - *Th17 cells:* important in autoimmune disease, produce IL-17.
- *Cytotoxic T cells:* CD8 T cells become αβ cytotoxic cells and kill cells expressing their specific antigen target, either by release of perforin and granzymes or by expression of Fas ligand which engages Fas on the target, provoking apoptotic cell death.
- *Regulatory T cells:* CD25 T cells inhibit target T cells, or release inhibitory cytokines such as IL-10 and TGF-β.

B cells

B cells are lymphocytes which use antibody as their antigen-specific receptor. They develop in bone-marrow from pro-B, to pre-B, to B cells and after encountering antigen a proportion differentiate into effector cells called plasma cells, devoted to synthesis and secretion of antibodies.

Antibody formation usually requires T-cell help but may be thymus independent.

A note on CD numbers

Cluster of **D**ifferentiation numbers identify cell-surface antigens distinguished by monoclonal antibodies. There are >300 CD numbers.

Antibodies

The antibody, or Ig molecule, plays the part of cell-surface receptor on B lymphocytes. The B-cell receptor (BCR) is also secreted into the blood.

- *Structure:* a typical antibody molecule has 12 domains arranged as 2 heavy and 2 light chains linked by disulfide bonds to form a Y shape (Fig 15.1). The domains may be variable or constant.
- *Classes:* 5 types of Ig heavy chain define the class or isotype of antibody: IgM, IgG, IgA, IgE, and IgD. IgG is further subdivided into subclasses IgG1–IgG4.
- *Synthesis:* antibody synthesis involves V (D)J recombination and class switching.

V (D)J recombination

The variable region is encoded by gene segments called variable (V), diversity (D), and joining (J) segments. Multiple copies exist, and each B cell assembles an Ig variable region by randomly selecting and combining V, D, and J segments.

Class switching

This allows different daughter cells from the same activated B cell to produce antibodies of different isotypes. Initially only cell-surface IgM and IgD are produced.

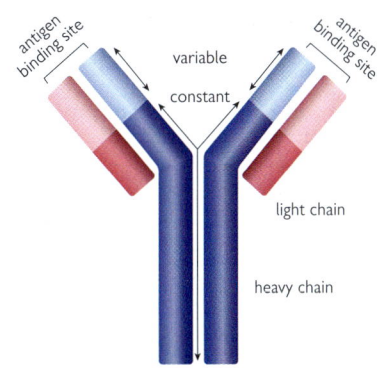

Fig 15.1 Antibody molecule: immunoglobulin. Reprinted by permission from Macmillan Publishers Ltd: Nature (421) 6921, The double helix and immunology; Nossal, © 2003.

15.2 Pathogens: infectious disease

Infectious or communicable diseases are caused by a small minority of the vast array of microbes that exist and by a handful of multicellular pathogens such as helminths.

Less than 1% of the estimated 3 billion microbial species have been identified, and only a few of these cause disease in otherwise healthy humans. Nevertheless, despite immunization and antibiotics, infections remain the major cause of morbidity and mortality in children worldwide, causing 70% of deaths in children <5 years.

Classification of pathogens

Infectious microorganisms are classified as:
- *Primary pathogens:* cause disease in normal, healthy hosts.
- *Opportunistic pathogens:* cause disease in a host with impaired defences.

The main biological categories of pathogens and their characteristics are shown in Table 15.1.

Table 15.1. Pathogens		
Organism	Structure	Visibility
Bacteria	Unicellular: prokaryotic	Light microscope
Viruses	Particles: nucleic acid and protein	Electron microscope
Protozoa	Unicellular: eukaryotic	Light microscope
Fungi	Uni- or multicellular	Naked eye
Worms	Metazoan	Naked eye
Prions	Protein, no nucleic acid	Electron microscope

Transmission

The modes of transmission include:

Human to human
- *Respiratory diseases:* contact with aerosolized droplets spread by sneezing, coughing, talking, kissing
- *Gastrointestinal (GI) diseases:* ingestion of contaminated food or water.
- *Sexually transmitted diseases:* contact with biological fluids.
- *Congenital infections:* transplacental transfer from mother to fetus in utero
- *Neonatal infection:* infection acquired during passage through birth canal
- *Breast-feeding:* transmission from mother to infant.

Zoonoses: animals to humans
- *Vector:* most vectors are arthropods. Transmission method may be mechanical, such as contaminated fly appendages, or biological by mosquito or tick bite. Lyme disease and leishmaniasis are vector borne
- *Contact:* tinea
- *Bite:* rabies
- *Ingestion of faeces:* toxoplasma, toxocara
- *Inhalation:* bird flu
- *Ingestion of animal:* prion disease, salmonellosis.

Pathogenicity

A pathogen is by definition a parasite that causes disease by inducing pathology. The symptoms and signs of infectious disease arise both from tissue damage caused by the pathogen and from the body's own immune response.

Pathogenic mechanisms include:

Direct tissue damage
- *Cytopathic infections:* many viruses cause cell lysis, as do intracellular organisms such as *Rickettsia*, *Chlamydia*, and mycoplasma. The malaria parasite causes lysis of hepatic and red cells.
- *Toxins:* bacteria may actively secrete 'exotoxins' or have 'endotoxins' as a component of their cell wall. Examples of bacterial exotoxins are listed in Table 15.2.

Table 15.2. Bacterial exotoxins		
Bacteria	Exotoxin	Action
Staphylococcus	Leukocyte Enterotoxin 'Toxic shock' toxin	Kills phagocytes Diarrhoea 'Superantigen': T-cell activation
Streptococcus	Streptolysin Streptokinase, hyalase	Kills phagocytes Tissue spread
Diphtheria	eEF2 inactivator	Inhibits protein synthesis
Pertussis	AB_5 toxin	G protein ribosylation
Clostridium tetani	Protease	Inhibits glycine, GABA release—spastic paralysis
Clostridium botulinum	Protease	Inhibits acetylcholine release—flaccid paralysis
Cholera vibrio	AB_5 toxin	
Shigella dysenteriae	Shiga toxin (Stx) AB_5 toxin	Inhibits protein synthesis
Escherichia coli	Enterotoxins AB_5 toxin: verotoxin	Diarrhoea Haemolytic uraemic syndrome

Endotoxins

The prototype endotoxin is the lipopolysaccharide (LPS) in the outer membrane of various gram-negative bacteria such as *Neisseria meningitis*. The lipid moiety, lipid A, is responsible for toxic effects and the polysaccharide chain is highly variable among different bacteria.

Endotoxins are released into the circulation when bacteria are lysed causing endotoxaemia and 'septic shock' by triggering release of inflammatory cytokines such as TNFα, IL-1, and IL-6 by mononuclear cells.

Immune response pathology

The immune response itself may harm the host: immunopathology. Mechanisms include:
- *Inflammation:* an acute inflammatory response involving the whole body causes fever and malaise.
- *'Shock':* toxins may mediate their ill effects via the immune system as described above causing signs of 'shock' or circulatory failure by two mechanisms:
  - *toxic shock:* a 'cytokine storm' provoked by activation of T-lymphocytes by superantigens
  - *septicaemic shock:* activation of macrophages by endotoxins and other microbial components

- *Immune-complex disease:* glomerulonephritis may occur from 'immune complex' deposition after infection by streptococci, malaria, or hepatitis B.
- *Postinfectious autoimmune disease:* the immune response to infection may cause autoimmune disease of the nervous system such as encephalomyelitis and Guillain–Barré syndrome or the heart in rheumatic fever.

Immunodeficiency
The pathogen may impair immune function. This occurs most conspicuously in HIV infection, but both measles and chickenpox cause immunosuppression, opening the door to secondary bacterial infection.

Microbial genome sequencing
Genomic technology has energized the field of microbial research. *Haemophilus influenza* was the first free-living organism for which the complete genome sequence was determined and complete genome sequences are now available for several hundred microbes including all the major human pathogens.

Anticipated benefits from microbial genome sequencing include:
- Discovery of microbial markers for pathogenicity, so called virulence genes
- Discovery of specific molecular targets for microbial identification and new diagnostic techniques
- Selection of candidates for rational development of new therapeutic agents and vaccines.

Epidemiology
Infectious diseases may follow any of several patterns in a population:
- *Sporadic:* occasional occurrence
- *Endemic:* regular cases often occurring in a region
- *Epidemic:* an unusual high number of cases occurring in a region
- *Pandemic:* a global epidemic.

A number of critical disease characteristics determine the transmission of infectious diseases. There is a complex relationship between virulence and transmission. Virulence may enhance transmission by causing higher infectiousness via explosive diarrhoea or sneezing, but a rapidly fatal disease may kill the host before the microbe is passed onto another host. An emerging pathogen is likely to be most virulent in its earliest victims.

Nosocomial infection
Nosocomial infections are infections acquired as a result of treatment in a hospital or health-care service unit (from the Greek *nosos* = disease, *komeo* = to take care of). Infections are classed as nosocomial if they first appear 48 h or more after hospital admission or within 30 days of discharge. The converse is *community acquired* infection.

Nosocomial infections are common for many reasons:
- Clustering of patients who may be infected and immunosuppressed
- Health-care staff moving from patient to patient provide a transmission route
- Medical procedures bypass natural protective barriers
- Selective pressure in hospitals for emergence of antibiotic-resistant pathogens.

Strategies for prevention of nosocomial infection include isolation of patients, hand-washing, and gloving. Correct hand-washing is the most important strategy. In addition, gloves may be worn to provide a protective barrier to prevent gross contamination of hands and to reduce likelihood of transmission.

Global epidemiology: the major killers
Worldwide, millions of children <5 years die each year from infectious diseases, many of which are vaccine-preventable deaths (VPDs). Among adults ~600 000 deaths per year are attributable to hepatitis B virus infections, the majority of which were acquired in childhood.

Immunization programmes have led to eradication of smallpox in 1980, elimination of measles and poliomyelitis from regions of the world, and reduction in mortality attributed to diphtheria, tetanus, and pertussis.

Estimates of deaths in children <5 years each year attributable to infection are shown in Table 15.3.

Table 15.3. Childhood deaths from infection.	
Pathogen/disease	Annual deaths
Acute respiratory infections	3.5 million
Gastro-enteritis/diarrhoea	2 million
Malaria	1 million
Measles	240 000
Pertussis	300 000
Haemophilus influenzae B	400 000
HIV/AIDS	300 000
Tetanus	200 000
Tuberculosis (TB)	500 000

Notifiable diseases
Doctors in England and Wales have a statutory duty to notify a 'proper officer' of the local authority of suspected cases of certain infectious diseases. The complete list of 30 diseases is available at the UK Health Protection Agency web site, and includes the following infections:
- *Viral:* measles, mumps, rubella, acute encephalitis, hepatitis
- *Bacterial:* dysentery and food poisoning, scarlet fever, typhoid fever, TB, meningitis, meningococcal septicaemia, whooping cough, ophthalmia neonatorum
- *Protozoal:* malaria.

15.3 The feverish child: aetiology and assessment

Feverish illness is the most common manifestation of infectious disease in childhood and one of the most common problems in clinical practice. The approach to clinical evaluation and management is described in this section.

Body temperature

Fever or *pyrexia* is an increase in internal body temperature to above normal, usually by 1–2 °C, due to a temporary elevation in the body's thermoregulatory set point.

Hyperthermia, in contrast, is an increase in body temperature above the thermoregulatory set point due to excessive heat production or failure of thermoregulatory mechanisms, e.g. in malignant hyperthermia or heat stroke.

Measurement and normal variation

Normal body temperature varies with location of measurement and shows diurnal variation. The normal oral human body temperature is 36.8 ± 0.7 °C.

Temperature measurement

The oral and rectal routes should not be routinely used to measure body temperature of children aged 0–5 years.

In babies <4 weeks an electronic thermometer in the axilla is used. In infants and children >4 weeks either an electronic or chemical dot thermometer in the axilla or infrared tympanic thermometer should be used by health-care professionals.

Compared to oral measurements, axillary or tympanic temperatures are 0.5–1.0 °C lower and rectal temperatures 0.5 °C higher. Reported parental perception of a fever should be considered valid and taken seriously.

Normal variation

Body temperature shows diurnal variation with lowest levels around 4 a.m. and highest levels in the evening at around 6 p.m. Temperature may increase after eating and with activities like playing, but this is not a fever as the set point is normal.

Pathophysiology of fever

Temperature is regulated by a centre in the hypothalamus which acts on thermoregulatory neurons to orchestrate heat effector mechanisms via the autonomic nervous system.

Substances that induce fever are termed *pyrogens* and may be exogenous or endogenous:

- *Exogenous pyrogens:* include components of infectious agents such as lipopolysaccharide (LPS)
- *Endogenous pyrogens:* include the cytokines which are part of the innate immune system and mediate the increase in thermoregulatory set point.

The sequence of events involved in fever generation is as follows:

- Exogenous pyrogen stimulates the innate immune system. This results in release of endogenous pyrogens, cytokines such as IL-1, IL-6, TNF-α which circulate to the brain, accessing the anterior hypothalamus.
- Pyrogenic cytokines activate the arachidonic acid pathway, generating prostaglandin E2 (PGE2). The enzymes phospholipase A2, cyclo-oxygenase-2 (COX2) and prostaglandin E2 synthetase mediate synthesis and release of PGE2. NSAIDs act at this point.
- PGE2 acts on the neurons in the preoptic area. These send fever signals to the dorsomedial hypothalamus.
- Hypothalamus stimulates the sympathetic system leading to increased heat production by shivering and non-shivering thermogenesis and increased heat conservation by peripheral vasoconstriction and tachycardia.

Feverish illness

Most feverish illnesses in childhood are caused by self-limiting viral infections but a significant few are caused by serious bacterial or other infections. A major challenge is to distinguish the two, and identify children in the early stages of a progressive and potentially lethal disease.

Fever is usefully classified according to grade or level, duration, and pattern.

Grade

- *Low grade:* <39.0 °C
- *Moderate:* 39.0–40 °C
- *High grade:* >40.0 °C

Duration

Most self-limiting febrile illnesses resolve within 5 days.

The term 'pyrexia of unknown origin' (PUO) is reserved for a febrile illness present for >10 days (definitions vary for duration from 1 to 3 weeks) with no apparent source despite evaluation including initial laboratory investigations. An acute febrile illness with no immediately apparent source should **not** be termed a PUO.

Pattern

- *Continuous fever:* does not fluctuate more than 1 °C in 24 h and is seen in pneumonia, urinary tract infection (UTI), and typhoid fever.
- *Remittent fever:* fluctuates >1 °C in 24 h; seen e.g. in infective endocarditis.
- *Intermittent fever:* temperature normal for some hours of the day, as occurs in malaria.

Causes of fever

In most cases fever is caused by an infection, but especially in prolonged fever other causes should be considered including autoimmune disease, malignancy and drug reactions.

Common and important causes of acute, <5 days and protracted fever in childhood are shown in the Boxes below. Note that causes of protracted fever such as Kawasaki disease should still be considered and even diagnosed during the acute phase.

> **Causes of acute fever, <5 days**
>
> - Bacterial:
>   - *focus on examination:* bacterial meningitis, pneumonia, upper respiratory tract infection, tonsillitis, otitis media, septic arthritis/osteomyelitis, appendicitis
>   - *no 'focus' on examination, with or without rash:* septicaemia, scarlet fever, staphylococcal scalded skin syndrome
> - Viral: fever and rash
>   - *adenovirus:* erythematous rash, respiratory, or GI symptoms.
>   - *herpes viruses:* HHV-1, gingivostomatitis, HHV-6 or 7, roseola infantum/exanthema subitum; EBV, glandular fever; VZV, chickenpox; CMV, glandular-fever-like illness.
>   - *enteroviruses:* coxsackievirus A16, hand, foot and mouth disease; Coxsackievirus A1–10, 16, 22, herpangina.

> **Causes of protracted fever, >5 days**
>
> *Infection*
> - Bacterial:
>   - *focus on examination:* abscess, osteomyelitis, endocarditis, urinary tract infection
>   - *no focus on examination:* TB, typhoid fever, leptospirosis, brucellosis, cat scratch disease
> - Viral: glandular fever, EBV or CMV
> - Protozoan: malaria
>
> *Inflammation*
> - Vasculitis: Kawasaki disease
> - Connective tissue disease: systemic onset juvenile idiopathic arthritis, SLE, inflammatory bowel disease
>
> *Malignancy*
> - Haematological: Hodgkin lymphoma, leukaemia
> - Solid tumours: Wilms tumour, neuroblastoma
>
> *Drug induced*
>
> *Fabricated or induced illness (FII)*

Clinical evaluation

System specific symptoms in the history such as cough, diarrhoea and vomiting, painful limp, sore throat, or dysuria may provide important clues to a focus of infection. Specific enquiry is made about medication and recent travel abroad.

Examination

The UK National Institute for Health and Clinical Excellence (NICE) guideline published 2007 for assessment of feverish illness in children <5 years suggests the following three-stage approach:

1 Identify any immediate life-threatening features: compromise of the **A**irway, **B**reathing, **C**irculation, or **D**ecreased level of consciousness.
2 Use the traffic light system for identifying likelihood of serious illness: see Section 15.4
3 Check for symptoms and signs associated with specific serious diseases:

- *Meningococcal disease (septicaemia):* non-blanching, purpuric rash with lesions >2 mm, CRT ≥3 s
- *Meningitis or encephalitis:* decreased level of consciousness, seizures, neck stiffness or bulging fontanelle
- *Pneumonia:* tachypnoea, crackles, recession, nasal flaring, oxygen saturation ≤95% in air
- *Urinary tract infection:* >3 months: vomiting, abdominal pain or tenderness, urinary frequency, dysuria, haematuria
- *Septic arthritis/osteomyelitis:* swelling or tenderness of a limb or joint, not using an extremity, non-weight-bearing
- *Kawasaki disease:* fever >5 days and four of the following:
  - bilateral conjunctival injection, polymorphous rash, cervical lymphadenopathy, mucous membranes (cracked lips, strawberry tongue), extremities (erythema, oedema, desquamation).

Note that the duration and height of fever does not alone predict the likelihood of serious illness. The blood pressure should be measured if there are any signs of circulatory compromise such as tachycardia or prolonged capillary refill time. Hydration status must be assessed carefully.

Protracted fever

Features in the history or examination may prompt consideration of certain diagnoses:

History

- *Travel abroad:* malaria, typhoid, arbovirus infection: yellow fever, dengue
- *Animal exposure:* cat scratch disease, brucellosis (animal contact or ingestion of unpasteurized milk), leishmaniasis, leptospirosis
- *GI symptoms:* giardiasis, Salmonella, Campylobacter infection, inflammatory bowel disease
- *Behavioural/psychosocial:* FII
- *Sore throat:* EBV or CMV

Examination

- *High, swinging fever:* malaria, brucellosis, abscess
- *Rash:* Kawasaki disease, systemic onset JIA, glandular fever, typhoid fever
- *Conjunctivitis:* Kawasaki disease, measles, adenovirus infection
- *Respiratory signs:* TB
- *Lymphadenopathy:* TB, EBV, lymphoma
- *Organomegaly:* hepatitis, EBV infection, leukaemia
- *Musculoskeletal signs:* juvenile chronic arthritis, inflammatory bowel disease
- *Bone tenderness:* leukaemia, osteomyelitis.

Management: immediate treatment

Children with fever and shock should be given an intravenous bolus of 0.9% sodium chloride (normal saline), 20 mL/kg body weight.

Parenteral antibiotics should be given to children with fever and shock or who are unrousable or showing signs of septicaemia. A 3rd generation cephalosporin, cefotaxime or ceftriaxone, is indicated, with the addition of amoxicillin to cover Listeria in infants <3 months.

IV aciclovir is indicated for children with fever and symptoms or signs suggestive of herpes simplex encephalitis.

Oxygen should be given to children with signs of shock or oxygen saturation of <92–95% in air.

15.4 The feverish child: management

Further management is guided by the age, with a threshold at 3 months, and the presence or absence of green, amber, or red features using the traffic light system, according to the following NICE guidelines.

Traffic light system

The traffic light system is a useful way of identifying the likelihood of serious illness.
The child is assessed according to:
- Colour
- Activity
- Respiratory signs
- Hydration
- 'Other' signs

and then assigned to one of three categories:
- *Green:* low risk
- *Amber:* intermediate risk
- *Red:* high risk.

Green: low risk

The criteria are as follows:

Colour
- Normal colour of skin, lips, and tongue.

Activity
- Responding normally to social cues
- Content and smiling
- Awake or awakens easily
- Strong normal cry.

Hydration
- Normal skin and eyes
- Moist mucous membranes.

Other
- Absence of amber or red symptoms or signs.

Amber: intermediate risk

The criteria are as follows:

Colour
- Pallor reported by parent or carer.

Activity
- Not responding normally to social cues
- Decreased activity
- No smile
- Wakes only with prolonged stimulation.

Respiratory
- *Nasal flaring*
- *Tachypnoea:*
  - RR >50 breaths/min (age 6–12 months)
  - RR >40 breaths/min (age >12 months)
- Oxygen saturation ≤95% in air
- Crackles on auscultation.

Hydration
- Poor feeding in infants
- Dry mucous membranes
- CRT ≥3 s
- Reduced urine output.

Other
- Fever for ≥5 days
- Swelling of a limb or joint
- Non-weight-bearing or not using an extremity
- A new lump ≥2 cm.

Red: high risk

The criteria are as follows:

Colour
- Pale or ashen
- Blue or mottled.

Activity
- No response to social cues
- Appears ill to a health-care professional
- Unable to rouse or if roused does not stay awake
- Cry weak, high pitched, or continuous.

Respiratory
- Grunting
- *Tachypnoea:* RR >60 breaths/minute
- *Chest indrawing:* moderate or severe.

Hydration
- Reduced skin turgor.

Other
- *Temperature:*
  - ≥38°C (age 0–3 months)
  - ≥39°C (age 3–6 months)
- Non-blanching rash
- Neck stiffness or bulging fontanelle
- Status epilepticus or focal seizures
- Focal neurological signs
- Bile-stained vomiting.

Further management (by a paediatric specialist)

Further management according to the guidelines depends on whether the patient is an infant or child younger or older than 3 months of age. Guidelines are not protocols (see Chapter 21.5) and the actual management of each individual case is a matter of clinical judgement.

Infant younger than 3 months

After assessment, observe and monitor vital signs:
- Temperature
- Heart rate
- Respiratory rate.

Initial investigations
- FBC and CRP
- Blood culture
- *Urine:* dipstick and culture
- *CXR:* if respiratory signs
- *Stool culture:* if diarrhoea present.

Lumbar puncture
Admit and perform lumbar puncture and start parenteral antibiotics if the infant is:
- <1 month old
- Age 1–3 months but unwell or with a total WBC either < 5 × 10^9/L or > 15 × 10^9/L.

Whenever possible, perform lumbar puncture before the administration of antibiotics.

Infant or child 3 months or older

Assess under the 'traffic light' system and proceed according to whether risk of serious illness is low, intermediate, or high.

Green: low risk
- Investigations: urine dipstick and send for microscopy and culture.
- Carefully assess for symptoms and signs of pneumonia.
- Do not perform blood tests or CXR as a 'routine'.

If no clinical diagnosis requiring admission to hospital is reached, children with 'green' features can be sent home with advice about antipyretics, regular fluids, and the need to seek further medical advice in the event of deterioration, a fit, a non-blanching rash, or persistence of fever >5 days.

Amber: intermediate risk
If no clear clinical diagnosis is apparent to guide management consider the following investigations:
- *Urine:* dipstick, microscopy and culture
- *FBC, CRP, and blood culture*
- *CXR:* if fever > 39 °C and/or total WBC ≥20 × 10^9/l
- *Lumbar puncture:* if infant <1 year old.

Consider admission to hospital according to clinical and social circumstances (see below).

If admission is unnecessary but diagnosis remains uncertain a 'safety net' should be provided for the carers in the form of information on warning symptoms and how to access health care and a follow-up review.

Red: high risk
If no clear clinical diagnosis is apparent to guide specific management the following investigations should be performed:
- FBC, CRP, and blood culture
- Urine dipstick, microscopy, and culture.

Depending on clinical assessment consider the following investigations:
- Lumbar puncture
- CXR (irrespective of temperature or total WBC)
- Urea and electrolytes
- Blood gases.

Admission to hospital

In addition to the child's clinical condition, factors to consider include:
- Social and family circumstances
- Parent's or carers' anxiety and 'instinct'
- Recent contact with serious infectious disease
- Recent travel abroad to high-risk area
- Previous family experience of serious illness
- Protracted, unexplained fever.

Antibiotic treatment of suspected bacterial infection

- Give immediate parenteral antibiotics (third-generation cephalosporin, for example, cefotaxime or ceftriaxone) to a child with fever
  - And signs of shock
  - Who is unrousable
  - And signs of meningococcal disease
  - Younger than 1 month
  - Aged 1–3 months with a white blood cell count less than 5 or greater than 15x10^9/litre
  - Aged 1–3 months who appears unwell.
- If serious bacterial infection is suspected and immediate treatment is required, give antibiotics against *Neisseria meningitidis, Streptococcus pneumoniae, E. coli, Staphylococcus aureus*, and *Haemophilus influenzae* type b (for example, a third-generation cephalosporin).
- Add an antibiotic active against Listeria if child is younger than 3 months of age (e.g. ampicillin or amoxicillin).
- Consider parenteral antibiotics in children with a decreased level of consciousness. Look for symptoms and signs of meningitis and herpes simplex encephalitis.
- If rates of antibacterial resistance are significant, refer to local guidelines.

15.5 Immunodeficiency

The immunodeficiencies are classified by aetiology into the primary immunodeficiency diseases (PIDs) and the secondary immunodeficiencies. Susceptibility to infection is the main clinical manifestation.

Primary immunodeficiency diseases (PIDs)

The PIDs are a heterogeneous group of genetic disorders with a frequency of up to 1/500 if common, mild varieties are included. Molecular geneticists have now identified more than 100 different genes responsible for PIDs but fortunately many are very rare.

A classification of the more important PIDs is given in the Box.

Primary immunodeficiency diseases

Adaptive immunity
- Antibody deficiencies:
  - common variable immunodeficiency (CVID)
  - selective IgA deficiency
  - transient hypogammaglobulinaemia of infancy
  - selective IgG subclass deficiency
  - X-linked agammaglobulinaemia
- Combined B and T cell defects:
  - severe combined immunodeficiency (SCID)
  - MHC class I or class II deficiency
  - hyper-IgM syndrome

Innate immunity
- Phagocytic cell defects
- Neutropaenias:
  - congenital neutropaenias: Kostman disease
  - Shwachman–Diamond syndrome
  - cyclic neutropaenia
- Neutrophil function defects:
  - chronic granulomatous disease
  - leucocyte adhesion defects
- Complement deficiency:
  - deficiencies of complement C1–C9
  - properdin deficiency
  - mannose-binding lectin deficiency
  - C1-inhibitor deficiency
- IFN-α associated immunodeficiency

Immunodeficiency syndromes
- Di George syndrome: with thymic defect
- Wiskott–Aldrich and Chediak–Higashi syndrome
- Hermansky–Pudlak syndrome
- DNA repair defects:
  - ataxia-telangiectasia
  - Bloom syndrome
  - Nijmegen breakage syndrome
- Chronic mucocutaneous candidiasis
- Hypohidrotic ectodermal dysplasia

Immune dysregulation diseases include familial haemophagocytic lymphohistiocytosis, X-linked lymphoproliferative syndrome, and autoimmune lymphoproliferative syndrome. Many of these disorders are X-linked and the most of the rest are autosomal recessive (AR). A minority are autosomal dominant (AD) or inherited as 'complex' traits. Individual PIDs are discussed in Section 15.6.

Secondary immunodeficiency

Secondary or acquired immunodeficiency is more common than primary and may affect any or all components of the innate or adaptive immune systems. Worldwide, malnutrition and infection are the most important cause. The main causes are shown in the Box.

Causes of secondary immunodeficiency

- Malnutrition
- Viral infections:
  - HIV
  - EBV infection
  - *measles*: inhibits IL-12 production
- Preterm birth
- Drugs:
  - cytotoxic
  - *immunosuppressive drugs*: corticosteroids, ciclosporin A, tacrolimus
- Radiation therapy
- Diseases affecting the immune system:
  - *malignancy*: leukaemia, lymphoma
  - nephrotic syndrome
  - protein losing enteropathy
  - sickle cell disease
  - *asplenia*: genetic or acquired
  - diabetes mellitus

Pathogenesis

The three main consequences of immunodeficiency are susceptibility to infection, autoimmune disease, and tumour development.

Susceptibility to infection

Pathogens which cause disease in hosts with weakened immune systems are termed *opportunistic*. Deficiencies in particular arms of immunity correlate to some extent with susceptibility to infection with specific pathogens, but the interactions within the immune system prevent strict correlation. Immune mechanisms most important for the main pathogenic microbes are:

Viruses
Interaction with receptors on the cell surface is necessary prior to intracellular replication. Rapid antigenic variation aids evasion of specific antibody responses. Viral immunity depends on neutralizing antibodies and cytotoxic T cells.

Bacteria
Bacterial virulence is enhanced by pili allowing adherence, flagella allowing motility, capsules which frequently have T-independent antigens, and the production of endotoxins and exotoxins.

Bacterial immunity depends on antibodies for neutralization of toxins, opsonization, and phagocyte function.

Fungi

T-cell function is important for immunity to fungi which rarely cause invasive disease in immunocompetent hosts.

The pathogens that typically cause infection in deficiencies of specific aspects of immunity are shown in Table 15.4.

Table 15.4. Immune defects and susceptibility to infection.

Adaptive immunity		
Antibody deficiencies	Bacteria	*Staphylococcus, Streptococcus* sp., *Haemophilus influenzae, Moraxella catarrhalis*
	Viruses	Enteroviruses
	Protoza	Giardia
T-cell deficiencies	Bacteria	*Mycobacterium, Listeria*
	Viruses	Herpesviruses, measles, respiratory syncytial virus, adenovirus
	Fungi	*Candida, Aspergillus, Pneumocystis*
Innate immunity		
Neutrophils	Bacteria	*Staphylococcus, E. coli, Klebsiella*
	Fungi	*Candida, Aspergillus*
Complement	Bacteria	*Neisseria, Staphylococcus*
	Fungi	*Candida, Aspergillus*

Clinical features

Frequent infections are a feature of normal childhood especially when children are first exposed to new microbes in daycare or school. Parents often have unnecessary concerns that their child's immune system is weak in some way.

Features which should raise the suspicion of immunodeficiency include:

- Recurrent severe infections
- Severe course of infection with organisms of low pathogenicity
- Failure to respond to appropriate therapy
- Infection with 'opportunistic' organisms
- *Family history:* consanguinity, unexplained infant death especially in boys for X-linked recessive disorders.

Additional features of immunodeficiency may include failure to thrive, diarrhoea, skin rashes, delayed separation of the umbilical cord, hepatosplenomegaly, or dysmorphic/syndromic signs.

Certain patterns of presentation are more common with specific defects:

- *Recurrent ENT and airway infections:* antibody deficiencies, neutropaenia, HIV infection, Wiskott–Aldrich syndrome
- *Recurrent pyogenic infections:* phagocyte deficiency, neutropaenia, or defects in phagocyte function
- *Recurrent infections with same pathogen:* depends on pathogen:
  - encapsulated bacteria: antibody deficiencies
  - encapsulated bacterial sepsis: asplenia
  - meningococci: complement or antibody deficiency
  - *Candida:* T-lymphocyte deficiency, chronic mucocutaneous candidiasis
- *Failure to thrive in infancy:* T-lymphocyte deficiency, e.g. HIV

- *Unusual infections/severe course:* T-lymphocyte deficiency in HIV, Wiskott–Aldrich syndrome, X-linked lymphoproliferative syndrome
- *Clinical features of a syndrome:* Di George syndrome, ataxia telangiectasia, Wiskott–Aldrich syndrome.

Management

Investigations

Initial screening tests are easily available and diagnose major abnormalities including SCID and AIDS.

- *Full blood count and differential:* neutropaenia, lymphopaenia, Howell–Jolly bodies in asplenia
- *Immunoglobulins:* IgG, IgA, IgM: Ig deficiencies
- *HIV test:* with appropriate counselling
- *CXR:* thymic shadow.

Further investigations are guided by the likely clinical diagnosis and the results of initial investigations in consultation with a paediatric immunologist. Examples of further investigation of specific components of the immune system are:

Antibodies

- *Antigen-specific antibodies:* to diphtheria, tetanus, Hib
- Isohaemagglutinins (>12 months).

Lymphocytes

- Lymphocyte subpopulations:
  - CD3+: T lymphocytes
  - CD3+/CD4+: helper T lymphocytes
  - CD3+, CD8+: cytotoxic T lymphocytes
  - CD19+, CD20+: B lymphocytes
- *Lymphocyte proliferation tests:* mitogen responses.

Neutrophil function

- Nitroblue tetrazolium test (NBT)
- Microbicidal assays
- Chemotaxis.

Complement deficiency

- Red cell haemolytic assays depending on CH50 (classical pathway) or AP50 (alternate pathway)
- *Immunoassays for:* C3, C1q, C2, C4, C5–9
- C1-inhibitor levels.

Molecular DNA studies

Treatment

Options are discussed under individual syndromes in Section 15.6 and range from prophylactic antibiotics to immunoglobulin replacement therapy and gene therapy.

15.6 Specific primary immunodeficiencies

Common variable immunodeficiency (CVID)

Common variable immunodeficiency (CVID) is a heterogeneous group of disorders characterized by a marked decrease in immunoglobulins in at least two of the three major isotypes—IgM, IgG, and IgA—and absent specific antibodies in response to vaccines.

A number of different molecular aberrations have been identified, including defective CD40 ligand expression and mutations in *TAC1* and *TNFRSF13B*, which can also cause selective IgA deficiency. T-cell numbers may be normal or low, and although B-cell numbers may be normal they fail to differentiate.

Onset is usually later in life, rarely <2 years, with recurrent bacterial infection of the respiratory tract. Autoimmune manifestations occur in 50% and there is an increased risk of lymphomas. Some patients have granulomatous disease of the gut, lung, and skin.

Treatment is supportive with immunoglobulin infusions and prophylactic antibiotics. Bone marrow transplantation has been undertaken in some patients.

Selective IgA deficiency (IGAD)

Selective IgA deficiency is the most common form of PID in the western world, affecting as many as 1/600 individuals. Most are sporadic but AD or multifactorial inheritance is recognized with a susceptibility locus at the MHC region.

It is usually asymptomatic but may be associated with recurrent sinopulmonary infection, autoimmune disorders, atopy, malabsorption, and malignancy especially if present in combination with IgG2 subclass deficiency.

Definitive diagnosis depends on demonstration of a serum IgA <0.07 g/L in a patient >4 years of age with normal IgG and IgM levels and no other cause for hypogammaglobulinaemia.

Transient hypogammaglobulinaemia of infancy (THI)

Delayed maturation of Ig production of unknown aetiology which resolves spontaneously by age 2–3 years. A minority progress to CVID or IGAD.

Presentation is usually with increased frequency of URTIs including otitis media. Diagnosis rests on concentrations of one or more Ig isotypes <2.5 SD for age on two or more occasions. Management involves prompt treatment of infections with antibiotics and prophylactic antibiotics, azithromycin or augmentin, over the winter months.

X-linked agammaglobulinaemia (XLA)

Bruton XLA is an X-linked immunodeficiency characterized by failure of B-cell maturation due to mutations in Bruton tyrosine kinase which prevent Ig heavy chain re-arrangement.

Male infants usually present in the 1st 2 years of life with recurrent bacterial infections of the respiratory tract, pneumonia, sinusitis due to encapsulated bacteria, diarrhoea caused by *Giardia* or *Campylobacter*, and enteroviral infections. Arthritis of large joints develops in 20%. Tonsillar tissue and lymph nodes are vestigial or absent, as is gut-associated lymphoid tissue (GALT).

B-cell CD19 percentages are low at <2% and IgG, IgA, IgM, and IgE are absent or very low.

Treatment is with regular IV or SC immunoglobulin monthly, aiming for target IgG trough levels of 8–9 g/L. Live vaccines should be avoided.

Severe combined immunodeficiency (SCID)

Severe combined immunodeficiency is a heterogeneous group of inherited disorders characterized by severe defects in both cellular and humoral immunity. The overall incidence is between 1/50 000 and 1/500 000. Males are affected more than females because of one X-linked type.

Aetiology

SCID is classified into those with or without B cells:
- *T-/B+ SCID:* X-linked due to mutations in *IL2RG* encoding a gamma chain common to receptors for IL2 and other interleukins, SCIDX-1 and *JAK3* (recessive).
- *T-/B- SCID:* mutations in *ADA*, encoding adenosine deaminase, and in *RAG1* or *RAG2* genes (including Omenn syndrome).

Over 10 additional gene defects have been discovered.

Clinical features

Infants with SCID usually present in the first 6 months of life with failure to thrive, persistent diarrhoea, respiratory symptoms and/or thrush, severe bacterial infection, and *Pneumocystis* pneumonia (Fig 15.2).

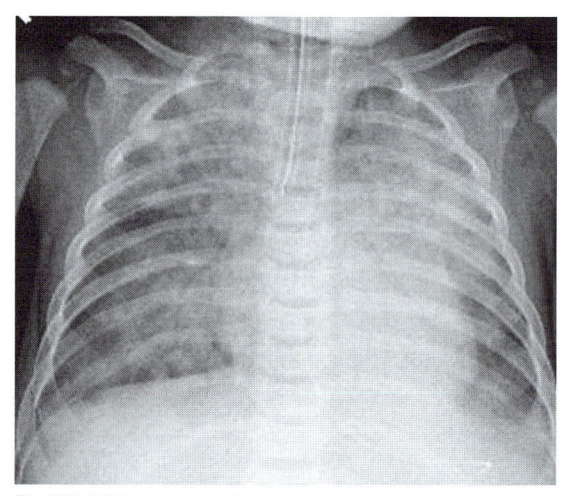

Fig 15.2 SCID: pneumocystis pneumonitis.

Disseminated BCG infection, BCGosis, may occur if given BCG at birth. Skin rash may be due to viral or fungal infection, maternal T cell engraftment or Omenn syndrome.

Diagnosis and management

The total lymphocyte count is low at $<3.0 \times 10^9$/L and total T-cell numbers are also low with CD3+ <20%.

Ig concentrations are variable as maternal IgG may still be present and defects in B cell and NK cell development are variable. A normal lymphocyte count does not exclude SCID.

If SCID is diagnosed or strongly suspected, immediate management involves:
- Move child to microbiological isolation
- All blood products used irradiated and CMV negative
- Prophylactic co-trimoxazole, 30 mg/kg twice weekly
- No live vaccines or contact with people who have recently received live vaccines.

Further management options include continued antibiotic prophylaxis, antiviral and antifungal prophylaxis, and attention to nutrition and skin care.

Prognosis is poor. Curative treatment options are bone marrow transplantation and gene therapy which has been used successfully for SCIDXI and SCIDADA. In the latter gene therapy is used together with enzyme replacement with PEG-ADA. Genetic counselling should be offered.

Hyper-IgM syndrome (HIGM)

HIGM is a rare inherited disease usually caused by recessive mutations in the X-linked gene *CD40LG*, but AR forms exist.

The CD40 ligand on T-cells interacts with CD40 on B-cells promoting their growth and differentiation and isotype switching. Defects in this pathway cause non-functional B-cells which produce excess IgM but no IgG, IgA, or IgE and impaired macrophage function.

HIGM presents in infancy with recurrent bacterial and opportunistic infections of the respiratory tract (*Pneumocystis*) and GI tract (*Cryptosporidium* spp.). Chronic neutropaenia may cause oral or rectal ulcers. Associated liver disease is an important cause of morbidity and mortality.

Neutropaenia

See section on white cell disorders in Chapter 13.10. Intrinsic, inherited neutropaenias may be isolated, *SCN1-4* including Kostmann disease, or occur in syndromes such as Shwachman–Diamond and Fanconi anaemia.

Chronic granulomatous disease (CGD)

Chronic granulomatous disease is a genetically heterogeneous PID in which neutrophils are unable to kill ingested microbes on account of defects in the NADPH oxidase membrane complex which generates the microbicidal 'respiratory burst'.

Gene defects have been identified for all of the phagocyte oxidase (phox) proteins which assemble to activate the oxidase. The most common, accounting for 70%, is in the X-linked gene *CYBB*, encoding P91-phox. The other defects are AR.

Patients develop deep-seated recurrent and chronic bacterial and fungal infections involving lungs, skin, liver, and bones. Organisms include *Staphylococci*, *E. coli*, *Serratia marcescens* and *Nocardia*. Fungi such as *Candida* and *Aspergillus* sp. cause severe infections.

The nitroblue tetrazolium test (NBT) is diagnostic and shows an impaired neutrophil respiratory burst.

Management includes prophylactic antibiotics, steroids for granulomatous disease, high dose antifungal treatment with ambisome and caspafungin for severe fungal infection with granulocyte infusions and IFN-γ therapy. Bone marrow transplantation has been used successfully and gene therapy attempted.

Complement component defects

Defects of many components of the complement cascade and related proteins occur. Most are AR and predispose to infection and autoimmune disorders.
- *MBL:* frequent infection in neonates and in context of other immunodeficiencies
- *C3 deficiency:* rare but severe risk of infection
- *C5–9:* causes recurrent infection with *Neisseria*
- *C2 deficiency:* causes pyogenic infections and a lupus-like syndrome with vasculitis and polymyositis
- *C1 inhibitor deficiency:* may be inherited in hereditary angio-oedema (see below) or acquired in diseases such as SLE.

Hereditary angio-oedema (HAE)

Hereditary angio-oedema is a rare genetic disorder associated with defective function of C1-esterase inhibitor (C1INH), a serine protease inhibitor (serpin) which normally inhibits the conversion of C1 to C1r and C1s and also inhibits various proteins of the coagulation cascade.

Three types are described:
- *Type I (85%):* decreased levels of C1INH
- *Type II (15%):* decreased function of C1INH
- *Type III:* mutations in the factor XII gene cause oestrogen-sensitive HAE in females. C1INH levels normal.

Clinical features are variable and include episodes which may be spontaneous or triggered and are caused by oedema most commonly in GI tract or neck, throat, and face. Abdominal attacks cause pain, vomiting, and watery diarrhoea. Oedema of the oropharynx and larynx may be life threatening. Failure to respond to antihistamines or steroids is a useful clinical clue to diagnosis.

C1-esterase inhibitor assay can be done but may be normal.

Prophylaxis options include danazol which stimulates hepatic synthesis of C1INH and fibrinolysis inhibitors such as tranexamic acid. C1INH concentrate is available for short term prophylaxis presurgery and for emergency treatment of an acute attack. Acdrenaline (epinephrine) is indicated for airway obstruction.

DiGeorge syndrome (DGS)

DiGeorge syndrome is one of the 22q11 microdeletion syndromes (see Chapter 12.6). The main features are cono-truncal cardiac defects, hypocalcaemia due to small or absent parathyroids, and immunodeficiency due to thymic aplasia or hypoplasia. T-cells are reduced in number and have impaired function giving increased susceptibility to systemic fungal infections and disseminated viral infections. Most children have a mild immunodeficiency phenotype and T cell numbers increase with age.

Wiskott–Aldrich syndrome (WAS)

Wiskott–Aldrich syndrome is an X-linked recessive immunodeficiency characterized by thrombocytopaenia, eczema, and recurrent infections. It is caused by mutations in the *WAS* gene at Xp11.22 which encodes the WAS protein. Defects in WASp cause defective polymerization of the lymphocyte actin cytoskeleton. Both T- and B-cell function are affected.

Recurrent bacterial and viral infections occur. EBV, varicella, and herpes simplex viruses are most troublesome. Autoimmune diseases occur and there is an increased incidence of leukaemia and lymphoma.

15.7 Measles, mumps, and rubella

Measles and rubella are viral exanthems. An *exanthem* is a rash that 'bursts forth' and is typically a widespread and symmetrical maculopapular rash which may be caused by viruses, bacteria, or drug reactions. An *enanthem* refers to the oral lesions such as Koplik spots that may accompany an exanthem.

Childhood exanthems were previously numbered 1–6 according to their historical order of description.

Measles

Measles or rubeola is a highly communicable, vaccine-preventable disease caused by a paramyxovirus. A licensed vaccine has been available since 1963 and the introduction of immunization programmes has lead to a 99% reduction in incidence in immunized developed world populations.

Epidemiology
The Measles Initiative, a global partnership between UNICEF, WHO, and other organizations, has led to mass vaccination campaigns with an estimated 500 million children receiving measles vaccine between 2000 and 2006. In this period, global measles deaths fell by 68% from 757 000 to 242 000 and measles deaths in Africa from 396 000 to 36 000.

In the UK, measles vaccine is given as part of the combined MMR vaccine, uptake of which fell following unsubstantiated reports of a link with autism in the early 2000s. A fall in rates from >90% to 79% has been associated with an increase in cases of measles to 740 in 2006 and 971 in 2007.

Aetiology and pathogenesis
Measles virus is spread via respiratory droplets, either by direct contact or by airborne aerosol transmission. Viral replication occurs locally in epithelial cells. Viraemia then disseminates the virus prior to the appearance of a rash.

Maternal antibodies play a significant role in protection against infection in infants <1 year.

Measles virus infection causes a generalized immunosuppression which persists for weeks or months and predisposes individuals to severe bacterial infections, particularly bronchopneumonia, a major cause of measles-related mortality. In individuals with deficient cellular immunity, measles causes a progressive and often fatal giant cell pneumonia.

Clinical features
The incubation period from exposure to onset of symptoms is 7–14 days. The prodromal phase is marked by:
- Malaise, fever, and anorexia
- *The 3 Cs:* conjunctivitis, coryza and cough.

This is followed by the eruptive phase marked by:
- *Fever:* often up to 40 °C, begins with prodrome and lasts 7–10 days.
- *Enanthem:* Koplik spots, like grains of sand on a red base on the buccal mucosa, appear 2 days before rash
- *Rash:* an erythematous, maculopapular rash starting on the head and spreading to cover most of the body and become confluent (Fig 15.3). Desquamation and brown 'staining' occurs after 1 week. The rash may be absent in patients with deficiency in cellular immunity.
- *Lymphoid involvement:* generalized lymphadenopathy and mild hepatomegaly.

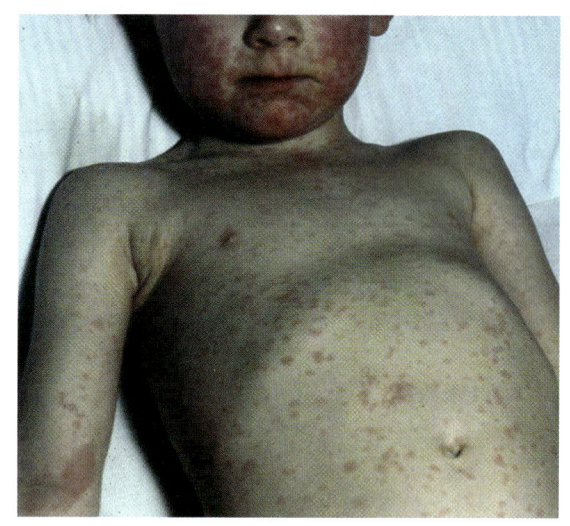

Fig 15.3 Measles: rash.

Complications
- *Respiratory:* otitis media, tracheitis, bronchopneumonia
- *Neurological:* acute encephalitis (1/1000); subacute sclerosing panencephalitis is now very rare (it does not occur with vaccine-related strains of virus).

Risk factors for severe measles include malnutrition, vitamin A deficiency, and immunocompromised hosts as in HIV infection or leukaemia.

Case fatality rates are higher in children<5 years or immunocompromised children. In healthy children, mortality rates are 1–3/1000.

Management
Diagnosis

Diagnostic tests for measles include:
- *Serology:* test for measles IgM antibody which may not be detectable until day 3 of rash
- *Viral culture:* isolation from nasopharyngeal swabs
- *Immunofluorescence:* identification of measles antigen.

Viral genotyping in a reference laboratory may determine whether the isolate is endemic or imported.

Prevention

In the UK, measles vaccine is given as part of the routine immunization programme as a component of MMR at 13 months and with the pre-school booster at 3 years and 4 months.

Treatment

Treatment is supportive as no specific antiviral therapy exists.

Vitamin A supplements are associated with reduction in morbidity and mortality and are recommended in malnourished or immunodeficient children. Antibiotics for otitis media or pneumonia.

Patients are contagious from 1–2 days before onset of symptoms to 4 days after the onset of rash and for the duration of the illness in immunocompromised patients.

Mumps

Mumps, or epidemic parotitis, is an acute generalized infection caused by a paramyxovirus and characterized by swelling of one or more salivary glands, usually the parotids.

Epidemiology

In the UK, infection was very common in childhood before the introduction of the MMR vaccine in 1987. It was almost completely eliminated in the 1990s, but a resurgence occurred with an outbreak from 2004–2006 of 70 000 cases in the UK. Most cases involved young adults attending college who were too old to have been vaccinated and too young to have been exposed to natural infection.

Aetiology and pathogenesis

Transmission is by direct contact, droplet spread, or contaminated fomites. Virus replication occurs in the upper respiratory tract mucosa and may remain localized. Transient viraemia leads to systemic viral spread most commonly but not always or necessarily affecting the parotids, the CNS, and the genitourinary tract.

Mumps virus has an affinity for glandular epithelium, including ductal epithelium leading to parotitis, pancreatitis, and orchitis. Subsequent testicular atrophy can occur. Virus enters CSF via the choroid plexus causing aseptic meningitis but primary encephalitis is rare.

Clinical features

Mumps has a long incubation period of 15–24 days with a median of 19 days. A child is infectious from 1–2 days before to 5 days after onset of parotid swelling.

One third of mumps infections are without recognizable symptoms. Clinically manifest infections start with fever, anorexia, malaise, and headache followed by painful swelling of the parotid glands, initially often unilateral (Fig 15.4).

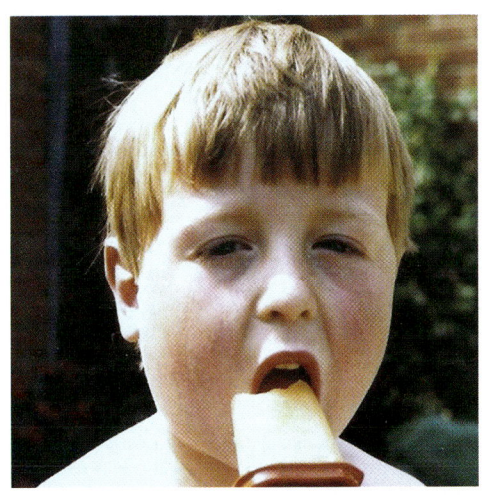

Fig 15.4 Mumps: parotitis (Series editor age 5 years in 1983).

The differential diagnosis of salivary-gland swelling includes other viral infections such as EBV, parainfluenza or adenovirus, drugs, salivary stones, and metabolic disorders. In the absence of parotid swelling mumps is in the differential diagnosis of viral encephalitis and torsion of the testis.

Complications

- *Epipidymo-orchitis and oophoritis:* epididymo-orchitis occurs in up to 30% of adult men, but is rare before puberty, and is bilateral in 30% of cases. Testicular atrophy may occur but sterility is rare. Oophoritis occurs in 5% of post-pubertal females.
- *CNS: aseptic meningitis:* CSF pleiocytosis occurs in 50% of cases, but clinically manifest meningitis in only 1–10% and encephalitis in 0.1%. Mumps meningitis is benign but sensorineural hearing loss is a recognized sequela of mumps.
- *Miscellaneous rare complications:* pancreatitis in 4%, myocarditis, arthritis, hepatitis, thrombocytopaenia, and glomerulonephritis.

Management

Diagnosis

- *Serology:* measurement of IgM antibody by ELISA
- *Immunofluorescence:* staining of specimens
- RT-PCR
- *Virus isolation:* from saliva, CSF, urine only within first week of illness.

Prevention is by vaccination as a component of MMR. Two doses are required.

Treatment

Treatment is supportive and symptomatic for what is usually a benign, self-limiting illness. Avoidance of acidic food such as fruit juices or ice-lollies (see Fig 15.4) minimizes pain caused by salivary stimulation. INF-α2b has been used for mumps orchitis.

Rubella

Rubella (Latin for 'little red'), commonly known as German measles, is a common mild childhood infection which occurs worldwide and since the introduction of vaccine in 1969 has become rare in countries with high uptake rates.

Its main importance is the devastating damage to the fetus caused by transplacental infection.

Aetiology and pathogenesis

Acquired rubella is transmitted via airborne droplet emission of the rubella virus, a togavirus. Viraemia occurs 5–7 days after infection, with transplacental transfer in pregnant women.

Clinical features

After an incubation period of 14–21 days the illness starts with low-grade fever, coryza, and tender posterior cervical lymphadenopathy. An erythematous, maculopapular rash starting on the face and spreading to the trunk appears 24–48 h later. Forcheimer's sign of red papules on the soft palate occurs in 20%. One third of females experience joint pains. Encephalitis is rare.

Congenital rubella syndrome (CRS)

Intrauterine infection during the 1st trimester may cause miscarriage, still birth, or CRS in survivors which may encompass cardiac defects: typically patent ductus, cataracts and deafness, low birthweight, hepatosplenomegaly, thrombocytopaenia, and 'blueberry muffin' skin lesions. See Chapter 1.8.

Management

Rubella virus specific IgM antibodies appear after the rash but can persist for over a year, so a positive result must be interpreted with caution.

Vaccination is part of the MMR vaccine given routinely in the UK. In children and adults the infection is mild and self-limiting. The prognosis for CRS is poor.

15.8 Enterovirus and parvovirus infection

Enteroviruses

Enterovirus infection is extremely common and responsible for a myriad of clinical syndromes from a mild upper respiratory tract infection to neonatal sepsis or paralytic poliomyelitis. Non-polio enteroviral infections are prevalent worldwide. Vaccination has eradicated wild polio from all but a handful of countries.

Aetiology and pathogenesis

Enteroviruses belong to the Picornaviridae family of small RNA viruses and are classified into:

- *Nonpolioviruses:*
  - coxsackie viruses: 24 group A, 6 group B
  - echoviruses : 34 types
  - enteroviruses (unclassified): 5 types
- *Polioviruses:* types 1, 2 and 3.

Pathophysiology

Spread is by faecal–oral or respiratory routes, fomites, and from mother to infant in the perinatal period. Initial replication occurs in local GI lymphatic tissue followed by a biphasic viraemia, mild on day 3 and major on days 3–7.

Different patterns of spread and replication account for the distinct clinical syndromes:

- *Coxsackie viruses:* pharynx (herpangina), skin (hand, foot, and mouth disease), myocardium (myocarditis), meninges (aseptic meningitis), lungs, and adrenals
- *Echovirus:* skin (viral exanthems), liver (hepatic necrosis), myocardium, meninges (aseptic meningitis), lungs, and adrenals
- *Poliovirus:* replicates in oropharynx and GI tissue and may then invades the motor neurons of the anterior horn cells of the spinal cord, causing direct cellular destruction. It can progress to the CNS.

Clinical features

In temperate climates, enteroviral infections are most common during summer and early autumn. 90% of enteroviral infections are asymptomatic or cause a non-specific febrile illness. Recognized syndromes are:

- *Hand, foot, and mouth disease:* non-painful vesicles in the oropharynx and painful vesicles on palms and soles appear after 1–2 days fever and with an exanthema (Fig 15.5). Most commonly coxsackievirus A16.

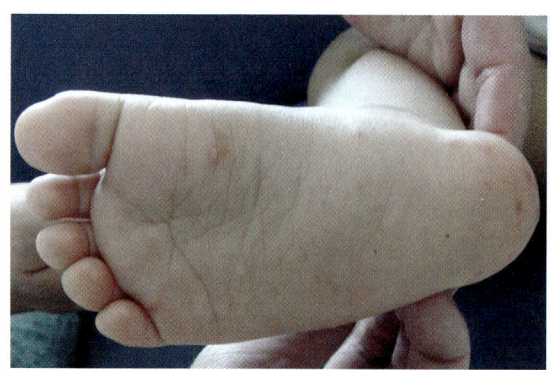

Fig 15.5 Hand, foot, and mouth disease: foot lesions.

- *Non-specific febrile illness:* duration 3–7 days
- *Herpangina:* painful vesicles on posterior pharynx and tonsils in children 3–10 years. Most commonly coxsackie A.
- *Viral exanthems:* pink, maculopapular blanching rash that mimics rubella and roseola. May appear after cessation of fever. Most commonly echoviruses
- *Myocarditis/pericarditis:* chest pain, dyspnoea, arrhythmias, cardiac failure. Most commonly coxsackie B5 or echoviruses. (Parvovirus can cause myocarditis in the immunocompromised.)
- *Aseptic meningitis:* headache, stiff neck, photophobia with non-specific rash. Most commonly coxsackie B and echovirus. Neurotropic strains, enterovirus 71 can cause fatal encephalitis
- *Bornholm disease:* severe muscular pain in chest, pleurodynia and abdomen (named after island of Bornholm).
- *Neonatal sepsis:* a serious 'sepsis like' infection by coxsackie B or echoviruses.
- *Poliovirus infections:* cause four clinical syndromes:
  1. *asymptomatic:* 90–96% of infections
  2. *abortive:* 5%, febrile illness with respiratory and GI tract symptoms
  3. *non-paralytic:* 2%, flu-like illness with signs of aseptic meningitis
  4. *paralytic:* febrile illness resolves and is followed by asymmetric flaccid paralysis. Involvement of brainstem or bulbar region impairs cardiac and respiratory activity (Fig 15.6).

Paralytic disease can also be caused by reversion of the oral vaccine virus to virulent form, so called vaccine-associated paralytic polio (VAPP).

The ratio of asymptomatic to paralytic infections is 1/1000 in children and 1/75 for adults.

Management

Diagnostic tests

- *Viral culture:* stool, rectal swab, and throat specimens give highest yield, but urine, blood and CSF also used. Cell culture is necessary (Fig 15.7)
- *RT-PCR:* rapid and sensitive and can detect all enteroviruses
- *Serology:* poorly standardized and lacks specificity.

Treatment

Prevention: inactivated polio vaccine (IPV) is part of the routine immunization schedule in the UK (Fig 15.8).

The Global Eradication of Polio initiative started in 1988, in which year 350 000 cases were reported worldwide. The number dropped to 784 in 1993. A resurgence in Nigeria in 2005–2006 has caused delay and polio remains endemic in a handful of countries: Nigeria, India, Pakistan, and Afghanistan.

There is no specific therapy for enteroviruses. IV immunoglobulin has been used in life-threatening infections in neonates and immunodeficient patients.

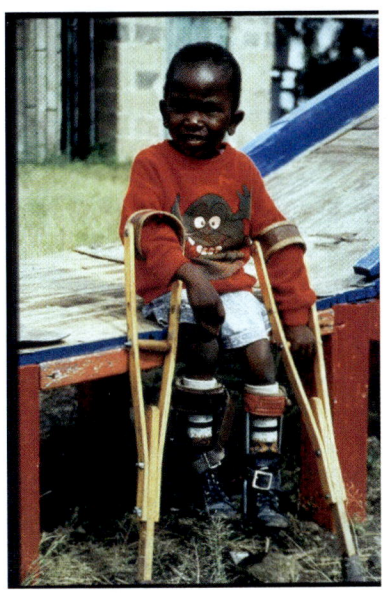

Fig 15.6 Paralytic polio: a devastating disease. Reproduced courtesy of the World Health Organisation.

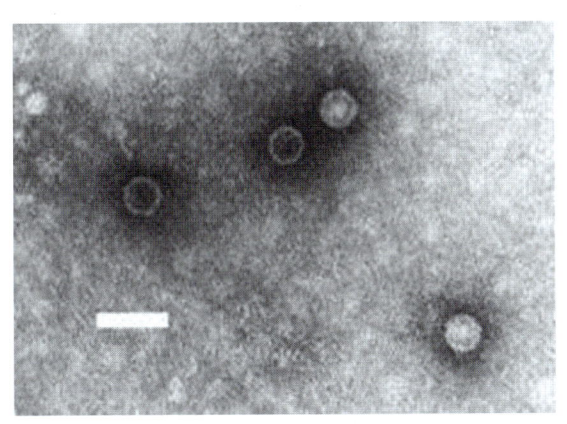

Fig 15.7 Poliovirus particles: transmission EM negative stain. *Source*: United States Environmental Protection Agency.

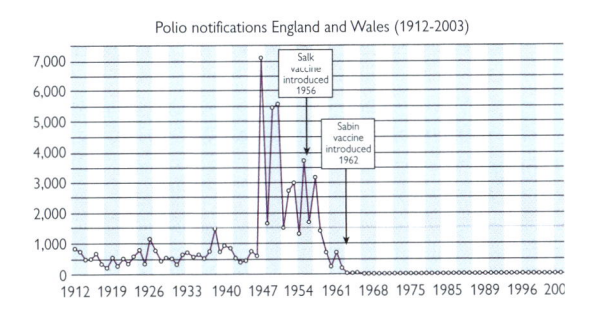

Fig 15.8 Eradication of polio in the UK. The last natural case was reported in 1982 and the last imported case in 1993.

Parvovirus B19, erythema infectiosum

Erythema infectiosum, 'slapped cheek syndrome' or 5th disease is caused by infection with human parvovirus B19. Outbreaks occur in nurseries and schools with epidemics every 3–4 years. Parvovirus B19 is a small DNA virus primarily spread by respiratory droplets. Transplacental transmission and transfer in infected blood products also occurs.

It is classified as an erythrovirus because of its capability of invading red cell precursors in the bone marrow.

Clinical features

The incubation period is 4–14 days. A child is contagious in the period before the rash appears.

About 20% of infected individuals are asymptomatic, but the disease starts with a viraemic phase causing fever and malaise and a facial rash described as 'slapped cheek' with erythema of cheeks sparing the forehead and nasolabial folds.

A week later 'lace-like' rashes on the torso and extremities appear which can last up to 5 weeks.

Additional features may include:

- *Aplastic crisis:* most patients have an arrest of erythropoiesis. In patients with chronic haemolytic anaemia such as sickle cell anaemia or hereditary spherocytosis and a red cell life span of a few days, this can cause severe anaemia requiring blood transfusion. Children with immunodeficiency may develop chronic anaemia. Parvovirus B19 infection in pregnant women before week 20 can cause hydrops fetalis due to severe fetal anaemia.
- *Arthritis:* a seronegative polyarthritis more common in females, usually lasting 1–3 weeks but persisting for months in 10–20%.

Parvovirus can cause myocarditil in immunocompromised patients, e.g. post heart transplant.

Management

Diagnosis is by IgM serology or PCR based assays.

There is no vaccine. Treatment is symptomatic. IV immunoglobulin may be beneficial in patients with immunodeficiency. Transfusion is often necessary for parvovirus-induced aplastic crises in patients with haemolytic anaemia.

15.9 Herpesvirus infections: HSV and VZV

The Herpesviridae are a family of double-stranded DNA, encapsulated viruses. The name comes from the Greek *herpein*, 'to creep', a reference to the skin rashes caused.

Eight viruses in this family cause disease in humans and are referred to as human herpes virus, HHV1–8 or by their original names (see Table 15.5).

Table 15.5. Human herpesviruses and their primary diseases

Type	Synonym	Diseases
HHV-1	Herpes simplex virus 1 (HSV-1)	Gingivostomatitis, encephalitis
HHV-2	Herpes simplex virus 2 (HSV-2)	Genital herpes
HHV-3	Varicella zoster virus (VZV)	Chickenpox
HHV-4	Epstein-Barr virus (EBV)	Infectious mononucleosis
HHV-5	Cytomegalovirus (CMV)	Congenital infection
HHV-6	Roseolavirus	Roseola infantum
HHV-7		Roseola infantum
HHV-8		Kaposi sarcoma

Herpesviruses all have large DNA genomes encased within a protein capsid wrapped in a lipid envelope forming the virion. After contact with CCD receptors the virion is internalized and viral DNA migrates to the nucleus where replication and transcription of viral genes occurs.

Common properties of herpesviruses include:

- *Neurovirulence*: capacity to invade and replicate in the nervous system
- *Lytic activity*: transcription of lytic genes leads to cell death
- *Latency*: transcription of 'latency associated transcript' allows the virus to persist in host cells indefinitely. Reactivation of latent virus may subsequently cause disease such as cold sores and shingles.

Herpes simplex viruses (HSV)

HSV are ubiquitous pathogens distributed worldwide and cause a wide variety of illnesses. Over 80% of infections are asymptomatic.

Aetiology and pathogenesis

Two types of HSV exist:

- *HSV-1 (HHV-1)*: transmitted by contact with infected saliva. Infection is common in children. By age 30 years 80% of individuals of low socio-economic status are seropositive. HSV-1 has the capacity for neurovirulence and becomes latent most commonly in the trigeminal ganglion. Dissemination occurs in people with impaired T-cell immunity.
- *HSV-2 (HHV-2)*: transmitted sexually or to the newborn from a mother's genital tract. Antibodies to HSV2 emerge at puberty and correlate with sexual activity.

Clinical features

The clinical course of disease depends on the age and immune status of the host, the site of infection, and the antigenic type of virus. Primary infections tend to be more severe and longer than recurrent episodes. There is overlap between clinical syndromes caused by HSV-1 and HSV-2 but HSV-1 usually causes orofacial lesions and HSV-2 genital and neonatal infections. Over 80% of infections are asymptomatic.

Acute herpetic gingivostomatitis

The most common manifestation of primary HSV-1 infection in children aged 6 months to 5 years. Incubation period is 3–6 days. Abrupt onset of high fever is accompanied by anorexia, swollen erythematous gums, and vesicles on oral mucosa, tongue, and lips which rupture and coalesce into ulcerated plaques. Acute disease lasts 5–7 days and symptoms subside in 2 weeks. The child refuses to eat or drink. The differential diagnosis is enteroviral infection which is less painful, Stevens–Johnson syndrome, and aphthous ulcers.

Recurrent herpes labialis ('cold sores')

The most common manifestation of recurrent HSV-1 infection. Unusual to have >2 recurrences per year.

Genital herpes

Primary genital herpes can be caused by both HSV-1 and HSV-2 and is asymptomatic in most patients. It is more common in sexually active adolescents. Reactivation and recurrence is common. In a young child it should raise the possibility of child abuse, although autoinoculation of HSV-1 from another site can occur.

Less common, serious clinical syndromes

- *Meningoencephalitis* (see Chapter 7.14): occurs in neonates as part of systemic HSV-2 infection or in older children. Untreated, the mortality is 70%.
- *Eczema herpeticum*: occurs in patients with eczema causing localized or disseminated infection which can be lethal.
- *Ocular herpes*: conjunctivitis, blepharitis, epithelial keratitis (dendritic ulcers). Urgent ophthalmic investigation and aggressive treatment is required.
- *Neonatal herpes*: neonatal HSV infection occurs in 1/0 000 live births and is caused by contact with infected genital secretions. 75% are caused by HSV-2 and the risk of transmission in primary vaginal infection is 50%. Infection may manifest as lesions localized to skin, eye, or mouth or disseminated visceral disease with or without encephalitis.

Management

Diagnostic investigations

- Electron microscopy or immunofluorescence of vesicular fluid
- PCR of HSV DNA e.g. in CSF in meningoencephalitis
- *Viral isolation in tissue culture*: positive in 2–5 days.

Treatment

Specific therapy is available. Aciclovir is a nucleoside analogue which selectively inhibits HSV DNA polymerase after phosphorylation by viral thymidine kinase. Oral, topical (including eye drops), and IV aciclovir is available. It must be given early when the virus is replicating and before cell lysis has occurred. Mild disease can be treated supportively. IV aciclovir is indicated for severe disease. Oral aciclovir reduces symptoms when given within 72 h of onset in gingivostomatitis.

Varicella zoster virus (VZV)

Primary infection with VZV causes chickenpox. Herpes zoster or shingles is caused by reactivation of latent virus. Chickenpox is usually mild and self-limiting but can be lethal in the newborn or immunocompromised patients.

VZV infection occurs worldwide and is endemic in most countries, tending to occur in seasonal peaks during winter and spring. Annual incidence in the UK is 48/10 000. Childhood infection is so common that 90% of adults are immune.

Aetiology and pathogenesis

Transmission is by direct contact or the respiratory route via airborne droplets. Viraemia occurs 4–6 days later. After primary infection VZV remains dormant in sensory roots for life. Infectivity is from 72 h before the rash appears until all spots have crusted over, usually within 7–8 days.

Severe disease occurs in neonates and immunocompromised hosts.

Clinical features

Chickenpox

The incubation period is 10–24 days, usually 10–14 days. Onset is usually with pyrexia of 38–39 °C for up to 4 days with headache, malaise, and abdominal pain.

Rash: crops of itchy papules and vesicles appear over 3–5 days initially on the scalp, head, and neck and spreading to the trunk but sparse on the limbs (Fig 15.9). Mucous membranes such as oropharynx and vulva are involved. Lesions evolve through stages of papule, vesicle, pustule, and crust.

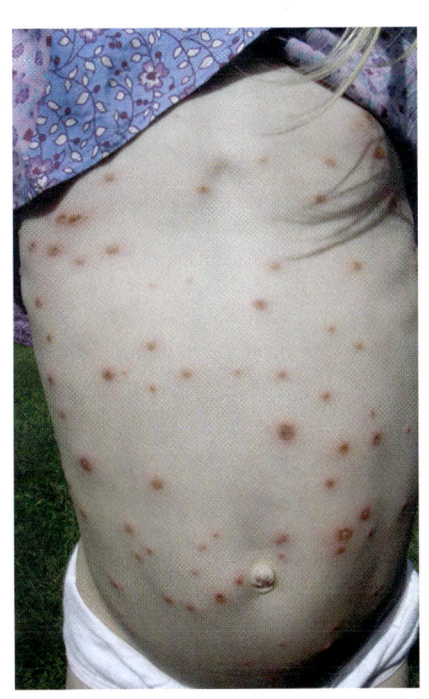

Fig 15.9 Chickenpox rash: lesions at different stages.

Complications include:
- *Secondary bacterial infection:* especially group A streptococcus. Necrotizing fasciitis is a recognized complication as lesions provide a route to the fascia
- *Pneumonia*

- *Post-infectious encephalomyelitis:* classically as acute cerebellar ataxia.
- *Thrombocytopaenia.*

In the newborn and the immunocompromised patient severe, disseminated, life-threatening haemorrhagic disease is a risk.

Herpes zoster (shingles)

A vesicular eruption occurs in the distribution of a sensory dermatome often in the thoracic region and usually unilateral (Fig 15.10). A prodrome of pain and tenderness in the affected dermatome with fever is less common in children than adults. Reactivation of virus in cranial nerve roots may cause:

- *Cranial nerve V:* corneal lesions
- *Cranial nerve VII:* Ramsay–Hunt syndrome of facial nerve paralysis with vesicles in the external ear.

Postherpetic pain is less common in children. Recurrent shingles should prompt suspicion of immunodeficiency.

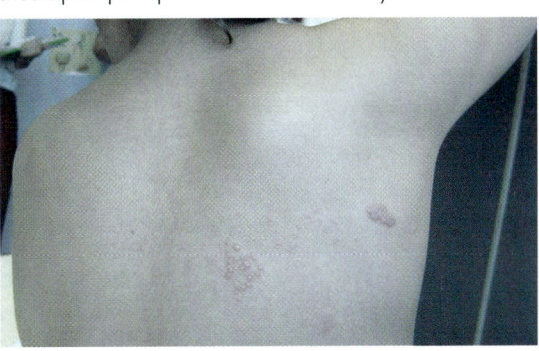

Fig 15.10 Varicella zoster: shingles of right thoracic dermatome.

Management

Diagnosis is clinical but confirmation may be sought by viral culture, serology, immunofluorescence assay, or PCR. Treatment is supportive for chickenpox in an immunocompetent child, but specific management is required in several situations and may include varicella vaccination, human varicella zoster immunoglobulin, and aciclovir.

Varicella vaccination

Live varicella vaccines are available and are part of routine immunization in some countries such as the USA, but not the UK for a variety of complex reasons. Varicella vaccine is recommended for:

- Non-immune health-care workers at risk of exposure
- Non-immune, healthy, close household contacts of immunocompromised patients.

Human varicella zoster immunoglobulin (VZIG)

VZIG prophylaxis is recommended for susceptible individuals at risk of severe varicella who have had significant exposure to chickenpox or shingles. This includes pregnant women, neonates, and immunosuppressed patients.

VZIG is recommended for newborns whose mothers develop chickenpox in the period 7 days before to 7 days after delivery.

Aciclovir

Aciclovir is indicated for neonates with chickenpox, severe chickenpox in adolescents within 24 h of onset of rash, immunocompromised patients, and patients with shingles.

15.10 Herpesviruses: EBV, CMV, and HHV-6, 7, and 8

Epstein–Barr virus (EBV)

The Epstein-Barr virus, or human herpesvirus 4 (HHV-4) infects >95% of the world's population. The most common clinical manifestation is infectious mononucleosis, but EBV is also a human tumour virus associated with several human malignancies.

Aetiology and pathogenesis

EBV is most commonly transmitted via saliva, hence the 'kissing disease', but aerosol transmission also occurs.

Virus replication in nasopharyngeal epithelial cells is followed by viraemia and infection of the lymphoreticular system including liver, spleen, and B lymphocytes in peripheral blood. Latent infection is established in B lymphocytes, a balance being struck between occasional reactivation and host immune surveillance.

The host immune response includes generation of CD8+ cytotoxic T-lymphocytes, the characteristic 'atypical' lymphocytes found in peripheral blood. Most acute clinical symptoms reflect T-cell proliferation and organ infiltration.

EBV and malignancy

- *Burkitt lymphoma*: most common childhood tumour in Africa is associated with EBV and malaria infection. Malaria causes reduced immune surveillance of EBV-immortalized B cells, allowing them to proliferate
- *Nasopharyngeal carcinoma*: occurs in southern China and Africa, linked to genetic factors and nitrosamine-rich diet of salted fish
- Non-Hodgkin lymphoma
- *Lymphoproliferative syndromes*: in immunosuppressed patients such as AIDS/HIV or post-transplant EBV-associated lymphoproliferative disorders occur.

Clinical features

The primary clinical syndrome is 'glandular fever'. The incubation period is 30–50 days in adolescents, but shorter in young children. Onset may be gradual with 1–2 weeks of fatigue and malaise or abrupt with sore throat, headache, fever, myalgia, and abdominal pain. Infants and young children with primary infection are usually asymptomatic.

Examination

- *Fever:* in 90%, up to 40 °C
- *Pharyngitis:* exudative in 30%, petechiae at palatal junction in 30–60%. Massive tonsillar enlargement can occur.
- *Lymphadenopathy:* posterior cervical, axillary, inguinal
- *Splenomegaly:* tender splenomegaly, 2–3 cm in 50%
- *Hepatomegaly:* common, but jaundice is rare (5%)
- *Rash:* erythematous, maculopapular rash in up to 15%, more common in young children. Treatment with ampicillin or amoxicillin causes a rash in 90% of patients.

Note that EBV accounts for 90% of cases of infectious mononucleosis but other viruses associated with a similar illness include cytomegalovirus, HSV-1 and 2, and rubella.

Complications

- Airway obstruction from pharyngotonsillar swelling
- *Splenic rupture:* spontaneously or from minor trauma.
- *CNS:* meningitis, encephalitis, Guillain–Barré syndrome
- Haemolytic anaemia, thrombocytopaenia
- Chronic-fatigue-like syndrome
- Lymphoproliferative syndromes in immunosuppressed patients and fatal primary infection in patients with X-linked lymphoproliferative syndrome.

Management

Diagnostic investigations

- *FBC:* atypical lymphocytosis. Total WBC 10–20 × 10^9/L with >50% lymphocytes. Usually 20% are 'atypical' (see Fig 15.11) Most are CD8+ cytotoxic T lymphocytes.

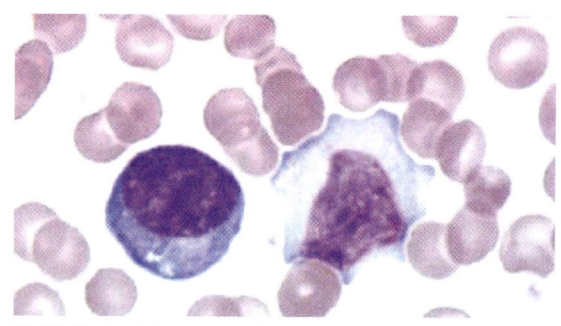

Fig 15.11 Atypical or reactive lymphocytes. Large with condensed chromatin pattern in nucleus and pale blue, basophilic cytoplasm. Seen in EBV infection and also CMV, toxoplasmosis, viral hepatitis, and streptococcal infection. Reproduced courtesy of New York State Department of Health, Wadsworth Center.

- *Heterophile antibody tests:* EBV heterophile antibodies agglutinate red cells from other species such as sheep after absorption with guinea pig cells. Tests include Paul–Bunnell, using tube dilution and Monospot by rapid slide agglutination which has low sensitivity
- *EBV serology:* viral capsid antigen-IgM measurable at symptom onset
- *PCR:* detects EBV DNA in plasma.

Treatment

This self-limited illness does not usually require specific therapy and isolation is not indicated as infectivity is low.

Steroids are indicated for significant upper airways obstruction or severe thrombocytopaenia or haemolytic anaemia. New therapies for EBV lymphoproliferative disease include antibodies to CD20 expressed on B cells and EBV specific cytotoxic T cells.

Cytomegalovirus (CMV)

Cytomegalovirus, or human herpesvirus-5 (HHV-5) infects up to 60% of the population by adulthood and is the virus most frequently transmitted to a fetus before birth, causing congenital CMV infection.

Aetiology and pathogenesis

Transmission occurs through body fluids—saliva, genital secretions, urine or breast milk—and also transplacentally and rarely via blood transfusion or organ transplantation.

Initial infection after birth is often asymptomatic but the virus establishes latent infection which may reactivate if the immune system is suppressed.

Lytically replicating virus disrupts the cytoskeleton causing massive cell enlargement, hence the name, and intranuclear 'owl's eye' bodies.

Clinical features

In normal hosts, most CMV infections (post-birth) are asymptomatic but CMV may cause an infectious mononucleosis/glandular fever like syndrome.

CMV is an important cause of congenital infection (see Chapter 1.10).

In immunocompromised patients CMV infection can cause severe disease including encephalitis, retinitis, pneumonitis, hepatitis, and colitis.

Management

Diagnostic investigations

- Detection of early antigen fluorescence foci, DEAFF test on urine or blood
- Intranuclear inclusions in biopsy specimens
- PCR.

Treatment

No treatment is necessary in healthy immunocompetent hosts.

In immunosuppressed patients options include ganciclovir or foscarnet, or cidofovir if CMV is resistant to ganciclovir.

Human herpesvirus 6 (HHV-6)

Human herpesvirus 6 (HHV-6) is an ubiquitous infection which classically causes roseola infantum (exanthema subitum) and accounts for up to 30% of all febrile seizures up to the age of 2 years.

Aetiology and pathogenesis

The mode of transmission is uncertain but is probably from saliva.

Infection is almost ubiquitous in infants, usually after maternal antibodies have waned at 6–24 months. HHV-6B accounts for 93% of infections.

HHV-6 infects and replicates in CD4+ lymphocytes primarily, but also in macrophages and epithelial cells. It causes direct cytolysis and lifetime latency is established in myeloid and bone marrow progenitors.

HHV-6 is a powerful inducer of cytokines and triggers the release of IL-Ib and IFN-α, hence the high-fever. HHV-6 may invade the CNS, infecting neural and glial cells.

Reactivation of HHV-6 in immunosuppressed individuals can lead to serious disseminated disease.

Clinical features

Primary infection with HHV-6 is frequently asymptomatic but may cause roseola infantum and febrile seizures in young infants. HHV-6 infection accounts for up to 20% of infant hospitalizations.

Roseola infantum

Abrupt onset of non-specific high fever for 3–5 days is followed by a maculopapular rash associated with a rapid decline of fever. Additional features may include:

- Cough or diarrhoea
- Papules on soft palate, Nagayama's spots.
- *Febrile seizures:* in 8%. HHV-6 infection accounts for up to 30% of febrile seizures in infants 5–24 months. Seizures tend to be clustered, prolonged, and focal.
- *Signs of meningoencephalitis:* bulging fontanelle and altered consciousness.

In the immunocompromised host HHV-6 reactivation causes severe disease including disseminated infection, interstitial pneumonitis, encephalitis, and graft versus host disease.
Rare primary infections occur in adults.

Management

Diagnostic tests are not well established. Options include viral culture, immunohistochemistry, serology, and PCR on CSF.

Treatment is supportive for roseola infantum. Antiviral therapy with ganciclovir or foscarnet is probably beneficial in immunosuppressed patients.

Human herpesvirus 7 and 8

HHV-7 is in the same subfamily of betaherpesviridae as HHV-6 and may cause a similar spectrum of disease.

HHV-8 is associated with Kaposi sarcoma in children with HIV infection.

15.11 Human immunodeficiency virus: HIV/AIDS

Human immunodeficiency virus (HIV) infection in childhood nearly all occurs by mother to child transmission (MTCT) and is now a preventable disease. Nevertheless, in 2007 almost half a million children aged <15 years were infected.

Epidemiology

Global
Since its recognition in 1981 HIV/AIDS is estimated to have resulted in about 25 million deaths. In 2007, UNAID/WHO statistics document 33 million people living with HIV including 2.5 million children <15 years of age. Of these children 1.8 million are in sub-Saharan Africa and 3000 in western and central Europe.

In 2007, UNAID estimate that there were approximately 400 000 new infections in children <15 years and 300 000 deaths, nearly all in sub-Saharan Africa. About 15 million children have been orphaned.

United Kingdom
At end 2006, an estimated 73 000 people were living with HIV in the UK, of whom one third are unaware of their infection. In 2007 there were >6000 new diagnoses of HIV including about 80 arising from MTCT. A total of ~1600 cases of HIV arising from MTCT have been diagnosed, about one half of whom were born in the UK.

The number of children born in the UK to HIV-positive mothers was 1139 in 2006, but the proportion of such babies infected with HIV has fallen sharply since the introduction of screening and preventive measures.

Aetiology and pathogenesis

Transmission
Most paediatric HIV infection occurs by vertical MTCT. Transmission occurs in utero, peripartum in two thirds and postnatally through breast-feeding.

Maternal viral load is a critical determinant of risk of transmission. Before the advent of interventions, transmission rates were 15–20% in Europe and USA compared to 30–50% in Africa. Transmission rates in women diagnosed antenatally and following recommended interventions has fallen to 1–2%.

Transmission via blood or blood products or via mucous membranes in sexual intercourse is uncommon in children.

Pathogenesis
HIV is an enveloped RNA retrovirus containing reverse transcriptase which allows it to copy its RNA into DNA which is integrated into host-cell genome as proviral DNA. Two types exist: HIV-1 which is widespread and HIV-2 found in West Africa.

HIV primarily affects CD4+ T-lymphocytes as well as macrophages and neurons and glial cells. Interaction with CD4 and the receptor CCR5 is required for cell infection. An immune antibody response (against core and envelope proteins p24, p41, and gp120) and CD8+ T-lymphocyte response is generated which keeps viral replication in check but is unable to eliminate the infection.

HIV disease arises from direct cell damage and from acquired immunodeficiency.

Immunodeficiency
The number of CD4+ T lymphocytes gradually falls leading to a failure of all types of T-dependent immunity. The T-suppressor CD8+ T lymphocyte count increases initially, accounting in part for the lymphadenopathy which develops. The B-lymphocyte count remains normal but dysgammaglobalinaemia develops with impaired humoral immunity.

Immunodeficiency leads to recurrent severe bacterial infection and opportunistic infections.

HIV itself causes an encephalopathy and failure to thrive.

Clinical features
Most families in the UK with HIV infection are of African origin, but a minority are families in which IV drug abuse is the risk factor. The most common clinical challenge is management of a newborn infant born to a HIV-positive mother. However, HIV infection in infants and children, usually in a child born abroad or in the UK before antenatal screening, may present in many different ways.

Perinatal HIV infection leads to two main categories of presentation: rapid progressors (30%) and slow progressors.

Rapid progression
These infants typically present with *Pneumocystis jiroveci* pneumonia at 10–14 weeks of age, or HIV encephalopathy with developmental delay or regression in the 1st year of life.

Slow progression
These children may present in many different ways with illness ranging from asymptomatic to severe and including:

- Generalized lymphadenopathy, hepatosplenomegaly or parotid enlargement (Fig 15.12)
- *Skin manifestation:* shingles, extensive molluscum, fungal nail infections.
- *Respiratory tract:* recurrent severe bacterial pneumonia, lymphatic interstitial pneumonitis (LIP)
- *GI tract:* unexplained diarrhoea, failure to thrive, wasting, hepatitis with steatosis, oral candidiasis after 6–8 weeks, gingivitis/stomatitis
- *Haematological:* unexplained pancytopaenia, anaemia, thrombocytopaenia
- *Opportunistic infections: Pneumocystis jiroveci* pneumonia, CMV, *Mycobacterium avium, Cryptosporidium, Toxoplasmosis, Giardia*
- *TB:* pulmonary or extrapulmonary
- *Malignancy:* children with HIV have a ×30 increased risk of malignancy. Although the risk of Kaposi sarcoma is almost removed by effective ART, the effect on the risk of lymphoma (×2500) in children is is unknown.

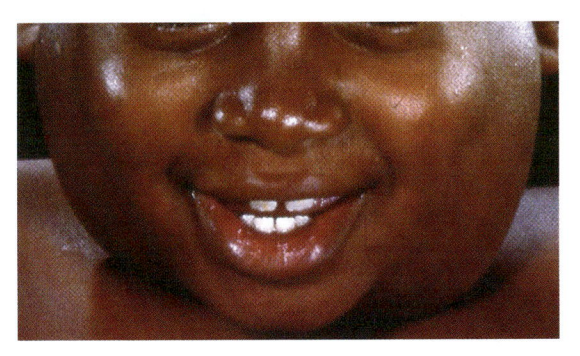

Fig 15.12 HIV infection: parotid enlargement. Often associated with generalized lymphadenopathy and LIP.

Management

Diagnostic investigations
During infancy this depends on detection of viral nucleic acid by PCR as all infants born to HIV-seropositive mothers have passively acquired maternal antibodies. After 18 months, detection of HIV antibodies indicates infection. Repeat testing is necessary in newborn infants (see below).

- *DNA:* PCR assay of DNA extracted from peripheral blood mononuclear cells. It can detect 1–10 copies of viral DNA. A single assay has a sensitivity of 95% and specificity of 97% on samples from infants 1–36 months of age.
- *Antibodies:* ELISA test for IgG antibodies to P24 antigen. Reliable and nationally available.

Prevention of vertical transmission
Antenatal testing for HIV is now routinely offered to all pregnant women in the UK. Women aware of their HIV infection at an early stage can choose the following interventions which reduce the risk of infection to ~1%:

- *Antiretroviral therapy (ART):* HAART and IV zidovudine to mother before delivery
- Consider elective Caesarean section at 38 weeks gestation. However,
  if viral load is controlled on HAART vaginal delivery is safe
- Counselling against breast-feeding.

Infant born to an HIV-infected mother

- **At birth:** 24–48h HIV-1 PCR/ P24Ag on baby's blood, not cord blood. False negatives occur.

Infected infants
- 30% positive at 48 h indicating *in utero* infection
- 93% positive at 2 weeks

Start ART, zidovudine and continue for 4 weeks.
- **6 weeks:** repeat HIV-1 PCR/P24Ag

Start cotrimoxazole prophylaxis for *Pneumocystis*.
- **3 months:** repeat HIV-1 PCR/P24Ag

If PCR is negative at 3–4 months then >99% sure infant is not infected and *Pneumocystis* prophylaxis stopped. Follow up until P24Ag antibody is negative at 18 months.

HIV-positive infants and children
Treatment depends on clinical category, immune status and viral load. It encompasses ART, specific therapy for opportunistic infections or complications, and family support.

Clinical categories/staging
WHO staging, 2006 (summary overview)

1. asymptomatic or persistent generalized lymphadenopathy
2. persistent parotid enlargement (Fig 15.12), hepatosplenomegaly, infections (warts, molluscum, herpes zoster, fungal nail, repiratory tract), papular pruritic eruptions
3. malnutrition, diarrhoea, TB, pancytopaenia, recurrent bacterial pneumonia, LIP, necrotizing ulcerative gingivitis/periodontitis.
4. severe wasting, recurrent severe bacterial infection, opportunistic infections (pneumocystis, CMV, fungi) malignancy (Kaposi's, NHL), encephalopathy (Fig 15.13), cardiomyopathy

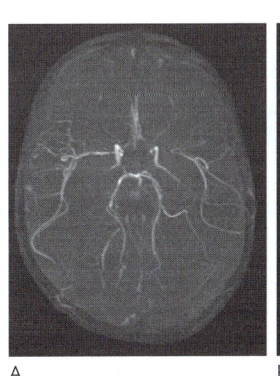

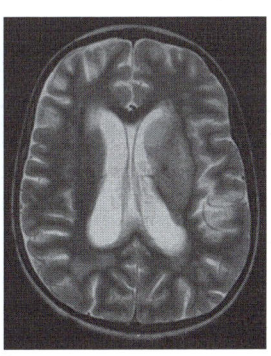

Fig 15.13 HIV encephalopathy: Cranial MRI. A. MR angiogram showing focal narrowing of left middle cerebral artery (arrow). B. MRI showing resulting left basal ganglia infarct with oedema.

Immune categories are best expressed as CD4+ lymphocyte percentages rather than absolute counts and are age dependent: at 3–5 years a CD4+ >25% is no immunodeficiency, 15–25% mild, and <15% severe.

Antiretroviral therapy (ART)
Highly active antiretroviral therapy (HAART) regimens usually comprise three antiretrovirals in combination. Children are treated according to the Paediatric European Network for Treatment of AIDS (PENTA) guidelines.
Three classes of compound are available:

- *Nucleoside reverse transcriptase inhibitors (NRTIs):* zidovudine, didanosine, lamivudine
- *Non-nucleoside reverse transcriptase inhibitors (NNRTIs):* efavirenz, nevirapine
- *Protease inhibitors:* ritonavir, kaletra, nelfinavir.

The standard regimen comprises two NRTIs and either a NNRTI or a protease inhibitor. Criteria for initiating HAART remains controversial. Adherence, side effects, and palatability are problems and children are managed by specialist multidisciplinary teams.

Vaccines remain a major hope but HIV is highly mutable and remains an elusive target.

15.12 Tuberculosis

Tuberculosis (TB) is an infectious disease caused by bacteria belonging to the *Mycobacterium tuberculosis* complex. It remains the most common cause of infection-related death worldwide with a global death rate of 1.6 million in 2006 and an estimated 14 million people living with TB disease.

Epidemiology

The WHO estimates that >9 million new cases of TB occur each year and that up to 40% of the world's population is infected with *M. tuberculosis*. TB occurs disproportionately among disadvantaged populations and a resurgence of the disease has been provoked by the HIV/AIDS epidemic, development of multidrug resistant (MDR) organisms and deterioration of the public health infrastructure for TB services. Children are under-reported, as few are sputum smear positive.

Prevalence shows a striking variation (Table 15.6).

Table 15.6. TB: approximate prevalence per 100 000	
Western Europe (e.g. UK)	10
Eastern Europe (e.g. Ukraine)	100
Indian subcontinent	400
Sub-Saharan Africa	500–1000

United Kingdom

In 2007, 8496 cases of TB were notified In the UK of whom 40% were living in London. In the UK, like other western European countries, the prevalence is low, with a large proportion of disease occurring in recent immigrants from high-burden regions such as sub-Saharan Africa. Other high-risk adult groups include the homeless, drug and alcohol users, and prisoners.

Paediatric TB in the UK represents 2.5% of notifications. Some areas of London have rates of >40/100 000 in children <16 years and the relative proportion of African children, mostly born abroad, has increased.

Aetiology and pathogenesis

Transmission

Infection occurs by inhalation of aerosolized particles containing *M. tuberculosis* following close contact with an individual, usually an adult, with active pulmonary TB. Ingestion of *M. bovis* is now rare. Infection follows exposure in only 10–30% of healthy people.

Pathogenesis

The subsequent course of infection depends on the bacterial load and the age, immune status, and nutritional status of the host. The natural history spans a spectrum from asymptomatic, dormant TB infection to disseminated TB disease. Progression to disease is more likely in young children <2 years.

TB infection: no disease (90%)

Inhaled bacilli are ingested by macrophages but continue to multiply and infected macrophages are carried to the regional lymph nodes. A cell-mediated immune response develops 2–3 weeks after infection and CD4+ helper T cells activate macrophages to kill intracellular bacterial with granuloma formation. IFN-γ and IL-12 pathways are important in host defence.

The lung lesion, Ghon, or primary focus together with enlarged regional lymph nodes form the primary complex. Bacilli may escape intermittently into the blood stream and lodge elsewhere in the body—in the CNS, bones, or kidneys—remaining dormant.

Tuberculin reactivity, detectable by skin test, develops 2–12 weeks after initial infection with a median of 3–4 weeks.

TB disease (10%)

Primary infection may progress to disease, especially in young children and adolescents, or disease may result from reactivation of dormant infection. TB disease is conveniently classified as pulmonary or extrapulmonary:

- *Pulmonary TB* (see Chapter 3): may manifest in several forms including endobronchial TB, progressive primary TB with pneumonia and caseation, or pleural effusion
- *Extra-pulmonary TB*: includes lymphadenopathy, miliary TB, tuberculous meningitis and vertebral or renal TB.

Clinical features

Tuberculosis infection

This is recognized by a positive tuberculin sensitivity skin test such as the Mantoux test. The CXR is normal or may show a healed 'primary complex'. Tuberculin hypersensitivity may manifest as erythema nodosum or phlyctenular conjunctivitis. TB infection may be diagnosed incidentally, on screening or during contact tracing.

TB disease

Depends on site involved: pulmonary or extrapulmonary.

Pulmonary TB (see Chapter 3.6)

Progressive primary pulmonary TB presents as a pneumonia with fever, cough, dyspnoea, anorexia, weight loss, night sweats, and lymphadenopathy.

Endobronchial disease or pleural effusion are associated with signs of bronchial obstruction and pleural fluid.

Extrapulmonary TB

- *Lymphadenopathy:* usually involves cervical or supraclavicular nodes (Fig 15.14). Nodes are firm and non-tender but may caseate and suppurate.

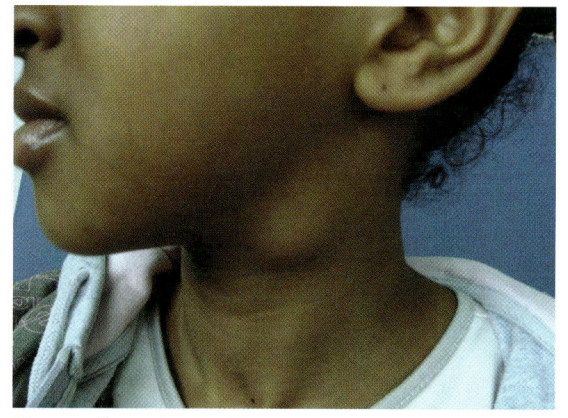

Fig 15.14 Extrapulmonary TB: cervical lymphadenopathy.

- *Miliary TB:* a complication of primary TB in young children. Manifests with low-grade fever, malaise, fatigue, weight loss. Examination may reveal lymphadenopathy (Fig 15.15), hepatosplenomegaly, respiratory signs, and retinal choroidal tubercles.
- *Tuberculous meningitis (TBM):* develops in 5–10% of children <2 years. A subacute, insidious onset 3–6 months after

infection is usual with progression to reduced consciousness, cranial nerve palsies, and death if unrecognized. Choroidal tubercles may be seen on fundoscopy (Fig 15.15). Tuberculomas may occur with or without TBM.

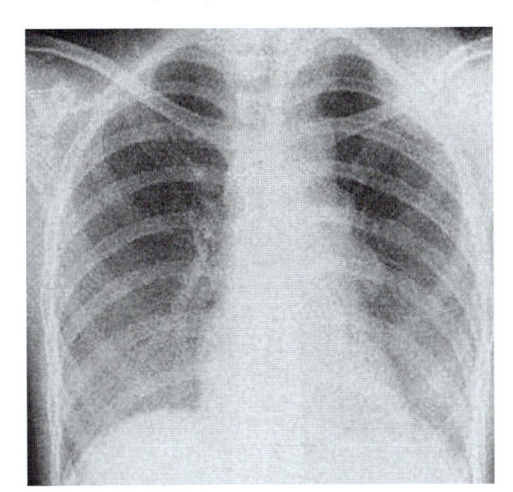

Fig 15.15 Hilar lymphadenopathy and miliary TB: CXR.

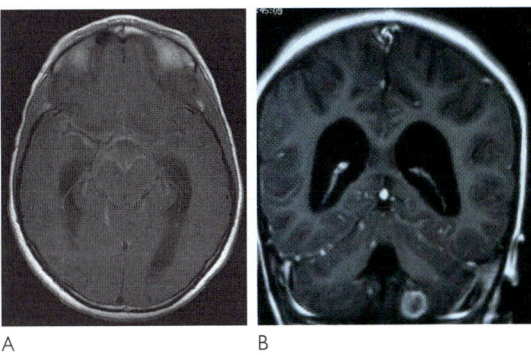

Fig 15.16 Tubercular meningitis: A. Bilateral dilated ventricles and meningeal enhancement. B. Hydrocephalus and cerebellar tuberculoma.

- *Congenital TB*: is rare and manifests during the 2nd or 3rd week of life with poor feeding, lethargy, fever, cough with hepatosplenomegaly, lymphdenopathy, and papular skin lesions.

Management

Diagnosis
Making a definitive diagnosis of TB in children is often challenging because of the difficulty in obtaining secretions or biopsy specimens for isolation of the organism. The main investigations used are tuberculin skin testing, microbiological tests (microscopy, cultures, histology), and CXR.

Tuberculin skin testing: Mantoux test
In the UK, 0.1 mL of 1/1000 (10 TU) is injected intradermally into the volar aspect of the forearm. The amount of induration (not erythema) is measured at 48–72 h, transverse to the long axis of the forearm. The threshold for a 'positive' test—5, 10, or 15 mm—depends on the clinical context.
- ≥15 mm: positive in any child >5 years
- 10–15 mm: children >5 years, patients who have not had BCG, high-risk immunosuppressed, or with increased risk of exposure
- ≥ 5 mm: close contact with known or suspected contagious case, immunodeficient children, e.g. HIV infection.

A history of BCG vaccination is not taken into account.

Note that a negative Mantoux test does not exclude TB infection or disease. False negatives may occur with incorrect technique or in the presence of anergy which may occur in 10% of normal population, the very young, in presence of miliary TB, or in some viral infections.

ESAT-6 and CFP-10 antigens: T-cells producing IFN-γ specific to these antigens can be measured by ELISA and this test holds promise as a diagnostic and monitoring tool used in Quantiferon gold or T SPOT TB.

Microbiological tests
Suitable specimens for microscopy and culture include sputum which is not usually available in young children, gastric lavage, bronchoalveolar lavage (BAL), early morning urines, and biopsy specimens of lymph node or bone marrow.

Ziehl–Neelsen stain to demonstrate acid-fast bacilli (AFB). Culture takes 4–8 weeks but allows typing and sensitivity testing. New culture techniques take 2–3 weeks. PCR-based tests currently have poor sensitivity (40–70%) and specificity.

Chest radiography
CXR is the classic diagnostic tool. Changes may be typical of (e.g. hilar lymphadenopathy) or consistent with pulmonary TB.

Prevention: BCG vaccination
Vaccination with Bacille Calmette–Guerin (BCG), a live attenuated strain of *M. bovis*, was introduced in 1921 and 14 billion doses have been administered. Its efficacy shows striking population variation. In the UK, BCG vaccination is given to newborn infants born to a high-risk group or in a high-risk location.

Complications include subcutaneous abscess, lymphadenitis, and disseminated disease if given inadvertently to immunodeficient children. Work is under way to develop new TB vaccines, e.g. BCG strains expressing additional antigens or which can be given orally.

Treatment
Anti-TB drugs are given as chemoprophylaxis or as chemotherapy.

Chemoprophylaxis
This is indicated for children with latent TB infection (positive Mantoux test only) to prevent progression to disease and for close contacts of smear-positive TB patients if they are HIV-positive or immunocompromised. Options are:
- Isoniazid for 6 months, plus pyridoxine for breast fed or malnourished infants
- Isoniazid and rifampicin for 3 months.

Chemotherapy
This is indicated for TB disease. The recommended regimen for pulmonary or extrapulmonary (non-meningitis) disease is:
- *Initial 2 months*: isoniazid, rifampicin, pyrazinamide and a fourth drug (ethambutol) if the risk of isoniazid resistance (6% in London) is high. The fourth drug can be omitted in patients with low risk of isoniazid resistance such as previously untreated, white, or HIV-negative.
- Further 4 months of isoniazid and rifampicin alone.

Expert advice is needed for multidrug resistance. New drugs include moxifloxacin, a quinolone antibiotic.

Corticosteroids are used in conjunction with anti-TB chemotherapy for 6–8 weeks in TB meningitis, pericarditis, military TB, or endobronchial disease with obstruction.

15.13 Staphylococcal and streptococcal infections

The syndrome of 'septicaemic shock' is considered in Chapter 2. Specific bacterial infections such as pneumonia, osteomyelitis, septic arthritis, infective endocarditis, and impetigo are considered in detail in other chapters.

Staphylococcal infections

Staphylococci are gram-positive bacteria which are divided into:
- *Coagulase-positive: Staphylococcus aureus*
- *Coagulase-negative (CONS)*: e.g. *Staphylococcus epidermidis*.

Epidemiology and transmission
- *Staph. aureus* colonizes the skin and mucous membranes of 30–50% of healthy children. The usual sites are anterior nares, throat, axilla, perineum, vagina or rectum.
- *Staph. epidermidis* is part of the normal 'resident' skin flora in everyone and is also found on mucosal surfaces.

Transmission
- *Staph. aureus* is most often transmitted by direct contact. Infection occurs when defences are compromised and many infections are caused by endogenous organisms.
- Methicillin-resistant *Staph. aureus* (MRSA) and methicillin-resistant CONS are an important cause of nosocomial infections. Health-care-associated MRSA infections result from the patient's own organism or from strains transmitted by the hands of health-care professionals.
- CONS are the commonest cause of infections associated with implanted foreign materials such as central venous lines and CSF shunts.

Pathogenesis
Staphylococci cause a variety of superficial infections, foreign body infections, and invasion beyond the skin may lead to localized suppurative adenitis or bacteraemia leading to septicaemia or deep-seated haematogenous infection: osteomyelitis, septic arthritis, acute endocarditis, or pneumonia. Invasive disease is more common in immunocompromised individuals. *Staph. aureus* expressing genes for Panton–Valentine leucocidin (pvl) cause severe disease.

Staphylococci produce three exotoxin-mediated syndromes: toxic shock syndrome, scalded skin syndrome, and food poisoning.

CONS are relatively low-pathogenicity species but cause indolent infections of implanted foreign materials which can only be cured by removal of the foreign body. CONS are the most common cause of sepsis in preterm neonates and immunocompromised individuals.

Clinical features
Superficial infections
Staph. aureus is the most common cause of hordeola (styes), boils, impetigo (bullous and nonbullous) (Fig 15.17), paronychia and wound infections. Secondary infection of eczema is common. Cellulitis, lymphadenitis, and periorbital cellulitis may all be caused by *Staph. aureus*.

Deep infections
Staph. aureus is an uncommon cause of septicaemia or pneumonia but remains the most important cause of osteomyelitis and septic arthritis.

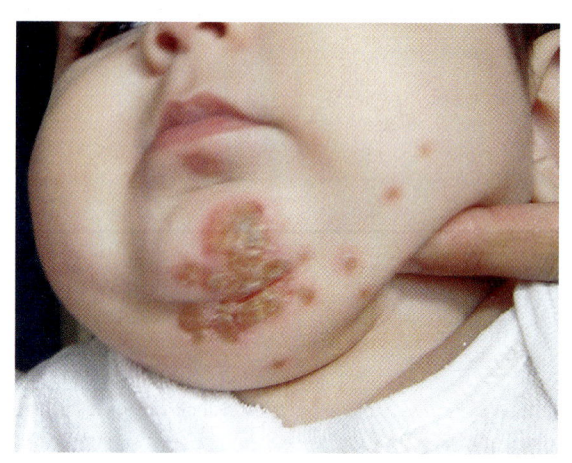

Fig 15.17 Impetigo.

Toxin-mediated syndromes
Toxic shock syndrome (TSS)
This is caused by exotoxins produced by *Staph. aureus*:
- *Enterotoxins B or C:* SEB, SEC
- *Toxin-shock syndrome toxin-1:* TSST-1.

A similar syndrome is caused by exotoxins of group A streptococci (see below).

Disease is triggered by the toxin acting as a superantigen which allows non-specific binding of MHC II with T-cell receptors resulting in polyclonal T-cell activation and a 'cytokine storm'.

The focus of infection is minor such as a skin abrasion. In the past it was associated with use of high absorbency tampons which provided an optimal aerobic environment for toxin production and absorption.

Diagnostic criteria:
- Body temperature >38.9°C
- Systolic blood pressure <90mmHg
- *Diffuse rash:* intense erythoderma ('boiled lobster') with subsequent desquamation
- *Involvement of three or more organ systems:* GI tract, renal failure, hepatitis, mucositis, DIC, CNS (confusion).

TSS can be fatal within hours, the mortality is 15%, and requires aggressive treatment in a PICU with initial IV fluids, antistaphylococcal antibiotics, and IV immunoglobulin.

Staphylococcal scalded skin syndrome (SSSS)
SSSS is caused by circulation of exfoliative toxins causing separation of skin through the stratum granulosum layer of the epidermis.

Manifestations are age related. In the neonate generalized exfoliation may occur. In older children, fever with a tender scarlatiniform eruption and localized bullae followed by peeling. Dehydration can occur. Treatment involves fluid management and IV antibiotics.

Staphylococcal food poisoning
Ingestion of food contaminated with preformed enterotoxins from *Staph. aureus*. Abdominal pain, vomiting with or without diarrhoea occurs after 1–6 h.

Management
Diagnostic investigations
Gram stain and culture of microbiological specimens are the standard tests. Phage typing and toxin identification may be useful in TSS and SSSS. Staph. aureus is almost never a contaminant when isolated from blood culture.

CONS from blood culture may be a contaminant or a pathogen in a preterm neonate, immunocompromised child, or patient with a prosthetic device.

Prevention
Strict hand-washing by health-care professionals is important in prevention of nosocomial infection, as is aseptic technique in insertion of central venous lines and other implants. Recurrent skin infection can be interrupted with topical antistaphylococcal agents such as chlorhexidine soap and nasal carrier cream.

Treatment
Most Staph. aureus strains are β-lactamase producers and penicillin resistant. Suitable antibiotics include flucloxacillin and co-amoxiclav. Other useful agents are sodium fusidate, gentamicin, clindamycin, rifampicin, and the glycopeptides vancomycin and teicoplanin.

Localized Staph. aureus infection such as lymphadenitis (Fig 15.18) or septic arthritis often requires surgical drainage.

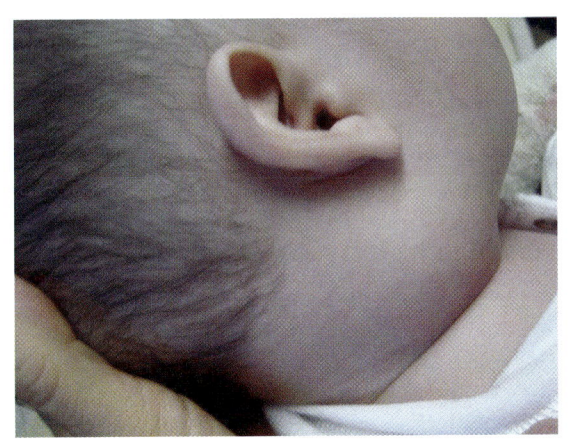

Fig 15.18 Acute bacterial cervical adenitis: an abscess has formed, requiring surgical drainage.

Streptococcal infections
The genus *Streptococcus* includes gram-positive organisms that are catalase negative and display chains in Gram stains. Streptococci are further classified into:

β-Haemolytic
- Group A: Strep. pyogenes: 100 distinct M-protein types of which 8 are associated with rheumatic fever and 4 with glomerulonephritis
- Group B: Strep. agalactiae: GBS are divided into 9 serotypes based on capsular polysaccharides.

α-Haemolytic
- Strep. viridans: 21 species, part of normal flora
- Strep. pneumoniae: the pneumococcus is encapsulated and there are at least 90 distinct serotypes (see next section).

Group A streptococci, Strep. pyogenes (GAS)
Streptococcal pharyngitis is more common in the autumn and winter months. Asymptomatic carriage of GAS in healthy children during outbreaks of pharyngitis is up 50%.

Pathogenesis
GAS cause disease by several mechanisms:
- *Toxin production:* streptolysin-O and circulating exotoxins responsible for scarlet fever and toxic shock like syndrome.
- *Autoimmune mechanisms:* cause rheumatic fever, glomerulonephritis, and paediatric autoimmune neuropsychiatric disorders associated with streptococcal infection (PANDAS).

Clinical features
- Acute infection causes several distinct syndromes:
- *Acute pharyngotonsillitis:* this is the most common GAS infection, associated with fever, malaise, sore throat, and a purulent pharyngotonsillitis usually in a child >3 years. Complications include otitis media, sinusitis, peritonsillar abscesses, and cervical adenitis (Fig 15.17).
- *Impetigo or pyoderma:* GAS skin infection is more common in tropical climates and complicates eczema. Streptococcal cellulitis is characterized by dark red induration of the skin.
- *Scarlet fever:* produced by an erythrogenic toxin, and is more commonly associated with pharyngitis than skin infection. A red, generalized rash occurs with punctate lesions, giving a 'sandpaper' texture. Face and forehead are involved with typical circumoral pallor.
- *Invasive infections:* invasive infection is more likely in infants and young children. Risk factors include varicella infection and diabetes mellitus. Examples include septic arthritis, osteomyelitis, necrotising fasciitis, pneumonia, and septicaemia.
- *Toxic-shock-like syndrome (TSLS):* occurs in association with skin infection with severe pain at the site and progression as described for TSS.

Management
Diagnosis
- *Throat swab:* culture is the most useful confirmation test in pharyngitis. Rapid antigen detection tests have high sensitivity and low specificity
- *Blood culture:* in suspected invasive infection
- *ASOT:* indicated in suspected poststreptococcal glomerulonephritis and suspected Kawasaki disease.

Treatment
Penicillin V for 10 days is used for GAS pharyngitis except in patients with penicillin allergy, in whom a macrolide or cephalosporin is a suitable alternative. Superficial infections such as cellulitis or adenitis in which staphylococci or streptococci may be the pathogen require broad spectrum cover with co-amoxiclav. Suspected necrotizing fasciitis is an emergency requiring urgent surgical exploration.

Group B streptococci (GBS)
Strep. agalactiae (GBS) is an important cause of perinatal bacterial infection. Clinical features and management are described in Chapter 1.9.

Strep. viridans
These organisms are part of the normal flora of mouth and upper airways. The Strep. mutans group is implicated in dental caries. Strep. viridans is a cause of infective endocarditis.

15.14 Pneumococcal and meningococcal infections

Pneumococcal infection

The pneumococcus or *S. pneumoniae* is a capsulated organism and an important cause of invasive infections including septicaemia, pneumonia, and meningitis. However, since the introduction of routine immunization with pneumococcal conjugate vaccines in the UK in 2006 it is anticipated that the pattern and frequency of infection caused by this organism will change.

Aetiology and pathogenesis

Of the 90 known serotypes, 7 cause most invasive childhood infections in the USA. *Pneumococci* are ubiquitous and many people carry the organism in the upper respiratory tract.

Transmission is from person to person by respiratory droplet contact. Invasive disease occurs in association with a viral upper respiratory tract infection or in the presence of a specially virulent serotype such as 1, 6, or 14. Infections are most prevalent in winter months.

High risk groups include children with:
- *Sickle cell disease:* hyposplenism
- Asplenia
- Varicella infection
- Nephrotic syndrome
- Immunodeficiency, cochlear implants, basal skull fracture with CSF fluid leak.

Clinical features

Pneumococcal infection may manifest as:
- *Upper respiratory tract infection:* otitis media, conjunctivitis, mastoiditis, periorbital cellulitis
- *Pneumonia:* usually lobar
- *Bacteraemia:* may cause febrile seizures
- *Invasive infections:* septicaemia, meningitis, septic arthritis, osteomyelitis, endocarditis.

Management

Diagnosis

Identification of gram-positive diplococci on Gram stain or culture from suitable samples from normally sterile sites such as blood, CSF, pleural, or joint fluid. Recovery of pneumococci from upper respiratory tract samples does not necessarily imply a pathogenic role.

Prevention

There are two types of pneumococcal vaccine:
- *Pneumococcal polysaccharide vaccine (PPV):* capsular polysaccharides, 23-valent.
- *Pneumococcal conjugate vaccine (PCV):* capsular polysaccharides, 7-valent. Conjugated to protein CRM_{197}.

Children <2 years show a poor response to PPV but the conjugated PCV is immunogenic from 2 months of age. PCV protects against pneumococcal meningitis, bacteraemia, pneumonia, and otitis media and is now part of the routine immunization programme in the UK.

In addition to PCV, at-risk children are offered a single dose of PPV. Prophylactic penicillin is given to children with nephrotic syndrome, sickle cell disease, asplenia, or HIV.

Treatment

Antibiotic options include penicillin, amoxicillin, macrolides (erythromycin, clarithromycin) and cephalosporins, e.g. cefuroxime.

Typical first line antibiotic choices for clinical syndromes consistent with pneumococcal infection are:
- *Lobar pneumonia:* IV cefuroxime, oral co-amoxiclav
- *Bacterial meningitis:* IV ceftriaxone
- *Cervical lymphadenitis:* IV or oral co-amoxiclav.

Penicillin, however, remains a suitable first line choice in areas of the world where penicillin resistance is uncommon.

Meningococcal infection

Meningococcal disease arises from systemic bacterial infection by *Neisseria meningitidis*, a gram-negative diplococcus. There are at least 13 serogroups based on surface capsular polysaccharide, of which groups B and C are most common in the UK.

Epidemiology

Meningococcal disease occurs worldwide. Attack rates are highest in infancy and a second peak occurs in adolescence at 15–19 years. In temperate climates infections are more common in winter and in the 'meningitis belt' of sub-Saharan Africa at the end of the dry season.

Most cases are sporadic but hyperendemic periods occur, for example during the world wars. Large epidemics have occurred linked to the hajj pilgrimage to Mecca (predominantly serogroup A and W135).

Since the introduction of routine immunization with a Men C conjugate vaccine in the UK in 1999, group C cases have fallen by over 90% and group B strains now account for 80% of UK cases.

Transmission and pathogenesis

Nasopharyngeal colonization varies with age. It is low in infants and young children, peaks at 25% in adolescence, and falls to 10% in adults. Transmission is by aerosol, droplets, or direct contact with respiratory secretions of a carrier and requires frequent or prolonged close contact.

Pathogenesis

Development of invasive disease depends on pathogen virulence factors and host factors and remains poorly understood. Virulence factors include capsulation, pilation aiding adherence, and membrane proteins that influence epithelial penetration.

Host risk factors increasing susceptibility include respiratory tract infection, smoking both active and passive, and impaired immunity in sickle cell disease, asplenia, and specific immunodeficiencies e.g. of complement components.

After invasion, the host response to infection may be important in determining the inflammatory cascade and rapid progression to purpura fulminans in some cases.

Invasive disease may lead to a spectrum of subsequent pathology and clinical manifestations, most commonly septicaemia or meningitis either alone or in combination. Less common are occult febrile bacteraemia or chronic meningococcaemia.

Clinical manifestations

Meningococcal disease usually presents as meningitis or septicaemia, or a combination of both. Rare presentations include arthritis, pneumonia, occult bacteraemia, endocarditis, chronic meningococcaemia, or conjunctivitis.

Onset varies from insidious, with mild coryza (due to a viral URTI) and fever lasting a few days, to fulminant disease with acute, overwhelming illness developing over a few hours.

Features of septicaemia or meningitis may occur in isolation or combination and are considered separately for convenience.

Meningococcal septicaemia

The characteristic rash is often non-specific initially, with a red, maculopapular appearance before evolving into the well known petechial or purpuric 'non-blanching' rash (Fig 15.19).

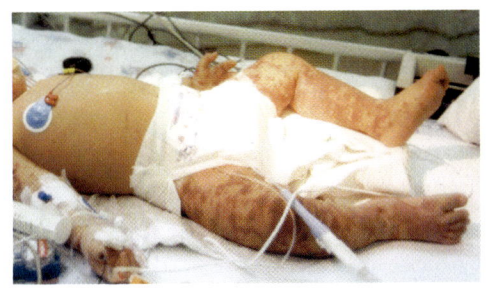

Fig 15.19 Meningococcal septicaemia: late stage rash.

Other features of septicaemic presentation may include vomiting, drowsiness, irritability, confusion, poor feeding, and high-pitched cry.

Signs of early 'compensated' shock are tachycardia and prolonged capillary refill time. The evaluation and management of septicaemia and septic shock is described in Chapter 2.8.

Bacterial meningitis

Neisseria meningitidis is now the most common organism causing acute bacterial meningitis outside the neonatal period. Features of meningitis are age dependent and non-specific in the early stages, especially in infants.

Symptoms may include fever, headache, and vomiting with increasing anorexia, lethargy, and drowsiness.

Examination reveals fever and a petechial rash in about 50% of those with meningococcal disease. Specific CNS signs reflect meningeal irritation and the accompanying encephalitis/encephalopathy.

- *Meningeal irritation:* in older children, neck stiffness and positive Kernig's sign. In infants, extended posture may be evident in an advanced case, but a tense or 'bulging' fontanelle is the most useful sign.
- *Encephalopathy:* altered consciousness, seizures.

The differential diagnosis of meningococcal disease is most difficult in the early stages, when the characteristic rash if present is non-specific or subtle. A localized petechial rash on face or neck can occur with vomiting or coughing and often causes unnecessary alarm. Children with immune thrombocytopaenic purpura or Henoch–Schönlein purpura are usually well and not difficult to identify.

Management

Diagnostic investigations

- *FBC and differential:* a neutrophil leucocytosis or neutropaenia render invasive bacterial disease likely
- *CRP:* a non-specific test, but a CRP <0.5 mg/dL renders sepsis unlikely
- Blood culture and culture of throat swab, skin and urine samples
- Blood for PCR detection of meningococcus
- Lumbar puncture (LP).

LP is not necessary in cases of septicaemia and contraindicated if there are signs of raised intracranial pressure such as reduced level of consciousness or focal neurology. In the absence of contraindications, LP, and examination of CSF is essential for confirmation of diagnosis and pathogen identification.

CSF is sent for:

- *Microscopy and culture:* organisms may be visible on microscopy and an excess of neutrophils, usually 300–2000/mm^2
- Bacterial antigen detection by latex agglutination
- PCR for bacterial and viral DNA
- Protein is increased to 1–5 g/L and glucose reduced to <66% of plasma glucose level.

Prevention

Men C conjugate vaccine is part of the immunization schedule in the UK but protects against group C only.

A quadrivalent (ACWY) polysaccharide vaccine provides protection against serotypes A, C, W135, and Y but protection is not long-lasting. It is recommended for travellers to regions with outbreaks due to these subgroups and is a visa entry requirement for hajj pilgrims to Saudi Arabia.

Chemoprophylaxis is indicated for household contacts of cases of meningococcal infection using a 2 day course of rifampicin. The disease is notifiable.

Treatment

If meningococcal disease is suspected, urgent antibiotic treatment is vital. In primary care, a single dose of benzylpenicillin given IV or IM is recommended. In hospitals, IV therapy with a 3rd generation cephalosporin such as ceftriaxone is initiated after blood cultures have been taken.

The management of septicaemia is described in Chapter 2.8.

Bacterial meningitis is treated initially with ceftriaxone or in infants under 3 months with cefotaxime and ampicillin to cover *Listeria*. Concurrent oral dexamethasone reduces the risk of sensorineural hearing loss. Additional management measures may include fluid restriction, antiepilepsy drugs, and measures to reduce intracranial pressure. Treatment duration is 7–21 days depending on age and organism.

Meningococcal disease has a mortality rate which is higher in septicaemia (10%) than in meningitis (2%).

Long-term sequelae are more severe in neonatal and pneumococcal meningitis, sensorineural deafness being most common. Limbs may be lost from ischaemia secondary to intravascular thrombosis in meningococcal septicaemia.

15.15 Zoonoses

A zoonosis is any infectious disease naturally transmitted from vertebrate animals to humans.

Many different wild and domestic animals act as reservoirs including cats and dogs, birds, cattle and sheep, monkeys, rodents, and deer. Transmission may occur by direct contact, respiratory spread, ingestion of animal tissue or body fluids, or via a vector: mosquitoes, fleas, ticks, bugs, or bats.

Over 50 zoonoses of potential paediatric importance are known and some of the more important are described here.

Avian influenza, 'bird flu'

Influenzavirus A is a genus of the Orthomyxoviridae family which contains one species, influenza A virus, which causes influenza in birds and some mammals including humans, pigs, horses, and dogs. Influenza A virus subtypes are labelled according to an H number, 1–16, for haemagluttinin and N number, 1–9, for neuraminidase.

Influenza A virus subtypes currently circulating among humans and pigs are:
- *H1N1*: caused 'Spanish flu' pandemic of 1918–19
- *H3N2*: caused 'Hong Kong flu' pandemic of 1968–69
- *H1N2*: resulted from re-assortment of genes between H1N1 and H3N2.

The current epizootic is caused by the avian influenza virus, H5N1, which can be transmitted from wild fowl to other birds, a variety of mammals, and humans. H5N1 has mutated into a variety of strains with differing pathogenic profiles. The mortality rate of highly pathogenic H5N1 avian influenza in humans is high (60%). A pandemic infection with influenza A H1N1 believed to originate from pigs (swine flu) was declared by the WHO in 2009.

Opinions differ sharply on whether a pandemic in humans killing 5–150 million people is possible or likely. Research is ongoing to develop vaccines and antivirals.

Brucellosis

Brucellosis or undulant fever, Malta fever is caused by gram-negative coccobacilli, *Brucella melitensis*, *B. suis*, *B. abortus*.

Humans contract the disease by contact with infected animals (cattle, sheep, pigs, goats) or their secretions or by ingesting unpasteurized milk or milk products. UK cases are usually acquired in the Mediterranean region.

The incubation period is up to 3 months. Clinical manifestations vary from mild to severe and include fever, chills, weight loss, and arthralgia. Hepatosplenomegaly may develop.

Diagnosis is by culture of blood, bone marrow, or urine and serological tests are available. Treatment of choice is doxycycline or co-trimoxazole in children <12 years for 3–6 weeks.

Cat-scratch disease

This uncommon infection occurs worldwide and is caused by a small, gram-negative bacillus, *Bartonella henselae*. Transmission occurs when a cat, usually a kitten, scratches a human usually <20 years of age.

A primary cutaneous papule appears 7–12 days after the scratch, followed by local lymphadenopathy 2–6 weeks later which may suppurate. Diagnosis is by serology for *Bartonella* antibodies or histology on lymph node biopsy. The differential is atypical mycobacterium infection.

Lymphadenitis usually recovers without treatment, but several oral antibiotic agents appear effective including azithromycin, rifampicin, and ciprofloxacin.

Cryptosporidiosis

Cryptosporidium is a protozoan parasite that infects humans and a wide range of domestic and wild animals. It is spread through the faecal–oral route and is one of the most common water-borne diseases.

Infection is more common in those in regular contact with bodies of fresh water (e.g. swimming pools), and several outbreaks have followed contamination of drinking-water supplies.

In children, the usual illness is watery diarrhoea with low-grade fever and abdominal pain lasting ~2 weeks. Serious or even life-threatening illness occurs in those with severe T-cell immunodeficiency (HIV/ADS or SCID). Diagnosis depends on microscopic examination of stools for oocysts.

In the immunocompetent child management is supportive. Immunodeficient children can avoid infection by drinking water that has been boiled and require treatment with an anticryptosporidial agent, e.g. azithromycin.

Leishmaniasis

Leishmaniasis is a vector-born zoonosis caused by parasitic protozoan species of *Leishmania* including *L. donovani* in the visceral form and *L. major* and others in the cutaneous form.

The reservoir is a variety of animals including dogs and rodents, and the vector is sandflies. Leishmaniasis is found in rural parts of 88 countries including most tropical and subtropical countries. The majority of cases occur in the Middle East, Indian subcontinent, Brazil, and Peru.

Three clinical forms exist:
- *Cutaneous leishmaniasis*: parasites proliferate locally leading to an erythematous papule where the bite took place, usually on an exposed area such as the face. This evolves to become a nodule and then a shallow ulcer (Fig 15.20). Satellite lesions and regional lymphadenopathy may occur. A scraping or punch biopsy sample is stained (Giemsa) for Leishman–Donovan (LD) bodies.

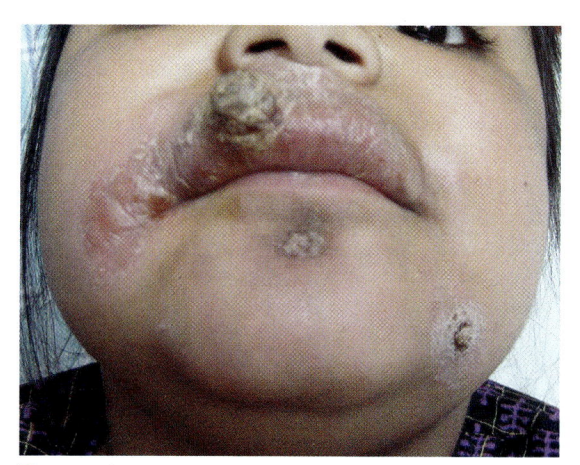

Fig 15.20 Cutaneous leishmaniasis.

- *Mucosal leishmaniasis, espundi:* following cutaneous infection, years later, spread to the mucosa of the oral or naso-pharynx occurs with eventual destruction of facial bones.
- *Visceral leishmaniasis, kala-azar:* L. donovani concentrate and multiply in bone marrow, liver, and spleen with malaise, fever, lymphadenopathy, and hepatosplenomegaly. Pancytopaenia develops with haemorrhage and secondary infection which may be fatal. Diagnosis is by visualization of Leishman–Donovan bodies in aspirates from bone marrow, spleen, or lymph nodes.

Liposomal amphotericin is the drug of choice for visceral leishmaniasis. Cutaneous and mucosal leishmaniasis may heal spontaneously but can be treated with topical paromomycin or liposomal amphotericin.

Lyme disease

Lyme disease or Lyme borreliosis is caused by a tick-borne spirochaete, *Borrelia burgdorferi*, and is named after the town of Lyme, Connecticut where it was first described in 1977.

Lyme disease is the most common tick-borne disease in the northern hemisphere. It is endemic in parts of the USA but uncommon in the UK. UK regions where infection has been reported include the New Forest and Exmoor.

Transmission is by ticks, *Ixodes* spp., which are found on deer in the UK. The ticks are tiny and their bites painless, and it is probably necessary for them to feed on humans for several hours to transmit the spirochaete (Fig 15.21).

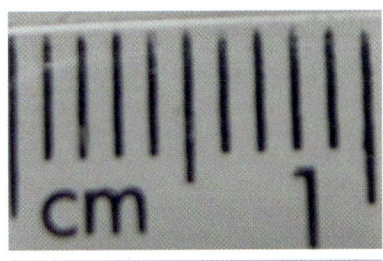

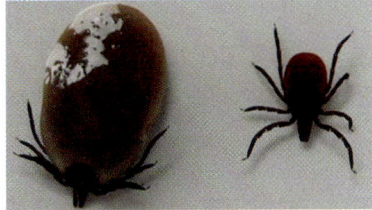

Fig 15.21 Adult tick after (and before) a blood meal. Courtesy of Lyme Disease Action.

The incubation period is 3–20 days. The clinical manifestations are divided into three stages:
- *Early localized:* a distinctive rash, erythema migrans, at the site of the tick bite. It begins as a red macule which expands to form a large annular lesion, sometimes with central clearing, a 'bulls eye' lesion. Fever, malaise, neck stiffness, myalgia, and arthralgia often accompany the rash.
- *Early disseminated:* multiple erythema migrans at distant sites. Other manifestations can include cranial nerve palsies especially VII, aseptic meningitis, conjunctivitis, carditis, and arthralgia.
- *Later disease:* recurrent pauci-articular arthritis.

Diagnosis may be made on clinical grounds. Culture is difficult, but serological tests are available as is PCR testing.

Treatment is with doxycycline for children >8 years and amoxicillin for children <8 years. for 3 weeks.

Leptospirosis

Leptospirosis is a zoonosis of worldwide distribution caused by spirochaetes of the genus *Leptospira*.

Humans are infected through contact with water, food, or soil contaminated by urine of infected animals. Primary hosts include rats, dogs, pigs, and dairy cattle. The usual port of entry is through abraded skin or mucous membranes.

Leptospirosis infection in humans can vary in severity from asymptomatic infection to severe Weil disease.

The disease is biphasic. An initial septicaemic phase characterized by fever, chills, and sometimes a rash is followed by a second immune-mediated phase with jaundice and renal failure. Pulmonary haemorrhage is a major complication.

Diagnosis is based on serology and detection of leptospires in blood or CSF by microscopy, culture of PCR. In the early stage treatment is with penicillin or erythromycin.

Salmonellosis

Salmonellosis is the term used for infection with nontyphoidal salmonella bacteria. These are gram-negative bacilli with a number of species and many serovars. Important species causing salmonellosis are *S. enteritidis* and *S. typhimurium*.

The principal animal reservoirs for non-typhoidal salmonella organisms are poultry, livestock, reptiles, and pets. The major mode of transmission is food of animal origin such as poultry, eggs, and dairy products, but other modes include ingestion of contaminated water and contact with infected pets such as turtles. Most cases are sporadic.

The incubation period is 6 h to 3 days. Infection may be asymptomatic but most commonly causes vomiting, watery diarrhoea, and abdominal cramps. Invasive disease can occur in immunocompromised patients.

Prevention depends on good hygiene and proper methods for food production, preparation, and cooking. Infected children should be excluded from daycare or school until risk of infection is minimal. Treatment is supportive and antibiotics are not recommended.

Transmissable spongiform encephalopathies (TSEs)

The TSEs are caused by prions which are unique amongst agents able to transmit disease in having no nucleic acid.

Variant Creutzfeld–Jacob disease (vCJD) is a TSE caused by transmission of the prion agent responsible for bovine spongiform encephalopathy (BSE). It is of particular interest and concern in the UK on account of the outbreak of BSE ('mad cow disease') which occurred in the UK, 1986–2000. Since 1990, there have been ~160 deaths from vCJD in the UK including ~6 in children. The mode of transmission is assumed to be consumption of beef products contaminated by nervous system tissue.

The human genotype at codon 129 of the prion protein gene, *PRNP*, plays an important role in susceptibility. All vCJD patients are homozygous for the methionine allele at this site. Heterozygotes at this site may be resistant and develop vCJD over a very long period of 30–50 years.

The disease prion promotes refolding of native protein into the diseased state. Insoluble misfolded protein increases exponentially, leading to cell death.

15.16 Malaria and typhoid

Malaria
Malaria is caused by infection with *Plasmodium* protozoa transmitted by a mosquito vector. Malaria (the term originates from medieval Italian: *mala aria* = bad air) remains a major scourge with an estimated 500 million infected annually and 1 million children <5 years dying each year in sub-Saharan Africa from *P. falciparum* infection.

Epidemiology
Malaria is endemic in a broad band around the equator, in areas of the Americas, many parts of Asia, and most of Africa, but it is in sub-Saharan Africa that 85–90% of malaria deaths occur. Mortality is highest in children <5 years, pregnant women, and non-immune travellers.

In the UK ~2000 cases occur each year in travellers returning from malaria-endemic countries, of which 10–20% are in children <16 years. Most infections (88%) are acquired in Africa and *P. falciparum* accounts for 75% of cases. A travel history is essential in all febrile children.

Aetiology and pathogenesis
In humans malaria is caused by four species of *Plasmodium*: *P. falciparum*, *P. malariae*, *P. ovale*, and *P. vivax*.

Mosquito vectors and the life cycle
The primary host and transmission vectors are female *Anopheles* mosquitoes. The mosquito is infected by taking a blood meal from an infected human, ingesting gametocytes which differentiate into gametes that fuse in the mosquito gut producing an ookinete. This produces an oocyst which releases sporozoites that migrate to the salivary glands ready to infect a new human host.

Malaria in humans develops in two phases: an hepatic and an erythrocytic phase (Fig 15.22). Sporozoites enter the bloodstream and migrate to the liver where they infect hepatocytes and multiply asexually for a period of 6–15 days. This yields merozoites which escape into the blood and infect red cells, beginning the erythrocytic phase.

In the erythrocytes, the merozoites develop into ring forms, trophozoites then schizonts, then merozoites again, rupturing the red cells and returning to infect more red cells. Several such cycles occur, waves of fever coinciding with simultaneous waves of merozoites escaping and reinfecting red cells. Only the ring forms circulate, the other red cells tending to adhere to endothelium of the small blood vessels.

Immunity
The outcome of infection depends on host immunity, the mechanisms of which remain poorly defined. The parasite is relatively protected within the liver and red cells and expresses many different and highly variable proteins at different stages of its life cycle. An important degree of natural immunity does develop, however.

Complications
Severe disease is typically seen with *P. falciparum*, because of its capacity to create high levels of parasitaemia and its capacity for sequestration in small postcapillary vessels. This allows evasion of circulation through and removal by the spleen and contributes to end-organ damage in the brain (causing cerebral malaria), placenta, lungs, and kidneys.

Clinical features
Symptoms usually appear 8–15 days after infection but patients infected with *P. vivax* may manifest up to 3 months after returning from an endemic area. A history of recent travel to an endemic area is a key to diagnosis in the UK.

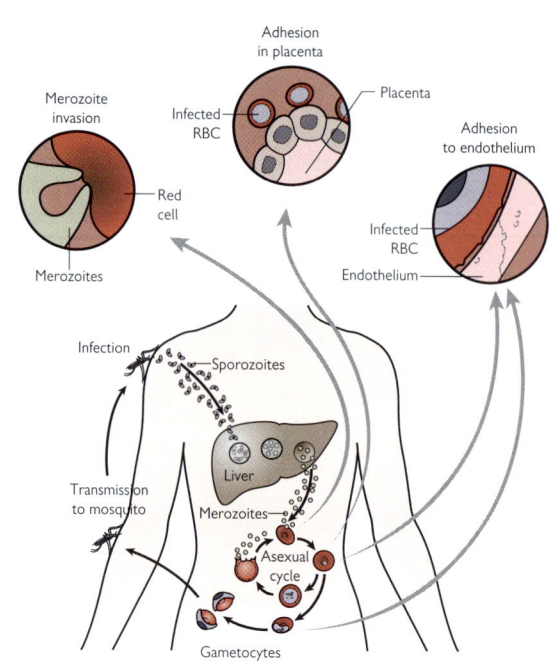

Fig 15.22 Malaria life cycle: human phases.

Presenting symptoms usually include fever, headaches, abdominal pain, arthralgia, vomiting and diarrhoea, malaise, fatigue, and muscle aches.

Signs depend on severity of illness which in turn depends on host immunity and parasite load. Fever may be the only physical finding but pallor and jaundice with splenomegaly may be present. Non-immune patients may become severely ill with any or all of several clinical syndromes:
- Severe anaemia with jaundice as a signs of haemolysis
- *Cerebral malaria*: decreased level of consciousness, confusion, coma, and seizures
- *Renal failure*: acute tubular necrosis caused by severe acute intravascular haemolysis and haemoglobinuria ('blackwater fever'). Rare in children
- *Pulmonary oedema*: uncommon in children
- *Hypoglycaemia*: from disease and caused by quinine.

Management
Diagnostic tests
Microscopy of thick and thin blood films
Thick films allow a higher volume of blood to be scanned in one microscopic field and are more sensitive for parasite detection. Thin films allow species identification and determination of parasitaemia levels (the % red cells harbouring parasites). Three sets of films 12–24 h apart are necessary to be confident of exclusion if clinical suspicion is strong.

Field tests
OptiMAL-IT detects parasite lactate dehydrogenase and can distinguish *P. falciparum* from other species. Parasite nucleic acids are detected using PCR.
Additional investigations include:
- *FBC*: anaemia and thrombocytopaenia are common; fewer then 5% of patients have a raised WBC
- Blood glucose, urea and electrolytes, LFTs

- Check G6PD status
- Blood culture: typhoid fever is in the differential for a febrile child returning from the tropics.

Prevention

- *Protection*: protective clothing from dusk to dawn as *Anopheles* feed at night, mosquito repellents, bed nets
- *Chemoprophylaxis*: taken for 1 week before departure and for 4 weeks after return. Options depend on pattern of chloroquine resistance:
  - *chloroquine-sensitive*: chloroquine weekly, proguanil daily.
  - *chloroquine-resistant*: mefloquine weekly, doxycycline daily
- *Vaccines*: vaccines for malaria remain under development.

Treatment

Depends on the species and severity.

- *P. falciparum malaria*: in the UK all are assumed to be chloroquine-resistant and treated with quinine until parasitaemia is cleared. Oral quinine is used unless the patient is severely ill with parasitaemia >2% in which case IV infusion is indicated. Monitor blood glucose for hypoglycaemia and ECG. This is followed by a single dose of pyrimethamine-sulfadoxine (Fansidar) or a 3 day course of atavaquone proguanil (Malarone). Exchange transfusion may be considered if parasitaemia is very heavy (>10%).
- *P. vivax, ovale, malariae*: oral chloroquine followed by oral primaquine to eradicate liver stage and prevent relapses. G6PD status must be checked before giving primaquine.

Typhoid fever

Typhoid fever or enteric fever is a systemic infection by *Salmonella typhi* (Fig 15.23) or the less virulent *S. paratyphi*. These are gram-negative bacilli of the genus *Salmonella*.

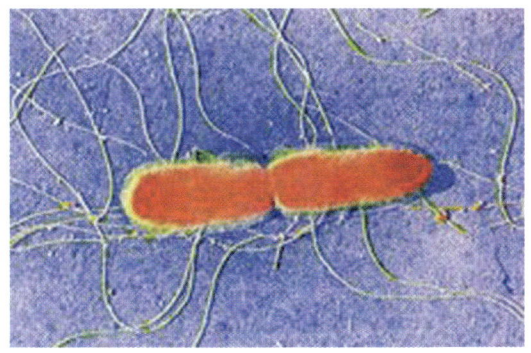

Fig 15.23 *Salmonella typhi*: flagellated motile bacterium. Reprinted by permission from Macmillan Publishers Ltd: Nature; 405; Smaglik; Bacterial AIDS vaccine ready for testing, © 2000.

Epidemiology

Typhoid and paratyphoid occur worldwide but are endemic in countries with poor sanitation and poor food hygiene. About 20 million cases per year occur worldwide with up to half a million deaths, mostly in children. In the UK, most cases are imported from India and Africa (300–400/year).

Both organisms can exist outside the body, but infection occurs almost exclusively in humans, so water or food contaminated by sewage can act as environmental reservoirs.

Aetiology and pathogenesis

Transmission is by food or water contaminated by faeces or urine from an infected person. Asymptomatic carriers with the organism in the biliary tree and excreted in the faeces are an important source. The most famous was 'Typhoid Mary', a cook in New York responsible for seven outbreaks.

After ingestion *S. typhi* invades the gut and multiplies in the mononuclear phagocytic cells of the RES. The infected macrophage travels through the mesenteric lymph nodes, into the thoracic duct to seed the liver, spleen, bone marrow, and lymph nodes. It then causes apoptosis of macrophages and escapes into the blood stream where the Vi antigen forms a capsule to protect the bacterium from phagocytosis. Bacteria re-enter the GI tract from the gallbladder via the bile and may also invade the urinary tract and appear in stool.

About 10% of patients excrete *S. typhi* for at least 3 months and 2–5% become long-term carriers.

Clinical features

The incubation period averages 1–3 weeks, shorter periods (1–10 days) being usual for paratyphoid infection. During this period a minority of patients have transient diarrhoea due to enterocolitis that resolves before the bacteraemia develops.

As bacteraemia develops there is slow onset of a sustained fever, with malaise, headache, anorexia, abdominal pain, and a dry cough. There may be constipation (due to obstruction at the ileocecal valve by swollen Peyer patches) or diarrhoea at this stage.

The physical findings evolve as the disease progresses and include:

- *Fever*: remittent week 1, peaks to 39–40°C in week 2.
- *Rose spots*: a subtle, sparse, blanching, maculopapular rash on the trunk caused by bacterial emboli occurs in a third of patients at the end of the first week. Relative bradycardia is common at this stage
- *Splenomegaly*: common in the 2nd week.

Unusual presentations include lobar pneumonia, arthritis, or neuropsychiatric manifestations. Untreated mortality is 20%.

Management

Diagnostic investigations

- *Culture*: isolation of the organism from blood, bone marrow, stool or urine provides definitive diagnosis, but the chance of isolation varies with time:
  - *1st week*: blood and stool cultures positive in 85–90%
  - *2nd week*: stool and urine
  - *bone marrow aspirate*: 90% sensitive at any time
- *FBC*: anaemia, thrombocytopaenia and relative lymphopaenia
- *LFTs*: transaminases and bilirubin levels are often elevated
- *Serology*: Elisa tests for specific IgM are available.

Prevention

Hygiene precautions are most important. Partially effective typhoid vaccines are available:

- *Vi polysaccharide vaccine*: children > 18 months. Injectable.
- *Oral vaccine Ty21a*: children > 6 years. Live, attenuated.

Vaccination is recommended for travellers to endemic areas. Cases, carriers, and close contacts may spread infection and may be considered for exclusion from work or school.

Treatment

Antibiotic treatment is started while the results of confirmatory tests are pending and is guided by regional sensitivity profiles. First line options are ceftriaxone and ciprofloxacin. Treatment should be for a minimum of 2 weeks or up to 6 weeks for abscesses, osteomyelitis, or immunocompromised patients. The disease is notifiable. Family and close contacts are screened for infection by stool specimens.

15.17 Allergy

Allergy and atopy

Allergy is a state of abnormal hypersensitivity acquired after exposure to an environmental substance (allergen) which is normally harmless. The hypersensitivity is usually a type I, immediate IgE-mediated reaction.

Allergy is common in individuals with atopy, a genetically determined propensity for developing IgE mediated reactions to environmental allergens. Important clinical manifestations of atopy include eczema, asthma, hayfever, and food allergy.

Epidemiology

The prevalence of allergy and atopy is highest in industrialized, developed countries and has increased over a time period of decades too short to be explained by population genetic changes. Several hypotheses have been proposed to explain this increase (see below).

Aetiology and pathogenesis

Genetic basis

Atopy and allergy are strongly familial. Concordance in monozygotic twins is 70% and in dizygotic twins 40%. Multiple genes have been implicated in asthma and asthma related traits (ASRT) such as atopy and atopic dermatitis.

Common mutations in the gene (*FLG*) for fillagrin, a protein important in skin barrier function, have recently been associated with atopic dermatitis and related phenotypes.

Pathogenesis

Th2 lymphocytes generate a family of cytokines, IL-4, IL-5, IL-13, that mediate allergic inflammation in part by promoting class switching of antigen-specific B cells to the production of IgE. The 'hygiene hypothesis' proposes that exposure to microorganisms in early life activates Th1 responses and that reduced exposure due to a 'hygienic' environment leads to persistence of the early skew towards Th2 cytokine generation.

Secreted IgE binds to an IgE-specific receptor, FcERI, on mast cells and basophils, sensitizing these cells to the allergen. On subsequent exposure, the allergen cross-links IgE and FcERI receptors causing degranulation of mast cells and basophils with release of histamine and other mediators.

Mast cells are found in epithelial tissue of skin, respiratory, and GI tract. Stored substances released on degranulation include histamine, tryptase, cytokines, and derivatives of arachidonic acid, prostaglandins, and leukotrienes. These mediators cause:

- Vasodilation
- *Capillary leak:* urticaria, angio-oedema, hypotension
- *Smooth muscle contraction:* bronchoconstriction, abdominal pain
- *Mucosal oedema:* laryngeal oedema, bronchial narrowing
- Mucous hypersecretion.

Late-phase response

This may follow 2–24 h after the initial immediate reaction and is caused by migration of neutrophils, eosinophils, CD4 lymphocytes, and basophils to the initial site.

Environmental factors

Environmental allergen exposure may occur via the skin, gut, or respiratory tract and allergens range from micro-organisms to food components.

Clinical features

Asthma, atopic eczema, and anaphylaxis are all discussed elsewhere. The atopic diseases of eczema, food allergy, asthma, and allergic rhinitis cluster together and tend to manifest in a progressive sequence which has been called the 'allergic march'.

The clinical manifestations of an allergic reaction vary with severity and systems involved but commonly include:

- *Cutaneous:* itchy, urticarial rash (hives)
- *Angio-oedema:* oedema of face, oral cavity, upper respiratory tract
- *Respiratory tract:* laryngeal oedema (stridor) and or bronchoconstriction (wheeze) with tachypnoea
- *GI tract:* abdominal pain and distension.

Management

Diagnostic investigations

Diagnosis of an allergic disease is primarily clinical, but several tests are available to aid in identifying causative allergens for IgE mediated reactions.

- *Skin prick test (SPTs):* these are readily available and inexpensive and can be performed on infants. Small amounts of suspected allergens or their extracts such as pollen, grass, peanut extract are introduced intradermally and any visible inflammatory response recorded. The mean diameter of any 'wheal' is recorded at 15 min. SPT has a low positive predictive value. Many patients with a positive result are asymptomatic. However, it has a high negative predictive value and a negative result renders IgE-mediated disease unlikely.
- *Specific serum IgE levels:* food-specific IgE levels can be measured using modifications of the radioallergenosorbent test (RAST) but false positive tests are common.

Prevention and treatment

Avoidance of allergen exposure is an obvious strategy but not always easy to achieve. Many pharmacotherapeutic agents are available for the treatment or prevention of allergic reactions including antihistamines, corticosteroids, antileukotrienes, and mast cell stabilizers.

Immunotherapeutic strategies such as desensitization may be considered in severe cases, and a monoclonal anti-IgE antibody which binds to free and B-cell associated IgE is now available (omalizumab).

Food allergy

Food allergy is an adverse response to food mediated by immune mechanisms. It is important to recognize that adverse reactions to food may occur via a number of non-immune mechanisms. These reactions are described as food *intolerance* and may be caused by:

- *Enzyme or transporter deficiencies:* lactose intolerance due to lactase deficiency, glucose/galactose malabsorption
- *Pharmacological mechanisms:* vasoactive amines triggering migraine, caffeine, monosodium glutamate
- *Inborn errors of metabolism:* urea cycle disorders
- *Psychological:* food aversion
- *Toxins:* food poisoning (staphylococcal), mushrooms.

Epidemiology

Food allergy is common, affecting 6–8% of children and is the most common cause of severe, anaphylactic reactions in children. Estimates of the frequency of severe reactions vary but severe nut allergy may have an incidence of up to 12/100 000 children. One third of children with moderate to severe atopy have IgE-mediated food allergy.

Aetiology and pathogenesis

Allergens

In children 'the big eight' causing 90% of food allergy are: milk, egg, peanut, tree nut, seafood, shellfish, soy, and wheat.

Cross-reactions can occur, e.g. between cow's milk and soya or goat's milk, and between peanuts and soybeans.

Immune mechanisms

There are three categories of allergic response mechanism:
- *Type 1 IgE mediated*: immediate onset.
- *Mixed IgE/non IgE mediated*: the eosinophilic inflammatory disorders. Onset is delayed
- *Non-IgE mediated/T-cell mediated*: food-protein-induced enteropathies such as coeliac disease.

These mechanisms lead to distinct pathophysiological responses and a distinct set of clinical syndromes.

Clinical features

Diagnosis of food allergy hinges initially on a detailed history which should include family or previous history of atopy and a description of the episodes: food suspected to have provoked adverse reaction, amount ingested, interval between ingestion and reaction, detailed description of reaction.

The spectrum of clinical manifestations depends on the immune mechanisms,

IgE-mediated type 1

Reactions usually occur within 2 h of ingestion and are usefully categorized by severity:
- *Mild*: local erythema, urticarial rash, pruritus
  - oral allergy syndrome: itching and tingling of lips, tongue, palate or oropharynx, usually provoked by fresh fruit or vegetable allergens such as apples, peaches, kiwi, celery, hazelnuts
- *Moderate*: generalized urticaria, angioedema, rhinoconjunctivitis, vomiting. Mild respiratory involvement
- *Severe*: multisystem reaction (anaphylaxis) with dyspnoea, hypotension, and loss of consciousness.

Mixed IgE/non-IgE mediated

The eosinophilic gastroenteropathies manifest according to the site of the inflammation and usually present in an indolent fashion at 1–18 months. Causative foods include cow's milk, soy, wheat and egg.
- *Eosinophilic oesophagitis*: vomiting, dysphagia, failure to thrive, abdominal pain. The clinical features may be indistinguishable from gastro-oesophageal reflux disease.
- *Eosinophilic gastroenteritis and gastroenterocolitis*: vomiting, abdominal pain, diarrhoea, failure to thrive, occult blood loss and anaemia, protein-losing enteropathy, constipation.

Non-IgE-mediated.

There are several distinct syndromes:
- *Cow's milk protein allergy*: this is the most common food allergy affecting 2.5–7.5% of children. Clinical features in 50% are those of non-IgE mediated reactions ranging from failure to thrive, vomiting, and colic to protocolitis and anaemia. Symptoms develop within 4 weeks of starting feeds. Most infants and children outgrow milk allergy by 2–4 years.
- *Proctocolitis*: as a result of cow's milk protein allergy. Usually presents in the first 6 months with mucousy, bloody stools. Up to 60% of cases occur in breast-fed infants (intact cow's milk proteins are in breast milk).
- *Coeliac disease*: gluten enteropathy.
- *Food protein-induced enterocolitis syndrome (FPIE)*: allergens include cow's milk protein and soy and multiple other foods. It does not seem to occur in breast-fed infants. Symptoms occur 2 h after ingestion and include vomiting, diarrhoea and lethargy severe enough in 20% to cause severe dehydration and circulatory collapse.
- *Lymphonodular hyperplasia*: this may be a normal finding or associated with a variety of features including abdominal pain, diarrhoea, and anaemia.

Management

Diagnostic investigations

These depend on the suspected immune mechanism. Skin prick testing or measurement of food specific IgE levels is indicated for IgE-mediated allergy.

Additional diagnostic strategies include atopy patch testing, trial of allergen avoidance, or elimination diets, and food challenges to determine if resolution has occurred. Diagnostic tools for evaluation of eosinophilic or non-IgE mediated reactions include endoscopy and biopsy.

Prevention and treatment

- Avoidance of the allergen by expert dietetic advice is the cornerstone of management. In the case of peanut or tree nut allergy the best advice is to avoid all nuts at all costs.
- Infants with cow's milk protein allergy who are not breast-fed should receive a dietary product based on extensively hydrolysed protein, or in some cases an amino acid mixture.
- School support and education. 'Medic Alert' identification.

Treatment of IgE-mediated reactions includes:
- Oral antihistamines
- Self-administered epinephrine (Epipen, Anapen).

Provision of self-administered epinephrine is a controversial issue. If prescribed, education and training is essential. Most would agree on the following indications:
- Previous history of life-threatening episode
- Co-existent asthma
- Parental request after informed discussion.
- Trace exposure has caused a mild-moderate reaction
- Allergy to nuts (90% of fatal reactions).

15.18 Henoch–Schönlein purpura and Kawasaki disease

Henoch–Schönlein purpura (HSP)

This is an IgA-mediated small-vessel vasculitis which occurs in all age groups but is most common in young children. 75% of cases occur in children <10 years and 50% in children <5 years.

HSP is the most common vasculitis of childhood with a reported incidence of 10–20/100 000 children and a male predominance of up to 2:1.

Aetiology and pathogenesis

The exact aetiology is uncertain but involves the vascular deposition of IgA immune complexes following an infectious trigger in genetically predisposed individuals.

HSP is more prevalent within Hispanic populations and uncommon in Afro-Caribbeans. The incidence is highest in autumn, winter, and spring. It is associated with HLA B35, HLA-DRB1*01, and heterozygous C2 complement deficiency.

An antecedent upper respiratory infection is reported in 50% of cases. Many organisms have been implicated:

- *Bacteria:* group A β-haemolytic streptococci, Mycoplasma pneumoniae
- *Viruses:* hepatitis A and B, varicella, EBV, parvovirus B19.

HSP has also followed vaccinations including MMR and hepatitis B and various drugs, although none of the latter has been proved to be associated in controlled studies.

Pathogenesis

Deposition of IgA immune complexes occurs in small vessels in the skin, kidneys, intestinal mucosa, and joints. IgA occurs as two isotypes:

- *IgA1:* serum IgA is predominantly monomeric IgA1.
- *IgA2:* 60% of IgA in secretions is polymeric IgA2.

In HSP polymeric IgA1 is mainly deposited. There is evidence that abnormal glycosylation of IgA1 is a factor.

Deposition of IgA1 complexes activates the alternative complement pathway leading to recruitment of polymorphonuclear leukocytes and inflammation and necrosis of vessel wells with concomitant thrombosis. This is manifest histologically as a leukocytoclastic vasculitis.

The clinical manifestations of HSP reflect small-vessel vasculitis in several organ systems.

Renal involvement is potentially the most important feature and varies from minimal change to crescentic glomerulonephritis. Henoch–Schönlein nephritis (HSPN) is histologically indistinguishable from IgA nephropathy (Berger disease) and may share a common immunogenetic pathway. Characteristically there is a focal and segmental glomerulonephritis and immunofluorescence reveals mesangial IgA with IgG, C3, and fibrin.

Clinical features

The hallmark is the classical palpable purpuric rash but an evolving picture may be present with other symptoms such as abdominal pain or arthralgia preceding the rash and making diagnosis more difficult.

The diagnostic criteria for HSP of the Paediatric Rheumatology European Society, superseding those of the American College of Rheumatology, are:

Palpable purpura (mandatory) in the presence of at least one of the following four features:

- Diffuse abdominal pain
- Acute arthritis or arthralgia
- *Renal involvement:* haematuria and/or proteinuria
- A biopsy showing predominant IgA deposition.

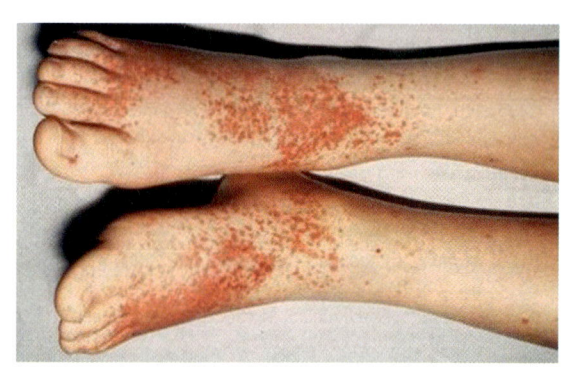

Fig 15.24 HSP: typical purpuric rash and distribution.

As many cases follow an URTI, onset may be accompanied by fever and malaise in addition to specific symptoms reflecting organ involvement:

- *Skin:* the classical rash is a palpable purpuric rash often symmetrical over the extensor, dependant surfaces of the lower limbs and buttocks. This may be preceded by urticarial or erythematous maculopapular lesions and may range from petechiae to large ecchymoses (Fig 15.24).
- *GI tract:* involved in 50–75% of cases, colicky abdominal pain being the most common symptom. Vomiting, GI haemorrhage, bowel wall perforation, or infarction may occur. Intussusception is an important complication. Protein-losing enteropathy, pancreatitis, and hydrops of the gallbladder have all been described.
- *Joints:* arthritis or arthralgia occur in up to 75% of patients and is the presenting complaint in 25%. Large joints of the lower limbs are most commonly affected (feet, ankles, knees) with pain and swelling. Permanent joint damage does not occur.
- *Renal:* renal involvement is present in up to 60% of cases. HSP nephritis may manifest as haematuria (macroscopic or microscopic) with or without proteinuria, or as nephritis, nephrotic syndrome, hypertension, or renal impairment. Severe renal disease is present in 5–7%. Renal involvement may be delayed, but has developed by 4 weeks in 80% and within 3 months in 97% of those affected.

Rare manifestations of HSP include:

- *Orchitis:* a swollen, tender scrotum, bilateral or unilateral, occurs in up to 24% of boys and may mimic torsion. Scrotal oedema may also complicate hypoalbuminaemia. Scrotal USS may be indicated or surgical exploration.
- *Neurological:* headache, encephalopathy, seizures, ataxia may occur.
- *Pulmonary:* diffuse alveolar haemorrhage may present as interstitial pneumonitis.

Children <2 years have less renal, GI, and joint involvement but more subcutaneous oedema.

The diagnosis is usually obvious on account of the characteristic rash, but an atypical presentation may cause difficulties.

Systemic lupus erythematosus may be associated with a similar vasculitic rash. The petechiae of septicaemia usually occurs in an unwell child and immune thrombocytopenic purpura is identified on the full blood count.

Management
Investigations
Diagnosis is clinical but investigations are aimed at excluding other possible diagnoses and assessing the extent of organ involvement, especially renal:
- *FBC*: thrombocytosis has been associated with severe disease, anaemia with blood loss
- *Coagulation screen*: normal
- *Renal biochemistry*: U&E, creatinine
- *Urinalysis*: dipstick and microscopy for haematuria and proteinuria.

Additional investigations are required in certain circumstances:
- *Systematically unwell child*: blood cultures, urine for culture, CXR
- *Diagnosis uncertain*:
  - *autoimmune profile*: antinuclear antibody, dsDNA, ANCA, Immunoglobulins: IgA↑ in 50%, C3, C4, ASOT, antiDNAse B titres
  - *Skin biopsy*: leucocytoclastic vasculitis with IgA deposits on direct immunofluorescence.
- *Severe GI tract symptoms*: ultrasound to exclude intussusception, endoscopy for severe haemorrhage.
- *Renal disease*: renal biopsy is considered if there is acute nephritis, impaired renal function, nephrotic syndrome, or nephrotic range proteinuria (UP:UC>250 mg/mmol) for 4–6 weeks.

Treatment
HSP is in most cases a self-limiting disease and treatment is supportive. Significant morbidity may be associated with GI or renal disease. Abdominal pain usually settles within a few days and joint pain is often managed with NSAIDs unless there is significant renal disease. Specific measures may include:
- *GI disease*: oral prednisolone, 1 mg/kg daily for 2 weeks and weaning over 2 weeks may reduce intensity of abdominal pain and its duration. IV methylprednisolone has been used for severe haemorrhage and for protein-losing enteropathy.
- *HSP nephritis*: long-term renal impairment occurs in 20% of those with nephrotic/nephritic syndrome and renal impairment. Decreased factor XIII activity, hypertension, renal failure, and crescents on renal biopsy have an unfavourable prognosis. The treatment of HSPN remains controversial but early referral to a paediatric nephrologist is appropriate as there is some evidence for benefit from aggressive treatment in those with rapidly progressive glomerulonephritis. Options include methylprednisolone, cyclophosphamide, oral prednisolone, dipyridamole, and plasma exchange.

Prognosis
In two thirds of cases resolution without morbidity occurs within 4 weeks. In one third, recurrence occurs between 6 weeks and 2 years after the initial episode. The long-term outlook is predominantly related to renal involvement. Children should be monitored closely (blood pressure and urine dipstick) for 3–6 months after the acute episode as renal involvement can occur late. 97% develop their renal involvement within 6 months.

50% of children with severe renal disease at presentation have renal insufficiency at 6 years follow-up and HSPN accounts for 2–3% of children with end-stage renal failure. All patients with HSPN require lifelong follow-up as late deterioration can occur especially during pregnancy.

Kawasaki disease (KD)
KD is a systemic vasculitis with a predilection for cardiac involvement which may be fatal. Worldwide the annual incidence varies from 3/100 000 in the UK to 100/100 000 in Japan. It affects predominantly children <5 years with a peak at 18 months. The cardiac features and management are discussed in Chapter 4.7.

Clinical features
Diagnosis is clinical. This disease evolves through three phases: acute, subacute, and convalescent.

Acute phase: day 1–10
Diagnostic criteria include a fever for at least 5 days together with at least four of the following:
1 *Rash*: diffuse, polymorphic, not vesicular, lasts 7 days (Fig 15.25)
2 *Conjunctivitis*: bilateral, no corneal ulceration (anterior uveitis may be present)
3 *Oral mucositis*: strawberry tongue, erythema/cracking of lips and tongue
4 *Cervical lymphadenopathy*: may be a solitary, painful gland
5 *Peripheral extremities*: erythema and oedema in first week.

Subacute phase: day 11–25
Fever, rash, and lymphadenopathy subside. Thrombocytosis develops. The tips of fingers and toes desquamate.

Convalescent phase
Starts once clinical signs disappear and lasts until inflammatory markers normalize.

Differential diagnosis includes toxic shock syndrome, staphylococcal scalded skin syndrome, scarlet fever, and viral infection such as enterovirus, measles, adenovirus, and EBV.

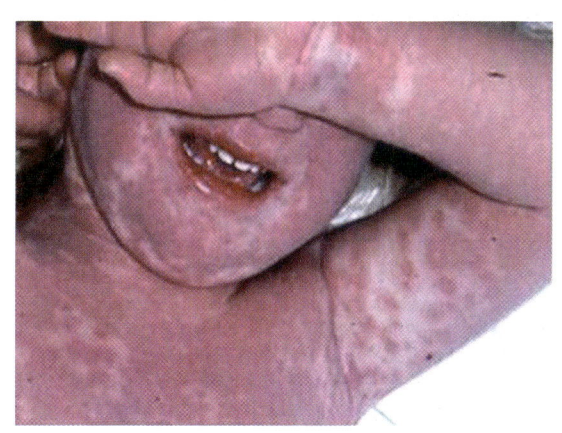

Fig 15.25 Kawasaki disease: polymorphous rash and red lips.

15.19 Case-based discussions

A child with an allergic reaction

A 14 month old boy attends a follow up outpatient clinic after attending the hospital emergency department with 'an allergic reaction'. On that occasion he developed an itchy rash all over his body, with swelling of face, lips, and eyes. His mother thinks it may have occurred as a result of eating some home-made cake. He was discharged home after 4 h of observation.

What further history is required?

The history of the episode is consistent with a mild allergic reaction: urticaria and angioedema. The history suggests that there was no involvement of the respiratory or cardiovascular system. In order to ascertain the severity and possible causes the following questions need to be asked:

- The ingredients of the cake, especially asking if nuts were present. Any other new foods given that day. Quantity ingested
- Interval between ingestion of food and reaction
- Speed of onset and duration of symptoms
- How long the symptoms lasted.
- Past medical history of atopy
- Family history of atopy including hay fever, eczema, asthma, and food allergies
- What medication was given during his 'allergic reaction'.

You find out the following:

After eating just a mouthful of cake the reaction happened within 20 min. He was treated with oral piriton. His mother says they measured his blood pressure and oxygen and they were normal. He has a previous history of atopic dermatitis. His brother has a peanut allergy and so he has never eaten peanuts as they do not have them in the house.

Was the management of this child in the emergency department appropriate?

This child had an immediate-type hypersensitivity reaction, probably to egg. The reaction should have been rated as mild, as there was no evidence of respiratory compromise (dyspnoea, wheeze, bronchospasm, stridor, hypoxaemia) or cardiovascular involvement (reduced BP, syncope, collapse).

If there had been evidence of involvement of respiratory or cardiovascular systems a diagnosis of anaphylaxis would have been appropriate and administration of IM adrenaline indicated.

If the reaction had been moderate or severe the child should not have been discharged home. After initial treatment and resolution of symptoms, 5% of children will go on to develop further symptoms. The second reaction usually occurs 4–10 h after the initial event. Children who have experienced significant allergic reactions should be observed for at least 12 h after treatment.

What is the further management?

IgE sensitivity tests by skin prick tests or allergen-specific IgE levels should be done. For this child, the results of skin prick tests were:

Egg white: strong reaction; peanut: medium reaction; wheat, negative; cow's milk, negative.

The overall PPV of SPTs is 50–65% but the negative predictive value of a negative test approaches 100%.

Advice on food avoidance should be given. Egg should certainly be avoided. A child who has had a severe reaction to cooked egg is likely to have a more severe reaction to the more immunogenic proteins in raw or lightly cooked egg.

This child also has a moderate skin reaction to peanuts, but his clinical response to peanuts is undetermined. It is not, however, uncommon for children to be sensitized to peanuts despite never having been known to ingest such products. He should be advised to avoid peanut products with further clarification of clinical sensitivity by formal in-hospital peanut challenge at aged 4–5 if the sensitization as determined by skin test persists. He should also be tested for sensitivity to other nuts.

A MedicAlert bracelet should be provided, and other carers such as the local nursery should be informed. He does not meet criteria for prescription of self-injectable adrenaline (EpiPen).

A child with chickenpox

A 7 year old girl is admitted with chickenpox. The rash developed 4 days previously and new lesions are continuing to appear. Concern has arisen on account of two painful, spreading lesions on her anterior chest wall (Fig 15.26).

On examination she is systemically unwell with high-grade fever and signs of early circulatory compromise: tachycardia and prolonged peripheral CRT.

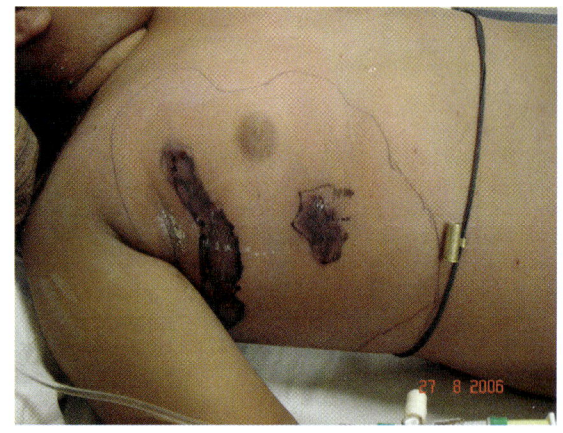

Fig 15.26 Anterior chest wall lesions.

What diagnosis should be considered?

Necrotizing fasciitis is a recognized complication of chickenpox and presents with tender erythematous mottled lesions which spread rapidly. Several factors contribute to pathogenesis. The vesicles create a full-thickness dermal lesion providing a route for bacteria to spread from the skin surface into the subcutaneous tissues. Causative organisms include GAS and *Staph. aureus*.

What is the management?

This is a life-threatening emergency requiring early aggressive surgical debridement. Immediate resuscitation and IV broad-spectrum antibiotics are indicated. Preoperative MRI can be helpful in differentiating necrotizing fasciitis from cellulitis and delineating the affected tissues to aid surgical planning. However, any delay in definitive surgical treatment is inadvisable.

Wound swabs grew a heavy growth of Staph. aureus and GAS. She survived after extensive surgical debridement and intensive care.

Chapter 16
Musculoskeletal disorders

16.1 Musculoskeletal system *346*
16.2 Musculoskeletal system: clinical skills *348*
16.3 Orthopaedics: congenital disorders *350*
16.4 Orthopaedics: acquired disorders *352*
16.5 Osteogenesis imperfecta and achondroplasia *354*
16.6 Osteopetrosis, osteoporosis, and rickets *356*
16.7 Juvenile idiopathic arthritis (JIA) *358*
16.8 Reactive arthritis and transient synovitis *360*
16.9 Systemic lupus erythematosus (SLE) *362*
16.10 Connective tissue disorders *364*
16.11 Osteomyelitis and septic arthritis *366*
16.12 Case-based discussions *368*

16.1 Musculoskeletal system

Development

Skeletal system
The skeletal system develops from mesenchyme, derived from mesoderm and the neural crest. Condensations of mesenchymal cells form models of the bones. In most bones, such as the long bones, the mesenchyme undergoes chondrification followed by endochondral ossification (see below). Some bones, such as the flat bones of the skull, develop by intramembranous ossification.

The appendicular skeleton develops from endochondral ossification of the cartilaginous bone models in the developing limbs. Joints develop from the interzonal mesenchyme between bone primordia.

Limbs
Embryogenesis of the limbs begins towards the end of the 4th week as elevations of the ventrolateral body wall, upper limb buds appearing ~2 days before the lower. The limb buds elongate by mesenchymal proliferation. Condensation into cartilage anlages forms the bone models. Myoblasts originating in the somites form the muscle masses. Differentiation of the limb elements is complete by 8 weeks. The majority of congenital limb anomalies arise during this early period.

Muscular system
The muscular system develops from mesoderm derived from the myotome regions of the somites and from myogenic precursor cells in the limb buds. Most skeletal muscles are distinct by the 8th week. Motor nerve development precedes that of sensory nerves and embryonic movements occur by the 6th week.

Bone
The infant human endoskeleton is composed of 300 bones of 5 main types: long, short, flat, irregular, and sesamoid (embedded in tendons).

Structure
The primary tissue of bone is osseous tissue, essentially a mineralized connective tissue composed of cells, a protein matrix, and mineral. Other tissues found in bone include marrow, endosteum and periosteum, nerves, blood vessels, and cartilage.

Bone is composed of two subtypes:
- *Woven bone:* formed when bone is laid down rapidly as in the fetus, healing fractures, or bone-forming tumours. It is disorganized and weak.
- *Lamellar bone:* formed when bone is laid down slowly. It is composed of an outer cortex of compact, dense bone (80%) and an inner porous network of trabecular, cancellous, or spongy bone (20%).

Osseous tissue is composed of cells and extracellular matrix.

Cells
- *Osteoblasts:* responsible for bone formation. They synthesize osteoid which is primarily type 1 collagen, alkaline phosphatase, and prostaglandins.
- *Osteoclasts:* responsible for bone resorption through secretion of proteolytic enzymes, matrix metalloproteinases, and hydrochloric acid. Activated by osteoblasts and prostaglandins and inhibited by calcitonin.
- *Osteocytes:* mature osteoblasts which are found in bone lacunae and have processes which react to mechanical stress, and contribute to matrix maintenance and calcium homeostasis.

Extracellular matrix
The matrix is the major constituent of bone and is composed of:
- *Organic constituents, 35%:* mostly type 1 collagen
- *Inorganic constituents, 65%:* calcium and phosphate as hydroxyapatite.

The matrix is initially laid down as osteoid by osteoblasts. Mineralization involves osteoblast secretion of vesicles containing alkaline phosphatase which cleaves the phosphate groups and allows calcium and phosphate deposition.

Function
Bones have several functions:
- Maintenance of body shape and structure
- Movement of individual parts or the whole body
- *Protection of internal organs:* skull and ribs
- *Blood production:* site of haematopoiesis
- *Mineral storage:* reserves of calcium and phosphorus.

Formation and growth
The main steps are:
- Development and growth of a cartilage model
- Primary ossification centres in the fetus form the diaphysis of cortical bone with an expanded metaphysis at either end, consisting of cancellous bone.
- Next to the metaphysis lies the cartilaginous growth plate, the physis.
- Secondary ossification centres develop in the epiphyses of the long bones.
- Skeletal maturation is reached when all the cartilage is replaced by bone, fusing the metaphyses and epiphyses together (physeal closure).

Bone remodelling, in which bone is resorbed and replaced with little change in shape, continues throughout life by the action of osteoblasts and osteoclasts controlled in part by paracrine signalling.

Joints
There are three main types of joint:
- *Synovial joints:* with a cavity and designed for movement
- *Fibrous joints:* without a cavity and designed to resist movement: sutures, syndesmoses
- *Cartilaginous joints:* bones attached by cartilage allowing a little movement: synchondroses and symphyses.

Synovial joints
Synovial joints achieve movement at the point of contact between articulating bones. A capsule surrounds the articulating surfaces and a lubricating synovial fluid is present within the capsule. Examples include ball and socket joints (shoulder, hip), hinge joints (knee, elbow between humerus and ulna), and gliding or planar joints (carpals of the wrist).

A synovial joint is composed of five tissue types: bone, cartilage, synovium, synovial fluid, and tensile tissues—ligament and tendon, attached at entheses.

- *Hyaline cartilage*: forms a thin layer on the end of the bone and is the smooth surface allowing gliding movement and bearing weight. It consists of cartilage matrix composed of collagen and proteoglycans in which are embedded the chondrocytes that secrete the cartilage matrix.
- *Synovium*: is the soft tissue that lines the non-cartilaginous surfaces within the joint cavity and the cavities of tendon sheaths and bursae. The outer layer or subintima may be fibrous, fatty, or areolar and the inner layer or intima is a layer of modified fibroblasts and macrophages.

Normal synovial fluid is clear and noticeably thick and viscous, like egg white. Its viscous and elastic properties are due to hyaluronan, a long-chain glycosaminoglycan. Lubrication is provided by a specialized glycoprotein, lubricin.

Ligaments hold bones together and tendons transmit muscle power to bones. The point where ligament, tendon, or aponeurosis joins bone is called an *enthesis*.

Connective tissue

Connective tissue, derived from mesoderm, is classified into:
- *Connective tissue proper*: areolar or fibrous
- *Specialized connective tissue*: blood, bone, cartilage, fat
- *Embryonic connective tissue*: mesenchymal or mucous.

Connective tissue proper

The extracellular matrix of connective tissue proper contains fibres composed of various structural proteins including collagen, elastin, and fibrillin. It is classified into:
- *Areolar*: loose connective tissue holding organs, and epithelia in place with fibres of collagen or elastin
- *Fibrous*: densely packed collagen fibres form ligaments and tendons.

The three important protein components, collagen, elastin, and fibrillin are considered in turn.

Collagen

Collagen is the most abundant protein in the human body, comprising 25% of the whole body protein content.

Collagen chains are synthesized as longer precursor procollagens which undergo post-translational glycosylation and hydroxylation before secretion into the extracellular space. The subunits form a triple-stranded helix which is secreted. The propeptides are then removed by procollagen peptidase to form tropocollagen. The tropocollagen subunits self-assemble into fibrils which are bundled into fibres (Fig 16.1).

The triple-helical structure arises from an unusual abundance of three amino acids: glycine, proline, and hydroxyproline which make up a repeating motif Gly-Pro-X.

Types of collagen

There are 16 different types of collagen encoded by >30 different genes. Over 90% of the collagen in the body is accounted for by collagens I, II, III and IV. Their locations can be remembered by the following:

Collagen I:	**ONE**	(b**ONE**):	bone
Collagen II:	**TWO**	(car**TWO**lage):	cartilage
Collagen III:	**THREE**	(re**THREE**cular):	reticular fibres
Collagen IV:	**FOUR**	(F|**OUR**e):	basement membranes.

- *Type I collagen*: gives bone its elasticity and strength. Each triple helix has two α_1 and one α_2 chains.
- *Type II collagen*: is the major collagen in cartilage.
- *Type III collagen*: is the main component of reticular fibres in the skin, muscle, and blood vessels.
- *Type IV collagen*: forms the network of all basal lamina.

Collagen is therefore the main protein component of bones and teeth as well as cartilage, ligaments, tendons, and fascia. Along with keratin it gives strength and elasticity to skin. It is present in the cornea and lens of the eye.

Elastin

Elastin is a specialized protein made by linking soluble tropoelastin molecules together.

Amorphous elastin is a component of elastic microfibrils in which it is deposited on a scaffold of microfibrillar-associated proteins. Microfibrils are bundled into elastic fibres which are found in the skin, lungs, arteries, veins, connective tissue proper, elastic cartilage, periodontal ligament, bladder, and intervertebral discs. Elastin synthesis stops at age 12 years.

Elastin is encoded by the elastin gene *ELN* on chromosome 2q. Deletions causing Williams syndrome usually include *ELN* and mutations in *ELN* cause supravalvar aortic stenosis.

Fibrillin

Fibrillin-1 is a major component of the microfibrils, forming a sheath around amorphous elastin. It is a large glycoprotein with cysteine-rich and calcium-binding domains. It is encoded by the *FBN-1* gene, defective in Marfan syndrome (MFS).

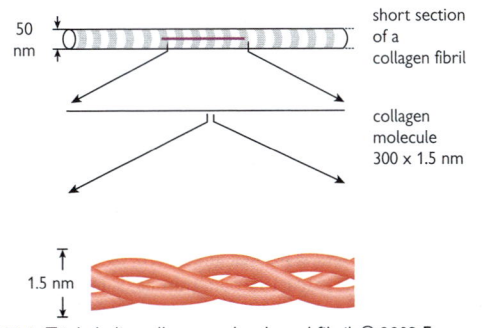

Fig 16.1 Triple helix collagen molecule and fibril. © 2003 From Essential Cell Biology, 2E by Alberts et al. Reproduced by permission of Garland Science/Taylor and Francis.

16.2 Musculoskeletal system: clinical skills

History
Musculoskeletal conditions often present with pain or alterations in any behaviour requiring mobility and locomotion.
Young children may of course have difficulty localizing pain, and the history is often inferred from a carer's observations. Enquiry should focus on the nature of any pain/preceding factors and the presence or absence of systemic symptoms.

Pain
- Is it localized or diffuse and multiple?
- Localized to long bone, joint, back, or muscle?
- Acute onset or trauma related?
- Related to activity or to period of rest (morning stiffness)?
- Mechanical joint pain often has an acute, trauma-related onset and is worse on activity and eased by rest. Inflammatory joint pain is more likely to be protracted and insidious, eased with activity and worse after rest (morning stiffness or 'gelling') and associated with immobility.
- Hip pathology may cause referred pain in the knee. Nocturnal pain is always significant and suggests inflammatory disease or malignancy.
- Nocturnal limb pains or 'growing pains' are a diagnosis of exclusion and characteristically occur in the age group 3–11 years. There is lower limb pain, often symmetrical, not present on awakening and with no limitation of physical activities or limp. Physical examination is normal except for hypermobility.

Recent history
Trauma or sporting activity or recent upper respiratory tract or gastrointestinal infection (reactive arthritis).

Systemic symptoms
Fever, malaise, weakness, anorexia, weight loss, or rashes.

Examination
Systemic examination is combined with
- *pGALS*, paediatric Gait, Arms, Legs, Spine: a musculoskeletal locomotor screening examination
- *pREMS*: paediatric regional examination of the musculoskeletal system based on the 'look, feel, move' principles.

A knowledge of normal variants of posture and gait at different ages is essential.

Systemic examination
- *Fever:* suggests inflammation or infection
- *Systemic toxicity:* suggests sepsis
- *Rash:* may be seen in systemic lupus erythematosus (SLE), Henoch–Schönlein purpura (HSP), dermatomyositis
- *Anaemia:* sickle cell disease, leukaemia
- *Abdominal examination:* tenderness or mass in inflammatory bowel disease (IBD), organomegaly in leukaemia.

pGALS
A modified paediatric version of the GALS system used in adult practice allows an initial screen of the locomotor system to be followed by detailed examination of the relevant area (pREMS). Gait, and the most common abnormality of gait, a limp, are considered in detail below.

For the screening manoeuvres, features assessed, and abnormalities detected, see Box.

> **pGALs screening procedure**
> - Observe standing from all sides for posture and habitus.
>
> **GAIT**
> Observe walking on tip-toe and heels. See below for details
>
> **ARMS**
> The following manoeuvres test function and movement at the joints of the shoulder, arm, and hands:
> - 'Put your hands behind your head'
> - 'Hold your hands straight out in front of you'
> - 'Reach up, touch the sky and look at the ceiling'
> - 'Turn your hands over and make a fist'
> - 'Pinch index finger and thumb together'
> - 'Put hands together palm to palm, then back to back'
> - Squeeze the metacarpophalangeal joints (MCPs) gently.
>
> **LEGS**
> Inspect while standing:
> - Normal quadriceps bulk and symmetry
> - Knee swelling or deformity
> - Foot: normal or abnormal foot arches.
>
> Examine while lying:
> - Feel for knee effusion, press on patella
> - Test active movement of knees, feel for crepitus
> - Test passive movement of hip flexion, internal rotation.
>
> **SPINE**
> - 'Open wide and put three of your fingers in your mouth' (tests temporomandibular joint)
> - 'Try and touch your shoulder with your ear'
> - 'Bend forward and touch your toes'.
>
> Ask the child to copy you in doing the manoeuvres, and look for non-verbal and verbal clues for discomfort. Checking for asymmetry allows early identification of subtle abnormalities.

Gait: detailed assessment
Gait refers to a manner of forward progress, which in humans includes walking, running, hopping, skipping, and crawling. A normal mature walking gait involves a cyclic loss and regaining of balance with an alternating and symmetrical swing, stance, and toe-off phase for each leg.

Ambulation begins with a broad base, arms outstretched for balance evolving into the reciprocal arm swing of a mature gait. Gait should be observed with the child wearing shorts and in bare feet, and the following noted:
- Symmetrical or asymmetrical?
- Reciprocal arm swing?
- Heel strike present or walking flat footed or on toes?

Gait patterns may be normal variants or pathological.

Normal variants in gait and stance
Bow legs (genu varum) is normal at birth to 18–24 months and knock knees (genu valgus) is common at 3–4 years, usually correcting by 7 years. Flat feet with normal arches evident on

tiptoeing resolve by 6 years. Rickets and Blount disease are pathological causes of bow legs.

Intoed gait

This arises from normal developmental variation at three sites in the feet, leg, and hip.
- *Feet*: metatarsus adductus: corrects by 2 years.
- *Leg*: internal tibial torsion: often associated with bow legs in Afro-Caribbeans. Corrects by 4–6 years.
- *Hip*: persistent femoral anteversion: hip joint internally rotates. Corrects by 8–10 years.

Tiptoed gait

This often represents a transient phase in development of normal gait. Pathological causes include limb shortening if unilateral, cerebral palsy with tight Achilles tendons, and muscular dystrophy if late onset and DDH. Idiopathic toe walking is a diagnosis of exclusion.

Pathological gait variants: limp

A limp, or asymmetrical gait, is the most common abnormality. Several types are recognized:
- *Antalgic limp*: pain on weight-bearing is minimized by shortening the stance phase. The extreme of this situation is refusal to weight-bear or walk.
- *Trendelenberg test*: when walking the pelvis drops rather than rises on the side opposite to that bearing the weight, usually due to abductor weakness. Occurs in unilateral chronic hip disease and cerebral palsy. Bilateral pathology causes a 'waddling' gait.
- *Unilateral foot-drop*: weak ankle dorsiflexors as in peroneal neuropathy leads to a high stepping gait.
- *Unilateral equinus gait*: limited ankle dorsiflexion caused by shortening of Achilles tendon or gastrocnemius tightening.

Causes of a limp

The causes of limping in children are legion. The age of the child, duration of the limp and presence or absence of pain are important guides.

The most important cause of acute painful limp at all ages is mechanical trauma followed by bone or joint infection, and joint inflammation which may be benign as in 'transient synovitis' or more serious as in juvenile idiopathic arthritis. Common causes by age are shown in the Box.

Causes of an acute painful limp

Toddler up to 5 years:
- *Infection*: septic arthritis, osteomyelitis, discitis
- *Mechanical trauma*: non-accidental injury, toddler's fracture

5–10 years:
- *Mechanical trauma*: overuse injuries, sports injuries
- Transient synovitis/ irritable hip
- Perthes disease
- *Less common*: juvenile idiopathic arthritis, malignant disease

10–17 years:
- *Mechanical trauma*: overuse injuries, sport injuries
- Slipped capital femoral epiphysis
- Juvenile idiopathic arthritis
- *Malignant disease*: leukaemia, lymphoma, bone tumour
- Idiopathic pain syndromes, conversion disorder.

---

pREMS: regional examination: 'look, feel, move'

If pGALS identifies a local problem the relevant region is examined by inspection, palpation and, if in a joint, assessment of active and passive movements.

Look: inspection

Inspect a joint for swelling, erythema, and evidence of muscle wasting (e.g. quadriceps atrophy in knee inflammation). A collagen disorder may show scarring and skin laxity. Inflamed joints are held in a position of comfort, usually flexion at the knee and flexion with external rotation at the hip.

Feel: palpation

Palpation of accessible joints will reveal warmth, swelling, or tenderness. The hip and sacroiliac joints are not of course accessible to palpation. Muscle tenderness may be present in inflammatory myopathies.

Movement

The range of movement, active and passive, should be tested and any reduction, painful or otherwise, noted.

Causes of a swollen joint

A swollen joint indicates arthropathy which may or may not represent inflammation (arthritis) and may or may not cause arthralgia (pain). The causes of a swollen joint are many and categorized according to pathological mechanism:
- *Trauma*: accidental or non-accidental
- *Infection*: septic arthritis, viral arthritis
- *Inflammation*: postinfectious arthritis, juvenile idiopathic arthritis (JIA), SLE, DM.
- *Vasculitis*: HSP
- *Haematological*: sickle cell disease, haemophilia
- *Malignancy*: leukaemia, Ewing sarcoma, osteosarcoma
- Drug reactions.

Investigations

Imaging dominates the investigation of musculoskeletal disorders and is considered here. Blood tests and microbiological samples are often required and the indications for specific tests are considered with each disease.

Imaging

- *Radiology*: plain radiographs provide clear views of bones and joints and useful information regarding soft tissues including joint effusions. If hip pathology is suspected, AP and frog-leg lateral views of the pelvis are required.
- *Ultrasound*: especially useful for imaging the hip joint. It is sensitive for detection of hip joint fluid but has low specificity for distinguishing pus, blood, and inflammatory effusion. It is the most useful initial investigation for detection of effusion or developmental dysplasia of the hip.
- *Radionuclide scan*: ^{99m}Technetium-labelled methylene diphosphonate is taken up at skeletal sites with increased bone turnover or blood supply.
- *Magnetic resonance imaging*: MRI is more sensitive than radiology in detecting bone or joint infection. It is the modality of choice for imaging the vertebral column and spinal cord.

16.3 Orthopaedics: congenital disorders

Arthrogryposis
Arthrogryposis is the term used for joint contractures, and occurs in a number of distinct syndromes.

Arthrogryposis multiplex congenital (AMC)
Contractures affecting multiple joints develop prenatally and are apparent at birth. Joint motion is essential for normal musculoskeletal development. Limb movement is normally apparent from 8 weeks and prenatal limitation of joint mobility leads to contractures. The incidence is 1/3000 live births.

Causes
- *Extrinsic:* fetal crowding or constraint due to oligohydramnios or multiple pregnancy.
- *Intrinsic:*
  - *neurological:* anencephaly, neural tube defects, anterior horn cell defects
  - *muscular:* congenital myopathy, myotonic dystrophy, myasthenia gravis
  - *skeletal:* synostosis, prenatal joint fixation.

Clinical features
It is usually symmetrical and involves all four limbs. In severe forms, jaw and back are affected. There is muscle weakness, fibrosis, and short tendons. Facies are normal, intelligence is unaffected, and the condition is non-progressive.

Management
Investigations are directed towards identifying an underlying cause, a genetic disorder being present in 30%. Treatment options include multidisciplinary assessment, physiotherapy, and occupational therapy. Surgical intervention may be required and attention is given to the psychosocial and emotional implications.

Distal arthrogryposis syndrome
Distal arthrogryposis syndrome is a rare, heterogeneous autosomal dominant (AD) disorder. Several different types exist. The hands and feet are predominantly affected, with overlapping fingers, ulnar deviation and flexion contractures of fingers, and foot deformities including talipes equinovarus and vertical talus. There may be webbing of soft tissues, so-called pterygia.

Congenital talipes equinovarus (CTEV)
In this deformity of the foot and ankle (*talipes*, Latin *talus* = ankle + *pes* = foot), also called 'club foot', the foot is held in a rigid equinovarus position (Fig 16.2). The foot is inverted and supinated and the forefoot is adducted. The incidence is 1/1000 live births and it is more common in boys.

Aetiology and pathogenesis
CTEV is distinguished from *positional talipes equinovarus* which can be passively corrected, i.e. the foot can be fully dorsiflexed to touch the front of the lower leg. This resolves spontaneously within 6–12 weeks.
True CTEV may be:
- *Idiopathic, primary:* there is multifactorial inheritance with a 20–30% risk for offspring of an affected parent and a 3% risk for sibling of an affected infant.
- *Secondary:* oligohydramnios, neuromuscular disorders such as spina bifida, arthrogryposis, malformation syndromes.

The main abnormality is subluxation of the talonavicular joint. The affected foot is shorter and the calf muscles, Achilles tendon, and tibialis posterior tendon are small and tight.

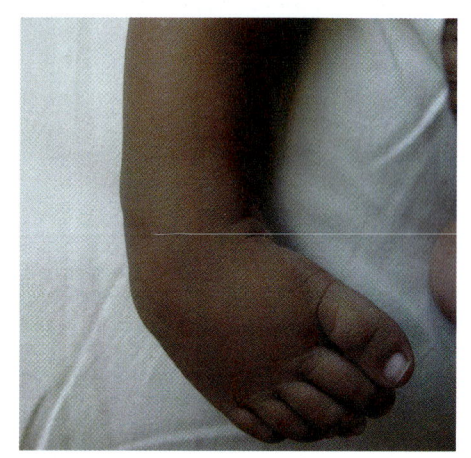

Fig 16.2 Congenital talipes equinovarus.

Clinical evaluation
Antenatal diagnosis may be made on ultrasound. The hind foot lies in equinus and varus with a supinated and adducted forefoot and deep skin creases. Positional talipes should be excluded and underlying causes sought.

Management
Referral is made to an orthopaedic surgeon. Early treatment improves prognosis. Conservative treatment encompasses the Ponseti technique:
- Manipulation and serial plaster casts.
- Percutaneous tenotomy of Achilles tendon under local anaesthetic at ~6 weeks.
- 'Boots and bars' treatment for first few years as necessary with further plastering if deformity recurs.

Corrective surgery may be required at 6–12 months of age if there is a failure to obtain or maintain reduction of the talonavicular joint and hindfoot/forefoot alignment. Soft tissue release and realignment of joints is carried out.

The prognosis for idiopathic club foot is good with a functional, pain free, supple plantigrade foot as the usual outcome. Surgery is more often required in the context of a neuromuscular disorder or syndrome and recurrent deformity is not uncommon.

Developmental dysplasia of the hip (DDH)
This condition includes a spectrum of abnormalities ranging from self-limiting neonatal hip instability, through subluxation or partial dislocation with acetabular dysplasia to complete hip dislocation.

The incidence of abnormal hips on neonatal screening is 6–15/1000 live births, but only 1–2/1000 have established dislocation requiring treatment.

Aetiology and pathogenesis
Risk factors include:
- *Female sex:* F:M ratio 5:1
- First-born child
- *Positive family history:* in 20% of affected infants
- Breech presentation.

The presence of the femoral head within the acetabulum is the stimulus for normal hip development. A combination of factors including joint laxity, poor muscle tone, and abnormal acetabular shape may lead to instability of the hip joint, or subluxation or complete dislocation.

Clinical evaluation

Screening for DDH is part of the routine neonatal examination (see Chapter 2). The Barlow manoeuvre tests for a dislocatable hip and the Ortolani test establishes whether a hip is dislocated and can be relocated into the acetabulum.

Ultrasound scan

A hip ultrasound scan is useful at 4–6 weeks of age. Most centres perform selective screening of at-risk infants with family history or breech delivery but the value of routine ultrasound screening of all infants is still being assessed.

Late presentation may manifest as delayed walking, abnormal gait, or 'stiffness' during nappy changing especially if bilateral. The Barlow and Ortolani tests are difficult to perform after the first few months in neurologically normal children. The clinical signs at this stage include:
- Limitation of abduction of the flexed hip
- Apparent shortening of the leg which lies in external rotation
- *Positive Galeazzi test:* one knee lower than the other when both hips and knees flexed to right angle
- *Abnormal gait:* there may be a waddling, Trendelenburg gait, unilateral toe walking or exaggerated lumbar lordosis particularly in bilateral dislocation
- Asymmetrical thigh skin creases.

Management

Investigations

Hip ultrasound scan is indicated if an abnormal hip is suspected on newborn examination or in at risk infants. After 4–6 months an AP pelvic radiograph is the optimal investigation. This may reveal delay in ossification of the femoral head, a broken Shenton's line and increased acetabular slope (Fig 16.3).

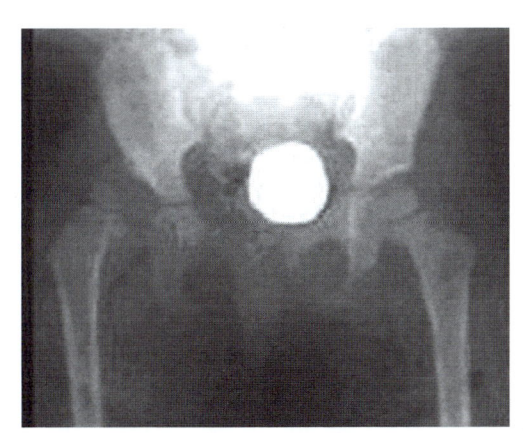

Fig 16.3 DDH: delayed ossification of femoral head and increased slope of acetabulum on right side at age 2 years with subluxation of the joint.

Treatment
Conservative

Most unstable hips detected at birth will resolve within the first few weeks of life. Clinical and ultrasound assessment is repeated at 2–3 weeks and treatment commenced for persistent instability or dislocation by 4–6 weeks at the latest using the Pavlik harness.

The Pavlik harness holds the hip in flexion and abduction encouraging the hip to reduce into the joint and reducing risk of dislocation by preventing adduction and extension. The femoral head gradually stabilizes within the acetabulum. Progress is monitored clinically and with ultrasound. The usual period in the harness is 6–12 weeks with a success rate of 85% or more.

Operative

Indications are failed conservative treatment or late presentation after 3 months. Options are closed reduction with release of tight adductor and psoas muscles or open reduction with release of the joint capsule as well as muscle releases. The reduced position is held with a plaster cast such as a hip spica for some months. In addition, a femoral and/or pelvic osteotomy may be required especially in those presenting after age 2 years.

Early identification and treatment of DDH confers a good prognosis. Avascular necrosis of the femoral head may occur secondary to treatment in 5%. Residual hip problems may lead to early onset degenerative arthritis.

Flat feet

A flat foot has no medial arch on weight-bearing. This is normal in babies partly due to fat masking the arch and partly because the arch only fully develops by age 4–6 years.

Flat feet are usefully classified as:
- *Flexible:* flat feet apparent on standing in full weight-bearing position but an arch appears when person stands on tip toe.
- *Rigid:* the arch is always absent due to pain, muscle spasm, or abnormal anatomy.

Flexible flat feet

Supple, flexible flat feet are very common and usually of no clinical significance. Risk factors include a family history and joint laxity which allows the foot to adopt a planovalgus position on weight-bearing.

Most flexible flat feet are asymptomatic and presentation is on account of parental concern. There may be aching discomfort in feet or calves, worse on activity.

Examination should exclude excessive joint laxity or a neuromuscular disorder. Flat feet improve with age as joint laxity lessens. Orthotic supports may improve symptoms.

Rigid flat feet

In this condition, the arch is absent even when the patient is not standing. Causes include:
- *Painful foot lesions:* infection, inflammation such as JIA
- *Tarsal coalition:* abnormal union of two or more bones in the hindfoot or midfoot: talocalcaneal, calcaneonavicular.

Pain on movement provokes muscle spasm and a stiff joint. Symptoms may include pain and stiffness with limping. Examination should exclude a generalized arthropathy and may reveal a stiff subtalar joint.

Management

Investigations and treatment depend on aetiology. Plain radiographs of the foot and a CT scan will identify a tarsal coalition and may exclude infection. Blood tests for inflammation markers are required for suspected infection or JIA.

For symptomatic tarsal coalition management depends on location and extent of the coalition. Conservative therapy is usually tried first: analgesia and anti-inflammatories, rest, below-knee walking cast. If this fails, surgical options include resection of the coalition and rarely arthrodesis.

16.4 Orthopaedics: acquired disorders

Perthes disease

Perthes disease or syndrome is a childhood hip disorder characterized by idiopathic avascular necrosis of the bony epiphysis of the femoral head. The incidence is 1–2/10 000 and boys are affected 3–5 times more often than girls. It usually affects children aged 4–8 years, range 2–12 years.

Aetiology and pathogenesis

The aetiology is unknown. The incidence is increased in boys, lower socio-economic groups and low birthweight children. Familial clustering indicates a genetic contribution.

(Avascular necrosis may also occur as a complication of sickle cell disease, treatment of developmental dysplasia of the hip, steroid therapy or infection).

Pathogenesis

Perthes disease is a dynamic process with several stages:
- Blood supply to the ossific nucleus of the femoral head is compromised
- Necrosis of the bone results in flattening and collapse and fragmentation of the femoral head
- The femoral head becomes revascularized over several months and the femoral head regrows and remodels over several years
- The femoral head may return to normal, or permanent deformation may cause incongruous joint movement.

The disease is bilateral in 10–20%.

Several staging schemes have been proposed, including the most commonly used Herring scheme based on the fragmentation stage of the lateral pillar of the femoral head.

Clinical features

The presenting symptom is pain which may be localized to groin, thigh, hip, or knee and is usually accompanied by a limp which is initially intermittent.

Examination findings depend on stage and severity:
- *Gait:* antalgic limp if unilateral
- *Limitation of hip joint movement:* loss of abduction and internal rotation with a fixed flexion deformity
- A short leg lying in external rotation
- Wasting of upper thigh muscles.

The differential diagnosis includes all causes of a painful limp in the older child and other causes of avascular necrosis. Multiple epiphyseal dysplasia is bilateral and symmetrical.

Management

Investigations

Plain radiography of the pelvis with AP and frog lateral views is the modality of choice (Fig 16.4). However, radiographs may be normal in early symptomatic disease. Bone scan is more sensitive in the early case. MRI is equally sensitive and allows more precise localization of involvement.

Treatment

Prognosis and treatment both depend on age and severity. At least half of all cases will resolve without deformity and without any treatment, especially children aged <5 years and milder cases.

Conservative management of mild cases aims to maintain the range of movement and contain the femoral head in the acetabulum and includes:

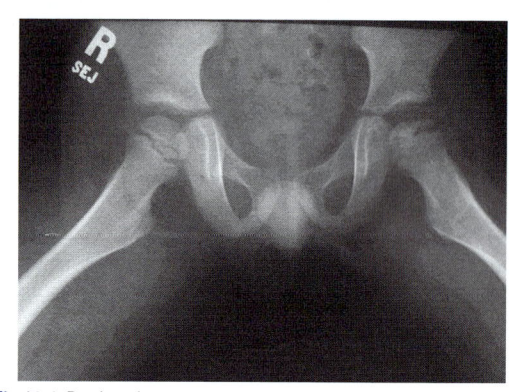

Fig 16.4 Perthes disease: unilateral left sided.

- *Maintaining range of movement:* physiotherapy, swimming uses hip joint in full range of movements, avoidance of wheelchair and crutches which favour stiff hip in flexion and adduction
- Analgesia
- Observation.

In more severe cases options may include:
- Bed rest or crutches if pain is severe
- *Surgery:* The indications for surgery remain controversial. Some recommend femoral or pelvic osteotomy in early Perthes to protect the vulnerable femoral head from deformational forces.

Children <5 years have a very good chance of full recovery, but if the process starts later and involves the whole head there is less time for remodelling of the joint and the prognosis is less good.

Osgood–Schlatter disease

This is a benign, self-limiting common cause of knee pain in active young adolescents resulting from inflammation at the site of insertion of the patellar tendon into the tibial tuberosity. It is more common in boys and bilateral in 25% of patients.

It arises from a combination of the rapid growth spurt and stress from activity, especially running and jumping. Stress from contraction of the quadriceps is transmitted through the patellar tendon on to a small portion of the partially developed tibial tuberosity.

Pain is the most common presenting symptom, together with swelling over the tibial tubercle. The differential diagnosis includes osteosarcoma, so-called chondromalacia patella or idiopathic anterior knee pain, and osteomyelitis. AP and lateral knee radiographs are indicated to exclude other pathology such as neoplasm or infection.

Treatment is conservative and includes analgesics and NSAIDs, ice applications, and rest. Full recovery is expected but may take time.

Slipped capital femoral epiphysis (SCFE)

The capital or upper femoral epiphysis slips off the femoral neck at the level of the cartilaginous growth plate or physis. The incidence is 2–10/100 000. It occurs in prepubertal boys and girls with a M:F ratio of 2.4:1.

Aetiology and pathogenesis

The cartilage physeal plate is weaker than the surrounding bone and affected patients have an expanded hypertrophic zone. Slippage occurs through this weakened area.
Risk factors include:
- *Gender and race:* common in Afro-Caribbean boys
- *Obesity:* places more shear forces on the growth plate
- *Hormonal changes:* associated with prepubertal period
- *Genetics:* family history in 5–7%
- *Trauma:* minor trauma may precede the slip.

In children <10 years bilateral SCFE may be associated with endocrine disorders: hypothyroidism, panhypopituitarism, growth hormone abnormalities.

Clinical features

The presenting symptom is aching pain in the thigh, knee, or groin which may follow an episode of trauma.

Examination may reveal:
- *Abnormal gait:* antalgic limp, inability to weight-bear
- Short and externally rotated leg
- Restricted hip movements.

SCFE is classified into:
- *Acute, chronic or acute on chronic:* symptoms for <3 weeks are acute and >3 weeks are chronic.
- *Stable or unstable:* based on ability to weight-bear
- *Grades of severity:* based on the % displacement of femoral head in relation to neck: mild <30%, moderate 30–50%, severe >50%.

Management

Diagnosis is based on AP and lateral radiographs of the pelvis and hips. The degree of slippage is estimated. In patients <10 years endocrine investigation should be considered.

Treatment

Surgery is usually required. Initial treatment includes analgesia and relief of weight-bearing. An acute, unstable hip is an orthopaedic emergency requiring operation within 24 h. The aim of surgery is to prevent further slippage until the physis has closed. Most hips do well. Complications include chondrolysis and avascular necrosis as complications of treatment and degenerative arthritis. 'Prophylactic' pinning of the normal hip is advised by some.

Scoliosis

This is a growth-related deformity of the spine in which there is abnormal lateral curvature and a rotational deformity of variable magnitude. The prevalence is 0.5–3%. It is most common in adolescent girls.

Aetiology and pathogenesis

Scoliosis is classified into postural and structural types:
- *Postural scoliosis:* this is fully correctable and is caused by leg length discrepancy or poor posture
- *Structural scoliosis:* there is a primary or 'fixed' curve compensated by one or more secondary curves. Left and right refer to the convexity of the primary curve.

Most structural cases are idiopathic. Adolescent idiopathic scoliosis accounts for most patients and has a genetic contribution to aetiology. The female to male ratio is 8:1 and 90% are right thoracic curves. Inheritance is AD with incomplete penetrance.

Structural scoliosis may also occur secondary to diseases which affect the neuromuscular support or vertebral anatomy such as cerebral palsy and muscular dystrophy, vertebral anomalies, trauma, radiotherapy, and genetic syndromes such as neurofibromatosis 1.

Curve progression is a key factor determining outcome and may be difficult to predict. Severe curvature will compromise cardiorespiratory function.

Clinical evaluation

Spinal curvature may be noted by a family member or on routine medical examination. It is usually asymptomatic but may be associated with back pain. Clinical examination focuses on evaluating whether any spinal curvature is postural or structural, and on identifying any underlying cause:

Spine examination

Observe standing if possible from front, side, and back. Check for asymmetry of shoulders and hips.

Perform Adams forward bend test: ask child to bend forward and place clasped hands between knees. Rib prominence is visible on side of the curve.

Palpate whole spine for tenderness, swelling, or muscle spasm. Assess lower limb lengths for true or apparent asymmetry and assess straight leg raise for root pain. General and neurological examination may identify a cause.

Management

Plain radiographs of the whole spine in AP and lateral view are required. MRI is advisable in all children <12 years and in any adolescent with a left thoracic curve, rapid progression, or neurological signs. Treatment options include observation, bracing, and surgery. Adolescent idiopathic scoliosis can be observed if the curve remains <25°, braced if 25–40°, and surgery considered if >40°.

16.5 Osteogenesis imperfecta and achondroplasia

Osteogenesis imperfecta (OI)

OI or brittle bone disease is a group of genetic disorders characterized by increased bone fragility and a spectrum of clinical phenotypes ranging from mild to severe and lethal. The overall incidence is 1/5000 and sex incidence is equal.

Aetiology and pathogenesis
OI types I–IV are caused by mutations in either of two genes encoding type I collagen chains:
- *COLIA1*: encoding the collagen type 1 pro-α_1 chain.
- *COLIA2*: encoding the collagen type 1 pro-α_2 chain.

Most cases show AD inheritance.

Molecular pathogenesis.
Type 1 collagen fibres are present in bone, but also in teeth, sclera, and ligaments. They are composed of triple-helical molecules formed by intertwining two pro-α_1 chains and one pro-α_2 chain.

Mutations that result in a reduction in *quantity* of type 1 collagen usually cause mild OI whereas mutations that lead to half the normal amounts of *defective* collagen cause severe OI by a dominant negative effect.

Additional rare syndromes resembling OI but not caused by mutations in *COLIA* genes have recently been described and designated OI types V–VIII.

Collagen gene disorders
Mutations in at least 22 different collagen genes cause diseases with phenotypes reflecting the distinct roles of different collagens in the body tissues. In addition to OI, collagen gene disorders include Ehlers–Danlos syndrome, epidermolysis bullosa, Alport syndrome, Stickler syndrome, and Bethlem myopathy.

Clinical features and evaluation
The phenotype is variable and classified into types I–IV.

Type I: mild. Incidence 1/30 000 live births
The most common and mildest type of OI. Inheritance is AD but new mutations occur so a family history of OI may be absent. Presentation is usually with fractures after minor trauma, most fractures occurring before puberty. Variable features include:
- *Hearing loss:* often begins in 3rd decade
- *Dentinogenesis imperfecta:* opalescent teeth in type IB, absent in type IA
- *Mitral valve prolapse:* in 50%.

Examination usually reveals:
- Normal stature
- Blue sclera (a blue-grey tint from choroidal veins)
- Kyphoscoliosis
- Easy bruising, joint laxity and muscle weakness.

Radiologic features
Wormian bones in skull. Thinning of long bones with thin cortices. Mild platyspondyly. Old fractures but usually no deformity of long bones.

Type II: very severe. Incidence 1/60 000 live births
An extremely severe form, often with early lethality. 50% are stillborn. All patients have *in utero* fractures and diagnosis may be made prenatally. There is short trunk and limbs, small chest with protuberant abdomen, soft calvarium, small nose, and micrognathia. Inheritance may be AD or AR.

Radiography shows multiple fractures, gross under-ossification, deformed (crumpled) long bones, and beaded ribs.

Most cases die within the 1st year due to severe respiratory problems from pulmonary hypoplasia or brain haemorrhage.

Type III: severe
A severe form with progressive deformity. *In utero* fractures are common. On examination there is short stature, limb shortening with progressive deformity, triangular face with frontal bossing, spinal curvature, and barrel-shaped thorax. Sclera have variable hues and there may be joint laxity and early hearing loss. Respiratory problems, constipation, and herniae occur.

Radiography shows severe osteoporosis, thin bowed long bones, biconcave vertebrae, Wormian bones.

Type IV: variable
This type is between types I and III in severity. Most fractures occur before puberty. Sclera are blueish at birth but become normal in colour. Slight short stature and a mild to moderate bone deformity occur. Brittle teeth and hearing loss are variable. Inheritance is AD.

Radiography shows osteopaenia and fractures.

Diagnostic investigations
Diagnosis is made on the clinical and radiographic findings. The differential diagnosis may include non-accidental injury (NAI), especially in mild OI. Differentiating features between OI and NAI include the type of fracture (metaphyseal corner fractures common in NAI, not in OI). OI does not account for certain non-skeletal manifestations if these are present. In OI, fractures continue while child is in a place of safety.

Unfortunately, OI and child abuse can coexist and definitive exclusion of OI by investigation is challenging. Available tests include:
- *Skin biopsy:* collagen synthesis analysis in cultured dermal fibroblasts. False negative rate is 15%
- *Bone mineral density:* dual-energy X-ray absorptiometry (DEXA) scan can be normal in OI
- *Bone biopsy:* bone histology is variable
- *Genetic testing:* mutation analysis of collagen genes is not readily available: the genes are large and each family harbours a unique mutation.

Treatment
Medical care
Treatment is directed towards preventing and treating fractures, maximizing independent mobility and weight-bearing and developing optimal bone mass and muscle strength. Strategies include:
- Optimal nutrition (calcium, vitamin D) and exercise
- Advice and counselling to parents on handling
- Use of wheelchairs, braces, and mobility aids, e.g. special shoes for valgus ankles
- *Bisphosphonates:* cyclical administration of IV pamidronate reduces bone pain and fracture rate and increases bone mineral density.

- *Fracture care:* fractures heal normally in 85% of patients but emphasis is on minimizing disuse osteoporosis and maintaining normal alignment.
- *Regular hearing tests:* every 3 years from age 7.
- Dental treatment.

Surgical treatment

Interventions may include:

- *Intramedullary rod placement:* metal rods inserted into long bones for internal fixation may improve weight-bearing in children with bowed long legs and assist in correcting limb alignment after fractures, especially of the femur.
- *Scoliosis surgery:* spinal fusion may be performed.

General anaesthesia is a risk in OI due to neck hypermobility, risk of basilar compression, and risk of hyperthermia.

Genetic counselling is usually as for AD inheritance. In type II OI the recurrence risk in siblings is 5%, reflecting the contribution of parental germ cell mosaicism.

Prognosis is variable. Most children and adults with OI lead productive and active lives although children with more severe forms are often wheelchair bound.

Achondroplasia

Achondroplasia is an AD genetic disease characterized by short stature with disproportionate shortening of the proximal limbs. The incidence is 1/15 000–45 000 worldwide. Sex incidence is equal.

Aetiology and pathogenesis

Achondroplasia is caused by gain of function, activating mutations in *FGFR3*, the gene for fibroblast growth factor receptor 3. Nearly all cases are caused by a mutation causing substitution of arginine for glycine at position 380 (G380R).

Inheritance is AD with full penetrance. 80% of cases are caused by *de novo* mutations, almost always in the paternal allele and associated with increased paternal age (>35 years).

Activation of the FGF3 receptor causes decreased endochondrial ossification and inhibited proliferation of chondrocytes in growth plate cartilage. This leads to failure of long bone growth and abnormal formation of skull and vertebrae.

Allelic variants

Different mutations in *FGFR3* cause distinct phenotypes: hypochondroplasia, thanatophoric dwarfism, and severe achondroplasia with developmental delay and acanthosis nigricans (SADDAN).

Clinical features

The diagnosis is usually evident at birth and prenatal diagnosis may be made on the basis of limb shortening evident on ultrasound during the third trimester of pregnancy. Features include:

- *Head and neck:* macrocephaly, frontal bossing, flat nasal bridge, contracted skull base (Fig 16.5)
- *Trunk:* normal length
- *Limbs:* rhizomelic (proximal) shortening, limited elbow extension. Trident hands and brachydactyly

Average adult height is ~130 cm. In the absence of CNS complications, intelligence and life expectancy are normal. Complications affect several systems:

- *CNS:* hydrocephalus in 5% due to stenosis of sigmoid venous sinus. An additional potential contributor to macrocephaly. Spinal cord compression, due to cervical instability, may cause sudden death in infancy
- *Musculoskeletal:* delayed motor milestones due to hypotonia. Waddling gait with exaggerated lumbar lordosis and bow legs. Premature degenerative joint disease and spinal disorders such as kyphosis
- *Obesity:* aggravates joint problems and CVS risks
- *Respiratory system:* otitis media: recurrent OM caused by abnormal anatomy. Sleep apnoea: caused by upper airway obstruction and central apnoea due to brainstem compression. Restrictive pulmonary disease.

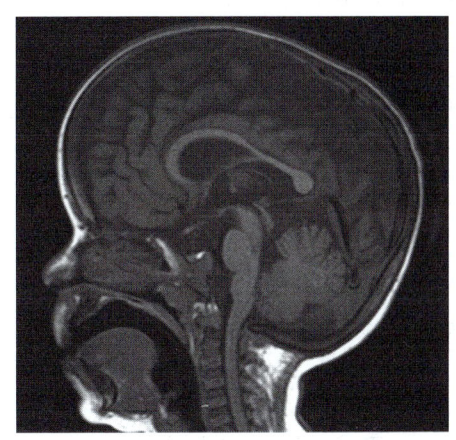

Fig 16.5 Achondroplasia. Sagittal T1 MRI: large cranial vault, small skull base, cervico-medullary kink, large suprasellar cistern. Image courtesy of Dr Laughlin Dawes, radiopaedia.org.

Diagnostic investigations

- *Genetic testing:* detection of the two common mutations is widely available
- *Imaging:* a skeletal survey at birth confirms the diagnosis. The features include:
  - large calvarium with narrow foramen and small skull base
  - vertebral bodies short with wide intervertebral discs, square-shaped long bones, irregular growth plates
  - *hands:* broad short metacarpals and phalanges and trident configuration.

In utero, fetal ultrasound shows progressive discordance between femur length and biparietal diameter and can distinguish homozygous (lethal) achondroplasia from heterozygous.

Treatment

Medical care includes:

- Cranial USS at birth and 2, 4, 6 months to identify hydrocephalus
- Monitor growth and head circumference
- Control weight to avoid obesity
- Treat ear infections and dental crowding.

Growth hormone is not recommended.

Surgical interventions may be required for limb lengthening, symptomatic bow legs or knock knees, spinal stenosis, kyphosis, and craniomedullary compression.

Genetic counselling is as for AD inheritance. If both parents have achondroplasia each child has a 1:4 chance of being homozygous affected, with perinatal lethality.

16.6 Osteopetrosis, osteoporosis, and rickets

Osteopetrosis
Osteopetrosis, or marble bone disease, is a group of rare genetic disorders characterized by abnormal osteoclast function and defective resorption of immature bone.

Aetiology and pathogenesis
Mutations in at least six genes including the chloride channel gene *CLCN7* and the gene encoding carbonic anhydrase II cause osteopetrosis. Defective osteoclast function leads to dense, brittle bone which encroaches on bone marrow causing defective haematopoiesis and compresses nerves in bony channels, including in particular the optic and facial nerves.

Clinical features
Several distinct clinical forms are recognized:
- *Malignant infantile osteopetrosis:* in this most severe form birth fractures are often sustained and hypocalcaemic seizures occur in the neonatal period. Marrow encroachment causes anaemia and thrombocytopaenia, and hepatosplenomegaly develops. Pressure on the optic nerve causes visual impairment by 6 months and deafness or hydrocephalus may occur. Untreated, survival beyond 10 years is unusual. Treatment with γ-interferon increases bone resorption and red cell production. Bone marrow transplantation offers the prospect of cure.
- *Osteopetrosis, renal tubular acidosis and retardation:* may be caused by mutations in the gene for carbonic anhydrase II. Calcium deposits occur in brain.
- *Adult benign osteopetrosis:* originally called Albers–Schonberg disease. Patients present with fractures in early adulthood and may develop deafness or facial nerve paralysis. Inheritance is AD.

Osteoporosis
Osteoporosis is a disease of the skeleton characterized by reduced bone mass and density with a reduction in both matrix and mineralization and deterioration of the microarchitecture. It is uncommon in children and teenagers.

Aetiology and pathogenesis
Bone density increases rapidly during growth spurts, peak bone mass being reached after puberty. Osteoporosis in childhood may be secondary or idiopathic.

Secondary osteoporosis is associated with:
- *Drugs:* systemic corticosteroids
- *Inflammatory disease:* JIA, IBD
- *Endocrine* disorders: Cushing's syndrome, hyperparathyroidism, hyperthyroidism
- *Renal disease*
- *Anorexia nervosa*
- *Osteogenesis imperfecta*
- *Immobility:* cerebral palsy, spinal cord injury.
- *Diet:* calcium and vitamin D deficiency.

Idiopathic juvenile osteoporosis occurs in children aged 8–14 years and usually resolves spontaneously.

Clinical features
Osteoporosis is often clinically silent until a fracture occurs. Juvenile idiopathic osteoporosis may cause lower back pain, hip and foot pain, kyphosis, or a limp.

Diagnostic investigations
Plain radiography may reveal osteopaenia but is relatively insensitive and changes may not be noticeable until 30% of bone mineral is lost.

Bone mineral density is best measured by DEXA scan. Bone biopsy may be considered. Serum calcium and phosphate levels are normal but alkaline phosphatase may be slightly elevated and there may be hypercalciuria.

Treatment
In addition to treating any underlying cause options include:
- *Diet:* adequate calcium and vitamin D intake
- Weight-bearing exercises
- Protection of spine from fractures
- Bisphosphonates.

Rickets
Rickets is the failure of osteoid to calcify in growing bone due to deficiency of vitamin D. A resurgence of nutritional rickets has occurred in breast-fed infants with pigmented skin living in temperate zones.

Aetiology and pathogenesis
Nutritional deficiency of vitamin D, from either inadequate oral intake or inadequate exposure to UV light, is the most common cause. Less common reasons for inadequate vitamin D action exist, and occasionally dietary deficiency of calcium or phosphate may produce the same end result.

Vitamin D
- *Vitamin D3, colecalciferol* is formed in the skin from 5-dihydrotachysterol under the influence of UV light. This is the main source of vitamin D.
- *Vitamin D2, ergocalciferol* is present in fish oils and is absorbed orally and converted to D3 in the skin. Breast milk contains little or no vitamin D.

Colecaciferol is hydroxylated in two steps:
- Hydroxylation at position 25 in the liver, producing *calcidiol*, 25-hydroxycolecalciferol
- Hydroxylation at position 1 in the kidney, producing *calcitriol*, 1,25-dihydroxycolecalciferol.

Calcitriol is the active form and acts on the vitamin D receptor. It acts like a hormone at three main sites:
- *Intestine:* promotes calcium and phosphorus absorption
- *Kidney:* promotes phosphate reabsorption
- *Bone:* promotes release of calcium and phosphate.

These actions increase concentrations of calcium and phosphate in extracellular fluid leading to calcification of osteoid, primarily at the metaphyses (see Chapter 10.9).

Pathophysiology of vitamin D deficiency
Calcitriol levels fall, hypocalcaemia develops, and parathyroid hormone release is stimulated. Excess parathyroid hormone produces renal phosphate loss, further reducing calcification potential. Early on, therefore, the serum calcium level is low but is restored by the parathyroid response, with a very low phosphate level. Alkaline phosphatase produced by active osteoblasts leaks into extracellular fluids and the serum level of this enzyme rises.

Changes in bone
Laying down of uncalcified osteoid at the physes leads to widening of these regions, producing characteristic clinical and radiological changes. Softening of the bones results in deformity. Weight-bearing causes bow legs, weak ribs lead to Harrison sulci and pectus carinatum.

Causes of rickets
- *Nutritional rickets:* risk factors include breast-feeding without vitamin D supplements, and skin pigmentation in temperate climes. Even in sunny areas, sunlight exposure may be inadequate if infants are deliberately covered and unexposed
- *Malabsorption:* inadequate calcium and phosphate intake
- Chronic renal failure
- *Genetic rickets:* rickets may be caused by defects in vitamin D hydroxylase enzymes, the vitamin D receptor causing end-organ unresponsiveness and the phosphate-regulating endopeptidase gene, *PHEX*, mutations in which cause X-linked hypophosphataemic rickets.

Clinical features
Rickets is often asymptomatic and a high index of clinical suspicion should be maintained in infants at risk. Rarely, an acute infection may precipitate hypocalcaemia and tetany as a presenting manifestation. The clinical stigmata depend on the stage of evolution and severity (Fig 16.6).

Skeletal
- *Skull:* frontal bossing and softening of the skull bones, especially along suture lines, craniotabes. Delayed closure of anterior fontanelle and wide sutures.
- *Thorax:* expansion at the costo-chondral junctions causes a 'rickety rosary'. Harrison's grooves, pectus carinatum, and kyphoscoliosis develop.
- *Limbs:* flared metaphyses apparent at distal radius at wrist, femur at the knee and tibia causing 'double malleoli' at the ankle. Weight-bearing causes bow legs or knock knees. Short stature develops.
- *Muscular:* generalized hypotonia with delayed walking
- *Nervous system:* irritability, tetany, apathy.

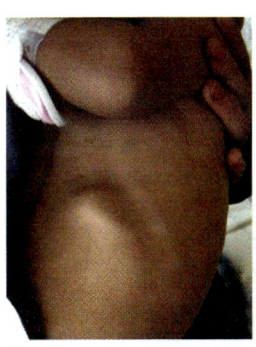

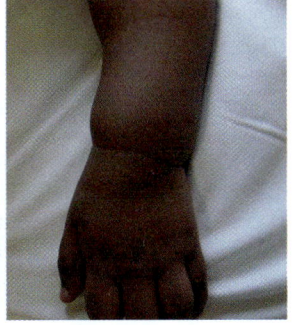

Fig 16.6 Rickets: A. Rickety rosary and Harrison groove. B. Metaphyseal expansion at wrist.

Diagnostic investigations
Imaging
A plain radiograph of the knee showing metaphyseal ends and epiphyses of the femur and tibia is the best single view in children <3 years. Growth is most rapid at this site, accentuating any changes. Flared, broadened and cupped metaphyses are apparent (Fig 16.7) together with generalized osteopaenia and coarsening of trabeculae.

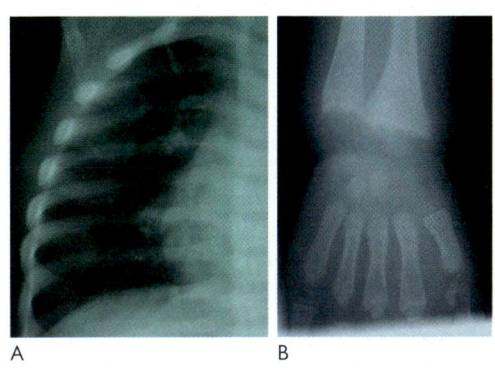

Fig 16.7 Rickets: radiological signs. A. Thorax: expansion of costo-chondral junctions. B. Wrist: flaring and cupping of metaphyses.

Bone biochemistry
Serum calcium, ionized fraction is low initially but often in normal range at presentation due to ↑PTH. Serum phosphate is low and alkaline phosphatase is raised.

Calcidiol levels are low and PTH levels raised, but these measurements are not necessary for diagnosis.

Medical care
Nutritional rickets is preventable and there is a compelling case for providing dietary supplementation of 200–400 iu (5–10 micrograms) of vitamin D daily to at-risk infants including breast-fed, dark-skinned infants in the UK.

For low-birthweight babies, <1500 g supplementation with vitamin D, calcium, and phosphate is required if breast milk is their primary dietary source.

Established nutritional rickets is treated with vitamin D, either as vitamin D2 (ergocalciferol) or vitamin D3 (colecalciferol). Treatment may be given daily over several months as 5000–10 000 iu (125–250 micrograms) daily or in a single day as 600 000 iu (15 000 micrograms) as 4–6 oral doses or as an IM injection. Vitamin D is well stored in the body and released gradually. Single-day therapy avoids compliance problems.

In nutritional rickets the phosphate rises and radiographic healing is evident in 7–8 days.

Oral calcium supplementation may be required if there is hypocalcaemia. Rickets secondary to genetic causes or other diseases such as chronic renal failure or hepatic disease may require a different approach. Alfa-calcidol is used in chronic renal failure. Orthopaedic correction may be required for severe deformities. Rickets in children in the 19th century was a major stimulus for the development of orthopaedic (from the Greek *orthos*, straight and *paidos*, child) surgery.

16.7 Juvenile idiopathic arthritis (JIA)

JIA is defined as arthritis of unknown aetiology beginning before the 16th birthday and persisting for at least 6 weeks in which other known conditions have been excluded. This term and a new classification have been introduced by the International League of Associations for Rheumatology (ILAR). The overall prevalence is 10–20/100 000.

JIA is a heterogeneous group of disorders which differ in their aetiology, pathogenesis, prognosis, and frequency. The ILAR classification, based on mode of onset in first 6 months, is shown in Table 16.1.

Table 16.1. ILAR classification of JIA	
Category	% JIA
Systemic onset	10
Oligoarticular	60
Polyarticular	30
Enthesitis related	<1
Psoriatic	5
Unclassified	<1

Aetiology and pathogenesis

JIA behaves as a complex genetic trait involving multiple genes related to immunity and inflammation. Trigger factors include infection, trauma, and possibly stress.
Certain HLA antigens are associated with an increased risk of JIA. Polymorphisms in genes encoding interleukin-6 and macrophage migration inhibitory factor may be associated with systemic-onset JIA.

Pathogenesis

Chronic inflammation of the synovium occurs. B lymphocyte, macrophage, and T-cell invasion may be found. Release of cytokines and vascular growth factors induces synoviocyte proliferation and angiogenesis with pannus formation. Cytokines associated with tissue destruction include interleukin-6 and tumour necrosis factor (TNF).

Clinical features

The clinical features, including age of onset and sex incidence, vary with subtype. JIA overall is more common in girls, but systemic-onset JIA occurs with equal frequency in boys and girls and enthesitis-related arthritis is more common in boys. Oligoarticular and systemic-onset JIA tends to occur in early childhood (1–5 years). Polyarticular, rheumatoid-factor-positive JIA is more common in adolescent girls.

Systemic-onset JIA (SOJIA)

SOJIA affects males and females equally and occurs throughout childhood, most commonly at age 1–5 years. The characteristic presenting features include:

- *Fever:* quotidian with 1–2 spikes >38.5 °C per day
- *Rash:* evanescent, salmon pink, non-pruritic rash on trunk and extremities (Fig 16.8)
- *Arthralgia:* symmetrical, affecting one or several joints. Frank joint swelling may not occur for months after onset.

Additional features include lymphadenopathy, dermographism, hepatosplenomegaly, and anaemia. Serositis may occur and manifest as pericarditis or abdominal pain.

The differential diagnosis is wide and includes viral infections, malignancy, Kawasaki disease, connective tissue disorders such as SLE, dermatomyositis and rheumatic fever.

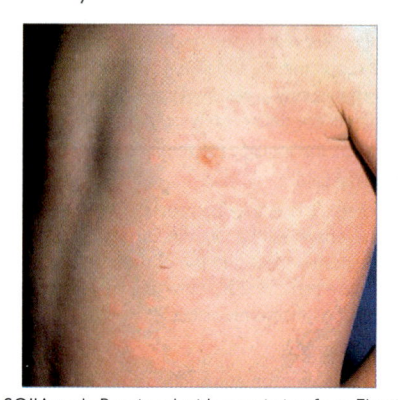

Fig 16.8 SOJIA: rash. Reprinted with permission from Elsevier (The Lancet 2007; 369: 767–778).

Investigations

- Full blood count:
  - anaemia, normochromic and microcytic
  - neutrophil leucocytosis
  - thrombocytosis >400 ×10^9/L
- *Inflammatory markers:* ↑ESR, ↑CRP, ↑ferritin
- IgM rheumatoid factor and ANA negative.

Prognosis is poor. Half remit in the first few years, but half have recurrent episodes and progressive arthritis occurs in one third, with osteoporosis and growth retardation. Amyloidosis in adult life is a risk if inflammation is not controlled.

Oligoarticular JIA

Oligoarticular JIA most commonly affects girls <6 years and is the most common and well-defined subtype. Arthritis affects 1–4 joints during the 1st 6 months, usually involving the lower limbs joints, knee (Fig 16.9), and ankle.

The disease may be 'limited', persisting in <4 joints or 'extended' if five or more joints are affected after 6 months.

An important feature is anterior uveitis which may be silent and sight threatening. It usually develops in the first 4 years and 3 monthly slit-lamp examination in the 1st 2 years is mandatory. Antinuclear antibodies (ANA) are often present and associated with uveitis.

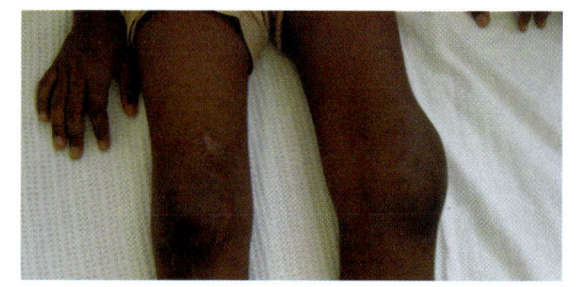

Fig 16.9 Oligoarticular JIA: knees.

Investigations

- *FBC:* normal
- *IgM rheumatoid factor, RF:* negative
- *ANA:* frequently positive.

Exacerbations and remissions occur. Prognosis is worse in the 'extended' form. Uveitis needs early treatment to prevent synechiae, cataracts, glaucoma, and blindness.

Polyarticular JIA
This may be rheumatoid factor positive or negative. Arthritis affects 5 or more joints in the first 6 months. Large and small joints can be involved, often symmetrically.

Polyarticular JIA, rheumatoid factor negative
Affects girls more than boys with a biphasic age distribution: early peak 2–4 years, later peak 6–12 years. Up to 50% are ANA positive and at risk of uveitis: there is overlap with oligoarthritis in young females. Cervical spine and temperomandibular joint involvement is common.

Investigations
- *FBC:* mild anaemia, mild neutrophil leucocytosis, moderate thrombocytosis
- *IgM rheumatoid factor:* negative
- *ANA:* positive in 20–40%.

The course is variable. 50% go into remission within 10 years. Recurrent episodes cause progressive deformity.

Polyarticular JIA, rheumatoid factor positive.
More common in girls with a peak in late childhood, >8 years or adolescence. An aggressive, symmetrical arthritis affects particularly the small joints of the wrists, hands (Fig 16.10), ankles, and feet. Knees and hips involved early with elbows and other joints later. The pattern is similar to adult rheumatoid arthritis. Rarely, rheumatoid nodules occur on pressure points and vasculitis may cause nail fold lesions.

Investigations
- *FBC:* moderate anaemia, ESR: elevated.
- *ANA:* might be positive.
- HLA DR4 associated.

Prognosis is poor, with severe joint destruction.

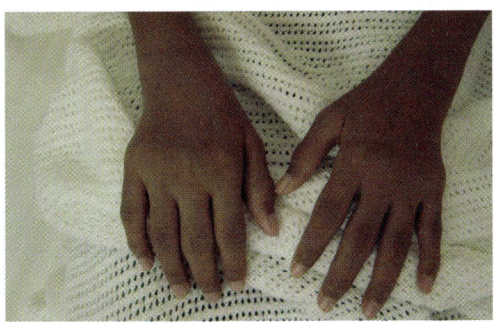

Fig 16.10 Polyarticular JIA: hands.

Enthesitis-related arthritis
Formerly called juvenile ankylosing spondylitis. There is male preponderance with onset >8 years. Asymmetrical lower limb arthritis occurs with enthesitis, inflammation of ligaments or tendon insertions, and tenosynovitis. Acute anterior uveitis may cause painful red eyes. Spinal and sacroiliac involvement is uncommon and occurs late. IgM rheumatoid factor is usually negative. HLA B27 +ve in 90%. The functional outcome is good in the majority.

Psoriatic arthritis
Arthritis and psoriasis, or arthritis and at least two of: dactylitis, nail pitting or onycholysis, or psoriasis in a first degree relative. There is a female preponderance. Uveitis and spondylitis can occur. Arthritis is asymmetrical and flexor tenosynovitis may occur. It may start with a single swollen digit. IgM rheumatoid factor usually negative but ANA may be positive. A remitting and relapsing course into adulthood is common.

Clinical evaluation of JIA
The differential diagnosis of JIA is wide and diagnosis can be challenging. Important differentials include:
- *A single swollen joint:* septic arthritis, reactive arthritis, and post-infectious arthritis
- *Systemic disease:* SLE, juvenile dermatomyositis (JDM), polyarteritis nodosa (PAN), or malignancy such as leukaemia or neuroblastoma can mimic JIA. In acute lymphoblastic leukaemia up to 60% have musculoskeletal symptoms.

Rheumatoid factor (RF) and ANA can be raised in healthy children or by intercurrent illness. RF positivity requires confirmation on 2 occasions 3 months apart. Thrombocytopaenia is rare in SOJIA and raises the possibility of SLE or ALL. A relative lymphocytosis is common in JIA, but lymphopaenia or neutropaenia raises the possibility of leukaemia.

New imaging modalities include MRI and ultrasound. Ultrasound is useful for joint effusions, synovial hypertrophy and tendon pathology. MRI shows synovial hypertrophy, articular cartilage, bone and bone marrow and overall joint integrity in great detail, especially when used with gadolinium DTPA which enhances inflamed synovium.

Treatment
A multidisciplinary, team approach is essential to provide care based on physical therapies and drug treatment. Psychological support is essential for patient and family, and social worker involvement may be required.

Physical therapies
- *Physiotherapy:* an active programme of exercises and stretching to maintain joint function and muscle strength. Patients should be encouraged to be as active as possible. Splinting may be necessary to prevent deformity and preserve function, but is now used less often.
- *Occupational therapy:* useful for hand problems.

Drug treatment
The main classes of drugs available include:

Anti-inflammatories
- *NSAIDs:* to control pain, inflammation, fever
- *Corticosteroids:* oral, IV, or intra-articular.

Disease-modifying antirheumatic drugs (DMARDs)
- *Methotrexate:* drug of choice for most JIA
- *Sulfasalazine:* useful for enthesitis-related JIA, or arthritis associated with IBD
- *Hydroxycholorquine:* useful for arthritis, especially in SLE.

Biological agents
Cytokine inhibitors: used under specialist supervision. Etanercept, infliximab, and adalimumab inhibit the activity of TNF and are used for patients in whom methotrexate has failed. Anakinra (anti-interleukin 1) can be helpful in SOJIA. Other agents include anti-IL6, rituximab (anti-CD20). Bone marrow transplantation is considered if these fail.

Monitoring of uveitis is essential to allow treatment with topical corticosteroids and mydriatics. This can prevent glaucoma and progression to band keratopathy and posterior synechiae causing blindness.

16.8 Reactive arthritis and transient synovitis

Reactive arthritis and post-infectious arthritis

Reactive arthritis is a transient, autoimmune-mediated arthritis which may follow a variety of bacterial or viral infections. The term was introduced to describe arthritis following enteric infection and as a component of what became known as Reiter syndrome in which arthritis was accompanied by urethritis and eye inflammation (uveitis and conjunctivitis). In this context there is an association with HLA-B27.

In childhood, the term reactive arthritis and postinfectious arthritis are ill defined and often used interchangeably to describe arthritis in the wake of infections, not just enteric, in which septic arthritis has been excluded.

Aetiology and pathogenesis

Infections in childhood causing reactive arthritis include:

- *Bacterial:* Shigella, Salmonella, Yersinia, Campylobacter, Chlamydia, Mycoplasma, Borrelia burgdorferi (Lyme disease pathogen)
- *Viral:* parvovirus B19, herpes, coxsackie.

The autoimmune mechanisms involved remain uncertain. Overlapping subsets of 'spondyloarthritis' have been proposed

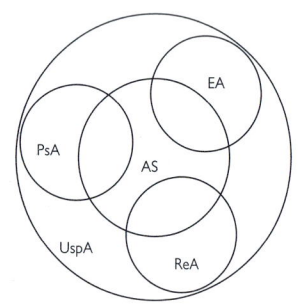

Fig 16.11 Spondyloarthritis subsets: AS, ankylosing spondylitis (enthesitis-related arthritis); EA, enteropathic arthritis; PsA, psoriatic arthritis; ReA, reactive arthritis; UspA, undifferentiated spondyloarthritis.

Clinical features

Arthritis is usually asymmetrical and affects the large joints of the lower limb such as the knee. In Reiter syndrome there is a triad of conjunctivitis, urethritis, and arthritis ('can't see, can't pee, can't climb a tree'). In addition, there may be fever, mouth ulcers, and pustules on palms, soles, toes. Onset of symptoms is ~10 days after the infection.

Management

Investigations

- *FBC:* Hb normal, mild neutrophil leucocytosis
- *ESR:* raised
- *IgM RF and ANA-negative*
- High incidence of HLA B27 +ve.

Treatment

Reactive arthritis is often self-limiting but may be chronic or progressive. Options include antibiotics if an organism is identified, physiotherapy, and NSAIDs.

Arthritis and inflammatory bowel disease

Arthritis is the most common extraintestinal complication of IBD, affecting an estimated 25% of all patients. The sex incidence is equal.

Aetiology and pathogenesis

Arthritis complicating IBD is one form of enteropathic enteropathy, an umbrella term for various patterns of inflammatory arthritis associated with a range of gastrointestinal pathologies. There is overlap with the seronegative spondyloarthropathies,, including reactive arthritis associated with enteric infection.

The pathophysiology is poorly understood. One possibility is abnormal permeability of the bowel to bacterial antigens. Genetic susceptibility, particularly HLA-B27 positivity, is important.

Clinical features

There are two main clinical groups:

- *Peripheral arthritis:* oligoarthritis affecting knees, ankles, wrists and elbows usually coincides with the course of the IBD but occasionally arthritis precedes the bowel symptoms. Prognosis is good if IBD is well controlled.
- *Spinal arthritis (spondylitis):* pain and stiffness in the joints of the spinal column, worse in the morning, appears months or years before onset of IBD. Acute iritis may occur, but is very rare.

Associated features may include erythema nodosum, pyoderma gangrenosum, and the features of IBD: mucosal ulcers, weight loss, and growth failure.

Management

Investigations

- *FBC:* a normochromic normocytic anaemia
- *Platelet count may be elevated*
- *ESR:* elevated
- *IgM RF and ANA negative*
- *HLA-B27:* positive.

Treatment

Peripheral arthritis responds to medication and exercises to improve range of motion. NSAIDs should be used with caution because of gastrointestinal side effects.

Spinal arthritis is treated with physiotherapy and NSAIDs.

Transient synovitis (TS)

Also called 'irritable hip', TS is a benign, self limiting inflammation of the synovium of the hip joint. It is twice as common in boys as in girls and is the most common cause of acute hip pain in the age range 3–10 years.

Aetiology and pathogenesis

No definitive cause is known. Minor trauma or preceding viral infection or vaccination may act as trigger factors in susceptible individuals.

A joint effusion occurs. There is non-specific inflammation and hypertrophy of the synovial membrane.

Clinical features

TS is most common in boys aged 3–10 years. The presenting symptom is unilateral hip pain, although in some the pain is referred to thigh or knee. In very young children the only symptom may be crying. A limp may be the presenting feature. In 50% there is a recent history of upper respiratory tract infection and there may be a history of minor trauma. Transient synovitis is a diagnosis of exclusion.

Examination reveals:
- Afebrile, or mild temperature elevation
- *Hip held flexed and turned outwards:* flexion, external rotation, abduction to maximize comfort
- *Hip examination:*
  - restriction of active and passive motion, especially internal rotation. The hip may be tender to palpation
  - the log roll: gently roll entire lower limb from side to side with patient supine. Involuntary muscle guarding may occur on the affected side.
- Antalgic limp.

The differential diagnosis includes all those causes of a painful hip in this age group. Septic arthritis or osteomyelitis are the most important conditions to exclude. Perthes disease occurs in the same age group and is more common in boys.

Diagnostic investigations

Blood tests

- White cell count, ESR, and CRP may all be slightly elevated. This is helpful in distinguishing from septic arthritis in which high fever is usually associated with ESR >40 mm/h and WBC >12 × 10^9/L.
- Blood culture.

Imaging

- *Ultrasound scan of hip:* Hip ultrasound is sensitive for detection of an intracapsular effusion with capsular distension >2 mm (Fig 16.12). An effusion is nearly always present in TS, but ultrasound scan cannot reliably distinguish between TS and septic arthritis. Absence of an effusion should prompt a continued search for the source of the pain.
- *Hip radiograph:* AP and frog lateral views of pelvis and both hips may show increased joint space. The main value is to exclude bone lesions such as occult fractures or osteoid osteoma, and slipped capital femoral epiphysis.

Aspiration

If septic arthritis remains possible on clinical grounds, needle aspiration is undertaken (under ultrasound guidance).

Treatment

Treatment options for transient synovitis are:
- *Bed rest:* avoid weight-bearing for a few days if necessary
- *Traction:* if discomfort is considerable, traction of the hip in a few degrees of flexion minimizes intracapsular pressure
- *NSAIDs:* control pain and shorten duration of symptoms.

If significant symptoms persist beyond 7–10 days the diagnosis should be reconsidered. A link between transient synovitis and subsequent Perthes disease remains controversial and unlikely.

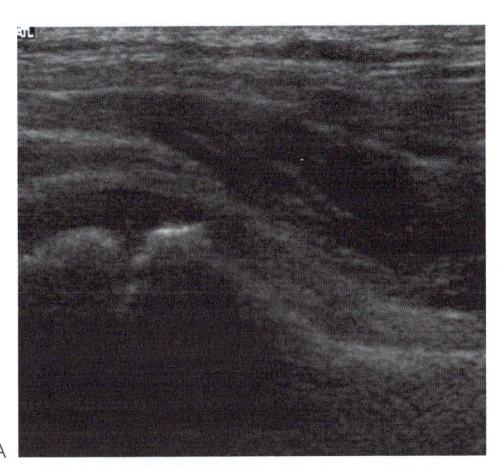

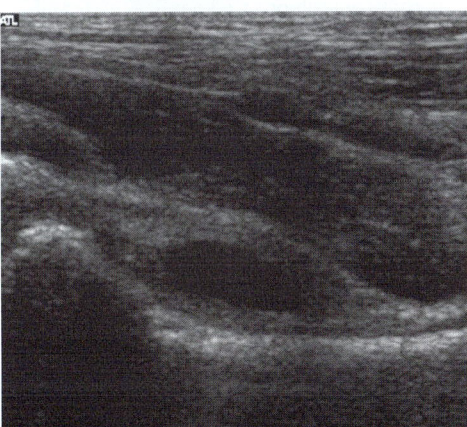

Fig 16.12 Hip ultrasound scan: A. Normal. B. Joint effusion.

16.9 Systemic lupus erythematosus (SLE)

SLE is a multisystem autoimmune disease characterized by the presence of antibodies directed against cell nuclei, in particular to double-stranded DNA (dsDNA). It is an uncommon disease with an overall childhood incidence of 0.5/100 000 per year, peaking at 5/100 000 per year in young adult females.

In young children the sex distribution is slightly skewed towards females but in adolescent and young adults the F:M ratio is 10:1. SLE is more common in certain ethnic groups: Afro-Caribbeans and Asians.

Aetiology and pathogenesis

The disease may be triggered by a variety of environmental agents in genetically predisposed individuals.

Genetic factors

A genetic predisposition to SLE exists. The concordance rate in monozygotic twins is 25–70%. If a mother has SLE, the risk to offspring is 1:40 for daughters and 1:250 for sons.

Available evidence indicates that SLE is a 'complex' trait influenced by multiple genes. At least 9 susceptibility loci are known (*SLEB1–9*), and separate loci identified for SLE with haemolytic anaemia (*SLEH1*) and with nephritis (*SLEN1–3*).

Genes involved encode proteins involved in MHC class II and early complement pathway components, Toll-like receptors, and protein tyrosine phosphatase non-receptor 22. Pathways of innate and acquired immunity are involved.

Exogenous factors

- *Sunlight:* photosensitivity is a precipitant of skin and systemic manifestations
- *Drugs:* minocycline, procainamide, hydralazine, and isoniazid. Sex ratios are equal and renal or CNS features uncommon.

Pathogenesis

An autoimmune reaction occurs to intracellular antigens, normally invisible to the immune system. Dysregulated apoptosis may contribute. Autoantibodies, circulating immune complexes, and T lymphocytes all contribute to the multisystem pathology in skin, kidneys, CNS, bone marrow, cardiovascular, respiratory and gastrointestinal system, and vascular endothelium.

Tissue deposition of immune complexes triggers complement activation and cytokine production.

Specific autoantibodies are found to:
- dsDNA
- *Extractable nuclear antigens (ENAs):*
  - anti-Smith (Sm), anti-RNP, anti-Ro, and anti-LA
  - anti-RNP is associated with mixed connective tissue disease and neonatal lupus is almost always caused by anti-Ro or anti-LA antibodies.
- *Rheumatoid factors:* an IgM antibody to IgG (in 30%).

Clinical features

The classical presentation is with fever, fatigue, erythematous malar rash, and polyarthritis with pain and stiffness more overt than swelling of joints. However, presentation may be with single-system disease dominating the manifestations, such as isolated thrombocytopaenia or nephritis.

It is reasonable to consider SLE in any child unwell for >1 week in whom no other cause can be found.

The criteria of the American College of Rheumatology are for classification and research purposes and more stringent than those needed for diagnosis in practice. They reflect the multisystem nature of the disease. If 4 of the following 11 criteria are fulfilled at any time the diagnostic specificity is 95%:

1. Malar (butterfly) rash
2. Discoid rash
3. Photosensitivity
4. Oral ulcers
5. *Arthritis:* non-erosive
6. *Serositis:* pleuritis or pericarditis
7. *Renal disorder:* proteinuria ≥0.5 g/day or cellular casts
8. *Neurological disorder:* seizures or psychosis
9. *Haematological disorder:* cytopaenia: anaemia, lymphopaenia, thrombocytopaenia
10. Positive immunoserology to:
    - dsDNA or Smith (Sm) nuclear antigen
    - phospholipids, based on anticardiolipin antibodies, lupus anticoagulant, or false positive syphilis serology for 6 months
11. Anti-nuclear antibodies (ANA).

Manifestations are protean and the disease follows a remitting and relapsing course.

Considering the manifestations by system in detail:

- *Systemic:* fever, fatigue, malaise, anorexia, nausea, weight loss
- *Arthritis:* arthralgia out of proportion to swelling, polyarthritis of small and large joints
- *Skin:* malar, butterfly rash over cheeks and bridge of nose (Fig 16.13), also involving chin and ears, but sparing nasolabial folds. Maculopapular rash on palms and soles of feet. Discoid rash in 20%. Photosensitivity. Raynaud's phenomenon
- *Mucous membranes:* ulcers of mouth, hard palate, nose
- *Renal:* nephritis or nephrotic syndrome may occur with haematuria, proteinuria, hypertension
- *CNS:* in 30% children. Encephalopathy (seizures, headache, stroke, cognitive dysfunction, psychosis), chorea, transverse myelitis, blurred vision (retinal vasculitis)
- *Cardiovascular:* pericarditis, myocarditis, Libman–Sacks endocarditis associated with antiphospholipid antibodies (rare).
- *Respiratory:* pneumonitis, pleuritis, haemoptysis (rare)
- *Haematological:* haemolytic anaemia and thrombocytopaenia
- *Gastrointestinal:* mesenteric arteritis, hepatitis, pancreatitis, hepatosplenomegaly.

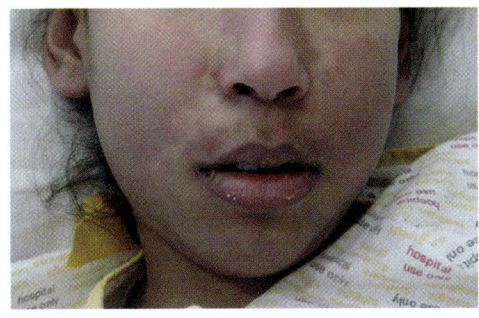

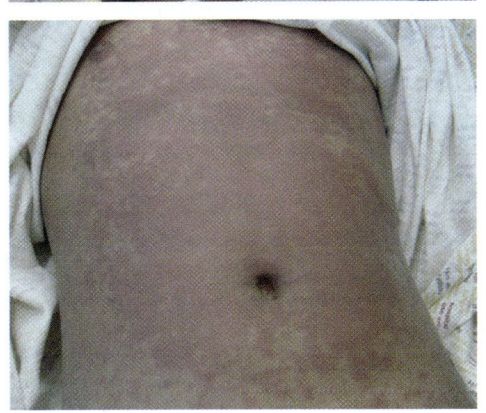

Fig 16.13 SLE rash: A. Butterfly malar facial rash. B. Truncal rash.

Management

Investigations at diagnosis
- *FBC:* normochromic normocytic anaemia, lymphopaenia, and thrombocytopaenia.
- *ESR:* raised in 90% with normal CR
- *Urinalysis:* microscopic haematuria or proteinuria in renal involvement
- *Autoantibodies:*
  - ANA: strongly positive, titre >1:160 in >95%. A negative ANA makes SLE very unlikely, but a positive ANA is very common in children without SLE
  - anti-dsDNA: highly specific, may reflect disease activity
  - anti-ENA: not very specific
  - RF: positive in 30%
  - Antiphospholipid antibodies: positive in 30%.
- *Complement C3, C4*: hypocomplementaemia often present. Raised complement is against the diagnosis of SLE.

Imaging such as chest radiograph, cardiac echo and cranial MRI depends on clinical findings.

Treatment
A multidisciplinary approach is required for this challenging disorder. General measures are important, in combination with drugs tailored to the disease severity and pattern of involvement in the individual child:

General measures
- *Diet and exercise:* avoid high calorie, high salt food to avoid steroid-induced weight gain, and encourage exercise
- *Sun-protection:* wear sunscreen >SP50 daily on all exposed skin.
- *Fatigue and sleep:* fatigue is common and affects school performance, and steroids may induce sleep disturbance.
- *Psycho-social issues:* education of child and family about SLE is essential. Poor school attendance may indicate psychosocial issues. SLE impacts on adolescence and vice versa. There may be denial, poor adherence, and reluctance to tell friends or teachers. Transition of control of disease management from parents to child is important.
- *Immunisation:* live vaccines are contraindicated in those on corticosteroids or immunosuppression, but pneumococcal vaccine at diagnosis and 5 yearly and influenza vaccine yearly is recommended.

Drug treatment
Medications used include:
- *Hydroxychloroquine:* this is standard first line treatment for mild disease (skin, joint, pulmonary disease) or as adjunctive treatment in more severe disease. Retinal damage is a risk, but minimal at a dose of <6 mg/kg per day. Annual monitoring (visual fields, colour vision) is done. It has been shown to be cardioprotective in studies in adults.
- *Corticosteroids:* are nearly always required at some stage. In severe, systemic disease IV methylprednisolone for 3 days is given initially, followed by oral prednisolone which is subsequently tapered. Side effects can be devastating and include poor growth, weight gain, mood swings, osteoporosis, hypertension, and avascular necrosis.
- *NSAIDS:* for musculoskeletal symptoms and serositis.
- *Anti-thrombotic agents:* low-dose aspirin is used in children with high levels of antiphospholipid antibodies and/or lupus anticoagulant or other anticoagulants (warfarin, heparin) after a thrombotic episode.
- *Immunosuppressive agents:* azathioprine or mycophenolate mofetil (MMF) is used for moderate/severe disease and cyclophosphamide for severe organ involvement.

A number of additional options exist for severe disease resistant to standard therapy:
- *Rituximab:* B cell depletion using this monoclonal antibody to CD20 has been used, especially for thrombocytopaenia.
- *Plasmapheresis,* splenectomy in severe refractory cytopaenia and autologous or allogeneic bone marrow or stem cell transplants have all been used.

Regular monitoring of disease activity scores (e.g. BILAG) and laboratory tests, FBC, ESR, CRP, C3/C4, LFTs, renal biochemistry are important.

The course and prognosis is variable. Ten year survival is now 85–90%. Infection is an important cause of mortality especially when disease is active. Cumulative disease damage causing end-stage renal failure, osteoporosis, and atherosclerotic cardiovascular disease occur as a consequence of the disease itself.

16.10 Connective tissue disorders

Dermatomyositis (DM)
Dermatomyositis is a rare inflammatory disorder affecting skin and muscle and sometimes other organs. Juvenile dermatomyositis typically has onset age 5–10 years and is more common in girls. Polymyositis with inflammation of muscles alone is very rare in childhood.

Aetiology and pathogenesis
The cause of DM is unknown although there is evidence for some genetic association with HLA types DR3, DR5, DR7. Trigger factors may include infectious agents such as viruses and toxoplasma and drugs including hydroxyurea, penicillamine, and statins.

Pathogenesis
An autoimmune-mediated inflammation of muscle and blood vessels is present. Circulating autoantibodies are common, including ANA and so-called myositis-specific antibodies. Muscle biopsy reveals perivascular and interfascicular inflammatory infiltrates with muscle fibre degeneration and regeneration.

In contrast to adult DM, there is no association with malignancy. Calcinosis of skin or muscle is commoner in children and is seen in 40%.

Clinical features
Onset is usually insidious but may be sudden. A prodromal phase may last for months with non-specific symptoms such as lethargy and irritability, before a rash and overt muscle weakness develops.

Examination may reveal:
- Fever
- *Rash:* the characteristic skin signs are a periorbital heliotrope eruption and Gottron papules
  - *Heliotrope rash:* a violaceous, reddish purple rash with or without oedema involving the periorbital skin
  - *Gottron papules:* elevated violaceous papules and plaques over bony prominences, particularly the MCP and IP joints
  - periungual telangiectases, facial erythema, poikiloderma (pigmentary and atrophic changes) on exposed skin
- *Muscles:* myositis is manifested as proximal muscle weakness and tenderness. Palatal involvement may cause dysphagia.

Signs of involvement of other organs may be present:
- *Arthralgia and joint swelling:* especially small joints of hand
- *Pulmonary disease:* pneumonitis, aspiration
- *Myocarditis:* with arrhythmias.
- Gastrointestinal dysfunction.

In time, muscle wasting, contractures, and calcinosis may develop. Calcinosis cutis can occur anywhere either as nodules or as sheets of calcium.

Management
Investigations
- *Muscle enzymes:* creatine kinase and lactate dehydrogenase elevated
- *Muscle MRI:* useful in assessing presence of an inflammatory myopathy and selecting a biopsy site. Has replaced electromyography which shows myopathic changes
- *Muscle biopsy:* perivascular inflammation, perifascicular atrophy, increased connective tissue.

Treatment
- *Activity:* physiotherapy to prevent contractures and strengthen muscles
- *Palatal and respiratory dysfunction:* avoiding supine posture and nasogastric tube feeding may be required.
- *Corticosteroids:* IV methylprednisolone followed by oral prednisolone 1–2 mg/kg per day
- *Cytotoxic agents:* methotrexate, cyclosporine and azathioprine have all been used
- *Skin disease:* sun-avoidance and sun-screens, hydroxycholoroquine or methotrexate.

High-dose IV immunoglobulin may benefit muscle and skin disease. Severe disease may require cyclophosphamide or anti-TNF agents.

Mixed connective tissue disease (MCTD)
MCTD is best considered as an undifferentiated connective disease the hallmarks of which are Raynaud phenomenon and anti-RNP antibodies. Its existence as a true separate disease entity remains controversial. It is more common in females (F:M 6:1) with a median age of onset of 12 years.

Specific causes remain undefined. The hallmark is the presence of autoantibodies to small nuclear ribonucleoproteins.

Clinical features
The most common presenting features are polyarthritis, general malaise, and Raynaud phenomenon. Multisystem disease may manifest with a plethora of features:
- *Cutaneous:* vasculitic rashes, Gottron papules, sclerodermatous skin, alopecia, rheumatoid nodules
- *Joints:* polyarthritis, sausage-shaped fingers
- *GI tract:* dysphagia, gastro-oesophageal reflux, parotitis
- *Serositis:* pleuritis, pericarditis
- Muscle weakness.

Management
Investigations
- *FBC:* leukopaenia, thrombocytopaenia, haemolytic anaemia common, ESR: elevated
- *ANA:* positive
- *RF:* occasionally positive
- *Anti-RNP antibodies:* positive in high titre (anti-Sm negative).

Treatment
Avoid cold exposure to minimize Raynaud symptoms. Mild disease can be managed with NSAIDs and/or hydroxychloroquine. Severe disease may require corticosteroids with or without cytotoxic agents. MCTD may evolve into recognizable syndromes: SLE, systemic sclerosis, or overlap syndromes.

Ehlers–Danlos syndrome (EDS)

This is a group of heritable disorders of connective tissue characterized by joint hypermobility and skin hyperextensibility. Other variable features occur in more severe types, including easy bruising and rupture of blood vessels or internal organs.

The overall incidence is 1/5000 births worldwide, but some types are much more common than others.

Aetiology and pathogenesis

EDS is caused by mutations in genes that alter the structure, production, or processing of collagen or proteins that interact with collagen. At least nine different disease genes have been identified, the most commonly involved being *COL5A1*, *COL5A2*, and *COL3A1*.

Clinical features: classification

A revised classification by Villefranche in 1997 proposed reduction of the number of major types to six and gave them descriptive names. This replaced the earlier classification EDS I–X. Only two varieties are at all common.

Hypermobile (EDS III): 1/10 000–15 000.
Caused by mutations in:
- *COL3A1* encoding collagen, type III, α1
- *TNXB* encoding tenascin-Xb.

However, in most families the basic defect is unknown. Inheritance is AD.

The major features are generalized joint laxity (hypermobility) with smooth, velvety, hyperextensible skin. Joint dislocations and subluxations are common and painful degenerative joint disease is a common complication. Mitral valve prolapse is an uncommon feature. There is overlap clinically with benign joint hypermobility syndrome.

Classical (EDS I and II, gravis and mitis): 1/25 000–50 000.
Caused by mutations in *COL5A2*, *COL5A1*, or *COL1A1*. Inheritance is AD and a family history is common.

Major features are soft, highly elastic, velvety skin which may tear, bruise, or scar easily and heal with 'cigarette paper' scars. There is mild joint laxity and there may be manifestations of tissue extensibility such as hernia or cervical insufficiency. Pregnancy can be life-threatening.

Vascular (EDS IV): 1/100 000
Most cases caused by mutations in *COL3A1* which can also cause hypermobility EDS.

The major feature is fragile blood vessel walls and organ membranes with a tendency to aneurysms or ruptures of arteries. Skin is thin and translucent and extensive bruising can occur and may be mistaken for NAI. Characteristic facial features are protruding eyes, small chin, lobeless ears.

Management

Diagnosis is based on clinical features and family history. Mutation analysis for most forms of EDS except hypermobility type is available. A skin biopsy may be taken to confirm the diagnosis and determine the type but is not routine practice.

There is no specific treatment, but patients can be helped by muscle strengthening.

Benign joint hypermobility syndrome (BJHS)

This is defined as the presence of joint hypermobility together with musculoskeletal pain. There is a validated score system, the *Brighton* criteria, incorporating the *Beighton* score (the names are confusingly similar), but it is less useful in children.

It must be remembered that the presence of joint hypermobility in itself does not equate to BJHS. Children have inherently more hypermobile joints than adults with a prevalence of 5–30% and hypermobility is associated with a variety of musculoskeletal symptoms including 'growing pains' and back pain. Up to 10% of school-age children have loose joints and occasional pain after exercise or at night.

Aetiology and pathogenesis

Hypermobility *per se* is probably a 'complex' genetic trait. BJHS displays AD inheritance. There is clinical overlap with Ehlers–Danlos syndrome, hypermobile type.

Clinical features

Joint pain is the most usual presenting complaint. Children typically have pain in multiple joints, most commonly in weight-bearing knee and ankle joints after physical activity or repetitive use. Back pain in adolescence and hip pain in gymnasts or dancers may occur.

There may be a history of flat feet, abnormal gait ('knock-knees'), 'double-jointedness' or shoulder or patellar dislocation. Unusual or bizarre hand postures may be assumed for writing tasks.

Examination

The Beighton score is done using five manoeuvres, four of which are done bilaterally to give a total possible score of 9.
1. Apposition of thumb to flexor surface of forearm
2. Passive dorsiflexion of MCP joint to 90°
3. Hyperextension of knee beyond 90° (neutral)
4. Hyperextension of elbow beyond 90° (neutral)
5. Forward flexion to put hands flat on floor with knees extended.

The Beighton score is used in the Brighton criteria. The major criteria (two required) are:
- Beighton score of ≥4.
- Arthralgia for >3 months in four or more joints.

A host of minor criteria reflect other manifestations of connective tissue disorder such as skin striae or extensibility, marfanoid habitus, hernia, or mitral valve prolapse.

Diagnosis of BJHS is one of exclusion, especially of inflammatory or infectious causes of arthralgia.

Management.

The prognosis is good in this non-inflammatory disorder, but sequelae are potentially significant and some question how 'benign' a syndrome is in which some patients develop chronic disabling pain. Education, avoidance of vigorous, repetitive activity, and exercise therapy to improve muscular stability and proprioception at specific joints are key management strategies. Osteopathic manipulative treatment may be useful additional treatment.

16.11 Osteomyelitis and septic arthritis

Osteomyelitis

Osteomyelitis is an inflammation of bone caused by infection, usually with pyogenic bacteria. Acute haematogenous osteomyelitis is more common in boys and in Afro-Caribbeans. 50% of cases occur in preschool children.

Aetiology and pathogenesis

The route of infection is haematogenous in most cases. However, cases secondary to a penetrating injury, open fracture, or infection in a contiguous site may occur.

Organisms

Staphylococcus aureus accounts for 70–90% of acute haematogenous osteomyelitis in children. *Haemophilus influenzae* type B (Hib) is now rare following introduction of vaccination.

Other organisms which may cause osteomyelitis at different ages include:

- *Neonate (0–2 months)*: Group B streptococcus, *E. coli.*
- *Child*: *Strep. pneumoniae*, Group A or group D streptococci, *Kingella kingae, E. coli.*

In children with sickle cell disease, osteomyelitis may be caused by *Salmonella, Strep. pneumoniae, Staph, aureus,* or gram-negative bacilli. *Pseudomonas aeruginosa* may cause osteomyelitis following penetrating wounds of the foot.

Mycobacterium tuberculosis causes chronic osteomyelitis.

Pathogenesis

Mild trauma may cause bone compromise allowing seeding of bacteria during transient bacteraemia. Contributory factors include host susceptibility, age-related vascular anatomy, and virulence of the infecting organism.

- *Host factors:* immunodeficiency from chronic illness or malnutrition, inherited disorders, or immunosuppressive drugs. The newborn is relatively immunodeficient.
- *Vascular factors:* vascular loops in the metaphysis create a sluggish circulation proving an environment conducive to bacterial growth. Under 18 months, vascular spread to the epiphysis may occur with septic athritis if the joint is entered. In sickle cell disease vascular-occlusion and hyposplenism contribute to susceptibility.
- *Virulence factors:* bacterial chemiadsorption to cartilage matrix of the growth plate.

Pathological phases

Haematogenous osteomyelitis evolves through five phases:

- *Inflammation:* acute inflammation increases the intraosseous pressure, causing pain and local tenderness.
- *Suppuration:* pus forms over 48–72 h, passes along Volkmann canals to the surface, elevating the periosteum. Pus may then burst into surrounding soft tissue or into a joint if the metaphysis is intra-articular.
- *Necrosis:* osteonecrosis occurs, creating a sequestrum of dead bone.
- *New bone formation:* at 10–14 days the periosteum lays down new bone. New bone forms an involucrum, ensheathing the sequestrum.
- *Resolution:* hastened by surgical drainage of pus.

Clinical features

Duration of symptoms is used to classify osteomyelitis into:

- *Acute:* acute illness with fever and localized bone symptoms, within 1 week
- *Sub-acute:* insidious onset over 1–4 weeks with fewer systemic features and more prominent local bone signs
- *Chronic:* lasts for >3 months and usually caused by infection from a contiguous site or with an unusual organism, e.g. TB.

Acute haematogenous osteomyelitis usually presents with fever and pain in infants. A history of minor trauma is present in 35% of cases.

Examination reveals an unwell, febrile child with pain and focal point tenderness. Overlying swelling and redness may be present with limp or refusal to weight-bear. Asymmetric movement of extremities (pseudoparalysis) is an early sign in newborns or infants. The metaphyses of long bones femur, tibia, or humerus are most commonly affected.

The differential includes trauma, bone tumour, bony infiltrates, and bone infarcts (in sickle cell disease) and in infants, CNS disease causing true paralysis, and inflicted injury.

Management

Investigations

- *FBC:* increased WBC in 50% with neutrophilia
- *ESR and CRP:* elevated in up to 98%, but non-specific
- *Blood cultures:* positive in 40–60%
- *Imaging:*
  - *plain radiographs:* usually normal as changes (periosteal elevation, radiolucent metaphyseal lesions) only develop at 7–14 days. Deep soft tissue swelling can appear by 3 days
  - *ultrasound:* may detect periosteal elevation or fluid within an affected adjacent joint. Peri-acetabular tissues should be included in the hip USS
  - *MRI:* detects changes well before radiographic changes apparent. Excellent for spine, pelvis, and limbs. However, differentiating oedema of infection from that of trauma or infarction may be difficult
- *CT scan:* superior to MRI for detection of sequestra.

Treatment

- *Antibiotics:* in children, *Staph, aureus* accounts for 80%, so initial treatment is with IV flucloxacillin ± fusidic acid. Alternative options include clindamycin, cefuroxime, and vancomycin. In the newborn, benzylpenicillin and cefotaxime is used to cover *Streptococci*. In a patient with sickle cell disease, flucloxacillin or ciprofloxacin to cover *Salmonella*. Positive blood or aspirated pus cultures may guide continuation treatment which is for 4–6 weeks depending on the organism, severity, and response judged by normalization of CRP and ESR. IV antibiotics are given for 3–7 days, changing to oral if response satisfactory.
- *Surgery:* bone aspiration or biopsy may be necessary. Associated septic arthritis, e.g. of the hip, requires incision and drainage. Recurrence may occur despite adequate treatment in 5–10%. Complications include disturbances in bone growth with limb-length discrepancies and angular deformity.

Variants of osteomyelitis

Neonatal osteomyelitis

The proximal femur is most common site with joint involvement in 76%, but multifocal osteomyelitis occurs. Group B streptococcus is the most common organism.

Epiphyseal osteomyelitis
From birth to 18 months the infection may spread into the epiphysis via blood vessels that cross the cartilaginous physis or growth plate. Septic arthritis may then develop.

Subacute osteomyelitis
Radiographic findings are usually present, but biopsy and curettage may be necessary as neoplastic and infiltrative disorders are difficult to exclude.

Vertebral osteomyelitis and discitis
Vertebral osteomyelitis is uncommon but may occur in sickle cell disease due to *Salmonella* infection. The aetiology and pathogenesis of discitis remains obscure. Infection or trauma may be responsible. A limp or refusal to walk is a common presentation. Diagnosis and localization is best achieved by MRI. Antibiotics may shorten the duration of discitis.

Chronic recurrent multifocal osteomyelitis (CRMO)
This is a benign, self-limiting, ill-defined disease of uncertain aetiology. Presentation is with symmetrical swelling over affected bones such as clavicle, spine, thorax, or pelvis. Anti-inflammatory medication is indicated.

Septic arthritis

Septic arthritis, a serious pyogenic infection within a joint, is a clinical emergency. It is relatively common in infancy and childhood although the exact frequency is uncertain. It is about twice as common as osteomyelitis and the incidence peaks in the early years of the first decade.

Aetiology and pathogenesis

Septic arthritis is haematogenous except in rare circumstances when it is caused by a penetrating wound, contiguous spread from an adjacent cellulitis, or decompression of osteomyelitis into joints such as the hip in which the capsule attaches to the metaphysis.

Haematogenous septic arthritis may develop directly through the synovial blood vessels.

Pathogens
Septic arthritis implies bacterial infection, although viral and fungal infection can occur, e.g. in preterm neonates. In all age groups the most common infecting organism is *Staph. aureus*. Other pathogens occur in distinct age groups:
- *Neonatal:* Group B streptococci, gram-negative organisms, *Candida albicans. Neisseria* sp. from an infected birth canal
- *<3 years:* Kingella kingae
- *Teenagers: Neisseria gonorrhoeae* can cause polyarticular septic arthritis in sexually active teenagers.

Pathogenesis
The joint space becomes a closed abscess. Damage to the joint occurs within hours by cartilage degradation by enzymes and bone ischaemia from increased joint pressure.

The potential result of a septic hip is complete destruction of the femoral head, destruction of the capsule with dislocation, and loss of 30% of the growth potential of the femur.

Clinical features

Developing septic arthritis is accompanied by fever, malaise, and localizing signs and symptoms at the affected joint including a limp or pseudoparalysis.

Examination reveals a fever >38 °C and local joint signs.

Superficial joints may display swelling, erythema, and tenderness but such signs are less evident with deeper joints.

The most consistent sign is pain with passive motion. The child appears comfortable while the joint is immobile in the position of maximal capsular volume.

Inability to weight-bear on a lower extremity or to spontaneously move any joint is suspicious of septic arthritis.

The differential diagnosis most commonly encountered is transient synovitis of the hip or postinfectious arthritis.

Management

Joint aspiration with a large-bore needle under imaging guidance is the most important diagnostic procedure. Pus is obtained (WBC >50 × 10^9/L, 80% neutrophils) and Gram stained. Additional initial investigations include:
- *FBC:* a normal WBC does not exclude septic arthritis
- *CRP, ESR:* CRP is more sensitive and responsive than ESR. A high fever (>38 °C), inability to weight-bear, and raised inflammatory markers (ESR >40 mm/h, CRP >2.0 mg/dL, and WBC >12 × 10^9/L) are predictive of septic arthritis
- *Blood cultures:* positive in 50% of cases.

Imaging
- *Plain radiographs:* no bony findings are likely but useful to exclude other conditions
- *Ultrasound scan:* this is most useful for identifying an effusion in the hip and also for guiding joint aspiration
- *MRI scan:* indicated in suspected psoas abscess and useful in defining an associated osteomyelitis.

Treatment
A septic joint requires drainage as well as antibiotics.
- *Medical therapy:* choice of antibiotic may be guided by Gram stain results or be empirical initially, based on age. Combination therapy is used. Options include flucloxacillin, aminoglycosides to cover gram-negative bacilli and *Pseudomonas*, clindamycin or vancomycin as cover for MRSA, cefotaxime for *K. kingae* or gonococcal arthritis. Initial therapy is IV, but switch to oral is acceptable after 3–7 days if clinical response is satisfactory. Duration of therapy is usually up to 2 weeks but treatment is not stopped until symptoms and signs resolve and WBC, CRP, and ESR return to normal.
- *Surgical therapy:* adequate drainage is essential. Options include percutaneous needle aspiration in peripheral joints or open drainage for the hip and for peripheral joints not responding to aspiration.

Rehabilitation is required to maximize residual joint function.

16.12 Case-based discussions

A boy with fever and rash
A 3 year old boy presents with a 3 week history of very high fever. He does not want to play, has a reduced appetite, and does not seem right according to his mother. There is no other specific or relevant history. He is usually well and takes no medications. He has not been abroad.

On examination, he is febrile at 39° C, and looks very unwell and miserable. He has a macular pink rash over his trunk. He is tachycardic and tachypnoeic at 45/min. He complains that his arms and legs hurt all over, but his limbs and joints are normal on examination. There is marked cervical lymphadenopathy and a slightly enlarged liver and spleen.

What is your differential diagnosis?
A child with protracted fever and a rash with lymphadenopathy and organomegaly might have an infective, malignant, or autoimmune disease as the underlying cause. Infective causes include glandular fever and several which would have required foreign travel, e.g. typhoid, *Brucellosis*. Infection of occult sites should also be considered. Malignancies such as lymphoma or leukaemia are possible. Autoimmune diseases should be considered, including JIA, SLE, and other vasculitides such as Kawasaki disease.

Initial investigations reveal:
Hb 9.0 g/dL Film: normocytic, normochromic anaemia
FBC: WCC 17.1 × 10^9/L, neut 12.4 × 10^9/L, plt 855 × 10^9/L
CRP 112 mg/L, ESR 94 mm/h
Ferritin 1084 μg/L

A decision is made to admit him for monitoring of his fever, but not to start any antibiotics. His fever chart over 48 h shows high regular spikes and intermittent slightly hypothermic temperatures. His mother tells you that every time he is hot, he has a spreading pink rash, which clears as the fever settles. The nurse looking after him corroborates this.

What does this suggest?
These findings are typical of systemic-onset JIA. This boy is a typical age for presentation, and, unlike many other autoimmune conditions, the incidence is equal in boys and girls. The high swinging fever with a salmon pink rash is typical. Children often have a history of malaise and anorexia. They may complain of joint pains, but joints frequently show no signs of arthritis at presentation. The anaemia, neutrophilia, and inflammatory response are characteristic.

What would you expect on his autoimmune screen?
Children with SOJIA tend to have negative rheumatoid factor, dsDNA, and ANA.

His fever and symptoms resolve with a course of methylprednisolone. He is discharged home for outpatient treatment with methotrexate and NSAIDs. Three weeks later he re-presents to the hospital emergency department. He is unwell, has a fever of 38.8 °C, and a blotchy rash. He is slightly hypotensive, tachycardic, and has a prolonged capillary refill time. He is also slightly dehydrated.

What is the differential of this presentation?
This could represent a flare-up of disease. However, this child is also profoundly immunocompromised as a consequence of his treatment, and severe systemic sepsis is a possibility, particularly as he has features of septic shock—hypotension and prolonged capillary refill time. Blood cultures should be taken and broad spectrum antibiotics should be administered. Infection must be excluded, by trial of clinical response to antibiotics and by blood cultures, before a disease flare is treated.

A girl with fever and rash
A 9 year old Asian girl presented with a 2 week history of fever. There had initially been some diarrhoea, without vomiting, which had resolved after 3 days. There was no significant previous history and no history of recent foreign travel.

On examination she was systemically unwell with a fever of 40 °C. There was a faint pink non-pruritic macular rash involving the face and trunk and reddish macules on the fingers and toes. Generalized lymphadenopathy was evident but no organomegaly (Fig 16.14)

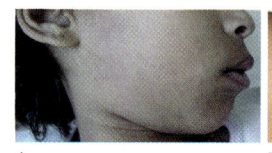

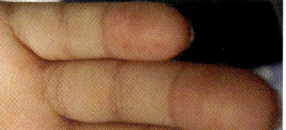

A   B

Fig 16.14

Investigations:
FBC Hb 8.9 g/dL, WCC 3.7 × 10^9/L, with lymphopaenia and thrombocytopaenia, platelets 96 × 10^9/L
ESR 126 mm/h, CRP 87 mg/dL.
Blood cultures: grew Salmonella enteriditis at 24 h
Urinalysis: proteinuria + and haematuria ++ on dipstick testing.

What is the differential diagnosis?
The most likely diagnosis is SLE. There is a well established association between SLE and non-typhoidal salmonellosis. Although this occurs most often in patients with active disease on intensified immunosuppression, *Salmonella* bacteraemia can occur at first presentation. It is hypothesized that patients with SLE have a specific immune defect predisposing to invasive disease.

What would you expect on her autoimmune screen?
She had strongly positive ANA and positive anti-dsDNA antibodies. She was ant-Ro and anti-La positive. There was marked hypocomplementaemia. The uncharacteristically raised CRP was ascribed to her bacteraemia.

She went on to develop severe lupus nephritis and required treatment with hydroxychloroquine and mycophenolate mofetil. Subsequently her general disease became active, especially in the skin. This was treated with rituximab.

Chapter 17

Mental health

17.1 Paediatric mental health *370*
17.2 Common emotional and behavioural problems *372*
17.3 Developmental disorders *374*
17.4 Attention deficit and conduct disorder *376*
17.5 Anxiety, depression, and psychosis *378*
17.6 Case-based discussions *380*

17.1 Paediatric mental health

Mental health

How the mind is functioning is reflected in how a child thinks, feels, and acts and mental health is manifested by normal activity in these three domains of cognition, emotions, and behaviour.

The obvious and striking difference between children and adults in respect of assessing mental health is the need in children to consider development and the way in which cognition, emotions, and behaviour change with age.

A mentally healthy child is able to:

- Develop psychologically, emotionally, and intellectually
- Initiate, develop, and sustain mutually satisfying personal relationships
- Develop a moral sense of right and wrong
- Become aware of and empathize with others
- Manifest emotional distress and maladaptive behaviour that is *within normal limits* for their age and the environmental context.

Normal development

Child development is considered in Chapter 18 and adolescent development in Chapter 19, but some aspects relevant to mental health are considered here. A knowledge of the wide normal ranges of development in each of three domains is a prerequisite for assessing a child's mental health.

Cognitive development

Cognition involves learning and memory, perception, attention, speech and language, and reasoning. Basic cognitive functions develop by 2–6 years. Specific functions include:

- *Speech and language:* communication in infants is non-verbal and achieved by crying, facial expression, gesture, and babbling. From 12–15 months children begin to use words to achieve specific outcomes and express preferences and by 24 months to express future intent. By age 3 years children use language for full communication and by 6 years have acquired an intelligible language system.
- *Memory:* by age 3 years short-term memory can hold two or three items of information and memory develops in parallel with language during the preschool years.
- *Attention:* attention depends on frontal lobe function and is also a learned activity. Its maturation is reflected initially in ability to focus on an external event such as playing with a toy and subsequently by the ability to inhibit or prevent inappropriate responses.

Emotional development

The development of language allows a child to describe their internal emotional experiences as the child learns the meaning of words like 'happy' and 'sad'. Early normal expressions of anxiety occur in response to strangers and to separation from parents. A fearful response to animals or the dark is also common and regarded as normal.

Behavioural development

Normal behavioural development allows increasing autonomy and acceptable patterns of bladder and bowel control, sleeping, feeding, socialization, and self-control. Normal development in these domains is discussed below.

Mental health disorders

The term 'paediatric mental health' has been introduced to encompass those mental health problems which come primarily within the remit of the paediatrician. See 'Child in mind' at the RCPCH. Child and adolescent mental health (CAMH) services deal with disorders requiring specialized expertise.

Diagnostic categories are less easily applied to disorders of the mind, and current classification schemes focus on the presenting features of each disorder (phenomenology) rather than on aetiology or pathogenetic mechanisms.

As discussed below, the aim of clinical evaluation is often to achieve a 'diagnostic formulation' rather than a categorical diagnosis.

Epidemiology

The latest UK data come from a survey by the Office for National Statistics: *Mental health of children and young people in Great Britain*, 2004.

Prevalence of mental disorders

1 in 10 children aged 5–16 had a clinically diagnosed mental disorder. The common disorders found were: anxiety or depression (4%), conduct disorders (6%), and hyperkinetic disorder (2%). Mental disorders are more common in boys than girls, and affect:

- 10% of boys, 5% of girls aged 5–10 years
- 13% of boys, 10% of girls aged 11–16 years.

The sex ratio varies markedly for certain problems:

- *Male excess:* autistic spectrum disorders, tic disorders, hyperactivity, conduct disorder, juvenile delinquency, completed suicide, nocturnal enuresis
- *Female excess:* specific phobias, deliberate self-harm and depression (postpubertal), anorexia nervosa and bulimia.

Many children have multiple diagnoses. For example, children with generalized anxiety disorder often have specific phobias. Children with hyperactivity often meet criteria for conduct disorders.

Early-onset disorders include autistic spectrum disorders, hyperactivity disorders, oppositional-defiant disorder, enuresis, and separation anxiety. Teenage onset is most commonly seen in depression, deliberate self-harm and suicide, anorexia nervosa and bulimia, panic attacks, substance abuse, and major psychoses. See Chapter 19 for adolescent disorders.

Diagnostic groupings

The two main classifications in current use are:

- *International classification of Diseases of the World Health Organization:* ICD-10
- *Diagnostic and Statistical Manual of the American Psychiatric Association:* DSM-IV.

The three main diagnostic groupings are:

- *Emotional disorders:* anxiety disorders, phobias, depression, obsessive-compulsive disorder (OCD), somatization
- *Disruptive behaviour:* hyperactivity disorders, oppositional-defiant disorder, conduct disorders
- *Developmental disorders:* autistic spectrum disorders; enuresis and encopresis.

Clinical assessment

Presentation: general aspects
It is essential to consider the mental health of every child who presents to a paediatrician. There are few disorders of any kind which do not have some impact on a child's mental health. Up to 40% of children with a chronic disorder are likely to have a co-morbid mental health problem.

Mental health problems: symptoms and impact
A significant mental health problem arises when the degree of distress or maladaptive behaviour is outside the normal limits for the child's age, development, and family context. The same problems may be considered trivial by one family but as a major difficulty by another.

A significant problem is present if the symptoms are having a substantial *impact* as judged from:
- *Social impairment:* family disruption, educational failure
- *Distress for the child:* children may be able to fulfil normal roles despite significant inner turmoil and anguish
- *Disruption for others:* antisocial behaviour, offending, family disruption. Conduct problems can cause major disruption without much distress for the child.

Behaviour as communication
It is useful to think of behaviour as an attempt to communicate. This applies to behaviour at all developmental stages. A crying infant, toddler having a tantrum, or self-harming adolescent, can all be seen as attempts at communication.

This model is more likely to lead to a shared understanding with parents than a model based on 'abnormality' which may imply parental incompetence or naughtiness of the child.

The consultation

Personal skills and attitudes
A good starting premise should be that all parents wish to do their best for their children and that your role is to build on any existing strengths and to remove obstacles to achieving resolution of the problems.

A respectful acceptance of parents' difficulties, empathy with the child's predicament, and a caring curiosity with good active listening skills will render the consultation therapeutic and help the family find solutions.

History
The mnemonic SIRSE can guide and expand the standard paediatric history if a significant mental health problem is suspected. Questions should be 'open' rather than 'closed', and specific information sought rather than generalizations.
- **S**ymptoms: What kind of problem is it? When did it start and how frequent is it? How is it managed and by whom?
- *Impact:* What social impairment, distress or disruption is being caused? How is day to day functioning affected? Who is most affected and in what way?
- **R**isk factors: **P**redisposing, **P**recipitating, and **P**erpetuating factors. See Diagnostic formulation, below.
- **S**trengths: What **P**rotective factors or assets are there to work with? See Diagnostic formulation, below.
- *Explanatory models:* What beliefs and expectations about the problem and its solution do the family have?

Parents may agree to a request for information from school. Teachers are generally excellent observers, but some symptoms may be missed or misconstrued. Anxiety, depression, or playground victimization may all be missed whilst inattention with hyperactivity may reflect learning difficulties.

Examination
Observing child and family
Observe the child's activity and attention, social interactions, developmental level, and play. Observe the interaction between parent and child: is it warm, sensitive, critical, supportive? Is the attitude of child to parent: distant, interrupting, ignoring, or challenging? Between the parents is there agreement, friction, accord, or discord? Are all children treated the same or are there family alignments?

Physical examination
General examination should take note of:
- *Dysmorphic features:* especially if a generalized learning disability is present. A clue may be gained to existence of a syndrome such as fragile X
- *Signs of abuse:* bruises, burns, bites.

A neurological examination is required if there is a history of seizures, regression, developmental delay, abnormal gait, dysarthria, asymmetrical hand use, or skin signs of a neurocutaneous disorder.

Diagnostic formulation

A 'diagnostic formulation' is more likely to lead to an appropriate management plan than a traditional 'diagnosis' focused on a biological abnormality. Mental health disorders are usually caused by a complex interaction of numerous factors involving both nature and nurture. This is expressed in the *biopsychosocial model*.

A diagnostic formulation considers biological, psychological and social factors under the 'four Ps' scheme which involves three risk factor types: **p**redisposing, **p**recipitating, and **p**erpetuating and **p**rotective factors which provide resilience. The diagnostic formulation is the summary of these factors.
Examples of each factor type include:

Predisposing factors: confer vulnerability
- *Biological:* genetic predisposition, chronic illness
- *Psychological:* sexual, physical, or emotional abuse
- *Social:* lone parent, homelessness, refugee status.

Precipitating factors: act as triggers
- *Biological:* acute illness
- *Psychological:* parental separation, bereavement
- *Social:* bullying, victimization, scapegoating, teasing.

Perpetuating factors: maintain the problem
These encompass predisposing factors but include new factors which may create a vicious circle that maintains the problem.

Protective factors: confer resilience
- *Biological:* calm temperament, average or higher intelligence
- *Psychological:* sense of self-mastery, positive attitude
- *Social:* good parenting style, external support system.

17.2 Common emotional and behavioural problems

Preschool children: <5 years

Emotional and behavioural problems in the preschool child are age dependent. Whether a family experiences the behaviour of their child as a problem is independent of whether the behaviour is within the normal range: many 'normal' behaviours are presented as a problem and 'abnormal' behaviour may not present.

Crying

A normal, healthy infant cries for 1–3 h in 24 h. The pattern changes with age:

- *1–3 months*: average 2 h/day. Crying episodes cluster in late afternoon and evening. 40% of total occurs between 6 p.m. and midnight
- *4–6 months*: average 1 h/day
- *6–12 months*: average 1 h/day with an increase in night-time crying.

Persistent crying is usefully defined as crying for more than 3 h/day on more than 3 days/week. This is found in 10–15% of infants in the 1st 3 months and whether it is considered excessive depends on parental response.

Health visitor support and advice on coping with a crying baby can be helpful. If persistent crying generates anger or frustration the baby should be placed in a safe place and a break taken away from the baby. Further advice is available from GP, health visitor, NHS Direct or the Cry-sis helpline in the UK.

Sleeping

The average newborn infant sleeps for 16–18 h in 24 h with the sleep–wake cycle lasting 3–4 h. By 3 months many infants show a stable diurnal wake–sleep cycle, and by 6 months many will sleep through the night. By 4–5 years most children sleep 10–12 h in 24 h in one sleep period. Between 5–10 years total sleep time gradually decreases.

Sleep problems
It has been said that it is parents rather than children who suffer from sleep problems. The problem may be with settling to sleep or night waking, or both. 50% of night-wakers have a problem settling. In confusional arousals the child cries out and thrashes around for 5–15 min.

Night waking in the first year of life is normal and can cause severe parental sleep deprivation. Difficulties in settling are common in infants and toddlers. Many health visitors run sleep clinics offering behavioural advice along the following lines:

- *Bedtime routine*: 'winding down' period, warm bath, snack, story. Be consistent.
- *Checking routine for night waking (>9 months)*: leave crying child for 5–10 min, check the child and leave. Repeat as necessary with increasing interval. If child gets out of bed, return him or her promptly and firmly. Do not give any rewards. A 'gradual retreat' method may be used in which you sit by the cot instead of leaving, gradually sitting further away each night.
- *Give positive reinforcement*: star charts
- Keep a sleep diary.

Feeding problems: food refusal and faddiness

Up to 20% of normal children undergoing the transition from milk to solids are reported to be slow or fussy eaters. Many children go through a period of food refusal at some time between the age of 2 and 5 years, in part as a means of asserting independence.

Food refusal and faddiness
About 10% of children go through a period of food refusal in their 1st 5 years. This often starts at the end of the 1st year and beginning of the 2nd. A baby who previously ate a wide range of foods happily may suddenly narrow the range of acceptable foods or refuse to eat anything at all.

This may trigger 'food wars' if the parents are confrontational and put pressure on the child to eat. Parents always lose food wars, especially if snacks or drinks are offered between meals by parents anxious that the child will starve. A child who is not hungry is even less inclined to eat the food on offer, but a child will always eat when hungry.

Management
Examination and perusal of a weight chart is important to exclude an underlying medical problem and confirm that the child is thriving.

A diary should be kept, all food between meals banned and positive encouragement given for mouthfuls eaten.
Important advice includes:

- Do not give your child *any* food, sweets, snacks, or sweet drinks between meals, however little your child eats at mealtime
- Offer a range of foods in small portions and avoid the consumption of too many drinks during the meal
- Offer meals without putting any pressure on your child to eat but remove any remaining food without comment after 20 min
- Eat with your child if possible, and praise your child if any food is eaten
- Try not to make a fuss about small matters such as the order of courses, finger feeding, or messiness.

Most children recover a normal range of food preferences.

Temper tantrums and oppositional behaviour

Tantrums are outbursts of annoyance or rage and are a normal part of childhood development. The peak of prevalence is between 18 months and 3 years, 'the terrible twos', coinciding with a period marked by curiosity and frustration when demands for instant gratification are not met.

Strategies for avoiding or dealing with tantrums are built on a foundation of positive attention. Children prefer negative attention to no attention at all, and negative attention merely reinforces undesirable behaviour. Helpful strategies to offer parents include:

- *Distraction*: interest the child in alternative behaviour if a tantrum appears imminent. Point out amusing item or picture, introduce a toy. Timing is crucial
- *Ignoring*: calmly continue with whatever you are doing without expressing any emotion
- *Pay attention to good behaviour*: reward or praise good behaviour. Praise includes verbal and non-verbal such as smiles or hug. Stop ignoring and praise when the screaming stops.

School-age children: 5–11 years

Sleep problems

In preadolescents, common sleep problems include nightmares, night terrors, and sleep-walking or somnambulism. Mental health disorders can cause sleep problems, and sleep problems may mimic or exacerbate mental health problems. Psychotropic medication or its withdrawal may induce sleep problems. The same risk factors may predispose to both mental health problems and sleep difficulties.

Sleep problems are common among children with generalized learning difficulties, physical disabilities such as cerebral palsy, blindness, generalized anxiety, and medical conditions which may worsen at night such as asthma and eczema.

Sleep problems usually present as difficulty getting to sleep or staying asleep, daytime somnolence, or episodic disturbance at night. Examples of the latter include the following:

Nightmares

These are a form of unpleasant dream and arise from REM sleep, making them more common in the second half of the night. The child wakes, frightened and alert, and is able to remember the dream and its content.

Nightmares at a frequency of <1 per week are common in the age range 5–10 years. Indicators for concern would be a high frequency, repetitive theme, or a child afraid to go to bed because of fear of the nightmares occurring.

Predisposing factors include stress such as bullying or abuse, and nightmares are a feature of post-traumatic stress disorder.

Night terrors and sleepwalking

These involve partial arousal out of deep non-REM, phase IV sleep and are therefore most common in the first couple of hours of sleep. Night terrors affect about 3% of children in the 4–10 year age range with a peak at 4–7 years.

In night terrors the child wakes abruptly, screaming or shouting and may rush around in an agitated state. The child appears terrified and agitated and is neither rousable nor consolable. After 10–20 min peaceful sleep is resumed. There is usually no recollection of the episode in the morning.

Sleepwalking (somnambulism)

This occurs in up to 17% of children with a peak age at 8–12 years. The child wanders around for up to 10 min with eyes wide open. Micturition may occur and there is significant risk of injury.

If these episodes occur at a regular time they may be prevented by 'scheduled awakening' 15–30 min before the episode is due. Safety measures such as securing doors or windows and placing a gate across the stairs may be necessary.

Somatization

Somatization is the communication of emotional distress through physical symptoms. It is estimated to be a factor in 50% of general paediatric consultations.

Aetiology

The aetiology is usually multifactorial and dominated by personality and family factors. Using the biopsychosocial model:

- *Biological*: previous illness or surgery, female sex
- *Psychological*: personality traits such as conscientious, sensitive, obsessional, or anxious
- *Social*: family factors: parental disharmony, overprotection, family members with somatic symptoms, emotional abuse, stress: bereavement, moving house, school problems: bullying, academic stresses.

Clinical features

Common forms of somatization include:

- *Recurrent pain*: abdominal and other sites
- *Fatigue*: isolated or with other symptoms
- Motor or sensory deficit without organic explanation.

In the primary school age group recurrent abdominal pain is the most common somatic symptom, peaking at age 9. Headaches, limb pain, dizzy spells, and fatigue become more common with increasing age. See Chapter 19.6.

Recurrent abdominal pain

Recurrent abdominal pain affects 10–20% of school-age children at some time. It is categorized as one of the functional gastrointestinal disorders: childhood functional abdominal pain. see Chapter 5.8. It may be associated with other symptoms such as headaches, nausea, vomiting, or limb pain. A full history and examination is important to exclude the 'alarm features' suggestive of an organic cause: see Chapter 5.8.

Management of somatization

A comprehensive, sympathetic, and non-confrontational approach will allow the child and parents to feel they have been listened to, understood, respected, and believed.

A medical or 'organic' diagnosis can usually be excluded with an adequate history and clinical examination. An endless search for a medical cause using investigations may make the symptoms more entrenched.

Management strategies include:

- Reassurance that assessment has ruled out serious organic disease and developing with the family and child a shared explanation that links symptoms and distress with stress.
- Helping the child develop techniques to control symptoms until they recede.
- Maintaining a focus on gradual resumption of normal activities with the aid of physiotherapy if necessary and discouragement of sick-role behaviour.

School refusal

The child refuses to go to school or sets out for school but returns home. Anxiety or fear of school attendance may be overt, with attempts to force attendance being met by tears, tantrums, or physical resistance. School refusal peaks on starting school, after school transfer, and in the early teens.

Factors contributing include:

- *Personality*: the children are usually of average intelligence and academic ability and are often conformist at school. It may be a feature of separation anxiety or specific phobias, or depression in teenagers.
- *Family factors*: poor organization or discipline, emotional overinvolvement with the child. Some children have to look after a sick parent.

Support, in close liaison with the school, for parents and child is necessary to achieve a return to school. In chronic cases a gradual reintegration may be necessary with a specific behavioural programme. Small tutorial classes facilitate anxiety management in older children.

17.3 Developmental disorders

Autism spectrum disorders (ASD)

This is an umbrella term used to cover both core autism and a broader range of autistic-like disorders. The hallmark of ASD is a deficit in some or all of three key areas:

- *Reciprocal social interactions*
- *Communication:* verbal and non-verbal
- *Flexibility of thinking and behaviour.*

Subcategories include autism and Asperger syndrome. Rett syndrome and childhood disintegrative disorder are two rare categories which are currently included within ASD as they have features in common with autism.

Epidemiology

Prevalence rates of both autism and ASD appear to have increased, in part due to more complete ascertainment and the broader definition of ASD. Prevalence rates vary depending on the diagnostic criteria used. Estimates for core autism are 0.6–2.0/1000 and for ASD 6–11.6/1000, or up to 1.2% in 9–10 year old children. Boys are 3–4 times more likely to be affected than girls overall.

Aetiology

10–15% of cases of autism occur in children with identifiable medical conditions including:

- *Tuberous sclerosis complex:* 20–60% have autism
- Fragile X syndrome
- Phenylketonuria
- Traumatic brain injury.

For most children with ASD, genetic factors are of primary importance. Concordance in identical twins is 60–80%, much higher than that in non-identical twins, indicating a heritability of 90%. The recurrence rate in siblings is 3% for narrowly defined autism and 10–20% for milder variants. The evidence is that ASD are inherited as 'complex' traits.

As yet, research has failed to identify any major environmental factor that contributes to causation.

Clinical features and diagnosis

Diagnosis of ASD is not straightforward. A formal diagnosis of core autism is made by a specialist who will apply one of the established clinical screeening instruments such as Checklist for autism for toddlers (CHAT) or Autism Diagnostic Interview—Revised (ADI-R). Early diagnosis of ASD is important, not least because of evidence that early intervention results in improved outcome.

The characteristic features of autism and Asperger syndrome are considered in turn.

Autism

The autistic end of the spectrum is characterized by the onset before age 3 years of symptoms in three domains:

- *Social impairment:* reciprocal interactions are impaired. Parents may report lack of social smiling, preference for playing alone, lack of interest in other children, being in his/her own world, failure to seek comfort when hurt. Examination may reveal an aloof child with poor eye contact.
- *Communication impairment:* speech development is markedly delayed and 30% never acquire useful speech. Speech if it emerges is deviant with echolalia, pronominal reversal, ('you' for 'I'), inverted words, stock phrases. The child talks at rather than with people. Gestures are reduced. The child does not point or wave goodbye.
- *Stereotyped behaviour:* activities and interests are restricted and repetitive features include resistance to change with insistence on routines and rituals. There can be stereotypies such as hand flapping or twirling, attachment to unusual objects, and consuming preoccupation with restricted subjects. Make-believe play is usually lacking.

Definite indicators for further evaluation include:

- No babbling by 12 months
- No gesturing, pointing or waving by 12 months
- No single words by 16 months or two-word phrases by 24 months
- Loss of language or social skills at any age.

Commonly associated features outside these three domains include abnormal sensory responses, early hyperactivity replaced later by underactivity, abnormal eating such as food fads and sleep problems.

Co-morbidity is extensive and includes:

- *Generalized learning disability:* this is present in the majority. In severe autism IQ ranges from 50–100. (In Asperger syndrome, see below, intelligence is normal or above average.)
- *Epilepsy:* seizures affect 25% with peak onset at 11–14 years
- *Emotional and behavioural disorders:* attention deficit hyperactivity disorder, temper tantrums, phobias, depression
- *Tourette syndrome.*

Asperger syndrome

This term is used for a group at the more able end of the spectrum of autistic disorders with regard to social and communication handicap. It is usually diagnosed between the age of 6 and 14 years but may go unrecognized into adulthood.

Asperger syndrome differs from core autism in the following respects:

- *Language development:* vocabulary and grammar develop normally but speech is often stilted and pedantic with abnormal intonation
- *Social interactions:* less aloof than in autism, but empathy is impaired
- *Behaviour:* circumscribed interests rather than motor stereotypies.

Management

A UK National Autism Plan for Children provides guidelines for investigation, early diagnosis, and intervention. Whole-population screening is not recommended, but identification of ASD can be improved by increased recognition of alerting signals to detect those requiring formal assessment.

A full physical examination should be undertaken and investigations done if clinically indicated including karyotyping and fragile X DNA analysis. Cognitive, speech and language assessments should be undertaken and observations made in more than one setting.

The mainstays of management are:

- Giving open, sensitive and repeated feedback about the diagnosis.
- Ensuring the family receive information about local parent groups, education and training, support services, and

social benefits. In the UK, the National Autistic Society is a well-recognized resource and advocacy group.
- Placing the emphasis on behavioural and educational approaches. Behavioural therapy can reduce tantrums, aggressive outbursts, fears, and rituals and foster normal development. The National Autism Plan for Children recommends access to ASD-specific educational opportunities for preschool and school-age children
- Using pharmacological intervention judiciously. It does not alter long-term prognosis but medication for specific associated symptoms may be required, e.g. antiepilepsy drugs, stimulants for hyperactivity (although repetitive behaviour may increase), and SSRIs for severe anxiety, depression, or self-injury.

Enuresis

Bladder and bowel control
85% of children are dry at night by age 5 years and 95% by age 7 years. 50% of 2 years olds are able to ask for and use a potty or toilet and most of the rest are capable of this before going to school at rising 5 years.

Enuresis is the involuntary passage of urine beyond the age at which bladder control is expected. It is categorized as:
- Nocturnal (night-time), diurnal (daytime), or both.
- Primary (continence never established) or secondary (loss of continence following at least 6 months of dryness).

Enuresis overall is twice as common in boys than girls but diurnal enuresis is more common in girls. Most children are dry by 3–4 years, but 15% of 5 year olds, 5% of 10 year olds, and 1% of 15 year olds are still wet at night.

Aetiology
- *Biological:*
  - *genetic predisposition:* a family history in 70%
  - *urinary tract infection:* in 5% of secondary enuresis
  - *urinary tract abnormalities:* small bladder capacity, incomplete bladder voiding, detrusor instability secondary to constipation
- *Psychological:* general developmental delay, associated psychiatric disorders in a minority
- *Social:* stressful life events such as trauma, separation, birth of a younger sibling, social disadvantage, family disorganization.

Clinical evaluation
A full history and examination should establish the category and exclude an organic cause. Urinalysis for glycosuria/ketonuria and culture should be undertaken.

Management
The Enuresis Resource and Information Centre (ERIC) has information for children, parents, and professionals on their website and provides a telephone helpline.

Secondary nocturnal enuresis in response to acute stress is the most common presentation and is usually self-limiting.

Advice for simple primary nocturnal enuresis includes:
- Parents should avoid a punitive attitude and avoid excess attention to the wetting.
- Emphasize common nature of problem and expectations that the child will grow out of it.
- *Simple measures:* omitting drinks in 4 h before bedtime, ensuring bladder emptying at bedtime, lifting child to repeat bladder emptying at parental bedtime.
- *Star charts:* document progress, reward achievement.

If these simple measures are unsuccessful, options used in an enuresis clinic include:
- *Enuresis alarms:* 'bell and pad' in children >6 years successful in 80–90% but high relapse rate.
- *Medication:* desmopressin, an antidiuretic, is available as nasal spray or tablets and useful in older children who have not responded to behavioural approaches. Useful for known responders for short-term relief.
- *Bladder training:* diurnal enuresis may be improved. The interval between voiding is gradually increased from hourly up to 3–4 h intervals.

Encopresis

Encopresis is the passage of faeces in an inappropriate place and is synonymous with functional faecal incontinence. The diagnosis is often reserved for children >4 years of age, when toilet training has usually been achieved. There is a close relationship with constipation, which is difficulty or delay in the passage of stools.

Encopresis is more common in boys (M:F ratio 4:1) and affects about 1% of school-age children.

Aetiology
- *Biological:* chronic constipation can cause retention with overflow, called retentive encopresis or soiling. The cause of chronic simple constipation is multifactorial but related to diet and developmental factors and may be triggered by dehydration or an anal fissure (see Chapter 5.9).
- *Psychological:* some children with serious emotional problems may intentionally pass stools inappropriately or smear them on sheets or walls.
- *Social:* non-retentive encopresis is associated with neglect and disadvantage and may be triggered by an external stressor. Co-morbid conditions include enuresis, hyperactivity, and behaviour disorders.

Clinical evaluation
A comprehensive assessment is indicated with a particular focus on identifying the presence or absence of constipation and identifying contributory emotional or social factors. Organic causes for constipation should be excluded.

Management
Constipation needs to be treated using diet and laxatives, and a routine of bowel opening established. Behavioural modification strategies include the use of positive reinforcement rather than punitive approaches and externalization. Parents and child are encouraged to objectify and personify the problem. Continued, consistent, and optimistic professional input is needed for a successful outcome.

17.4 Attention deficit and conduct disorder

Attention deficit hyperactivity disorder

Attention-deficit hyperactivity disorder (ADHD) is a disorder characterized by levels of inattention, hyperactivity, and impulsiveness inconsistent with the level of development.

ADHD is defined in DSM-IV and a more severe form, hyperkinetic disorder (HKD) is defined in ICD-10. HKD requires pervasiveness in all three areas and an early age of onset. Attention deficit disorder (ADD) is also recognized.

The UK prevalence of ADHD is 3–5% and of HKD 1–3%. The M:F ratio is about 3:1.

Aetiology and pathogenesis

Family, adoption, and twin studies indicate that genetic factors make a major contribution. Susceptibility genes include those for specific dopamine transporters and receptors.

Neuropsychological and neuroimaging studies implicate frontal networks and frontostriatal dysfunction as the underlying neurobiological dysfunction.

Psychosocial factors are important, as indicated by links with deprivation and institutional care, family and social dysfunction such as domestic violence, parental substance abuse, child abuse. There is evidence supporting an adverse effect of food additives on hyperactive behaviour in the general population of children, not just those with ADHD.

ADD or ADHD has an increased frequency, >20% in certain conditions, perhaps implying a causal relationship:
- Prenatal exposure to alcohol or heroin
- *Low birthweight/very low birthweight infants:* 10% have ADHD
- *Genetic syndromes:* neurofibromatosis type 1, Angelman syndrome, fragile X syndrome
- Traumatic brain injury.

Co-morbidity

ADHD is associated with numerous neuropsychiatric and developmental disorders. The majority of children have one or more co-morbid conditions including:
- Very frequent:
  - oppositional defiant or conduct disorder
  - developmental coordination disorder
  - *specific learning difficulties:* dyslexia, dyscalculia
- Frequent:
  - tics and Tourette syndrome
  - anxiety
- Less frequent:
  - autistic spectrum disorder
  - generalized learning difficulties.

Clinical features

The clinical picture is shaped by the developmental psychopathology, co-morbidity, and psychosocial factors. The manifestations change with age and vary with context, i.e. home, school, clinic. The symptoms fall into three main groups:
- *Inattention:* brief attention span, easily distracted, switches from one activity to another, avoids sustained effort, forgetful, loses things
- *Hyperactivity:* fidgets (fine motor restlessness), always 'on the go' (gross motor restlessness), cannot play quietly, leaves seat in class, talks excessively
- *Impulsiveness:* acts without reflection, blurts out answers, interrupts others, does not wait their turn in games.

Formal diagnostic criteria vary. ICD-10, DSM-IV require:
- *Chronicity:* symptoms present for at least 6 months
- *Early onset:* some symptoms before age 7 years
- *Pervasiveness:* symptoms evident in two or more settings, e.g. home and school
- Six or more symptoms across the three domains of inattention, hyperkinesis, and impulsivity
- *Absence of another mental disorder:* a child with ASD or Tourette syndrome with hyperactivity and inattention is not given a second diagnosis of ADHD.

Assessment and diagnosis

Assessment is focused on the three main domains and identification of associated features and co-morbid disorders. Age of onset and information from the school is important as behaviour in clinic may not be typical.
- *Attention:* assess how long the child persists when engaged in various tasks such as playing or reading
- *Hyperactivity:* proportion of time fidgeting, how long sitting down when performing tasks, frequency of running off
- *Impulsiveness:* rash behaviour, frequent interrupting.

Associated features

It is not uncommon for these children to have defiant, aggressive, and antisocial behaviour, problems with social relationships, specific developmental delays, or learning problems (e.g. language, reading), and clumsiness.

Differential diagnosis

A multidisciplinary assessment is essential to distinguish ADHD from similar symptoms in the context of various co-morbid disorders or as a variant of normality.
- *Normality and situational hyperactivity:* most children are inattentive, hyperactive, or impulsive on occasion, particularly when tired, bored, hungry, upset, or receiving little adult attention. Some intolerant parents complain of behaviours well within the normal range.
- *Emotional and behavioural disorders:* severe anxiety or depression and attachment disorders or abuse can cause restlessness or inattention. Misdiagnosis in such cases is potentially damaging to the child. Conduct or oppositional disorders may be mixed with hyperactivity or mimic hyperactivity.
- *Tics and dyskinesias:* may be mistaken for fidgeting, but children with tic disorders are often hyperactive.
- ASD
- *Generalized learning disability:* hyperactivity is more common but may be at a level appropriate for mental age.

Management

ADHD cannot be cured, but the symptoms and associated impairments can be helped by a multimodal treatment approach: educational support, behavioural and psychological interventions, pharmacotherapy, and dietary manipulation.
- *Educational support:* close liaison with school is vital. Special learning problems may need remedial help and teaching needs to allow for the limited attention span.
- *Psychological/behavioural interventions:* education of child and family about the condition, emphasizing that the problems are not wilful naughtiness and that they are not the fault of child

or parent. Parent-training programmes for younger children (3–8 years) in which parents are seen in groups and given advice about child-management appear of limited use.

- *Pharmacotherapy:* stimulant medication is a well-tested treatment and can be useful for children aged 6 years and above. Options include methylphenidate and dexamfetamine. Non-stimulant drugs sometimes used include atomoxetine, an inhibitor of noradrenaline uptake. NICE guidelines recommend these three where drug treatment is considered appropriate, within their licensed indications.
  - *methylphenidate,* a dopamine stimulator, has a good efficacy and safety profile. It is useful as part of a comprehensive treatment programme for children of 6 years and over with severe ADHD. Treatment must be monitored and stopped if there is no effect. New, extended long-lasting preparations such as Concerta XL or Equasym XL provide a smoother profile of benefit and better compliance. Stimulant treatment is usually well tolerated but common side effects include appetite suppression with weight loss and delayed sleep onset.
  - *atomoxetine* may be useful for children not adequately responding to stimulants or with intolerable side effects. It is particularly useful for children whose ADHD is more prominent at home than at school.
- *Diet:* dietary treatment is popular with parents and is probably more effective for younger children. It comes in two forms: exclusion and supplementation. Exclusion diets are worth considering if parents have noticed a reaction to certain foods such as additives, oranges, milk, or wheat products. There is some evidence that supplementation with essential fish oils may improve symptoms in children with developmental coordination disorder.

Prognosis
Two-thirds of children take some symptoms into adult life. Overactivity wanes in adolescence, but inattention and restlessness persists with academic underperformance and increased risk of antisocial and delinquent behaviour.

Conduct disorder (CD)
This is characterized by persistent failure to control behaviour appropriately within socially defined rules, resulting in impairment in everyday functioning.

The overall prevalence is about 4% with a predominance of boys, although rates in adolescent girls are rising.

CD usually involves defiance, aggression, and antisocial behaviours. It remains debatable whether it is a mental health problem.

Aetiology: risk factors
CD clusters in families, and evidence indicates that shared environment is more important than shared genes in causation. Environmental factors associated with CD include:
- *Family:* parental psychiatric disorder or criminality, parental discord, poor child-rearing practices: lack of warmth, lack of supervision, inconsistent discipline
- *School:* poorly organized, unfriendly schools
- *Social environment:* socio-economic disadvantage, deviant peer culture with kudos for stealing or violence.

Clinical features
Manifestations change with age. Younger children manifest oppositional-defiant disorder (ODD) and older children CD.

Oppositional defiant disorder (ODD)
Characterized by disobedience, temper outbursts, angry or spiteful behaviour, deliberately annoying behaviour.

Vignette (© Youthinmind)
He just will not do what he is told. He answers back and throws huge temper tantrums if he cannot get his own way. He winds others up, particularly his brothers, and is glad when he gets other children into trouble because he has provoked them into shouting at him or hitting him. He is just the same at school. He is so stroppy, it does not take much to set him off.

Conduct disorder
Typical behaviour includes: telling lies, fighting, bullying, staying out late, running away from home, playing truant, cruelty to people or animals, criminal behaviour such as robbery or rape. This category includes 'well-adjusted criminals' who are not regarded as deviant within their subculture.

Vignette (© Youthinmind)
She used to bunk off school with her friends to go shoplifting, and they sold what they stole to buy drugs, alcohol, and cigarettes. Once she started secondary school, I lost all control over her. When she did go to school she was constantly in trouble because she would swear at teachers and refuse to do any work. She was finally permanently excluded from school because she was caught selling drugs. She was first in contact with the police for trespassing when she was 12 years old.

Vignette (© Youthinmind)
He has never had any friends, and he doesn't like school. He walks out if he doesn't like a lesson and wanders round town on his own. He was horribly bullied when he was younger, and now he gets into trouble for bullying younger children. He has also tried setting fire to a shed in the local park.

Associated features of CD include low mood, specific reading disorder, and poor interpersonal relationships.

The differential diagnosis includes:
- *Adjustment disorder:* transitory <6 months problems after a psychosocial stressor such as bereavement, trauma, or abuse
- *ADHD:* hyperactivity and CD may coexist.

Management
The strong environmental causation gives some grounds for therapeutic optimism. Behavioural modification strategies are focused on the child, family, school, and community. About 40% of children with CD become delinquent young adults.

17.5 Anxiety, depression, and psychosis

Fears, worries, and misery often cluster together and have been lumped together into a broad category of 'emotional disorders of childhood'. This broad group is now divided into many more specific disorders, although many children do not fit within precise diagnostic categories.

Anxiety disorders

Anxiety is a feeling of threat experienced in anticipation of an undesirable event which may be unknown or specified. Fear is a feeling of threat in the actual presence of a particular person, situation, or object.

Significant anxiety disorders affect around 4–8% of children and adolescents.

Table 17.1. Classification and epidemiology of anxiety disorders	
Anxiety disorders	Prevalence
Generalized anxiety disorder	2–6%
Separation anxiety disorder (SAD)	4%
Specific phobias	2–3% (more common in girls)
Social phobias	1%
Panic disorder, avoidant disorder including school refusal, and post-traumatic stress disorder (PTSD) are less common.	

Aetiology
Normal development of anxiety
Infants and toddlers cannot of course easily talk about emotions. It is assumed that they experience fear, but limited capacity to imagine the future probably protects against anxiety. Fear of strangers and separation anxiety peaks at ~18 months.

In early childhood fears appear in response to animals, the dark, and imagined situations. From 6–11 years fear of illness, parental death, and losing control are common. Adolescence brings new anxieties related to peer comparisons and social settings.

The onset of pathological anxieties tend to parallel these age-related changes.

Nature and nurture
Anxiety disorders run in families and twin studies have shown that genetics and non-shared environmental factors contribute equally to familial clustering.

Prospective studies show that temperamentally shy, inhibited, timid infants and toddlers are at increased risk of anxiety disorders in later childhood.

Anxiety disorders can be related to adverse life events, especially if several events occur in combination.

Clinical features
Generalized anxiety disorder
This disorder is characterized by unrealistic or excessive, persistent, generalized anxiety about past, present, or future everyday events and situations. It is more common in adolescents than in prepubertal children.

Anxiety is accompanied by physical symptoms such as restlessness, fatigue, muscular tension, and somatic complaints such as headaches or stomach aches.

Vignette (© Youthinmind)
I can't think of anything that he doesn't worry about. If it's not worry about his health, it's worry about whether he might have upset people at school, or about his homework, or about asteroids hitting the Earth. He'll worry himself sick about the slightest little thing, like whether he might have made a spelling mistake in a school essay he's just handed in.

Separation anxiety disorder (SAD)
Normal anxiety about separation from attachment figures emerges at ~6 months and wanes as the child acquires the ability to keep attachment figures 'in mind' when not physically present.

SAD is diagnosed if intensity of anxiety is developmentally inappropriate and leads to social impairment. Affected children worry unrealistically that their parents will leave and not return, or come to harm, or that they will get lost or taken away. SAD may manifest as school refusal.

Vignette (© Youthinmind)
He gets frantic if left on his own at all. He follows me from room to room, he doesn't want me to have my own life. He won't stay with his friends or even stay the night with his Gran like all his cousins do. He won't even stay over with his dad (we're divorced and I've remarried). It is not always easy to get him to go to school. He has to phone me at lunch time to check up on me. He gets upset if I want to go out with my new husband, and needs to know when I'll be back.

Specific phobias
Specific fears are common in childhood with different fears peaking at different ages: animals 2–4 years; the dark 4–6 years; death or war, adolescence.

The fear is classified as a phobia if it results in substantial distress or in avoidance that interferes with everyday life. Phobias involve unreasonable and exaggerated fears.

Vignette (© Youthinmind)
He is really terrified of dogs. I know lots of children are afraid of big dogs or aggressive dogs, but this is different. He is afraid of any dog, no matter how friendly or well-behaved it is. He doesn't want one to come near him and if one does, then he screams and grabs me tight or tries to run away.

Social phobia
This condition is an exaggeration and persistence of the normal phase of stranger anxiety which is prominent up to 30 months in normal children.

Affected children are anxious about meeting new or large groups of people, eating, reading or writing in front of others, or speaking in class. The child may be able to socialize with family members and familiar adults but shows marked avoidance of contact with unfamiliar people due to fear of embarrassment.

Social anxiety disorder is seen in children and may evolve into social phobia in adolescents. It is more than just shyness as there is dysfunction and disrupted relationships.

Vignette (© Youthinmind)
She doesn't like being with people she doesn't know, she is extremely shy. Once she's used to people, she's all right with them, just so long as she's with them one-to-one. But she doesn't even like family parties with her cousins and uncles and aunts, even though she's OK with them individually.

Treatment
- *Generalized anxiety disorder:* parental counselling, stress reduction, cognitive behaviour therapy
- *Separation anxiety disorder:* parental counselling, family therapy, operant techniques to alter balance of rewards and disincentives
- *Specific phobias:* parents can be taught to provide graded exposure to achieve desensitization. Child and parent counselled to understand that avoidance increases anxiety and exposure reduces it
- *Social phobia:* parental counselling, social skills training, cognitive behaviour therapy.

Sensitive and timely onward referral is required for most of these disorders.

Depression
The term depression can be used to refer to:
- A single emotional symptom (misery or sadness)
- A syndrome or cluster of symptoms including cognitive and behavioural symptoms
- A disorder fulfilling additional criteria of severity and persistence.

Epidemiological figures obviously depend on diagnostic criteria, but recent figures suggest that depressive disorder affects ~2% of prepubertal children and 5% of adolescents, with a female preponderance among adolescents. The prevalence of childhood depression has risen and the average age of onset fallen in recent decades.

Aetiology
Developmental considerations
Children <6 years have difficulty identifying and verbalizing feelings of sadness but may manifest symptoms and signs seen in depression such as passivity, unresponsiveness, tears, altered sleep and appetite. From 7–8 years children develop the ability to maintain sustained beliefs about themselves, including negative beliefs.

Risk factors for depression include:
- *Biological:* depression increases after puberty with a female preponderance in adolescence. Genetic factors are suggested by twin and family studies. Children with a parent or sibling with depression have a risk 10 times higher than the population risk. Chronic, severe, or life-threatening medical conditions predispose to depression.
- *Psychological:* chronic anxiety or a vulnerable temperament with low self-esteem or negative thinking style.
- *Social:* family dysfunction, abuse, or bereavement.

Clinical features
Many children may feel sad or miserable on occasion but are not considered to be depressed.

A depressive disorder is diagnosed on the basis of a cluster of symptoms in four domains which are persistent for more than 1–3 weeks and cause distress and social incapacity:
- *Emotional:* sadness, misery, anhedonia (loss of enjoyment), fearfulness
- *Cognitive:* loss of interest, poor concentration with deterioration in school work, feelings of worthlessness, guilt and hopelessness, thoughts of death, suicidal ideation
- *Behavioural:* inactivity, agitation or retardation, self-harming, social withdrawal
- *Biological:* change in sleep pattern (sleeping more or less), change in appetite (decreased or increased), reduced energy levels with tiredness after slight effort.

Comorbidity is common, with 50% of depressed children having at least one other psychiatric disorder.

Vignette (© Youthinmind)
This last month or so she seems really down in the dumps. She has been crying about the slightest little thing. A few times I've heard her being really grumpy with her friends when they have called up to speak to her. She used to have many interests, like her favourite soap operas, listening to her music. But now she's just not interested in any of it. She just stays in her room and only comes down if we insist. She is waking up really early in the morning and she's stopped eating even her favourite meals. She doesn't have her usually energy any more. I doubt if she gets much homework done since she's tired and she can't seem to focus on anything.

Treatment
Treatment is the remit of CAMH services. General advice is given on the benefits of regular exercise and sleep, a healthy diet, and how to access self-help materials.

For mild or moderate depression support and stress reduction may be sufficient, followed if necessary by cognitive-behavioural therapy, in a group or individualized, or interpersonal therapy. The cognitive part increases self-esteem and coping skills and the behavioural part encourages involvement in rewarding activities.

In the treatment of moderate severe depression there can be a role for medication combined with psychological therapy. Based on its efficacy and risk profile fluoxetine is the drug for choice.

Psychosis
Psychosis refers to a cluster of symptoms and signs which reflect a breakdown in the appreciation of reality.
Clinical features may include:
- *Hallucinosis:* a breakdown in perception of perceptual reality leading to hallucinations
- *Delusional thinking:* a breakdown in appreciation of reality in terms of holding ideas and beliefs that others of the same cultural background would consider false
- *Thought disorder:* breakdown in connectedness and coherence between one thought process and the next.

Psychosis may be a feature of:
- *Psychotic disorders:* schizophrenia, bipolar disorder
- *Delirium/acute confusional states:* consciousness is also usually clouded. Causes include high fever, viral encephalitis, substance abuse especially ecstasy and cannabis), substance withdrawal, steroid withdrawal.

Visual hallucinations suggest an organic confusional state. Schizophrenia is uncommon <13 years of age.

Admission to a paediatric ward is usually necessary initially for joint paediatric and mental health assessment. It is easy to underestimate how much parents and young people value the general support and attentive care provided by the non-specialist in addition to the highly specialized management required for an organic psychosis.

17.6 Case-based discussions

A toddler with tantrums

A mother aged 23 years brings her first child, a boy aged 3, for review of his mild asthma. She mentions at the end of the consultation her concern that he has always been very active and disobedient and in the last few months has had tantrums on several occasions. These occur if he does not get his way and involve shouting and screaming until he becomes exhausted. In addition, he has taken to hitting and even biting a neighbour's child who comes round to play.

What further information should be sought?
Enquire about developmental milestones, any previous medical history or current medications, the family situation, and parenting styles.

There is a history of delayed speech and he has only just begun to say two words together. His mother is separated from the biological father and until recently lived with maternal grandmother. Now they live in a second floor flat some distance away. She misses her mum's support. The last time her son had a tantrum she lost her temper and slapped him.

What is your diagnostic formulation?
Consider this behavioural problem using the biopsychosocial model and applying the four Ps:
- **P**redisposing factors include developmental delay which may cause frustration, lack of secure attachment figures, the family structure, and negative parenting style.
- **P**recipitating factors may include the recent separation from father and the loss of maternal grandmother's support.
- **P**erpetuating factors include parenting style, isolation from major supports, and lack of access to outdoor play space.
- **P**rotective factors include the fact that some aspects of the behaviour are within the realms of normal development and seeking help is a positive feature.

What advice and help can you give?
Advice is required on good parenting in general and on dealing with tantrums in particular. Be aware that it will be easier to dispense advice than it will be for this isolated young mother to act on it. Liaison with the family's health visitor is essential to provide support and oversight.

Advice on parenting
- *Be consistent:* it is important to stick to any rules and not give in if the rule is ignored on any occasion.
- *Give lots of praise:* let your children know when they have done something well and when you are pleased with them. 'Catch them being good' and then praise and reward them.
- *Be calm:* be calm and clear with commands. Keep commands short and simple. Avoid a continual stream of nagging with vague instructions.
- *Play with your child:* playing for a period each day is the most effective way of improving relationships.
- *Set consistent consequences for disobedience:* consequences should be immediate but not punitive.

Dealing with tantrums
- *Avoiding tantrums:* anticipate tantrum situations and try to prevent them by distraction using favourite books and toys. Store favourite sweets or biscuits out of sight. Avoid the child becoming tired or hungry by well-timed naps or snacks.
- *Coping with tantrums:* stay calm and do not get upset. Remember that this is normal behaviour. Ignore the tantrum and praise the child as soon as you see signs of calming down.

These strategies are all part of behaviour therapy.

What do you know about behaviour therapy?
Behavioural methods are based on the idea that behaviour can be 'unlearned'. They have been used for tackling bodily functions such as eating, sleeping, enuresis, encopresis, antisocial behaviour in prepubertal children, hyperactivity, specific phobias, and obsessive-compulsive disorder. Emotional disorders such as school refusal and recurrent pain may also respond.

A functional A, B, C analysis is performed first:
- *Antecedents:* analysing the immediate 'stimulus' factors preceding the behaviour
- *Behaviour:* detailed description of behaviour including frequency, severity, duration
- *Consequences:* impact on siblings and parents, attainment of child's goals.

The goals of therapy are negotiated with the child and parents. The main goal is promotion of desired behaviour in the hope that unwanted behaviour fades away. Target behaviours should be specified precisely.

Techniques include those to increase desired behaviours and those to reduce negative, undesired behaviours.

To increase desired behaviours
- *Positive reinforcement:* reward through praise and rewards, e.g. star charts. A prize can be given when an agreed number of stars has been earned
- *Negative reinforcement:* remove aversive stimulus when behaviour has occurred
- Remove interfering conditions.

To reduce negative behaviour
- *Stimulus removal:* remove antecedent stimuli.
- *Remove positive reinforcement:* remove previous reward such as attention associated with the behaviour. This may cause a transitory worsening of behaviour: the 'extinction burst'.
- *Time out:* take the child away from the context where the behaviour occurred to a dull, quiet place for a few minutes: 1 min per year of age. The child must know what behaviour has led to the time out. The child stays until he or she has been quiet for a minute. Time out is difficult to carry out, and must not be used over-punitively.
- *Punishment:* usually a telling-off or verbal criticism. Use of smacking is never a recommended part of therapeutic programmes.

A full range of psychiatric disorders illustrated by assessment of a fictitious teenager is available at www.dawta.com/f1.html.

Chapter 18

Community child health

18.1 Community child health *382*
18.2 Child public health *384*
18.3 Child health promotion *386*
18.4 Immunisation *388*
18.5 Immunisation: the vaccines *390*
18.6 Child development *392*
18.7 Neurodevelopmental disorders *394*
18.8 Hearing loss and communication disorders *396*
18.9 Child maltreatment *398*
18.10 Child physical abuse *400*
18.11 Emotional abuse, sexual abuse, neglect, and FII *402*
18.12 Management of suspected child maltreatment *404*
18.13 Case-based discussions *406*

18.1 Community child health

Community child health services

Community child health is the field of paediatrics in which the health and well-being of the individual child is promoted and disease prevented within the child's social, physical, environmental, and physiological context. It also includes organized efforts to develop good public health policies.
Community child health encompasses:

Child public health: global and UK
- Child health statistics
- Determinants of health
- Difficult circumstances and vulnerability.

Child health promotion and disease prevention
- Screening and surveillance
- Immunisation
- Health promotion and injury prevention.

Children with chronic disorders
- Neurodisability and developmental disorders
- Chronic, complex conditions
- Special educational needs
- Emotional and behavioural disorders.

Safeguarding children
- Child protection
- Vulnerable children, children in need
- Looked-after children (adoption and fostering).

The organization and delivery of community child health services within the UK Children's National Service Framework are considered here together with children's rights, UK law including the Children Acts 1989 and 2004 and the Human Rights Act 1998.

Children's rights: UNCRC

The United Nations Convention on the Rights of the Child (UNCRC) is an international human rights treaty that grants all children and young people aged 18 and under a comprehensive set of rights. The UK signed the convention in 1990 and it came into force in 1992. The convention gives children rights in the following areas:
- *General:* life, survival, and development
- *Civil rights and freedoms:* name and nationality, freedom of expression, protection from torture
- *Family environment:* right to live with and have contact with both parents or to appropriate alternative care
- *Health:* right to good quality health care and food, clean water and environment, special care and support if disabled
- *Welfare:* right to a standard of living good enough to meet their physical and mental needs, privacy, reliable information
- *Education and leisure:* right to education and to play, leisure, and participation in cultural life and the arts.

Governments agree to ensure that: children are cared for and protected from violence, abuse, and neglect by parents or anyone who looks after them, and that they are protected from harmful or dangerous work, dangerous drugs, or abuse.

National Service Framework (NSF)

The UK NSF for children, young people, and maternity services was published in 2004. It is divided into three parts and promotes the delivery of high quality, integrated, patient-focused care. The standards encompass:

Part I
- Promoting health and well-being, identifying needs, and early intervention and support for parenting
- Child, young person, and family-centred services
- Growing up into adulthood and safeguarding welfare of children and young people (<15 years).

Part II
- Services for children and young people in respect of illness, hospitalization, disability or complex health needs, mental health disorders, medicines.

Part III
- Maternity services.

Children Act 1989 and 2004

The Children Act 1989 contains several important principles that influence the attitude to children today. It was the first time in law that the welfare of the child became paramount. The Act also reflects the principle that it is better for children to be brought up by their families, and introduced the idea of parental responsibility.

The 2004 Act reformed children's services and it establishes for England:
- A Children's Commissioner to champion the views and interests of children and young people
- A duty on Local Authorities to:
  - promote cooperation between agencies
  - set up Local Safeguarding Children Boards
  - draw up a 'Children and Young People's Plan'
  - appoint a Director of Children's Services
- A duty on key agencies to safeguard and promote the welfare of children
- Provisions relating to foster care and education of children in care and the creation of an integrated inspection framework and the conduct of reviews to assess progress.

Every child matters: change for children

Every child matters: change for children, based on the Children Act 2004, is a new approach to the well-being of children and young people in the UK. The aim is for every child, whatever their background or circumstances, to have the support they need to:
- Be healthy
- Stay safe
- Enjoy and achieve
- Make a positive contribution
- Achieve economic well-being.

Everyone delivering services for children and young people has an important role in working towards these outcomes: childcare, schools, health services, social care, youth services, the police and criminal justice system, and culture, sports, and play organizations.

The NHS will have a central role in achieving the outcomes and the Children's NSF delivery strategy will be aligned to 'Change for Children' which combines guidance in *Every child matters* and the NSF.

Common assessment framework 2008

The Common assessment framework (CAF) is a key part of delivering front line services that are integrated and focused around the needs of children and young people. The CAF is a standardized approach to conducting an assessment of a child's additional needs and deciding how they should be met. The CAF is shown in Fig 18.1.

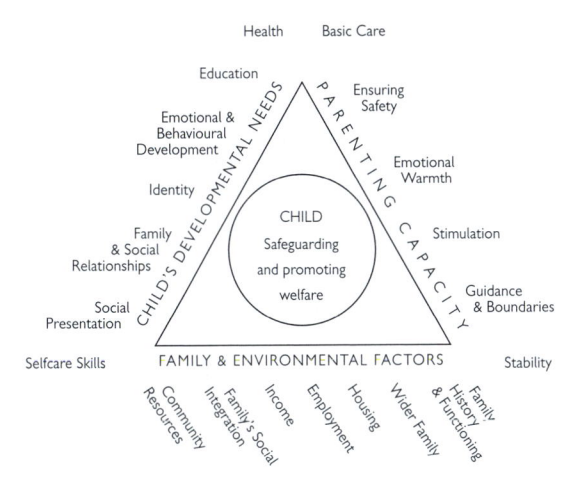

Fig 18.1 Common assessment framework.

The structure of the CAF form reflects the three main categories within which assessment of the unborn baby, infant child, or young person is undertaken.

CAF assessment summary: strengths and needs are assessed for whichever of the following elements are appropriate:

Development
- *Health:* general health, physical development, speech, language and communication.
- Emotional, social and behavioural development
- Identity, including self esteem, self-image
- Family and social relationships
- Self-care skills and independence
- *Learning:* understanding, participation in learning, education and employment: special educational needs or disability.

Parents and carers
- Basic care, ensuring safety and protection
- Emotional warmth and stability
- Guidance, boundaries and stimulation

Family and environmental
- Family history, functioning and well-being (illness, bereavement, violence, substance misuse, criminality, relationship breakdown, mental health, abusive behaviour.)
- *Wider family:* support networks, wider roles.
- Housing, employment and financial considerations (including entitlement to and receipt of benefits)
- Social and community resources, including education.

Looked-after children: adoption and fostering

Adoption

Adoption is the legal act of placing a child with a parent or parents other than the birth mother or father. An adoption order has the effect of severing the parental responsibilities and rights of the birth parent (s) and transferring them to the adoptive parent (s). The Adoption and Children Act 2002 (England and Wales) places the needs and welfare of the child, not the prospective parents, at the centre of the process.

About 2000 children a year are adopted in England, most being >4 years of age. Most children are adopted from local authority care and have experienced abuse and neglect.

Adoption: the process

In England and Wales social services and voluntary organizations act as adoption agencies. The following steps occur:

- *Consent by natural parents:* this requires an infant to be at least age 6 weeks.
- *Assessment of prospective adoptive parents:* single people, cohabiting couples, and same-sex couples can all adopt. Adopters must be over 21, or over 18 if one of a couple is the birth parent. Disabled adults are encouraged to adopt. Choice of family ideally reflects birth heritage including ethnic origin. Certain criminal offences disqualify.
- Application for adoption order and adoption hearing.

Prior to the adoption a medical history and examination aim to provide prospective parents with all the information relevant to their decision about adopting the child. There are no medical conditions which absolutely contraindicate adoption.

Fostering

Fostering is the provision of parental care and nurture to children not related through legal or blood ties. It does not provide legal permanency, as parental rights remain with the natural parents, local authority, or courts.

At any one time around 39 000 children in England are placed with foster carers by social services departments. Fostering is usually short term, but may be long term.

Reasons for foster care include:
- Care of babies awaiting adoption
- Child maltreatment
- Family problems (e.g. hospitalization).

Private fostering is defined in the Children Act 1989 as a child under the age of 16 years, or 18 years if disabled, being placed for 28 days or more in the care of someone who is not the child's guardian or close relative (i.e. parent, step-parent, aunt, uncle, grandparent), by private arrangement. Such children are potentially vulnerable and there is now a legal requirement that children's social care services are informed that a child is being privately fostered.

18.2 Child public health

Global child health

The health of children and young people in developing countries presents quite different problems and challenges to that in a developed country such as the UK. Of the world's 1 billion children, 85% live in the developing world. A third of annual global deaths occur in children <5 years. This equates to 11 million deaths annually or 30 000 each 24 h. 98% of these deaths occur in developing countries.

Causes of mortality and morbidity
Mortality

Neonatal mortality: the burden of neonatal disease in the developing world is huge. Of the 130 million infants born each year, ~4 million die in the first 4 weeks of life and a similar number are stillborn. The main causes of death are preterm birth (27%), infections (26%), and birth asphyxia (23%).

The indices most commonly used to compare different regions and monitor progress over time are:
- *Infant mortality rate (IMR):* neonatal (death of liveborn infant up to 28 days) and postneonatal (28 days–12 months) deaths per 1000 live births.
- *Under-5 mortality rate, U5MR:* deaths of under-5 year old children per 1000 live births.

The global causes of childhood death (2002), in order of magnitude, are:
- Perinatal and neonatal disorders
- Diarrhoeal disease
- Acute respiratory infection (ARI)
- Malaria
- HIV/AIDS
- Measles.

The emergence of HIV/AIDS in sub-Saharan Africa has had a major impact, with half a million children dying each year from complications of HIV/AIDS.

Morbidity

The burden of disease for various conditions worldwide in order of magnitude for the Disability Adjusted Life Years (DALYs) is: infectious and parasitic disease, injuries, perinatal conditions, neuropsychiatric conditions, nutritional deficiency, malignant conditions, and congenital anomalies.

Determinants of global child health

Poverty is the main determinant of child mortality and morbidity, associated as it is with malnutrition, lack of access to sanitation and clean water, ignorance, and absence of health care.

Improvements in global child health therefore depend on improvements in nutrition, sanitation, education, and health services. In addition, there are programmes targeted at specific health issues, including:
- Expanded Programme on Immunisation (EPI)
- Control of Diarrhoeal Disease (CDD)
- Acute Respiratory Infection (ARI).

These are being combined into a broader WHO strategy for the Integrated Management of Childhood Illness (IMCI). The IMCI involves:
- Training health workers to assess sick children systematically and identify children who can be managed at home, require out patient treatment or urgent assessment.
- Improving health systems and family and community practice in relation to child health.

The Millennium Development Goals (MDGs)

All the UN's Millennium Development Goals (see Box) are intimately linked to child health.

Millennium Development Goals
Goal 1. Eradicate extreme poverty and hunger.
Goal 2. Achieve universal primary education.
Goal 3. Promote gender equality and empower women.
Goal 4. Reduce child mortality.
Goal 5. Improve maternal health.
Goal 6. Combat HIV/AIDS, malaria, and other diseases.
Goal 7. Ensure environmental sustainability.
Goal 8. Develop a global partnership for development.

Children in difficult circumstances (CDC)

The term 'children in difficult circumstances' encompasses children in a host of circumstances including street children, working children, orphans, children living with HIV, refugees, child soldiers, and children being sexually abused or exploited.

In some countries the category also includes children in custodial care, children of inadequate parents (substance-abusing, learning difficulties, teenage), and child carers. There is considerable overlap between groups. For example, orphans are more likely to become street children or to be engaged in child labour.

Global estimates for the number of children classified as CDC are unreliable, but are in the order of:
- *Child labour (hazardous):* 100 million
- *Street children:* 10–100 million
- *HIV/AIDS orphans:* 14 million.

Child labour is defined as all economic activities carried out by persons aged <15 years excepting household work. The percentage of children primarily involved in work varies by region: sub-Saharan Africa (40%), Asia (25%), Latin America (12%).

Street children are further divided into two types:
- *Children on the streets (90%):* work on the streets but go home to sleep.
- *Children of the streets (10%):* live in the streets (abandoned, orphans, runaways).

Numbers of street children vary by region: Latin America (40 million), Asia (30 million), Africa (10 million). Boys predominate by 10:1. The health risks are high and include malnutrition, violence, infectious disease (STIs, HIV), and substance abuse.

UK child public health

In 2001 there were 13.5 million children aged <18 years in the UK of whom 3.4 million were <5 years. The proportion of children <16 in the population has fallen from 25% (1971) to 20% (2001). Pensioners now outnumber children.

Causes of mortality and morbidity

The health of children in the UK has improved significantly in the last century mainly due to the effect of better nutrition, immunisation, and antibiotics in reducing the impact of infectious disease.

Child mortality

Causes of child death in the UK vary with age and sex.

The infant mortality rate is 6/1000 live births and the death rates for under 5s are ~10% of the worldwide average at 5000 deaths per year. In children aged 1–4 years the rate is 0.3/1000; in children aged 5–14 years it is 0.12/1000. The rate rises after age 15 years (with an excess of boys) because of an increased risk of road traffic injuries.

Infant mortality, half of which occurs in the first month of life, accounts for 70% of all deaths in children up to age 14 years. Infant mortality is accounted for by congenital anomalies, prematurity and low birthweight, sudden unexplained death in infancy (SUDI), and infection.

The leading causes of death beyond infancy are injury and poisoning, nervous system disease such as cerebral palsy, respiratory disease, infections, and cancer.

Child morbidity

Major child health problems in the UK now include:
- *Social and health inequalities:* child poverty remains a major determinant of ill health
- *Childhood obesity:* in 2000, 20% of boys and 27% of girls were overweight
- *Mental health disorders:* ~10% of children aged 5–15 years have a mental health problem
- *Accidents and injuries:* the UK has high rates for injuries to child pedestrians
- *Child abuse and neglect:* ~50–100 fatal cases per year
- *Adolescent health:* teenage pregnancy and sexually transmitted infection, substance abuse, suicide and self-harm, delinquency
- *Chronic illness and neurodisability:* increase in prevalence of cerebral palsy due to increased survival rates and increased survival of preterm infants. Increase in prevalence of non-malignant life-threatening conditions such as cystic fibrosis and chronic renal failure.

Determinants of health in children

The determinants of health act at various levels, and a common model (Dahlgren and Whitehead) is one where the child is at the centre and the factors that influence health are placed in a series of four concentric circles. Ultimately health is the interaction of genetics, health behaviours, and the environment.

Age, gender, genetics (hereditary factors)

These are factors over which we have no individual control. Genetic susceptibility exists for many common childhood disorders including, obesity, asthma, epilepsy, and attention deficit hyperactivity disorder (ADHD).

Lifestyle and health behaviours

- *Nutrition:* breastfeeding, unhealthy diets. The Barker hypothesis proposes that *in utero* and early life environment influences susceptibility to adult diseases
- *Smoking:* smoking in pregnancy increases risk of low birth weight, stillbirth, and infant death. Passive smoking increases risk of SUDI and respiratory problems
- *Exercise:* the 'obesogenic' environment
- *Risk-taking behaviour:* substance misuse, early sexual activity, accidents.

Social and family environment

- Relatives, friends, and community support have a huge influence on well-being, and have a positive influence particularly for vulnerable children
- *Parenting and child-parent relationships:* ranging from good care, nurture, and clear boundaries to neglect
- *Families:* impact of conflict, domestic violence, parental divorce (affects 150 000 children a year in the UK)
- *Family structure:* 23% of dependent children live in single-parent households. 8% of babies born to teenage mothers, 40% outside marriage.

Social/environmental

- *Social environment:* quality of housing, neighbourhood, air quality, work, education, living conditions and facilities, much of which is linked to income level.
- *Child poverty:* poverty and deprivation in themselves may make good parenting more challenging and put children at an emotional and educational disadvantage. Social and environmental constraints may make healthy lifestyles more difficult to achieve. Social inclusion or exclusion, school environment, access to services.
- *Society* national economy, health service provision, global pollution, growth or otherwise in the labour market all influence an individual or community's ability to be 'healthy'.

Health inequalities

Health inequalities are differences in mortality and morbidity between population groups and are increasing in the UK child population. They are caused by variation in the determinants of child health described above. A substantial proportion is related to poverty. Certain groups of children can be identified as vulnerable and at risk of poor health:

- *Socio-economic groups:* there is a clear socio-economic class gradient for most of the leading causes of morbidity and mortality in UK children. The infant mortality and child mortality rates, prevalence of mental health disorders and death rate from injury are all higher in social class V.
- *Ethnicity:* numerous factors reduce the health and well-being of children from minority ethnic groups in the UK:
  - *genetics:* sickle cell disease and thalassaemia are more common in certain populations; consanguineous marriage increases the incidence of autosomal recessive (AR) disorders
  - *cultural factors:* differences in child-rearing, absence of familiar food, cultural and language barriers to health service access
  - *environment:* pigmented skin, lack of sunlight, and late weaning increase the incidence of rickets.

18.3 Child health promotion

Child health promotion includes any activity designed to improve health by intervening 'upstream' to tackle determinants of health at an individual, community, or public policy level. The Children's NSF in the UK launched a Child Health Promotion Programme which has replaced the Child Health Surveillance Programme.

Definitions of health
- *Health is the absence of disease:* this so-called 'deficit' model ignores the positive aspects of good health.
- *Health is a state of complete physical, mental, and social well-being:* this World Health Organization definition is broader and more appropriate for the field of health promotion.

Disease prevention
Prevention may be:
- *Primary:* stopping occurrence of the disease e.g. immunisation
- *Secondary:* screening or preventing further episodes
- *Tertiary:* e.g. managing diabetes mellitus, cystic fibrosis.

Child health promotion
Health promotion is usually achieved by a combination of health education and related organizational and economic programmes designed to support changes in behaviour and in the environment that will improve health. It operates at three levels: individual, community, and public policy:

Individual level
- *Providing information and health education:* education is often delivered to individuals in groups such as schools or antenatal classes and aims to build skills as well as providing information. It can only succeed with active participation if behaviour and lifestyle is to change.
- *Empowerment:* empowerment is the process of helping people to develop a sense that they can take charge of their own or their children's health.

Community level
- *Community development:* working with a community such as a village, school, or young offenders institution to identify areas of concern and improve health and well-being.
- *The National Healthy Schools Programme:* a Healthy School is defined as one that 'promotes the health and well being of pupils and staff through a well-planned taught curriculum in a physical and emotional environment that promotes learning and healthy lifestyle choices'. The core themes are education concerning relationships, drugs, healthy eating, physical activity, and emotional well-being.

Policy level
National (government) and international public policies have a significant impact on health in relation to:
- Services for health, transport, education, fiscal matters.
- Advertising and media influences
- Environmental safety.

Paediatricians may influence policy level health promotion by advocacy, speaking out in support of children, and lobbying to put pressure on governments.

In infancy and early childhood lifestyle choices influencing health are largely made by parents, e.g. breast-feeding, diet, sleeping position, passive smoking, parenting style. In later childhood there is increasing scope for children to make their own decisions about school meals, physical exercise, or substance abuse but these choices are strongly influenced by parental example, peer pressure, and cultural norms.

Disease prevention

Levels of prevention
There are three levels of prevention: primary, secondary, and tertiary.
- *Primary prevention:* stopping occurrence of disease. Examples include:
  - *immunisation:* described in detail in section 18.4 below
  - 'Back to Sleep' campaign to prevent sudden unexplained death in infancy
  - folic acid supplementation to prevent neural tube defects
  - contraceptive advice and health education to prevent unwanted teenage pregnancies.
- *Secondary prevention:* mitigating effects of disease by early detection. Examples include screening and surveillance or preventing further episodes, e.g. of child abuse.

These two strategies are considered in detail below.
- *Tertiary prevention:* slowing progress or consequences of established disease. Examples include optimizing management of chronic disease such as cystic fibrosis or diabetes mellitus and support for children with complex disabilities, e.g. cerebral palsy.

Screening
Screening is the process of trying to prevent disease by testing a population or targeted group to detect a disease in its early presymptomatic stage. There is a difficult balance between potential harm caused by anxiety and any potential benefits from reducing the risk of the disease or its complications.

Responsibility for screening programmes and policy in the UK rests with the National Screening Committee.

A screening programme requires careful evaluation and design in order to maximize the benefit and minimize the risk of harm. The following criteria are applied:
- *The disease or condition:* the condition should be a significant health problem and there should be a detectable latent or early symptomatic stage. The natural history should be understood.
- *The test:* simple, safe, precise, validated and acceptable.
- *The intervention:* an effective treatment or intervention with evidence that early treatment leads to better outcomes.
- *The programme:* evidence from RCTs that the programme is effective in reducing mortality or morbidity and is more cost-effective than other options for managing the condition.

The benefits should outweigh any physical or psychological harm caused by the test, diagnostic procedures or treatment. Disadvantages are significant for false positives (anxieties, further interventions with risks) and false negatives (false reassurance and possible worse outcomes).

Surveillance

The term 'surveillance' in child health is used to mean 'close observation' of children by knowledgeable health professionals with the aim of detecting problems early and intervening appropriately'.

Child Health Promotion Programme (CHPP)

A new updated CHPP was introduced in the UK in 2008. It builds on the Children's NSF and covers pregnancy and the 1st 5 years of life. The aims are to:
- Place greater emphasis on health promotion in early life.
- Support a model of 'progressive universalism': core programme for all, extra services for those with specific needs an targeting of vulnerable groups..
- Encourage partnership between agencies to develop local services such as GPs and Children's Centres.
- *Focus on public health priorities:* breast feeding, obesity, social and emotional development.

It is anticipated that effective implementation of the CHPP should lead to:
- Increased rates of breastfeeding.
- Positive parenting that improves children's social and emotional well-being.
- Prevention of specific serious and infectious diseases.
- Early detection of developmental delay, growth disorders and congenital anomalies.
- A reduction in obesity.

The main core components of the CHPP at each stage are described below

Core CHPP programme

Preconceptual counselling
Nutrition, adverse effects of smoking and alcohol, need for vitamin and folic acid supplements.

Antenatal
- *Screening:*
  - all pregnant women: anaemia, blood group, rhesus D status, atypical antibodies, hepatitis B, HIV, rubella immunity, syphilis, bacteriuria, risk factors for pre-eclampsia
  - at-risk populations: sickle-cell disease, thalassaemia
  - fetal abnormalities: Down syndrome screening, fetal anomaly ultrasound scan at 18–20 weeks
- *Disease prevention:* fetal surgery
- *Health promotion:* advice on breast-feeding, alcohol, smoking, parentcraft.

Newborn
- *Screening:*
  - physical examination including immediate physical examination at birth and full examination at 24–72 h with emphasis on eyes for cataracts, hips for developmental dysplasia, heart, and undescended testes in boys
  - newborn blood spot screening test at 5–8 days
  - tests for hypothyroidism, PKU, cystic fibrosis, medium chain acyl-coA dehydrogenase deficiency (MCADD), haemoglobinopathies
  - an oto-acoustic emissions hearing test by 4–5 weeks
- *Disease prevention:* administration of vitamin K
- *Health promotion:* advice on breast-feeding, sleeping position, passive smoking. Assess need for BCG and Hep B immunisation.

10 day postnatal visit
Care of the infant passes from midwife to health visitor who will check the emotional health of the mother for postnatal depression and give advice on feeding and sleeping.

6–8 weeks
- *Screening:* physical examination with emphasis on heart, hips, eyes, and testes in boys. Also check for jaundice, organomegaly, dysmorphism, hernias, tone, spine, palate. Record length, weight, occipitofrontal head circumference.
- *Health promotion:* advice on immunisation, dental health, car safety, and injury prevention.

2, 3, and 4 months
Immunisation, weight check, and health promotion as for 6–8 weeks.

By one year
Systematic assessment of physical, social, and emotional development and family needs by health visiting team.

Age 12–15 months
- *Immunisation:* 1st MMR
- *Health promotion:* advice on injury prevention (stair gates, fireguards, toys, etc.).

Age 3–4 years
- *Immunisation:* 2nd MMR and DT booster
- *Health promotion:* road safety, healthy diet.

Age 4–5 years
A review before or at school entry by the school nurse of:
- Height and weight
- Immunisation status
- *Vision:* preschool orthoptist-led screening being introduced.
- *Hearing:* preschool sweep test.
- Physical, developmental, emotional, or specific health problems e.g. special educational needs, disability.

Personal child health record (PCHR)

The PCHR or 'red book' is given to all mothers at the 10 day postnatal visit. It is a record of the child's growth and development from birth to 5 years. It includes details of the birth and subsequent checks and a record of immunisations. There are growth charts and pages to record the child's milestones and outpatient visits. There is a special red book for infants with Down syndrome.

It is valued by parents and enhances communication between parents and professionals and between professionals.

18.4 Immunisation

Immunisation is the process of protecting individuals from infection by inducing passive or active immunity. Passive immunity is induced by administering antibodies and active immunity by stimulating the adaptive immune system using a vaccine. The terms vaccine and vaccination originate from the use of the cowpox virus *Vaccinia* (from latin *vacca* = cow) to protect against smallpox.

After access to clean drinking-water, immunisation is the most effective public health measure for promoting health and has saved millions of lives. Vaccination led to the eradication of smallpox in 1980 and a similar programme has almost eradicated polio.

Rationale of vaccines and timing

The adaptive immune system has a memory so that immunity is generated to specific pathogens that a host has encountered. Active immunisation relies on stimulating the immune system with a vaccine which mimics the pathogen but does not cause the disease.

A vaccine may be:
- *Inactivated:* tetanus toxoid, virus protein subunits, acellular pertussis vaccine, inactivated organism, capsular polysaccharides
- *Attenuated live organisms:* e.g. measles, mumps vaccines.

If vaccination is performed too early the immune system may not be mature enough to respond and high levels of maternal antibody may blunt the response. Vaccination after the time of likely exposure to natural infection is clearly too late.

UK immunisation programme

The aim of the routine childhood immunisation programme is to protect all children against the following 10 infections:
- Diphtheria, tetanus, and pertussis
- Polio
- Haemophilus influenzae type b (Hib)
- Meningococcal serogroup C (MenC)
- Pneumococcal
- Measles, mumps, and rubella

The schedule is shown in Table 18.1.

Primary immunisation with diphtheria, tetanus, pertussis, polio, and Hib vaccine (DTaP/IPV/Hib) is given at 2, 3, and 4 months of age. Pneumococcal conjugate vaccine (PCV) is given at 2 and 4 months and MenC vaccine at 3 and 4 months. Measles, mumps, and rubella (MMR) with a further dose of PCV is given at 13 months and MMR booster pre-school.

Further booster doses are given as indicated at 3 years 4 months to 5 years and 13–15 years.

Selective immunisation is provided at birth to protect against:
- *Tuberculosis:* BCG given to babies who are more likely to come into contact with TB than the general population
- *Hepatitis B:* to babies whose mothers are hepatitis B positive.

Preterm infants are immunized by chronological age.

Table 18.1. The UK immunisation programme (2008)

Age to immunize	What vaccine is given	How given
2 months	Diphtheria, tetanus, pertussis, polio and Hib (DTaP/IPV/Hib)	1 injection
	Pneumoccocal (PCV)	1 injection
3 months	DTaP/IPV/Hib	1 injection
	MenC	1 injection
4 months	DTaP/IPV/Hib	1 injection
	MenC	1 injection
	PCV	1 injection
12 months	Hib/Men C	1 injection
~13 months	Measles, mumps, and rubella (MMR)	1 injection
	PCV	1 injection
3 years 4 months to 5 years	Diphtheria, tetanus, pertussis, and polio (DTaP/IPV or dTaP/IPV)	1 injection
Preschool	MMR	1 injection
13–18 years	Tetanus, diphtheria, and polio (Td/IPV)	1 injection

Adverse events following immunisation (AEFIs)

Research in advance of vaccine introduction may not detect problems that are rare or manifest after a long latent interval. In the UK, the Medicines and Healthcare Products Regulatory Agency (MHRA) monitors vaccine safety using the voluntary Yellow Card reporting scheme.

The WHO classifies AEFIs into four types:
- *Programme related:* wrong dose, wrong timing, contaminated vaccine
- *Vaccine induced:* reactions caused by a specific vaccine or its components
- *Coincidental:* apparent link only on account of coincidental timing
- *Unknown:* unclassifiable AEFIs.

Vaccine-induced AEFIs

Common
- *Pain, swelling, or redness at site of injection:* local adverse reactions, mild and self-limiting
- *Systemic reactions:* fever, malaise, headache, anorexia,

Examples include local reactions and fever within 48 h of DTaP/IPV/Hib, rash and fever 7–10 days after MMR, parotitis 3 weeks after MMR.

Rare

Rare vaccine-induced AEFIs include seizures, hypotonic-hyporesponsive episodes (HHE), idiopathic thrombocytopaenic purpura within 30 days of MMR, acute arthropathy, and anaphylaxis. The differential diagnosis of anaphylaxis is fainting and panic attacks.

Unfounded suggestions of links between pertussis vaccine and brain damage and between MMR and autism and inflammatory bowel disease led to major falls in uptake levels of corresponding vaccines in the UK.

Contraindications to immunisation

Almost all individuals can be safely vaccinated with all vaccines. If in doubt, seek advice before withholding or advising against immunisation. Withholding immunisation may have serious consequences for both the child and the public.

Contraindications

- *A confirmed anaphylactic reaction* to a previous dose of a vaccine containing the same antigens or another component of the vaccine e.g. neomycin, streptomycin, polymyxin B.
- *Live vaccines:* may be temporarily contraindicated in individuals who are immunosuppressed (see below) or pregnant.
- *Egg allergy:* a previous anaphylactic reaction to egg contraindicates influenza and yellow fever vaccines. MMR vaccine can be given safely to most children with egg allergy, but should be done under controlled conditions in those with a history of anaphylaxis.
- *Acute illness with fever or systemic upset:* immunisation should be postponed until recovery. Minor illness does not require postponement.
- *Children with an evolving neurological condition:* immunisation should be deferred until the condition has resolved or stabilized and a diagnosis has been made.

Live vaccines and immunosuppression

Live vaccines such as BCG and MMR are contraindicated in the following infants and children with defective immunity:

- Children treated for malignant disease with chemotherapy or radiotherapy either currently or within the last 6 months.
- *Transplant patients:* all solid organ transplant patients on immunosuppressant drugs or patients who have had a bone marrow transplant until 12 months after finishing immunosuppressive treatment.
- Children who have received high-dose steroid treatment within the previous 3 months, i.e. oral or rectal prednisolone 2 mg/kg per day for a week or 1 mg/kg per day for 1 month.
- Children who have received immunosuppressant drugs (e.g. azathioprine, methotrexate) alone or in combination with steroids within the previous 6 months.
- Patients with severe primary immunodeficiency, e.g. SCID, Wiskott–Aldrich syndrome, di George syndrome.
- *Children with HIV infection:* HIV-positive children can receive MMR unless there is severe immunosuppression when measles vaccine is a risk. They should *not* receive BCG, yellow fever, or oral typhoid vaccines. Inactivated polio virus vaccination is preferable.

False 'contraindications'

The following are *not* contraindications to immunisation:
- *Personal or family history of:*
  - seizures (febrile or afebrile) with no evidence of neurological deterioration
  - autistic spectrum disorder or inflammatory bowel disease
  - asthma or hay fever
- Pregnancy of child's mother
- Previous history of neonatal jaundice, natural pertussis, measles, mumps, or rubella immunisation
- Being under a certain weight, surgery, or anaesthesia
- *Stable neurological conditions:* cerebral palsy, Down syndrome.

Parental concerns

Common parental concerns which should be allayed because they are unfounded include: vaccines are ineffective, multiple vaccines 'overload' the immune system, vaccines cause long-term side effects, vaccines cause disease.

A current concern is the belief, despite evidence to the contrary, that MMR vaccination is associated with autism. If appropriate, parents should be advised to consult: http://www.mmrthefacts.nhs.uk. See Box.

MMR: truths and myths

Top 10 truths

- MMR is the safest way that parents can protect their children against measles, mumps, and rubella.
- >500 million doses of MMR have been used in >90 countries in the last 30 years. WHO states it is safe.
- No country recommends MMR vaccine as three separate doses.
- Unimmunized children increase the chance of others getting diseases.
- There is no evidence that MMR vaccine causes autism or inflammatory bowel disease. Many studies show it does not.
- The *Lancet* study of 1998 stated: 'we did not prove an association between MMR vaccine and the syndrome described'.
- Single vaccines in place of MMR put children and their families at unnecessary risk.
- MMR vaccine was thoroughly tested before being introduced.
- Two doses are necessary to give the best protection.
- Very few children have a contraindication to MMR vaccine.

Top 10 myths

- Getting protection by catching the diseases is better than having the vaccine.
- Giving three viruses at once overloads the immune system.
- Other countries give MMR as separate vaccines.
- Immunisation is unnecessary because the diseases are rare.
- MMR causes autism and bowel disease.
- A scientific paper showed a real link between MMR and autism and bowel disease.
- Giving the MMR vaccines separately reduces side effects.
- The vaccine was not properly tested before introduction.
- One dose is sufficient.
- Boys do not need protection against rubella and girls do not need protection against mumps.

18.5 Immunisation: the vaccines

Diphtheria

Diphtheria is caused by infection with *Corynebacterium diphtheria* in the pharynx or skin. The introduction of immunisation against diphtheria in the UK in 1940 led to a dramatic fall in number of notified cases and deaths from the disease.

Diphtheria vaccine: D, d

The vaccine is a cell-free purified toxin treated with formaldehyde to form toxoid and absorbed on to an adjuvant. It is produced in two strengths: D (30 iu) and d (2 iu). The low dose of vaccine is used for primary immunisations in children >10 years and in the booster at 13–15 years.

Diphtheria vaccine is available only in combined products.

Tetanus

Tetanus is an acute disease caused by tetanus toxin released following infection by *Clostridium tetani*, the spores of which are present in soil or manure.

Maternal and neonatal tetanus due to infection of the umbilical stump remains an important cause of death in many countries. In 2006, 8376 cases were reported worldwide.

Tetanus immunisation was introduced in the UK in 1961.

Tetanus vaccine: T

Tetanus vaccine is a cell-free purified toxin treated with formaldehyde to form toxoid and absorbed on to an adjuvant. It is given only as part of combined products.

Pertussis

Pertussis (whooping cough) is caused by infection with *Bordetella pertussis*, or less commonly by *B. parapertussis*. Severe complications such as bronchopneumonia and cerebral hypoxia or death are most common in infants <6 months. Before introduction of immunisation in the 1950s annual UK notifications were >120 000.

Pertussis vaccine: aP

Whole-cell pertussis vaccines have been replaced in the UK by acellular vaccines, aP, made from highly purified selected components of the organism which are treated with formaldehyde and absorbed on to adjuvants. Three- and five-component vaccines are available. A five-component vaccine, Pediacel, is used for primary immunisation in the UK programme and does not attenuate the response to Hib.

The pertussis vaccines are given only as part of combined products.

Poliomyelitis

Poliomyelitis is an acute illness caused by infection by one of the three polio virus serotypes, types 1, 2, and 3. The paralytic form causes asymmetric flaccid paralysis.

During the 1950s epidemics of poliomyelitis occurred each summer with as many as 8000 annual notifications of paralytic poliomyelitis in the UK. Routine immunisation with inactivated poliomyelitis vaccine, IPV-Salk, was introduced in 1956 and replaced by live attenuated oral polio vaccine, OPV-Sabin, in 1962. However, the live attenuated vaccine virus can itself revert to a virulent form and cause paralytic disease: vaccine associated paralytic polio (VAPP).

Following the introduction of immunisation in the UK, cases fell to a low level. The last case of natural polio infection acquired in the UK was in 1982. A Global Eradication of Polio Initiative was started in 1988 and polio is now endemic in just a handful of countries: see Chapter 15.8.

Polio vaccine: IPV

Since 2004 inactivated polio vaccine, IPV, has been used for routine primary immunisation. IPV is made from three poliovirus strains, Salk serotypes 1, 2, and 3, treated with formaldehyde and absorbed on to adjuvants. It is given only as part of combined products.

Haemophilus influenzae type b (Hib)

Haemophilus influenzae can cause serious invasive disease, especially in young children. Invasive disease is usually caused by encapsulated strains of which there are six typeable serotypes, a–f. Type b was the most prevalent strain. Invasive Hib diseases include meningitis, septicaemia, septic arthritis, osteomyelitis, and pneumonia.

Asymptomatic carriage of Hib in nose and throat occurred in 4% of preschool children before introduction of immunisation.

Vaccines containing purified capsular polysaccharides were introduced in the 1970s but failed to protect younger children, in whom the risk was highest, due to poor immunogenicity. Development of highly effective conjugate Hib vaccines, first licensed in 1987, overcame this problem.

Since the introduction of Hib conjugate vaccine into the UK immunisation schedule, disease incidence has fallen sharply. Between 1991 and 1998 cases <5 years fell from 803 to 21, and <1 year from 300 to 7. This is attributable both to direct protection and to an indirect effect due to the prevention of nasopharyngeal carriage.

Hib vaccine

Hib vaccines are made from capsular polysaccharides conjugated either with CRM_{19}, a non-toxic diphtheria toxin, or tetanus toxoid. The vaccines are given as part of a combined product.

Meningococcal disease

Meningococcal disease is caused by systemic infection by *Neisseria meningitidis*. There are 13 serogroups of which groups B and C are most common in the UK. Asymptomatic nasopharyngeal carriage occurs in 25% of adolescents, 5–11% of adults, and a low percentage of infants and young children.

Meningococcal infection presents as meningitis, septicaemia, or a combination of both. Overall mortality remains about 10%. Epidemics caused by group A infections coincided with both world wars and subsequent hyperendemic periods occurred in 1972–1975, 1985, and 1995–96.

Vaccines based on the serogroup C polysaccharide proved inadequate and a new MenC conjugate vaccine was introduced into the UK routine immunisation programme in 1999. Confirmed group C cases subsequently fell by 90% in all age groups immunized, and group B strains now account for 80% of laboratory-confirmed isolates.

MenC conjugate vaccine, MenC
MenC conjugate vaccines are made from capsular polysaccharides extracted from cultures of group C *Neisseria meningitidis* and conjugated with either CRM_{197} (a non-toxic diphtheria toxin) or tetanus toxoid. MenC vaccine confers no protection against other serogroups such as B, A, or W135.

Pneumococcal disease

Pneumococcal disease is caused by infection with *Streptococcus pneumoniae*, the pneumococcus. Only capsular types are virulent. Invasive pneumococcal disease is a major cause of morbidity and mortality causing septicaemia, meningitis, and pneumonia. The very young and those with an absent or non-functioning spleen are at high risk.

Currently the pneumococcus is one of the most frequently reported causes of bacteraemia, meningitis, and community-acquired pneumonia.

Pneumococcal vaccines: PPV and PCV

- *Pneumococcal polysaccharide vaccine (PPV)* contains purified capsular polysaccharide from each of 23 capsular types, accounting for 96% of isolates causing serious infection in the UK.
- *Pneumococcal conjugate vaccine (PCV)* contains polysaccharide from 7 common capsular types conjugated to CRM_{197}, 7-valent PCV.

PPV has been recommended for at-risk groups since 1992. In 2006 PCV was added to the routine childhood immunisation programme.

Measles, mumps, and rubella

These three viral diseases are discussed in detail in Chapter 15. Before the introduction of measles vaccine in 1968 annual notification of measles varied between 160 000 and 180 000 with peaks every 2 years and ~100 deaths each year. Between 1968 and 1988, when MMR was introduced, coverage was low and measles remained a major cause of morbidity and mortality in the UK.

Mumps caused 1200 hospital admissions each year and was the commonest cause of viral meningitis before the introduction of MMR. The most important consequence of rubella infection is fetal loss or congenital rubella syndrome (CRS) due to maternal rubella infection. Selective rubella immunisation of prepubertal girls and non-immune women of childbearing age was introduced in the UK in 1970.

Measles, mumps, and rubella vaccine: MMR
MMR vaccines are freeze-dried preparations of live, attenuated strains of measles, mumps, and rubella viruses.

Following the introduction of the MMR vaccine in 1988 and the achievement of coverage levels >90%, measles notification fell to low levels. Mumps cases fell dramatically, but an increase in mumps cases occurred in 1999 and 2004 in those born in 1980–87 (mainly in higher education institutions) who had not received immunisation.

CRS is now mainly seen in minority ethnic groups who have not been infected or immunized before coming to the UK.

Tuberculosis

The disease is discussed in detail in Chapter 15.12. Notifications of TB in the UK declined over most of the last century, from 117 139 new cases in 1913 to 5086 in 1987. Since then there has been a resurgence of new cases to 7000 in 2004.

The epidemiology has changed. TB is now a disease which occurs predominantly in specific population subgroups and communities. BCG immunisation was introduced in the UK in 1953 and has undergone several changes. It is now a risk-based programme, the key part of which targets newborns at risk of exposure to TB.

The Bacillus Calmette–Guerin vaccine: BCG
The BCG vaccine contains a live attenuated strain derived from *M. bovis*.

BCG immunisation is offered to:
- All infants (aged 0–12 months) living in areas of the UK with an annual incidence of TB ≥40/100 000.
- Children with a parent or grandparent born in a country with an annual incidence of TB ≥40/100 000 including:
  - infants aged 0–12 months
  - previously unvaccinated children aged 1–5 years
  - previously unvaccinated, tuberculin-negative children aged 6–16 years
  - previously unvaccinated tuberculin negative contacts of cases of respiratory TB
  - previously unvaccinated tuberculin negative new entrants under 16 years who were born in or lived in (>3 months) in a country with an annual TB incidence of ≥40/100 000.

Hepatitis B

Hepatitis B is an infection of the liver caused by the hepatitis B virus (HBV). The disease is described in Chapter 5. Chronic HBV infection is defined as persistence of HbsAg in the serum for 6 months or longer. WHO estimates that 350 million people worldwide are chronically infected with HBV. Patients who are HbsAg and HbeAg positive are most infectious. The prevalence of chronic HBV infection in antenatal women in the UK is 0.14% overall but rises to 1% in some inner city areas.

Hepatitis B vaccine
The hepatitis B vaccine contains HbsAg adsorbed on to an adjuvant. It is an inactivated vaccine.

Hepatitis B immunoglobulin
Specific hepatitis B immunoglobulin (HBIG) provides passive and temporary immunity and is given concurrently with hepatitis B vaccine.

Recommendations for use specific to paediatrics include:

Post-exposure immunisation
- Babies born to mothers who are chronically infected or who have had acute hepatitis B during pregnancy. These infants should receive a complete course of vaccination in most cases including HBIG in addition to hepatitis B vaccine.
- Families adopting children from countries with a high or intermediate prevalence of hepatitis B in whom the hepatitis status is unknown.

18.6 Child development

Normal development follows a recognized sequence and the range of expected ages or 'milestones' at which particular development skills are attained is well established.

Categories of development

Development is usefully grouped into four categories but there is of course considerable overlap:
- *Gross motor*: sitting, walking, running
- *Fine motor and vision*: hand skills, visual development
- *Speech, language and hearing*: communication skills both verbal and non-verbal, hearing development
- *Social behaviour and play*: feeding, toileting, dressing, social relationships.

Development of cognition and emotion is described in Chapter 17.

Normal development

Gross motor

Development proceeds in a head to toe direction. Head, neck, and trunk control is obviously a prerequisite for sitting. Moving into the prone position, kneeling on all fours and crawling usually precede standing and walking.

Table 18.2. Gross motor milestones (average)	
3 months	Lifts head and shoulders off floor in prone position. Little or no head lag on pull to sit
6 months	Rolls front to back and usually back to front
8 months	Sits independently without support
10 months	Crawls, pulls to stand
12 months	Walking independently
18 months	Squats to pick up object, kicks a ball
2 years	Runs and jumps
3 years	Stands on one leg momentarily
4 years	Hops

Fine motor and vision

Fine motor skills require visual skills and the two are closely integrated.

Table 18.3. Fine motor and vision milestones (average)	
3 months	Watches own hands, fixes and follows object through 90° laterally
4 months	Reaches and grasps an object, holds with palmar grasp
6 months	Transfers objects between hands
10 months	Mature pincer grasp, bangs bricks in imitation
5 months	Builds 2-brick tower
18 months	Builds 3-brick tower, to and fro scribble
2 years	Builds 6-brick tower, circular scribble, builds train with chimney
3 years	Copies a 3-brick bridge, draws circle
4 years	Draws a person with head, body, legs. Builds 6-brick steps

Speech, language, and hearing

- *1st year (prelingual)*: non-verbal communication and comprehension begins in the 1st year. Vocalizations start as open vowel sounds, followed by double-syllable babble and variation in pitch and volume with facial expression. Receptive language precedes expressive language.
- *2nd year*: comprehension of single words begins. Expressive language develops with sound labels, e.g. 'mama','dada' followed by single words to label or request. Next comes ability to join two words together.

Table 18.4. Speech and language milestones (average)		
	Comprehension	Expression
3–6 months	Responds to speech	Babbling, cooing
9 months	Responds to name Imitates: lip smacking	Babbles with two syllables ('da-da')
12 months	Plays 'peek a boo', waves	Imitates, points, 1–2 words
18 months	Understands simple commands. Objects by name	6–20 words
2 years	Understands two word commands (e.g. 'feed teddy')	50 words. Joins two words. Joins in nursery rhymes
2.5 years	Asks questions	200 words. Uses pronouns ('I', 'me')
3 years	Understands three word commands (e.g. 'give me a doll, teddy, and cup'). Understands prepositions	Tasks in short (3–4 words) sentences. Asks 'what' and 'who' questions
4 years		Asks 'why', 'when', 'how' questions Counts up to 20 by rote

Social behaviour and play

The development of self-help skills such as feeding and dressing is influenced by family environment.

Table 18.5. Social behaviour and play milestones (average)	
6 weeks	smiles in response
3 months	expresses pleasure on cuddling
9 months	stranger awareness
12 months	helps with dressing, waves bye-bye, plays peek-a-boo
18 months	takes off socks, hat, spoon-feeds self
2 years	plays alongside other children
3 years	eats with fork and spoon, joins in make-believe play
4 years	can dress and undress, except for shoe laces.

Developmental assessment

The first aim is to determine whether a child's development is within the normal range for age. If not, the degree of abnormality and possible causes are assessed.

Assessment may be a general screening designed to establish whether a set of age-appropriate tasks can be accomplished. This may be informal or formal with a test such as the Denver screening test.

Alternatively, it may be a more detailed assessment to identify the exact level of attainment in each developmental domain. The assessment may be informal, or formal using a standardized assessment with a scoring system such as:
- *Griffiths mental development scales:* for children up to 8 years
- *Bayley scales of infant development:* for children up to 42 months.

General principles:
- Use a systematic, structured approach
- Start with tasks below the expected level of attainment
- Avoid long gaps between tasks, maintain interest (see Fig 18.2)
- Do gross motor testing last
- Ensure optimal positioning:
  - <18 months: seated on carer's lap at table
  - 2–5 years: seated at small table opposite you.

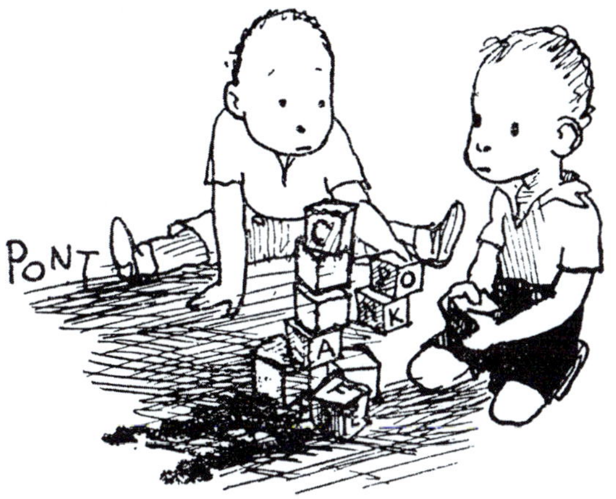

"THERE ARE TIMES WHEN I REALLY BEGIN TO WONDER IF ALL THIS IS WORTH WHILE."

Fig 18.2 *Punch,* 1 December 1937. Reprinted courtesy of *Punch.*

Useful general questions include: Any concerns about development? Age of attainment of key milestones? Differences between child and siblings or peers? Family history of vision, hearing, developmental problems?

Scheme of assessment

Infant: <12 months
Equipment: cubes, cup, cloth, sock, shoe, brush, coloured small toy, small object (e.g. raisin), paper and pencils.

Fine motor and vision
- *Fine motor:* place raisin in front of each hand, offer cube to observe reach, grasp, and manipulation from 4 months. Test with cubes: imitation of banging, grasp, and hold. Observe for hand preference or asymmetry.
- *Vision:* Useful questions: Does the child look at you, look at a bright light (from birth), follow you (from 1/12), reach for objects (4/12), pick up small objects (9/12), point to objects at a distance (12/12)?

- *Vision testing:* observe visual behaviour, fixing and following, detection of small objects, preferential looking acuity system (e.g. Keeler cards), cover test from 8 months.

Speech, language, and hearing
- *Hearing:* useful questions: Does the child startle, blink or cry to a loud noise (from birth), notice sounds in home e.g. vacuum cleaner (from 1/12), quieten, smile, or turn to voice (4/12), turn immediately to sounds on each side (7/12), listen, search for quiet sounds out of sight (9/12), respond to name, 'no', 'bye bye' (12/12)?
- *Hearing tests:* otoacoustic emissions screening (neonatal). Health visitor history at 8 months.
- *Speech and language:* observe non-verbal communication (facial expressions, gestures), turn taking, encourage imitation of hand clapping, waving 'bye bye', call name and give simple instructions, examine single-word recognition with familiar objects: 'Where's the cup?'.

Social behaviour and play
Ask about self-feeding, observe behaviour and interactions.

Gross motor
Lie infant supine on mat and encourage to roll, pull to sitting position and place in sitting position. Pull to stand or bear weight, observe stepping, walking. Hold in ventral suspension, place in prone position.

Toddler: 1–4 years
Equipment: small table and chairs, 12 1-inch cubes, paper and pencils, doll, teddy, picture book, ball, toys, real objects (cup, spoon, etc.), access to stairs.

Fine motor and vision
- *Fine motor:* offer 1-inch cubes: encourage tower building. Build bridge, train, or steps for child to imitate. Offer paper and pencils: observe spontaneous drawing. Draw shapes for child to copy, ask child to draw a person. Observe manipulation and coordination (beads and puzzles)
- *Vision:* Useful questions: does the child bump into things, does the child recognize you across a room?
- *Vision testing:* visual acuity >24 months: single optotype (Sheridan–Gardener cards). >30 months: linear letter matching (e.g. Sonksen–Silver chart). When children can recognize letters, use a standard Snellen chart.

Speech and language and hearing
- *Hearing screen:* speech discrimination: >2 years. Child is asked to choose a toy from a set of pairs with similar names, e.g. 'tree' and 'key'.
  - play audiometry assessment: >2–3 years. Child is conditioned to perform a task in response to a sound
  - pure tone audiometry: >3 years. A pure tone audiogram is delivered to each ear separately via headphones. Each sound is loud at first and reduced to establish the hearing threshold
- *Speech and language:* observe non-verbal communication, check understanding at single-, two-, and three-word level and then use of prepositions, adjectives, and verbs.

Social behaviour and play:
Ask about self-help skills and play, observe social interactions throughout.

Gross motor
Observe gait: walking, running, jumping. and hopping. Stand on one leg, pick object up from floor, go up and down stairs.

18.7 Neurodevelopmental disorders

Concepts of neurodisability
It is useful to be clear about the terminology used and to appreciate that many technical terms have become stigmatizing by common usage, such as 'spastic', 'retarded', 'mental'.

The following new definitions for classification are proposed by the WHO ICIDH 2:
- *Impairment:* abnormality or loss of psychological, physiological or anatomical structure or function.
- *Activity (replacing disability):* nature and extent of functioning at the level of the person. Activities may be limited.
- *Participation (previously handicap):* the nature and extent of the person's involvement in life situations. Participation may be restricted.

Examples corresponding to specific disorders are shown in the Box.

Disorder	Impairment	Activity	Participation
Congenital hemiplegia	Unilateral weakness of arm and leg	Uses one hand, other supports	Plays piano with only one hand
Retinopathy of prematurity	Severe visual impairment	Able to walk with help	Reads using Braille
Epilepsy	Recurrent seizures	Episodic falls	Rides a tricycle

Cultural attitudes to neurodisability vary widely. In familial deafness, a deaf child may be preferred to a hearing child.

Epidemiology
Reliable estimates of the prevalence of childhood disability are difficult to obtain, not least because of variation in the way that childhood disability is defined and recorded. Using broad definitions, the prevalence is between 3% and 7%.

The prevalence of physical and multiple disabilities in childhood is estimated to be ~1–2%.

Classification
Neurodevelopmental disorders and disabilities are often multiple but can be grouped into the following categories:
- *Global developmental delay:* learning disability
- *Gross motor delay:* physical disability
- Vision impairment
- Hearing impairment
- *Communication disorders:* speech and language delay, autistic spectrum disorders.

Global delay: learning disability
Global delay is defined as significant (2 standard deviations below the mean) delay in two or more developmental domains. Many such children are later found to have significant learning disability.

A child has a learning disability if he or she has greater difficulty in learning than the majority of children of the same age.

It is defined by WHO as a state of arrested or incomplete development of the mind. This includes a significant impairment of intellectual functioning and adaptive social functioning. It is present from childhood and not acquired.

Using IQ as a quantitative measure, with an average of 100 and standard deviation of 15, the ICD-10 categories are:
- *Mild:* IQ 50–69
- *Moderate:* IQ 35–49
- *Severe:* IQ 20–34
- *Profound:* IQ <20.

Measurements in the lower range are difficult; a simpler division is severe <50 and mild/moderate 50–69.

Aetiology
A clear aetiology is more likely to be identified in severe learning disability. It is important to distinguish global developmental delay due to a static lesion of the CNS from a progressive neurodegenerative condition (see Chapter 7). The latter causes a progressive loss of skills or regression which can be hard to recognize because development is occurring in parallel.

Severe learning disability is seen in a very wide range of conditions in which cerebral hemisphere structure and function is disturbed. Causes are usefully divided into genetic and acquired.

Genetic
- *Chromosomal disorders:* Down syndrome, Williams syndrome
- *X-linked disorders:* fragile X syndrome (FXS) in boys
- *Rett syndrome (RS):* in girls
- *Imprinted gene disorders:* Angelman syndrome, Prader–Willi syndrome
- *Autosomal dominant disorders:* neurofibromatosis, tuberous sclerosis complex
- *Cortical malformations.*

Acquired

Prenatal:
- congenital infections
- fetal alcohol syndrome
- iodine deficiency
- *Perinatal:*
  - hypoxic–ischaemic encephalopathy
  - hypoglycaemia
  - bilirubin encephalopathy
  - preterm birth
- *Postnatal:*
  - *intracranial infection:* meningitis, encephalitis
  - *traumatic brain injury:* accidental, non-accidental
  - *asphyxia:* cardiac arrest, drowning
  - hypothyroidism.

Clinical assessment
History should establish
- *Birth history:* perinatal brain insults
- *Family history:* consanguinity, previous pregnancy loss
- *Developmental history:* global or specific delay, evidence of regression.

Examination

In addition to developmental assessment, examination may identify:

- *Dysmorphic features:* stigmata of a syndrome, e.g. Down, fragile X, Williams, Rett syndromes
- *Cutaneous stigmata:* neurocutaneous syndromes
- *Microcephaly or macrocephaly*
- *Organomegaly:* in storage disorders
- *Fundus abnormalities:* retinopathy, 'cherry-red' spot.

Management

Investigations are directed towards establishing a specific diagnosis which may allow more precise prognosis, allow genetic counselling, and on occasion reveal a treatable condition.

First line screening tests

- Karyotype
- Fragile X screening
- Thyroid function tests.

Second line investigations

These are indicated if clinical evaluation suggests a specific diagnosis and may include:

- *Neuroimaging:* cortical malformations
- *Neurophysiology:* EEG
- *Metabolic investigations:* plasma and urine amino acids, organic acids
- *Specific genetic testing:* FISH, DNA testing.

Gross motor delay

Presentation may be as the floppy infant with poor head control, delayed sitting, or delayed walking. The upper limit of normal age for walking is 18 months. 3% of children walk after 18 months but only 3% of these have an underlying problem. See Chapter 7.

Causes of a floppy infant

- *Central neurological disorders:* cerebral palsy, cortical malformations
- *Neuromuscular disorders:* e.g. spinal muscular atrophy.

Causes of delayed walking

- *Cerebral palsy:* spastic diplegia
- *Muscular dystrophy:* Duchenne muscular dystrophy
- *Spinal disorders:* spina bifida occulta
- Developmental dysplasia of the hip
- Global developmental delay
- *Bottom-shuffling:* a normal variant associated with a later average age of walking. It can, however, be associated with conditions such as cerebral palsy and careful examination is indicated
- *Benign hypermobility:* hypotonia and ligamentous laxity.

Visual impairment

This is discussed in Chapter 8. It is important to recognize that visual impairment may arise from defects in visual pathways or cortex despite normal ocular anatomy and function.

Services for disabled children

Child Development Team (CDT)

In the UK each area has a CDT, usually housed in a Child Development Centre, which provides:

- Assessment, diagnosis, and management of neurodevelopmental disability
- Advice and support to parents, teachers, child care staff and others
- *Expertise for schools:* special schools and children in mainstream schools
- Information for the disability register for planning services.

Services in a Child Development Centre include:

- *Health services:* for medical diagnosis and treatment, nursing care, and long-term disability; palliative care for the dying child with a disability
- *Multidisciplinary staff:* community paediatrician, clinical psychologist, specialist health visitor, physiotherapy, occupational therapy, speech and language therapy, nurses, play therapy, and the child and adolescent mental health team
- *Social care:* advise on grants and allowances, respite care facilities, leisure and day care facilities. The Disability Living Allowance is an allowance for a child who has needs in excess of those of a non-disabled child of the same age
- *Education services:* preschool home teaching, educational assessment, peripatetic teachers for visually and hearing impaired, educational psychologist, educational welfare officer, nursery nurse and teachers
- *Voluntary organizations:* parent support. In some areas there is Portage—developmental guidance for disabled children, play facilities, educational opportunities, support services, respite care.

Special educational needs (SEN)

A child with learning difficulties or disabilities when compared to a child of the same age who requires different or extra help in school is said to have special educational needs. About 20% of children will have SEN at some point.

Children seen by the child development team may need help when starting school. Such children will enter mainstream nursery or a special needs nursery with extra support and/or a statement of educational need. Today there are far fewer special schools and many children <5 years start in mainstream schools or schools with a special unit e.g. for the hearing impaired or visually impaired.

A child with a less severe disability may come to the attention of the school via the parent or the teacher. There is a specialist educational needs coordinator (SENCO) to help in every school. First the child has an Individual Education Plan (IEP) that identifies the problem and gives the child the help required. If there are still difficulties the child can have an Early Years Action Plus or School Action Plus. Very few children will require a statutory assessment and then a statement of educational needs. At 14 years there is transition planning to adult services in health and social care, ready for leaving full-time education between 18 and 20 years of age.

School health service

The school health service is important in the management of children with a health component to their special needs. As well as the delivery of individual care such as tube feeding in a mainstream school, there will be an important role in coordinating health care and ensuring the children also receive routine health promotion.

18.8 Hearing loss and communication disorders

The ear is the organ of both hearing and balance. It receives and amplifies sound and converts it into neural impulses.

Sound

Sounds are vibrations transmitted through an elastic solid, liquid or gas capable of detection by the human organ of hearing. Sounds are characterized by:
- *Pitch (frequency)*: measured in Hz (cycles per second). A sound of single frequency is a pure tone
- *Loudness (intensity)*: measured in decibels (dB) (Table 18.6).

The decibel is a unit for expressing relative loudness or intensity of sound on a logarithmic scale. 0 dB is the usual human auditory threshold at 2 kHz. The threshold of pain is 100 db.

Table 18.6. Loudness of some sounds	
Source	dB
Calm breathing	10–20
Speech	40–60
Radio or TV	60
Dog barking	80
Overhead jet	110–140
The Who: live pop concert 1976	126
Rifle shot at 1 m	140

Hearing impairment

Hearing loss is defined at the following thresholds:
- *Mild*: 20–30 dB
- *Moderate*: 30–50 dB
- *Severe*: 50–70 dB
- *Profound*: 70–90 dB.

Classification and causes
- *Conductive*: a problem in the external or middle ear
- *Sensorineural*: a problem in the cochlea or eighth nerve
- *Mixed*: combination of conductive and sensorineural.

Conductive hearing loss
Up to 30% of children in the first few years of life may have an episode of conductive hearing loss of up to 60 dB.

Causes include:
- Acute otitis media
- Otitis media with effusion (OME)
- Ear wax.

Otitis media with effusion (OME)
There is an accumulation of fluid behind an intact tympanic membrane in the absence of acute infection. Prevalence peaks at 1 year and again at 3–5 years.

Risk factors include season (winter), smoke exposure, bottle-feeding, and anatomical abnormalities such as cleft palate, craniofacial abnormalities, Down syndrome.

Hearing levels fluctuate from normal (<20 dB) to <45 dB and this fluctuation may contribute to speech and language delay.

Tympanometry measures middle ear volume and compliance: a flat compliance or impedance curve is obtained.

Treatment options include adenoidectomy, grommets, and hearing aids.

Sensorineural hearing loss (SNHL)
SNHL is most often caused by hair cell damage in the cochlea. It is less common than conductive hearing loss with a prevalence of ~1.2/1000 live births and 3/1000 schoolchildren. The prevalence increases with age as at least a third are acquired and progressive forms. Most is irreversible.

Causes
Genetic (50% of congenital deafness)
Inherited forms of hearing loss are categorized as non-syndromic or syndromic:
- *Non-syndromic (70%)*: dominant (DFNA) or recessive (DFNB) and mitochondrial forms exist. The most common is DFNB1 caused by mutations in *GJB2* which encodes the gap junction protein connexin-26, CX26.
- *Syndromic (30%)*:
  - *dominant*: Stickler syndrome, Waardenburg syndrome
  - *recessive*: Pendred syndrome, Usher syndrome.

In addition, hearing loss is a component of a complex phenotype in a number of syndromes including Jervell–Lange–Neilsen syndrome and Treacher–Collins syndrome.

Acquired
- *Prenatal*: congenital infection, fetal alcohol syndrome
- *Perinatal*: hyperbilirubinaemia, birth asphyxia
- *Postnatal*:
  - infection: meningitis, measles, mumps.
  - head injury
  - drugs, e.g. aminoglycosides.

Mixed hearing loss
Mixed hearing loss occurs when a conductive loss is imposed on a sensorineural loss. Hearing assessment shows air conduction thresholds to be poorer than the abnormal bone conductive thresholds.

Clinical assessment of hearing

Universal neonatal screening will lead to earlier identification of congenital hearing impairment which has an incidence of 1/1000 live births. Hearing impairment affects the linguistic, social, and emotional development of a child and it is essential to test hearing in any child with speech and language delay. Parents usually notice hearing impairment.

Strategies for testing hearing are described in section 18.5. Pure-tone audiometry can be used when a child is old enough to perform an action in response to a sound and will accept earphones, i.e. from ~2.5 years. Pure tone audiometry response allows distinction between conductive, sensorineural. and mixed patterns of hearing loss (Fig 18.3). The aim is to ascertain the degree, nature and cause of any hearing loss. Children with hearing impairment frequently have complex needs: 40% have an additional disability. Visual problems are four times more common, mental health problems are more common and there is a higher prevalence of child abuse. Dysmorphic features or a positive family history are indicators for a genetic referral.

Treatment options include hearing aids and cochlear implantation which can provide hearing for children who are profoundly deaf and can deliver hearing sensation at levels of 30–45 dB across frequencies that allow speech to be heard.

Communication disorders

- *Communication* may be verbal or non-verbal
- *Language* is a system for communicating thoughts and emotions using voice sounds, written symbols, or gestures and has two components: expressive and receptive
- *Speech* is the oral transmission of language using articulated sounds. It is just one aspect of expressive language.

Development of communication

Speech and language development is influenced by a host of environmental factors as well as innate capacities.

Environmental factors

- *Family structure and size:* the first child in a family often speaks earlier and children in large families speak later
- *Multiple births:* twins and triplets often speak slightly later than singletons
- *Bilingualism:* in the UK 8% of children starting primary school have English as a second language. Delay of expressive language is usually ~3 months in bilingual children.
- *Neglect:* severe social and linguistic deprivation.

Intrinsic factors

- *Familial:* a family history is common
- *Gender:* boys speak later than girls and have a higher incidence of speech and language problems (M:F 2:1)
- *Hearing impairment:* this hinders comprehension and acquisition of spoken language
- *Learning disability:* generalized learning difficulties is a common cause of speech and language problems. Cognitive function is important for comprehension and communication.

Classification

Communication disorders may occur in isolation, e.g. delay in expressive language or in the context of other disorders such as autistic spectrum disorder or learning disability.

Disorders of speech production

- *Dysarthria:* neuromuscular disorders such as cerebral palsy impair ability to articulate sounds and are often associated with feeding and breathing difficulties
- *Dysphonia:* vocal cord abnormalities
- *Dysfluency:* stammer/stutter normally affects 4% of children between 2–4 years. It is usually transient but may persist. More common in boys (M:F 4:1)
- *Structural problems:* cleft lip and palate
- *Dyspraxia:* inability to coordinate speech muscles.

Specific language impairment

- *Expressive language delay:* may occur in isolation or in the context of other neurodevelopmental disorders including autistic spectrum disorders and learning disability. Autistic spectrum disorders all include deficits in some or all of reciprocal social interactions, communication, flexibility of thinking, and behaviour and are considered in Chapter 17.
- *Receptive aphasia:* inability to comprehend
- *Loss of speech and language:* in neurodegenerative disorders
- *Landau–Kleffner syndrome:* acquired epileptic aphasia.

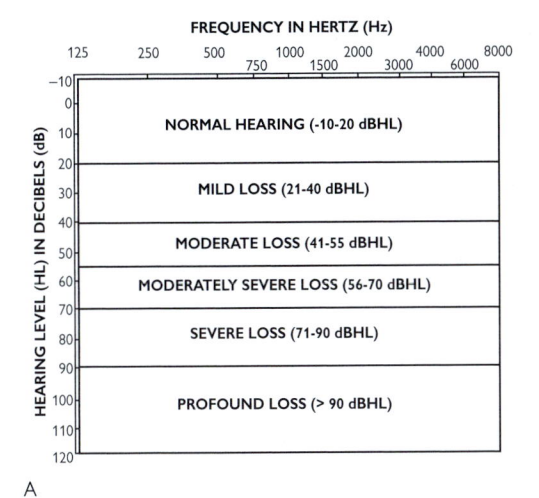

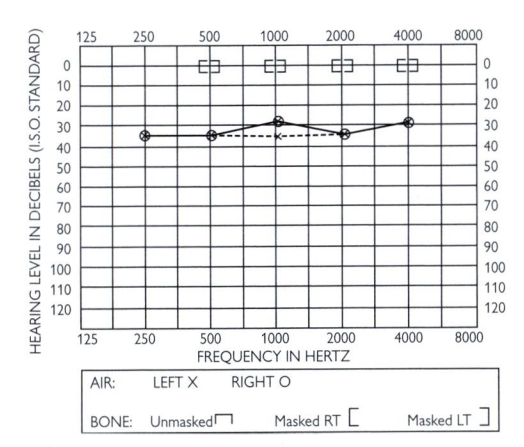

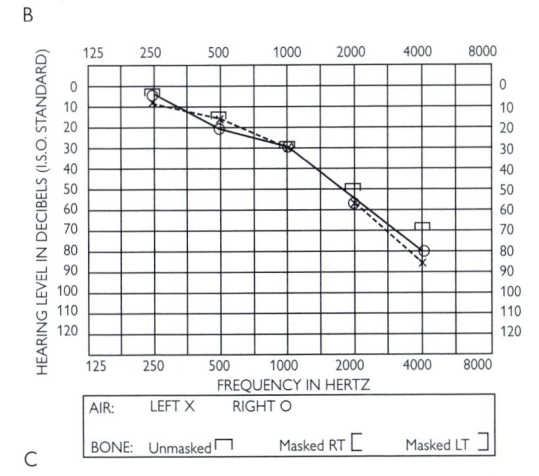

Fig 18.3 Audiograms: A. Levels of hearing loss. B. Mild bilateral conductive hearing loss. C. Mild–severe bilateral sensorineural hearing loss.

Management

It is anticipated that the >800 babies born each year with significant permanent hearing loss will be identified on screening and will benefit from early intervention.

Management is multidisciplinary and may include ENT and genetic referral, audiologist, speech and language therapists, teachers, and social workers.

18.9 Child maltreatment

Child abuse and neglect
Society has been slow to recognize child abuse and neglect and to acknowledge it as a problem. The idea of child abuse runs counter to most people's perception of 'good enough' parenting and the belief that parental care at home is an optimal environment.

History
In the distant past, UK society viewed children as parental possessions and parents were at liberty to treat children in any way they wished. Although abuse was observed and reported, it was accepted unless extreme and physical chastisement was accepted as a disciplinary necessity: 'spare the rod and spoil the child'. Society was reluctant to accept that carers could deliberately harm children for whom they were responsible.

Medical recognition that children needed protection dates from the work of Caffey and Kempe who described what was termed 'battered child syndrome' between 1946 and 1962. Professional recognition of child sexual abuse followed about two decades later.

The first organized professional response to child abuse in the UK led to the National Society for Prevention of Cruelty to Children being established in 1890. The development of legal and professional strategies and systems to safeguard children remains an ongoing process.

Definitions and classification
Abuse and neglect are forms of child maltreatment and are defined as inflicting harm or failing to act to prevent harm. Harm includes impaired health and development caused by ill treatment or the absence of a reasonable standard of parental care, i.e. neglect. Significant harm is harm which reaches the threshold to justify a child protection enquiry.

Working together, 2006 classifies forms of maltreatment as:
- Physical abuse
- Emotional abuse
- Sexual abuse
- Neglect
- Fabricated or induced illness (FII).

These forms of maltreatment often overlap. A child who is physically harmed will suffer emotionally. Sexual abuse may involve physical coercion. Neglect may lead to physical injury. The degree and motivation of maltreatment ranges from passive to deliberate, providing a parallel categorization:

- *Neglect*: sustained failure to meet the needs of a child, due to ignorance in some cases
- *Mild ill-treatment*: mild, acknowledged ill-treatment by loving parents often as part of 'disciplining' a child and culturally dependent, e.g. smacking
- *Impulsive ill-treatment*: unpremeditated ill-treatment by parents under pressure and often ignorant of the extent of potential damage by the impulsive act. The perpetrator often shows shame and remorse
- *Premeditated, deliberate abuse:* sustained ill-treatment undertaken for gain by disturbed, dangerous, and manipulative individuals. This is a serious, rare criminal activity which occurs in all countries and cultures.

Epidemiology
The true prevalence of child maltreatment is difficult to ascertain in part because of difficulties in definition. Defining what is child abuse remain a subject of debate and varies between societies. The appropriateness of smacking children to enforce discipline, for example, remains controversial. It is against the law in 24 countries, excluding the UK. Culture should not be used to justify maltreatment, for example female genital mutilation.

It is estimated that between 4–16% of children experience physical abuse and 1 in 10 neglect or emotional abuse. In 2007 in the UK about 1.5% of children were referred to social care for suspected abuse and about 3% of these referrals were investigated. In 2007 there were 25 per 10,000 children on the child protection register, those under 1 yr having the highest rate. The percentage in each category were:

- Neglect   46%
- Physical injury   12%
- Sexual abuse   7%
- Emotional abuse   27%
- Mixed   9%.

Non-accidental head injury had an incidence of 2.1/10 000 infants <1 year according to a population-based study. Children <1 year are most vulnerable to physical abuse and are at greater risk of serious harm: they are four times more likely to be killed than the average person in England and Wales.

It is estimated from mortality statistics produced by the Office of National Statistics that 50–100 children die from child abuse each year in the UK.

Aetiology: risk factors
It is well established that certain personal, social, and family attributes predispose to child abuse and neglect. Knowledge of these risk factors must be considered in the identification of children at risk of harm, especially in the presence of clinical concerns. Several risk factors are often present.

Risk factors can be categorized as follows:
- Child factors
- Parental factors
- The family
- Community and environment.

Child factors
The following children are vulnerable:
- *Unwanted:* unplanned, wrong gender
- *Born preterm or low birthweight*: separation or hospitalization disrupts attachment
- *Physical or learning disabilities*
- *Behavioural problems:* difficult temperament or personality, soiling or wetting, crying interminably or inconsolably.
- Looked-after children or those not attending school.

Parental factors
Parents or carers may be vulnerable if they have:
- *Mental health problems:* neurosis, psychosis, low IQ
- *Health problems:* poor physical health or disability

- *No support:* lone parents
- *History:* of abuse or neglect as a child, in care.
- *Immaturity:* teenage parents are more likely to neglect
- *Personality disorder:* parents with unrealistic expectations or negative attitudes to their child's behaviour, rigid or antisocial personalities, impulsive or aggressive.

Family factors
Families may be vulnerable if there is:
- Drug and/or alcohol abuse
- *Domestic violence:* current or previous violence towards other family members or animals
- *Social isolation:* lack of social constraints and weak supportive networks
- *Poverty:* can be associated with stress and poor family relationships, inadequate housing, homelessness, unsafe or violent neighbourhoods.

All health-care workers have a responsibility to safeguard children from prevention of child abuse to its recognition, through monitoring the health and development of children who have been maltreated to therapeutic intervention and prevention of further abuse.

Paediatricians have an important role in safeguarding children as part of a multiagency team. This section focuses on the duties and responsibilities of paediatricians in relation to child protection including the legal framework, the approach to paediatric assessment, and the strategies for management.

Safeguarding children

Working together to safeguard children (HM Government, 2006) is a guide to interagency working to safeguard children and promote their welfare. It emphasizes that:
- Agencies and professionals need to work in partnership with each other and should work openly and collaboratively with children and families.
- Information must be shared between agencies.

This document reflects the principles contained within the United Nations Convention on the Rights of the Child (see section 18.2), takes into account the European Convention on Human Rights, and is informed by the requirements of the Children Act 1989 and the Children Act 2004.

The legal framework
The main relevant principles of the Children Act 1989 and the Children Act 2004 include:
- The welfare of the child is paramount
- Children should remain within their own families wherever possible
- Children in danger should be kept safe
- Children should be informed about what is happening to them and their wishes and feelings taken into account considering their age and understanding.
- Parents continue to have parental responsibility even if their children are not living with them.

Note that legal procedures differ across the UK and procedures and terminology in England may differ from those in Scotland, Wales, and Northern Ireland.

Local organizational framework
Each NHS Trust has a named doctor, usually a consultant paediatrician, and a named nurse for child protection. Each local authority is required to have a Local Safeguarding Children's Board (LSCB) made up of all agencies with responsibility for services to children: social services, health, education, police, probation and the voluntary sector.

Each area has a designated doctor and nurse for safeguarding children who work closely with the named professionals.

Terminology
It is useful to know the definition of common terms with legal definitions.

Child in need
A child is taken to be in need if:
- He or she is unlikely to achieve a reasonable standard of health or development without the provision of services by a local authority
- He or she is disabled.

Significant harm
Significant harm is the threshold which justifies compulsory intervention in family life. The threshold is reached when ill-treatment or absence of a reasonable standard of parental care impairs the health (physical or mental) or development (physical, intellectual, social, or behavioural) of a child.

Impairment is significant if the health or development is less than could reasonably be expected of a similar child receiving reasonable parental care.

Parental responsibility
Parental responsibility is the right, duty, responsibility, and authority which in law a parent has in relation to their child and his property.

The birth mother has parental responsibility from birth, but the birth father has parental responsibility jointly with the mother only if they marry, at any time before or after conception.

Parental responsibility may be shared by a number of people and may be acquired by:
- *Other adults such as unmarried father, grandfather, or step-parents:* by a court order
- *Local authority:* by making a care order
- *Adoptive parents:* adoption confers parental responsibility
- *Birth father:* by a formal agreement with the mother or by putting his name as the father on the birth certificate.

Foster parents do not have parental responsibility. Only those with parental responsibility can give consent for medical procedures such as immunisation.

18.10 Child physical abuse

Physical abuse may involve hitting, shaking, throwing, burning, scalding, suffocating, or drowning a child. It may occur as a component of factitious or induced illness (see below) and physical injury may arise from neglect by failure to provide adequate supervision or protection.

The dangers are age-related: the younger the child the more at risk they are of serious or fatal injury from physical abuse.

The Welsh Child Protection Systematic Review Group maintains a useful database of literature and reviews at http://www.core-info.cf.ac.uk

Clinical evaluation

History
Confident diagnosis of inflicted injury can be especially difficult, as a false history is often given by the perpetrator and a young infant or child may be unable to disclose the abuse. However, certain features of the history and certain patterns of injury should raise concern about inflicted injury:

- Vague, unwitnessed, inconsistent, discrepant history between parents or carers
- History does not make sense, inconsistent with injury, inappropriate to child's development
- History of inappropriate child response such as 'did not cry' or 'felt no pain'
- *Unusual behaviour by parent/carer:* delay in seeking medical advice, lack of concern, unduly friendly or hostile response to professionals
- Unexplained injury noted by others, e.g. at school or day nursery
- Not accompanied by parent/carer without good reason
- Child fearful and wary of adults
- Multiple injuries of different ages, previous history of unusual injury.

It should be remembered that infants of any age may fall from elevated surfaces or be dropped. Short vertical falls of less than 1 m do not usually cause severe injury, but the impact surface is also important.

Examination
The aim of examination is to make a diagnosis of probable or possible abuse or accidental injury, to exclude medical conditions with similar features, and to screen for other health problems.

Bruises, burns and scalds, fractures, oral injuries, or bites are the most common external signs of injury and in each case there are features that may allow a distinction between inflicted and accidental injury.

Bruises
Bruising is the most common sign in children who have been physically abused, but children also sustain bruises from everyday play and accidents.

Bruising in a baby who is not independently mobile is very uncommon (<1%). In mobile children bruising is common on shins and knees, and most accidental bruises occur over bony prominences on the front of the body.

Patterns of bruising suggestive of abuse include:
- *Bruising on babies:* 'those who don't cruise rarely bruise'
- Bruising in a child who is not independently mobile
- Bruises away from bony prominences
- Bruises to face, back abdomen, arms, ears, buttocks, or hands
- Multiple bruises in clusters
- Multiple bruises of uniform shape
- *Bruises carrying imprints of implement or ligature or hand:* a positive image of implement
- Bruises with surrounding petechiae: a negative image of implement.

Buttock bruises may be punishment related, and on inner thigh or genital area they may suggest sexual abuse.

A bruise should never be interpreted in isolation. There is no adequate published evidence to support accurate ageing of bruises from naked eye assessment or photographs. A full blood count including platelets and coagulation screen is essential before ascribing excessive bruising to abuse.

Fractures
Accidental fractures are common in children, affecting up to 66% of boys and 40% of girls by their 15th birthday. Most accidental fractures occur in children >5 years of age, most non-accidental fractures in those <3 years of age.

However, fractures can be indicative of abuse and indicate serious assault. Fractures are found in up to 25% of physically abused children and most usually (80%) in children <18 months. Many abusive fractures are occult and may only be revealed by radiography. Fractures, especially of the ribs, may not be associated with bruising.

Features suspicious of abuse include:
- Any fracture in the 1st year with no clear history.
- *Rib fractures:* single or multiple are highly indicative of abuse from squeezing, shaking or direct blows.
- *Metaphyseal fractures:* fragment of bone separated from distal long bone, 'bucket-handle' on radiograph. Caused by gripping, twisting, or shaking injury.
- *Spiral fracture of long bone in a child <15 months:* highly suggestive of abuse in immobile children. Caused by a twisting force. >15 months, a transverse femoral fracture is the most common accidental or abusive femoral fracture. A fractured femur in a child not yet walking is suspicious. Supracondylar fractures of humerus are usually accidental.
- Multiple fractures of different stages of healing.
- *Periosteal new bone formation:* damage to the periosteum by gripping or twisting raises it from the shaft and new bone appears 7–10 days later.

In infants <1 year, a skull fracture is as likely to be accidental as to result from abuse. In either case a linear, parietal fracture is the most common variety.

Fractures with minimal force can occur in osteogenesis imperfecta, rickets, osteomyelitis, and malignancy.

Thermal injuries
Thermal injuries encompass scalds from hot liquids, contact burns from hot objects such as an iron, burns from flames, and chemical or electrical burns. Most burns are accidental.

Accidental scalds are common and are usually 'spill injuries' where a toddler reaches out and pulls a hot drink or cooking liquid over themselves, or from turning on a hot tap. Accidental scalds are usually asymmetrical, irregular, and involve upper trunk, face or arms. Five seconds exposure to water at 60 °C will cause a scald. In many homes hot water is at 60 °C, although 54 °C is recommended.

Features suspicious of inflicted thermal injuries include:

Scalds
- Immersion scalds usually affect limbs in a 'glove' or 'stocking' distribution and tend to be of uniform depth with a clear demarcation line
- Splash burns from hot water thrown at or poured over a child.

Contact burns
- Burns to unusual areas such as back, shoulders or buttocks, lips, or genitalia. Burns often multiple. Margins may reflect shape of a hot object.
- Cigarette burns are circular with a central cratered lesion 1–2 cm in diameter. Accidental brushing against a cigarette rarely makes such marks and leaves a 'tail'.
- Burns may be inflicted deliberarely as punishment.

Oral injuries and bites
Accidental injuries to the mouth are very common and are usually caused by falls or sporting injuries. In physical abuse, the head and face are areas of the body most commonly injured and cuts or bruises to the lips are the most common abusive oral injury.

For a long time it was believed that injury to the upper labial frenum was diagnostic of abuse. The evidence does not support this view. A torn labial frenum in isolation is not diagnostic of abuse. It can occur accidentally from a fall or accidental blow to the face.

Bites
If an adult bites a child hard enough to leave a mark, it is an assault. A bite leaves an oval or circular mark with two symmetrical opposing U-shaped arches which may include puncture wounds, indentations, or bruises. A forensic dentist should be consulted to assist in distinguishing a child's bite from an adult's. An animal bite is narrower and tends to tear the skin and leave deep puncture wounds.

Non-accidental head injury (NAHI)

Traumatic brain injury is the most common cause of death in physical child abuse, and 95% of severe brain injury in the 1st year of life is inflicted.

NAHI is most commonly seen in infants <6 months of age and has a mortality of 30% with residual disability of varying severity in half of the survivors.

Aetiology and pathogenesis

The exact mechanism and minimal forces necessary to produce the injuries found are unknown. The assaults are rarely witnessed, perpetrator confessions are rare, and experiments on biomechanics have limitations.

Available evidence suggests that vigorous, repetitive shaking with or without impact, causes the triad of encephalopathy, subdural haemorrhage and retinal haemorrhage, hence the old term 'shaken baby syndrome'. Of course, other causes exist for each of these features *in isolation*, but the suggestion that the triad can arise from normal handling or transitory obstruction to breathing (the 'Geddes hypothesis') was rejected by the Court of Appeal in 2005.

Brain damage arises from several mechanisms:
- Traumatic shearing injury
- *Hypoxic–ischaemic injury:* damage to the cervicomedullary junction causes apnoea and hypoxia
- *Subdural haemorrhage:* rotational forces rupture subdural veins causing subdural haematomas which are usually bilateral over the convexity of the cerebral hemispheres. Acutely they are small and cause no mass effect.

Clinical features

Infants with NAHI present with a wide variety of symptoms which usually fall into one of four categories. The diagnosis should be considered in any infant or young child who collapses inexplicably.

Hyperacute encephalopathy (6%)
Extreme 'whiplash' forces cause cervicomedullary damage with acute respiratory failure and cerebral oedema.

Acute encephalopathy (53%)
Characterized by coma, fits, raised intracranial pressure, apnoea, hypotonia, and shock with widespread retinal haemorrhages. Investigation reveals anaemia and bilateral subdural haematomata. There may or may not be coexistent other injuries: fractures or bruises and additional signs of impact injury to the head: scalp injury, skull fracture, subgaleal haemorrhage.

Subacute non-encephalopathic (19%)
The brain injury is less intense, without swelling or clinical encephalopathy.

Chronic subdural haematomata (22%)
Infants present with signs and symptoms of isolated chronic expanding subdural haematomas: failure to thrive, vomiting, hypotonia, and an expanding head circumference. Retinal haemorrhages have cleared by time of presentation, but additional features of abuse such as rib fractures may be present.

Coagulation results may be abnormal immediately after the event but recover rapidly if the child survives. Haemoglobin often falls due to blood loss.

There may be no signs at all of external injury.

18.11 Emotional abuse, sexual abuse, neglect, and FII

Emotional abuse

Emotional abuse arises from a relationship between child and parent or carer which is characterized by harmful interactions which impair a child's psychological and emotional health and development.

Emotional abuse is the most difficult form of abuse to identify and is probably under-recognized. It frequently coexists with other forms of abuse and its impact is cumulative, serious, and long term.

Key features

Children at risk of emotional abuse may be:
- *Unwanted:* wrong sex, disabled, rejected
- Seen as ill or difficult
- *In difficult family circumstances:* marital discord, separation, domestic violence
- *Born to vulnerable parents:* alcohol or drug misusers, depressed, mentally ill.

Parental responses are sustained, repetitive, and inappropriate. They convey negative emotions such as criticism, threats, or ridicule and make the child feel unloved and unwanted. These responses may or may not be deliberate. The child may be rejected, isolated, terrorized, ignored, or corrupted.

Key features include:
- Emotional unavailability, unresponsiveness, and neglect
- *Persistent negative attributions:* denigration, belittling, blaming, criticizing
- *Unrealistic expectations:* failure to protect or overprotection, exposure to distressing behaviour such as domestic violence
- *Failure to recognize child's individuality and psychological boundaries:* use of child as friend and confidant, use to fulfil parent's ambitions, fabricated or induced illness (FII)
- *Failure to promote child's social adaptation:* depriving child of opportunity to develop peer relationships, intellectual deprivation, encouragement to misuse drugs or to be involved in criminal activity.

Clinical features: indications of impairment

Emotional abuse causes anxiety and low self-esteem. The symptoms and signs are non-specific and vary with age:
- *Infant:* feeding difficulties, crying, poor sleep patterns, delayed development. Irritability, apathetic, non-demanding. Failure to thrive.
- *Toddler or preschool child:* spectrum from overactive to apathetic. Head-banging, bad-temper, 'clingy'. Developmental delay in language and social skills.
- *School child:* wetting and soiling, rejection by peers. Poor school performance. Antisocial behaviour, victims and perpetrators of bullying.
- *Adolescent:* depression, self-harm, substance abuse, eating disorders, low self-esteem, oppositional, aggressive, delinquent and criminal behaviour.

Sexual abuse

Child sexual abuse is the forcing or enticing of a child or young person to take part in sexual activities including prostitution, whether or not the child is aware of what is happening. The sexual activities may involve physical contact, penetrative or non-penetrative acts or non-contact activities such as watching sexual activities, the production of images, or encouragement to act in sexually inappropriate ways.

Key features

Responsibility rests with the perpetrator who gains sexual gratification from the abuse. In most cases the perpetrator is a family member (intrafamilial abuse). Less commonly it occurs as a random attack, prostitution, or via a paedophile network (stranger abuse). Most commonly fathers, stepfathers, or maternal boyfriends abuse daughters, but boys can also be victims.

Perpetrators may be male or female but are more likely to be male. They may commit a large number of offences and there is a high likelihood of re-offending. Most deny the abuse and refuse to participate in treatment programmes.

Clinical features

Child sexual abuse may present in a wide variety of ways which are highly age dependent. Physical signs are absent in most abused children and are more likely after a recent sexual assault.

Presentation may include:
- Allegation by child
- Allegation by sibling or another person
- *Physical complaints:* UTI, vulvovaginitis (low specificity)
- Behavioural abnormalities
  - sexualized behaviour through words, play, or drawings, precocious knowledge of adult sexual behaviour
  - difficulty learning, unexplained changes in school performance and concentration
  - lack of trust in familiar adults.
  - young people may present with mental health problems, psychosomatic complaints or self-harm
- Pregnancy or sexually transmitted diseases outside the period for vertical transmission.

Note that children can develop complex coping mechanisms to accommodate the abuse and may even seem to encourage or provoke a sexual response in the perpetrator. Adjustment may include secrecy, helplessness, self-blame, and guilt, all of which lead to delayed disclosure.

Physical signs

Diagnostic signs include pregnancy and presence of semen in vagina, anus, or external genitalia of an under-age child. The latter is only likely after an acute assault, i.e. in the previous 3 days in girls <13 years and all boys or previous 7 days in 13–16 year old girls.

The significance of other signs within the anogenital area such as changes in hymen or anus lie within the province of a doctor with specific forensic expertise and training.

Neglect

Neglect is the most prevalent form of child maltreatment, accounting for almost one half of children and young people referred to social care for suspected abuse in the UK. It is a persistent failure to meet a child's basic physical and psychological needs, resulting in serious impairment of health and development.

Key features

Neglect is defined through acts of parental omission, a form of 'passive' abuse. Many parents who neglect their children lack resources and motivation to be good enough parents.

Deliberate deprivation of basic requirements such as food, warmth, protection, and affection is best regarded as an active form of 'deprivational abuse' rather than neglect.

Neglect may take many forms, including failure to:
- Provide adequate food, shelter, and clothing on account of abandonment or exclusion from home
- Protect from physical harm or danger
- Ensure access to appropriate medical care
- Provide opportunity for social, emotional, and cognitive development
- Send child to school
- Provide age-appropriate and consistent limit-setting.

Neglected children are at risk of growing up into inadequate and neglectful parents, giving rise to a 'cycle of deprivation'.

Recognition of neglect

The impact of neglect varies according the age, temperament and coping mechanisms of the child. Risk factors for neglect in the parents and family include:

Parents/caregivers
- Learning difficulties, mental illness, substance abuse
- History of neglect or abuse, being in care or in prison
- Poor parenting skills, parents put their needs first.

Family
- Domestic violence, social isolation, poor housing.
- Poverty, financial problems (debts, unemployment)
- Lack of supervision, inappropriate carers (open house)
- Failure to keep appointments, poor school attendance.

Clinical features

Indicators of neglect vary with age:

0–2 years
- *Physical:* failure to thrive, frequent accidents, frequent hospital admissions, late presentation with physical symptoms
- *Development:* late attainment of milestones, failure to attend for immunisations, development checks
- *Behaviour:* attachment disorders (avoidant, inconsolable). lack of social responsiveness, self-stimulatory behaviour: rocking, head banging

2–5 years: preschool children
- *Physical:* failure to thrive, stunted growth; unkempt and dirty; frequent accidents, e.g. ingestions. Untreated infections, e.g. otitis media or conditions, e.g. squints. Malnutrition: iron deficiency anaemia. Poor dental hygiene.
- *Development:* speech and language delay. Social and emotional immaturity
- *Behaviour:* overactive, aggressive, impulsive. Indiscriminate friendliness, lack of skills for cooperative play. Seek physical contact from strangers.

5–16 years: school-age children
- *Physical:* short stature, underweight, or obese. Poor hygiene, unkempt appearance, poor general health
- *Development:* Learning difficulties, poor concentration, low educational attainment. Low self-esteem, poor coping skills. Social–emotional immaturity
- *Behaviour:* Soiling and wetting. Self-stimulating or self-injurious behaviour. Conduct disorders, poor social relationships, delinquency. Poor school attendance, truanting, runaways.

Fabricated or induced illness (FII)

This term describes a form of abuse and has replaced Munchausen syndrome by proxy.

FII encompasses a very wide spectrum of behaviours in which the parent or carer either fabricates or exaggerates the history or induces illness by direct means. FII can have fatal consequences and explains some rare cases of sudden unexplained death. The exact incidence is uncertain.

Key features

Motivation clearly varies, but certain characteristics of fabricators or illness inducers are apparent:
- The child's mother is the perpetrator in 89% of cases
- Previous 'paramedical' training is present in 20%
- A distant, passive, or absent father may be evident
- Perpetrator has history of abuse as a child in 25%, previous contact with mental health agencies in 30%.

Harm to the child may be emotional, indirect via unnecessary investigations by doctors or unnecessary surgery, or direct via the actual induction of illness.

Clinical features

FII should be considered under the following clinical circumstances:
- Inconsistent or unexplained symptoms and signs
- Mismatch between symptoms described and those observed by medical attendants
- Recurrent presentation for assessment and care
- Family history of unexplained illness or death
- Problems occurring only in presence of parent/carer
- Acute symptoms and signs ceasing when child is separated from parent/carer
- Treatment which does not produce expected effect.

Verbal and non-verbal fabrications

These often relate to paroxysmal conditions in which diagnosis depends on history. Symptoms reported include bleeding, choking, headache, vomiting, abdominal pain, seizures, recurrent infections. Non-verbal fabrication includes adding blood to urine and heating thermometers to fabricate a fever.

Induced illness

Withholding nutrients by inappropriate dietary restrictions or diluting feeds, induction of fever, poisoning (low toxicity: emetics, laxatives, diuretics; high toxicity: insulin, salt). Smothering may result in apparent life-threatening episodes or in sudden unexplained death in infancy (SUDI).

18.12 Management of suspected child maltreatment

Health-care workers may become aware that a child is being maltreated or is at risk of maltreatment in several ways:
- *Observation:* direct observation of symptoms and signs of abuse or neglect
- *Allegation:* reports made by a child or another person not directly involved of abuse or neglect.

Although it is useful to classify the types of abuse for purposes of description, there is commonly overlap and coexistence of several types. A NICE guideline on child maltreatment was issued in July 2009.

Paediatric assessment

If a doctor becomes concerned that a child is being neglected or abused they should first discuss those concerns with the more senior doctor responsible for the child.

History taking, examination and investigations specific to suspected *physical abuse* are discussed here.

History
A full history should include:
- Duration, frequency and timing of any alleged abuse or accident
- Behavioural and emotional problems
- *Social history:* current members of household and child-care arrangements, previous child protection concerns. Contact details of any professionals involved with the family.
- *Family history:* including safety and well-being of siblings
- Personal or family history of bleeding disorder.

In accidental falls both the height of the fall and the impact surface such as grass or concrete are important. Short vertical falls of <1 m rarely cause serious injury.

Examination
- *Height, weight, and head circumference:* plot centiles
- State of cleanliness, clothing
- Developmental status
- Top to toe external examination including scalp, fontanelle, fundi, inside of mouth, behind ears, genitalia, anus, and soles of feet
- Demeanour and response to carer
- *Injuries:* document site, size, colour, stage of healing. Measure and draw on body charts.

Documentation and recording is of particular importance and may be reviewed in court. Clear, legible notes with diagrams are essential, and must always be dated and signed.

A search for untreated medical conditions is wise, as abused children may be neglected as well.

Consent
A child of 16 years and over can give their own consent, but exceptions include the learning disabled. Children <16 can give their own consent provided they understand the value and purpose of what is involved. This is called 'Fraser competence' after the judge in the Gillick case.

Discussion with a child depends on age. It is unnecessary in a baby, good practice in a young child, and essential with an older 'Fraser competent' child. A child can be examined without consent if in need of urgent treatment.

Additional consent is recommended for colposcopy, genital and anal examination, photographs, and investigations such as radiography, blood tests, and forensic samples.

Acute management

Investigations
Investigations may identify occult injury such as fractures and subdural haematoma and exclude medical conditions in the differential diagnosis, e.g. bleeding diathesis. Investigations depend on injuries but some are required in most cases. Local practice varies.

Skeletal survey
A skeletal survey should be performed in all children <2 years in whom physical abuse is suspected. There is a high yield of occult abusive fractures. Over 2 years the decision to do a skeletal survey depends on clinical context but is indicated if there is:
- A fracture suggesting abuse
- Unexplained neurological symptoms or signs
- Older children with severe soft-tissue injury

The standard survey is shown in the Box.

Standard skeletal survey
- Skull:
  - AP, lateral, and Townes view (if clinically indicated)
  - skull radiographs should be taken as part of the skeletal survey even if a CT scan has been done or is planned.
- *Chest:* AP including clavicles. Left and right oblique views
- *Abdomen:* AP including pelvis and hips
- *Spine:*
  - AP of any region not seen on chest and abdomen
  - lateral of cervical, thoracic, and lumbar regions
- Limbs:
  - AP of all four limbs
  - PA of hands
  - DP of feet

Further radiographs after 2 weeks may increase detection of fractures by demonstrating them in a more advanced stage of healing. A bone scan is an alternative.

Neuroimaging
If non-accidental head injury (NAHI) is suspected following an acute presentation, cranial CT should be undertaken as soon as the child is stabilized. If the initial cranial CT is abnormal, or if abnormal neurology or encephalopathy persists with an apparently normal CT, MRI should be done on day 3–5.

Non-acute presentation requires neuroimaging by CT or MRI depending on age and availability.

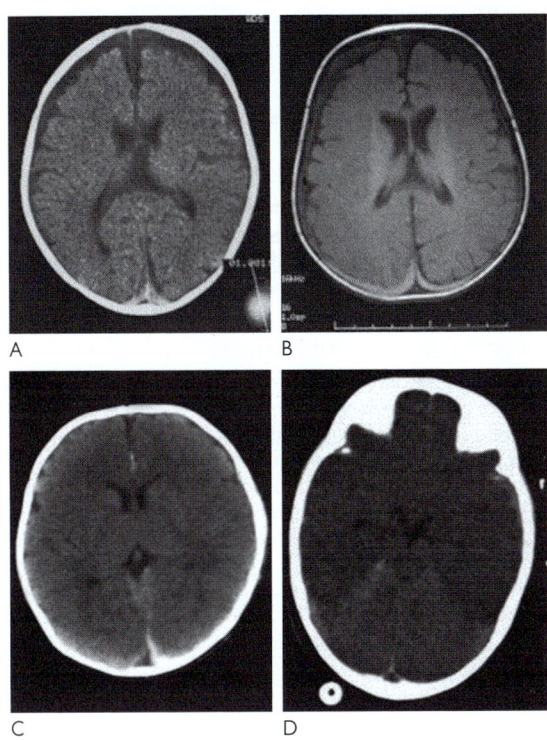

Fig 18.4 Neuroimaging in NAHI: A. Cranial CT and B. MRI showing bilateral posterior subdurals and prominent frontal extra-axial fluid collections. C. Cranial CT with bilateral shallow interhemispheric acute subdural haematomas and normal brain parenchyma. D. Cranial CT showing small volume interhemispheric blood and reduced attenuation of hemispheres with 'reversal' sign (cerebellum higher attenuation than hemispheres). Reprinted from Clinical Radiology, 60 (1), Stoodley, Neuroimaging in non-accidental head injury: if, when, why and how, 2005, with permission from Elsevier.

Blood tests

Bony injury

- *Blood culture, FBC:* for osteomyelitis
- *Calcium, phosphate, alkaline phosphatase:* for rickets
- *Serum copper, caeruloplasmin:* copper deficiency (rare).

Bruising, bleeding, or purpura

Immune thrombocytopenic purpura (ITP) is the bleeding diathesis most likely to be mistaken for non-accidental injury.

- *Haematological investigations: first line:*
  - full blood count and film, including platelet count
- *Coagulation screen:*
  - prothrombin time (PT)
  - activated partial thromboplastin time (APTT)
  - thrombin time
  - fibrinogen.

These investigations may be normal in Henöch–Schonlein purpura, von Willebrand disease, and in some rare disorders: platelet function defects, factor XIII deficiency, and Ehlers–Danlos syndrome. Second line investigations include von Willebrand factor, factor VIII and IX assays, platelet aggregation studies, PFA-100, lupus anticoagulant.

Further management

Confidentiality

Personal information about children and families is subject to a legal duty of confidentiality and should not normally be disclosed without consent of the subject. However, personal information must be disclosed without consent if you believe that disclosure is in the child's best interests.

Doctors should share information with other agencies on a 'need to know' basis. Confidentiality must not stand in the way of child protection.

Duty of care

A paediatrician has a duty of care towards the patient who is the child. There is *no* competing duty of care owed to the child's parents or carers, but the doctor is of course required to act reasonably and in good faith in a competent and professional manner and to comply with any statutory requirements.

Further actions

After the initial assessment a senior doctor will discuss concerns with the child if appropriate for age and the parents, unless such a discussion would place the child at risk of significant harm. A referral to children's social care should be made within 24 h.

Hospital admission may be required for medical treatment, further investigation, or to ensure the child's immediate safety. Consideration should be given to safety of siblings.

Social care are the lead agency for child protection and will coordinate the interagency response. A strategy discussion or meeting involving social services, police, health, and other agencies will take place within 24 h and a child protection conference is held if the child is judged to be at continuing risk of significant harm.

Child protection conference

The role of this conference is to:

- Share all relevant information about child and family
- Assess risk to child
- Decide about need for child protection plan
- Appoint a key worker and core group.

A child protection plan is then developed and implemented by the key worker and core group members.

Orders to protect children

- *Emergency protection order:* granted by a court if a child is likely to suffer significant harm if not removed or the local authority does not have access to the child. Lasts for 8 days.
- *Protection order:* used in extreme emergency, e.g. if parents are threatening to take an injured child from the ward. It can be taken out by the police for 72 h.
- *Wardship:* can be used when urgent medical treatment is needed and parental consent is withheld.
- *Care order:* the responsibility for the child is taken over by the local authority who will work in partnership with the parents but prioritize the welfare of the child.
- *Supervision order:* gives social services power and duty to visit the family and impose conditions on parenting.

18.13 Case-based discussions

Disease prevention and health promotion: examples

Childhood injuries
Accidents and injuries to children remain a common cause of morbidity and mortality for which there is a strong social class gradient.

Health promotion
- *Individual level:* advice to parents and children, access to safety equipment
- *Community level:* action by local authorities to improve road safety, soft surfaces in playgrounds
- *Public policy level:* legislation on seat belts, speed limits in built-up areas.

Prevention measures
- *Primary prevention:* use of safety equipment, fluorescent clothing for cyclists, cycle proficiency training, traffic calming, safe areas to play
- *Secondary prevention:* seat belts, cycle helmets
- *Tertiary prevention:* effective emergency services, neurological units, rehabilitation facilities.

Childhood obesity
Obesity in children in the UK is rising fast. If this increase continues children's life expectancy will be less than their parents', with obesity the chief cause of premature death. A screening programme for childhood obesity is not recommended as there is no intervention of proven effectiveness.

Health promotion
- *Individual level:* education about healthy eating, exercise prescriptions
- *Community level:* better access to local leisure facilities and sports clubs, outdoor play spaces; local food cooperatives for cheap, fresh produce.
- *Policy level:* nutritional standards for school catering, labelling to identify healthy food, 'safe routes to school' to encourage walking to school; research into production of lower-fat foods.

Sudden unexplained death in infancy (SUDI)
The rate of SUDI was > 2/1000 live births in the UK until 1991. Risk factors are well known and include sleeping prone, parental smoking, co-sleeping, and male gender. There is a social class gradient and an increased incidence in boys and low-birthweight babies.

Health promotion: SUDI prevention
Appropriate advice to parents has lead to a 75% reduction in the SUDI rate. This includes putting babies on their backs to sleep ('Back to Sleep') with head uncovered and feet placed to foot of cot, avoiding overheating, stopping smoking in pregnancy, and avoiding co-sleeping on sofa or armchair. Action is taken at:
- *Individual level:* advice from health professionals
- *Community level:* communication via antenatal and prenatal groups
- *Policy level:* clear guidance to health professionals, media campaigns, leaflets.

A case of SUDI
A 4 month old baby is bought by ambulance to the hospital emergency department, having been found in his cot blue and not breathing 30 min previously. The parents tried mouth-to-mouth resuscitation when they found him while waiting for the ambulance to arrive. After 20 min there has been no response to resuscitation.

When and what samples do you collect?
This will be defined as a sudden unexplained death in infancy (SUDI) and the Department of Health guidelines in Working Together 2006 need to be followed (see Box).

If possible, take specimens before the child is declared dead. If not, get the permission of the coroner.

Blood samples can be taken from a venous or arterial site. A larger gauge needle may be necessary. The femoral vein can be used for sampling blood. Cardiac puncture should be avoided if possible as this may damage intrathoracic structures and make post-mortem findings difficult to interpret. Record the site from which all samples were taken. Document all samples taken.

Whom do you inform?
- Coroner's officer
- Police
- Hospital or duty social work team
- General practitioner
- Health visitor
- Designated doctor for SUDI.

What happens to the parents?
Good practice is a joint police/paediatric home visit within 24 h, preferably with the consultant paediatrician. If the police visit alone, then the health visitor or a community nurse may visit a few days later. Support, advice and information for parents may include details of Foundation for the Study of Infant Deaths (FSID): www.sids.org.uk/fsid, Child Death Helpline, and Cruse: Bereavement Support and Advice

The consultant should arrange to meet the parents a few days after the post-mortem has been performed to provide preliminary results, and meet them again 2 months later to provide his/her views on the cause of death.

Samples in SUDI	
Sample	Test
Blood	Toxicology
Blood	Culture and sensitivity
Blood	Chromosomes
Blood	Inherited metabolic disease
Cerebrospinal fluid (CSF)	Microscopy, culture, and sensitivity
Nasopharyngeal aspirate (NPA)	Viral cultures, immunofluorescence, and DNA amplification techniques
Nasopharyngeal aspirate (NPA)	Culture and sensitivity
Swab any lesions; also throat swab	Culture and sensitivity
Urine (if available from suprapubic aspiration)	Toxicology
Urine (if available from suprapubic aspiration)	Organic acids, amino acids

Chapter 19
Adolescent medicine

- 19.1 Adolescence: from child to adult *408*
- 19.2 Clinical skills in adolescent medicine *410*
- 19.3 Adolescent health *412*
- 19.4 Adolescent health promotion *414*
- 19.5 Depression, suicide, and self harm *416*
- 19.6 Somatic symptoms and fatigue *418*
- 19.7 Eating disorders and obesity *420*
- 19.8 Sexual health and substance misuse *422*
- 19.9 Case-based discussions *424*

19.1 Adolescence: from child to adult

Adolescence: time of transition

What is adolescence?
Adolescence (from the Latin *adolescere*, to grow up) is the period of transition from childhood to adulthood. This transition involves biological, psychological, and social domains.

The chronological age spanned by adolescence shows individual biological variation and is also determined by social and cultural factors. The World Health Organization (WHO) defines adolescents as young people aged between 10 and 19 years, that is up to the 20th birthday. It is useful to differentiate between early, middle, and late adolescence.

'Adolescent' and 'teenager' are often used as synonyms, but it should be remembered that 'teen' is merely an artefact of English-language number terminology and does not occur in most other tongues. The group noun 'young people' is generally preferred.

Adolescent medicine
In adolescence, all aspects of clinical medicine are played out against a background of the most rapid physical, psychological, and social developmental changes since early infancy. These changes produce specific disease patterns, unusual symptom presentations, and above all, unique communication and management challenges.

Most paediatricians encounter adolescents in their clinical practice and require knowledge in the following important areas:
- The basics of adolescent development
- Communication skills
- Ethical, consent, and confidentiality issues
- Generic chronic illness management skills
- Health promotion
- Substance misuse and sexual health.

In childhood, parents are largely responsible for all aspects of a young person's health, from the most basic routines of cleaning teeth to the intricacies of chronic illness management. By the end of adolescence, all of these will be almost entirely the responsibility of the individuals themselves.

The challenge of working with adolescents is to maintain an effective clinical relationship during this transition. Communication skills are needed to take an accurate history, bearing in mind new life domains not applicable to children, e.g. sex, drugs, and employment.

Physical examination of adolescents require consideration of privacy and personal integrity as well as requiring additional skills such as pubertal assessment.

The effective treatment of illness in adolescence requires knowledge of development in order to adeptly manage issues regarding adherence, identity, consent and confidentiality, and relationships between the young person and their family.

Adolescent development
During adolescence, young people will go through puberty and the completion of growth, take on a sexually dimorphic body shape, develop new cognitive skills including abstract thinking capacities, elaborate a clearer sense of personal and sexual identity, and develop a degree of emotional, personal, and financial independence from their parents. Clinical interactions with adolescents must be seen against this ever-changing background. Adolescent development takes place in distinct but inter-related biological, psychological, and social domains (see Box).

Puberty and cognitive development are biologically determined, but the greater part of psychological and social development will vary depending on environmental and socio-cultural contexts. For adolescents in some cultures, social development may be dramatically foreshortened, consisting of brief initiation ceremonies.

> **Bio-psycho-social development in adolescence**
>
> *Biological*
> - *Puberty:* growth spurt, body dimorphism
> - Bone mineral accretion, enzyme maturation
>
> *Psychological*
> - Concrete to abstract thinking
> - Body image and sexual identity
> - Self-esteem and self-efficacy
>
> *Social*
> - Independence from family and parents
> - Educational and vocational capacity
> - Financial independence

Biological development:
Biological elements of adolescent development include puberty, completion of height growth and maturation in all other organ systems, particularly cardiovascular, liver, renal, and muscle and bone growth, together with maturation of enzyme systems such as cytochrome P450 systems, accretion of peak bone mass, and the development of sexually dimorphic adult patterns in blood lipids, haemoglobin, and red cell indices.

Puberty
Both boys and girls pass through identifiable stages of development of secondary sex characteristics, commonly known as the Tanner stages 1–5 (Fig 19.1).

Puberty may occur over as little as 18 months or as long as 5 years. At 13 years, boys can manifest the entire range from completely prepubertal to entirely masculinized.

Boys
The earliest sign in boys, increasing testicular volume (>4 mL), begins at a mean age of 12 years, about a year after the development of breast buds in girls at 11 years.

The commonest concerns regarding puberty in adolescence are delayed puberty and short stature, particularly in boys. The 97th centile for developing testicular volume is 15 years, thus ~2% of boys will still be prepubertal and short at 15 years. This is almost always a normal variant, so called constitutional delay of puberty and growth and is often familial. Those with no signs of puberty by age 15 should be referred to a paediatric endocrinologist for further investigation. See Chapter 10.5.

Girls
Girls usually appear significantly more developed earlier as the female growth spurt occurs early in puberty (mean age

11–12 years) compared with later in puberty (mean age 14 years) in boys. The defining event of puberty in girls is menarche. The mean age at menarche showed a decline in most developed countries through the first half of the 20th century, stabilizing in the 1960s at ~13 years for white girls and 12.5 years for black girls in most developed countries.

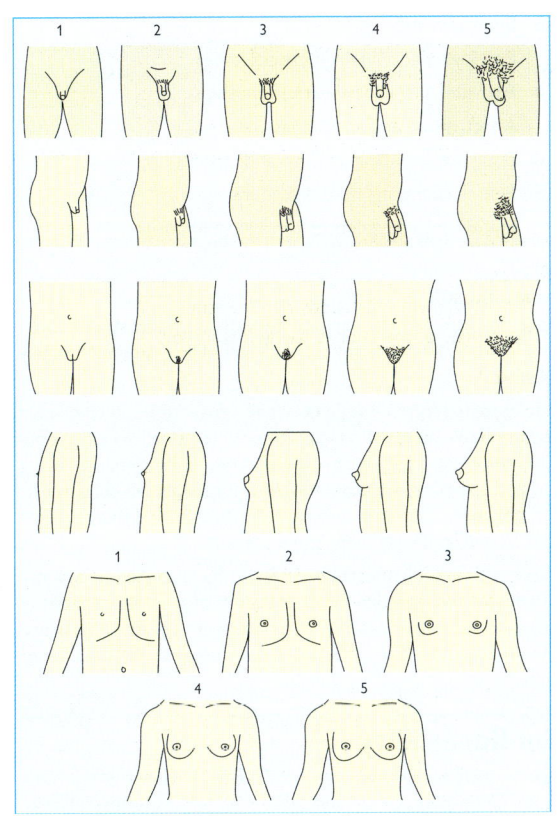

Fig 19.1 Tanner stages 1–5.

Psychological development:
Enhanced cognitive capacity drives the development of abstract thinking—the ability to use internal symbols or images to represent reality. This contrasts with the more childish concrete thinking, in which there is a need for objects to represent 'things' or 'ideas'. Abstract thinking capacities facilitate the acquisition of complex mathematical and language abilities, but also drive the search for identity which in many senses characterizes adolescence.

Being able to visualize many possible future selves drives adolescent questioning of identity in many domains, from basic self-efficacy and self-esteem to specific questions about sexual identity, religion, and morality.

The capacity for abstract thinking is essential in order to give informed consent to treatment and to independently manage chronic illness regimens.

It is also important to recognize the interactions of psychological developments with puberty, particularly in the context of a developing sense of sexuality and body image. Body image and self-esteem are vulnerable to both differences in the timing of puberty compared with peers and the physical effects of chronic illnesses.

Social changes:
Key social changes during adolescence include
- Changing relationships with family and peers
- Development of intimate relationships
- Transition to work or higher education.

Changing relationships: independence
Adolescence is often characterized as a time of developing 'independence' from parents and family, with the challenge of forming intimate relationships one of the key elements of developing adulthood. In early adolescence, young people form close but large peer groups, often with similar behaviours, dress, and speech. By mid-adolescence, further identity development results in socialization in small groups, with the beginnings of more intimate relationships. Relationships with parents are renegotiated at each stage.

As adolescents start to redefine themselves in relationships to others, they begin to move to a central position where they define other people relative to themselves! This can make it hard to understand the impact of behaviour on others, or to feel concern for how others might be affected by behaviour. There is often a strongly held view that no other person can have a clear understanding of how the young person feels.

As the ability to think in abstractions develops, it interacts with this sense of uniqueness and creates both an awareness of outcomes for others and a belief in personal invulnerability: being 'bulletproof'. This can lead young people to take significant risks, believing that negative outcomes will not apply to them.

The timing of changes and the point at which successful completion is expected varies greatly between cultures. In many Western societies, adolescence commonly extends over many years, with its end-points marked by relative financial independence after the completion of education. In contrast, in some societies, the social rights and responsibilities of adulthood may be conferred at initiation ceremonies or rites.

Family dynamics
Most adolescents are part of a family, the functioning and dynamics of which will have an important impact on their development. In reciprocal fashion, adolescent physical and mental problems will impinge on the family.

The concept of family is evolving, and it is important to be aware of the diversity existing today. In addition to the 'classical' nuclear or extended family, single parent, second marriage, and same-sex parental relationships exist.

Family functioning styles range from rigid, structured, and enmeshed to chaotic, flexible, and disengaged. The two important positive determinants of adolescent socialization in family functioning are a high level of parental involvement and the setting of clear boundaries and controls.

Common stressors on family functioning may include alcoholism, divorce, family restructuring, mental illness, unemployment, and major losses.

19.2 Clinical skills in adolescent medicine

Online resources
New online adolescent health educational materials exist, created by the UK Department of Health and the Royal College of Paediatrics and Child Health. These can be accessed via the following link:

http://www.rcpch.ac.uk/Education/Adolescent-health-project

Communication
Working with adolescents is the only time in clinical practice when health professionals do not deal directly with an adult. Instead, there is the challenge of communicating with a personality undergoing rapid psychological and social changes who may not share an adult's understanding of society nor adult cognitive abilities to decide between treatment alternatives in the light of future health risks.

In addition, complexities arise in relation to adolescents' competence to seek, consent to, or refuse medical treatment, and their rights to confidentiality.

Communication with adolescents requires an understanding of their cognitive and social development level and a non-judgemental understanding of the social contexts of their health behaviours. Remember how thinking styles change from concrete to abstract:

Concrete thinking
'You said I would get ill if I missed my asthma inhalers. But I forgot them for several days and remained fine. Therefore I don't need then any longer'.

Abstract thinking
'I missed my asthma inhalers for a few days and was fine. However, I think that was because I was not doing any exercise and the weather was warm. I think I will need them in the future when I start doing exercise and the weather gets cold'.

Practical tips for effective consultation
- *Assure confidentiality:* both in the individual clinical interaction and the clinic structure
- *Provide a safe environment:* a gender balance amongst staff facilitates emotional 'safety'
- *See adolescents by themselves:* parents should not be excluded, but should be informed that adolescents are also routinely seen by themselves
- *Be empathetic, respectful, and non-judgemental:* particularly when discussing 'exploratory' or 'risk-taking' behaviours
- *Be yourself:* young people want a knowledgeable doctor, not someone trying to be cool or hip
- *Explain concepts in a developmentally appropriate fashion:* for young adolescents use only 'here-and-now' concrete examples and avoid abstract 'if, then' discussions.

History and examination
History
A full psychosocial history is usually the key component in consultations with adolescents and is focused on the most common health issues. The HEADS protocol provides a systematic approach (see Box).

HEADS protocol

- **H** **H**ome life, including relationship with parents
- **E** **E**ducation and
  Employment, including financial issues
- **A** **A**ctivities, including sports, friendships
  Affect, mood and its fluctuations
- **D** **D**rug use, including tobacco and alcohol
- **S** **S**ex, including any risk behaviours
  Suicide, including depression and self-harm

Examination
Basic skills are generally applicable, with the addition of a focus on growth including height and weight and assessment of pubertal stage.

Adolescents require even more than usual attention to privacy and confidentiality and it is appropriate to ask all young people whether or not they wish their parents to be present during physical examination, especially of the genitals. Be sensitive to the possibility that they may have difficulty telling their parents that they do not wish them to be present.

Many, but not all, adolescents prefer to be examined by a same-sex doctor. A chaperone for examination of an adolescent of the opposite sex is mandatory. Tanner stages to assess puberty are shown in Fig 19.1 and signs of substance misuse are considered elsewhere.

Confidentiality
Adolescents consistently rate confidentiality as one of the most important aspects of medical care. It underpins future relationships with professionals and is based on mutual trust. Full confidentiality can and should be assured to young people, but they should be informed of the circumstances in which disclosure is required for the purpose of protecting the adolescent or others from risk or serious harm.

Issues for which confidentiality may be especially important include:
- *Sexual health:*
  - request by an unaccompanied young person for contraception or abortion
  - sexually transmitted infections
- *Substance misuse:* particularly of illicit drugs
- Mental health disorders.

Practical strategies to ensure confidentiality include education of staff about the professional duty of confidentiality and ensuring that adolescents are aware of confidentiality practices and policies, e.g. through displayed posters.

Confidentiality should *not* be kept, and disclosure may be required by law, in the following situations:
- *Significant risk of harm to the adolescent:* sexual abuse, suicidal intent, or significant self-harming behaviour.
- *Significant risk of harm to others:* for example, disclosure of homicidal intent.

In such circumstances attempts should be made to persuade competent adolescents to consent to disclosure and adolescents should be informed of the intention to disclose (if necessary without consent) unless to do so would place them at further risk of harm.

Issues of competence and confidentiality may coexist, particularly in relation to matters of sexual health such as contraception and abortion, and it may be necessary to seek legal advice.

Competence and consent

Ethical and legal principles
All professionals have an ethical duty to act in the best interests of their patients. They are also required to act within the law and there are legal principles underpinning provision of health care in the UK which are defined by statutes such as the Children Act and the UK Human Rights Act and by 'common law' which derives general principles from specific cases.

Competence
Legally, an adolescent's right to make decisions for themselves depends on their 'competence'. Competence refers to their ability to make such decisions which of course depends on their cognitive abilities (understanding and intelligence), rationality, experience, and self awareness.

Competence is context dependent and may fluctuate. Pain, environment, and mental state may all reduce competence, but experience of illness may actually increase it. Assessment of competence must be done in situations that maximize competence.

The legal criteria and age limits for competence differ between countries. In the UK, competence is presumed over the age of 18 years. Between 16 and 18 years adolescents are legally presumed competent to *consent* to treatment (see below), but not necessarily to *refuse* life-saving treatment. Under 16 years, adolescents are legally presumed incompetent unless they show otherwise. In practice it is appropriate to presume competence from age 12 years if the following criteria are satisfied:
- Understanding of nature, purpose and necessity of proposed actions
- Understanding of benefits, risks, alternatives and effects of no action
- Believe the information applies to them
- Retains information long enough to make a choice.

This is sometimes referred to as 'Fraser competence' (see below) and was in the past called 'Gillick competence'.

In law, assessing competence is the doctor's responsibility, though others may assist in the task.

Consent for medical treatment
To be legally valid, consent must be informed and be freely given by a person who is competent to do so. A young person >16 years is legally presumed to be competent to consent to treatment. A minor, <16 years, may be judged (by a doctor) to be competent 'if and when the child achieves sufficient understanding and intelligence to understand fully what is proposed' (Gillick *v.* West Norfolk and Wisbech Area Health Authority, 1985, judgement by Lord Fraser). Consent can therefore be given by the competent minor rather than the parents in these circumstances.

Fraser guidelines
In his judgment on the Gillick case in 1985, Lord Fraser said that a doctor can give contraceptive advice or treatment to a person <16 years without parental consent providing the doctor is satisfied that:
- The young person understands the doctor's advice
- The doctor cannot persuade the young person to inform his or her parents or allow the doctor to inform the parents that he or she is seeking contraceptive advice
- The young person is very likely to begin or continue having sexual intercourse with or without contraceptive treatment
- The young person's physical or mental health or both are likely to deteriorate if he or she does not receive contraceptive advice or treatment
- The young person's best interests require the doctor to give contraceptive advice or treatment, or both, without parent consent.

Refusal of treatment
Adolescents between 16 and 18 years can consent to treatment but cannot necessarily legally refuse life-saving treatment. Obviously, refusal is especially problematic if the proposed treatment will clearly prevent death or significant harm, but if the risks and benefits are more evenly balanced wider consideration of best interests is required and legal intervention may be necessary if an unresolvable dispute arises: Courts have overturned adolescents' refusal of blood transfusion in leukaemia and heart–lung transplantations.

Every effort should be made to understand reasons for refusal and, if possible, to remedy them. Forcing adolescents to have treatments they do not want can produce psychological harm and further lack of cooperation. Overriding an informed, sustained refusal by a competent adolescent is justified only in extreme circumstances. If a minor or elective procedure is refused, it should be postponed to allow further discussion.

19.3 Adolescent health

Epidemiology

Adolescents constitute a significant fraction of the population, have a distinct pattern of health and illness, and have experienced minimal or no improvement in overall health status in the last four decades.

Demographic factors

The WHO classifies young people as those aged 10–24 years, encompassing adolescence (10–19 years) and youth (15–24 years). In the developed world adolescents account for 13–15% of the population. In mid-2000 there were 7.6 million adolescents in the UK, making up 12.7% of the population, approximately equal to the proportion of children.

Patterns of disease

Adolescent mortality has fallen little in comparison to the drop in deaths in young children. Morbidity rates show adverse trends in key priority areas such as mental health (male suicide), sexual health (teenage pregnancy and sexually transmitted infections, STIs), cardiovascular risk (smoking, obesity, type 2 diabetes), and substance abuse.

Mortality

Death rates in 15–19 year olds are now higher than in the 1–4 year age group (Fig 19.2). Gains from conquering infectious diseases have been offset by rising mortality from 'social' causes including injuries (especially road traffic accidents) and suicide.

Road traffic accidents, mainly motor vehicle collisions, account for 27% of deaths in 15–24 year olds, with an excess of these deaths in young men. These injuries are associated with risk factors such as alcohol, depression, and social disruption, rendering transport patterns an important potentially modifiable determinant of adolescent mortality.

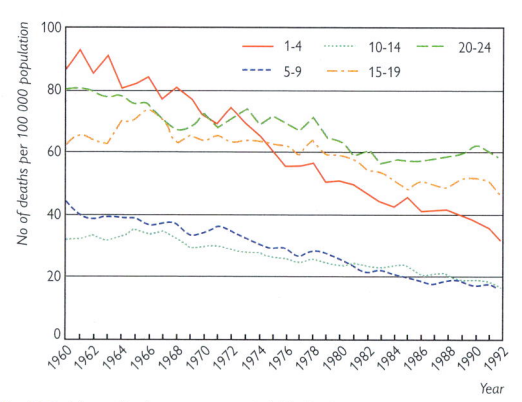

Fig 19.2 Mortality by age group in UK 1960–92.

In the UK the suicide rate for older male teenagers almost doubled between 1970 and 1988 and remained high during the late 1990s, falling slightly in the early 21st century.

Morbidity

Key public health indicators in the adolescent age group have almost uniformly shown adverse or no change in the last two decades. The health areas of particular concern in adolescence include chronic illness, mental health, obesity, sexual and reproductive health, and substance abuse.

Chronic illness

Up to 30% of teenagers have a chronic illness, defined as one that lasts >6 months, and up to 10% report having a chronic condition that limits their daily life or requires extended periods of care.

The burden is increasing for several reasons: over 85% of children with congenital or chronic conditions (e.g. cystic fibrosis, congenital heart disease) are now surviving into adolescence and the prevalence of certain chronic disorders seen in adolescence such as asthma, diabetes and obesity has increased (Table 19.1).

Table 19.1. Prevalence of certain chronic conditions in mid-adolescence (per 1000 adolescents aged 12–18 years).

	Prevalence
Serious mental health problems	~120
Asthma	100
Skin conditions	32
Cerebral palsy	15
Epilepsy	4
Diabetes types 1 and 2	4
Cystic fibrosis	0.1

Mental health

Mental health problems encompass the continuation of childhood-onset problems such as attention deficit hyperactivity disorder and conduct disorder, the emergence of new disorders such as depression and eating disorders, and the early onset of 'adult' disorders such as schizophrenia.

A recent UK survey of 11–15 year olds found serious mental health problems in 13% of boys and 19% of girls.

Obesity

Obesity now overshadows all other chronic illnesses in adolescents. Estimates based on new definitions from the International Obesity Task Forces suggest that almost a quarter of UK 10–15 year olds are overweight and a further 7% are obese. A shift towards eating more calorie-dense foods and taking less exercise (the 'obesogenic environment') is held responsible, and strategies for tackling this major public health problem remain the subject of lively debate.

Sexual and reproductive health

Sexual health becomes a new health priority in early adolescence. 'Risk-taking' behaviours are common when adolescents become sexually active and the adverse consequences of unsafe behaviour of course include unwanted pregnancy and STIs including HIV.

Teenage pregnancy

Rates in the UK are among the highest in western Europe. This is a long-established problem: the rate of under 18 conceptions has been 40/1000 for >30 years (Fig 19.3) with minimal improvement in recent years. Under 16 pregnancies make up a relatively small proportion (20%) of all under 18 conceptions. Poverty is the strongest risk factor for teenage pregnancy, but others include low educational expectations, poor parental supervision, and lack of access to services.

Although teenage pregnancy can be a positive life choice for some young women in specific ethnic or social groups, for most the adverse outcomes are costly. Teenage mothers have poorer antenatal health, and are less likely to finish their education and get a good job. They are more likely to become single parents and live in poverty and their children are at greater risk of poor health.

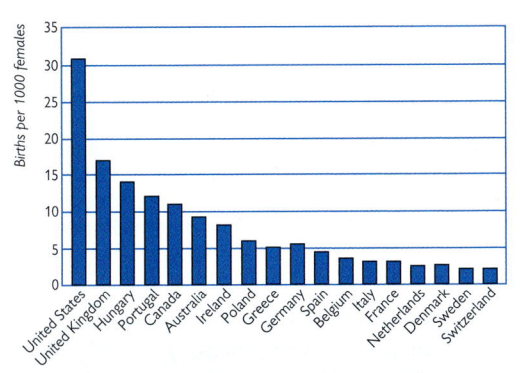

Fig 19.3 Births per 1000 age 15–17, OECD countries, 1998. Courtesy of Trust for the Study of Adolescence.

Sexually transmitted infections
Rates of STIs increased significantly among teenagers in the late 1990s. The overall rate of diagnosis of uncomplicated *Chlamydia* in the 16–19 year old age group almost trebled in males and more than doubled in females in the UK. Gonorrhea and to a lesser extent genital herpes rates have shown similar increases. The highest STI rates are currently found in Black Caribbean and Black African young people, suggesting that cultural and socio-economic factors play a role, including immigration.

Substance misuse: alcohol, tobacco, and other drugs
Alcohol and tobacco are the most commonly used drugs in adolescence and account for 95% of the morbidity and mortality related to substance misuse in this age group. Illicit drugs pose more serious health risks, but are much less commonly used. Regular alcohol drinking rises from 3% of 11 year olds to 40–50% of 15 year olds and 70% of 17 year olds. The proportion of regular smokers rises from 1% of 11 year olds to 26% of girls and 21% of boys aged 15 years in the UK.

Cannabis is the most common drug of misuse in Western countries. In the UK, 30–50% of 16–17 year olds report having tried cannabis and ~10% report weekly use.

Chronic illness in adolescence

The burden of chronic illness in adolescence is increasing as larger numbers of children with chronic diseases survive beyond the age of 10 years and the prevalence of disorders such as diabetes, obesity, and asthma increases.

Chronic illness impacts on adolescence and adolescence impacts on many chronic illnesses and their management.

Impact of disease on adolescence
Chronic illness impacts on many domains of development and has repercussions on the family unit.

Physical development
Short stature and pubertal delay are common sequelae of chronic illness, and conditions that limit physical activity contribute to obesity. Visible signs of disability or treatment may mark young people out as different. These physical effects have emotional consequences if they lead to a negative self-image and reduced self esteem.

Emotional development and mental health
Young people with chronic illness do not have an increased rate of mental illness. They are, however, likely to be unhappier than their healthy peers, and stress from managing their condition may trigger depression, anxiety, and adjustment disorders. This may manifest as behavioural problems or declining school performance.

Social aspects: school, work, and family
Alienation from the peer group and absence from school cause social isolation and may ultimately lead to educational and vocational disadvantage and failure. It is essential to think proactively from an early stage about encouraging the development of independent adult living and vocational skills.

Chronic illness can exacerbate normal parenting issues. Progress towards autonomy may be hindered, prolonging dependence on parents. Parents may experience anxiety, guilt, and frustration and siblings may miss out on parental attention.

Impact of adolescence on disease
These include the physiological effects of puberty and growth on some diseases, and the impact of adolescent behavioural traits on disease and its management.

Physiological effects
Endocrine changes of puberty may destabilize diabetes or epilepsy, and lung function in cystic fibrosis often deteriorates during adolescence, especially in girls.

Behavioural effects
The consequences of adolescent 'exploratory' behaviours may be amplified in those with chronic illness. Smoking worsens health outcomes in asthma and cystic fibrosis; diabetes control is more difficult if alcohol consumption and energetic partying become part of the lifestyle; disrupted sleep may destabilize epilepsy.

Adherence and concordance
Young people are often perceived as 'non-compliant'. However, there is little evidence that they are worse than adults in adhering to medical regimes. Poor adherence is developmentally almost 'appropriate', arising in part from immature abilities to imagine future consequences, allied with the concept of being 'bulletproof'. Medical advice may be rejected as part of a young person's growing independence from parents, and regimes manipulated as part of conflict with parents or other authority figures.

Strategies for improving treatment adherence should be:
- *Educational:* provide information and explanation at an appropriate level
- *Negotiated:* a treatment plan, with short-term goals and perceived immediate benefits wherever possible should be negotiated with the young person ('concordance') ensuring that they see it as achievable and consistent with their routines and priorities
- *Practical:* written instructions should be jargon free
- *Family based:* enlist the support of parents in addition to dealing with the young person independently
- *Reviewed:* regular review is essential.

Maximizing adherence in itself is not the main measure of success. It can be achieved if regimes are tailored to goals which entirely ignore long-term health outcomes.

19.4 Adolescent health promotion

Health promotion includes the science and art of helping people change their lifestyle to move towards a state of optimal health.

In this context lifestyle refers to a range of behaviours which impact on health, and health itself is defined as not merely the absence of disease but an optimal state of physical, emotional, and social well-being.

Adolescent health behaviours

Aspects of adolescent development generate a set of behaviours which, although not unique to this age group, certainly dominate the agenda: a penchant for drugs and unsafe sex is not the major concern in the geriatric population. Cognitive changes during adolescence also influence the responsiveness of this age group to the style and content of health promotion messages.

Challenges

The following features of adolescence provide unique challenges and opportunities in the field of health promotion.

Exploratory behaviour

Young people explore the diversity of adult behaviours open to them, including smoking, drinking, drug use, driving, violence, and sexual activity. Many of these involve health risks and are therefore often designated 'risk-taking' behaviours. Risk may arise from ignorance, exuberance or the tendencies of young people to feel 'invulnerable' or 'bulletproof'.

Concrete thinking

In early adolescence, concrete thinking predominates, with young people able to understand linear concrete relations between cause and effect. For example, a message that smoking causes lung cancer may have low impact as they perceive that friends who smoke do not have lung cancer.

Clustering of behaviours

Behaviours conferring a risk to health tend to cluster in adolescence. For example, those who smoke are also more likely to drink alcohol, take drugs, engage in unsafe sex, and be the victims or perpetrators of violence. This arises in part because many of these problems have risk factors in common, many of which reflect the socio-economic circumstances in which young people are raised.

Adverse trends

Adolescent mortality and morbidity show worrying trends in several priority areas such as mental health, sexual health, and cardiovascular risk.

Opportunities

A focus on health promotion in young people could have important benefits, for several reasons.

Adolescent behaviours track into adult life

This is a time when new health behaviours are laid down which often continue into adulthood and influence health and morbidity throughout life. Evidence challenges earlier hopes that young people 'grow out of' health risk behaviours and mental health problems. The opportunity exists to disrupt the initiation of health risk behaviours or to prevent their long-term persistence. Good habits in relation to exercise and nutrition are laid down at this time: adolescent obesity predicts adult obesity, which is strongly predictive of cardiovascular risk. Unhealthy sexual behaviours begun in adolescence can persist for many decades.

Resilience

This term is used for a variety of concepts, but probably best describes the process of resistance to adopting risky behaviour. Adolescents have the capacity to exhibit resilience and this can be promoted by encouraging assets within the individual (competence, coping skills, self-efficacy) and providing external resources that help youth overcome risk, such as adult mentoring or community organizations.

Health promotion areas

The major areas in which health promotion for adolescents is important include:
- Health risk behaviours: substance misuse (tobacco, alcohol, drugs), sexual health
- Mental health
- Vaccination, e.g. HPV vaccination
- Violence
- Nutrition and exercise
- Parent-adolescent communication
- Health inequalities and social exclusion.

Strategies for health promotion

Principles

General principles worth adopting include the following:
- Health promotion messages should begin in early adolescence and use concrete motivators with a focus on 'here and now'
- Strategies should be on behalf of adolescents as well as directed at adolescents
- Interventions should focus on increasing adolescents' overall self-esteem and self empowerment
- The most relevant and up to date evidence based information should be provided using methods and language deemed appropriate by the adolescents themselves
- Using 'stages of change' model. This model of behaviour change envisages stages from pre-contemplation to contemplation, preparation, action, and maintenance. Action-orientated advice for those who are not ready to change may be unhelpful and even entrench unhealthy behaviour.

Levels of health promotion

Health promotion strategies may be implemented at several different levels.

Individual level

Peer interventions, youth recreation programmes, mentoring programmes. Individual approaches by health professionals exhorting adolescents to behave in healthy ways, don't smoke, use contraception, etc., are relatively ineffective. However, brief health promotion discussions during routine clinical interactions with young people are encouraged.

Community level
- *Local*: environmental changes such as policing policy for violence prevention

- *Schools:* the school is a vital environment for health promotion for such risk behaviours as substance misuse, unplanned pregnancy, abnormal eating patterns, and bullying
- *Family:* Parent training and family intervention.

Public policy level

Health promotion by society as a whole on behalf of adolescents. This might include creation of greater socio-economic equality, social marketing, banning cigarette advertising, or reorganization of services, e.g. making emergency contraception available over the counter.

Examples of health promotion

Teenage pregnancy

In 1999 the UK government's Social Exclusion Unit published a Teenage Pregnancy Report which identified factors contributing to the high rate of conception in girls <18, including ignorance about contraception and the tasks of parenthood.

A Teenage Pregnancy Strategy was implemented at local and national level aiming to cut pregnancy rates among 15–17 year olds by 15% (2004) and 50% by 2010. Some overall progress has been made, with local success achieved in areas in which there was active engagement of all mainstream partners, a well-publicized contraception and sexual health advice service centred on young people, and a strong focus on targeted interventions with high-risk groups.

Evidence indicates that inconsistent use of contraception combined with earlier and increased sexual activity contribute to slow progress. Some argue that enhancing young people's negotiation skills to resist pressure and enable them to postpone sexual debut would help.

In Uganda, a government-led **ABC** campaign (**A**bstinence, **B**e faithful, and if not use a **C**ondom) was effective.

Obesity

Obesity represents a prime example of a condition in which contributory factors are easy to identify and health promotion should have an important role. Yet motivating people to eat a healthier diet and adopt a more active lifestyle is not easy. The television, games console, and car cannot be uninvented, and strong commercial pressures combined with natural appetite drive the consumption of calorie-dense foods high in sugar, fat, and salt.

To screen or not?

Obesity fulfils most of the criteria for a condition that justifies screening, except for the fact that no effective intervention has yet been identified. A recent government initiative to weigh and measure all primary school-children at age 6 and 11 years and provide routine feedback to parents about BMI values has generated controversy over whether this is justifiable screening.

Health promotion strategies for obesity include:

Individual level

- *Physical activity:* walk or cycle to school, encourage active play and an active lifestyle in the whole family, use stairs rather than lifts, decrease TV viewing and sedentary behaviours
- *Dietary suggestions:* a balanced, varied diet for the whole family, regular meals (avoid snacking and grazing), smaller portions, low-calorie drinks and less energy-dense food; grill, boil or bake food rather than frying.

Community level

- *Physical activity:* increased access to sport and recreation facilities within schools and communities, more choice in the style of activities offered (not all children like competitive sports)
- *Diet:* food education and cooking skills as part of the school curriculum.

Public policy level

- *Physical activity:* 'exercise on prescription', reduced-cost access to local authority sports centres, protection of school playing fields from sale, improving safety for play, sport, and cycling or walking to school
- *Diet:* nutritional standards for school food, subsidized fruit and vegetables, ban on advertising unhealthy foodstuffs, endorsements of healthy products by celebrities, mandatory clear and accurate labelling of all foods (e.g. the 'traffic light' system), food pricing and packaging policies that favour healthy rather than unhealthy foods
- *Research:* research to increase evidence base for effectiveness of interventions.

Teenage Health Freak website

This website (www.teenagehealthfreak.org) promotes health in a user-friendly way to teenagers.

Transitional care

Ensuring that young people transfer seamlessly from paediatric to adult services is now a central part of chronic illness management. It entails a significant change from family-centred paediatrics, which frequently infantilizes the adolescent, to an adult medical culture which acknowledges patient autonomy and addresses reproduction and employment issues, but also may neglect growth, development, and family concerns. It also entails the loss of well-known and valued paediatric caregivers and the necessity of trusting new and unknown adult carers. It requires more than a simple referral letter.

This transition period is particularly dangerous in those diseases for which adult services or skills are poorly developed, such as metabolic diseases or congenital heart disease. It is important for all paediatric specialist clinics to have transition guidelines, and those where larger numbers of adolescents are transferring should develop an active transition programme with the receiving adult service. Preparation for transition should begin in early adolescence, and the move depends on more than just chronological age.

19.5 Depression, suicide, and self harm

Adolescent mental health

Mental health problems in adolescence have increased, driven in part by social changes such as disruption of family structures and growing unemployment. It can be difficult to distinguish normal behaviours from more serious mental disorders. The latter are persistent and have greater impact. Common mental health problems include depression, self harm and suicide, somatic symptoms, and fatigue. Attention-deficit/hyperactivity disorder, the autistic spectrum disorders, conduct disorders, anxiety disorders, depression, somatization and the psychoses are considered in Chapter 17. Eating disorders and substance misuse are considered elsewhere.

Epidemiological studies suggest that the prevalence of severe depression in adolescents is as high as 10%, rendering the recognition and treatment of depression and related self-harming behaviour, including suicide, the highest priority in adolescent mental health.

Depression

This is considered in more detail in Chapter 17. Risk factors include a family history of depression, bereavement, physical and sexual abuse, and trauma or severe stress.

Signs and symptoms are similar to those in adults and must persist for at least 2 weeks before major depression is diagnosed. These include sad mood, loss of energy and interest in activities once enjoyed, difficulty concentrating, sleep disturbance, recurrent thoughts of death or suicide.

Masked presentations such as behavioural problems, school failure, and occasional school phobia and somatic symptoms are common in early adolescence, particularly in boys. Potential suicide risk should be assessed.

Suicide

Rates are higher in males than females (Fig 19.4) and suicide is very rare <15 years. Risk factors include broken homes and substance misuse. A psychiatric disorder, usually depression, is present at the time of death in most. There is a strong association with previous self harm, which is reported in up to half of those committing suicide.

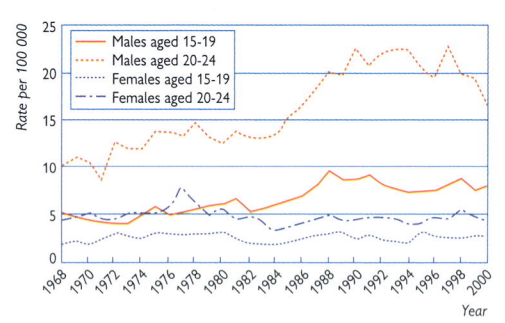

Fig 19.4 Suicide and undetermined deaths in England and Wales in 15–19 year olds and 20–24 year olds between 1968 and 2000. data source: Office for National Statistics, 2003.

Self-harm

Definitions

Self-harm is defined as self-poisoning or injury irrespective of the purpose of the act. Obviously in young children this encompasses accidental self-poisoning, but from age 11 years upwards any self-harm is commonly to some extent intentional.

The term 'deliberate' is best avoided as it implies an intention which may be absent, and the older term 'parasuicide' implied a component of suicidal intent which is not usually present.

The most common forms of self-harm are self-poisoning and self-cutting.

Epidemiology

This is one of the most common adolescent problems presenting to general paediatricians responsible for acute admissions from hospital emergency departments. In a community study of mental health, 6.5% of girls and 5% of boys in the age range 11–15 years reported trying to harm themselves. Self-harm becomes more common with increasing age up to 17 years and girls outnumber boys, especially amongst younger adolescents. The repetition rate in the first year is up to 10%. The risk of completed suicide is uncertain, but may be as high as 4% in older male teenagers.

Aetiology

Risk factors are similar to those for suicide, and there is increasing recognition of the importance of depression in non-fatal self-harm by adolescents.

The reported motivation often arises from a desire to:
- Escape from troubling situations
- Express distress to others
- Change the behaviour of others
- Make others feel guilty
- Seek help or gain inner relief.

Common preceding problems or trigger factors include:
- Disputes with parents, peers, siblings, boyfriends, or girlfriends
- School problems, including bullying
- Abuse
- Physical ill health
- Depression or low self-esteem
- Awareness of self-harm by others.

Clinical assessment

Most acts of self-harm in adolescents inflict trivial injury (e.g. self-cutting) and do not come to the attention of medical services. Self-poisoning makes up 90% of cases referred to hospital and usually involves readily available over-the-counter substances such as paracetamol.

Approach

Self-harming patients need respect, understanding, and attention to the feelings that have led to the self-harm. The temptation to regard young people who harm themselves as wasting professional time and as a nuisance should be resisted. It is helpful to accept self-harm as a response to emotional pain and a way of dealing with distress, rather than 'attention seeking' or 'manipulative' behaviour.

History

This should include:

- *Events surrounding the self-harm:* a factual account of what happened:
  - details of any overdose
  - any attempt to avoid detection?
  - impulsive or pre-meditated?
- *Predisposing factors:* family discord, abuse, previous history of self-harm, or psychiatric disorder. The current family situation should be explored in detail such as who is at home, who is the main confidant, is there a lot of conflict?
- *Precipitating factors:* row with a boyfriend, bullying, loss of a beloved relative or animal, interpersonal crisis, awareness of self-harm by others, house move, an assault
- *Perpetuating factors:* poor family communication, hopelessness
- *Protective factors:* friend or family confidant, resilient personality.

Assessment of suicidal intent and risk of suicide

This can be difficult to establish, as a denial of intent may be unreliable and the physical severity of the harm done is not a reliable indicator of suicidal intent. Toxicity of injected or ingested substances may be underestimated. Asking about suicide does not make it more likely to occur. Useful questions include:

- Did you plan this, or was it an impulse?
- Did you expect that this might kill you?
- What was in your mind when you did it?
- Did you try to avoid being found out?
- Did you tell anyone or leave a note?
- Who would have minded most if you had died?

Features suggesting high suicidal intent include a premeditated rather than impulsive act, conducted in isolation with precautions to avoid discovery, and preparations anticipating death such as a suicide note or message.

In addition, the PATHOS questionnaire for overdoses, scored out of five, can help to estimate risk (see Box).

> **PATHOS questionnaire**
> - **P**roblems for >1 month?
> - **A**lone in the house when overdose occurred?
> - **T**hree hours or more spent planning the overdose?
> - **H**opeless feelings about the future?
> - **S**ad feelings for most of the time before the overdose?

Risk of further self-harm

Factors associated with repeated self harm include depression, alcohol or drug misuse, abuse, disturbed family relationships, and social isolation.

It may also be necessary to talk to the carers, usually the parents. Discuss with the patient what they may want to be shared and whether they wants to be present when you see their parents. See section 19.2 for guidance on confidentiality.

Examination

Physical examination is directed initially towards any medical consequences of the self-harming behaviour. Observation will provide information about mood and self-esteem, relationship with parents and staff, capacity to express feelings.

Management

The majority have self-harmed without suicidal intent and in response to an interpersonal crisis, and can be discharged to outpatient treatment. Inpatient treatment is required for the minority with a severe depressive or psychotic disorder and an ongoing risk of suicide, or those with a major psychosocial crisis.

Treatment options for the former category include problem-solving therapy which can be extended to involve the whole family or done in groups. Problem-solving techniques can be taught, coping strategies rehearsed, and an attempt made to improve cognitive and social skills. Liaison with the school may be important, for example if bullying is a factor, and an emergency contact option in anticipation of future crises.

Self-cutting

Self-cutting may be quite minor or a cause for serious concern.

- Minor superficial cutting in association with transient mood change and no history to suggest an eating disorder or past abuse has a benign prognosis.
- Deep cuts and scars with persistent depression and anxiety in the context of a history of abuse and overdosing or eating disorders is of serious concern.

The important principle of initial management is to give attention to the feelings underlying the cutting behaviour and the least possible attention to the cuts themselves.

19.6 Somatic symptoms and fatigue

Fatigue and recurrent headache, backache, or abdominal pain are common symptoms in adolescence and rarely have an identifiable organic basis. The latter are often grouped together as 'somatic symptoms' and may occur with or without fatigue.

The two presentations are considered separately here, but there is substantial overlap especially in the approach to management. In most cases, the symptoms are believed to reflect an imbalance between the increased educational, social, and physical demands on young people and the physiological demands of puberty and growth.

Somatic symptoms

In surveys ~1/10 teenagers report daily headaches or backache (Fig 19.5), and most of these symptoms do not trigger medical consultation. Abdominal pain is more common in younger adolescents. Features suggesting a more significant somatiform disorder include multiplicity (e.g. headaches, muscle aches, and fatigue), chronicity with duration >3 months, increasing school absence, social isolation, and a history of recent psychological stress at home (e.g. divorce) or school (e.g. bullying).

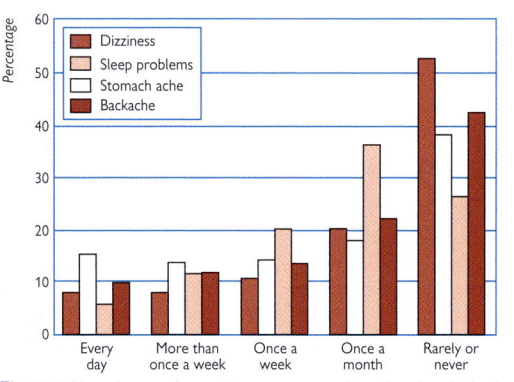

Fig 19.5 Prevalence of somatic symptoms other than headache in the previous 6 months in 11–17 year olds in Europe. Adapted from WHO, *Health behaviour in school-age children*, 1997–1998. Calverton, MD: macro International, 2002.

Clinical assessment

It is important to take an adequate history, including social, school, and family issues and consider the extent to which bullying, depression, or family conflict may be precipitating or maintaining factors.

A careful physical examination is as important as investigation in excluding an organic basis. Pressures for extensive, prolonged investigations are best resisted as a endless searching for an organic 'answer' can delay and interfere with rehabilitation.

Briefly assessing the young person's mood is also important. Significant concerns should be raised where symptoms are associated with depressed mood (e.g. flat or constrained affect, being tearful and feeling hopeless, loss of interest in friends and school) or with significant loss of quality of life or with failure to attend school.

Headaches

Headaches are the most common chronic symptoms in adolescence after fatigue. Features favouring an organic cause include an abrupt onset or recent change in severity, morning headaches, or headaches that wake the patient from sleep.

Examination must include inspection of the fundi and measurement of blood pressure. Trivial organic causes include sinusitis, refractive errors and excess caffeine consumption. Ordering a brain scan without examining the patient carefully is bad practice. Tension type headaches are more common than migraine, which only affects ~2% of adolescents. See Chapter 7.10.

Abdominal pain

Recurrent abdominal pain in adolescents is most likely to be functional. Features suggesting an organic cause include weight loss and alterations in bowel habit. In girls it is important to consider gynaecological causes. See Chapter 5.8.

For the organic differential diagnosis, see Box.

Abdominal pain: differential diagnosis
Common causes
• Constipation
• Recurrent UTIs
• Non-ulcer dyspepsia/*Helicobacter pylori* infection
• Dysmenorrhea
Uncommon causes
• Peptic ulcer disease
• Irritable bowel syndrome
• Pelvic inflammatory disease
• 'Mittelschmerz'
Rare causes
• Inflammatory bowel disease
• Renal or biliary calculi
• Ovarian cyst

Management of somatic symptoms

After excluding common organic pathology, a useful common approach to somatic symptoms is to be guided by the impact of the symptom on school, family, and social life as well as the degree of distress it causes. Labelling symptoms as psychological often alienates the family. The reality of the symptoms, despite lack of identifiable cause, should be acknowledged and simplistic 'mind–body' splits avoided.

A pragmatic, two-pronged rehabilitative approach is most useful based on improving function while controlling symptoms. Prospects of success are enhanced if this includes:

- Engagement of the patient and family
- Ownership of the management programme by the young person
- *Multidisciplinary approach:* physical (physiotherapist, occupational therapist), psychologist (family therapy, cognitive behavioural therapy), and social (return to school programme or home tuition) elements are all useful
- Goal setting and frequent reviews.

Fatigue

In normal usage, fatigue is defined as a subjective state in which there is a temporary loss of strength and energy, and a feeling of exhaustion, resulting from hard physical or mental work. In this sense it is synonymous with tiredness or weariness, but should be distinguished from drowsiness which is a manifestation of the need to sleep. Acute fatigue is a normal response to exertion and is relieved by rest. There in no commonly accepted definition of fatigue in the context of health and illness.

Fatigue is almost a 'normal' part of adolescence. However, the difficulty most adolescents have in waking early is not a manifestation of fatigue: a survey of chronotypes in 25 000 people showed that children are natural early risers but sleep later as they enter adolescence. Maximum lateness occurs at around 20 years and the trend then reverses.

Acute fatigue syndromes

Acute fatigue syndromes associated with viral illness are very common among teenagers, with ~10–20% of adolescents suffering a major acute fatigue syndrome after certain viral infections such as Epstein–Barr virus (mononucleosis or glandular fever). Epstein–Barr virus infection is predominantly an illness of teenagers. Few reach their third decade without seroconversion and about 10% are estimated to develop severe acute fatigue syndrome after infection.

Chronic fatigue syndrome (CFS)

The definition of CFS, sometime known as myalgic encephalomyelitis (ME), has been much debated. There is no doubt, however, that it occurs in children and adolescents albeit less commonly than in adults. The UK prevalence is estimated at 50–100/100 000 with a preponderance of girls. Most cases are mild or moderate.

The cause of CFS is unknown, but theories abound. It is likely that CFS is caused by a combination of physical and psychological factors including genetic susceptibility, viral infections, and traumatic events such as bereavement.

Clinical features and diagnosis

There are no widely accepted diagnostic criteria for CFS in children and young people. Criteria similar to those used in adults can be applied but diagnosis should be considered after a shorter symptom duration of 3 rather than 6 months. Characteristic features include:

Debilitating fatigue

This is the hallmark symptom. Fatigue is both physical and mental and not merely secondary to exercise or activity. Activity is often reduced to <50% of premorbid levels.

Additional symptoms

These may be:
- **Common:** malaise, sleep disturbances, poor memory and concentration, recurrent or persistent pain, sore throat, myalgia, arthralgia, headaches, abdominal pain, tender or swollen lymph nodes
- **Infrequent:** dizziness, photophobia, hyperacusis, feeling hot and cold, diarrhoea.

Onset may be sudden or gradual, and some patients report a preceding acute illness. Psychiatric co-morbidities may present such as depression in ~30% of young people.

History and examination

The severity, onset, and course of all symptoms should be established and family dynamics explored if there appear to be potential emotional dimensions to the illness.

A complete physical examination is required to identify other underlying illnesses. Examination may reveal anaemia, muscle wasting, lymphadenopathy or organomegaly, chronic sinusitis, postural hypotension, or hypothyroidism.

The differential diagnosis includes a number of conditions which may not be evident clinically and a set of 'routine' investigations is advisable (Table 19.2).

Table 19.2. Investigations in suspected CFS	
Full blood count	Anaemia (iron deficiency, leukaemia)
ESR, CRP	Autoimmune disease (SLE, IBD) Chronic infection (TB)
Urea and electrolytes	Renal failure Hypocalcaemia
Thyroid function tests	Hypothyroidism
Liver function tests	Hepatitis
Creatine kinase	Myopathy
Urine dipstick	Nephritis, diabetes, UTIs

Management

There is no cure, no single approach suitable for all patients and a limited evidence base for most proposed interventions. The paediatrician should establish an empathetic rapport with the patient and family and implement a comprehensive management plan based on a multidisciplinary team approach. The plan should include:

Activity management advice

An activity diary allows a 'baseline' level of activity to be established and a plan for gradual, graded increase in exercise and activity made which the patient feels is achievable. The idea is that inactivity itself, with physical deconditioning, can maintain the illness. Pacing is a strategy designed to avoid a vicious cycle of overactivity and setbacks.

Advice and symptomatic treatment

This may include advice on diet, sleep, pain, and mood. Behavioural and cognitive interventions may promote a better sleep regime. If simple analgesics are ineffective, a psychologist may help with perception and management of pain. If mood or emotional disorders such as depression coexist, referral for psychiatric advice and specific treatment is indicated.

There is no evidence to support recommendation of the use of immunoglobulins, magnesium injections, essential fatty acids, high-dose vitamin supplements, interferon, steroids, anticholinergic drugs, staphylococcus toxoid, or anti-viral therapies.

The prognosis is probably better in young people than in adults. Evidence is limited, but studies with an extended follow up show recovery in >80% with an average illness duration of 2–3 years. A minority remain incapacitated by persistent debilitating illness.

Florence Nightingale (1820–1910), a founder of the nursing profession, may have had a form of CFS in later life.

19.7 Eating disorders and obesity

Adolescence is characterized by significant gains in body weight of up to 15 kg. Disorders related to eating habits, nutrition and exercise are common in adolescence and range from anorexia nervosa to obesity.

Table 19.3. Prevalence of eating behaviour problems in the UK

Eating behaviour	Prevalence (%)	Sex ratio (F:M)
Dieting	35	1.5 : 1
Anorexia nervosa	0.4	9 : 1
Bulimia nervosa	1.0	30 : 1
Obesity	7–10	1.3 : 1

Eating disorders

Dieting is common in adolescents. About 40% of girls and 23% of boys begin to diet for a variety of reasons, and 6–12% of adolescents choose to become vegetarian. Abnormal eating behaviours include extremely selective (faddy) eating and food phobias.

The eating disorders anorexia nervosa (AN) and bulimia nervosa are characterized by a morbid preoccupation with body weight and shape and manifested by distorted or chaotic eating behaviour. They occur in all ethnic groups and 90% of cases are female.

Anorexia nervosa (AN)

Surveys suggest that up to 1% of females aged 15–25 years may have AN. It is very uncommon in prepubertal girls. About 25% of cases occur in boys. There is no single cause for anorexia, but a number of biological, psychological, and social factors contribute:

- *Biological factors:* genetic factors contribute 50% to the variance for development of an eating disorder, and AN shares a genetic risk with depression. Genes can influence eating regulation, and personality.
- *Psychological factors:* there is a tendency for those who develop AN to have certain personality traits including obsessionality and perfectionism. Co-morbid disorders include anxiety and depression, and obsessive compulsive disorder. Low self-esteem is common.
- *Social factors:* The promotion of thinness as the ideal female form by the media in Western industrialized nations is believed to contribute. Eating disorders are rare in societies that do not equate thinness with sexual attractiveness, and more common in those with jobs in which body image or shape is important (dancers, models). Families of young people with anorexia tend to be high-achieving with high expectations and excessive parental control. Trigger factors can include divorce or separation, sexual or physical abuse, bereavement, bullying, sport, or the stress of exams.

Diagnosis

This can be difficult as the patient may deny that they are ill and rarely seeks help, concern being raised by a family member (see Box). The diagnosis should be considered in any adolescent with severely abnormal eating attitudes, rapid weight loss, or a failure to attain or maintain a healthy weight for age, but formal criteria include:

- Refusal to maintain body mass at or above 85% of expected minimum for age, i.e. a body mass index (BMI) lower than the 2nd centile. A BMI of <17.5 is almost diagnostic of AN in adults.
- Low weight self-induced by avoidance of 'fattening foods' and one or more of: vomiting, purging, exercise, appetite suppressants, or diuretics.
- Intense fear of gaining weight or becoming fat.
- Abnormal influence of body shape or weight on self evaluation with denial that body weight is abnormally low and denial that low body weight is unhealthy.
- Endocrine disturbance.
- Delay or arrest of puberty or amenorrhoea in postmenarcheal females.

Key questions (how much would you like to weigh? how do you feel about your weight? are you or anyone else worried about your eating or exercising?) asked in a non-judgemental way can help in deciding about further assessment. Anger or distress at these questions, or a secretive or evasive response, should heighten concern.

Physical signs emerge as the disorder progresses. These may include loss of scalp hair with lanugo on face and body, cold hands with mottled peripheries, hypothermia, hypotension, and bradycardia.

Warning signs of anorexia nervosa
- Deliberate self-starvation with weight loss
- Denial of hunger and refusal to eat
- Fear of gaining weight
- Constant exercising
- Sensitivity to cold
- Absent or irregular periods

Management and prognosis

Assessment and management requires a multidisciplinary approach, tackling medical, nutritional, and psychological aspects of care. Early intervention and family involvement is essential. Outpatient care is usually possible in mild or moderate cases and may include psychotherapy strategies such as cognitive behavioural therapy (CBT).

Criteria for considering hospitalization include very rapid or severe weight loss, a high suicide risk, or signs of significant physical compromise: severe dehydration, bradycardia (resting HR ≤45/min) or hypotension (diastolic BP ≤40 mmHg). If there is an immediate threat to life, admission to hospital may be arranged against the patient's wishes under the Mental Health Act or Children Act.

Anorexia has the highest mortality rate of any psychiatric disorder, with up to 10% dying due to related causes. Approximately 20% may remain chronically anorexic.

Bulimia nervosa

Episodes of binge eating alternate with starvation, self-induced vomiting, or purgative abuse. There is a morbid dread of fatness and there may be a previous history of AN. Weight may be normal. There is an association with depression, self-harm, and substance abuse. Up to 60% respond to treatment.

Obesity

Epidemiology
Rates of overweight and obesity have increased substantially among children and adolescents in almost all developed countries over the last two decades (see section 19.3).

In the UK, an estimated 7–8% of adolescents of both sexes are seriously obese and a further 15% seriously overweight (see below for definitions). If trends continue at least one third of adults, one fifth of boys, and one third of girls will be obese by 2020. Most obesity is primary in origin due to long-term imbalance between nutritional intake and energy expenditure.

Health risks
Being overweight restricts body activity, damages health, and shortens life. It also harms self-esteem and social life. Obesity in adolescence is of concern because it is associated with current and future health problems (see Table 19.4).

Table 19.4. Health risks associated with obesity	
Current	Type 2 diabetes mellitus
	Insulin resistance (metabolic) syndrome
	Polycystic ovarian syndrome
	Non-alcoholic steatohepatitis
	Asthma, sleep apnoea
	Low self-esteem, depression
Future	Excess mortality:
	cardiovascular risk
	(hypertension, hyperlipidaemia)
	type 2 diabetes mellitus
	cancer
	Social and economic disadvantages

Assessment: definitions of overweight and obesity
Obesity is an increased body weight caused by excessive accumulation of fat. The BMI (weight/height^2) is widely used in adults, with cut-off points of 25 and 30 kg/m^2 for overweight and obesity. BMI in childhood changes with age but centiles have been created which pass through these points at 18 years and provide corresponding points from 2–18 years (Fig 19.6).

Clinical assessment
The history should establish the 'obesity trajectory' and the family risk profile. The birthweight, early feeding history, and age and rate of onset of obesity should be established to identify periods of rapid weight gain or loss. A family history of obesity and related problems such as diabetes and cardiovascular disease should be sought. Physical activity levels, diet, and eating patterns should be documented.

In addition to documenting BMI and waist circumference, physical examination is directed towards identifying rare secondary cases of obesity and the presence or absence of complications. Dysmorphic features, short stature, precocious or late puberty, or learning disability should trigger concern.

Identified monogenic syndromes and secondary causes of obesity are rare and account for <1% of community adolescent obesity. They include endocrine disorders such as hypothyroidism, Cushing disease, growth hormone deficiency, and genetic syndromes (Prader–Willi, Bardet–Biedl).

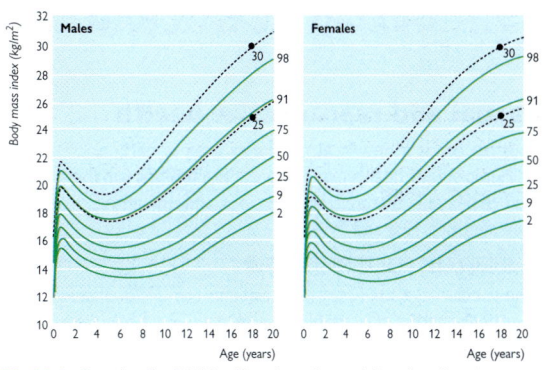

Fig 19.6 Centiles for BMI for British males and females showing extra-centile curves giving cut-off points for overweight and obesity corresponding to adult values of 25 and 30 kg/m^2. Cole TJ et al. *BMJ* 2007;320, 1240. Adapted by permission from BMJ.

Minimal investigations are indicated if high risk is established and include basic biochemistry, fasting insulin, glucose and lipid levels, and thyroid function tests.

Management
Prevention is ideal, using both macroeconomic and local interventions designed to promote healthy eating and increased physical activity (see section 19.4).

Management of the individual patient depends on the degree of overweight and corresponding level of risk, and the age and the level of commitment to change of the young person and their family. Risks in the psychological domains include emotional overeating, parental psychological health, and, rarely, child protection concerns.

A multidisciplinary plan involving the family should be implemented, designed to promote exercise and change eating habits. The aim in adolescents who are still growing is to maintain weight static as height increases. Rapid weight loss from strict dieting is difficult to achieve and overambitious targets can undermine motivation. If adolescents have stopped growing, a weight loss of ~0.5 kg/week is a reasonable target but ideally treatment should be initiated before the end of the pubertal growth spurt. The team may include family physician, practice nurse, health visitor, school nurse, dietitian, clinical psychologist, and paediatrician.

Advice and information offered should include:
- *Physical activity:* walk or cycle to school, take up active play and activities, reduce sedentary activities
- *Diet:* regular meal times, avoid grazing and snacks, grill, boil or bake food rather than fry, low-calorie drinks (preferably water), five portions of fruit and vegetables per day, reduce intake of sweets, crisps, biscuits, cakes.

Realistic goals should be negotiated and regular monitoring planned. If there are major psycho-social issues, counselling or specialist services can assist in the development of coping strategies. Keep a positive attitude and aim for small incremental changes towards a sustainable healthy lifestyle. No drugs for the treatment of obesity in childhood are currently licensed in the UK. Treatment with metformin for insulin resistance may be used in specialist centres.

19.8 Sexual health and substance misuse

Sexual and reproductive health

This becomes a new health priority area in early adolescence with important health promotion opportunities for the prevention of sexually transmitted infections and unwanted pregnancy (see sections 19.3 and 19.4.)

Adolescent sexual behaviour

The median age for first intercourse in the UK dropped during the 1990s and is now stable at ~16 years for both sexes. Early sexual debut is associated with unsafe sex through ignorance, lack of access to contraception, and the frequency with which it is likely to accompany the use of intoxicants such as alcohol which may diminish rationality and negotiating skills.

Sexually transmitted infections (STIs)

As described in section 19.3, there has been a significant rise in STI rates in the over-16 age group in the UK creating a major public health concern. Risk factors for STIs in adolescence include:

- Unsafe sex
- Multiple partners: sequential or concurrent
- Mental health problems
- Substance misuse
- Physiological immaturity (*Chlamydia* infects the immature cervix more easily).

Clinical presentations of STIs in adolescents are similar to those in adults. It is important to note that *Chlamydia*, commonly asymptomatic in older adolescent girls and women, usually presents with a symptomatic vaginal discharge in young adolescent girls. Gonorrhoea is asymptomatic in up to 80% of females, although again girls aged <13 years usually have vaginal discharge. In males, urethritis and discharge are common.

Early detection and treatment of curable STIs can stop further complications, including infertility and ectopic pregnancy. With highly sensitive new nucleic acid amplification tests on voided urine widely available, all sexually active adolescent females attending primary care and genitourinary medicine and family planning clinics should be screened, regardless of symptoms.

Teenage pregnancy: contraception

As described above, the United Kingdom has the highest rate of teenage pregnancy in western Europe and prevention of unwanted teenage pregnancy is a major focus of health promotion in adolescence. Risk factors are well established and include poverty, low educational achievement, being 'in care', being the child of a teenage mother, and mental health problems. Protective factors which reduce risk include:

- Higher levels of connectedness with school and family
- Postponement of sexual activity
- Stable relationship with a partner
- Strong religious beliefs
- Access to: adequate sex education and information, sexual health services that are 'adolescent friendly', training in assertiveness and decision-making skills.

Contraception

Clearly, the effective use of contraception can prevent unwanted pregnancy and barrier methods provide additional protection against STIs. Teenagers are relatively poor users of both barrier and hormonal contraceptives, and condoms remain the contraceptive of choice of young people; >75% reported that they used condoms at their last intercourse, with 15% using the oral contraceptive, 1% injectable contraception, and 6% emergency contraception.

The most appropriate contraceptives for most young people are generally condoms and the contraceptive pill. However, adolescents have a relatively high failure rate with both these methods because of condom failure and irregular pill use. Because of this, many countries promote the 'double Dutch' method for adolescents: using condoms plus oral contraception to protect against both pregnancy and STIs.

Emergency contraception is not a substitute for regular contraception and does not protect against STIs. Access to emergency contraception, however, is an important and effective preventive measure against an unwanted pregnancy. In the UK, knowledge of emergency contraception is low among young people. For example, less than half know about the 72 h 'window of opportunity.' Young women aged 16 and over can obtain emergency contraception over the counter at pharmacies. However, for girls <16, such contraception is available only on prescription either from doctors or, in exceptional circumstances, from approved pharmacists.

Measures that promote contraception which can be deployed in primary care include:

- Provision of condoms without counselling or appointments
- Provision of health promotion information which is accessible, includes information about emerging contraception and legal rights
- Advice to use 'double Dutch' method: condoms plus oral contraception.

The UK Department of Health has best practice guidelines on the provision of advice and treatment to young people under 16 on contraception and sexual and reproductive health.

Substance misuse

Misuse of alcohol, tobacco, and other drugs (ATOD) is a major international health problem amongst adolescents. Alcohol and tobacco account for 95% of morbidity and mortality in this age group. Although other drugs (cannabis, inhalants, opiates) may pose more serious immediate health risks, their use is less common (see section 19.3).

Risk and protective factors

These include individual personality traits and social environment factors, and frequently cluster within an individual. Risk factors include:

- *Intrinsic factors:* there is probably a genetic predisposition towards sensation-seeking behaviour and dependence on mood-altering substances. Antisocial behaviour, ADHD, conduct disorder, and depression are all associated with ATOD misuse.
- *Environmental factors:* family attitudes and parental modelling of substance misuse are important. Poor social connections combined with peer use of substances are strong predictors of substance misuse.

Misuse and dependence

Substance misuse (the term abuse is judged too judgemental by some) is defined as a maladaptive pattern of use leading to

clinically significant impairment or distress as manifested by one or more of the following over a 12 month period:
- *Physical ill health:* hepatic dysfunction, bronchitis
- *Mental ill health:* depression, cognitive impairment
- *Adverse social effects:* failure to fulfil role at home, school or work, irresponsible behaviour (e.g. drunk driving), substance related legal problems.

Criteria for dependence include the above with the addition of evidence for development of tolerance and withdrawal symptoms. Typically there is a strong desire to take the drug, impaired control over its use, persistent use despite harmful effects, and a higher priority given to drug access and use than to other activities and obligations.

Not all young people who use substances in the ATOD group proceed to levels that bring health problems. They may even be beneficial for recreational purposes or self-medication, The 'gateway' theory that tobacco and alcohol lead to the use of illicit drugs does not hold in adolescents. A minority go on to problematic high-dose use with clinical harm and dependence (Fig 19.7).

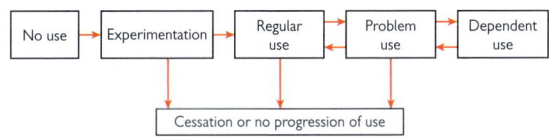

Fig 19.7 The spectrum of misuse. Printed by permission of Blackwells.

Specific harmful drugs
In the UK, harmful drugs are classified as follows:
- *Class A:* opiates, cocaine, hallucinogens (LSD), methadone, methylenedioxymethamphetamine (MDMA, ecstasy)
- *Class B:* amphetamine, dihydrocodeine (DF118), methylphenobarbitone
- *Class C:* benzodiazepines, cannabis.

Any Class B drug prepared for injection becomes Class A. Inhalants include paint, glue, petrol, and nitrous oxide (laughing gas). These substances are more commonly used by younger, high-risk adolescents as they are readily available and their purchase and possession are not illegal.

Clinical assessment
History
The history in a young person in whom substance abuse is suspected should encompass the following domains:
- *Substance misuse:* quantity, frequency, duration, route of administration. Enquire specifically about each substance as concurrent multiple substance is common
- *Related behaviours:* intoxication, bingeing, overdosing, unsafe sex, drunk driving
- *Dependence:* difficulty limiting use, tolerance or withdrawal symptoms
- *Complications:* infections (hepatitis, HIV), seizures
- *Psychological history:* ask about co-morbid psychiatric disorders (depression, etc.) and living environment, family support, relationships, trouble with the law.

Examination
Examination is directed towards identification of specific signs of substance misuse and complications of misuse. These may be acute and transitory or chronic and vary of course with the substance concerned:

Acute signs of intoxication
- *Amphetamines:* jaw grinding, cardiac arrhythmias
- *Cocaine:* muscle twitching, psychosis, cardiac arrhythmias
- *Opiates:* respiratory depression, pin-point pupils
- *Alcohol:* respiratory depression, hypoglycaemia

Acute signs of withdrawal
- *Alcohol:* tremor, high blood pressure
- *Amphetamines:* agitation, restlessness
- *Opiates:* dilated pupils, high blood pressure, rhinorrhea.

Alcohol or solvents may be smelt on the breath, and paint stains may be visible around the mouth. A serious case may be underweight, anaemic, or jaundiced with hepatomegaly and venepuncture marks and old scars on limbs or neck. A urine screen may be useful.

Management
Prevention of substance misuse by adolescents requires programmes which encourage acquisition of skills, promote social inclusion, and are developmentally appropriate. Strategies need to encourage moderation rather than just abstinence. Young people require information about safe levels of alcohol consumption, the hazards of drunk driving, and the health risks of drugs.

Helping a young person to reduce or stop substance misuse requires the development of a trusting relationship and good rapport combined with an open-minded and non-judgemental approach. The 'stages of change' model is relevant, and clearly options vary depending on the clinical context. Motivational conversations designed to counter misuse of alcohol and tobacco can explore:
- *Advantages/disadvantages:* 'Drinking makes you relax, but being drunk can look ugly'. 'Giving up smoking does not cause weight gain'.
- *Perspectives on risks:* consequences of unsafe sex while intoxicated.

Strategies for more serious cases are implemented by specialist services and include:
- *Counselling:* including cognitive behaviour therapy
- *'Detoxification':* drug withdrawal in a residential setting or as an outpatient
- Pharmacotherapy
- *Rehabilitation:* reintegration into education or employment and into healthier activities such as sport. A relapsing course is common. Reassurance that relapse is normal may reduce a demotivating sense of failure.

19.9 Case-based discussions

An adolescent with cuts

A 14 year old girl presents to the hospital emergency department with multiple superficial lacerations to her forearms. This is her second presentation with the same problem in the last 6 months. She lives at home with a younger sister and her mother who separated from her father a year ago. She had a row with her boy friend 2 days ago. She is accompanied by her grandfather.

On examination she appears well nourished and not unkempt. There are no signs suggesting substance misuse. She is alert and coherent. There are several minor superficial scratches on both forearms.

What is the diagnosis?
The most likely diagnosis is self-harm by self-cutting. The cuts are minor and there is no immediate evidence of serious injury. The term 'deliberate' self-harm is best avoided, as it implies intention which may not be the case.

How will you assess the patient?
First of all it is essential to establish the diagnosis of self harm. Although this can be straightforward, some adolescents may try to conceal it by claiming it was accidental.

History
A detailed account of events surrounding the self harm is followed by an exploration using the four Ps approach:
- **P**redisposing factors: previous history of self harm or psychiatric disorder, current family situation
- **P**recipitating factors: recent rows, recent losses, awareness of self harm by others
- **P**erpetuating factors: substance misuse, poor family dynamics
- **P**rotective factors: support network, resilient personality.

Examination should include a search for evidence of substance misuse and observation of mood and interactions with relatives and staff. Evidence of depression, anxiety, or psychosis should be sought. The possibility of pregnancy should be considered.

Investigations
Paracetamol and salicylate levels, urine toxicology, and a pregnancy test should be considered.

She attends school regularly and is academically successful. Although her parents are separated she is in regular contact with her father and has a good relationship with both grandparents who live nearby. Her mood appears good and she is polite and helpful to staff. Two of her school friends recently cut themselves after breaking up with their boyfriends.

What protective factors are present?
These include: positive peer relationships, being particularly good at something, good school attendance and academic achievement, positive plans for the future, close relationship with a positive role model, and good communication within the family. She has several of these, including good school performance and some good family relationships.

Is there any risk of suicide?
Assessment of suicide risk or intent can be very difficult. This appears to have been an impulsive act and not one likely to be fatal. No major risk factors for suicidal intent are evident. These include current suicidal ideation, psychiatric illness or personality disorder, severity of overdose or injuries, previous attempts, feelings of hopelessness, alcohol or drug dependence, early parental loss, neglect or abuse as child, social crisis, and physical illness, especially chronic painful disorders.

What is the further management?
After attending to her wounds and ensuring she is up to date with her tetanus immunisation, further assessment should be continued away from the emergency department.

She should be admitted overnight to the paediatric ward or ideally an adolescent ward. This enables time for an assessment by the psychiatrist from the Child and Adolescent Mental Health Services alongside the social worker. From the above history it seems unlikely that she will need one-to-one observations, but if necessary this can be put in place. If on the other hand she was seen to be of significant risk, an admission to a specialist adolescent unit would be appropriate.

What long-term measures are appropriate?
Reassurance and correction of any environmental adversity is the key to managing these problems. If there are features of depression these should be assessed and monitored by the psychiatrist. Again, if there are drug or alcohol problems then a specialist referral would be required.

If the social worker's assessment identifies significant family issues then family therapy may be of benefit. Liaison with the school can also help identify issues such as bullying and also help in monitoring the progress of this patient.

For continuity of care it is also essential to inform her GP and, if younger children are present within the family, the health visitor. Voluntary organizations such as Childline, Change our Minds, and Self Harm Alliance may also be useful.

Chapter 20

Pharmacology

20.1 Clinical pharmacology *426*
20.2 Paediatric prescribing *428*
20.3 Gastrointestinal and musculoskeletal systems *430*
20.4 Cardiovascular and respiratory systems *432*
20.5 Central nervous system *434*
20.6 Antibiotics *436*
20.7 Antifungals, antivirals, and antiprotozoals *438*
20.8 Endocrine system *440*
20.9 Malignancy, immunosuppression, and blood *442*
20.10 Nutrition *444*
20.11 Fluids and electrolytes *446*
20.12 Case-based discussions *448*

20.1 Clinical pharmacology

The way in which the body responds to a drug varies with age for many reasons, including in particular changes in body size and composition and liver enzyme maturation.

Important differences therefore exist between neonates, children, and adults in both the pharmacokinetics and the pharmacodynamics of medications prescribed.

It is worth being clear about some of the terms used:
- *Pharmacokinetics:* what the body does to a drug
- *Pharmacodynamics:* what a drug does to the body
- *Pharmacogenetics:* how variation in single genes gives rise to differing responses to drugs
- *Pharmacogenomics:* the new study of how genome-wide variation in numerous genes influences drug responses.

Pharmacokinetics

Pharmacokinetics is generally divided into four phases, summarized as ADME:
- **A**bsorption: the process of the drug entering the body
- **D**istribution: distribution and dispersion of a drug throughout the tissues and fluids of the body
- **M**etabolism: transformation of the parent compound into metabolites
- **E**xcretion: elimination of the substances from the body.

An important factor determining the pharmacokinetics of a drug is its chemical *polarity*. Water is a polar compound and therefore polar compounds tend to be water soluble and non-polar compounds lipid soluble.

> **Pharmacokinetics glossary**
> - *Drug clearance:* (rate of elimination)/ (plasma concentration)
> - *Zero-order kinetics:* drugs are metabolized at a constant rate; occurs when enzymes are saturated
> - *First-order kinetics:* drugs are metabolized as a constant percentage of the plasma concentration; occurs when enzymes are not saturated
> - *First-pass metabolism:* metabolism in the intestine or liver following initial absorption of a drug taken orally
> - *Half-life ($t_{1/2}$):* the time required for half of the absorbed dose of a drug to be cleared from the body. A 'steady state' is reached after 4–5 half-lives
> - *Bioavailability:* the fraction of the administered dose that reaches the circulation.

Absorption

Factors affecting absorption obviously depend on the route of administration, which is usually oral in children but may also include topical administration via the skin (transdermal) or mucous membranes of the nose or buccal cavity and inhalation into the respiratory tract. IM injection is rarely used and IV injection provides direct access to the circulation, bypassing the process of absorption.

Absorption after oral administration

Solid formulations must first be dissolved in the GI tract. The major factors then influencing absorption of drugs given orally are lipid solubility and gastric emptying. The former is pH dependent as unionized molecules are more lipid soluble than ionized. The pK_a is the pH at which a drug is 50% ionized. Acidic drugs are most highly ionized at low pH (acidic environment) and bases are most highly ionized at high pH (alkaline environment).

Drugs with an acidic pK_a such as aspirin and penicillin V are mainly unionized in the acid stomach and therefore easily absorbed. Weaker acids such as phenobarbital are better absorbed in the more alkaline intestine.

Developmental changes

Neonates, especially preterm infants, have reduced gastric acid secretion. Acid secretion is increased by 24 h and a mature value is reached by 3 years. Gastric emptying is prolonged in the 1st 24 h and peristalsis in the newborn is slow. Drug absorption in the stomach may be increased and in the intestine may be delayed.

Absorption of ampicillin and penicillin V is increased and of phenobarbital and paracetamol is decreased in newborns.

Transdermal absorption is increased in preterm infants due to the thinner stratum corneum and higher water content of the dermis.

Distribution

The drug is distributed around the body via the circulation from where it penetrates the tissues. Distribution depends on:
- *Lipid solubility:* determines passage across cell membranes
- *Binding to plasma proteins:* drugs vary in protein-binding capacity
- *Body composition:* relative size and water content of the body compartments such as circulating blood volume, fat and tissue compartments
- *Blood flow:* tissues with high blood flow receive the drug first
- *Blood–brain barrier (BBB):* unionized lipid-soluble drugs cross the BBB easily.

Developmental changes

At birth, the total body water and extracellular fluid volume are high so larger doses of water-soluble drugs (on a bodyweight basis) are required.

Neonatal protein-binding capacity is reduced, especially in preterm infants. Plasma albumin levels are low (adult levels reached by 1 year), binding capacity is reduced, and endogenous substances such as bilirubin compete. This leads to increased levels of active free drug for highly protein-bound drugs such as phenytoin. The BBB is functionally incomplete in the newborn and there is increased penetration of some drugs such as opiates.

Metabolism

Drug metabolism occurs mainly in the liver and usually has the effect of converting the drug into metabolites which are both less active and more polar (hydrophilic) and hence more easily excretable by the kidneys.

However, sometimes the metabolites are more active and pro-drugs are inactive until metabolized to the active drug (e.g. aciclovir, levodopa).

First-pass metabolism occurs in the bowel wall and liver for oral medications. This is useful for pro-drugs activated in the liver, such as enalapril, but means large doses are required for drugs with high first-pass metabolism such as propranolol. Metabolism is divided into phase I and phase II reactions:

- *Phase I:* biotransformation to a more polar metabolite by oxidation, reduction or hydrolysis. Oxidations are catalysed by an important class of enzymes called the cytochrome P450s
- *Phase II:* these reactions usually occur in the liver and involve conjugation of the drug or its phase I metabolite with an endogenous substance. Conjugation may be with glucuronide, sulfate, or glutathione.

Cytochrome P450 oxidases (CYP450s) are a class of oxidative enzymes found in bacteria, plants, and animals. About six CYP450 isoforms account for most hepatic drug metabolism. These enzymes may be induced or inhibited by some drugs and natural products, a phenomenon which accounts for many important drug interactions. Genetic variations in their activity account for variations in drug responsiveness.

Developmental changes
Hepatic metabolism is reduced at birth but increases rapidly during the first few weeks of life and reaches a peak exceeding that of adults in the 2nd year. Oxidation, hydroxylation, and glucuronidation reactions are more reduced than sulfation and methylation reactions. Drugs such as diazepam which are extensively metabolized by the liver have a greatly extended half-life in newborn infants.

Excretion
Excretion is primarily renal and depends on glomerular filtration rate, tubular reabsorption, and tubular secretion. Renal clearance is determined by polarity and water solubility. Polar drugs or drug metabolites are freely excreted by the kidneys.

Developmental changes
The kidney is functionally and anatomically immature in the newborn. The neonatal kidneys receive only 6% of the cardiac output, compared to 15–20% in the adult. Renal function approximates adult values by 6–8 months. Drugs which rely mainly on renal excretion, such as gentamicin, have a prolonged half-life.

Pharmacodynamics glossary

- *Effective dose 50 (ED_{50}):* dose producing desired therapeutic response in 50% of patients
- *Effective concentration 50 (EC_{50}):* plasma concentration at which 50% of maximum response is seen
- *Lethal dose 50 (LD_{50}):* the dose which is lethal in 50% of animals tested
- *Therapeutic index (TI):* a measure of relative safety: $TI = LD_{50}/ED_{50}$
- *Therapeutic range:* a range of acceptable plasma concentrations in which positive therapeutic results without undesirable side effects or toxic responses are anticipated
- *Maintenance dose:* the dose necessary to maintain therapeutic levels, based on the drug half-life and clearance rate

---

Drug targets
A few drugs act by virtue of their physico-chemical properties (e.g. activated charcoal, osmotic diuretics) but most have a specific action on a 'target' molecule. The majority of important drugs act on molecules which can be categorized into four types:

Receptors
Molecules normally activated by endogenous messengers such as transmitters, hormones, or cytokines. A drug may be an *agonist*, which activates the receptor, or an *antagonist*, which combines with and blocks the receptor. There are four classes of receptor:
- Ligand-gated ion channels
- G-protein-coupled receptors
- Enzyme associated receptors
- Transcription factor receptors.

Ion channels
Drugs may bind to accessory sites or may block the channel physically. Ion channels are usually selective for particular ions, e.g. sodium, potassium, calcium.

Enzymes
Many drugs target enzymes and may act as a competitive inhibitor (reversible or irreversible) or as a false substrate, subverting the normal metabolic pathway.

Transporters
Transport of polar ions and small organic molecules across lipid membranes usually requires a carrier protein transporter. A family of these transporters exists responsible for such diverse processes as transport of glucose and amino acids into cells, transport by the renal tubule and gut epithelium, and uptake of neurotransmitters.

Other targets include cytosolic proteins (e.g. tubulin, immunophilins), DNA, and cell wall constituents.

Pharmacogenetics
Pharmacogenetics is the study of how genetic variation gives rise to differing responses to drugs. Clinically important inherited variations affecting drug metabolism were the first to be recognized, but inherited variation in drug transporters or other drug targets also occurs.

Phase I metabolism
Genetic variation of several phase I enzymes are important Most intensively studied is *CYP2D6*. Most variants cause reduced activity, but some individuals have extra copies of the gene associated with enhanced activity. Others with variants include *CYP2C9*, *CYP2C19*, and *CYP3A5*.

Variation in butyrylcholinesterase, the enzyme that metabolizes succinylcholine, was one of the first pharmacogenetic effects to be recognized. It causes slow recovery from surgical paralysis. Variation in dihydropyrimidine dehydrogenase puts patients at risk for toxic effects from standard doses of fluorouracil.

Phase II metabolism
Variation in the *N*-acetylation of isoniazid was recognized many years ago. A polymorphism in *NAT2* divides people into 'slow' and 'fast' acetylators, and shows striking ethnic variation.

Mercaptopurine and the pro-drug azathioprine are metabolized in part by the enzyme thiopurine *S*-methyltransferase (TPMT) which can be assayed in red cells. Individuals with low or no TPMT activity have a greatly increased risk of life-threatening myelosuppression at normal dosage levels.

A Genechip test is now available which uses microarray technology to determine variants of *CYP2D6* and *CYP2C19*.

20.2 Paediatric prescribing

If in doubt consult the *BNF for Children* (BNFC), the essential resource for clinical use of medicines in children. Available online at bnf.org, the BNFC presents essential practical information to help health-care professionals prescribe, monitor, supply, and administer medicines for childhood disorders.

Rules for safe prescribing

In the UK, legal responsibility lies with the doctor who signs the prescription. See the Box for rules that should be followed in writing a prescription.

> **Rules for writing prescriptions**
> - Write legibly in capitals, sign legibly, date in black ink
> - *Avoid decimal points:*
>   - 3 mg **not** 3.0 mg
>   - 500 mg **not** 0.5 g
>   - 100 micrograms **not** 0.1 mg
> - If a decimal point is unavoidable, a zero must be written in front of the decimal point if there is no other number:
>   - **0.5 mL not** .5 mL
>
> Remember **'death by decimal point'**. An error of **1** decimal point will alter the dose given by a **factor of 10**.
> - Do not abbreviate milligrams, micrograms, nanograms, or units
> - *State dose as mass of active drug:* units of volume (e.g. 5 mL) or tablets (e.g. 1 tablet) should be avoided **except** for compound preparations.
> - Approved generic titles for drugs and preparations should be used and not abbreviated.
> - Strengths of liquid preparations should be clearly identified, e.g. 125 mg/5 mL.
> - *Controlled drugs:* These are indicated by CD in the BNF for children. They include morphine, temazepam, and barbiturates.
>   - The prescription must state in the prescriber's own handwriting: name and address of patient, the form and strength of any preparations, the total quantity in both words and figures, and the dose.

Formulation and dosing

Formulation

This refers to the preparation of a drug and is intended to optimize delivery and bioavailability.

Drugs for oral administration can be formulated as an aqueous solution, aqueous suspension, capsule, or tablet. Young children often prefer medicines in liquid form and this may necessitate crushing of tablets if the product is not available in liquid form. This may change bioavailability, depending on whether the tablet dissolves or disperses.

An excipient is an inactive substance used as a carrier for the active ingredients of a medication. Excipients include bindings, coatings, flavourings, and sweeteners. Palatability is a key issue in compliance, and taste preferences change with age. Oral liquid preparations that do not contain fructose, glucose, or sucrose are described as 'sugar free' in the BNFC.

Drugs for nasal or respiratory tract absorption may be formulated as dry powders or solutions for nebulization.

Dosage

Most children's doses are standardized by weight. The dose is determined by multiplying this by the bodyweight in kilograms. Take note as to whether the dose refers to individual single doses or to a total daily amount to be given in divided doses. Failure to distinguish these two options causes many errors.

Body surface area (BSA) estimates are more accurate than body-weight since most physiological phenomena correlate better with BSA. This can be calculated from nomograms based on height and weight which are available in the BNFC.

- In a very overweight child, dose should be calculated for an 'ideal weight' related to height and age.
- Doses are usually expressed for specific age ranges.
- Depending on the therapeutic index, doses may or may not be rounded to a convenient amount.

Unlicensed and off-label prescribing

The regulatory bodies that licence pharmaceutical companies to market their drugs include the Medical and Healthcare products Regulatory Agency (MHRA) in the UK, European Medicines Agency (EMA) in the European Union, and the Food and Drug Administration (FDA) in the USA.

Many children currently require medicines which are:
- *Unlicensed:* not specifically licensed for paediatric use
- *Off-label:* licensed medicines used for unlicensed applications such as a different disease or age group.

New draft European legislation and the UK Medicines for Children Research Network should address the present lack of data to support evidence-based prescribing.

The Medicine Act 1968 prohibits promotion of medicines outside their license limits, but does not prohibit their off-license prescription and use. Legal responsibility lies with the prescriber, but prescription of these products is not a breach of duty if it is supported by guidance from a respected body of medical opinion.

Drug monitoring

For most drugs measuring levels in the blood is unnecessary as their effect can be measured by clinical response (e.g. blood pressure, peak expiratory flow rate) or tests for pharmacodynamic effect.

Monitoring may be required in drugs with a narrow *therapeutic window*, i.e. a small gap between the concentration giving maximum efficacy and the toxic range and in cases of poisoning (aspirin, paracetamol). It may also be useful for checking compliance and to determine the effects of an interacting medication or change in renal or hepatic function.

Drugs for which monitoring may be indicated and for which levels can be measured include:
- *Antibiotics:* gentamicin, vancomycin
- *Antiepilepsy drugs:* phenytoin, carbamazepine
- *Cardiac drugs:* digoxin, antiarrhythmics
- *Others:* theophylline, ciclosporin, warfarin.

Drug interactions

Drug interactions are listed in Appendix 1 of the BNFC and may be:

- *Pharmaceutical:* for preparations administered parenterally, e.g. mixing heparin and hydrocortisone inactivates the heparin
- *Pharmocodynamic:* between drugs which act synergistically or antagonistically
- *Pharmacokinetic:* one drug affects the absorption, distribution, metabolism or excretion of another.

Pharmacokinetic interactions

- *Absorption:* drugs that increase (e.g. metaclopramide) or decrease (e.g. atropine) the rate of gastric emptying may affect absorption.
- *Distribution:* drugs bound to plasma albumin may be displaced by a second drug. This can be important for drugs that are >90% bound, e.g. warfarin, phenytoin.
- *Metabolism:* induction or inhibition, especially of CYP450 enzymes in the liver, represents a very important class of interactions:
  - *CYP450 inducers:* important inducers include phenytoin, phenobarbitone, carbamazepine, rifampicin, and sulfonylureas. This decreases the efficiency of drugs metabolized by the same enzyme and increases efficacy when the inducer drug is stopped.
  - *CYP450 inhibitors:* drugs which inhibit enzymes act more rapidly, with maximal inhibition occurring after five half-lives. Important inhibitors include omeprazole, cimetidine, sodium valproate, erythromycin and ketoconazole, isoniazid, sulphonamides.
- *Excretion:* drugs may share the same transport system in the proximal tubules, e.g. probenecid and penicillin. Potassium-sparing diuretics combined with angiotensin converting enzyme (ACE) inhibitors can cause hyperkalaemia.

Adverse drug reactions

These can be divided into dose-related (type A) and non-dose related (type B). In addition, some drugs lead to adaptive effects with unwanted withdrawal effects when stopped (e.g. corticosteroids and acute adrenal insufficiency) and some are associated with an increased incidence of birth defects (teratogens) or tumours (carcinogens).

Type A: dose-related adverse reactions

These are predictable and caused by an excess of the desired pharmacological effect (e.g. hypoglycaemia, bleeding) or by a drug's parallel unwanted action (e.g. respiratory depression). They are more common with drugs that have a steep dose-response curve or a low therapeutic index. They are caused by incorrect dosage or altered pharmacokinetics.

Type B: non-dose-related adverse reactions

These idiosyncratic reactions are unpredictable and rare but have a considerable mortality. Several inherited diseases predispose affected individuals to drug toxicity:

- *Glucose-6-phosphate dehydrogenase (G6PD) deficiency:* a large number of oxidative drugs including antimalarials, antibiotics, analgesics, and antipyretics will induce a severe haemolytic reaction
- *Malignant hyperthermia:* a life-threatening condition triggered by volatile anaesthetics or suxamethonium chloride which induce an uncontrolled increase in skeletal muscle oxidative metabolism. Due to mutation of the *RYR1* gene.
- Mitochondrial 1555A > G Mutation: risk of sensori-neural hearing loss with aminoglycosides even at drug levels in therapeutic range.

Most are allergic drug reactions, which are of four types:
- *type I:* anaphylaxis
- *type II:* cytotoxic reactions (blood dyscrasias)
- *type III:* serum sickness
- *type IV:* delayed hypersensitivity.

Reporting adverse drug reactions

In the UK, suspected adverse drug reactions are reported on the Yellow Cards provided in the BNFC or online (www.yellowcard.gov.uk). All serious and minor adverse reactions in children should be reported. If in doubt, report.

Prescribing in special circumstances

Pregnancy and breast feeding

In early pregnancy, teratogenesis is the main concern. However, functional development of certain organ systems can be affected during the 2nd and 3rd trimesters, and late in pregnancy neonatal toxicity or withdrawal effects are of concern. The BNFC identifies drugs which may have a harmful effect in pregnancy, and indicates the trimester of risk, as well as those not known to be harmful in pregnancy.

The UK National Teratology Information Service provides a 24 h service on all aspects of toxicity of drugs and chemicals during pregnancy.

Most drugs will enter the breast milk, but the dose received by the infant is usually very low (<10%). However, hypersensitivity reactions may occur even with small doses. Drugs that are contraindicated during lactation include chloramphenicol, ciprofloxacin, thiazides, and aspirin.

Prescribing in organ impairment

Dysfunction of most major organ systems influences pharmacokinetics and must be taken into account:

- *GI tract:* delayed gastric emptying (e.g. in trauma, raised intracranial pressure) or increased emptying (gastroenterostomy, coeliac disease). Steatorrhea reduces absorption of fat-soluble vitamins.
- *Renal impairment:* drugs that are renally excreted will accumulate in renal impairment and the dose regime may need to be adjusted either by reducing the size of individual doses or by increasing the dose interval For most drugs, any loading dose is unchanged. Doses are adjusted according to the severity of renal impairment which is divided into mild, moderate, or severe based on serum creatinine and GFR.
  - Potentially toxic drugs with a small margin of safety in renal impairment include aminoglycosides and digoxin.
  - Nephrotoxic drugs should obviously be avoided.
- *Hepatic impairment:* modification of prescribing is usually unnecessary except in certain circumstances including:
  - *severe liver failure:* opioids and benzodiazepines may accumulate and cause CNS depression with respiratory depression. Diuretics may cause hypokalaemia and precipitate encephalopathy
  - *cholestatic jaundice* impairs elimination of drugs excreted in bile, such as rifampicin and fusidic acid.

20.3 Gastrointestinal and musculoskeletal systems

Drugs used in gastro-oesophageal reflux disease and laxatives are described.

Gastro-oesophageal reflux disease

Compound alginate preparations

Alginates are polysaccharides derived from brown seaweeds (Fig 20.1). They form a 'raft' that floats on the surface of the stomach contents, reducing reflux and protecting the oesophageal mucosa. Alginate-containing antacids are used for mild gastro-oesophageal reflux disease.

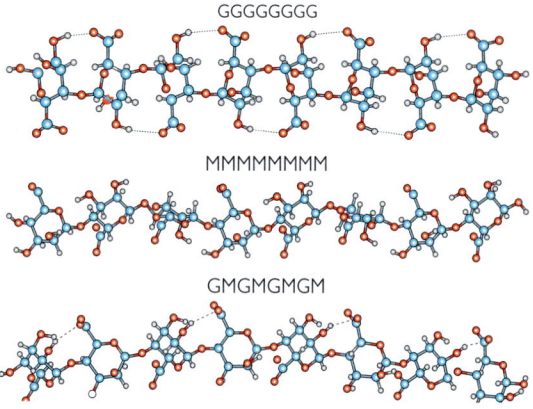

Fig 20.1 Alginates are linear unbranched polymers containing linked D-mannuronic acid (M) or L-guluronic acid, (G) residues. Reproduced with permission from London South Bank University.

One commonly used preparation (Gaviscon Infant) contains a mixture of sodium and magnesium alginate with colloidal silica and mannitol.

- *Contraindications:* not to be used in preterm neonates or where excessive water loss is likely (e.g. fever, diarrhoea, vomiting). Should not be used in combination with thickening agents.

H_2-receptor antagonists

Gastric parietal cells are stimulated to secrete acid by histamine acting on H_2-receptors. H_2-receptor antagonists act by reducing gastric acid secretion as a result of H_2-receptor blockade. Examples include cimetidine and ranitidine.

- *Indications:* healing of gastric and duodenal ulcers and relief of symptoms in gastro-oesophageal reflux disease
- *Interactions:* cimetidine inhibits CYP450 enzymes, reducing metabolism of several drugs including warfarin, phenytoin, and theophylline. Ranitidine does not have this effect.

Proton-pump inhibitors (PPIs)

PPIs inhibit gastric acid secretion by blocking the hydrogen–potassium ATP enzyme system or proton pump of the gastric parietal cell. Proton pump inhibition is irreversible, so the effect of a single dose lasts 2–3 days until new enzymes are synthesized. Omeprazole is licensed for use in children.

- *Indications:*
  - Severe GORD or in peptic ulcer disease complicated by stricture, ulceration or haemorrhage
  - Prevention and treatment of NSAID-associated ulcers. In children who need to continue NSAIDs after an ulcer has healed full dose should be continued to prevent asymptomatic ulcer recurrence.

Laxatives

Laxatives include bulk-forming agents, stimulants, stool softeners, and osmotic laxatives. Some laxatives act by more than one mechanism.

Bulk-forming laxatives

These stimulate peristalsis by increasing faecal mass. Examples include unprocessed wheat bran, ispaghula husk, and methylcellulose. They are of particular value in constipated children with small hard stools and insufficient fibre in the diet. They are useful in management of children with haemorrhoids, anal fissure, or irritable bowel syndrome.

- *Contraindications:* faecal impaction, colonic atony, or intestinal obstruction. Adequate fluid intake should be encouraged and carers advised that the full effect may take several days to develop.

Stimulant laxatives

Increase intestinal motility, probably through an effect on the myenteric plexus. Examples include senna, bisacodyl, and docusate sodium. They are useful in simple constipation in conjunction with an osmotic laxative or stool softener. Adverse effects can include abdominal cramps and diarrhoea with prolonged usage.

Senna tablets are not licensed for use in children <6 years and senna syrup is not licensed for children <2 years.

Osmotic laxatives

These act by increasing the amount of water in the large bowel, either by drawing fluid into the bowel or by retaining the fluid they were administered with. Examples include:

- *Lactulose:* a semi-synthetic disaccharide which is not absorbed from the GI tract. Side effects can include flatulence and abdominal discomfort.
- *Macrogols:* an effective non-traumatic means of evacuation in children with faecal impaction, and also useful in long-term management of constipation. Contraindications include intestinal obstructions or perforation, paralytic ileus, or severe inflammatory bowel disease. Side effects include abdominal pain and distension and a dehydrating effect which can be avoided by giving extra fluids.

Drugs used in rheumatic diseases are described including non-steroidal anti-inflammatory drugs (NSAIDs), corticosteroids, and disease modifying anti-rheumatic drugs (DMARDs).

Non-steroidal anti-inflammatory drugs (NSAIDs)

The NSAIDs have analgesic, antipyretic, and anti-inflammatory effects that are mediated by inhibition of the enzyme cyclo-oxygenase which catalyses the formation of prostaglandins and thromboxane from arachidonic acid derived from the phospholipid bilayer by phospholipase A_2.

There are three isoenzymes of cyclo-oxygenase: COX-1, COX-2, and COX-3. Selective inhibitors of COX-2 have been developed, but unfortunately some appear to increase the risk of myocardial infarction. There is evidence that paracetamol acts in part by inhibiting COX-3.

Table 20.1. NSAIDs

Salicylates	Aspirin
Arylalkanoic acids	Diclofenac
	Indometacin
2-Arylpropionic acids	Ibuprofen
	Naproxen
Fenamic acids	Mefenamic acid
Oxicans	Piroxicam
	Meloxicam

NSAIDs are classified according to chemical structure (Table 20.1). Differences in anti-inflammatory activity between them are small, but there is considerable variation in individual patient tolerance and response. Pain relief starts after the first dose and the full analgesic effect is normally obtained within a week. A clinically discernible anti-inflammatory effect may not be obtained for up to 3 weeks, or as long as 4–12 weeks in juvenile idiopathic arthritis (JIA).

Indications
- Treatment of JIA and other rheumatic diseases
- Management of children with soft-tissue injuries and strains and musculoskeletal disorders. Paracetamol should be used first for pain relief, but may be used in combination with a NSAID if relief is inadequate.

Side effects
The main adverse drug reactions associated with NSAIDs involve the GI tract and kidneys.

NSAIDs cause a dual insult to the GI tract. The acid molecules directly irritate the gastric mucosa, and inhibition of COX-1 reduces the levels of protective prostaglandins. The effects are dose related and children appear to tolerate NSAIDs better than adults. However, abdominal discomfort, nausea, bleeding, and ulceration may occur.

Renal effects occur in part because NSAIDs block the prostaglandin-mediated vasodilatation of the afferent arterioles of the glomerulus which maintains normal glomerular perfusion. Fluid retention and raised blood pressure may occur and renal failure may be provoked in patients with pre-existing renal impairment.

NSAIDs used in children

Ibuprofen
A derivative of 2-arylpropionic acid which inhibits COX-1 and COX-2. It is licensed for use in children >6 months of age and bodyweight >7 kg for relief of pyrexia, pain, and inflammation in rheumatic diseases and soft tissue disorders and for treatment of patent ductus arteriosus (PDA) in preterm neonates.

At low doses it has the lowest incidence of GI side effects. Its anti-inflammatory properties are relatively weak. It should be avoided in severe hepatic impairment.

Indometacin
Indometacin is a member of the arylalkanoic class of NSAIDs which includes diclofenac. Its high incidence of side effects precludes first line use in children. However, it is used as an alternative to ibuprofen for treatment of PDA in preterm neonates.

Corticosteroids

Systemic steroids
In children with rheumatic diseases corticosteroids are reserved for specific circumstances and used only under the supervision of a specialist.

Systemic corticosteroids are considered in JIA in systemic disease or when several joints are affected and in severe, possibly life-threatening episodes of systemic lupus erythematosus (SLE), systemic vasculitis, or dermatomyositis. In severe conditions, short courses of high-dose IV methylprednisolone may provide rapid relief with fewer adverse effects.

Long term corticosteroids may cause osteoporosis and there is a particular risk of osteopaenia in those unable to exercise.

Steroid injections
Local corticosteroid injections are used in inflammatory conditions of the joints, soft tissue, and tendons.

Triamcinolone hexacetonide is preferred for intra-articular injection as it is almost insoluble and has a long-acting depot effect. Other preparations used include triamcinolone acetonide, methylprednisolone, and hydrocortisone acetate. An acute inflammatory reaction to the microcrystalline suspension used may occur and needs to be distinguished from infection.

Disease modifying anti-rheumatic drugs (DMARDs)

DMARDs include drugs such as:
- *Antimalarials*: hydroxychloroquine sulphate
- *Immunomodulators*: methotrexate, azathioprine
- *Cytokine inhibitors*: etanercept, infliximab.

They are used under specialist supervision and require 4–6 months of treatment for a full response. Hydroxychloroquine may be useful in SLE and sarcoidosis. Methotrexate is the DMARD of choice in JIA. Etanercept, which inhibits tumour necrosis factor (TNF), is recommended in children aged 4–17 years with active, polyarticular JIA who have not responded to methotrexate.

20.4 Cardiovascular and respiratory systems

Drugs used in control of cardiac failure, arrhythmias, hypertension, and circulatory failure are discussed.

Diuretics

Diuretics act on the kidney to increase excretion of water and sodium chloride and are used for a variety of conditions in children including pulmonary oedema in respiratory distress syndrome or chronic lung disease of prematurity, cardiac failure, and hypertension. There are three main classes: thiazides, loop diuretics, and potassium-sparing diuretics.

Thiazides
These moderately potent diuretics inhibit sodium reabsorption at the beginning of the distal convoluted tubule. They are used in combination for management of pulmonary oedema or in lower doses for management of hypertension in association with cardiac disease.

Chlorothiazide is most commonly used.

Loop diuretics
These powerful diuretics inhibit reabsorption of sodium, potassium, and chloride from the ascending limb of the loop of Henle. Indications include pulmonary oedema, congestive heart failure, and hypertension.

Examples include furosemide and bumetanide.
Hypovolemia should be corrected before using in oliguria. High doses may be required in renal impairment.
- *Side effects:* include hypotension, hyponatraemia, and hypokalaemia. At high dose, changes in the electrolyte composition of the endolymph may be associated with deafness. Prolonged use may cause hypochloraemic alkalosis and increased calcium excretion with a risk of nephrocalcinosis especially in neonates.

Potassium-sparing diuretics
These act on the aldosterone-responsive segments of the distal neuron. Examples include the aldosterone antagonist spironolactone and amiloride which blocks the epithelial sodium channel (ENac).
- *Spironolactone:* often combined with other diuretics to reduce potassium loss. It is useful in long-term management of Bartter syndrome and control of ascites in infants with neonatal hepatitis
- *Amiloride:* a weak diuretic on its own but can be used as an alternative to potassium supplements with thiazide or loop diuretics.

Potassium supplements should not be given with potassium-sparing diuretics and they can cause severe hyperkalaemia if given with an ACE inhibitor or an angiotensin-II receptor antagonist.

Anti-arrhythmic drugs

The most common arrhythmias encountered in general paediatric practice are the supraventricular tachycardias, for which IV injection of adenosine is the initial treatment of choice.

Adenosine is a nucleoside composed of adenine attached to a ribose moiety. It acts by causing transient block of conduction in the AV node.

Incremental IV doses are given every 2 min until the tachycardia is terminated, up to a maximum single does of 500 micrograms/kg. The half-life is extremely short, so injection should be rapid over 2 s into a central or large peripheral vein followed by a rapid sodium chloride 0.9% flush. Cardiac monitoring should be in place.

Adenosine is not negatively inotropic and does not cause significant hypotension. It may be used safely in children with impaired cardiac function. Side effects can include facial flushing and bronchospasm.

Calcium-channel blockers

This class of drugs block the transfer of calcium into cells via voltage-gated calcium channels (VGCCs). Therapeutic effects show great variation, as individual calcium-channel blockers differ in their selectivity across the large range of channels which exist.

Principle actions are on the myocardial cells, conducting cells of the heart, and vascular smooth muscle in which prevention of calcium entry confers a negative inotropic effect, negative chronotropic effect (lowering of heart rate), and relaxation of vascular smooth muscle. Decreased cardiac output and decreased peripheral resistance combine to lower blood pressure.

Two important classes of calcium-channel blockers with important differences in action are the phenylalkylamines (e.g. verapamil) and the dihydropyridines, all identified by the suffix '-pine' (e.g. nifedipine).
- *Verapamil:* very negatively inotropic and reduces cardiac output, slows heart rate, and may impair A-V conduction. It should be avoided in heart failure and should not be used with β-blockers.
- *Nifedipine:* relaxes vascular smooth muscle and dilates coronary and peripheral arteries. In contrast to verapamil it has more influence on blood vessels and less on myocardium, and has no anti-arrhythmic activity. Modified-release preparations are available for long-term management of hypertension. Nifedipine is also used for angina due to coronary artery disease in Kawasaki disease and in the management of Raynaud syndrome.

Angiotensin-converting enzyme (ACE) inhibitors

These inhibit the conversion of angiotensin I to angiotensin II. Examples include captopril and enalapril. Treatment should be initiated only under specialist supervision. Indications include heart failure, hypertension, and diabetic nephropathy.

ACE inhibitors need to be used with care in children on diuretics as they can cause a rapid fall in blood pressure in volume-depleted children. Very low doses should be used, or the diuretic discontinued in advance.
- *Side effects:* profound hypotension, renal impairment, persistent dry cough. They are contra-indicated in children with critical renovascular disease in whom they may cause renal failure.

The angiotensin-II receptor antagonist losartan is an alternative for treatment of hypertension.

Bronchodilators, inhaled corticosteroids, leukotriene receptor antagonists, and oxygen are all important drugs used in the management of common respiratory disorders.

Bronchodilators

There are three main classes of bronchodilator:
- *Adrenoceptor agonists:* salbutamol, terbutaline, salmeterol
- *Antimuscarinics:* ipratropium bromide
- *Theophylline:* aminophylline.

Adrenoceptor agonists

These include short acting β_2-agonists such as salbutamol and terbutaline and long-acting β-agonists (LABA) such as salmeterol. Bronchial smooth muscle is strongly dilated by β_2-agonists.
- *Salbutamol:* this is usually administered by inhalation. Duration of action is 3–5 h. It should be prescribed as required rather than on a regular basis in children with mild or moderate asthma. A short-acting β_2-agonist inhaled immediately before exercise reduces the risk of exercise-induced asthma. Intravenous salbutamol may be useful in children with severe of life-threatening acute asthma.
- *Salmeterol:* administered by inhalation, the duration of action is ~12 h. It may be used in the management of chronic asthma, but is not indicated for immediate relief of acute attacks. Existing corticosteroid therapy should not be reduced or withdrawn. There is a potential for paradoxical bronchospasm which is an indication for discontinuation and alternative therapy.

β_2-Agonists should be used with caution in diabetes, hyperthyroidism, cardiovascular disease, arrhythmias, and hypertension. Side effects include fine tremor, headache, and tachycardia. Hypokalaemia is a risk after high doses.

Antimuscarinic bronchodilators

Ipratropium, a quaternary ammonium compound, is administered by inhalation and relaxes bronchconstriction caused by parasympathetic stimulation.

After aerosol inhalation it has a maximum effect after 30–60 min and a duration of action of 3–6 h. It is generally safe and well tolerated and can be used with short-acting β_2-agonists in acute asthma.

Side effects include dry mouth and tachycardia and acute angle-closure glaucoma has been reported.

Theophylline

Theophylline is dimethylxanthine and acts by inhibiting phosphodiesterase, producing an increase in intracellular cyclic AMP. Theophylline is given by injection as aminophylline, a mixture of theophylline and ethylenediamine which is more soluble, less potent, and shorter acting than theophylline alone.

It should be administered by very slow IV injection as a loading dose over at least 20 min followed by IV infusion. The therapeutic index is low and serious side effects include convulsions and arrhythmias.

Leukotriene receptor antagonists

Leukotrienes are synthesized in the cell by 5-lipoxygenase. A subgroup, the cysteinyl leukotrienes (LTC_4, LTD_4, LTE_4, LTF_4), are of particular importance in asthma as they are potent constrictors of smooth muscle, cause an increase in mucus production, and recruit leucocytes to sites of inflammation. They act at specific cell-surface receptors, CysLT1 and CysLT2.

Montelukast is an oral leukotriene receptor antagonist used for maintenance treatment of asthma in conjunction with an inhaled corticosteroid. It may be of benefit in those with exercise-induced asthma and in those with concomitant rhinitis.

Churg–Strauss syndrome, characterized by a vasculitic rash, eosinophilia, and worsening pulmonary symptoms, has been associated with the use of leukotriene receptor antagonists.

Oxygen

Molecular oxygen first appeared in the Earth's atmosphere 2 billion years ago as a product of the metabolism of early anaerobes, and its abundance has gradually increased due to its synthesis by photosynthetic organisms.

Oxygen is the third most abundant element in the universe by mass after hydrogen and helium. Its role as the principle electron acceptor for the generation of ATP by oxidative metabolism renders a continuous supply essential for the life of aerobic organisms.

Oxygen should be regarded as a drug and its use (flow-rate and concentration) documented for each patient in a hospital setting. High concentrations of oxygen can cause pulmonary epithelial damage, convulsions, and retinal damage, especially in preterm neonates.

Acute oxygen therapy

In infants, oxygen is usually given via nasal cannula if the concentration required is less than 50%. A humidified head-box is necessary to deliver concentrations of 60% or higher.

In children with chronic pulmonary conditions low-concentration oxygen therapy (24–28%) may be used to maintain target blood-oxygen saturations of at least 92%.

Domiciliary oxygen

Domiciliary oxygen can be prescribed for intermittent use (e.g. children at risk of nocturnal hypoxaemia) or continuous long-term use (e.g. chronic lung disease of prematurity). Oxygen concentrators are more economical than oxygen cylinders when oxygen is required for long periods.

Children and their carers should be advised of the fire risks when oxygen is being administered from a cylinder or an oxygen concentrator.

20.5 Central nervous system

The most commonly prescribed and important medications affecting the CNS are the analgesics and antiepileptic drugs.

Hypnotics

Hypnotics are not used in children except on rare occasions for night terrors or somnambulism.

Melatonin has been used for treatment of disordered sleep in children with visual impairment, cerebral palsy, chronic fatigue syndrome, and autism. Treatment should be initiated by a specialist as the long-term safety and efficacy has yet to be established.

Chloral and derivatives

Chloral hydrate and triclofos are now mainly used for sedation during diagnostic procedures and in intensive care units.

They accumulate during prolonged use and should be avoided in severe renal or hepatic impairment. Chloral has an unpleasant taste and requires dilution with plenty of water or juice.

Analgesics

Non-opioid analgesics, paracetamol, and ibuprofen and other NSAIDs are suitable for mild to moderate pain especially in association with fever, whereas opioid analgesics are more suitable for moderate to severe pain, especially of visceral origin. NSAIDs are considered elsewhere.

Chronic neuropathic pain is generally managed with a tricyclic antidepressant or carbamazepine which blocks sodium channels in nociceptive pathways.

Non-opioid analgesics

Paracetamol (acetaminophen)

The names acetaminophen and paracetamol come from the chemical names: N-**acet**yl-para-**aminophen**ol or **para**-**acet**yl**am**inophen**ol**.

Paracetamol is a potent analgesic and antipyretic drug but has no demonstrable anti-inflammatory activity. It appears to block a variant of the COX enzyme (see above) which is only expressed in the brain and spinal cord and is now referred to as COX-3. Its antipyretic effects are mediated by inhibition of prostaglandin E2 synthesis.

Paracetamol is metabolized in the liver where 60–90% of a therapeutic dose is converted to inactive compounds by conjugation with sulfate and glucuronide.

A small portion, 5–10%, is metabolized via the CYP450 system, generating the hepatoxic metabolite NAPQ1 which is immediately inactivated by conjugation with glutathione. It is generation of excessive amounts of NAPQ1 that accounts for the dose-related hepatotoxicity of paracetamol.

In overdose (>200 mg/kg in children) the conjugation pathways are saturated and more paracetamol is shunted to the CYP450 system to produce NAPQ1. Hepatocellular supplies of glutathione become exhausted, leaving NAPQ1 free to cause acute hepatic necrosis after a delay of ~24 h.

The antidote acetylcysteine acts by supplying sulfhydryl groups, mainly in the form of glutathione, to react with the toxic NAPQ1 metabolite. The antidote should be given as soon as possible after ingestion, preferably within 8 h.

Opioid analgesics

An opioid is a chemical substance that has a morphine-like action in the body. The term comes from opium, an extract of the poppy *Papaver somniferum*, which has been used for social and medical purposes for thousands of years. Morphine was the first alkaloid isolated from opium.

Opioids act by binding to opioid receptors found in the CNS and gut. There are four main classes of opioids:

- *Endogenous opioid peptides:* β-endorphin, met-enkephalin, dynorphin
- *Opium alkaloids:* morphine, codeine
- *Semi-synthetic opioids:* diacetylmorphine (heroin)
- *Fully synthetic opioids:* pethidine, methadone.

There are 17 major classes of opioid receptor, of which 3 are of principle importance:

- *μ (mu) receptors:* responsible for most analgesic effects (μ1) and respiratory depression (μ2)
- *κ (kappa) receptors:* contribute to analgesia at the spinal level and may elicit sedation and dysphoria. Produce few unwanted effects and do not cause dependence
- *δ (delta) receptors:* more important in the periphery but may contribute to analgesia.

All opioid receptors are G-protein-coupled receptors acting on GABA-ergic neurotransmission. They also facilitate opening of potassium channels and inhibit opening of calcium channels.

Opioid analgesics are used to relieve moderate to severe pain particularly of visceral origin (e.g. vaso-occlusive sickle cell crisis, postoperative pain, palliative care). They share many side effects including nausea and vomiting, constipation, and drowsiness with respiratory depression and hypotension in larger doses.

Morphine

This remains the most valuable opioid analgesic for severe pain. In addition to relieving pain it confers a state of euphoria and mental detachment. It is available as morphine sulfate for oral use and IV infusion.

It is the opioid analgesic of choice for the oral treatment of severe pain in palliative care, given regularly every 4 h (or every 12–24 h as a modified-release preparation). Morphine should be avoided in acute respiratory depression and in raised intracranial pressure or head injury as it affects pupillary responses vital for neurological assessment.

Antiepilepsy drugs (AEDs)

Valproate or carbamazepine are the first line AEDs of choice for the majority of common childhood epilepsies, and benzodiazepines are important for the acute control of status epilepticus. There are in addition a host of new AEDs available such as lamotrigine, topiramate, vigabatrin, and levetiracetam.

Control of epilepsy with a single AED (monotherapy) is preferred, but combination therapy with two or more may be necessary. The latter is complicated by drug interactions which may enhance toxicity. Interactions are usually caused by hepatic enzyme induction or inhibition.

The mechanism of action of many AEDs is uncertain and complex, although all must alter the balance between excitatory and inhibitory influences within the brain.

Two mechanisms are well established: blocking of neuronal sodium channels by carbamazepine, phenytoin, and lamotrigine (see Fig 20.2) and enhancement of GABAergic inhibition by benzodiazepines.

Valproate

Valproate is a fatty acid, 2-propylpentanoic acid, and is used either as the acid or its sodium salt, sodium valproate. It is effective for generalized epilepsies including idiopathic generalized, absence, and myoclonic epilepsies.

Side effects include liver toxicity, increased appetite and weight gain, transient hair loss, pancreatitis, and blood dyscrasias.

Liver dysfunction (including fatal hepatic failure) has occurred in association with valproate, especially in children <3 years of age; those with metabolic or degenerative disorders, organic brain diseases, or severe seizure disorders associated with learning difficulties; and in those on multiple AEDs. It usually occurs in the 1st 6 months of therapy. Liver function should be monitored in the 1st 6 months especially in children most at risk.

Valproate is teratogenic, causing congenital anomalies in ~5% of pregnant users. Its use should generally be avoided in children <2 years, overweight patients, and females of child-bearing age.

Carbamazepine

Carbamazepine stabilizes neuronal sodium channels in the inactivated state, thereby rendering brain cells less excitable. The same mechanism acting on sodium channels in peripheral nerves explains its efficacy in trigeminal neuralgia and neuropathic pain.

Carbamazepine is the drug of choice for partial seizures and for tonic-clonic seizures secondary to a focal discharge. It can exacerbate myoclonic and absence seizures. It is essential to initiate carbamazepine therapy at a low dose and build up slowly in increments every 2 weeks.

Common side effects include drowsiness and motor incoordination. Less common side effects include double vision, bone marrow depression, and cardiac arrhythmias.

Benzodiazepines

Benzodiazepines have anxiolytic, hypnotic, muscle relaxant, antiepileptic, and amnesic actions. They act by enhancement of activity at $GABA_A$ receptors. Important benzodiazepines in paediatric practice include diazepam, lorazepam, and midazolam. They are active orally and metabolized by hepatic oxidation although they are not hepatic enzyme inducers.

Diazepam remains an important drug for the control of convulsive status epilepticus, although lorazepam (IV) and midazolam (buccal) are useful alternatives. Diazepam is highly lipid soluble and is widely distributed throughout the body after administration. Respiratory depression is the most important side effect of its use in the acute control of convulsive seizures.

Newer AEDs

Lamotrigine

Lamotrigine is used for partial seizures and primary and secondarily generalized tonic-clonic seizures. It is also used for seizures in Lennox–Gastaut syndrome. It is licensed for monotherapy in children >12 years and as combination therapy in children >2 years.

Valproate increases plasma lamotrigine concentrations.

Side effects include serious skin reactions (Stevens–Johnson syndrome).

Topiramate

Topiramate is licensed as monotherapy in children >6 years with newly diagnosed epilepsy with generalized tonic-clonic seizures, or partial seizures with or without secondarily generalized seizures. It is licensed as combination therapy for children >2 years who are inadequately controlled on first-line AEDs and who have partial seizures with or without secondarily generalized seizures or Lennox–Gastaut syndrome.

Vigabatrin

Indications for vigabatrin are limited to adjunctive use only when all other appropriate AED combinations have proved ineffective or poorly tolerated. This is because one third of adults treated with vigabatrin have developed visual field defects which may be severe.

Vigabatrin has been used as monotherapy in the treatment of infantile spasms (West syndrome) as an alternative to steroids.

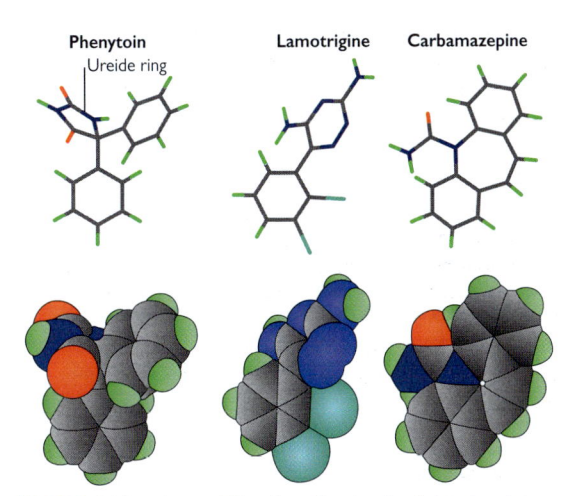

Fig 20.2 Stick and space-filling views showing the diphenyl moiety (ureide ring) common to three sodium channel blocking AEDs: phenytoin, lamotrigine, and carbamazepine.

20.6 Antibiotics

Drugs used for treatment of infection (antimicrobials) are categorized according to the nature of the pathogen into:
- Antibiotics (antibacterials)
- Antifungals
- Antivirals
- Antiprotozoals
- Anthelminitics.

Antibiotics

The term 'antibiotic' was originally used for drugs that kill or prevent the growth of bacteria and which were derived from living organisms in contrast to synthetic agents. It now encompasses all antibacterial drugs regardless of origin.

Antibiotic prescribing

Choosing a suitable antibiotic regimen requires consideration of:
- *The child*: age, ethnic origin, history of allergy, renal and hepatic function, whether immunocompromised
- *The organism*: the likely organism and its sensitivity.

Before starting antibiotic therapy the following considerations are good practice:
- *Is an antibiotic necessary?* probable viral infections should not be treated with antibiotics but they are helpful for controlling secondary bacterial infection (e.g. acute necrotizing ulcerative gingivitis secondary to herpes simplex stomatitis)
- *Microbiological samples*: should if possible be taken for culture and sensitivity testing. Blind prescribing for unexplained pyrexia is best avoided
- *Prevalent organisms*: knowledge of these and their sensitivities should be taken into account
- *Dose*: should be adjusted according to severity of infection. Use of a 'standard' dose in serious infections may not be adequate
- *Route of administration*: depends on severity of infection. Life-threatening infections require IV therapy
- *Local guidelines*: should be followed.

The duration of treatment should be the minimum required for effective treatment. If the patient's clinical condition is improving a change in antibiotics is generally not required, but the diagnosis and choice of antibiotic should be reviewed after 72 h if there has been no improvement. Prolonged treatment is necessary for certain infections such as tuberculosis or osteomyelitis.

Mechanisms of action

Antibacterials have three principal modes of action:
- *Inhibition of cell wall synthesis*: penicillins and cephalosporins
- *Inhibition of protein synthesis*: macrolides and aminoglycosides
- *Inhibition of DNA synthesis*: trimethoprim and quinolones.

Antibiotic resistance

This may be innate or acquired.
- *Innate resistance*: refers to an innate characteristic of the bacteria. Gram-negative bacteria possess an outer phospholipid membrane that confers resistance to certain penicillins
- *Acquired resistance*: antibiotic usage, especially broad-spectrum antibiotics, acts as an environmental selective pressure favouring resistant strains. Biochemical mechanisms include:
  - production of enzymes: e.g. β-lactamase
- alteration of drug binding sites: e.g. alteration of ribosome structure leading to erythromycin resistance.

Penicillins

The penicillins act by interfering with bacterial cell wall synthesis. They are bactericidal and diffuse well into body tissues and fluids with the exception of cerebrospinal fluid (CSF). Penetration into CSF is poor except when the meninges are inflamed.

Penicillins include:
- Benzylpenicillin and phenoxymethyl penicillin
- *Penicillinase-resistant penicillins*: flucloxacillin
- *Broad-spectrum penicillins*: ampicillin, amoxicillin, co-amoxiclav
- *Antipseudomonal penicillins*: piperacillin, ticarcillin
- *Mecillinams*: pivmecillinam.

The most important side effect of penicillins is hypersensitivity, which causes rashes or anaphylaxis and can be fatal. Allergic reactions occur in 1–10% of patients but anaphylaxis in fewer than 1/2000 (0.05%). There is cross-sensitivity to all penicillins and cephalosphorins.

Children with a history of a minor rash (local, non-confluent) or a rash occurring >72 h after administration are probably not allergic, and penicillin should not be withheld for a serious infection if there is no alternative.

Benzylpenicillin and phenoxymethylpenicillin

Benzylpenicillin (penicillin G) remains an important and useful antibiotic for susceptible infections (throat infections, otitis media, pneumonia, cellulitis) but is inactivated by bacterial β-lactamase and by gastric acid.

Phenoxymethylpenicillin (penicillin V) is gastric acid stable so suitable for oral administration. It is indicated principally for upper respiratory tract infections in children and for prophylaxis against streptococcal infections following rheumatic fever, after splenectomy, or in sickle cell disease.

Penicillinase-resistant penicillins

Flucloxacillin is effective in infections caused by *Staphylocci*, most of which now produce pencillinase.
- *Indications*: include cellulitis, osteomyelitis, acute endocarditis, and prophylaxis in cystic fibrosis.

It should be used with caution in patients with hepatic impairment. Cholestatic jaundice and hepatitis can occur up to several weeks after treatment.

Broad spectrum penicillins

Ampicillin and amoxicillin

These antibiotics are active against gram-positive and gram-negative bacilli but are inactivated by penicillinases. Amoxicillin is better absorbed by mouth, producing higher plasma and tissue concentrations. Ampicillin is also active against *Listeria* spp. and enterococci.
- *Indications*: the treatment of community-acquired pneumonia and middle ear infections, urinary tract infections, endocarditis, and *Listeria* meningitis.

Maculopapular rashes are common with both antibiotics and are not usually a reflection of true penicillin allergy. They are common in glandular fever and in children with lymphocytic leukaemia or cytomegalovirus infection.

Co-amoxiclav
This consists of a mixture of amoxicillin and clavulanic acid, a β-lactamase inhibitor which renders the combination active against β-lactamase-producing strains resistant to amoxicillin including resistant strains of *Staph. aureus, E. coli,* and *H. influenzae* as well as many *Bacteroides* and *Klebsiella* spp. The proportions are expressed in the form x/y (e.g 125/31) where x and y are the amounts in milligrams of amoxicillin and clavulanic acid respectively.

Antipseudomonal penicillins
These antibiotics are used mainly for the empirical treatment of septicaemia in immunocompromised children. For *Pseudomonas* septicaemia, they are given with an aminoglycoside since the two act synergistically.

Ticarcillin
Ticarcillin is active against *Pseudomonas aeruginosa* and has activity against other gram-negative bacilli including *Proteus* spp. and *Bacteroides fragilis*. It is available only in combination with clavulanic acid. The combination (timentin) is active against β-lactamase-producing bacteria.

Piperacillin
Piperacillin is more active than ticarcillin against *Pseudomonas aeruginosa* and is available in combination with the β-lactamase inhibitor tazobactam (as tazocin). The spectrum of activity of tazocin and timentin is comparable to that of the carbapenems, imipenem and meropenem.

Cephalosporins

Cephalosporins are broad-spectrum β-lactam containing antibiotics. They are bactericidal and have the same mechanism of action as penicillins: disruption of the peptidoglycan layer of bacterial cell walls. They are used for the treatment of septicaemia, pneumonia, meningitis, peritonitis, and urinary tract infections.

Cephalosporins are grouped into 'generations' by their antimicrobial properties. Each newer generation has greater activity against gram-negative organisms, in most cases with decreased activity against gram-positive organisms.

The main side effect is hypersensitivity and about 10% of penicillin-sensitive patients will be allergic to the cephalosporins. Their broad spectrum can encourage superinfection with resistant bacteria or fungi.

- *First generation:* cefalexin is orally active and useful for urinary tract and respiratory tract infections
- *Second generation:* cefuroxime is usually given IV and is useful for pneumonias and urinary tract infections
- *Third generation:* ceftriaxone has a longer half-life and can be given once daily. Indications include severe infections such as septicaemia, pneumonia, and meningitis. It is contraindicated in neonates with jaundice, hypoalbuminaemia, or acidosis as it may displace unconjugated bilirubin from albumin Ceftazidime has good activity against *Pseudomonas* and other gram-negative bacteria.

Sulphonamides and trimethoprim

These act by inhibition of nucleic acid synthesis. Sulphonamides have largely been replaced by more active and less toxic antibiotics. However, sulphamethoxazole and trimethoprim in combination (as co-trimoxazole) is synergistic and is the drug of choice in *Pneumocystis* pneumonitis. It is also indicated for toxoplasmosis.

Trimethoprim can be used alone for urinary and respiratory tract infections and for shigellosis and invasive salmonella.

Macrolides

These inhibit protein synthesis by binding to the ribosome. They are bacteriostatic at usual doses, but bactericidal in high concentrations. The antibacterial spectrum is similar to, but slightly wider than the penicillins. Macrolides are therefore a common substitute in patients with a penicillin allergy. However, unlike penicillins, macrolides are effective against *Mycoplasma, Mycobacteria,* and some *Chlamydia* and *Rickettsia*.

Macrolides include erythromycin, clarithromycin, and azithromycin.

- *Indications*: an alternative to penicillin in allergic patients, respiratory tract infections especially if *Mycoplasma pneumonia* infection suspected, otitis media, skin and soft tissue infections
- *Side effects:* include GI upset (nausea, vomiting, and diarrhoea). Erythromycin is a motilin agonist and its use in the perinatal period has been associated with an increased incidence of pyloric stenosis.

Clarithromycin has slightly greater activity than erythromycin and is given twice daily. Azithromycin has slightly less activity than erythromycin against gram-positive bacteria but enhanced activity against some gram-negative organisms including *H. influenzae*. It has a long tissue half-life and once-daily dosage is recommended. Both these derivatives cause fewer GI side effects than erythromycin.

Aminoglycosides

Aminoglycosides inhibit protein synthesis by binding to bacterial ribosomal subunits, causing misreading of mRNA. They must be given by injection. Excretion is renal. All are bactericidal against some gram-positive and many gram-negative organisms including *Pseudomonas, Acinetobacter,* and *Enterobacter*.

Examples include gentamicin, amikacin, neomycin, netilmicin, streptomycin, and tobramycin.

The most common usage of aminoglycosides is empiric therapy for serious infections such as septicaemia or complicated intra-abdominal or urinary tract infections. They are used in conjunction with β-lactam antibiotics in streptococcal infections for their synergistic effects, especially in neonates. Streptomycin was the first effective treatment for tuberculosis.

Side effects are dose related and include ototoxicity and nephrotoxicity. The interval between doses must be increased in children with renal impairment. Serum concentration monitoring is necessary to avoid toxicity and ensure efficacy. Samples are taken 1 h after IM or IV injection (peak level) and just before the next dose (trough level).

Quinolones

Quinolones inhibit bacterial DNA synthesis by binding to DNA gyrase.

- *Nalidixic acid:* is only used for urinary tract infection resistant to other antibiotics in children >3 months of age.
- *Ciprofloxacin:* has moderate activity against gram-positive bacteria but is particularly active against gram-negative bacteria including *Salmonella, Shigella, Campylobacter, Neisseria,* and *Pseudomonas*. It is also active against *Chlamydia* and some *Mycobacteria* but not most anaerobes.

Ciprofloxacin is licensed for pseudomonas infections in cystic fibrosis (in children >5 years). Other unlicensed uses in children include treatment of typhoid fever and prophylaxis of meningococcal disease.

20.7 Antifungals, antivirals, and antiprotozoals

Antifungal drugs
Fungal infections, or mycoses, can be divided into superficial (affecting skin, nails, scalp, or mucous membranes) and systemic (affecting deeper tissue and organs). The latter are more common in immunocompromised patients.
Three main groups of fungi cause human disease:
- *Moulds:* filamentous fungi such as the *dermatophytes* and *Aspergillus fumigatus*
- *True yeasts:* unicellular fungi, e.g. *Cryptococcus neoformans*
- *Yeast-like fungi:* similar to yeast but may form long, non-branching filaments, e.g. *Candida albicans*.

Antifungal drugs include the following main groups:
- *Polyene antifungals:* amphotericin, nystatin
- *Azoles:*
  - *imidazoles:* clotrimazole, ketoconazole, miconazole
  - *triazoles:* fluconazole, itraconazole, voriconazole
- *Echinocandins:* caspofungin
- *Other:* flucytosine, griseofulvin.

Amphotericin
Amphotericin is a macrolide antibiotic of complex structure active against most fungi and yeasts.

It is given by IV infusion, is highly protein bound and has poor tissue penetration. Oral absorption is poor but it can be used for intestinal candidiasis. When given parentally amphotericin is toxic (nephrotoxicity) and side effects are common. Lipid formulations are available which are less toxic and licensed for use in children.

Nystatin and miconazole
Nystatin is useful for the treatment of oral candidiasis in infants. Miconazole is used for the prevention and treatment of oral and intestinal fungal infections.

Antiviral drugs
Specific antiviral drugs are now available for viral infections and are of particular value in the immunocompromised. These antiviral drugs act by a variety of mechanisms (see Table 20.2). Antivirals are available for:
- HIV infection
- Herpesvirus infections
- Viral hepatitis
- Influenza
- Respiratory syncytial virus.

HIV infection
There is no cure for HIV infection. Treatment is aimed at suppressing viral infection for as long as possible and should be started before the immune system is irreversibly damaged. Drug treatment for HIV disease in children is undertaken by specialists within a formal paediatric HIV clinical network (see Chapter 15.6).

Antiretroviral drugs for paediatric use include:
- *Nucleoside reverse transcriptase inhibitors (NRTIs):* abacavir, lamivudine, didanosine, stavudine, combivir, tenofovir, zalcitabine, zidovudine (AZT)
- *Non-nucleoside reverse transcriptase inhibitors (NNRTIs):* efavirenz, nevirapina
- *Protease inhibitors (PIs):* lopinavir–ritonavir, nelfinavir, amprenavir, ritonavir.

Metabolic effects associated with antiretroviral treatment (ART) include fat redistribution, insulin resistance, and dyslipidaemia, collectively termed the *lipodystrophy syndrome*. It is particularly associated with regimens including protease inhibitors.

- *NRTIs:* should be used with caution in children with hepatitis B or C and in hepatic or renal impairment. Life-threatening lactic acidosis with hepatomegaly and hepatic steatosis has been reported with NRTIs.
- *PIs:* associated with hyperglycaemia and should be used with caution in diabetes, hepatic impairment and haemophilia.

Herpesvirus infections
Aciclovir

Aciclovir is a guanosine derivative which inhibits viral DNA polymerases. It must first be converted to the monophosphate by thymidine kinase which occurs most effectively by the virus specific enzyme. Phosphorylation is therefore limited primarily to infected cells. Host cell kinases then convert the monophosphate to the triphosphate that inhibits viral DNA polymerase.

Aciclovir is active against herpesvirus, but does not eradicate them. It can be given orally, IV, or topically. It is indicated for systemic treatment of varicella zoster in immunocompromised hosts and the systemic and topical treatment of herpes simplex infections of the skin, mouth, and eye. Unwanted effects are minimal. Extravasation during IV infusion can cause local inflammation.

Ganciclovir

This is related to aciclovir but it more active against cytomegalovirus (CMV) and much more toxic. It is indicated for life-threatening or sight-threatening CMV infections in immunocompromised patients only.

Viral hepatitis
Treatment for viral hepatitis should be initiated by a specialist. Management of uncomplicated acute viral hepatitis is largely symptomatic. Interferon alfa, peginterferon alfa, and oral ribavirin are used in the treatment of chronic hepatitis C in adults, but experience in children is limited.

Influenza
Vaccination remains the most effective way of preventing illness from influenza viruses. Oseltamivir and zanamivir reduce replication of influenza A and B viruses by inhibiting viral neuraminidase. This prevents new viruses from emerging from infected cells. They are most effective for treatment of influenza if started within a few hours of onset of symptoms and are licensed for use within 48 h of the first symptoms.

Table 20.2. Antivirals: mechanisms of action	
Inhibition of penetration of host cells	Amantadine, immunoglobulins
Inhibition of host-cell exit	Zanamivir, Oseltamivir
Inhibition of nucleic acid synthesis	
Viral DNA polymerase inhibitors:	Aciclovir, ganciclovir
Reverse transcriptase inhibitors:	Nucleoside-Zidovudine, Non-nucleoside-Nevirapin, efavirenz
Protease inhibitors	Amprenavir, atazanovir
Immunomodulators	Interferon alfa

In children 13–18 years, oseltamivir is also licensed for prophylaxis when used within 48 h of exposure to influenza and when influenza is circulating in the community and in exceptional circumstances to prevent influenza in an epidemic.

The effect of these drugs on hospitalization or mortality is not clear in those at risk of serious complications (chronic respiratory disease, cardiovascular disease, immunosuppression). Oseltamivir has been used in the treatment of H5N1 avian influenza ('bird flu') but higher doses and longer duration of treatment are required. It was widely used during the H5N1 avian influenza epidemic in South-East Asia in 2005. Concerns exist that oseltamivir may cause psychological side effects including delirium, hallucinations, and unusual behaviour in some children and teenagers.

Respiratory syncytial virus

- *Palivizumab*: a monoclonal antibody for the prevention of respiratory syncytial virus infection in infants at high risk during the infections season. This includes infants <6 months born at <35 weeks gestation, children <2 years treated in the last 6 months for chronic lung disease, and children <2 years with significant heart disease.
- *Ribavirin*: a synthetic nucleoside which interferes with synthesis of viral mRNA and inhibits a wide range of DNA and RNA viruses. It is licensed for treatment of severe bronchiolitis caused by RSV in infants but there is no clear evidence that it produces clinically relevant benefit.

Antiprotozoal drugs

These encompass antimalarials (Table 20.3), amoebicides, trichomonacides, anti-giardial drugs, leishmaniacides, trypanocides, drugs for toxoplasmosis and for pneumocystis pneumonia.

Antimalarials

Recommendations for the prophylaxis and treatment of malaria reflect guidelines by UK malaria specialists, and specialist advice should be sought.

Table 20.3. Antimalarials

Class	Examples
Quinolines	
Aminoquinolines	Chloroquine, primaquine
Methanolquinolines	Quinine, mefloquine
Naphthalenes	Atovaquone
Biguanides	Proguanil
Diaminopyridines	Pyrimethamine
Artemisinin group	Artemisinin, artemether
Others	Lumefantrine

Most antimalarials are toxic to the erythrocyte schizonts. Proguanil and pyrimethamine are effective schizonticides but act too slowly to be useful in acute attacks. Rapidly acting schizonticides include chloroquine but in most areas of the world *P. falciparum* is resistant to this drug. Quinine, mefloquine, malarone (proguanil with atoraquone), or riamet (artemisinin with lumefantrine) are used orally to treat *P. falciparum* infections. A course of quinine is complemented by a dose of fansidar (pyrimethamine with sulfadoxine) as an adjunct.

Quinine

Quinine is extracted from the bark of the South American cinchona tree and was isolated and named by French researchers in 1817. Before that the bark was first dried, ground to a fine powder, and mixed with liquid (wine usually) for oral administration. A Jesuit brother, originally trained as an apothecary, observed the Quechua Indians of Peru using the bark to treat shivering and sent a small quantity to Rome where it was first tested for treating malaria in 1631.

Quinine is used for the treatment of *P. falciparum* malaria, or if the infective species is not known, or the infection is mixed. Quinine is a very basic compound and always used as a salt. Quinine sulfate is the most common oral preparation and quinine hydrochloride is used for IV infusion. Quinine is not licensed for IM or PR use in the UK.

Oral quinine is not well tolerated: it tastes very bitter and may cause vomiting.

- *Side effects*: include *cinchonism* (tinnitus, headache, visual disturbance) but this is usually mild.

Quinine IV can cause cardiac arrhythmias and hypoglycaemia. Blood glucose and electrolytes should be monitored. It causes haemolysis in G6PD deficiency.

Quinine provides the flavour in tonic water, bitter lemon, and vermouth: the gin and tonic cocktail was invented when British colonials in India mixed their antimalarial quinine with gin to disguise the bitter taste.

20.8 Endocrine system

Drugs used in diabetes mellitus

- *Type 1 diabetes mellitus (T1DM)*, or insulin dependent diabetes mellitus (IDDM), is due to a deficiency in insulin following autoimmune destruction of pancreatic β cells.
- *Type 2 diabetes (T2DM)*, or non-insulin dependent diabetes mellitus (NIDDM), is caused by a combination of reduced insulin secretion and peripheral resistance to the action of insulin. The incidence of T2DM in children is increasing.

Insulins

Insulin is a 51 amino acid polypeptide arranged in two chains linked by disulfide bridges. All children with T1DM require insulin. There are differences in amino acid sequence between animal (pork, beef), human and human insulin analogues. Insulin is usually given by SC injection. There are three main types of insulin preparation:

- *Short acting:* soluble insulins have rapid onset (30–60 min), peak action at 2–4 h, and duration of action of up to 8 h
- *Intermediate acting:* have onset of action at 1–2 h, maximum effect at 4–12 h, and duration of 16–35 h, e.g. isophane insulin, insulin zinc suspension
- *Long acting:* have times of onset, peak and duration at the higher end of the intermediate range, e.g. insulin detemir and insulin glargine (Fig 20.3).

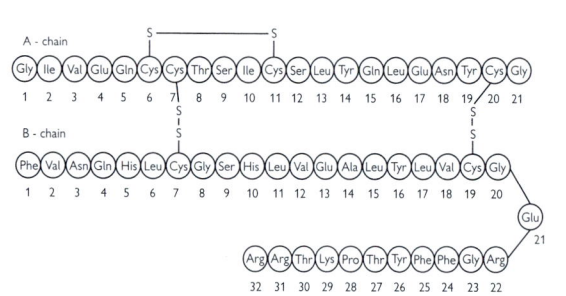

Fig 20.3 Insulin glargine. Asparigine at position A21 is replaced by glycine and two arginines are added to the C-terminus of the B-chain. This human insulin analog is soluble at pH 4 but has low solubility at neutral pH. After SC injection the acidic solution is neutralized with formation of microprecipitates from which insulin glargine is slowly released.

Insulin regimens

Most prepubertal children require ~0.6–0.8 units/kg per day. Initiation of insulin may be followed by a partial remission phase (honeymoon period) when insulin requirements fall. During puberty up to 1.5–2 units/kg per day may be required, especially during growth spurts. Higher than average requirements may reflect a very sedentary life style, poor compliance, or poor absorption from injection sites (e.g. due to lipohypertrophy).

A multiple injection regimen is commonly used: either soluble insulin or a rapid-acting insulin before meals and a long-acting insulin (e.g. insulin glargine) at bedtime.

Short-acting insulins can also be given by continuous subcutaneous infusion using a portable infusion pump. A pump may be appropriate for children who have recurrent hypoglycaemia or marked morning hyperglycaemia despite optimized multiple-injection regimens. High motivation, careful monitoring, and expert training, advice, and supervision is necessary for children on SC insulin infusion.

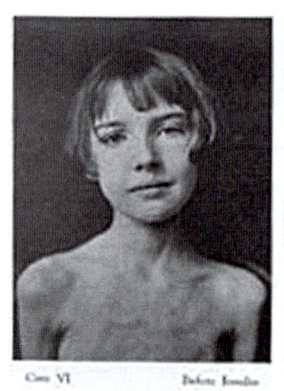

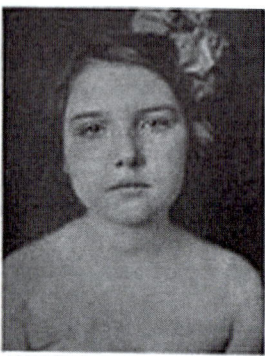

Fig 20.4 The miracle of insulin: before and after insulin treatment of a T1DM patient after its discovery in 1922.

Oral antidiabetic agents

Oral antidiabetic agents are used in the treatment of T2DM to augment the effects of diet and exercise, not to replace them. They include sulphonylureas (e.g. tolbutamide), biguanides (e.g. metformin), and others (e.g. acarbose).

Metformin is the drug of first choice in children in whom dieting has failed, as there is most experience with this drug in children. Metformin uncommonly causes hypoglycaemia and there is a lower incidence of weight gain. GI side effects are common. It may provoke lactic acidosis especially in children with renal impairment, in whom it is contraindicated.

Thyroid and antithyroid drugs

Thyroid hormones

The thyroid gland secretes two iodinated hormones:
- Tri-iodothyronine (T3)
- Thyroxine (levothyroxine, tetra-iodothronine) (T4).

Their release is controlled by thyrotropin (TSH). Both hormones act on receptors in the plasma membrane, mitochondria, and nucleus.

Thyroid hormones are used in juvenile hypothyroidism, diffuse non-toxic goitre, Hashimoto thyroiditis and congenital or neonatal hypothyroidism. Levothyroxine sodium is the treatment of choice for maintenance therapy. In severe hypothyroid states, including hypothyroid coma, liothyronine sodium provides a more rapid response, because it is less protein bound.

Antithyroid drugs

Antithyroid drugs are thionamides that competitively inhibit the reactions necessary for iodine organification. Onset of action is delayed (3–4 weeks) until preformed hormones are depleted.

Antithyroid drugs are used to prepare children for thyroidectomy or for long-term management of hyperthyroidism. Carbimazole is most commonly used. Its most important side effect is bone marrow suppression with neutropaenia and agranulocytosis. Children and their carers should be asked to report symptoms and signs suggestive of infection, especially sore throat.

Corticosteroids

The adrenal cortex secretes two main classes of steroid hormones:
- *Glucocorticoids:* hydrocortisone (cortisol)
- *Mineralocorticoids:* aldosterone.

Glucocorticoids diffuse into target cells and bind to a cytoplasmic glucocorticoid receptor. The receptor–hormone complex enters the nucleus and binds to steroid response elements on target DNA molecules, causing induction or repression of expression of specific genes.

In deficiency states, physiological replacement is best achieved by a combination of hydrocortisone and fludrocortisone. Hydrocortisone alone does not provide sufficient mineralocorticoid activity. However, the mineralocorticoid activity of cortisone and hydrocortisone makes them unsuitable for long-term therapeutic use as anti-inflammatory agents. Synthetic corticosteroids (e.g. prednisolone) are used for this purpose.

Replacement therapy

In Addison disease or following adrenalectomy, hydrocortisone by mouth is given in 2–3 divided doses. A higher dose is given in the morning and a lower dose in the evening to simulate the normal diurnal rhythm of cortisol secretion. Glucocorticoid therapy is supplemented by fludrocortisone. In acute adrenocortical insufficiency hydrocortisone is given IV.

In congenital adrenal hyperplasia hydrocortisone is used to suppress corticotropin, adjusting the dose according to clinical response and measurement of adrenal androgens and 17-hydroxyprogesterone. Salt-losing forms require mineralocorticoid replacement as well.

Glucocorticoid therapy

Synthetic glucocorticoids used for therapy rather than as hormone replacement include prednisolone, betamethasone, dexamethasone, and methylprednisone. Potency, duration of activity, and extent of mineralocorticoid activity varies. Steroids may be given systemically or locally in a wide range of conditions. Examples of the use of corticosteroids include:
- *Oral prednisolone:*
  - acute asthma
  - nephrotic syndrome
  - *autoimmune disorders:* juvenile idiopathic arthritis, systemic lupus erythematosus, autoimmune hepatitis
  - inflammatory bowel disease
  - epilepsy (e.g. infantile spasms)
  - acute leukaemia
- *Oral dexamethasone:* croup, raised intracranial pressure
- *IV hydrocortisone:* acute anaphylaxis, acute asthma
- *Topical hydrocortisone:* atopic eczema
- *Inhaled steroids:* chronic asthma.

Adverse effects of corticosteroids

Whenever possible local treatment (topical, intra-articular injection, inhalation, eye-drops, enemas) is preferable to systemic treatment, the side effects are listed in Table 20.4.

Table 20.4. Adverse effects of corticosteroids

Growth suppression	
Mineralocorticoid effects	Hypertension, sodium and water retention, potassium loss
Glucocorticoid effects	Diabetes, osteoporosis, psychosis, muscle wasting
Cushing's syndrome	moon face, striae, acne
Adrenal suppression	
Immunosuppression	increased susceptibility and atypical course of infections. Children who have not had chickenpox are at risk of fulminant, severe disease
Cataracts	

Every patient prescribed a systemic corticosteroid should receive the patient information leaflet supplied by the manufacturer and where appropriate a steroid treatment card. Gradual withdrawal of systemic corticosteroids is necessary in patients who have received >3 weeks of treatment.

Hypothalamic and pituitary hormones

Anterior pituitary hormones

Tetracosactide (tetracosactrin)

This analogue of corticotropin (ACTH) is used to test adrenocortical function. Failure of plasma cortisol concentration to rise after administration of tetracosactide indicates insufficiency. It should be used with caution in patients with allergic disorders, e.g. asthma, as there is a risk of anaphylaxis.

Growth hormone

Growth hormone is used to treat:
- Growth hormone deficiency
- Gonadal dysgenesis (Turner syndrome)
- Prader–Willi syndrome
- Chronic renal insufficiency (before puberty).

It can also be used (unlicensed) for Noonan syndrome and idiopathic short stature under specialist management. Synthetic human growth hormone, somatropin, produced by recombinant DNA technology has replaced growth hormone of human origin (somatotrophin).

Posterior pituitary hormones

Arginine vasopressin (antidiuretic hormone, ADH), and its analogue desmopressin, is used in the treatment of pituitary diabetes insipidus. Desmopressin is more potent and has a longer duration of action than vasopressin, and has no vasoconstrictor effect. Desmopressin can be given intranasally, orally, or by injection. Other uses include:
- *Vasopressin:* adjunct in acute massive haemorrhage of GI tract or oesophageal varices
- *Desmopressin:* indications include
  - investigation of suspected diabetes insipidus.
  - primary nocturnal enuresis (if urine-concentrating ability normal).
  - mild to moderate haemophilia and Von Willebrand disease.

20.9 Malignancy, immunosuppression, and blood

Cytotoxic drugs

In the UK, cytotoxic drugs are almost always administered to children in the context of a formal protocol in a specialist regional centre or shared care unit. These protocols are developed by the UK Children's Cancer Study Group (UKCCSG) together with other national and international organizations.

Cytotoxic anticancer drugs are classified according to their mechanism of action into:

- *Alkylating drugs:* prevent cell division by cross-linking DNA
- *Cytotoxic antibiotics:* block RNA production or degrade DNA by forming free radicals
- *Antimetabolites:* inhibit purine or pyrimidine synthesis
- *Vinca alkaloids:* inhibit mitosis by binding to microtubular proteins.

Cytotoxic drugs are toxic to both tumour cells and proliferating normal cells especially in the bone marrow, GI epithelium, and hair follicles. Side-effects common to most cytotoxic drugs therefore include:

- Extravasation causing local tissue irritation and necrosis
- Oral mucositis and secondary *Candida* infection
- Nausea and vomiting—may be acute, delayed, or anticipatory
- Bone-marrow suppression (exceptions are vincristine and bleomycin)
- Alopecia
- Thromboembolism.

Alkylating drugs

Examples include chlorambucil, cyclophosphamide, ifosfamide, and melphalan. Specific problems associated with these drugs include:

- Adverse effect on gametogenesis: most males sterile with prolonged use
- Increase in incidence of secondary tumours and leukaemia
- Fluid retention and hyponatraemia in young children
- Urothelial toxicity with haemorrhagic cystitis.

Chlorambucil is used in Hodgkin disease, cyclophosphamide in a wide range of malignancies including acute lymphoblastic leukaemia and Wilms tumour, ifosfamide in rhabdomyosarcoma and Ewing tumour.

Cytotoxic antibiotics

Examples include bleomycin, daunorubicin, and doxorubicin. Simultaneous use of radiotherapy should be avoided as toxicity is enhanced. The anthracycline antibiotics (daunorubicin, doxorubicin) are associated with cardiac toxicity which may be either idiosyncratic and reversible or related to total cumulative dose and irreversible. Cardiac function should be monitored before and at regular intervals throughout treatment.

Antimetabolites

These include methotrexate, cytarabine, and mercaptopurine.

- *Methotrexate* inhibits the enzyme dihydrofolate reductase, essential for the synthesis of purines and pyrimidines. It is given orally, IV, IM, or intrathecally. It is contra-indicated in significant renal or hepatic impairment. Methotrexate causes myelosuppression, mucositis, and (rarely) pneumonitis.
- *Cytarabine* interferes with pyrimidine synthesis and is a potent myelosuppressant.
- *Mercaptopurine* is used in maintenance therapy for acute lymphoblastic leukaemia and also in the management of inflammatory bowel disease (azathioprine is metabolized to mercaptopurine).

Vinca alkaloids

- *Vincristine* is used in the treatment of acute leukaemia, lymphomas and some paediatric solid tumours
- *Vinblastine* is used in treatment of Hodgkin disease and other lymphomas.

Neurotoxicity, usually as a peripheral or autonomic neuropathy, occurs with all vinca alkaloids and is a limiting side effect of vincristine. Vinblastine is less neurotoxic but causes more myelosuppression (vincristine causes negligible myelosuppression). Vinca alkaloids may cause reversible alopecia, and constipation is common.

Vinblastine and vincristine are for IV administration only.

Intrathecal administration is usually fatal. In the UK, a Health Service Circular (HSC 2003/010) provides guidance on safe practice for administration of intrathecal chemotherapy. This includes provision of a designated area for provision of intrathecal chemotherapy, a register of personnel trained to prescribe and administer intrathecal chemotherapy and labelling of vinca alkaloids: '*For IV use only—FATAL if given by other routes*'.

Other neoplastic drugs

Etoposide

This is used to treat acute leukaemias, lymphomas, and some solid tumours. It is usually given by slow IV infusion; concentrated infusions are associated with anaphylaxis and rapid infusions with hypotension.

Platinum compounds

Cisplatin and its derivative carboplatin are used in the treatment of a variety of paediatric malignancies. They interfere with mitosis by cross-linking DNA.

- *Cisplatin* is used in osteogenic sarcoma, stage IV neuroblastoma, some liver tumours, and infant brain tumours. Dose-related side effects include nephrotoxicity, neurotoxicity, and ototoxicity. Intensive IV hydration is required to control potential hypokalaemia and hypomagnesaemia. It causes severe nausea and vomiting.
- *Carboplatin* is used in a wide variety of solid tumours. It is much better tolerated than cisplatin and can be given IV in an outpatient setting. Nausea and vomiting are less severe and toxicity less of a problem. It is, however, more myelosuppressive than cisplatin.

Drugs affecting the immune response

Immunosuppressants are used to suppress rejection in organ transplant recipients and to treat a number of chronic inflammatory and autoimmune diseases. They include antiproliferative immunosuppressants, corticosteroids, calcineurin inhibitors, monoclonal antibodies, and interferon alfa.

Antiproliferative immunosuppressants

Aziathioprine is widely used for transplant recipients and in autoimmune conditions, usually when corticosteroids alone prove inadequate. Blood tests and monitoring for signs of myelosuppression are essential in long-term treatment. The risk of myelosuppression is increased in those with low activity of the enzyme thiopurine methyltransferase (TPMT) which metabolizes azathioprine. It is a prodrug, metabolized in the body to the active metabolite 6-mercaptopurine.

Mycophenolate mofetil is increasingly used in organ transplantation as it is associated with less bone marrow suppression, fewer opportunistic infections, and a lower incidence of acute rejection.

Calcineurin inhibitors

Ciclosporin is a fungal peptide composed of 11 amino acids. It binds to the cytosolic protein cyclophilin (immunophilin) of immunocompetent lymphocytes, forming a complex which inhibits calcineurin, responsible for activating the transcription of interleukin-2 (IL-2).

It is a potent immunosuppressant, virtually non-myelotoxic, but markedly nephrotoxic. It is used for prevention of organ rejection in transplantation and has been used in the treatment of nephrotic syndrome, inflammatory bowel disease, severe psoriasis, and severe eczema. Hypertrichosis is a notable side effect.

Tacrolimus (FK-506), a macrolide lactose discovered in a soil fungus in Japan, has a similar mode of action and side effects. It is used after liver transplantation and a topical preparation is available for severe atopic eczema.

Monoclonal antibodies

Basiliximab and the similar daclizumab are chimeric mouse–human monoclonal antibodies to the IL-2Rα receptor of T cells. By saturating the receptor they prevent T cell activation and proliferation and are used for prophylaxis of acute rejection in allogeneic renal transplantation. Their use is confined to specialist centres.

Rituximab and alemtuzamab are monoclonal antibodies which cause lysis of B lymphocytes. Rituximab is used in the treatment of aggressive lymphomas and severe cases of resistant immune-modulated disease including haemolytic anaemia, SLE, and refractory rheumatoid disease. Infusion-related side effects including cytokine release syndrome are common and occur predominantly during the first infusion. Alemtuzamab is used in the treatment of chronic lymphocytic leukaemia and T-cell lymphoma, and in some conditioning regimens for bone marrow and renal transplantation.

Interferon alfa

Interferon alfa (available as alfa-2a or alfa-2b) may have a role in inducing early regression of life-threatening corticosteroid-resistant haemangiomas of infancy. Interferon alfa preparations are also used in treatment of chronic hepatitis B and C, usually in combination with ribavirin. Side effects include myelosuppression and depression.

Anaemias and neutropaenias

It is essential to determine the aetiology before initiating treatment. Iron salts, for example, may be harmful if iron deficiency is not the cause of the anaemia.

Iron-deficiency anaemia

Prophylaxis is justifiable in individuals with risk factors for iron deficiency, e.g. preterm infants and those with malabsorption. Ferrous salts of iron are better absorbed than ferric salts. Choice of preparation is determined by formulation, palatability, incidence of side effects, and cost.

The dose of elemental iron to treat deficiency is 3–6 mg/kg per day. The dose should be specified in terms of elemental iron and iron salt (see Table 20.5)

Table 20.5. Iron content of different iron salts

Iron salt	Dose	Ferrous iron content
Ferrous sulfate	300 mg	60 mg
Ferrous gluconate	300 mg	35 mg
Ferrous fumarate	200 mg	65 mg
Sodium feredetate	190 mg	27.5 mg

Prophylactic iron supplementation of elemental iron 5 mg daily may be required in babies of low birthweight who are solely breast-fed. It is started 4–6 weeks after birth and continued until mixed feeding is established.

Iron salts may cause GI irritation and may be associated with constipation. Accidental overdose is potentially life threatening: as little as 20–30 mg/kg of elemental iron can be fatal.

Renal anaemias

Erythropoietin is a glycoprotein hormone produced by the kidney which regulates red blood cell production.

Epoietin, recombinant human erythropoietin, is used for the treatment of anaemia associated with chronic renal failure. Other contributing factors such as iron or folate deficiency should be corrected first. Epoitin alfa and beta are clinically indistinguishable. Epoitin beta is also used for the prevention of anaemia in preterm infants.

Neutropaenia

Granulocyte colony stimulating factor (G-CSF) is a glycoprotein cytokine produced by a number of different tissues (endothelium, macrophages) which stimulates the bone marrow to produce granulocytes and stem cells. The natural human glycoprotein exists in two isoforms, the 174 amino acid protein being more abundant and more active.

Recombinant human granulocyte-colony stimulating factor (rhG-CSF) is available in two varieties:

- *Filgrastim*: synthesized in *E .coli*, it differs slightly from the natural human sequence and is unglycosylated
- *Lenograstim*: synthesized in Chinese hamster ovary (CHO) cells it is glycosylated and identical to the natural human 174 amino acid isoform.

Most studies have been done with filgrastim, but there are no comparative studies. Indications have included cytotoxic-induced neutropaenia, severe congenital neutropaenia and neonatal neutropaenia. Side effects include hypersensitivity reactions and pulmonary infiltrates.

20.10 Nutrition

Oral nutrition

Foods for special diets
These encompass foods that have been modified to eliminate a particular constituent or nutrient mixtures formulated as a substitute. Certain of these foods share the characteristics of drugs and are termed 'borderline substances'. In the UK, the Advisory Committee on Borderline Substances advises on which substances can be regarded as drugs and therefore prescribed. A list is found in Appendix 2 of the BNFC.

Enteral nutrition
Enteral tube feeding has a role in both short- and long-term nutritional management in paediatrics. It may be used as primary therapy, in which the enteral feed derives all necessary nutrients or as a supplement to oral feeds. Most children receiving tube feeds should be encouraged to take oral food and drink.

A number of nutritionally complete foods are available, most containing protein from milk or soya. Those containing protein hydrolysates or free amino acids are only appropriate for patients unable to digest protein. Extra minerals may be required if GI secretions are being lost, and additional vitamins may also be needed.

Complete enteral feeds

- *Child 0–12 months:* term infants with normal GI function are given either breast milk or normal formula during the 1st year. If weight gain is inadequate, energy intake may be increased by supplementing or concentrating the feed but care is required to avoid an excessive osmotic load which may cause diarrhoea. Average intake 150–200 mL/kg per day.
- *Child 1–6 years (8–20 kg):* nutritionally complete, ready to use feeds based on caseinates, maltodextrin, and vegetable oils (with or without added medium-chain triglyceride oil or fibre) are available. Energy content may be 0.75 kcal/mL, 1.0 kcal/mL, or 1.5 kcal/mL. They contain residual lactose. Administered at a rate of 85–115 mL/kg per day.
- *Child 7–12 years:* feeds are available at 1.0 kcal/mL and 1.5 kcal/mL, also based on caseinates, maltodextrin, and vegetable oils (with or without fibre). Depending on clinical condition and nutritional requirements they are given at a rate of 50–70 mL/kg per day.
- *Child 13 years and over:* adult formulations used.

Feed thickeners
Carob-based thickeners may be used for children <1 year and starched-based thickeners for children >1 year of age. Pre-thickened formula is a casein-based formula containing small quantities of pre-gelatinized starch: the feeds only thicken when exposed to acid pH in the stomach.

Vitamins
Vitamins are defined as essential nutrients which the body cannot synthesize on its own and must therefore be obtained from the diet. The exceptions to this rule are vitamin D, which can be synthesized in the skin, and vitamin B3 (niacin) which is synthesized in small amounts in the liver from tryptophan.

The identification and biochemical characterization of the 13 human vitamins was a triumph of early 20th century biochemistry and medicine. By convention, letters of the alphabet were assigned sequentially followed by numbers (B1, B2, etc.), but many of the factors discovered later proved not to be vitamins, hence the gap between E and K and the missing B numbers (4, 8, 10, 11).

The 13 human vitamins are classified into:
- *4 fat-soluble vitamins:* A, D, E, K
- *9 water-soluble vitamin:* C and eight B vitamins.

Vitamin deficiencies may be primary, due to inadequate intake, or secondary, due to an underlying disorder such as liver disease. Storage of individual vitamins varies widely, influencing the duration of dietary deficiency necessary to induce a deficiency condition. Vitamins A, D, and B12 are generally stored in significant amounts.

Dietary reference values for vitamins are available. The use of vitamins as general 'pick-me-ups' is of no proven value, and excessive intake of certain vitamins is harmful, especially vitamin A and vitamin D.

Vitamin A
Vitamin A exists in several forms, including an alcohol (retinol), an aldehyde (retinal), and an acid (retinoic acid). The animal form, retinol, is a fat-soluble, antioxidant important in vision and immune function.

Deficiency is associated with xerophthalmia and increased susceptibility to infection. It is rare in the UK, but children with cholestatic liver disease are at risk and may require supplementation with monthly IM vitamin A. Preterm infants are given vitamin A as part of an oral multivitamin preparation once enteral feeding is established.

Vitamin B group
The eight water-soluble B vitamins are collectively referred to as the 'vitamin B complex' in supplements containing all eight (see Table 20.6).

Table 20.6.	B vitamins	
Vitamin	**Name**	**Deficiency disease**
B1	Thiamine	Beriberi
B2	Riboflavin	Ariboflavinosis
B3	Nicotinamide (niacinamide)	Pellagra
B5	Pantothenic acid	
B6	Pyridoxine	
B7	Biotin	
B9	Folic acid	
B12	Cyanocobalamin	Pernicious anaemia

Deficiency of the B vitamins is rare in the UK, but deficiency of B6 may occur during treatment with isoniazid or penicillamine and certain B vitamins are used in the treatment of metabolic disorders. Folic acid supplementation is important in haemolytic anaemias and is recommended during pregnancy.

Vitamin B: thiamine
Deficiency causes beriberi. It is used in the treatment of maple syrup urine disease and congenital lactic acidosis.

Vitamin B3: niacin (niacinamide)
Vitamin B3 encompasses niacin (also known as nicotinic acid) and the corresponding amide, niacinamide (nicotinamide).

The liver synthesizes niacin in small amounts from tryptophan. Dietary deficiency causes pellagra and occurs in areas where corn is the staple diet. Niacin has been used for the treatment of dyslipidaemias.

Vitamin B6: pyridoxine
Vitamin B6 deficiency is characterized by peripheral neuritis and may complicate isoniazid therapy or penicillamine treatment. Oral pyridoxine is used for prophylaxis or treatment. High doses of pyridoxine are also given in hyperoxaluria, cystathioninuria, and homocystinuria. Rare patients with onset of seizures in the neonatal period or early infancy respond to pyridoxine treatment.

Vitamin C: ascorbic acid
Vitamin C or L-ascorbate is an essential nutrient for higher primates and guinea pigs; most animals and plants synthesise their own vitamin C. It acts as an electron donor for eight enzymes, three of which participate in collagen hydroxylation and are essential for its triple helical structure. The other enzymes are involved in synthesis of carnitine, noradrenaline, and peptide hormones and in tyrosine metabolism.

Scurvy is caused by prolonged deficiency of vitamin C intake, resulting in defective collagen synthesis with defective formation of osteoid matrix and fragile blood vessels. It is now extremely uncommon in the paediatric population, but may occur in children with severely restricted diets attributable to psychiatric or developmental problems. Infantile scurvy (Barlow disease) was common in the 1950s until formula milks were fortified with vitamin C. Scurvy is sometimes included in the differential diagnosis of infants with unexplained bruising and fractures, as an alternative explanation to inflicted injury.

Ascorbic acid is also used to enhance excretion of iron 1 month after starting desferrioxamine therapy and in certain metabolic disorders (tyrosinaemia type III, transient tyrosinaemia of the newborn, and glutathione synthase deficiency).

Vitamin D
The term vitamin D is used for a range of compounds:
- *Vitamin D1:* molecular compound of ergocalciferol and lumisterol
- *Vitamin D2:* ergocalciferol (calciferol), derived from plant sources
- *Vitamin D3:* colecalciferol, derived from animal sources and synthesized in the skin from 7-dehydrocholesterol. It is hydroxylated in the kidney and liver to its active forms:
  - *calcidiol:* 1α-hydroxycolecalciferol (alfacalcidol)
  - *calcitriol:* 1, 25-dihydroxycolecalciferol.

Synthesis and function of vitamin D
Colecalciferol (vitamin D3) is produced photochemically from 7-dehydrocholesterol in the epidermal layer of the skin, specifically in the stratum basale and stratum spinale. This requires UV light at wavelengths of 270–290 nm. Melanin reduces UVB penetration and reduces the efficiency of synthesis. Natural sources of vitamin D are very limited but include fish oils, fatty fish, and eggs.

Calcitriol acts as a hormone, mediating its biological effects via the vitamin D receptor (VDR). VDR activation in intestine, bone, kidney, and parathyroid glands leads to regulation of calcium and phosphorus levels in the blood and maintenance of bone content. Vitamin D also appears to have a role in immunomodulation.

In childhood, deficiency of vitamin D causes rickets. Nutritional deficiency is uncommon, but infants from certain ethnic groups are at risk especially if breast-fed. The amount of vitamin D in breast milk is low and breast-fed babies, particularly if preterm, born to vitamin-D-deficient mothers or with high skin melanin content may become deficient. Most formula milks contain adequate vitamin D.

Simple vitamin D deficiency can be prevented by oral supplementation of 200–400 units of ergocalciferol (vitamin D2). Nutritional deficiency is treated with ergocalciferol (or colecalciferol) 3000–10 000 units daily depending on age. Deficiency caused by malabsorption or chronic liver disease requires pharmacological doses of ergocalciferol (or colecalciferol) up to 1 mg (40 000 units) daily.

Alfacalcidol or calcitriol are used for patients with severe renal or cholestatic liver disease, persistent neonatal hypocalcaemia, or vitamin D dependent rickets.

Vitamin E: tocopherols
Natural vitamin E exists in eight different isomers: four tocopherols and four toctrienols. α-Tocopherol is the most active form of vitamin E in humans and is a powerful antioxidant. Daily requirements are not well defined.

Vitamin E supplements are indicated in children with fat malabsorption including those with cystic fibrosis and cholestatic liver disease. Very low birthweight infants may be deficient in vitamin E and some neonatal units administer a single IM dose of vitamin E to preterm neonates at birth.

Vitamin K
Vitamin K is the group name for a cluster of naphthoquinone derivatives, including:
- *Vitamin K1:* phytomenadione, phylloquinone
- *Vitamin K2:* menaquinone.

Its biological function is in the carboxylation of glutamate to γ-glutamyl carboxylase (Gla) in a number of so-called Gla proteins. These include several blood coagulation factors (II, VII, IX, and X) and two proteins involved in the calcification of bone, osteocalcin, and matrix Gla protein.

Vitamin K deficiency leads to a haemorrhagic tendency and occurs in patients with fat malabsorption. Neonates are relatively deficient in vitamin K and in the UK it is recommended that all newborn infants receive vitamin K to prevent vitamin K deficiency bleeding. Vitamin K (as phytomenadione) 1 mg may be given as a single IM injection at birth, and this is recommended for all newborns especially those at particular risk (birth asphyxia, mothers with liver disease). Alternatively, in healthy babies, vitamin K may be given orally. A water-soluble preparation, menadiol sodium phosphate, is used in patients with fat malabsorption, especially if due to hepatic disease.

20.11 Fluids and electrolytes

Oral preparations
Oral rehydration therapy (ORT) using a variety of oral rehydration solutions (ORS) is of central importance in saving the lives of millions of children with diarrhoeal disease. Sodium and potassium salts may also be given by mouth to prevent or treat specific deficiencies, and oral bicarbonate may be required for the treatment of metabolic acidosis.

Oral rehydration solutions (ORS)
Oral rehydration therapy is indicated in the treatment of gastroenteritis, especially in infants in whom there is a risk of rapid and severe dehydration. Glucose (or other carbohydrates such as rice starch) is included to enhance intestinal absorption of salt and water.

Oral rehydration solutions used in the UK are lower in sodium concentration (50–60 mmol/L: 75 mmol/L) and higher in glucose concentration (90 mmol/L: 75 mmol/L) than those formulated by the WHO.

Oral sodium and water
Oral supplements of sodium chloride may be required in states of sodium depletion, e.g. preterm neonates in the 1st weeks of life, salt-losing bowel or renal disease, children with cystic fibrosis especially in warm weather. The requirement is generally 1–2 mmol/kg daily in divided doses.

Oral potassium
Oral supplements of potassium chloride may be necessary in the following situations:
- Chronic diarrhoea causing potassium loss in the faeces
- Secondary hyperaldosteronism e.g. renal artery stenosis, nephritic syndrome
- Long term corticosteroid treatment
- Patients taking digoxin or other anti-arrhythmic drugs in whom potassium depletion may cause arrhythmias.

Potassium salts cause nausea and vomiting and poor compliance is a limitation. Small divided doses minimize gastric irritation, but where appropriate potassium-sparing diuretics are preferable, e.g. in patients on loop diuretics.

Oral bicarbonate
Sodium bicarbonate is given by mouth for chronic acidotic states such as uraemic acidosis or renal tubular acidosis. It may affect the stability or absorption of other drugs and if possible 1–2 h should be allowed before other drugs are administered orally. In hyperchloraemic acidosis associated with potassium deficiency it may be appropriate to give oral potassium bicarbonate.

Intravenous fluids

Electrolytes and water
Solutions of electrolytes in water, sometimes termed crystalloids, are given IV to meet normal requirements or replenish deficits or continuing losses when it is not desirable or possible to use the enteral route. Fluids can also be administered SC or via the intraosseous route.

A variety of fluids are available (see Table 20.8) which contain different concentrations and mixtures of sodium chloride and glucose (as dextrose). In addition there are special solutions such as Hartmann (Ringer–lactate) which also contains sodium lactate, potassium chloride, and calcium chloride. A critical feature of an IV fluid is its osmolality (compared to plasma) and its tonicity (with reference to cell membranes).

Osmolarity and tonicity—what's the difference?
- *Osmolarity* is a measure of the osmotically active particles in a solution, independent of any membrane.
- *Tonicity* is a measure of the effective osmolality or osmolarity of a solution with reference to a membrane which is impermeable to some or all of the particles. In practice tonicity is defined in reference to a cell membrane by comparing the tonicity of the solution with that inside the cell.

Dextrose (D-glucose) is rapidly metabolized and although it contributes to the osmolarity of the infused solution it does not contribute to tonicity after infusion.

Plasma osmolarity is determined by the concentration of sodium, chloride, potassium, urea, and glucose in the blood. The main contributor is sodium and chloride, the concentrations of which are vastly higher than those of the other substances. Normal plasma osmolarity is 280–300 mOsmol/L.

Sodium chloride 0.9%, with a sodium and chloride content of 154 mmol/L each and osmolarity 308 mOsmol/L, is isosmolar (with plasma) and isotonic (with reference to the cell membrane). Glucose 5% has an osmolarity of 278 mOsmol/L and is isosmolar (with plasma) but is hypotonic, because the dextrose is rapidly metabolized leaving free water.

Maintenance fluid requirements
These are determined by bodyweight because of the relationship between body weight and metabolic rate. The volumes required beyond the neonatal period are shown in Table 20.7.

Table 20.7. Maintenance fluid requirements per 24 h in infants and children >1 month of age

Bodyweight (kg)	Fluid requirement per 24h
<3	150 mL/kg
3–10	100 mL/kg
10–20	1000 mL
	plus
	50 mL/kg for each kg >10kg
>20	1500 mL
	plus
	20 mL/kg for each kg >20kg

Maintenance requirements are usually met by using a standard solution of sodium chloride and glucose. Dilutional hyponatraemia is a risk with fluids such as sodium chloride 0.18% with dextrose 4%, especially in the postoperative period, and this is not recommended for maintenance fluids. Most children can be safely administered sodium chloride 0.45% or 0.9% with glucose 5% or 2.5% (there is currently little evidence to recommend a particular strength of glucose).

Sodium chloride 0.45% contains more than the maintenance requirement of sodium chloride (7.5 mmol/kg per 24 h if given at 100 mL/kg per 24 h) whereas 0.18% sodium chloride contains the usual maintenance requirement (3.1 mmol/kg per 24 h if given at 100 mL/kg per 24 h).

Potassium chloride is added to a concentration of 20 mmol/L to meet the usual potassium requirements, but adjustments may be needed if there is abnormal renal function or continuing extrarenal losses.

Replacement fluid requirements

Intravascular volume depletion is managed using bolus doses of 10–20 mL/kg of sodium chloride 0.9%. Replacement of continuing losses from severe diarrhoea or persistent vomiting is achieved with sodium chloride 0.9% with glucose 5% and added potassium as appropriate, or Hartmann/Ringer–lactate solutions.

Plasma and plasma substitutes

Human albumin solutions (HAS)

These contain protein derived from plasma, serum, or normal placentas, 95% of which is albumin. They contain no clotting factors or blood group antibodies and may be given without regard to the recipients blood group.

Available solutions may be isotonic (HAS 4.5% or 5%), or concentrated (HAS 20%). Isotonic HAS is used in hypovolaemic shock due to septicaemia. Concentrated albumin is used in hypoalbuminaemic patients with nephrotic syndrome as an adjunct to diuretic therapy if the latter is indicated.

Hypersensitivity reactions including anaphylaxis may occur.

Plasma substitutes

Slowly metabolized macromolecular substances such as dextrans and gelatin may be used to expand and maintain blood volume in shock arising from conditions such as burns and septicaemia. They may be of value initially, but are not used to maintain plasma volume There is a risk of fluid overload and plasma substitutes are used under specialist supervision in an intensive care setting. Dextran 70 (dextrans of average MW, ~70 000) is used predominantly for short term blood volume expansion. Dextran 40 (dextrans of MW ~40 000) is used in conditions associated with poor peripheral blood flow and ischaemia disease of the limbs. Gelatin (e.g. Gelofusine) is used for hypovolaemic shock, burns, and cardiopulmonary bypass.

Minerals

Calcium

Hypocalcaemia may be caused by vitamin D deficiency or hypoparathyroidism.

Mild asymptomatic hypocalcaemia may be managed with oral calcium supplements but severe symptomatic hypocalcaemia requires an IV infusion. Persistent hypocalcaemia requires oral calcium supplements. Calcium salts are available as oral and parental preparations.

- *Oral preparations*: calcium gluconate, lactate, and carbonate preparations are available as elixirs or effervescent or chewable tablets
- *Parenteral preparations*: Calcium gluconate 10% is available (0.22 mmol/mL). For IV infusion it should be diluted but it may be given undiluted via a central line or in an emergency. Extravasation causes severe tissue necrosis and it should not be given by IM injection. A continuous infusion for 24–48 h may be required, but the oral route should be used as soon as possible due to the risks of extravasation.

Magnesium

Hypomagnesaemia is uncommon but may be associated with secondary hypocalcaemia particularly in neonates, and magnesium deficiency may occur with excessive losses of GI fluid in diarrhoea or with a stoma or fistula. Magnesium sulphate may be given by IV infusion or IM injection (painful).

Maintenance therapy can be given orally using magnesium glycerophosphate. IV magnesium sulphate is also used in acute severe asthma, persistent pulmonary hypertension, and certain severe arrhythmias, especially in the presence of hypokalaemia.

Phosphorus

Oral phosphate supplements may be required in addition to vitamin D in children with hypophosphataemic vitamin D deficiency rickets. Diarrhoea is a common side effect.

Phosphate deficiency may occur in very low-birthweight infants and may compromise bone development if not corrected. IV phosphate is used for severe hypophosphataemia.

Table 20.8. Features of commonly used IV fluids in the UK				
Solution	Osmolarity (mOsmol/L)	Sodium content (mmol/L)	Osmolarity (compared to plasma)	Tonicity (with reference to cell membrane)
Sodium chloride 0.9%	308	154	Isosmolar	Isotonic
Sodium chloride 0.45%	154	77	Hyposmolar	Hypotonic
Sodium chloride 0.45% with glucose 5%	432	75	Hyperosmolar	Hypotonic
Glucose 5%	278	–	Isosmolar	Hypotonic
Glucose 10%	555	–	Hyperosmolar	Hypotonic
Sodium chloride 0.9% with glucose 5%	586	150	Hyperosmolar	Isotonic
Sodium chloride 0.45% with glucose 2.5%	293	75	Isosmolar	Hypotonic
Sodium chloride 0.18% with glucose 4%	284	31	Isosmolar	Hypotonic
Hartmann's solution	278	131	Isosmolar	Isotonic
4.5% human albumin solution	275	100–160	Isosmolar	Isotonic

20.12 Case-based discussions

A newborn with dehydration

A male infant age 9 days is referred to the hospital emergency department on account of lethargy and weight loss. He was a full-term normal delivery at home to a primiparous mother with no perinatal problems. He is breast-fed with no history of vomiting but has been reluctant to feed for 48 h and stool frequency had fallen. Seen once on day 6 by the community midwife, no concerns were noted. Birthweight was 3500 g.

On examination, the infant is crying and active. Markedly icteric. Temperature 37.5 °C Weight 2975 g. Normal skin turgor. Abdomen soft with no organomegaly. No murmurs. Normal tone. Fontanelle normal.

What is the differential diagnosis?

The loss of 15% bodyweight in a breast-fed but apparently well infant suggests a diagnosis of breast-feeding associated dehydration with hypernatraemia. In most cases the mother is primiparous. Infants with hypernatraemic dehydration have better-preserved extracellular volume and therefore often have less-pronounced clinical signs of dehydration. Clinical examination is therefore very variable. Jaundice is the most common presentation. Sepsis is an important differential.

Investigation results:
Na 158 mmol/L
K 6.0 mmol/L
Urea 12.0 mmol/L Creatinine 14 μmol/L
Bilirubin 220 μmol/L, conjugated 12 μmol/L
Glucose 5.0 mmol/L
Hb 20 g/dL, WCC 12.0×10^9/L, Neut 6.0×10^9/L
Platelets 450×10^9/L
CRP 1.0 mg/L

What is the further management?

The results confirm the suspected diagnosis. Initial treatment depends on clinical condition and degree of hypernatraemia. The hypernatraemia has developed slowly and must be corrected slowly.

Oral rehydration can be tried with expressed breast milk and additional formula milk. Alternatively, IV fluids such as 0.45% NaCl/ 4% dextrose can be given at a rate not exceeding 100 mL/kg per 24 h, aiming to correct the deficit over 48 h.

After 3 days of slow oral rehydration his sodium returned to normal and he gained weight. He was discharged home with a feeding plan and close follow-up was arranged with the health visitor and paediatrician.

What do you know about this condition?

The incidence is ~2.5/10 000 live births. A majority are born to primiparous mothers and presentation is at ~10 days (range 3–21 days).

It is thought to be secondary to lactation failure. The infant becomes dehydrated while the kidneys are mature enough to retain sodium ions. High sodium concentrations in the breast milk may be contributory.

Weight loss (>10% in the 1st week) and inadequate stooling are sensitive indicators of dehydration. Other points include feeding frequency and length, adequacy of milk flow, and frequency of urination. As in this case presentation is often with either jaundice or symptoms consistent with sepsis, such as fever and lethargy.

The most important complication is seizures which are more likely at sodium concentrations >165 mmol/L. Seizures may be caused by hypernatraemia or by the too rapid correction of hypernatraemia during treatment.

Less common serious complications include cavernous sinus thrombosis, permanent brain damage, disseminated intravascular coagulation, and acute renal failure. Deaths have been reported.

Chapter 21
Statistics and evidence-based medicine

21.1 Statistics: describing data and testing confidence *450*
21.2 Statistics: differences, relationships, risk, and odds *452*
21.3 Statistics: clinical test analysis and study design *454*
21.4 Evidence-based medicine (EBM) *456*
21.5 EBM: critical appraisal and implementation *458*
21.6 Critical appraisal exercise *460*

21.1 Statistics: describing data and testing confidence

Statistics is the science of collecting, organizing and analysing data from populations. It is based on:
- *Statistical theory:* a branch of applied mathematics concerned with the collection and interpretation of quantitative data
- *Probability theory:* used to estimate parameters and analyse relationships between variables.

A *population* is a large number of items (e.g. patients, subjects) each carrying an attribute which is studied to generate data (e.g. blood group, blood pressure). A sample of the population is studied and assumed to be random and therefore representative. The attribute which goes with each item is the *variate* of the population.

Describing data

Data is either
- *Qualitative* (categorical)
- *Quantitative* (non-categorical).

Qualitative data can be *nominal* or *ordinal*, and quantitative data can be *continuous* or *discrete* (interval). Examples are shown in Table 21.1.

Table 21.1. Types of data		
Qualitative		
Nominal	Gender, Eye colour	Binary if 2 variables
Ordinal	Satisfaction rating, pain scales	>2 categories; numerical but not continuous
Quantitative		
Continuous	Heart rate, BP, blood sugar	Can take any value
Interval/discrete	Number of antibiotic courses, age ranges	Set range of values

Measures of centre
- *Mean:* the sum of values divided by the number of values
- *Median*: the central value of the data series when the values are lined up in order of magnitude. Half the values will be above and half below the median
- *Mode*: the most frequently observed value in the data series. It is not always representative of the true central value.

Measures of spread
Frequency histogram
A frequency histogram is commonly presented. The symmetrical, bell-shape shown by this distribution, and by the line joining the bars, is known as the *normal* (or Gaussian) distribution (Fig 21.1A).

In a normal distribution, the mean, median, and mode are the same value and lie at the midpoint of the curve.

If the curve looks asymmetrical it is said to be *skewed*. The skew is described in the direction of the tail, so a longer tail to the right means the data is positively skewed, and to the left means the data is negatively skewed.
- *Range*: the difference between the largest and smallest value. It does not allow assessment of the values between the ranges but relies on the extreme data values.
- *Percentile* or *centile*: the value below which a certain percentage of values fall. The value at the 50th percentile means that half the data is above and half below that value.
- *Interquartile range:* usually describes the data which fall between the 25th and 75th percentile.

Standard deviation (SD)
This is a measure of the spread of values about the mean. Subtracting the mean from all values gives the deviations, but they are both positive and negative. More useful is the variance which is the average of the squared differences between each value and the mean The SD is the square root of the variance.

The SD can therefore be defined as the root mean square deviation of the values from their arithmetic mean. If the data points are all close to the mean, then the SD is close to zero. SD should only be used when the data has a normal distribution

The exact percentage of values that lie within defined intervals can be expressed, if the data has a normal distribution.

These are worth learning, and are shown in Fig 21.1B.
- ± 1 SD includes 68.27%
- ± 2 SD includes 95.45%
- ± 3 SD includes 99.73%

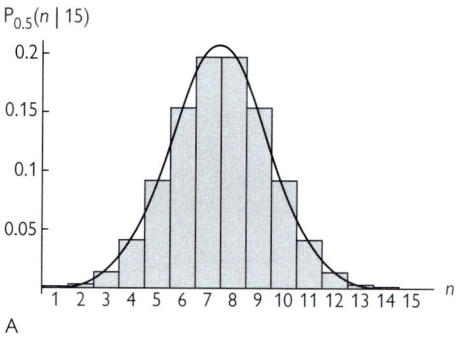

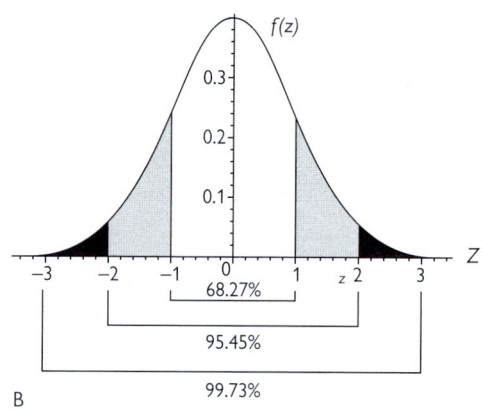

Fig 21.1 A. Normal (Gaussian) distribution. B. Standard deviation (SD) intervals.

Standard error of the mean (SEM)
It is clearly impossible to sample a whole population. Population statistics are therefore inferred from an estimate from a sample

population. The means of several sample populations will cluster around the true population mean, but will only ever approximate it. The *standard error of the mean* (SEM) describes how likely it is that a single sample mean estimates the true population mean. Contrast this with the standard deviation, which quantifies the scatter of the data.

$$SEM = SD/\sqrt{n}$$

Therefore as the sample size (n) increases, the standard error of the mean decreases, i.e. the estimation of the true mean becomes more accurate.

Testing confidence

Tyep 1 and type 2 errors

In order to decide the significance of a result or value, a hypothesis is constructed: the *null hypothesis*. This assumes that there is no (i.e. null) difference between groups, or no effect in the intervention being compared, i.e. that any difference is simply a result of chance. A significance test is chosen according to the type of data being analysed.

- *Type 1 error (false positive):* rejection of the null hypothesis when it is true (i.e. assuming that there is a difference between data sets when in fact there is not)
- *Type 2 error (false negative):* Accepting the null hypothesis when it is not true (i.e. assuming that there is no difference when there is one).

P-values

Once the null hypothesis is described, we can then calculate the probability of it being true. This is the P-value, and takes a value between 0 and 1.

The smaller the value (nearer to 0) the less likely the null hypothesis is to be true, suggesting that there is likely to be a difference between groups or as a result of the intervention under study. The value never is actually zero so we never totally disprove the hypothesis.

If the P-value is large, nearer to 1, we can say the sample is consistent with the null hypothesis, in other words that it is likely that no difference exists between the groups.

- *P = 0.05:* means that the probability of the difference having happened by chance is 1 in 20 or 5%. By convention this is frequently quoted as '*statistically significant*'
- *P = 0.01:* means that the difference will only have happened by chance 1 in 100 times or 1%. This is considered to be '*highly significant*'
- *P = 0.001:* means that the difference will have happened by chance 1 in 1000 times and is usually considered to be '*very highly significant*'.

However, a clinical context is always required for useful interpretation. Statistical significance is not the same as clinical relevance or significance. A large study may find a statistically significant difference that is too small to have any clinical relevance. A small study may fail to find a statistically significant result for a real and clinically relevant effect.

Confidence intervals (CI)

The confidence interval (CI) is a range of values in which we are fairly confident the true population value lies.

A confidence interval therefore gives an estimated range (interval) of values which is likely, with a defined degree of confidence, to include an unknown population parameter. It is usually reported as 95% CI: we can be 95% confident that the population value lies within those limits.

The range is estimated from a set of sample data, and the range refers to the 'true' value in the population. The confidence limits are the lower and upper boundaries which define the range, and the confidence level is the associated probability value, usually expressed as a percentage.

A confidence level of 95% is usually calculated (±1.96 SD includes 95% of the data). The interval width is an indicator of the degree of uncertainty about the unknown parameter.

A CI may be calculated for a mean value or for the difference between two means. If the latter interval includes zero we can say that there is no significant difference between the means of the two populations, at a given level of confidence. A CI can be calculated for the result of almost all statistical tests (Fig 21.2).

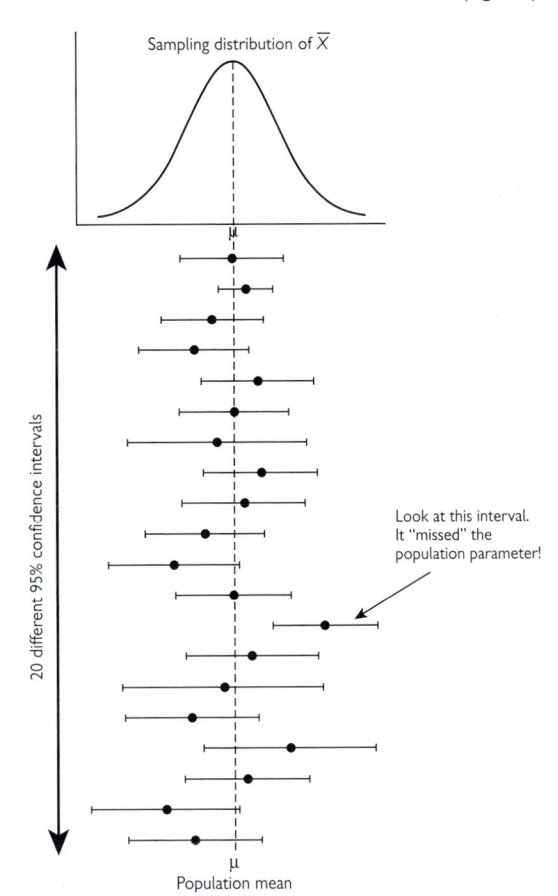

Fig 21.2 A sampling distribution of the mean based on all possible samples of size 100 and an illustration of the 95% CI for 20 possible samples. The means and intervals differ because they are different samples of different size. The CI includes the true population mean with 95% confidence. 1 out of 20 (5%) fails to capture the true mean. Reproduced courtesy of Burke Johnson.

Sample size and power

The *power* of a study is the probability that it will allow detection of a statistically significant difference, and is usually expressed as a percentage.

It is possible to predict the *sample size* that is needed to achieve a desired power. This calculation uses the standard deviation and a constant value obtained by describing the desired acceptable level of significance (P-value) for the study. Power can be increased by increasing the duration of the study or the precision used to detect outcomes.

21.2 Statistics: differences, relationships, risk, and odds

Testing differences
Two types of test, parametric and non-parametric, are used to compare estimates of sample means or proportions.
- *Parametric tests:* used to compare data which is normally distributed.
- *Non-parametric tests:* used for non-normally distributed data.

Some non-normally distributed data sets are 'transformed' prior to application of some of the tests of statistical significance. This usually involves taking the logarithm of the data, and enables it to fit into a normal distribution and be analysed using a parametric test.

Parametric tests
Student's t-test
This is typically used to compare just two samples and test the probability that the samples come from a population with the same mean value. A P-value will be given which can be interpreted as described above to prove or reject the null hypothesis of no difference between the groups.

The t-test may be paired or unpaired. A paired test is used when samples in the two groups are paired to each other, e.g. pre-and post-intervention results from the same group of patients.

Chi-squared (χ^2)
This test is a measure of the difference between the actual and expected frequencies (proportions or percentages).

The null hypothesis is that there is no difference between the sets of results, so the closer the value is to 0, the more probable it is that the null hypothesis is true. A corresponding P-value is provided. The χ^2 value is calculated based on the number of values in the data set (known as *degrees of freedom*). This affects the P-value.

Fisher's exact test is a better choice for analysis of contingency tables, particularly if the numbers are small. A contingency table shows the observed frequencies of data elements classified according to two variables, with the rows indicating one variable and the columns indicating the other variable.

ANOVA (analysis of variance)
This is a set of techniques used to compare the means of more than two samples. They can also allow for independent variables which may affect the outcome.

Non-parametric tests
Mann–Whitney U test, Wilcoxon rank sum test
These tests are used when the data is not normally distributed. In order to compare the values, the raw data is ranked and the ranking is then compared. When data takes the same rank, the average ranks for these values are taken. P-values are obtained allowing interpretation of the statistical significance of the test.

Analysing relationships
Correlation
Correlation exists if there is a linear relationship between two variables, e.g. height and weight in children.
The strength of the relationship is denoted by the Pearson correlation coefficient, denoted by *r*.
- A *positive* correlation means that as one variable increases the other also increases in value. If plotted, the graph slopes up from left to right (Fig 21.3).
- A *negative* correlation means that as the value of one variable increases the other decreases. The graph slopes down from left to right.

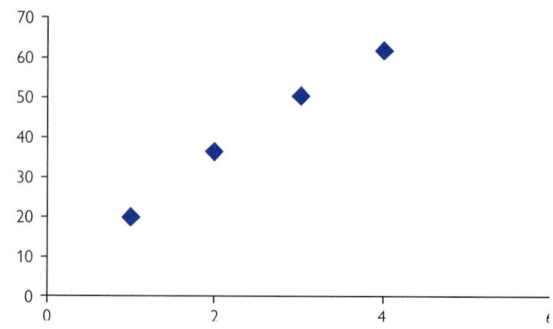

Fig 21.3 Positive correlation.

The value of *r*, whether positive or negative, lies between 0 and 1: 0 implies no correlation and +1 or −1 represents perfect positive or negative correlation.

Different values have different implications for the strength of the relationship (see Box), but cannot imply cause and effect.

Correlation and its implications

r value	Strength of relationship
0.0–0.2	Very weak, probably meaningless
0.2–0.4	Low, might warrant investigation
0.4–0.6	Reasonable
0.6–0.8	Strong
0.8–1.0	Very strong

The same values for strength of relationship apply to negative correlations. A P-value may be provided.

As with all statistical tests, the correlation must be interpreted according to the clinical context.

For normal distributions a Pearson correlation coefficient is calculated. For non-normal distributions, the Spearman correlation coefficient is used.

Causality
Association tells you nothing about causality. Meaningless associations abound, e.g. stork populations and human birth rate.
The following questions should be posed before causality can be proposed (Bradford Hill criteria):
- Is there a strong, specific and consistent association?
- Does the association make epidemiological and biological sense?
- Does the postulated cause precede the postulated effect?
- Is there a dose–response gradient?
- Is there supporting experimental evidence in humans?

Regression
Regression analysis is used to find how one set of data relates to another.

Linear regression is used to describe and predict the relationship where one data set (*y*) changes dependently and predictably with the other one (*x*).

The equation representing how *y* changes with any given change of *x* can be used to construct a straight line on a scatter plot. The regression line is the 'best fit' line through the data points on a graph (Fig 21.4). The regression line is given by the equation:

$$y = mx + c$$

where *c* is the *regression constant,* i.e. the value where the line intercepts the *y* axis, and *m* is the *regression coefficient,* i.e. the slope of the line, representing a positive or negative correlation.

This can be used to predict what value *y* may take for a given value of *x* (since *m* is the amount by which *y* changes, and *c* adds the difference when *y* is not at the baseline).

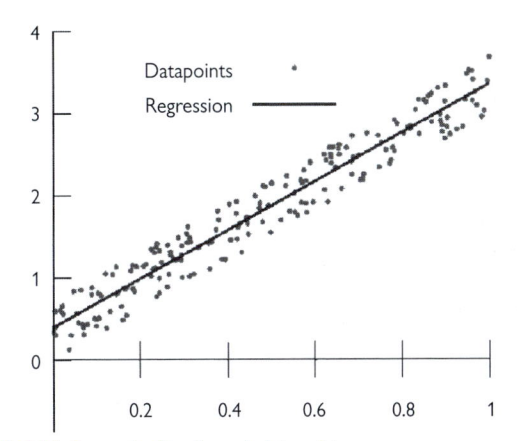

Fig 21.4 Regression line through data points.

Other types of regression include logistic regression (each case in the sample can only belong to one of two groups) and Poisson regression.

Correlation and regression are easily confused:
- Correlation measures the *strength* of the association between variables.
- Regression *quantifies* the association and should only be used if one of the variables is thought to precede or cause the other.

Risk and odds

Definitions

Risk is the probability that an event *will* happen.

As one boy is born for every two births, the risk (probability) of giving birth to a boy is 1/2 or 0.50.

If one in every 100 patients suffers a side effect from a treatment the risk is 1/100 or 0.01.

Odds are calculated by dividing the number of times an event happens by the number of times it does not happen. For every two births, one boy is born and one boy is not born. The odds of giving birth to a boy are 1/1 = 1, or 50:50.

If one in every 100 patients suffers a side effect from a treatment the odds are 1/99 or 0.0101

Odds and risk give similar values for rare events but may be very different for common events.

Absolute risk is a basic, non-comparative measure of risk equivalent to incidence. Incidence is usually expressed as the number of new cases of a condition over a given time (the rate) as a percentage of the population.

Risk and odds ratios

The *risk ratio* or *relative risk* is the risk of an event in the treated or exposed group (EER) divided by that in the control or unexposed group (CER).

A risk ratio of 1 indicates no difference in risk between groups. Risk ratios are often quoted with their 95% CI. This should not include 1 if the ratio is statistically significant, as 1 implies equal risk.

Measures of risk are often used in cohort studies which follow a group over a period of time to investigate the effect of a treatment or other risk factor.

- The *relative risk reduction* (RRR) is the proportion or percentage by which an intervention reduces the event rate:

  RRR = (CER − EER)/CER.

- The *absolute risk reduction* (ARR) is the difference between the event rate in the experimental group and the control group:

  ARR = CER − EER.

This is a more meaningful measure of the effect of a treatment and is the same as the *attributable risk* or the *excess risk*. ARR and RRR may be quoted as a percentage or proportion e.g. 20% or 0.20

Odds ratios are calculated by dividing the odds of having been exposed to a risk factor by the odds in a control group. An odds ratio of 1 indicates no difference in risk between the two groups. A CI should be provided. For a statistically significant ratio, the CI should not include 1.

Odds ratios are used in case-control studies.

Number needed to treat (NNT) and number needed to harm (NNH)

The *number needed to treat* (NNT) is the number of patients who need to be treated for one to gain benefit. It is the reciprocal of the ARR and is more meaningful than the RRR for assessing the efficacy of a treatment. RRR is constant regardless of risk, whereas NNT is likely to be higher in low risk groups. If the ARR is expressed as a percentage:

NNT = 100/ARR

The *number needed to harm* (NNH) is calculated in the same way to determine the number of patients treated for one to develop side effects. In this case of course the ARR is the percentage increase in deleterious events in the treated group.

21.3 Statistics: clinical test analysis and study design

Analysing clinical tests

Tests may be undertaken on patients (diagnostic) or on a population which may or may not be at increased risk of the disease (screening). In screening tests the prevalence of the disease may be low and this affects the conclusions which can be drawn from a positive or negative result.

Sensitivity and specificity

These concepts are useful in determining the value of tests for disease.

A 'two-by-two' table is produced, in which true positives and negatives are determined by the gold standard test:

Test result	Disease	
	Present	Absent
Positive	A: true positive	B: false positive
Negative	C: false negative	D: true negative

Sensitivity
Describes the proportion of patients with the disease who have a positive test, $A/(A + C)$. In other words, how likely the test is to pick up people who truly have the disease.

Specificity
Describes the proportion of patients who do not have the disease when the test is negative, $D/(B + D)$. In other words, how likely the test is to correctly identify patients without the disease.

Positive predictive value (PPV)

Describes the chance of a patient having the disease if the test is positive, $A/(A + B)$. In other words, how likely a positive test is to reflect a positive diagnosis.

This is dependent on prevalence: as prevalence increases, so does the predictive value of a positive test. Therefore, the more common a disease is, the more likely a positive test result will indicate accurately a positive disease status. This means that tests which are useful in clinical settings, where prevalence of a disease is high, may be much less useful in population screening, where prevalence of the disease is lower.

Negative predictive value (NPV)

Describes the chance of a patient being disease free if the test is negative, $D/(D + C)$. In other words, how likely a negative test is to reflect the absence of disease.

Predictive values are most relevant in a clinical setting, because the information you have available is the patient's test status, rather than their definitive disease status. A perfect test would have a high sensitivity, specificity, PPV and NPV, all of 1 (or 100%).

Likelihood ratio (LR)

This is the likelihood of obtaining a given result in a patient with the disease compared to the likelihood of that same result in a patient without the disease. (Likelihood refers to past events; probability refers to future events.) It gives a value for how much more likely the patient is to have the disease if the test is positive.

It is mainly used in the application of a diagnostic test with a known sensitivity to a target population with known prevalence of disease. The likelihood ratio incorporates both the sensitivity and specificity of the test and provides a direct estimate of how much a test result (either positive or negative) will change the odds of having a disease.

- *Likelihood ratio for positive test:* sensitivity/(1 − specificity)
- *Likelihood ratio for negative test:* (1 − sensitivity)/specificity.

Pre-test probability
This is the likelihood that a patient would have the disease in the first place. If the patient has no special risk factors, this is equivalent to *prevalence*.

Pre-test probability (prevalence) is calculated by

$$(A + C)/(A + B + C + D)$$

If the patient has particular risk factors, the pre-test probability can be adjusted for this.

Pre-test odds are the odds that the patient has the disease after the test is carried out. It is calculated by: prevalence/(1 − prevalence).

Multiplication of the pre-test odds and the likelihood ratio gives the *post-test odds*. This represents the chance that the patient actually has the disease, and factors in information about prevalence and risk factors (pre-test odds) and information about the test itself (likelihood ratio).

Study designs

Research study designs

There are a number of different study designs which researchers can use to gather their information and answer their question using statistical methods.

These include:

- Randomized controlled trials (RCTs)
- Cohort studies
- Case-control studies
- Cross-sectional surveys.

Such studies may be experimental/interventional or observational. Most quantitative studies fall within certain specific fields of research, each of which has a generally preferred study design:

- *Therapy:* RCT
- *Diagnosis:* cross-sectional survey
- *Screening:* cross-sectional survey
- *Causation:* cohort or case–control study.

Randomized controlled trials (RCTs)

RCTs are the gold standard in medical research for questions relating to interventions and are therefore mainly concerned with therapy or prevention.

Participants in the trial are randomly allocated to either one intervention (e.g. drug treatment) or another (e.g. placebo). Allocation should be concealed. The person enrolling should be unaware of which group the next patient would enter. Ideally the trial should be 'double blind', i.e. neither the participants nor the investigators know which arm the participants are in.

Advantages include:

- Rigorous evaluation of a single variable
- Prospective design avoids recall bias

- Selection and manipulation bias avoided
- Allows for meta-analysis.

There are situations when an RCT may be unnecessary or impractical, for example when a clearly successful intervention for an otherwise fatal condition is discovered (e.g. parachutes to prevent death related to gravitational challenge on exiting from aeroplanes during flight).

Cohort studies
Two or more groups of subjects are selected on the basis of their exposure or lack of exposure to a particular risk factor or agent and followed up to see how many in each group develop a particular disease or other outcome. Multiple exposures can be studied.

Disadvantages include the large numbers required for rare outcomes, and problems of drop-out bias and changes in practice during long follow-up periods. Cohort studies are used for determining the outcome of infants born prematurely.

Case–control studies
Patients with a particular disease or condition are identified and 'matched' with controls without the condition in question. Data are then collected on previous exposure to a possible causal agent. These studies are concerned with aetiology rather than treatment.

Advantages include relative ease and low cost, applicability to rare diseases and those with long latencies, and to investigation of exposures or effects which cannot be randomized.

Disadvantages include liability to bias in selection, diagnostic, and recall processes, and inability to demonstrate causality.

Clinical questions for which this design is appropriate might include whether prone sleeping reduces the risk of sudden unexpected death in infancy.

Cross-sectional surveys
A representative sample of participants or patients is studied to answer a specific clinical question at a single point in time. The data collected may refer to events in the past. This design allows determination of prevalence or relative risk (but not incidence) and is relatively quick and low-cost. An example of use would be determination of the current prevalence of cystic fibrosis in a population of adolescents.

Meta-analyses
A meta-analysis is a statistical synthesis of the numerical results of several studies which all addressed the same question. It may form one component of a systematic review It is based on primary research studies which in themselves individually may not have given a statistically significant result. The advantage of a meta-analysis is that the increased sample size may allow statistical significance to be achieved and increased confidence in the result.

The results of meta-analyses tend to be presented in standard format: the forest plot.

Forest plot
At the bottom of the chart there is a horizontal line showing a scale measuring the intervention effect. A vertical line through 1 signifies no difference in the effect being studied. To the left of the vertical line, the scale is less than 1, meaning a reduction and to the right an increase in effect.

The results of component studies are shown as squares centred on the point estimate of the result. The size of the square is proportional to the percentage weight contributed by that study to the overall analysis. A larger study has greater weight.

A horizontal line runs through the square to show the CI (usually a 95% CI).

A diamond shape, usually at the bottom near the baseline, gives the pooled analysis result. The widest part is located at the calculated point estimate, and the horizontal width is the confidence interval of the pooled data. If the confidence interval crosses the vertical line of no effect, there was no statistical significance between the interventions.

Study validity
Good study design reduces bias and confounding effects and enhances validity.

Bias
A *biased sample* is one in which members of the statistical population are not equally likely to be chosen.

Systematic bias is anything that erroneously influences the conclusions about groups and distorts comparisons.

Bias may occur during selection, recall, observation, and publication.

Confounders
A confounder is any circumstance other than the desired exposure which makes one population different from another. Gender, for example, can be a confounding factor.

Cheating

Certain manipulations applied before data are analysed or published can influence the results or conclusions.

These are difficult for readers to detect, but include:
- Failure to test whether data has a normal distribution
- Excluding drop-outs and non-responders
- Leaving outliers in or excluding them depending on whether they support your conclusions
- Leaving out confidence intervals which overlap zero difference between groups.

21.4 Evidence-based medicine (EBM)

Evidence-based medicine (EBM): what it is and is not

EBM can be defined as the conscientious explicit, and judicious use of current best evidence in making decisions about the care of individual patients.

More specifically, EBM is the use of *quantitative* estimates of the risk of benefit and harm, derived from good-quality research on population samples, to inform clinical decision-making about the management of individual patients.

The defining feature of EBM is therefore the use of numbers derived from research on *populations* to inform decisions about *individuals*.

An authority has said that EBM is *not* old hat, impossible to practise, cost-cutting, or cookery-book medicine. Nor is it an attempt by numerate young medical academics to browbeat experienced clinicians using a combination of epidemiological jargon and impenetrable statistical concepts.

EBM: a glossary

- *Study designs:* see section 21.3 for definitions of several study designs: RCTs, cohort studies, case–control studies, cross-sectional surveys.
- *Case series:* a report on a series of patients with a outcome of interest. No control group is involved.
- *Crossover study:* the administration of two or more experimental therapies one after the other in a specified or random order to the same group of patients.
- *Systematic review:* a summary of the medical literature that uses explicit methods to perform a comprehensive literature search and critical appraisal of individual studies and that uses appropriate statistical techniques to combine these valid studies.
- *Cost–benefit analysis:* assesses whether the cost of an intervention is worth the benefit by measuring both in the same units; monetary units are usually used.
- *Clinical practice guideline:* a systematically developed statement designed to assist clinician and patient decisions about appropriate health care for specific clinical circumstances.

How to practice EBM

The practice of EBM involves the following steps:
- *Step 1:* formulating the problem by converting the need for information into an answerable question
- *Step 2:* tracking down the best evidence to answer the question by searching the literature
- *Step 3:* critically appraising the evidence for its validity, impact and applicability
- *Step 4:* integrating the valid evidence with clinical expertise and the patient's unique biology, values and circumstances
- *Step 5:* evaluating our effectiveness and efficiency in executing steps 1–4 and seeking ways to improve them both.

Alternatives to EBM

Alternative but unsatisfactory personality-based approaches in the absence of evidence have been suggested by Isaacs and Fitzgerald (*BMJ* 1999; 319, 1618). These are not recommended but are worth looking out for.

- *Eminence based:* used by senior colleagues with faith in clinical experience (defined as making the same mistake again and again with ever increasing confidence)
- *Vehemence based:* a loud and vigorous expression of opinion is substituted for evidence. Popular with surgeons.
- *Diffidence based:* inaction based on a sense of despair. Better than the wrong action ('First, do no harm')
- *Nervousness based:* over-investigation and over-treatment based on a misplaced fear of missing something and subsequent complaints or litigation.

Formulating the problem

The first task is to formulate an answerable clinical question in response to a clinical encounter. Such foreground questions usually concern assessment, investigation, treatment or prognosis. A well-constructed question has four components, summarized by the acronym **PICO**:
- The specific **P**atient, **P**opulation, or **P**roblem of interest
- The main **I**ntervention: treatment, diagnostic test, etc.
- The **C**omparison intervention or exposure
- The clinical **O**utcome of interest.

Example: an ex-premature neonate now at term corrected is in nasal prong oxygen at 200 mL/min. The Hb is 7.9 g/dL and reticulocytes are 2.1%. You consider whether or not a blood transfusion is indicated.
- **P**atient: term corrected ex-prem in low-flow oxygen
- **I**ntervention: blood transfusion
- **C**omparison: wait and see
- **O**utcome: reduced time in oxygen, or reduced time to discharge, or reduction in episodes of desaturation or apnoea.

Searching the literature

Consider the '4S' approach to accessing evidence-based information. This is a pyramidal, hierarchical structure best accessed via the Internet (Fig 21.5).

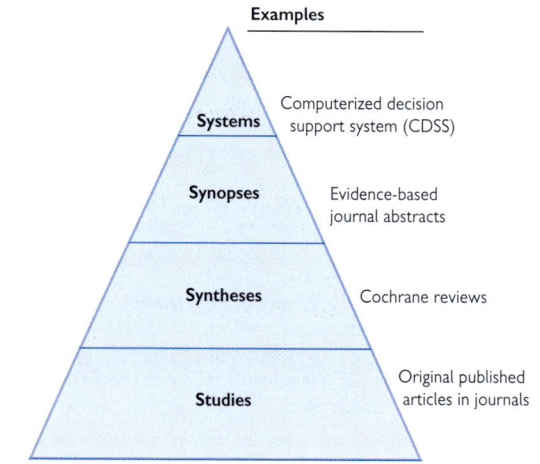

Fig 21.5 The '4S' approach to information.

Systems

The perfect ideal system of the future will integrate and summarize all relevant evidence about a clinical problem and automatically link to a patient's electronic medical record. At present a limited range of such systems are available and it is important to check that they are regularly revised and appraise evidence in an explicit way.

Examples
- *Clinical Evidence:* www.clinicalevidence.com
- *Evidence-Based Medicine Reviews (EBMR):* www.ovid.com
- *Evidence-Based Paediatrics and Child Health:* www.evidbasedpediatrics.com

Synopses

The perfect synopsis of a review or original article would provide exactly enough information to inform a clinical decision, but no more. Examples are available at:
- *ACP journal club:* www.acpj.org
- *Evidence-Based Medicine:* www.ebm.bmjjournals.com
- *Clinical Knowledge Summaries (CKS):* part of the National Library for Health: www.cks.library.nhs.uk/home

Systematic reviews (syntheses)

A systematic review is an overview of primary studies which contains a statement of aims and methods and has been conducted according to an explicit, transparent and reproducible methodology.

This systematic approach to reviewing published evidence usually includes:
- Stating objectives and defining criteria for inclusion
- Comprehensively searching for all relevant studies
- Assessing and tabulating characteristics and methodology of each study
- Applying eligibility criteria and justifying exclusions
- Assembling the most complete data set available
- Analysing results using meta-analysis of statistical data if appropriate
- Comparing alternative analyses if appropriate
- Preparing a critical summary of the review.

Systematic reviews have many advantages over 'journalistic' reviews which selectively include or exclude data according to some preconceived hypothesis and represent a seriously flawed variety of secondary research.

Databases of systematic reviews are available, e.g. the Cochrane Library (www.cochranelibrary.com)

A new online journal is also available: www.evidence-basedchild-health.com

Cochrane Library
Named after the epidemiologist Archie Cochrane, this library also includes information about the Cochrane Collaboration and its subject based review groups and methods. This includes two databases of synthesized evidence:
- *Cochrane Database of Systematic Reviews (CDSR):* 4000 systematic reviews
- *Database of Abstracts of Reviews of Effectiveness (DARE):* 5000 systematic reviews.

Studies: original publications

The Internet has revolutionized access to the primary literature by providing access to databases and to the World Wide Web via search engines.

Databases: PubMed
The huge MEDLINE database compiled by the US National Library of Medicine indexes >5000 journals and holds >16 million citations. It is accessible free online via Ovid or PubMed, one of the Entrez retrieval systems developed by the National Centre for Biotechnology information (NCBI): www.ncbi.nlm.nih.gov/PubMed/.

Pubmed features sophisticated search capabilities, links to full-text articles as well as abstracts, and links to other NLM search systems. PubMed BASICS: a tutorial and FAQs are available on the home page.

Searching Pubmed
To search PubMed, type a word or phrase into the query box then click on the Go button. The search may be by terms or key concepts, author, journal name, or specific citation.

Articles are indexed using a powerful vocabulary called Medical Subject Headings (MeSH). The MeSH database link on the sidebar allows you to find suitable Mesh terms, but 'autocompletion' will convert your amateurish efforts into MeSH terms automatically (e.g. 'bad breath' becomes 'halitosis'). Putting a * at the end of a truncated word will find all variations of ending. Neonat*, for example searches for neonatology, neonate, and neonatal.

Search terms can be combined with connector (Boolean) words AND, OR, or NOT, which should be entered in upper-case letters.

PubMed features tabs
Placed below the query box, these include Limits and Details. *Limits* allows your search to be focused according to publication features (full text/abstracts, language, date, journal group, type—clinical trial, editorial, etc.) or features of the subjects studied (species, gender, age). *Details* provides information on how PubMed ran the search.

Clinical queries
This section (on the blue sidebar) makes it easier to find applied clinical research. The three options include: Clinical study category, Find systematic reviews, and Medical genetics.

Clinical study categories include aetiology, diagnosis, therapy.

Search engines
Google (www.google.com) and Google Scholar (www.scholar.google.com) are incredibly fast and effective search engines which also provide access to electronic textbook chapters and resources such as E-medicine. Google gives access to >3 billion articles on the web.

Searching with well-selected terms performed well in a recent trial of solving diagnostic problems posed by case descriptions of rare conditions published in *NEJM* (search Google using search term 'Googling for a diagnosis').

21.5 EBM: critical appraisal and implementation

Critical appraisal: how to read a paper

This is the process of systematically assessing the information presented in a research paper to decide whether it is valid and could be used to inform practice. The aims of the study, how the researchers set about doing it, whether sense can be made of the results, and whether the conclusions are appropriate all must be assessed.

The Centre for Evidence Based Medicine (CEBM) in Oxford (www.cebm.net) suggests three questions to ask about a piece of research:

- Is it valid?
- Is it important?
- Is it applicable to the patient?

The CEBM has developed worksheets, which are available on their website, to help you work through the study. Available trials may not be ideal, but the best available should be reviewed with awareness of any limitations.

Points to consider under each question vary with the type of study: diagnostic, prognostic, harm/aetiology therapy, systematic reviews. The validity of a study determines whether it is worth taking into account. Validation checklists exist for different types of study design and are included below.

Selected important points under each question are considered in turn for each type of study.

Diagnostic studies
Validity
- Independent blind comparison with reference diagnostic standard?
- Evaluation in appropriate spectrum of patients?

Importance
- Does the test have the ability to distinguish between those with and without the disease?
- See section on specificity and sensitivity and likelihood ratios. If a test has a high sensitivity, a negative result rules out the diagnosis (SnNout).
- If a test has a high specificity, a positive test rules in the diagnosis (SpPin).

Applicability
- Cost-effective, available, and consequential?
- Were the methods for performing the test described in sufficient detail to permit replication?
- Can you estimate pre-test probability for your patient and will the post-test probability affect management or help your patient?

Prognostic studies
Validity
- Defined, representative sample of patients assembled at a common (early) point in their disease?
- Follow up long and complete?
- Objective outcome criteria applied in a 'blind' fashion?
- Sub-groups identified?
- Validation in an independent test-set of patients?

Importance
- How likely are the outcomes over time and what time-scale was used?
- How precise are the prognostic estimates?
- What were the CIs for the measures of prognosis?

Applicability
- Were the study patients similar to your own?
- Will the evidence make a clinically important impact on what you offer or tell the patient?

Harm/aetiology studies
Validity
- Clearly defined groups of patients similar in all important ways other than exposure to the putative agent?
- Outcome measures objective or blinded (to exposure) and applied in same fashion in both groups?
- Follow-up complete and long enough?
- Do the results satisfy tests for causation (see Bradford Hill criteria, above)?

Importance
- Are the size and confidence limits of the results presented and significant?
- For randomized trial or cohort study the relative risk (RR) and for case–control study the odds ratio (OR) is calculated. Has the number needed to harm (NNH) been calculated?

Applicability
- Can the study results be extrapolated to your patient?
- What are your patient's risks of the adverse outcome (patient's expected event rate)?
- What are your patient's preferences and expectations and what alternative treatments are available?

Therapeutic studies
Validity
- Was the study randomized and blinded?
- Was follow up complete and were patients analysed in the groups to which they were randomized, i.e. was analysis based on an 'intention to treat' principle? In an 'intention to treat' analysis all patients randomly assigned to one of the treatments are analysed together, regardless of whether or not they completed or received that treatment.

Importance
- What is the treatment effect and is it impressive?
- What are the values for RRR, ARR, NNT and their CIs?

Applicability
- How similar is your patient to those in the trial?
- How great would the potential benefit of therapy actually be for your patient?
- Will your patient's values and preferences be satisfied?

Integration: implementing EBM

The final step involves integrating the critical appraisal of the evidence with our clinical expertise and the patient's unique biology, values, and circumstances.

The patient's perspective should be incorporated into an evidence-based treatment choice. A patient's preferences may depend on value judgements, for example about the relative severity of the bad outcome therapy is intended to prevent and the adverse events which therapy may cause. This may be especially problematic in paediatric practice in which the patient may not be capable of communication.

For common clinical scenarios the practice of EBM may be facilitated by the use of evidence-based guidelines and patient information leaflets.

Guidelines

A guideline is defined as a systematically developed statement to assist practitioner decisions about appropriate health care in specific clinical circumstances.

Guidelines are quite different from *protocols*, which are instructions on what to do in particular circumstances. Protocols leave less room for individual judgement and are produced either for less experienced staff or for situations in which eventualities are predictable.

Guidelines may be local, national, or international and may be clinical, organizational, or ethical. They are not intended to force the abandonment of common sense or clinical judgement but merely provide a course of action to be considered.

Writing a local guideline
Local guidelines are not intended to re-invent the wheel but allow local practicalities to be taken into account if national guidelines exist. Simple rules include:
- Choose a common and important topic
- Involve all relevant stakeholders
- State a clear aim
- Adopt a national guideline if available
- Make it clear and unambiguous
- Use flowcharts and algorithms
- Make it evidence based
- Plan a review date.

Useful resources for guidelines include the following:
- *National Institute for Clinical Excellence* (www.nice.org.uk) is an independent organization responsible for providing UK national guidance on promoting health and preventing and treating ill health.
- *National Library for Health* (www.library.nhs.uk) is a digital library for UK NHS staff, patients and the public with links to common and useful resources.
- *Children's Acute Transport Service* (www.cats.nhs.uk). The website contains a number of useful clinical guidelines
- *Royal College of Paediatrics and Child Health* (www.rcpch.ac.uk). The website houses appraised and published national guidance.
- *National Guideline Clearinghouse™* (www.guideline.gov): a comprehensive database of evidence-based clinical practice guidelines and related documents. It provides guidelines and other material, mainly from American sources.
- *Education and Practice Edition of Archives of Diseases in Childhood* (www.adc.bmjjournals.com) contains best practice reviews, guideline reviews and updates.

Guidelines for good guidelines
The AGREE collaboration
The Appraisal of Guidelines Research and Evaluation (AGREE) collaboration is an international collaboration of researchers who work to establish a shared framework for the development, reporting and assessment of guidelines. The AGREE instrument has been developed to allow appraisal of the process used in development of a guideline. AGREE consists of 23 items organized into 6 domains, each of which captures a separate dimension of guideline quality:
- Scope and purpose
- Stakeholder involvement
- Rigour of development
- Clarity and presentation
- Applicability
- Editorial independence.

A simple set of questions which allow assessment of the content, process and presentational aspects of a guideline include the following:
- Did preparation involve a significant potential conflict of interest?
- Does it involve an appropriate topic and state clearly the target group to whom it applies?
- Did the guideline development panel include an expert in the topic area and a specialist in the methods of secondary research?
- Have any subjective judgements (e.g. guiding principles, values, ethical frameworks) been made explicit?
- Have all the relevant data been scrutinized and rigorously evaluated?
- Has the evidence been properly synthesized?
- Is the guideline relevant, comprehensive and flexible?
- Does the guideline include recommendations for its own dissemination, implementation and regular review?

Implementation
Any guideline will fail to improve patient care if not implemented. This involves an interplay of cultural and organizational factors which vary depending on the level at which the guideline is produced. When used wisely guidelines have the potential to benefit patients and health-care systems. The decisions of many clinicians remain informed by so-called *'mindlines'*: collectively reinforced, internalized processes informed by experience, interaction with colleagues and patients, and brief reading.

Patient (parent) information leaflets
These should be concise, free of jargon and acronyms and age appropriate. Useful sources are:
- *Great Ormond Street Hospital for Children:* www.gosh.nhs.uk
- *Clinical Knowledge Summaries (CKS):* patient information leaflets can be found at www.cks library.nhs.uk.

21.6 Critical appraisal exercise

Publication to appraise
Wakefield AJ, Murch SH, Anthony A, et al. Ileal–lymphoid nodular hyperplasia, non-specific colitis, and pervasive developmental disorder in children. *Lancet* 1998; 351: 637–641.

Type of publication
- *Primary study*: reporting original observations.
- *Harm/aetiology study*: it proposed by implication a putative adverse effect of a vaccine (MMR) and a putative aetiology for both bowel inflammation and autism.
- *Observational study*: described results of clinical observations and investigations in a group of 12 patients and proposed a new syndrome (chronic-enterocolitis/neuropsychiatric dysfunction or autistic enterocolitis). It was an extended case-report or short case-series, i.e. anecdotal.

The three main questions in appraisal
- Are the results valid?
- If valid, are they important?
- Are they applicable to my patient?

Are the results valid?
The first problem in this paper is the absence of a clearly stated research hypothesis. Several hypotheses are implied:

1. A specific syndrome exists in which bowel inflammation coexists with neuropsychiatric dysfunction.
2. This syndrome is caused by environmental triggers including, by implication, the MMR vaccine.
3. Vitamin B12 deficiency may have contributed to the neuropsychiatric dysfunction, as manifested by developmental regression.

Assuming these were the hypotheses tested, the study design is not appropriate and is clearly flawed, precluding the generation of valid results. Considering the first two hypotheses:

- *The syndrome*: selection bias undermines the hypothesis that this syndrome is real. As the authors state: 'Intestinal and behavioural pathologies may have occurred together by chance, reflecting selection bias in a self-referred group'. The sample was highly selected. The authors focused on a tiny number of children who had been referred to a major specialist centre because they had both bowel symptoms and an autism-like syndrome. The fact that these rare conditions occurred together proved nothing at all.
- *The causal link with MMR*: the study design is not appropriate for examining whether MMR vaccination is either associated with or causes either of the features of the putative syndrome. The appropriate study design is a large-scale epidemiological study with either a prospective cohort design or a case–control design to assess harm. In so far as the study attempts to address this hypothesis it is flawed in the following respects:

Design flaws
- No case-control design. No control group, numbers very small, and no power calculations.
- No clearly defined groups of patients similar in every respect except exposure to the MMR vaccine. The patient group was subject to selection bias and there was no control group for testing MMR as a causal agent. The control group for colonoscopy findings was poorly described and heterogeneous.
- Outcome measures poorly defined and subjective.
- No suggestion of 'blinding'. The investigators who examined the children and analysed the specimens all knew that the children had received MMR and that a link with autism and bowel disorder was proposed. Observer bias is possible.

In addition to these flaws the criteria for causality, even if a significant association had been demonstrated, were not addressed or met. These include the following:

- *Did the exposure precede the onset of the outcome?* This is a necessary condition for causality, but not a sufficient one. In this universe, cause must precede effect, but such a temporal relationship does *not* prove causality. In this study, the temporal association of symptoms to vaccination was based on recall by the child's parents or their physician. No steps were taken to guard against 'recall bias' (remembering a closer association between two events than actually occurred). In so far as the 'leaky bowel' was proposed to trigger the behavioural problems, the temporal relationship between bowel and behavioural symptoms does not suggest a causal link. In 6/12 cases the sequence is not known and in 5/12 the behavioural symptoms preceded or were simultaneous with the bowel symptoms.
- *Does a causal link make biological sense?* The first problem with MMR as a cause of intestinal inflammation is the failure to detect measles virus in the bowel. A paper reporting this failure appeared in the same edition of the *Lancet*. It was proposed that a dysfunctional intestine might permit increased permeability to exogenous peptides which exerted central opioid effects, a hypothetical speculation at best. The statements that intervals of 24 h to 2 weeks occurred between exposure (vaccination) and behavioural symptoms (autism) is biologically implausible. The observations on urinary methylmalonic acid concentrations do not strongly support a contribution of vitamin B12 deficiency to the developmental regression.

Dose–response gradients, dechallenge-challenge studies, and consistency between studies cannot be applied in this case.

Are the valid results important?
The results are not valid and cannot therefore be important in making evidence-based decisions. Of course, even valid results may not be important if the effect described is negligible in clinical practice.

Are the results applicable to my patient?
If appraisal of a study indicates that the results are invalid, the study should be ignored: it does not form part of the evidence base. The correct approach to a parent asking for advice about whether or not MMR should be given to their child in 1998 would have been to refer to the strong epidemiological evidence available at that time showing a high benefit-to-risk ratio and no association between MMR and chronic bowel or behavioural problems, as pointed out in the Commentary accompanying the *Lancet* paper. All subsequent research in this area would have vindicated your advice. See Chapter 18.4, Parental concerns.

Index

A

ABCDE 32
abdomen, acute 295
abdominal mass 118, 306
abdominal migraine 110
abdominal pain
 adolescence 418
 functional 110
 recurrent 373
abdominal wall defects 98–9
ABO incompatibility 22
ABO system 276
absence seizures 158
abuse 398–405
accidents and emergencies 29–52
ACE inhibitors 432
acetaminophen 434
achondroplasia 355
aciclovir 438
acid–base balance 25, 31, 123, 333
acne 204
acrodermatitis enteropathica 199
activated partial thromboplastin time (APTT) 273
acute abdomen 295
acute disseminated encephalomyelitis (ADEM) 172
acute fatigue syndrome 419
acute gastroenteritis 102–3
acute hepatitis 117
acute herpetic gingivostomatitis 324
acute inflammatory demyelinating polyradiculoneuropathy (AIDP) 172
acute kidney injury (AKI) 130
acute laryngotracheobronchitis (croup) 42, 43, 60
acute leukaemias 296–7
acute liver disease 117
acute liver failure (ALF) 117
acute lymphoblastic leukaemia (ALL) 296
acute motor axonal neuropathy (AMAN) 172
acute motor-sensory axonal neuropathy (AMSAN) 172
acute myeloid leukaemia (AML) 297
acute nephritis (AN) 127
acute otitis media (AOM) 58
acute pharyngotonsillitis 333
acute stridor 60, 72
acute viral encephalitis 170
acute viral hepatitis 117
adaptive immunity 309
Addison's disease 224
adenohypophysis 212
adenosine 432
adherence 413
adolescence 407–24
 chronic illness 412, 413
 communication 410
 competence 411
 confidentiality 410–11
 consent 411
 development 408–9
 eating disorders 420–1
 epidemiology 412–13
 fatigue 419
 health behaviours 414
 health promotion 414–15
 history and examination 410
 mental health 416–17
 obesity 421
 seizures 156
 sexual and reproductive health 412–13, 422
 somatic symptoms 418
 substance abuse 413, 422–3
 transition to adult services 415
adolescent rumination syndrome 109
adoption 383
adrenal disorders 224–5
adrenal gland 222–3
adrenocorticotrophic hormone (ACTH) 212
adrenoleucodystrophy (X-ALD) 152, 243
adverse drug reactions 429
adverse events following immunization (AEFIs) 388
adverse transfusion reactions 277
afterload 30, 74
AGREE collaboration 459
AIDS 328–9
airway obstruction 42–3, 60–1

Alagille syndrome 78, 115
Albers–Schonberg disease 356
albinism 188, 190, 207
Albright's hereditary osteodystrophy 226
alcohol
 adolescent misuse 413, 422–3
 maternal intake 3
 poisoning 41
aldosterone 121, 222
alemtuzamab 443
Alexander disease 152
alginates 430
alkylating drugs 442
alleles 249
allergic conjunctivitis 184
'allergic march' 340
allergic rhinitis 58
allergy 340–1, 344
alopecia 206
α-haemolytic streptococci 333
α_1-antitrypsin deficiency 115
Alport syndrome (AS) 138
amblyopia 181
ambulatory blood pressure monitoring (ABPM) 140
amiloride 432
amino acid metabolism 234–5, 240–1
aminoacidopathies 240
aminoglycosides 437
amoxicillin 436
amphotericin 438
ampicillin 436
anaemia 274
 aplastic 279
 Diamond–Blackfan 279
 Fanconi 279
 haemolytic 280–1
 iron deficiency 278, 443
 preterm infants 17
 renal 443
analgesics 434
 poisoning 41
analysis of variance (ANOVA) 452
anaphylactoid reactions 46
anaphylaxis 46–7
anaplastic large-cell lymphoma (ALCL) 299
anencephaly 148
aneuploidy 250
Angelman syndrome (AS) 266, 267
angiokeratoma corporis diffusum 245
angiotensin I/II 121
angiotensin-converting enzyme (ACE) inhibitors 432
anion gap 33
aniridia 180, 190
anisocoria 179
anisometropia 181
anophthalmia 190
anorexia nervosa 420
anterior segment dysgenesis (ASD) 180, 190
anti-arrhythmic drugs 432
antibiotics 436–7
 cytotoxic 442
antibodies 309
anticoagulation 273
antidepressant poisoning 41
antiepilepsy drugs (AEDs) 157, 434–5
antifungals 438
antimalarials 439
antimetabolites 442
antimotility drug poisoning 41
antiproliferative immunosuppressants 442–3
antiprotozoals 439
antiretroviral therapy (ART) 329, 438
antithrombin (AT) 273
antithyroid drugs (ATDs) 221, 440
antivirals 438
anus, imperforate 8, 27
anxiety disorders 378–9
aortic arch interruption 83
aortic stenosis (AS) 82–3
Apgar score 5
aphthous ulcers 206
aplastic anaemia 279
apnoeas 17
apparent life threatening events (ALTE) 42
appetite control 95, 212
arginine vasopressin (AVP) 213, 441

arrhythmias 90–1
arterial circulation 30
arterial thromboembolism 287
arthritis
 enthesitis-related 359
 inflammatory bowel disease 360
 juvenile idiopathic (JIA) 358–9, 368
 post-infectious 360
 psoriatic 359
 reactive 360
 septic 367
arthrogryposis multiplex congenital (AMC) 350
Asperger syndrome 374
asphyxia at birth 10
aspiration 71
aspirin poisoning 41
asplenia 275
astatic (atonic) seizures 158
asthma 66–7
astigmatism 181
asymmetric crying facies 11
asystole 35
ataxia 160–1
ataxia telangiectasia 160, 191
ataxic cerebral palsy 154
athlete's foot 203
atopic dermatitis 200–1
atopic eczema 200–1
atopy 340
atrial septal defects (ASD) 79, 80
atrioventricular (AV) block 91
atrioventricular (AV) connections 74
atrioventricular septal defects 81
attachment 9
attention deficit hyperactivity disorder (ADHD) 376–7
audiometry 396–7
auscultation
 heart 75
 respiratory system 56
autism spectrum disorders (ASD) 374–5
autoimmune disease
 conjunctivitis 184
 postinfectious 311
 pregnancy 3
autoimmune hepatitis 116
autoimmune thrombocytopaenia 3
automatisms 158
autosomal dominant (AD) diseases 251, 252
autosomal dominant polycystic kidney disease (ADPKD) 136
autosomal recessive (AR) diseases 251, 252
autosomal recessive polycystic kidney disease (ARPKD) 136
auxology 217
avian influenza 336
AVPU scale 33
azathioprine 442
azithromycin 437

B

bacteria 310
bacterial conjunctivitis 184
bacterial infection
 neonates 18–19
 skin 202
bacterial meningitis 335
bacterial sepsis 18–19
bacterial tracheitis 60
bad news 9
band heterotopias 150
Bardet–Biedl syndrome 136
Barlow manoeuvre 8
Bartter syndrome 137
basal skull fracture 38
basiliximab 443
bathing trunk naevus 198
Battle's sign 38
B cells 309
BCG vaccination 331, 391
Beau's lines 206
Becker muscular dystrophy (BMD) 169
Beckwith–Wiedemann syndrome (BWS) 267
behavioural development 370
behavioural problems 372–3

Bell's palsy 174
benign childhood epilepsy with centrotemporal
    spikes 159
benign joint hypermobility syndrome (BJHS) 365
benign myoclonus 156
benzodiazepines 435
benzylpenicillin 436
Berger disease 126, 127
Bernard–Soulier syndrome 289
β-haemolytic streptococci 333
bias 455
bile acid synthetic disorders 115
biliary atresia 114–15
bilirubin 22, 95, 114
bilirubin encephalopathy 22
binocular single vision 182
biophysical profile score (BPS) 2
biotinidase deficiency 241
bird flu 336
birth 4–5
    asphyxia 10
    changes at 4–5, 74
    injuries 11
birthmarks 198
birthweight 4, 96
bites 401
bladder exstrophy 134
bleach poisoning 41
bleeding disorders 275
bleomycin 442
blepharitis 184
blindness 181
Bloch–Sulzberger syndrome 199
blood–brain barrier (BBB) 145
blood cells 270–1
blood group 276
blood pressure 6, 30–1, 33, 140
blood products 277
blood transfusion 276–7
    adverse reactions 277
    jaundice 23
    preterm anaemia 17
blood volume 6
blue breath-holding 156
blue spots 198
body size and proportions 30
body temperature 6, 312
body water
    neonates 7
    total body water 121
bonding 9
bone 346
bone marrow transplantation (BMT) 277, 295
bone marrow trephine and aspiration 276
bone tumours 304
Bornholm disease 322
bovine spongiform encephalopathy (BSE) 337
Bowman's capsule 120
brachial plexus injury 11
bradyarrhythmias 90
bradycardia 33
bradypnoea 32
brain
    development 144
    imaging 147, 157
    perfusion 33
    traumatic injury 38, 171
    tumours 300
brainstem glioma 300
breastfeeding 9, 96
    prescribing 429
breast milk jaundice 23
breathing
    effort of 32
    noisy 56
    patterns 30, 54
Bristol Stool Form Scale 111
bronchial hyper-reactivity (BHR) 71
bronchiectasis 70–1
bronchiolitis 64
bronchodilators 433
Brown syndrome 182
brucellosis 336
Brugada syndrome 91
bruising
    excessive 290
    physical abuse 400
buffers 31
bulimia nervosa 420–1
Burkitt lymphoma 299, 326
burns 36–7, 400–1
bypass surgery 79

C

café-au-lait macules 207
calcineurin inhibitors 443
calcitonin (CT) 226
calcium-channel blockers 432
calcium disorders 226–7
calcium preparations 447
calcium stones 141
calculi 141
caloric intake, recommended 97
Canavan disease 152
cancer
    aetiology 292–3
    emergencies 295
    epidemiology 292
    genetic syndromes 292
    infection 295
    palliative care 295
    presentation 293
    red flags 293
    treatment 294–5
    see also specific cancers
candidiasis 203
caput succedaneum 11
carbamazepine 435
carbimazole 440
carbohydrate
    digestion and absorption 95
    metabolism 234, 238
carboplatin 442
cardiac anatomy and physiology 74–5
cardiac arrhythmias 90–1
cardiac catheterization 76–7
cardiac development 74
cardiac failure 74, 75, 92
cardiac investigations 76–7
cardiac output 30, 74
cardiac surgery 79
cardiac symptoms 75
cardiogenic shock 32
cardiology 73–92
cardiomyopathies 90
cardiopulmonary arrest 34–5
cardiopulmonary resuscitation (CPR) 34–5
cardiovascular system 30–1
    assessment in seriously ill child 32–3
    neonates 6
carotid bruit 75
carrier testing 253
case–control studies 455
catabolism 235
cataract 186
catecholamines 223
cat-scratch disease 336
causality 452
CD numbers 309
cefalexin 437
ceftriaxone 437
cefuroxime 437
cell division 248
cellular immunity 18, 308, 309
cellulitis 202
    orbital 185
    periorbital (preseptal) 185, 192
centile 450
centile charts 217
central core disease 167
central nervous system (CNS)
    development 144
    infections 170
    tumours 293, 300–1
central sleep apnoea (CSA) 59
cephalhaematoma 11
cephalosporins 437
cerebral blood flow (CBF) 145
cerebral palsies (CP) 154–5
cerebral perfusion pressure (CPP) 31, 145
cerebrohepatorenal syndrome 243
cerebrospinal fluid (CSF) 145
CFAP syndrome 110
chalazion 184
Charcot–Marie–Tooth disease type 1 and 2 166
CHARGE syndrome 26, 180, 261
chemotherapy 294
chest compressions 10, 34
chest expansion 32
chest pain 75
chest radiographs (CXR) 57, 76
chickenpox 21, 325
child abuse 398–405
child development 392–3
Child Development Team (CDT) 395

child health promotion 386–7, 406
Child Health Promotion Programme (CHPP) 387
childhood absence epilepsy (CAE) 159
childhood functional abdominal pain (CFAP) 110
child in need 399
child protection 399, 405
child public health 384–5
Children Act (1989/2004) 382
children in difficult circumstances (CDC) 384
children's rights 382
chi-squared (χ^2) 452
Chlamydia trachomatis 18
chloral hydrate 434
chlorambucil 442
choanal atresia 26
choking 42–3
cholelithiasis 113
cholestatic jaundice 7, 115
cholesterol 235
chromosomal disorders 250
chromosomes 248
chronic fatigue syndrome (CFS) 419
chronic granulomatous disease (CGD) 319
chronic kidney disease (CKD) 131
chronic liver disease 116–17
chronic lung disease of prematurity (CLD) 70
chronic stridor 61
chronic suppurative otitis media (CSOM) 58
ciclosporin 443
ciprofloxacin 437
circulatory changes at birth 4–5
cisplatin 442
clarithromycin 437
class switching 309
clavicle fracture 11
cleft lip and palate 26
clinically isolated syndrome (CIS) 172
club foot 350
cluster headaches 163
CNS
    development 144
    infections 170
    tumours 293, 300–1
coagulation cascade 272–3
coagulation disorders 284–7
coagulation screening tests 273
co-amoxiclav 437
coarctation of the aorta (COA) 82, 83
cobblestone dysplasia 150
cocaine 3
coeliac disease 104–5
cognitive development 370
cohort studies 455
cold sores 324
colic 108
collagen 347
collodion baby 199
coloboma 180, 188
colour vision 177
coma 31, 51
common arterial trunk (CAT) 85
common assessment framework (CAF) 383
common cold 58
common variable immunodeficiency (CVID) 318
communication
    adolescence 410
    behaviour as 371
    disorders 397
community-acquired pneumonia (CAP) 62–3
community child health 381–406
compensated shock 33
competence 411
complement component defects 319
complement system 308
compliance 30
compound analgesics, poisoning 41
computerized tomography (CT) 147
concomitant strabismus 182
concordance 413
conduct disorder (CD) 377
confidence intervals (CI) 451
confidentiality 410–11
confounders 455
congenital adrenal hyperplasia (CAH) 225, 232
congenital anomalies
    craniofacial 26
    gastrointestinal 26–7, 98–9
    nails 206
    orthopaedics 350–1
    respiratory tract 27
    urinary tract 132–3
congenital diabetes insipidus 215
congenital heart disease (CHD) 78–85

congenital hypopituitarism 214
congenital hypothyroidism 220–1
congenital infection 18, 20–1, 184
congenital muscular dystrophies 168
congenital myasthenic syndromes (CMS) 167
congenital myopathies 167
congenital nephrotic syndrome 128, 138
congenital rubella syndrome 20, 184, 321
congenital talipes equinovarus (CTEV) 350
congenital TB 331
conjugated hyperbilirubinaemia 23, 114–15
conjunctivitis 18, 184
connective tissue 347
connective tissue disorders 191, 364–5
CONS 332–3
conscious level, decreased 51
consent 404, 411
constipation, functional 111
continuous positive airway pressure (CPAP) 13
contraception 422
contrast sensitivity 177
convulsive status epilepticus (CSE) 31, 50
co-phenotrope poisoning 41
co-proxamol poisoning 41
Cori disease 238
cornea
 developmental anomalies 180
 inflammation 184
Cornelia de Lange syndrome (CdLS) 261
correlation 452
cortical dysplasias 150
cortical malformations 150
corticosteroids 222–3, 431, 441
coryza 58
co-trimoxazole 437
cough 56, 71, 72
cover tests 182–3
cow's milk protein allergy 341
Coxsackie viruses 322
cranial imaging 147, 157
cranial nerves
 palsies 183
 rapid screen 146
cranial vault abnormalities 150–1
craniofacial abnormalities 26
craniofacial syndromes 191
craniopharyngioma 300
craniosynostosis 151
crescentic glomerulonephritis 126
cri-du-chat syndrome 259
Crigler–Najjar syndrome 114
critical aortic stenosis 82–3
critical appraisal 458, 460
Crohn's disease (CD) 106–7
cross-matching 277
cross-sectional surveys 455
croup 42, 43, 60
Crouzon syndrome 260–1
crying 372
cryoprecipitate 277
cryptorchidism 134
cryptosporidiosis 336
Cushing's triad 31
Cushing syndrome 224
cutaneous leishmaniasis 336
cyanosis/cyanotic spells 12, 28
cyanotic heart defects 79, 84–5
cyclic vomiting syndrome 109
cyclophosphamide 442
cystic disease of the kidney 136
cystic fibrosis (CF) 68–9
cystinosis 138
cystinuria 136
cytarabine 442
cytomegalovirus (CMV) 21, 184, 327
cytotoxic drugs 442

D

dacryocystitis 185
Darier's sign 197
data types 450
daunorubicin 442
daydreaming 156
decompensated shock 33
decreased conscious level 51
deformational plagiocephaly 151
dehydration
 categorization 102
 neonates 7, 448
Dejerine–Sotas syndrome 166
delayed puberty 219
dendritic cells 308
depression 379, 416
dermatographism 197
dermatology 193–208
dermatomyositis 364
dermatophytosis 203
dermis 194
dermoscopy 197
desmopressin 441
determinants of health 385
development, normal 370, 392, 408–9
developmental assessment 392–3
developmental dysplasia of the hip (DDH) 8, 350–1
developmental milestones 392
diabetes insipidus 215
diabetes mellitus
 neonates 25
 type 1 (T1DM) 3, 228–9, 440
 type 2 (T2DM) 230, 440
diabetic ketoacidosis (DKA) 48–9
diabetic retinopathy 188
diagnostic formulation 371
dialysis 131
Diamond–Blackfan anaemia (DBA) 279
diaphragmatic hernia 27
diarrhoea 109, 142
diastematomyelia 148
diazepam 435
DIDMOAD 215
dietary fat, digestion and absorption 95
diffuse large B-cell lymphoma (DLBL) 299
diffuse neonatal haemangiomatosis 198
DiGeorge syndrome (DGS) 78, 226, 258–9, 319
digestion 94–5
dilated cardiomyopathy (DCM) 90
diphtheria 390
diphtheria vaccine 390
dipstick testing 125
disease modifying anti-rheumatic drugs (DMARDs) 431
disease prevention 386–7, 406
disseminated intravascular coagulation (DIC) 286
distal (type 1) renal tubular acidosis 137
distal arthrogryposis syndrome 350
diuretics 432
DNA 249
dopa responsive dystonia 161
dosage 428
Down syndrome (DS) 78, 191, 254–5, 268
doxorubicin 442
Dravet syndrome 159
'drop attacks' 158
drowning 39
drug abuse, adolescence 413, 422–3
drug interactions 429
drug monitoring 428
drug prescribing 428–9
dry eye 178
Duane syndrome 182
Dubin–Johnson syndrome (DJS) 115
Duchenne muscular dystrophy (DMD) 168–9
ductus arteriosus 5, 79
duodenal atresia/stenosis 26, 98
duplex kidney 134
dyschezia 109
dyskinetic cerebral palsy 154
dyspepsia 110
dyspraxia 148
dysraphism 148
dystonia 161
dystonia muscularis deformans (dystonia 1) 161
dystrophic epidermolysis (DEB) 199
dystrophinopathies 168–9

E

ear, nose and throat (ENT) 58–9
eating disorders 420–1
echocardiography 76
echovirus 322
Ecstasy poisoning 41
ectopia lentis 180
ectopic kidney 134
eczema 200–1
eczema herpeticum 324
Edwards syndrome 191, 255
effort of breathing 32
Ehlers–Danlos syndrome (EDS) 191, 365
elastic equilibrium volume (EEV) 54
elastin 347
electrocardiography (ECG) 77
electroencephalogram (EEG) 157
electrolytes 7, 121, 122–3, 446–7
electro-oculography (EOG) 177
electroretinography (ERG) 177

embryology
 cardiac system 74
 gastrointestinal tract 94
 haemopoiesis 270
 musculoskeletal system 346
 nervous system 144
 respiratory system 54
 urinary system 120
Emery–Dreifuss muscular dystrophy (EDMD) 169
emotional abuse 402
emotional development 370
emotional problems 372–3
empyema 63
encephalitis 170
encephalocele 148
encephalomyelitis 170
encopresis 375
endocrinology 209–32
endotoxins 310
endotracheal intubation 10, 51
enteral nutrition 7, 444
enteric nervous system (ENS) 94
enteroviruses 322–3
enthesitis-related arthritis 359
enuresis 375
eosinophilic granulomas 305
ependymomas 300
epicanthal folds 180
epidemic parotitis 321
epidermis 194
epidermolysis bullosa (EB) 199
epidermolysis bullosa simplex (EBS) 199
epiglottitis 42, 43, 60
epilepsies 156–9
epilepsy syndromes 158–9
epileptic seizures 156, 158
epispadias 134
epistaxis 58
epoietin 443
Epstein–Barr virus (EBV) 326
Erb's palsy 11
erysipelas 202
erythema infectiosum 323
erythema multiforme (EM) 205, 206, 208
erythema nodosum 205
erythromycin 437
erythropoiesis 270
erythropoietin (EPO) 121
escharotomy 37
esotropias 182
espundi 337
essential hypertension 140
etoposide 442
Every child matters: change for children 382–3
evidence-based medicine (EBM) 456–9
Ewing sarcoma family of tumours (ESFT) 304, 306
exanthum subitum 327
exotoxins 310
expiratory reserve volume (ERV) 54
external cardiac compressions 10, 34
extraocular muscles 182
extremely low birthweight 4
eye
 alignment 177
 anatomy 176
 developmental anomalies 180
 dry 178
 examination 176
 genetic disease 190–1
 infections and inflammations 184–5
 movements 177, 182–3
 red 178
 size abnormalities 178, 180
 watering 178, 192
eyelids
 developmental anomalies 180
 ptosis 179

F

fabricated or induced illness (FII) 403
Fabry disease 245
facial palsy 11, 174
faddiness 372
faecal disimpaction 111
faint 156
familial hypercholesterolaemia (FH) 239
familial hypertrophic cardiomyopathy (HCM) 90
Fanconi anaemia (FA) 279
Fanconi syndrome 137
fascioscapulohumeral muscular dystrophy (FSHMD) 169

INDEX

fat
  digestion and absorption 95
  metabolism 235, 239
fatigue, adolescence 419
fatty acids 235
feeding
  appetite regulation 95, 212
  infants 96
  neonates 9
  problems 372
feed thickeners 444
feet
  club foot 350
  flat feet 351
fetal alcohol syndrome 3
fetal growth and development 2
fever 312
feverish child 312–15
fibrillin 347
fibrinogen disorders 286
fibroblast growth factor (FGF) 216
filgrastim 443
FISH 253
Fisher's exact test 452
FK-506 443
flat feet 351
floppy infants 164–5, 395
flow–volume curves 55
flucloxacillin 436
fluids 446–7
  burns 37
  neonates 7
fluorescence in situ hybridization (FISH) 253
focal and segmental glomerulosclerosis (FSGS) 126, 128
focal epileptic seizures 158
folate deficiency 97, 279
follicle stimulating hormone (FSH) 212–13
Fontan procedure 79
food, digestion and absorption 94
food allergy 340–1, 344
food poisoning 332
food protein-induced enterocolitis syndrome (FPIE) 341
food refusal 372
foramen ovale 5
foreign body airway obstruction (FBAO) 42–3
Forest plot 455
formula milk 9
formulation 428
fostering 383
fourth nerve palsy 183
fractures
  basal skull 38
  clavicle 11
  physical abuse 400
  skull, at birth 11
fragile X syndrome (FXS) 264–5
Fraser guidelines 411
free fatty acids 235
frequency histogram 450
fresh frozen plasma (FFP) 277
Friedreich ataxia 160
fructose-1,6-bisphosphatase deficiency 238
fructose intolerance (HFI) 238
Fukuyama-type muscular dystrophy (FCMD) 150
functional abdominal pain 110
functional constipation 111
functional diarrhoea 109
functional dyspepsia 110
functional residual capacity (FRC) 54
fungal infections 203, 438
fungi 310
fused kidney 134

G

gait 146–7, 348–9
galactokinase deficiency 238
galactosaemia 238
gallstones 113
ganciclovir 438
gastroenteritis 102–3
gastrointestinal (GI) tract
  anatomy and physiology 94–5
  bleeding 107
  congenital anomalies 26–7, 98–9
  functional disorders (FGIDs) 108–9
gastro-oesophageal reflux (GOR) 100
gastro-oesophageal reflux disease (GORD) 100, 156, 430
gastroschisis 98
Gaucher disease 245

Gaussian distribution 450
generalized anxiety disorder 378
generalized epileptic seizures 158
genetic counselling 253
genetic disease 250–1
genetics 247–68
genetic tests 253
genital herpes 324
genomics 249
genotype 250
germ cell tumours (GCT) 301
germinal matrix–intraventricular haemorrhage (GM-IVH) 15
giant congenital melanocytic naevus 198
giardiasis 103
Gilbert syndrome (GS) 114
Gitelman syndrome 137
glandular fever 326
Glanzmann thrombasthenia 289
Glasgow Coma Score (GCS) 51
glaucoma 187
glioma 300
global child health 384
global delay 394–5
globe size 178, 180
glomerular filtration rate (GFR) 7, 120–1
glomerulonephritis 126–7
glomerulus 120
glucagon 228
glucocorticoids 222, 441
gluconeogenesis 234
glucose homeostasis 228
glucose metabolism 24, 234
glucose-6-phosphate dehydrogenase (G6PD) deficiency 22, 281
glutaric aciduria type 1 241
gluten 104
gluten-free diet 105
glycine encephalopathy 240, 241
glycogen metabolism 234
glycogen storage diseases (GSDs) 238
GM2-gangliosidosis type 1 245
Goldenhar syndrome 261
gonadotropins 212–13
gonococcal eye infection 18
Gower's sign 168
G-protein coupled receptors (GPCRs) 211
granulocyte colony stimulating factor (C-CSF) 443
Graves disease 221
grey matter disorders 152
group A streptococci (GAS) 333
group B streptococci (GBS) 19, 333
growth 216–17
growth factors 216
growth hormone (GH) 213, 216, 441
grunting 32, 56
guidelines 459
Guillain–Barré syndrome (GBS) 172–3
gums 206, 207
gut 94; see also gastrointestinal tract
gut-associated lymphoid tissue (GALT) 94

H

haematology 269–90
haematuria 127
haemoglobin 270–1
haemolytic anaemia 280–1
haemolytic uraemic syndrome (HUS) 138–9
haemophilia 284–5
Haemophilus influenzae type b (Hib) 390
haemopoiesis 270
haemorrhagic disease of the newborn (HDN) 286
haemorrhagic parenchymal venous infarction (HPI) 15
haemostasis 272–3
hair 194, 206
hand, foot and mouth disease 203, 322
Hand–Schuller–Christian disease 305
head
  abnormal shape and size 151
  birth injuries 11
  injury 38
  non-accidental injury (NAHI) 401
headache 162–3, 174, 418
head lice 203
HEADS protocol 410
health, definitions 386
health behaviours 414
health determinants 385
health inequalities 385
health promotion 386–7, 406, 414–15
healthy eating 96
hearing 392, 396–7

heart failure 74, 75, 92
heart murmurs 75
heart rate 31, 33
heart sounds 75
heart surgery 79
height measurement 217
Helicobacter pylori 101
Henoch–Schönlein purpura (HSP) 342–3
Henoch–Schönlein purpura nephritis 126, 127, 343
heparin-binding growth factors (HBGF) 216
hepatitis, acute 117
hepatitis, acute viral 117
hepatitis, autoimmune 116
hepatitis A 117
hepatitis B 20, 117, 391
hepatitis B vaccine 391
hepatitis C 20
hereditary angio-oedema (HAE) 319
hereditary fructose intolerance (HFI) 238
hereditary motor and sensory neuropathies (HMSN) 166
hereditary spherocytosis (HS) 22, 280–1
hernia
  diaphragmatic 27
  inguinal 27
  umbilical 8
herpangina 322
herpes labialis 324
herpes simplex encephalitis (HSE) 170
herpes simplex virus (HSV) 20, 184, 202, 324
herpesvirus infections 202–3, 324–7, 438
herpes zoster 325
herpetic whitlow 206
heterotopias 150
Hib vaccine 390
high-frequent oscillatory ventilation (HFOV) 13
highly active antiretroviral therapy (HAART) 329
hip
  developmental dysplasia (DDH) 8, 350–1
  irritable hip 361
  neonatal examination 8
Hirschberg test 182
Hirschsprung disease (HSCR) 99
hirsutism 206
histiocytosis 305
HIV 20, 328–9, 438
Hodgkin lymphoma (HL) 298
Holt–Oram syndrome 78
homocystinuria 240–1
hordeolum 184
hormone receptors 211
hormones 210–11
Horner's syndrome 179
H_2-receptor antagonists 430
HSP nephritis 126, 127, 343
human albumin solution (HAS) 447
human genome 249
human herpesviruses 202–3, 324–7, 438
human herpesvirus keratitis 184
human immunodeficiency virus (HIV) 20, 328–9, 438
human karyotype 248
human varicella zoster immunoglobulin (VZIG) 325
humoral immunity 18, 308, 309
Hunter syndrome 244, 245
Hurler syndrome 244–5
hydrocephalus 149
hydrogen ions 31
hydronephrosis 132
hygiene hypothesis 340
hypercalcaemia 227
hyper-IgM syndrome (HIGM) 319
hyperinsulinaemic hypoglycaemia, familial (HHF) 231
hyperkalaemia 123
hyperlipidaemias 239
hypermetropia 181
hypermobile joints 365
hypernatraemia 122
hyperoxaluria 141
hyperphenylalaninaemia (HPA) 240
hyperpigmentation 207
hypertension 140–1
  pregnancy 3
hyperthermia 312
hyperthyroidism 221
  maternal 3
hypertrichosis 206
hypertriglyceridaemias 239
hypertrophic cardiomyopathy (HCM) 90
hyperviscosity syndrome 295
hypnotics 434
hypocalcaemia 226–7
hypoglycaemia 24, 230–1, 246
hypokalaemia 33, 123

hypomagnesaemia 227
hypomelanosis 207
hyponatraemia 122
hypopigmentation 207
hypopituitarism 214
hypoplastic left heart syndrome (HLHS) 82
hypospadias 135
hypothalamus 212
hypothermia
 drowning 39
 neonates 6
hypothyroidism 220–1
hypoxic–ischaemic encephalopathy (HIE) 10, 14

I

iatrogenic hyperglycaemia 25
ibuprofen 431
 poisoning 41
icthyoses 199
idiopathic intracranial hypertension (IIH) 163
idiopathic ketotic hypoglycaemia 231
ifosfamide 442
IgA nephropathy 126, 127
immune-complex disease 311
immune-mediated encephalomyelitis 172
immune system 18, 308–9
immune thrombocytopaenic purpura (ITP) 288
immunization 388–91
immunization programme 388
immunodeficiency 65, 311, 316–19
immunodeficiency syndromes 316
immunopathology 310–11
immunosuppressants 442–3
imperforate anus 8, 27
impetigo 202, 333
impetigo neonatorum 198
imprinted gene disorders 266–7
inborn errors of metabolism (IEMs) 25, 236–44
incomitant strabismus 182
incontinentia pigmenti (IP) 191, 199
indometacin 431
induced illness 403
inequalities in health 385
infant dyschezia 109
infantile colic 108
infantile haemangioma 198
infantile hypertrophic pyloric stenosis (IHPS) 101
infantile nephropathic cystinosis 138
infantile seborrheic eczema 201
infantile spasms 159
infant mortality rate (IMR) 4, 384
infection
 cancer 295
 congenital 18, 20–1, 184
 epidemiology 311
 eye 184–5
 immunodeficiency 311, 316–17
 intracranial 170
 nails 206
 neonates 18–21
 pathogens 310–11
 skin 18, 198, 202–3
 transmission modes 310
 urinary tract (UTI) 124–5, 132–3
infectious mononucleosis 326
infective endocarditis (IE) 88
infestations 203
inflammatory bowel disease (IBD) 106–7, 360
inflammatory myopathies 167
influenza 336, 438–9
inguinal hernia 27
inguinoscrotal disorders 27, 134–5
inhaled foreign bodies 42–3
inhalers 67
inheritance 252–3
innate immunity 308
innocent murmurs 75
inspiratory capacity (IC) 54
inspiratory reserve volume (IRV) 54
insulin
 changes at birth 5
 synthesis and action 228
insulin-like growth factors (IGF) 216
insulin preparations and regimens 229, 440
interferon alfa 443
intermittent positive pressure ventilation (IPPV) 13
interquartile range 450
interrupted aortic arch 83
intersex 219
interventional cardiology 79
intoed gait 349
intracranial haemorrhage 11, 15

intracranial infections 170
intracranial pathology 38
intracranial pressure (ICP), raised 31
intraocular pressure (IOP) 187
intrauterine growth restriction (IUGR) 2
intravenous fluids 446–7
intraventricular haemorrhage 15
intubation 10, 51
intussusception 103
iodine deficiency 97
ion channels 144
ipratropium 433
iris 180
iron deficiency 97
iron-deficiency anaemia (IDA) 278, 443
iron poisoning 41
irreversible shock 33
irritable bowel syndrome (IBS) 109
irritable hip 361
isovaleric acidaemia 241
IV fluids 446–7

J

jaundice 7, 22–3, 114, 115
jitteriness 156
joints 346–7
 hypermobile 365
 swollen 349
junctional epidermolysis bullosa (JEB) 199
juvenile dermatomyositis 167
juvenile idiopathic arthritis (JIA) 358–9, 368
juvenile myoclonic epilepsy 159

K

kala-azar 337
karyotyping 253
Kasai porto-enterostomy 114–15
Kawasaki disease (KD) 86–7, 343
Kayser–Fleischer rings 116
keratitis 184
kernicterus 22
kidney
 acute injury 130
 anatomy 120
 chronic disease 131
 cystic disease 136
 duplex 134
 ectopic 134
 fused 134
Klinefelter syndrome 257
Klumpke's palsy 11
Koebner's phenomenon 197
koilonychia 206
Krabbe disease 152
Kugelberg–Welander disease 166
kwashiorkor 97
kyphoscoliosis 71

L

lamotrigine 435
Landau–Kleffner syndrome 159
Langerhans cell histiocytosis (LCH) 305
language development 392, 397
laryngomalacia 61
laxatives 430
learning disability 394–5
Leber congenital amaurosis (LCA) 190
left-to-right shunts 79, 80–1
Leigh's syndrome 243
leishmaniasis 336–7
Lennox–Gastaut syndrome 159
lenograstim 443
lens 180, 186
leptospirosis 337
Letterer–Siwe disease 305
leucocytes 271
leuconychia 206
leukaemias 293, 296–7
leukocoria 179
leukodystrophies 152
leukotriene receptor antagonists 433
Liddle syndrome 137
lids
 developmental anomalies 180
 ptosis 179
likelihood ratio (LR) 454
limb–girdle muscular dystrophies (LGMD) 169
limp 349
lips, swollen 208

lissencephaly 150
Listeria monocytogenes 19
listeriosis 19
live birth 4
liver disease
 acute 117
 chronic 116–17
 coagulation disorders 286
 neonates 114–15
liver failure, acute 117
liver functions 95
liver glycogenoses 238
local guidelines 459
long-chain deficiencies 239
long QT syndrome (LQTS) 91
looked-after children 383
loop diuretics 432
Loop of Henle (LoH) 121, 137
loose anagen syndrome 206
low birthweight 4
low vision 181
lumbar puncture (LP) 51
Lund and Browder chart 37
lung
 capacities 54
 changes at birth 4
 development 6, 54
 volumes 54
lung function tests 54–5
lupus nephritis 127
luteinizing hormone (LH) 212–13
Lyme disease 337
lymphocytes 309
lymphomas 293, 298–9
lysosomal storage diseases 244–5

M

macrocephaly 151
macrolides 437
mad cow disease 337
magnesium 447
magnetic resonance imaging (MRI) 147
malaria 338–9
malnutrition 97
malrotation and volvulus 27, 98
maltreatment 398–405
mandibulofacial dysostosis 261
Mann–Whitney U tests 452
Mantoux test 65, 331
maple syrup urine disease (MSUD) 240
marasmus 97
Marfan syndrome (MFS) 78, 191, 260, 268
Maroteaux–Lamy syndrome 244
mast cells 308
maternal attachment 9
maternal blood tests 3
maternal disorders 3
maternal mortality 4
McArdle disease 238
McCune–Albright syndrome 207
MDMA poisoning 41
mean 450
mean pressure 31
measles 337
measles, mumps and rubella (MMR) vaccine 389, 391
Meckel–Gruber syndrome 136
meconium aspiration 12
median 450
medium-chain acyl-CoA dehydrogenase deficiency (MCADD) 239
medullary cystic kidney disease (MCKD) 136
medullary sponge kidney 136
megalencephaly 151
megaureter 132
meiosis 248
melanin 207
MELAS 242
melatonin 434
melphalan 442
membranoproliferative glomerulonephritis (MPGN) 126, 128
membranous glomerulonephritis 126
MenC conjugate vaccine 391
Mendelian single-gene disorders 251
meningitis 170
meningocele 148
meningococcal disease 44, 45, 334–5, 390–1
meningococcal septicaemia 44, 45, 335
mental health 369–80, 412, 416–17
mercaptopurine 442
MERRF 242–3
meta-analyses 455

INDEX

metabolic acidosis 25, 33, 123
metabolic alkalosis 25, 33, 123
metabolic disorders 24–5, 191
metabolic myopathies 167
metabolic pathways 234–5
metachromatic leukodystrophy (MLD) 152
metformin 440
methotrexate 442
methylmalonic acidaemia 241
MHC molecules 309
miconazole 438
microbes 310
microbial genome sequencing 311
microcephaly 150, 151
microdeletion syndromes 258–9
mid-parental height 217
migraine 162–3
　abdominal 110
miliary TB 330
Millennium Development Goals (MDGs) 384
Miller–Fisher syndrome 172
mineralocorticoids 222
minerals 447
minimal change glomerulonephritis 126
minimal change nephrotic syndrome (MCNS) 128
mitochondrial encephalomyopathy, lactic acidosis, stroke-like episodes (MELAS) 242
mitochondrial respiratory chain disorders 242–3, 266
mitosis 248
mixed connective tissue disease (MCTD) 364
mixed sleep apnoea 59
MMR vaccine 389, 391
Mobitz type I/II block 91
Mobius syndrome 182
mode 450
molluscum contagiosum 202
monoamine oxidase inhibitor poisoning 41
monoclonal antibodies 443
monosomy 250
montelukast 433
morbidity 4, 384, 385, 412
morphine 434
Morquio syndrome 244
mortality 4, 384, 385, 412
mosaicism 250
motor delay 395
motor development 392
motor system examination 146–7
mouth ulcers 206
movement disorders 160–1
mucopolysaccharidoses (MPS) 244–5
mucosal leishmaniasis 337
multicystic dysplastic kidney (MCDK) 136
multifactorial disorders 250, 251
multiple carboxylase deficiency 241
multiple pregnancies 2–3
multiple sclerosis, ADEM 172
mumps 321
murmurs 75
muscle–eye–brain disease (MEB) 150
muscle glycogenoses 238
muscular dystrophies 168–9
musculoskeletal disorders 345–68
musculoskeletal system 346–9
mutation 249
mutation analysis 253
myasthenia gravis (MG) 167
　maternal 3
myasthenic syndromes 167
mycophenolate mofetil 443
mycoses 438
myelinated nerve fibres 188
myelination 144
myelomeningocele 148
myocardial contractility 74
myocarditis 89
myoclonic epilepsy with ragged-red fibres (MERRF) 242–3
myoclonic seizures 158
myopathies 167
myopia 181
myotonic dystrophy (MD1) 169
myotubular (centronuclear) myopathy 167

N

naevi 198
nail patella syndrome 206
nails 195, 206
nalidixic acid 437
napkin dermatitis (nappy rash) 201
nasolacrimal duct 180
National Service Framework (NSF) 382

natural killer (NK) cells 308
neck injuries 11
necrotizing enterocolitis (NEC) 16
necrotizing fasciitis 202, 344
negative predictive value (NPV) 454
neglect 398, 403
nemaline (rod) myopathies 167
neonatal abstinence syndrome 3
neonatal mortality rate (NMR) 4
neonates 1–28
　adaptation to extrauterine life 4–5, 74
　bacterial infection 18–19
　care 9
　congenital infection 18, 20–1, 184
　dehydration 7, 448
　dermatology 198–9
　examination 8
　feeding 9
　herpes 20, 324
　HIV 20, 329
　hypoglycaemia 24, 231
　hypopituitarism 214
　jaundice 7, 22–3, 114, 115
　liver disease 114–15
　metabolic disorders 24–5
　mortality 4, 384
　neurological disorders 14–15
　nutrition 7
　osteomyelitis 366
　parental support 9
　physiology 6–7
　respiratory disorders 12–13
　resuscitation 5, 10
　screening 9, 69
　seizures 15, 28
　stroke 28
　thrombocytopaenia 3, 288–9
　viral infection 20
　vitamin K deficiency 9, 97, 286, 445
nephritic syndrome 126
nephritis, acute (AN) 127
nephroblastoma 302, 306
nephrocalcinosis 141
nephrogenic diabetes insipidus 137
nephrology 122–3
nephron 120
nephronophthisis (NPHP) 136
nephrotic syndrome 128–9
　congenital 128, 138
nervous system
　development 144
　examination 146–7
　presenting symptoms 146
　seriously ill child 31, 33
neural tube defects (NTDs) 148
neuroblastoma 303
neurodegeneration 152–3
neurodevelopmental disorders 394–5
neurodisability 71, 394
neurofibromatosis type 1 191, 262
neurofibromatosis type 2 191
neuroglycopaenia 24
neurohypophysis 213
neuroimaging 147, 157
neurology 14–15, 143–74
neuromuscular disorders 164–7
neuronal death 10
neutropaenia 289, 319, 443
Niemann–Pick disease 115, 245
nifedipine 432
nightmares 373
night terrors 156, 373
Nikolsky's sign 197
nits 203
NK cell receptors 309
noisy breathing 56
non-accidental head injury (NAHI) 401
non-alcoholic fatty liver disease (NAFLD) 116–17
non-epileptic attack disorder 156
non-Hodgkin lymphoma (NHL) 299
non-opioid analgesics 434
non-parametric tests 452
non-proliferative glomerulonephritis 126
non-shivering thermogenesis 6
non-steroidal anti-inflammatory drugs (NSAIDs) 431
　poisoning 41
Noonan syndrome (NS) 78, 261
normal distribution 450
Norwood procedure 79
nosebleeds 58
nosocomial infection 311
notifiable diseases 311
nuchal translucency 3

nuclear receptor superfamily 211
number needed to harm (NNH) 453
number needed to treat (NNT) 453
nutrition 96–7, 444
　neonates 7
　puberty 218
nutritional support 97
nystagmus 183
nystatin 438

O

obesity 412, 421
obstructive heart defects 79, 82–3
obstructive sleep apnoea (OSA) 59
ocular herpes 324
odds 453
odds ratio 453
oesophageal atresia 98
oesophageal 24 h pH study 100
off-label prescribing 428
oligohydramnios 3
omphalocele 99
oncogenes 292
oncology 291–306
onychomycosis 203
open-heart surgery 79
ophthalmia neonatorum 18
ophthalmology 175–92
opioid analgesics 4343
　poisoning 41
opportunistic infections 316–17
oppositional behaviour 372
oppositional defiant disorder (ODD) 377
optic disc swelling 188–9
optic nerve 180, 188–9
optic neuropathy 189
oral allergy syndrome 341
oral rehydration solution (ORS) 102, 446
oral ulcers 206
orbital cellulitis 185
organic acidaemias 241
orofaciodigital syndrome 136
Ortolani manoeuvre 8
oseltamivir 439
Osgood–Schlatter disease 352
osmotic equilibrium 121
osteogenesis imperfecta (OI) 191, 354–5
osteogenic sarcoma 304
osteomyelitis 366–7
osteopaenia of prematurity 17
osteopetrosis 356
osteoporosis 356
osteosarcoma 304
otitis media 58
otitis media with effusion (OME) 58, 396
oxalate stones 141
oxygen delivery 30
oxygen therapy 13, 433
oxytocin 213

P

paediatric advanced life support 35
paediatric autoimmune neuropsychiatric disorders associated with streptococcal infections (PANDAS) 172
paediatric basic life support (BLS) 34
pain 36, 348
palivizumab 439
palliative care 295
pallid syncope 156
palpitations 75
pancreas 228
pancreatic insufficiency 113
pancreatitis 112–13
pancytopaenia 290
panda eyes 38
PANDAS 172
panhypopituitarism 214
papilloedema 188–9
papular urticaria 203
paracetamol 434
　poisoning 41
parametric tests 452
parasitic infestations 203
parathyroid hormone (PTH) 226
parental responsibility 399
parenteral nutrition 7, 97, 115
Parkland formula 37
paronychia 206
paroxysmal disorders 156
paroxysmal dyskinesias 161

parvovirus B19 21, 323
Patau syndrome 191, 255
patch testing 197
patent ductus arteriosus (PDA) 16–17, 79, 81
pathogen-associated molecular patterns (PAMPs) 308
pathogens 310–11
PATHOS questionnaire 417
patient triggered ventilation (PTV) 13
pediculosis 203
pedigrees 252–3
Pelizaeus–Merzbacher syndrome 152
pelvi-ureteric junction (PUJ) obstruction 132
penicillin G 436
penicillins 436–7
penicillin V 436
penile abnormalities 135
peptic ulcer disease (PUD) 101
percentile 450
pericarditis 89
perinatal mortality rate (PMR) 4
periorbital cellulitis 185, 192
periorbital swelling 192
peripheral circulation 30
periventricular leukomalacia (PVL) 15
periventricular nodular heterotopia (PNH) 150
peroxismal biogenesis disorders (PBDs) 243
persistent hyperplastic primary vitreous (PHPV) 180
persistent pulmonary hypertension of the newborn 12
personal child health record (PCHR) 387
Perthes disease 352
pertussis 63, 390
pertussis vaccine 390
Peutz–Jeghers syndrome 207
pGALS 348
pH 31
phaeochromocytoma 225
phagocytes 308
phakomatoses 191
pharmacodynamics 427
pharmacogenetics 427
pharmacokinetics 426–7
pharmacology 425–48
pharyngitis 333
phenotype 250
phenoxymethylpenicillin 436
phenylketonurias (PKU) 240, 246
phobias 378
'phone first' or 'phone fast' 34
phorias 182
phosphate supplements 447
photophobia 178
phototherapy 22–3
physical abuse 400–1
physiological jaundice 22
piebaldism 207
Pierre Robin sequence 26
pigmentation disorders 207
piperacillin 437
pituitary gland 212–13
pityriasis versicolor 203
placenta 2
plasma osmolality 121
plasma substitutes 447
platelet concentrate 277
platelets 271, 288–9
play milestones 392
pleural effusion 63
Plumber's lines 206, 207
pneumococcal disease 334, 391
pneumococcal vaccines (PPV/PCV) 391
pneumonia 12, 62–3
pneumothorax 13
poisoning 40–1
poliomyelitis 390
polio vaccine 390
poliovirus 322–3
polycystic kidney disease 136
polyhydramnios 3
polymicrogyria 150
Pompe disease 238
population 450
port wine stain 198
positive predictive value (PPV) 454
positive pressure ventilation 13
possetting 100
posterior urethral valves 132
post-infectious arthritis 360
post-infectious autoimmune disease 311
post-infectious encephalomyelitis 172
post-infectious glomerulonephritis 126
post-neonatal mortality rate 4
post-term 4

post-test odds 454
potassium (K^+) 123
potassium-sparing diuretics 432
power 451
Prader–Willi syndrome (PWS) 266–7
precocious puberty 218
predictive tests 253
pregnancy
  high/low risk 2
  maternal disorders 3
  multiple 2–3
  prescribing 429
  teenagers 412, 422
preimplantation genetic diagnosis (PGD) 253
preload 30, 74
prematurity
  chronic lung disease (CLD) 70
  osteopaenia 17
  retinopathy of prematurity (ROP) 188
pREMS 349
prenatal screening and diagnosis 3, 69, 254
prepregnancy care 3
prescribing 428–9
preseptal cellulitis 185, 192
preterm 4, 6, 7, 16–17
pre-test odds 454
pre-test probability 454
prevention of disease 386–7, 406
primary craniosynostosis 151
primary dystonias 161
primary haemostasis 272
primary hypertension 140
primary immunodeficiency diseases (PIDs) 316
primary peptic ulcer disease 101
primary renal anomalies 134
primary survey 36
primary vesicoureteric reflux 132
primitive neuroectodermal tumours (PNETs) 300
prions 310, 337
proctocolitis 341
progressive familial intrahepatic cholestasis (PFIC) 115
prolactin 213
proliferative glomerulonephritis 126
prolonged jaundice 23
propionic acidaemia 241
proptosis 178
protein
  digestion and absorption 95
  metabolism 234–5
  neonatal intake 7
  synthesis 249
protein C (PC) 273
protein–energy malnutrition 97
proteinuria 127
prothrombin time (PT) 273
proton pump inhibitors (PPIs) 430
protozoa 310
proximal (type 2) renal tubular acidosis 137
pseudo-epileptic seizures 156
pseudohypoaldosteronism (PHAI) type 1 127
pseudohypoparathyroidism 226
pseudo-proptosis 178
psoriasis 204
psoriatic arthritis 359
psychosis 379
ptosis 179
pubertal growth spurt 216
puberty 218–19, 408–9
PubMed 457
pulmonary atresia 84
pulmonary flow murmur 75
pulmonary haemorrhage 13
pulmonary interstitial emphysema (PIE) 13
pulmonary stenosis 83
pulmonary tuberculosis 65, 330
pulseless electrical activity (PEA) 35
pulse volume 33
pupils 179
pure tone audiometry 396–7
p-values 451
pyloric stenosis 26, 33, 101
pyoderma 333
pyrexia 312
pyrexia of unknown origin (PUO) 312
pyridoxine-dependent seizures 159
pyruvate kinase deficiency (PKD) 281

Q

quiet tachypnoea 32
quinine 439
quinolones 437

R

radiographs, chest (CXR) 57, 76
radiotherapy 294
raised intracranial pressure (ICP) 31
randomized controlled trials (RCTs) 454–5
range 450
rapid clinical assessment 32
rare factor deficiencies 286
Rastelli procedure 79
rattle 56
reactive arthritis 360
receptor tyrosine kinase 211
recession 30, 32
recovery position 35
recurrent aspiration 71
red blood cell isoimmunization 3
red blood cells 270–1
'red book' 387
red cell concentrate 277
red eye 178
reflex anoxic seizures 156
reflux nephropathy (RN) 132
refractive errors 181
Refsum disease 243
refusal of treatment 411
regression 452–3
regurgitation 100
rehydration 102
relative risk 453
renal agenesis 134
renal anaemia 443
renal anatomy 120
renal anomalies 134
renal biopsy 123
renal dysplasia 133
renal failure 130–1
renal function 120
renal pelvis dilation (RPD) 132
renal perfusion 33
renal replacement therapy 131
renal transplantation 131
renal tubular acidosis 137
renal tubule 120, 121, 136–7
renin–angiotensin–aldosterone system 121
rescue breaths 34
research study designs 454–5
residual volume (RV) 54
respiratory acidosis 33
respiratory alkalosis 33
respiratory distress 12, 43
respiratory distress syndrome (RDS) 6, 12–13
respiratory emergencies 42–3
respiratory failure 43
respiratory muscle weakness 71
respiratory noises 56
respiratory rate 32
respiratory support 6, 13
respiratory syncytial virus 439
respiratory system 30
  anatomy and physiology 54–5
  assessment in seriously ill child 32
  examination 56
  history 56
  investigations 56–7
  neonatal disorders 12–13
  neonates 6
restriction syndromes 182
restrictive cardiomyopathy 90
resuscitation 34–5
  birth asphyxia 10
  neonates 5
  when to stop 35
reticulocyte count 273
retina
  acquired retinopathies 188
  degenerations 190
  developmental disorders 188
  dysplasia 180, 188
  haemorrhages 188
retinitis pigmentosa (RP) 190
retinoblastoma 301
retinopathy of prematurity (ROP) 188
Rett syndrome 265
re-warming 39
rhabdomyosarcoma 303
Rh blood group 276
rheumatic fever (RF) 86
ribavirin 439
rickets 356–7
ringworm 203
risk 453
risk ratio 453

rituximab 443
RNA 249
Romano–Ward syndrome 91
roseola infantum 327
rotavirus 102
rubella 321
  congenital 20, 184, 321
rubeola 320
'rule of nines' 37
rumination 109

S

safeguarding children 399
salbutamol 433
salicylate poisoning 41
salmeterol 433
salmonellosis 337
salmon patch 198
salt, recommended intake 96
sample size 451
Sanfillipo syndrome 244
scabies 203
scalds 36–7, 400–1
scarlet fever 202, 333
Scheie syndrome 244
schizencephaly 150
school health service 395
school refusal 373
Schwartz formula 120
sclera, blue 191
scoliosis 353
screening 386
  cystic fibrosis 69
  Down syndrome 254
  neonates 9, 69
  neural tube defects 148
  PKU 240
  prenatal 3, 69, 254
secondary dystonias 161
secondary haemostasis 272–3
secondary headache 163
secondary hypertension 140
secondary immunodeficiency 316
secondary peptic ulcer disease 101
secondary survey 36
secondary vesicoureteric reflux 132
Segawa syndrome 161
seizures 15, 28, 31, 156, 158
selective IgA deficiency (IGAD) 318
selective serotonin re-uptake inhibitor (SSRI)
  poisoning 41
self-harm 416–17, 424
sensitivity 454
sensorineural hearing loss (SNHL) 396
separation anxiety disorder (SAD) 378
sepsis 18–19, 37, 44–5
septicaemia 44–5
septicaemic shock 310
septic arthritis 367
septic screen 19, 44
septic shock 33, 44–5
serious injury 36
seriously ill child 30–3
'setting sun' sign 149
severe combined immunodeficiency (SCID) 318–19
sex determination 219
sex steroids 216, 222
sexual abuse 402
sexual and reproductive health 412–13, 422
sexually transmitted infections 413, 422
shingles 325
shock 32–3, 310–11
  septic 33, 44–5
shockable rhythms 35
short bowel syndrome (SBS) 105
short stature 217, 232
shoulder injuries 11
Shwachman–Diamond syndrome (SDS) 113, 279
sickle-cell disease (SCD) 282–3
significant harm 399
Silver–Russell syndrome (SRS) 267
single gene disorders 250, 251
sinus arrhythmia 90
sinus bradycardia 90
sinus tachycardia 33, 90
SIRSE 371
situs ambiguus 74
situs inversus 74
situs solitus 74
sixth nerve palsy 183
skewed 450

skin
  anatomy 194
  biopsy 197
  descriptions of abnormalities 196–7
  development 195
  failure 195
  function 195
  infections 18, 198, 202–3
  infestations 203
  inflammatory disease 204–5
  neonates 198–9
  perfusion 33
  pigmentation disorders 207
skin prick tests (SPTs) 340
skull
  basal fracture 38
  birth fracture 11
  development 150–1
sleep apnoea 59, 71
sleeping 372, 373
sleepwalking 156, 373
slipped capital femoral epiphysis (SCFE) 353
Sly syndrome 244
small for gestational age (SGA) 2
Smith–Magenis syndrome 259
smoking 3, 413, 422–3
snoring 56, 59
snuffles 56
social behaviour development 392
social phobia 378
sodium (Na$^+$) 122
soft tissue sarcoma (STS) 303
solid tumours 293
somatic symptoms 418
somatization 373
spastic cerebral palsy 154
special educational needs (SEN) 395
specificity 454
specific phobias 378
speech and language disorders 397
speech development 392, 397
sphingolipidoses 245
spina bifida cystica 148
spina bifida occulta 148
spinal cord
  compression 295
  development 144
  injury 171
  tumours 301
spinal muscular atrophy (SMA) 166
spine, neonatal examination 8
spinocerebellar ataxias (SCA) 161
spirometry 55
spironolactone 432
splenomegaly 275
stability genes 293
standard deviation (SD) 450
standard error of the mean (SEM) 450–1
staphylococcal infection 18, 332–3
staphylococcal scalded skin syndrome 198, 202, 332
Staphylococcus aureus 332–3
statistics 450–5
stem cells 295
steroid injections 431
steroid-sensitive nephrotic syndrome (SSNS) 129
'sticky eyes' 18
stillbirth and stillbirth rate 4
Still's murmur 75
stool form 111
storage disorders 191
storage pool disorders 289
strabismus 182–3
streptococcal infections 202, 333
stridor 32, 56
  acute 60, 72
  chronic 61
stroke 28, 173
stroke volume 30
Student's t-test 452
study designs 454–5
Sturge–Weber syndrome 191
stye 184
subacute necrotizing encephalomyopathy 243
subaponeurotic haemorrhage 11
subarachnoid haemorrhage 11
subcortical band heterotopia spectrum 150
subdural haemorrhage 11
subgaleal haemorrhage 11
subglottic stenosis 61
substance misuse 3, 413, 422–3
sudden unexplained death in infancy (SUDI) 52, 406
suicide 416

sulphamethoxazole and trimethoprim 437
sulphonamides 437
supraventricular tachycardia (SVT) 91
surfactant 4, 6
surfactant therapy 13
surveillance 387
SVC obstruction 295
sweat glands 194
sweat test 69
synchronous intermittent mandatory ventilation (SIMV) 13
syncope 75
syndrome of inappropriate ADH secretion (SIADH) 215
synovial joints 346–7
synovitis, transient (TS) 361
syphylis, congenital 21
systematic reviews 457
systemic lupus erythematosus (SE) 362–3, 368
  maternal 3
systemic perfusion 33
systemic steroids 431

T

tachyarrhythmias 90
tachycardia 92
tachypnoea 32
tacrolimus 443
talipes equinovarus 350
tall stature 217
Tanner stages 409
Tay–Sachs disease 245
T-cell lymphoblastic lymphoma 299
T-cell receptors 309
T cells 309
teenage pregnancy 412, 422
teeth 206
temperature measurement 312
temper tantrums 372, 380
tension-type headache 162, 163
term infants 4
tertiary survey 36
tetanus 390
tetanus vaccine 390
tetracosactide (tetracosactrin) 441
tetralogy of Fallot (TOF) 84
thalassaemia 283
theophylline 433
thermal injuries 36–7, 400–1
thiazide diuretics 432
third nerve palsy 183
thrombin time (TT) 273
thrombocytes 271
thrombocytopaenia 3, 288–9
thrombophilia 287
thrombotic thrombocytopenic purpura (TTP) 138, 287
thrush 203
thyroid disorders 220–1
  maternal 3
thyroid function tests 220
thyroid hormones 220, 440
thyroid-stimulating hormone (TSH) 212
thyrotoxicosis 221
thyroxine 216
ticarcillin 437
tics 161
tidal volume (TV) 54
tinea 203
tiptoed gait 349
tissue factor pathway 272
tissue factor pathway inhibitor (TFPI) 273
tobacco use, adolescence 413, 422–3
toddler diarrhoea 109
tonic–clonic seizures (GTCS) 158
tonsillitis 59
topiramate 435
TORCH syndromes 184
total anomalous pulmonary venous drainage (TAPVD) 85
total body water 121
total burn surface area (TBSA) 37
total lung capacity (TLC) 54
total parenteral nutrition (TPN) 7, 115
TOXBASE 40
toxic megacolon 106
toxic shock 310
toxic-shock-like syndrome (TSLS) 333
toxic shock syndrome (TSS) 37, 332
toxoplasmosis 21, 184
tracheitis, bacterial 60
traffic light system 314

transforming growth factors (TGF) 216
transfusion reactions 277
transfusion-related acute lung injury (TRALI) 277
transient hypogammaglobulinaemia of infancy (THI) 318
transient neonatal myasthenia 167
transient synovitis (TS) 361
transient tachypnoea of the newborn (TTN) 4, 12
transitional care 415
translocations 250
transmissable spongiform encephalopathies (TSEs) 337
transplantation
  bone marrow 277, 295
  renal 131
transposition of great arteries (TGA) 85
trauma 36
traumatic brain injury (TBI) 38, 171
Treacher–Collins syndrome 261
Trendelenberg gait 349
tricarboxylic acid (TCA) cycle 234
triclofos 434
tricuspid valve abnormalities 84
tricyclic antidepressant poisoning 41
triglycerides 235
trimethoprim 437
trisomy 250, 254–5
tropias 182
truncus arteriosus 85
tube feeding 7, 444
tuberculin skin test 65, 331
tuberculosis (TB) 65, 330–1, 391
tuberculous meningitis (TBM) 330–1
tuberous sclerosis (TSC) 136, 263
tuberous sclerosis complex 191
tubulopathies 136–7
tumour lysis syndrome 295
tumour-suppressor genes 292–3
Turner syndrome 78, 191, 256–7
twins 2–3
twin–twin transfusion syndrome (TTTS) 2–3
type 1 and type 2 errors 451
type 1 diabetes mellitus (T1DM) 3, 228–9, 440
type 2 diabetes mellitus (T2DM) 230, 440
typhoid fever 339
tyrosinaemia type 1 115, 240

U

ulcerative colitis (UC) 106–7
ultrasound
  cranial 147
  fetal 3
ultraviolet light 197
umbilical hernia 8
umbilical infections 18
unconjugated hyperbilirubinaemia 23, 114
under-5 mortality rate (U5MR) 384
United Nations Convention on the Rights of the Child (UNCRC) 382
unlicensed prescribing 428
upper airway obstruction 42–3, 60–1
urea cycle 235
urea cycle disorders (UCDs) 241
ureterocoele 132

uric acid stones 141
urinalysis 123, 125
urinary system
  anatomy and physiology 120–1
  history and examination 122
urinary tract
  calculi 141
  congenital anomalies 132–3
  infection (UTI) 124–5, 132–3
urine
  dipstick testing 125
  haematuria 127
  osmolality 121
  proteinuria 127
urolithiasis 141
urticaria 203, 205
urticaria pigmentosa 207
uveitis 185

V

vaccines 388, 390–1
VACTERL 98
valproate 435
variant Creutzfeld–Jacob disease (vCJD) 337
varicella zoster virus (VZV) 21, 202, 325
vascular rings and slings 61, 83
vasovagal syncope 156
V(D)J recombination 309
venous circulation 30
venous hum 75
venous thromboembolism (VTE) 287
ventricular septal defect (VSD) 79, 80–1
ventriculoarterial (VA) connections 74
verapamil 432
vernix caseosa 195
very low birthweight 4
vesicoureteric junction (VUJ) obstruction 132
vesicoureteric reflux (VUR) 132–3
vigabatrin 435
vinca alkaloids 442
vinblastine 442
vincristine 442
viral conjunctivitis 184
viral encephalitis 170
viral hepatitis 117, 438
viral myositis 167
viral skin infections 202–3
viral warts 202
viruses 310
visceral leishmaniasis 337
visceroatrial situs 74
vision assessment 176–7
visual acuity (VA) 176–7
visual development 177, 392
visual evoked potential (VEP) 177
visual fields 177
visual impairment 181
vital capacity (VC) 54
vitamin A 97, 444
vitamin B 444–5
vitamin B12 deficiency 279
vitamin C 445

vitamin D 97, 121, 226, 356–7, 445
vitamin E 97, 445
vitamin K 9, 97, 286, 445
vitamins 444–5
vitamin supplementation 96
vitiligo 207
vomiting 118
  cyclic vomiting syndrome 109
  differental diagnosis 26
  episodic 109
von Gierke disease 238
von Hippel–Lindau syndrome 136, 191
von Willebrand disease (vWD) 285

W

Waardenburg syndrome (WS) 207
WAGR syndrome 180
waiter's tip position 11
Walker–Warburg syndrome (WWS) 150
walking, delayed 395
warts 202
water
  gut absorption 95
  neonatal loss 7
  total body water 121
water deprivation test 215
watering eye 178, 192
weaning 96
Werdnig–Hoffmann disease 166
West syndrome 159
wheeze 32, 56
white blood cells 271, 289
white cell concentrate 277
white matter disorders 15, 152
whooping cough 63, 390
Wilcoxon rank sum test 452
Williams syndrome 78, 259
Wilms tumour (WT) 302, 306
Wilson disease 116
Wiskott–Aldrich syndrome (WAS) 319
Wolff–Parkinson–White (WPW) syndrome 91
Wolf–Hirschhorn syndrome 259
Wolfram syndrome 215
Wood's light 197
Working together to safeguard children 399
worms 310
writing prescriptions 428

X

X chromosome 264
X-linked agammaglobulinaemia (XLA) 318
X-linked dominant (XLD) diseases 251, 252–3
X-linked hypophosphataemic rickets 136–7
X-linked recessive (XLR) diseases 251, 252

Z

Zellweger syndrome (ZWS) 243
zinc deficiency 97
zoonoses 310, 336–7